Complementary to this volume:

SIDE EFFECTS OF DRUGS ANNUALS 1–22 (1977–1999)
Edited by M.N.G. Dukes (Annuals 1–15) and J.K. Aronson (Annuals 16–22)

MEYLER'S SIDE EFFECTS OF DRUGS, 14th EDITION (2000)
Edited by M.N.G. Dukes and J.K. Aronson

UNWANTED EFFECTS OF COSMETICS AND DRUGS USED IN DERMATOLOGY, 3rd EDITION (1994)
A.C. de Groot, J.W. Weyland and J.P. Nater

DRUGS AND HUMAN LACTATION, 2nd Edition (1996)
P.N. Bennett

PHARMACOLOGICAL AND CHEMICAL SYNONYMS, 10th Edition (1994)
E.E.J. Marler

A MANUAL OF ADVERSE DRUG INTERACTIONS, 5th Edition (1997)
J.P. Griffin and P.F. D'Arcy

A DICTIONARY OF PHARMACOLOGY AND ALLIED TOPICS (1998)
D.R. Laurence and J. Carpenter

DRUG SAFETY IN PREGNANCY (2001)
C. Schaefer et al.

The Website of Side Effects of Drugs Annual 23, edited by Jeffrey K. Aronson, can be viewed at http://www.elsevier. com/locate/isbn/0444502122

SIDE EFFECTS OF DRUGS ANNUAL 23

A worldwide yearly survey of new data and trends in adverse drug reactions

EDITOR

J. K. ARONSON M.A., D.PHIL., M.B., F.R.C.P.

Clinical Reader in Clinical Pharmacology
University Department of Clinical Pharmacology
Radcliffe Infirmary, Oxford, United Kingdom

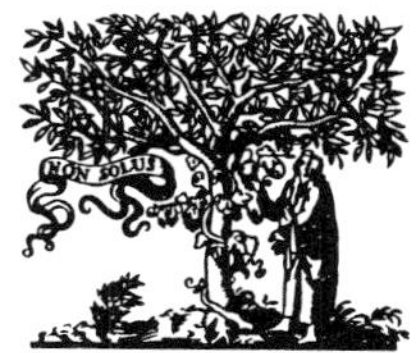

2000
ELSEVIER
Amsterdam – London – New York – Oxford – Paris – Shannon – Tokyo

ELSEVIER SCIENCE B.V.
Sara Burgerhartstraat 25
P.O. Box 211, 1000 AE Amsterdam, The Netherlands

First edition 2000

Library of Congress Cataloging in Publication Data
A catalog record from the Library of Congress has been applied for.

ISBN: 0-444-50212-2
ISSN: 0378-6080

∞ The paper used in this publication meets the requirements of ANSI/NISO Z39.48-1992 (Permanence of Paper).

Printed in The Netherlands.

Contributors

J.K. ARONSON, MA., M.B.CH.B., D.PHIL., F.R.C.P.
University Department of Clinical Pharmacology, Radcliffe Infirmary, Woodstock Road, Oxford, OX2 6HE, U.K. E-mail: jeffrey.aronson@Clinical-Pharmacology.oxford.ac.uk

I. AURSNES, M.D.
University of Oslo, Department of Pharmacotherapeutics, P.O. Box 1065 Blindern, N-0316 Oslo, Norway. E-mail: i.a.aursnes@ioks.uio.no

A. BAUER, M.D.
Friedrich-Schiller-University, Department of Dermatology and Allergology, Erfurter Strasse 35, D-07740 Jena, Germany.

A.G.C. BAUER, M.D.
Havenziekenhuis, Haringvliet 2, 3011 TD Rotterdam, The Netherlands.
E-mail: abauer@euronet.nl

P.J. BOWN, M.A., M.B., B.S., M.R.C.PSYCH.
East Surrey Hospital, Bletchingley Ward, Canada Avenue, Redhill, Surrey, RH8 9LH, U.K.
E-mail: pbown@bb45.freeserve.co.uk

C.N. BRADFIELD, M.B.CH.B.
The University of Auckland, Faculty of Medicine and Health Science, Department of Anaesthesia, Private Bag 92024, Auckland, New Zealand. E-mail: charles@kiwilink.co.nz

P.W.G. BROWN, F.R.C.S., F.R.C.R.
Northern General Hospital NHS Trust, Department of Diagnostic Imaging, Sheffield, S5 7AU, U.K.

A. BUITENHUIS, M.D.
Academic Medical Center, Department of Clinical Pharmacology and Pharmacotherapy, Meibergdreef 9, 1105 AZ Amsterdam, The Netherlands

H. CARDWELL, M.B.CH.B.
University of Auckland, Discipline of Anaesthesiology, Faculty of Medicine and Health Sciences, Private Bag 92019, Auckland, New Zealand. E-mail: hestercardwell@hotmail.com

A. CARVAJAL, M.D., PH.D.
Instituto de Farmacoepidemiologia, Facultad de Medicine, 47005 Valladolid, Spain.
E-mail: carvajal@ife.uva.es

C. CHIOU, M.D.
Immunocompromised Host Section, Pediatric Oncology Branch, National Cancer Institute, National Institutes of Health, Bldg 10, Rm 13N240, 10, Center Drive MSC, Bethesda, MA 20891, U.S.A. E-mail: chiouc@mail.nih.gov

N.H. CHOULIS, M.D., PH.D.
University of Athens, School of Pharmacy, P.O. Box 4315, Athens 102 10, Greece

P. COATES, M.B.B.S., F.R.A.C.P.
Royal Adelaide Hospital, Department of Endocrinology, North Terrace, South Australia 5000, Australia. E-mail: Pcoates.USERS.RAH_01@mail01.rah.sa.gov.au

J. COSTA, M.D.
Universitat Autònoma de Barcelona, Hospital Universitari Germans Trias I Pujol, Clinical Pharmacology Department, Ctra de Canyet, 08916 Badalona, Spain. E-mail: jcosta@cablecat.com

P.J. COWEN, M.D.
University Department of Psychiatry, Warenford Hospital, Oxford, OX3 7JX, U.K.
E-mail: phil.cowen@psychiatry.oxford.ac.uk

S. CURRAN, B.SC., M.B.CH.B., M.MED.SC., M.R.C.PSYCH., PH.D.
Fieldhead Hospital, Cader Unit, Wakefield, WF2 3SP, U.K.
E-mail: steve.curran@wpch-tr.northy.nhs.uk

M.D. DE JONG, M.D., PH.D.
Academic Medical Center, Department of Medical Microbiology, Room L1-104, Meibergdreef 9, 1105 AZ Amsterdam, The Netherlands. E-mail: m.d.dejong@amc.uva.nl

H.J. DE SILVA, M.B.B.S., M.D., D.PHIL, F.R.C.P., F.R.C.P.E., F.C.C.P.
University of Kelaniya, Department of Medicine, Faculty of Medicine, P.O. Box 6, Ragama, Sri Lanka. E-mail: hjdes@sunx86.lanka.net

F.A. DE WOLFF, M.D.
Leiden University Medical Centre, Toxicology Laboratory, Department of Clinical Chemistry, Pharmacy and Toxicology, P.O. Box 9600, 2300 RC Leiden, The Netherlands.
E-mail: F.A.de_Wolff@lumc.nl

A. DEL FAVERO, M.D.
Istituto di Medicina Interna e Science Oncologiche, Policlinico Monteluce, 06122 Perugia, Italy.
E-mail: delfa@unipg.it

J. DESCOTES, M.D., PH.D., PHARM.D
Hôpital Edouard Herriot, Centre Antipoison—Centre de Pharmacovigilance, 5 Place d'Arsonval, 69347 Lyon cedex 03, France. E-mail: jacques.descotes@chu-lyon.fr

S. DITTMANN, M.D., D.SC.MED.
International Immunization Consulting, 19 Hatzenporter Weg, 12681 Berlin, Germany.
E-mail: sd.internat.immun.consult@t-online.de

I.R. EDWARDS, M.B., F.R.C.P., F.R.A.C.P.
Uppsala Monitoring Centre, The WHO Collaborating Centre for International Drug Monitoring, Stora Torget 3, S-753 20 Uppsala, Sweden.

H.W. EIJKHOUT, M.D.
Central Laboratory of the Netherlands Red Cross, Blood Transfusion Service, Plesmanlaan 125, 1066 CX Amsterdam, The Netherlands. E-mail: H_Eijkhout@CLB.nl

C.J. ELLIS, M.D., F.R.C.P.
East Birmingham Hospital, Department of Communicable and Tropical Diseases, Bordsley Green East, Birmingham, B9 5ST, U.K.

P. ELSNER, M.D.
Friedrich-Schiller-University, Department of Dermatology and Allergology, Erfurter Strasse 35, D-07740 Jena, Germany. E-mail: elsner@derma.uni-jena.de

E. ERNST, M.D., PH.D.
University of Exeter, School of Postgraduate Medicine and Health Sciences, Division of Community Health Science, Department of Complementary Medicine, 25 Victoria Park Road, Exeter, EX2 4NT, U.K. E-mail: E.Ernst@ex.ac.uk

M. FARRÉ, M.D.
Universitat Autònoma de Barcelona, Institut Municipal d'Investigació Mèdica, Unitat de Farmacologia, Doctor Aiguader 80, 08003 Barcelona, Spain. E-mail: mfarre@imim.es

P.I. FOLB, M.D., F.R.C.P.
University of Cape Town Medical School, Department of Pharmacology, Groote Schuur Hospital, Observatory 7925, South Africa. E-mail: pfolb@uctgsh1.uct.ac.za

J.A. FRANKLYN, M.D., PH.D, F.R.C.P., F.MED.SCI.
University of Birmingham, Queen Elizabeth Hospital, Department of Medicine, Edgbaston, Birmingham, B15 2TH, U.K. E-mail: j.a.franklyn@bham.ac.uk

M.G. FRANZOSI, PH.D.
Istituto di Ricerche Farmacologiche "Mario Negri", Department of Cardiovascular Research, Via Eritrea 62, 20157 Milan, Italy. E-mail: franzosi@irfmn.mnegri.it

A.H. GHODSE, M.D., PH.D., F.R.C.P., F.R.C.PSYCH.
St. George's Hospital Medical School, Centre for Addiction Studies, 6th Floor, Hunter Wing, Cranmer Terrace, London, SW17 0RE, U.K. E-mail: h.ghodse@sghms.ac.uk

A.I. GREEN, M.D.
Harvard Medical School, Commonwealth Research Center and Massachusetts Mental Health Center, Department of Psychiatry, 74 Fenwood Road, Boston, MA 02115, U.S.A.
E-mail: alan_green@HMS.harvard.edu

A.H. GROLL, M.D.
Immunocompromised Host Section, Pediatric Oncology Branch, National Cancer Institute, National Institutes of Health, Bldg 10, Rm 13N240, 10, Center Drive MSC, Bethesda, MA 20891, U.S.A. E-mail: grolla@mail.nih.gov

K.Y. HARTIGAN-GO, M.D.
Philippine National Drug Policy Programme Office, Bldg. 12, Department of Health, San Lazaro Compound, Rizal Avenue, Manila, Philippines. E-mail: hartigan@doh.gov.ph

J.W. JEFFERSON, M.D.
Healthcare Technology Systems, 7617 Mineral Point Road, Madison, WI 53717, U.S.A.
E-mail: jeffj@healthtechsys.com

H.M.J. KRANS, M.D.
Leiden University Medical Center, Department of Endocrinology and Metabolic Diseases, Building 1 C4-R, Postbus 9600, 2300 RC Leiden, The Netherlands.
E-mail: h.m.j.krans@endocrinology.medfac.leidenuniv.nl

S. KRISHNA, B.A., D.PHIL., F.R.C.P.
St. George's Hospital Medical School, Department of Infectious Diseases, Department of Cell and Molecular Sciences, Cranmer Terrace, London, SW17 0RE, U.K.
E-mail: s.krishna@sghms.ac.uk

R. LATINI, M.D.
Istituto di Ricerche Farmacologiche "Mario Negri", Department of Cardiovascular Research, Via Eritrea 62, 20157 Milan, Italy. E-mail: latini@irfmn.mnegri.it

M. LEUWER, M.D.
The University of Liverpool, University Department of Anaesthesia, University Clinical Department, The Duncan Building, Daulby Street, Liverpool. L69 3GA, U.K.
E-mail: mleuwer@liv.ac.uk

P. MAGEE, B.SC., M.SC., M.R.PHARM.S.
Director of Pharmaceutical Sciences, Walsgrave Hospitals NHS Trust, Clifford Bridge Road, Walsgrave, Coventry, CV2 2DX, U.K. E-mail: Robmcrorie@aol.com

A.P. MAGGIONI, M.D.
Istituto di Ricerche Farmacologiche "Mario Negri", Department of Cardiovascular Research, Via Eritrea 62, 20157 Milan, Italy. E-mail: maggioni@irfmn.mnegri.it

L.H. MARTÍN ARIAS, M.D., PH.D.
Instituto de Farmacoepidemiologia, Facultad de Medicina, 47005 Valladolid, Spain.
E-mail: lmartin@ife.uva.es

G.T. McINNES, B.SC., M.D., F.R.C.P., F.F.P.M.
University of Glasgow, Department of Medicine and Therapeutics, Western Infirmary, Glasgow G11 6NT, Scotland.

R.H.B. MEYBOOM, M.D.
Netherlands Pharmacovigilance Foundation LAREB, Goudsbloemvallei 7, 5237 MH 's-Hertogenbosch, The Netherlands. E-mail: R.Meyboom@wxs.nl

T. MIDTVEDT, M.D., PH.D.
Karolinska Institutet, Laboratory of Medical Microbial Ecology, Box 60 400, S-171 77 Stockholm, Sweden. E-mail: Tore.Midtvedt@cmb.ki.se

S.K. MORCOS, F.R.C.S., F.F.R.R.C.S.I., F.R.C.R.
Northern General Hospital NHS Trust, Department of Diagnostic Imaging, Sheffield, S5 7AU, U.K. E-mail: Sameh@northngh-tr.trent.nhs.uk

S. MUSA, M.B.CH.B., M.R.C.PSYCH.
Fieldhead Hospital, Chantry Unit, Ouchthorpe Lane, Wakefield, WF1 3SP, U.K.
E-mail: shabirm@wpch-tr.northy.nhs.uk

A.N. NICHOLSON, O.B.E., D.SC., M.D.(H.C.), F.R.C.P. (EDIN. & LOND.), F.R.C.PATH., F.F.O.M, F.R.AE.S.
Centre for Human Sciences, Defence Evaluation and Research Agency, Farnborough, Hampshire, GU14 0LX, U.K.

S. OLSSON, M.SCI.PHARM.
Uppsala Monitoring Centre, The WHO Collaborating Centre for International Drug Monitoring, Stora Torget 3, S-753 20 Uppsala, Sweden.

J.K. PATEL, M.D.
Harvard Medical School, Commonwealth Research Center and Massachusetts Mental Health Center, Department of Psychiatry, Boston, MA 02115, U.S.A.
E-mail: jkpatel@HMS.harvard.edu

J.W. PATERSON, B.SC., M.B.B.S., F.R.C.P., F.R.A.C.P., F.R.C.P.A.
University of Western Australia, Department of Pharmacology, Nedlands, WA 6907, Australia.
E-mail: jpaterson@receptor.pharm.uwa.edu.au

K. PEERLINCK, M.D.
University of Leuven, Center for Molecular and Vascular Biology and Division of Bleeding and Vascular Disorders, Herestraat 49, B-3000 Leuven, Belgium.
E-mail: Kathelijne.peerlinck@med.kuleuven.ac.be

E. PERUCCA, M.D., PH.D.
University of Pavia, Clinical Pharmacology Unit, Piazza Botta 10, 27100 Pavia, Italy.
E-mail: perucca@unipv.it

B.C.P. POLAK, M.D.
Free University Hospital, Department of Ophthalmology, P.O. Box 7057, 1007 MB Amsterdam, The Netherlands. E-mail: oogheelk@azvu.nl

P. REISS, M.D., PH.D.
University of Amsterdam, National AIDS Therapy Evaluation Centre and Department of Infectious Diseases, Tropical Medicine and AIDS Academic Medical Center, P.O. Box 22700, 1100 DE Amsterdam, The Netherlands. E-mail: p.reiss@amc.uva.nl

H.D. REUTER, PH.D.
Siebengebirgsallee 24, D-50939 Köln, Germany. E-mail: ges-phyto@t-online.de

I. RIBEIRO, M.D.
St. George's Hospital Medical School, Department of Infectious Diseases, Department of Cell and Molecular Sciences, Cranmer Terrace, London, SW17 0RE, U.K.
E-mail: Iribeiro@aol.com

M. SCHACHTER, M.D.
Department of Clinical Pharmacology, Imperial College School of Medicine, National Heart and Lung Institute, St. Mary's Hospital, London, W2 1NY, U.K. E-mail: m.schachter@ic.ac.uk

A. SCHAFFNER, M.D.
University Hospital of Zurich, Department of Medicine, Medical Clinic B, Rämistrasse 100, CH-8091 Zurich, Switzerland. E-mail: klinsar@usz.unizh.ch

S. SCHLIEMANN-WILLERS, M.D.
Friedrich-Schiller-University, Department of Dermatology and Allergology, Erfurter Strasse 35, D-07740 Jena, Germany. E-mail: Sibylle.Schliemann-Willers@med.uni-jena.de

S.A. SCHUG, M.D., F.A.N.Z.C.A., F.F.P.M.A.N.Z.C.A.
University of Auckland, Discipline of Anaesthesiology, Faculty of Medicine and Health Sciences, Private Bag 92019, Auckland, New Zealand. E-mail: s.schug@auckland.az.nz

R.P. SEQUEIRA, PH.D.
Arabian Gulf University, College of Medicine and Medical Sciences, Department of Pharmacology and Therapeutics, P.O. Box 22979, Manama, Bahrain. E-mail: sequeira@ns1.agu.edu.bh

T.G. SHORT, MB.CH.B., M.D.
The University of Auckland, Faculty of Medicine and Health Science, Department of Pharmacology and Clinical Pharmacology, Private Bag 92019, Auckland, New Zealand.
E-mail: TimS@ahsl.co.nz

A. STANLEY, PH.D., M.R.PHARM.S.
Birmingham Oncology Centre, St. Chad's Unit, City Hospital, Dudley Road, Birmingham, B18 7QH, U.K. E-mail: andrew.stanley@cityhospbham.nhs.uk

W.G. VAN AKEN, M.D.
Central Laboratory of the Netherlands Red Cross, Blood Transfusion Service, Plesmanlaan 125, 1066 CX Amsterdam, The Netherlands. E-mail: H_van_Aken@clb.nl

C.J. VAN BOXTEL, M.D., PH.D.
Academic Medical Center, Department of Clinical Pharmacology and Pharmacotherapy, Meibergdreef 9, 1105 AZ Amsterdam, The Netherlands

G.B. VAN DER VOET, M.D.
Leiden University Medical Centre, Toxicology Laboratory, Department of Clinical Chemistry, Pharmacy and Toxicology, P.O. Box 9600, 2300 RC Leiden, The Netherlands.
E-mail: G.B.van_der_Voet@lumc.nl

R. VERHAEGHE, M.D.
University of Leuven, Center for Vascular and Molecular Biology, Herestraat 49, 3000 Leuven, Belgium. E-mail: Raymond.Verhaeghe@uz.kuleuven.ac.be

J. VERMYLEN, M.D.
University of Leuven, Center for Molecular and Vascular Biology and Division of Bleeding and Vascular Disorders, Herestraat 49, B-3000 Leuven, Belgium.
E-mail: jozef.vermylen@med.kuleuven.ac.be

T. VIAL, M.D.
Hôpital Edouard Herriot, Centre Antipoison—Centre de Pharmacovigilance, 5 Place d'Arsonval, 69347 Lyon cedex 03, France. E-mail: thierry.vial@chu-lyon.fr

T.J. WALSH, M.D.
Immunocompromised Host Section, Pediatric Oncology Branch, National Cancer Institute, National Institutes of Health, Bldg 10, Rm 13N240, 10, Center Drive MSC, Bethesda, MD 20891, U.S.A. E-mail: walshtj@mail.nih.gov

R. WALTER, M.D.
University Hospital of Zurich, Department of Medicine, Medical Clinic B, Rämistrasse 100, CH-8091 Zurich, Switzerland. E-mail: roland.walter@dim.usz.ch

E.J. WONG, M.D.
Harvard Medical School, Massachusetts Mental Health Center, Department of Psychiatry, Boston, MA 02115, U.S.A. E-mail: Ewong88@juno.com

J.Q. WONG, M.D., M.S.
Pharmacoepidemiology and Pharmacoeconomic Section, Philippine National Drug Policy Programme, Building 12, Department of Health, San Lazaro Compound, Rizal Avenue, Manila, Philippines. E-mail: johnw@mydestiny.net

C. WOODROW, M.D., M.R.C.P.
St. George's Hospital Medical School, Department of Infectious Diseases, Department of Cell and Molecular Sciences, Cranmer Terrace, London, SW17 0RE, U.K.
E-mail: cwoodrow@sghms.ac.uk

F. ZANNAD, M.D., PH.D., F.E.S.C.
Clinical Pharmacology and Cardiology Department, Centre d'Investigation clinique INSERM-CHU, Hôpital Jeanne d'Arc, Dommartin les Toul, Université Henri Poincaré de Nancy, 54000 Nancy, France. E-mail: f.zannad@chu-nancy.fr

O. ZUZAN, M.D.
Hannover Medical School, Department of Anesthesiology, D-30625 Hannover, Germany.
E-mail: Oliver.Zuzan@t-online.de

Contents

Special reviews

Cumulative index of special reviews, Annuals 16–22

Index of drugs

Note: the format 19.211 refers to SEDA 19, p. 211.

Index of side effects

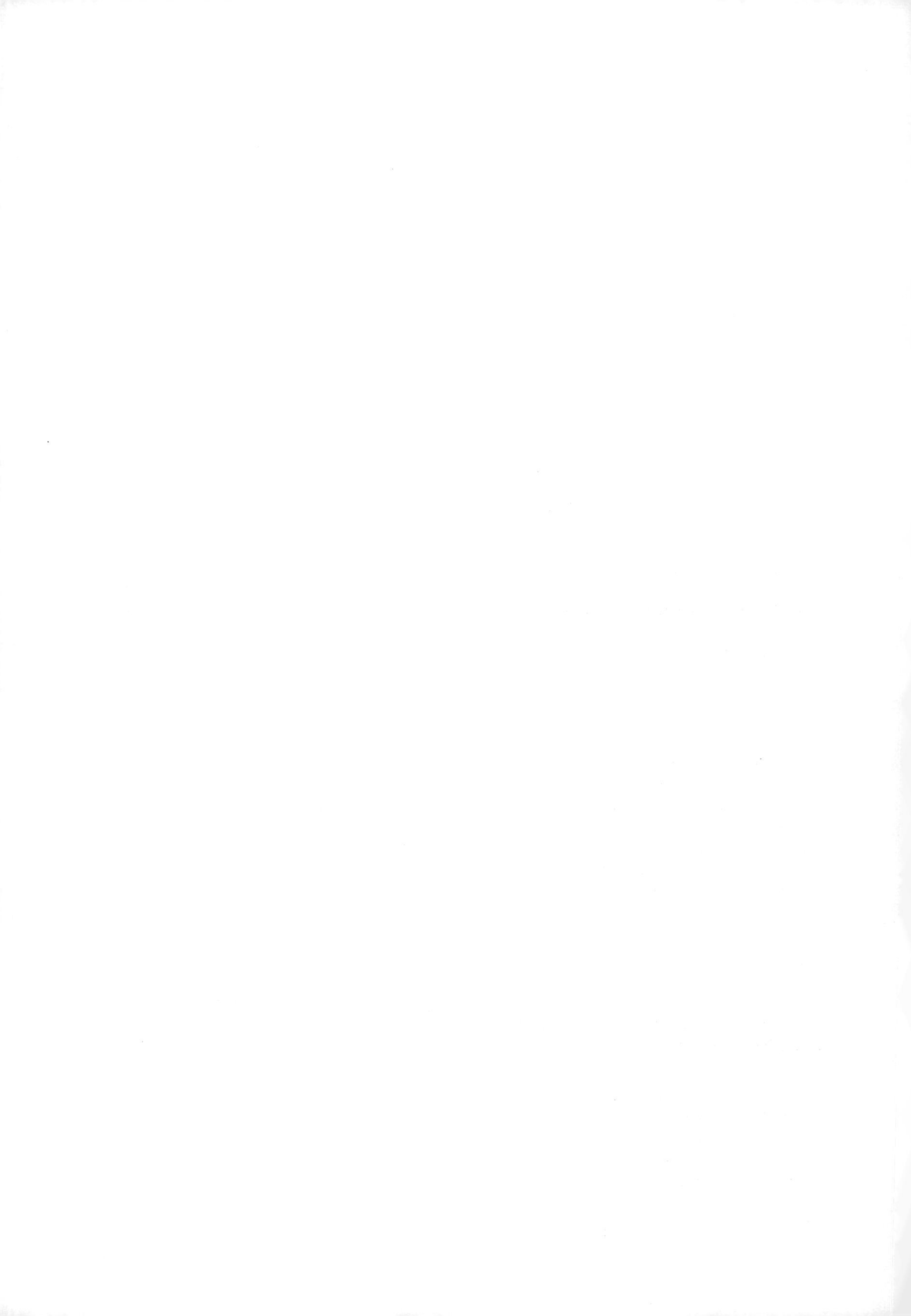

How to use this book

THE SCOPE OF THE 'ANNUAL'

The Side Effects of Drugs Annual has been published each year since 1977. It is designed to provide a critical and up-to-date account of new information relating to adverse drug reactions and interactions from the clinician's point of view. The *Annual* can be used independently or as a supplement to the standard encyclopedic work in this field, *Meyler's Side Effects of Drugs*, the 14th edition of which was published in November 2000.

SPECIAL REVIEWS

As new data appear, older findings may be discredited and existing concepts may require revision. The 'special reviews' deal critically with such topics, interpreting conflicting evidence and providing the reader with clear guidance. Special reviews are identified by the traditional prescription symbol and are printed in italic type. Older papers cited in these reviews are either listed by name or via cross-references to previous Annuals or past editions of Meyler's Side Effects of Drugs, which can be found in most medical libraries.

SELECTION OF MATERIAL

In compiling the *Side Effects of Drugs Annual* particular attention is devoted to those publications which provide essentially new information or throw a new light on problems already recognized. In addition, some authoritative new reviews are listed. Publications which do not meet these criteria are omitted. Readers anxious to trace all references on a particular topic, including those which duplicate earlier work, are advised to consult *Adverse Reactions Titles*, a monthly bibliography of titles from approximately 3400 biomedical journals published throughout the world, compiled by the Excerpta Medica International Abstracting Service.

PERIOD COVERED

The present *Annual* reviews all reports presenting significant new information on adverse reactions to drugs from January 1998–March 1999. During the production of this *Annual*, more recent papers have been included.

CLASSIFICATION

Drugs are classified according to their main field of application or the properties for which they are most generally recognized. In borderline cases, however, some supplementary discussion has been included in other chapters relating to secondary fields of application. Fixed combinations of drugs are dealt with according to their most characteristic component.

DRUG NAMES

Drug products are in general dealt with in the text under their most usual non-proprietary names; where these are not available, chemical names have been used; fixed combinations usually have no proprietary connotation and here trade names have been used as necessary.

SYSTEM OF REFERENCES

References in the text are coded as follows:

R: In the original paper, the point is *reviewed* in some detail with reference to other literature.

r: The original paper *refers* only briefly to the point, on the basis of evidence adduced by other writers.

C: The original paper presents *detailed original clinical evidence* on this point.

c: The original paper provides *clinical evidence*, but only *briefly or anecdotally*.

The code has not been applied to animal pharmacological papers.

The various Editions of *Meyler's Side Effects of Drugs* are cited in the text as SED-13, SED-14 etc.; *SED Annuals 1–22* are cited as SEDA-1, SEDA-2 etc.

INDEXES

Index of drugs: this index provides a complete listing of all references to a drug for which side effects and/or interactions are described.

Index of side effects: this index is necessarily selective, since a particular side effect may be caused by very large numbers of compounds; the index is therefore mainly directed to those side effects which are particularly serious or frequent, or are discussed in special detail. Before assuming that a given drug does not have a particular side effect, one should consult the relevant chapters.

For *interactions*, the reader should refer to the *Index of drugs* where all interactions are listed under the drugs concerned, irrespective of the chapter in which they appear.

It should be borne in mind that American spelling has been used throughout, e.g. anemia, estrogen etc. (instead of anaemia, oestrogen etc.).

A tribute to Graham Dukes

The history of *Meyler's Side Effects of Drugs* and its accompanying annual volumes (*Side Effects of Drugs Annuals*) is reflected in the history of two men, Leopold Meyler and Maurice Nelson Graham Dukes. Meyler founded the series in 1951 and Dukes assumed his mantle in 1973. This year, following the publication of the 14th edition of *Meyler's Side Effects of Drugs*, Graham Dukes has retired from its editorship after 25 years of leading the field in the clear and comprehensive presentation of information on adverse drug reactions, or, as I prefer to call them, adverse reactions to medicaments. Indeed, not only has he led the field—he has prepared the course.

Leopold Meyler was a physician who caught tuberculosis during the war while interned in a Nazi concentration camp. After the war he received drug treatment and experienced adverse effects. According to Professor Wim Lammers, writing a tribute in Volume VIII (1975), Meyler got a fever from para-aminosalicylic acid, but based on information from Meyler's widow, Graham Dukes has written elsewhere that it was deafness from dihydrostreptomycin; perhaps it was both. Meyler discovered that there was no single text to which medical practitioners could look for information about the unwanted effects of drug therapy. He therefore determined to make such information available and persuaded the Netherlands publishing firm of van Gorcum to publish a book (in Dutch) entirely devoted to the descriptions of the adverse effects that drugs could cause. He went on to agree with the Elsevier Publishing Company, as it was then called, to prepare and issue an English translation. The first edition of 192 pages (*Schadelijke Nevenwerkingen van Geneesmiddelen*) appeared in 1951 and the English version (*Side Effects of Drugs*) was published a year later.

The book was a great success, and a few years later Meyler started to publish what he called surveys of the unwanted effects of drugs. Each survey covered a period of two to four years (Table 1). They were labelled as volumes rather than editions, and after Volume IV had been published Meyler could no longer handle the task alone. For subsequent volumes he recruited co-authors, such as Andrew Herxheimer. In September 1973, Meyler died unexpectedly and Elsevier invited Graham Dukes to take over the editing of Volume VIII.

Graham Dukes was born in Barnsley, UK, in 1930. After school he went to St John's College, Cambridge, and simultaneously studied law and medicine—a surely unparalleled feat. In 1952, the year in which the first English edition of *Side Effects of Drugs* was published, he gained the degree

Table 1. The publishing history of the editions of the *Side Effects of Drugs* written or edited by Leopold Meyler

Volume	Date of publication	Years covered
First edition	1951 (Dutch)*	Up to 1951
	1952 (English)	
I	1957	1955–1956
II	1958	1956–1957
III	1960	1958–1960
IV	1963	1960–1962
V	1966	1963–1965
VI	1968	1965–1967
VII	1972	1968–1971

* Several updates to the Dutch volume were subsequently published.

Table 2. The publishing history of the editions of *Meyler's Side Effects of Drugs* and the *Side Effects of Drugs Annuals* edited by Graham Dukes

Volume	Date of publication	Years covered
Meyler's Side Effects of Drugs		
VIII	1975	1972–1975
Ninth edition	1980	*
Tenth edition	1984	*
Eleventh edition	1988	*
Twelfth edition	1992	*
Thirteenth edition	1996	*
Fourteenth edition†	2000	*
Side Effects of Drugs Annuals		
Volumes 1–11	1977–1987	1976–1986
Volumes 12–14‡	1988–1990	1987–1989
Volumes 15–16§	1991–1992	1990–1991

At various times, full or shortened editions of volumes in the Side Effects series have appeared in French, Russian, Dutch, German, and Japanese.
* Encyclopaedic editions.
† Co-editor-in-chief J.K. Aronson.
‡ Co-editor L. Beeley.
§ Co-editor J.K. Aronson.

of Bachelor of Laws, and in 1955 Master of Arts (Law). Only one year later he took his medical degree at University College Hospital, London. He was later to extend his studies in both these subjects by taking his MD at the University of Leiden (1963) and the degree of Master of Laws in International Law in Cambridge (1984). He then worked for 17 years in the pharmaceutical industry, first as the Medical Director of Richardson-Merrell Pharmaceuticals (Benelux) (1957–1961), and then with Organon International (1961–1972), where he ultimately became Research Manager. In 1972, he left the industry and joined the Netherlands National Drug Approval Agency as its Vice Chairman—a post he held until 1982, when he became the Head of the European Regional Pharmaceuticals Programme of the World Health Organization. He remained there until 1991 and simultaneously held the chair of Drug Policy Studies at the University of Groningen.

Graham accepted with relish the challenge of producing Volume VIII and transformed the enterprise. A comparison of Volume VII (1972) with Volume VIII (1975) is instructive:

- Volume VII was called simply *Side Effects of Drugs*; Graham called Volume VIII *Meyler's Side Effects of Drugs*, in memory of the man whose vision had started the enterprise;
- Volume VIII was 50% larger than Volume VII (1132 versus 758 pages), despite the fact that both covered four-year periods;
- Volume VII had two indexes (proprietary names and a subject index); Volume VIII had three (synonyms, drugs, and side effects);
- and finally, in Volume VIII Graham introduced a unique system of referencing in which each reference was accorded a modifier that indicated whether it was a clinical paper, major or minor (C or c), and whether it was a review, extensive or limited (R or r).

At this stage Dukes persuaded Elsevier that attempting to present both an overall view and detailed updates in a single volume every four years was inadequate, and he suggested that annual update volumes should be introduced. The four-yearly volume could then concentrate on providing a complementary critical encyclopaedic survey of the entire field. The first *Side Effects of Drugs Annual* was published in 1977 (Table 2). The first encyclopaedic edition of *Meyler's Side Effects of Drugs*, which appeared in 1980, was labelled the ninth edition, and since then a new encyclopaedic edition has appeared every four years (Table 2); the latest edition has just been published.

Table 3. Highlights from the curriculum vitae of Graham Dukes

Special interests
Pharmaceutical and health legislation
Pharmaceutical policies and planning
Drug information
Medical risk management and assessment
Adverse drug effects and responsibility for drug-induced injury
Drug litigation
Ethics of the pharmaceutical industry
Pharmacoeconomics

Current and recent positions
Emeritus Professor of Drug Policy Studies, University of Groningen, The Netherlands (1985–1997)
Adviser on Drug Policy Studies, Institute of Pharmacotherapy, University of Oslo, Norway (1997 onwards)
Senior Consultant on Drug Policies, The World Bank, Washington DC (1991, continuing)
Editor, The International Journal of Risk and Safety in Medicine (1990 to date)

Principal books
Patent Medicines and Autotherapy (1963)
Non-Steroidal Anti-Inflammatory Drugs (1964)
Antidepressant Drugs (1966)
Meyler's Side Effects of Drugs (1976–2000) (Table 2)
Side Effects of Drugs Annuals (1977–1993) (Table 2)
De Toelating van Geneesmiddelen (1981)
The Effects of Drug Regulation (1985)
Responsibility for Drug Induced Injury (1988, 1998)
Side Effects of Drugs Essays (1991)
Vitamins and Minerals: A Policy Outline (1992)
Drug Utilization Studies (1993)
Drugs and Money (6th edition 1991; 7th edition, 1999)

Distinctions
Chairman, Commission on "Gaps in Pharmaceutical Technology", Organization for European Co-operation and Development, Paris 1967–1969
Chairman, Committee on Abuse of Medicaments, Council of Europe, Strasbourg, 1972–1974
Chairman, Committee on Clinical Standards, Commission of the European Communities, Brussels, 1978–1982
Chairman, Commission on Clinical Pharmacology, Netherlands Health Council, 1977–1982
Chairman, Commission on Future Scenarios for Drugs, Netherlands Ministry of Health, 1990–1993
Team Leader, reform of Medicines Legislation and Control System in South Africa, WHO for South African Ministry of Health, 1998–1999
Honorary Consul of the Republic of Yemen in Norway, Government of Yemen, 1998 Officer of the Order of the Orange Nassau, 2000

Another innovation that Graham introduced was to list the addresses of all the National Centres participating in the WHO drug monitoring scheme in each volume. The list of addresses first appeared in the ninth edition and was prefaced with a note about international pharmacovigilance, which Graham wrote himself. Later he passed the authorship of this section to members of the WHO Collaborating Centre for International Drug Monitoring in Uppsala, Sweden—Kjell Strandberg in the eleventh edition and Ralph Edwards in subsequent editions. Graham also introduced into the Annuals the feature of special reviews—short articles, typographically distinguished from the rest of the text, and marked by the prescription symbol of the eye of Horus—dealing in depth with a specific topic of current interest. And he instituted the Side Effects of Drugs Essay, usually written by a guest author but sometimes (seven times in all) by Graham himself.

I have been privileged to have been associated with the Side Effects series since 1978, first as an author and then as Graham's co-editor (Table 2). It has been an extraordinary experience and a real education. Graham's mild manner conceals a razor-sharp mind that penetrates to the heart of the matter, whatever it is. His knowledge of people and developments in the field of pharmacovigilance is encyclopaedic and he is universally respected. His prose is elegant and is underpinned by an extensive cultural knowledge. A selection of highlights from his curriculum vitae, including some of the distinctions that he has received during his long career (Table 3), demonstrates his eminence more eloquently than I can.

On Saturday 23 September 2000, after a special symposium to honour Graham, organized in Verona under the auspices of Elsevier Science and the European Society of Pharmacovigilance, Elsevier Science hosted a private dinner party to say goodbye. After the first course the surprise guest, the Dutch Consul to Northern Italy, rose to give a speech. He outlined Graham's distinguished career, highlighted his work on the Side Effects series, and ended by saying that he had been commanded by Queen Beatrix of the Netherlands to present Graham with the insignia of an Officer of the Order of Oranje Nassau, the highest honour that the Queen can confer and one that is rarely awarded. It was an extraordinary moment. The astonished look on Graham's face was matched only by the loudness of the applause that greeted the richly deserved award.

Graham's presence in the Meyler camp will be sorely missed, but I hope that he will continue to give advice to the project as it moves into the electronic era. He has been an inspiration not only to the Side Effects series, but to the whole field of pharmacovigilance. I expect that he will continue to be influential for some time to come.

Jeffrey K. Aronson
Oxford, October 2000

Inclusion of therapeutic failures as adverse drug reactions

Kenneth Y. Hartigan-Go and John Q. Wong *

Introduction

Background and significance

An adverse drug reaction (ADR) is defined by the World Health Organization (WHO) as any response to a drug that is noxious and unintended and which occurs at doses normally used in man for the prophylaxis, diagnosis, and therapy of disease, or for the modification of physiological function (1). This definition excludes accidental or deliberate excessive dosage or maladministration. An ADR is often suspected, but rarely proven with certainty.

It has been estimated that 3–5% of hospitalizations can be attributed to ADRs. There is also a 30% chance that once patients are hospitalized, they will have some untoward experiences relating to drug therapy. The risk of a serious or life-threatening drug event is about 3% per patient in hospital (2).

Global concerns for the safety of drugs arose dramatically in the 1960s, after limb defects were observed in children born to mothers who took thalidomide (3).

International efforts to promote adverse drug reactions monitoring and reporting

The World Health Organization, through the Uppsala Monitoring Centre in Sweden, formerly the WHO Collaborating Centre for International Drug Monitoring (see Chapter 50), actively promotes awareness and educational programs in the recognition, monitoring, and analysis of ADRs. Furthermore, the Uppsala Monitoring Centre provides member countries of the WHO with a system for reporting ADRs. Their database contains upwards of 2 million reports from some 60 countries. These are analysed and causality is assessed. The information gained from such analysis then benefits government regulatory authorities and industry in the promotion of pharmacovigilance and drug safety.

In current training programs, health care providers are ideally instructed and reminded to report the following:

- suspected reactions to new drugs;
- suspected drug-drug interactions;
- ADRs that cause death;
- ADRs that are life-threatening;
- ADRs that cause admission to hospital;
- ADRs that cause a prolonged stay in hospital;
- ADRs that cause birth defects.

During the 16th annual meeting of national centers that monitor ADRs, held in Geneva in September of 1993, drug dependence and withdrawal were also considered as possible ADRs, because it was deemed that the process of ADR reporting might capture harmful effects from the use of drugs that have abuse and dependence potential.

However, there has as yet been no effort to include therapeutic failures as an ADR term. Nevertheless, from the standpoint of drug safety, ADR reporting is a potential mechanism for detecting 'bad' drugs, in particular counterfeit medicines. If all other measures to curb illicit and fake drugs fail, ADR reporting can

* This year's guest authors are Kenneth Hartigan-Go, MD, MD (UK), and John Wong, MD, MS. Dr Hartigan-Go is Deputy Director of the Bureau of Food and Drugs and Manager, Philippine National Drug Policy Programme Office, Department of Health, Philippines; Dr Wong is Consultant, Philippine National Drug Policy Program Office, Department of Health, Philippines.

play a significant role in detecting counterfeit medicines, because this is the last hurdle by which these may be detected.

Traditionally, ADRs have been classified as follows:

Type A—dose-related effects (Augmented).
Type B—non-dose-related effects (Bizarre).
Type C—dose- and time-related effects (Continuous or Chronic).
Type D—time-related effects (Delayed).
Type E—withdrawal effects (Ending of use).

This classification arises from the original classification into two types, A and B (4), which were later extended to four (5), and then to five (6).

There may be merit in considering the introduction of a new type of ADR, type F, representing *failure of treatment*, to help create an awareness that ADRs, or more appropriately, the more inclusive term 'adverse drug events' (ADEs) (7), can result from the use of fake, substandard, or adulterated medicines. In other words, that therapeutic failure can occur through a poor drug formulation. Suppose ventricular arrhythmias develop after the use of an antiarrhythmic drug, would a doctor suspect that the arrhythmia was the direct consequence of the medicine or therapeutic failure? This step was necessary to address real problems of therapeutic inefficacy seen in some cases in the Philippines (8).

Because ADR monitoring can identify other problem areas of drug usage, in this essay we shall also consider some of the other reasons for therapeutic failure, such as inadequate dosage, the wrong medicine, or the wrong diagnosis, resulting in the use of the wrong medicine. These reasons are not in the same category as pharmaceutical production problems.

What is therapeutic failure?

Therapeutic failure: definition and classification

Therapeutic inefficacy or failure of treatment refers to the lack of desired effect from the administration of a medicine. This happens when a prescribed medicine, intended to cure or prevent an illness or to modify a physiological function, does not work. Although therapeutic failures probably occur in daily medical practice, they may not be readily recognized.

The factors that account for therapeutic failures can be grouped into four categories:

1. ***Medical***
   (a) inappropriate medication for the disease;
   (b) underdosing;
   (c) poor patient compliance.
2. ***Pharmacological***
   (a) inappropriate route of administration;
   (b) drug interactions (pharmacokinetic or pharmacodynamic);
   (c) antimicrobial resistance;
   (d) tolerance.
3. ***Pharmaceutical***
   (a) counterfeit and/or substandard medicines;
   (b) manufacturing errors, toxic excipients, and preservatives;
   (c) expired medicines and improper storage conditions;
   (d) pharmaceutical interactions.
4. ***Medication errors (SEDA-22, xxiii)***
   (a) errors in planning (mistakes);
   (b) errors in the execution of correctly-planned actions (slips and lapses).

Clinicians have a significant role to play in helping to recognize this threat and in reporting their suspicions. The following sections contain some practical guidelines to help doctors understand the reasons for therapeutic failures and to be in a position to prevent consequent ADRs.

Medical reasons for therapeutic failure

Inappropriate medication for the disease

Assuming that the doctor has made a correct diagnosis, he may sometimes prescribe an inappropriate medication. For example: the prescription of captopril to treat hypertension related to hyperthyroidism, for which β-blockers would be more ideal; or the giving of antibacterial agents for viral illnesses. In neither case would the patient respond to the treatment.

Elderly people are often subjected to inappropriate prescribing practices. Because of their changing physiology and pathology, they sometimes do not respond to drugs in the same way as younger adults. In one study the most frequently prescribed potentially inappropriate medications were amitriptyline, chlordiazepoxide, diazepam, dipyridamole, and propoxyphene (9).

Empirical antibiotic therapy is often given inappropriately. The inappropriateness is proven prospectively by in vitro sensitivity tests. This phenomenon tends to occur more often in hospital-acquired bacteremia, in children aged 1–5 years, with cytotoxic drug therapy, and if an intravenous central line is present (10).

Self-medication can also account for inappropriate use of drugs. For example, when topical antifungal drugs became available over the counter in the US, there was a tremendous increase in their sales. An analysis of this phenomenon showed that most women misdiagnosed their symptoms and consequently used over-the-counter antifungal drugs inappropriately (11).

Inappropriate use of drugs through self-medication can occur as a result of medical advice columns. An evaluation of a sample of Canadian medical advice columns showed that a significant percentage of these articles contain inappropriate or even potentially dangerous advice (12).

Underdosing

When the dosage of a drug is insufficient, treatment failure can occur. Although this is not normally considered an adverse drug reaction, it is a common therapeutic problem. For example, chloramphenicol is usually given in a dosage of 500 mg every 6 hours for Gram-positive organisms, including anerobes; however, in treating meningitis and typhoid fever, the adult dose should not be less than 4 g/day.

In practice, most physicians begin treatment with most drugs with a low dose, measure physiological or pathological variables, and titrate the dosage to achieve a specific therapeutic effect. They do this in order to avoid dose-related adverse effects; however, they fail to see that sometimes this under-dosing will not produce the desired therapeutic effect (13).

In nursing homes, elderly patients who have heart failure and no contraindications to ACE inhibitors are often given dosages that are too low (14).

Drugs that are self-prescribed and those that are taken on the advice of drug vendors are often also used in doses that are too low.

Poor patient compliance

When a prescribed drug does not appear to be working, it is important to check patient compliance; a patient may not take the necessary medications properly for a number of reasons (15).

In chronic diseases, such as hypertension, in which it has been estimated that only about 50–60% adhere well to their prescribed regimens (16), knowledge of patient compliance is important. Ignoring this factor in explaining persistent hypertension can result in unwarranted, even potentially dangerous, prescribing of more of the drug. If the patient is not regularly taking the medication, but starts to do so after the increase in dosage, toxicity can occur.

Indicators that can be used to measure compliance can be classified as shown in Table 1. For example, one simple way to check if a patient is taking his rifampicin is to check the color of his urine; orange-colored urine suggests good patient compliance.

Table 1. *Indicators for measuring compliance*

Type of measure	Examples
Health outcomes	Blood pressure (antihypertensive drugs) Hospitalization
Surrogate markers	Weight change (diuretics) INR (anticoagulants) Drugs or markers measured in blood and urine
Indirect indicators	Tablet count Refill records Electronic monitors
Subjective reports	Reports by patients or others
Use of services	Appointment making Keeping and use of other services (17)

Pharmacological reasons for therapeutic failure

Inappropriate route of administration

The beneficial effects of intravenous insulin and subcutaneous insulin are completely different at times of diabetic ketoacidosis. This is because the disease can affect drug kinetics.

Chloramphenicol has a different effect when given intravenously and intramuscularly, because it precipitates at the site of intramuscular injection; this also happens with phenytoin.

Procaine penicillin should always be given intramuscularly and never intravenously; therapeutic mishaps, such as anaphylactic reactions, have been observed after inadvertent intravenous or intra-arterial administration.

Drug interactions

When two or more drugs are given together, there may be some antagonism of drug effects or inactivation of one or both of the drugs. Easy-to-use reference charts for drug interactions have been constructed (18, 19).

Therapeutic failure can occur as a result of drug interactions or drug incompatibilities. Examples are given in Table 2.

Table 2. *Examples of drug interactions leading to reduced effects*

Mechanism	Examples
Reduced drug absorption	Chelation of tetracycline with polyvalent cations (aluminum, iron, calcium, zinc) (20–23)
Increased metabolism	Reduced efficacy of oral contraceptives when used with enzyme inducers (e.g. rifampicin, carbamazepine, phenytoin) (24, 25) Reduced efficacy of oral anticoagulants when used with enzyme inducers (20, 26)
Reduced enterohepatic recirculation	Reduced efficacy of oral contraceptives when used with broad-spectrum antibiotics (e.g. ampicillin, tetracycline)
Increased excretion	Weakly acidic drugs (e.g. aspirin or phenobarbital) in an alkaline urine or weakly basic drugs (e.g. quinidine) in an acidic urine (20)
Pharmacological antagonism	Reduced bronchodilator effects of β-adrenoceptor agonists when used with non-selective β-blockers (20)

Antimicrobial resistance

Antimicrobial drugs can be selected empirically, according to the most common pathogens suspected to be causing the infection. This therapy can then be modified when a microorganism is cultured and its sensitivity to drugs is identified. When doctors prescribe antimicrobial drugs, they should suspect that the medication is not working if there is no improvement by the second or third day. Improvement can take the form of lysis of fever, improvement in the signs and symptoms of infection, improvement in laboratory evidence of infection (e.g. white cell count, C reactive protein concentration, radiography), or failure of progression of the infection. If these conditions do not occur, antimicrobial resistance should be suspected. However, there are exceptions to the rule that fever should abate within 2–3 days, particularly typhoid fever, in which fever may persist after the use of appropriate antimicrobial agents; even then, the patient may experience subjective improvement. One should also remember that persistent fever may itself sometimes be an adverse drug reaction.

Among the risk factors for the development of antimicrobial resistance are the use of antimicrobial agents in animals reared for food, previous antimicrobial therapy in chronic infections, a high rate of use of antimicrobial drugs in some settings (e.g. intensive care units), previous hospital admissions, injudicious or irrational antibiotic use due to patient pressure or suboptimal diagnosis and treatment, over-the-counter availability of antimicrobial drugs without prescription, international travel and commerce (leading to widespread transmission of resistant organisms), microbial adaptation and change, and breakdown of public health measures.

Tolerance

Some drugs cause tolerance. In other words, higher doses of the drug are needed to reach the same desired effects. Examples of drugs that produce tolerance include narcotic analgesics, the benzodiazepines, and nitrates (27). This means that after an initial therapeutic response the therapeutic efficacy of the drug wanes. Alternatively, certain diseases can lead to reduced tissue sensitivity to a drug. An example of this is hyperthyroidism, which causes reduced cardiac sensitivity to digoxin and is also associated with increased renal digoxin clearance, through increased glomerular filtration. Conversely, in the presence of hypothyroidism digitalis toxicity can occur at normal doses.

Although it is not necessary to report suspected drug inefficacy due to pharmacological tolerance, reports of tolerance to certain pharmaceutical agents may be a signal that the drug has abuse potential or can cause dependency.

Pharmaceutical reasons for therapeutic failure

Counterfeit or substandard medicines

Counterfeit or fake drugs are drugs that are deliberately and fraudulently mislabelled with respect to identity and/or source. They may be products with correct or wrong ingredients, products that contain no active ingredients or insufficient quantities of active ingredients, or products with fake packaging (28). They can be either branded or generic products. The patients who take these drugs, the doctors who prescribe them, the pharmacists who dispense them, and the nurses who administer them may not realize this.

It is the experience of the drug regulatory authority in the Philippines, the Bureau of Food and Drugs (BFAD), that some counterfeit drugs are packaged so professionally that they cannot be distinguished from the real drug by mere visual inspection. It then becomes the responsibility of the doctor to detect these fake drugs and to report them when suspected. The doctor may be in the best position to know whether or not a patient is responding to the drug.

Substandard formulations contain the correct active ingredients but in insufficient quantities. The WHO has initiated programs to prevent the distribution of substandard formulations and has drafted guidelines for testing bioequivalence, based on internationally accepted reference products, and has introduced compliance guidelines for the drug industry on good manufacturing practice (GMP).

Manufacturing errors, toxic excipients, and preservatives

A pharmaceutical product may be inadvertently prepared in the wrong way during manufacturing or compounding. It is therefore important to note the batch and lot numbers when an adverse reaction is suspected or when the drug does not seem to work within a reasonable time. In the past, toxic excipients detected in some formulations have led to deaths. An example of this was when diethylene glycol was used as a solvent in the preparation of paracetamol syrup instead of propylene glycol (29, 30).

Another example is that of lidocaine for use as an anesthetic. In some formulations of lidocaine that contain adrenaline, metabisulfite, a preservative, is included but is not always labelled. Metabisulfite can reduce the anesthetic efficacy of lidocaine. Furthermore, it can cause hypersensitivity reactions in individuals who have a history of asthma or allergies. Other agents that alter the pH of the solution can also reduce the efficacy of the anesthetic effects of lidocaine.

Preservatives used in moistened toilet tissues and in cosmetics can cause contact allergy (31). Nebulization of bacteriostatic saline solution containing benzyl alcohol, and even sterile saline, can cause bronchitis and pharyngitis in adults. Doctors who prescribe nebulized medications should be aware of the bronchodilator diluent used (32). In one study 26% of preserved saline solutions for contact lenses became contaminated with Gram-positive bacteria, most frequently coagulase-positive staphylococci (33).

Expired medicines and improper storage conditions

All medicines have shelf-lives and expiry dates. If drugs are used beyond the recommended dates, they may not work; even worse, the breakdown of these drugs and their excipients into toxic compounds may lead to bizarre and unpredictable adverse drug reactions. An example is the occurrence of the Fanconi syndrome (aminoaciduria, glycosuria, acetonuria, albuminuria, pyuria, and photosensitivity) after the use of outdated and degraded tetracyclines, due to the formation of toxic breakdown products (34, 35).

Improper storage conditions, such as extreme heat, humidity, and light, can destroy the efficacy of drugs. Product labels and pharmaceutical reference books should always be consulted for the proper methods of storing drugs.

Pharmaceutical interactions

Physicochemical drug incompatibilities during administration to the patient can also lead to therapeutic failure. For example, ciprofloxacin solution formulated for direct infusion is incompatible with furosemide, heparin, teicoplanin, and perhaps metronidazole (36).

The organic solvents and surfactants used in some drugs can leach diethylhexylphthalate (DEHP) from polyvinyl chloride (PVC) bags. Drug products that contain surfactants include ciclosporin, miconazole, and teniposide; the DEHP-leaching vehicles include those used in formulating taxol and taxotere. Thus, drugs that leach DEHP should be prepared in non-PVC containers and administered through non-PVC tubing (37).

Aztreonam and vancomycin hydrochloride are incompatible and unstable in high-concentration admixtures, resulting in microcrystalline precipitation (38).

Many drugs flocculate and precipitate with contrast agents (39).

Medication errors

Medication errors, which were reviewed in SEDA-22 (pp. xxiii–xxxvi), can also cause therapeutic failures. Errors can result from actual or potential administration of the incorrect medication to the patient. These errors may be due to inaccuracies in prescribing, transcribing, communication, dispensing, or drug administration. In the US between August 1991 and April 1993 there were 568 reports of medication errors (40). Nurses, pharmacists, and physicians were implicated in a majority of these incidents. The most commonly involved drugs were adrenaline, heparin, lidocaine, and potassium chloride. The most frequent causes of these errors were related to the drug products themselves (e.g. similar packaging, incomplete labelling); on the other hand, cognitive error was the most important factor in deaths.

Conclusion

There is a need to increase the awareness of health professionals in reporting ADRs. ADR reporting must be objective, specific, and accurate, and ADRs must be reported in a timely fashion in order for the reports to be useful. There is also a need to educate health-care workers on how to evaluate therapeutic inefficacy, as it is not always due to a product defect. But when there is a suspected fake or adulterated product, this should be sent to the local regulatory authorities for further analysis.

Therapeutic failures or inefficacy should form a new category of adverse drug reactions. Not only do they result in prolongation of the pathological state, they also result in increased costs, extended patient disability or incapacity, and longer stays in hospital. Efforts to prevent or minimize the medical and pharmacological causes of therapeutic failures should involve education and behavioral and attitudinal changes among doctors, nurses, pharmacists, and patients. There is also a need to examine existing health-care systems to see how they contribute to these causes. Epidemiological research, molecular, clinical, and social, can help to explore these causes further and to provide solutions. Lastly, appropriate regulatory action is necessary to correct the pharmaceutical causes of therapeutic failure, including quality assurance of the medicinal product.

REFERENCES

1. World Health Organization Scientific Group on Monitoring Adverse Reactions, Geneva 22–28 November 1964 (WHO document PA/8.65) and The WHO Collaborating Centre for International Drug Monitoring Guide to Participating Country (version September 1993), Uppsala, Sweden.
2. Nies AS, Spielberg SP. Principles of therapeutics. In: Hardman JG, Limbird LE, editors. Goodman and Gilman's The Pharmacological Basis of Therapeutics, 9th edition. New York: McGraw Hill, 1996:43–62.
3. Wiholm B, Olsson S, Moore N, Wood S. Spontaneous Reporting Systems Outside of the United States. In: Strom BL, editor. Pharmacoepidemiology. 2nd edition. West Sussex, England: John Wiley & Sons, 1994:139–55.
4. Rawlins MD, Thompson JW. Pathogenesis of adverse drug reactions. In: Davies DM editor. Textbook of Adverse Drug Reactions. Oxford: Oxford University Press, 1985:12–38.
5. Grahame-Smith DG, Aronson JK. The Oxford textbook of clinical pharmacology and drug therapy. Chapter 9. Adverse drug reactions. Oxford: Oxford University Press, 1984:132-57.
6. Laurence D, Carpenter J. A dictionary of pharmacology and clinical drug evaluation. London: UCL Press, 1994.
7. Bates DW, Cullen DJ, Laird N, Peetersen LA, Small SD, Servi D, Laffel G, Sweitzer BJ, Shea BF, Hallisey R, Vander-Vliet M, Nemeskal R, Leape LL. Incidence of adverse drug events and potential adverse drug events. Implications for prevention. ADE Prevention Study Group. J Am Med Assoc 1995;274:29–34.
8. Hartigan-Go K. Working methods for the Adverse Drug Reaction Monitoring Program in the Philippines. Drug Inform J 1998;32:85–92.
9. Aparasu RR, Fliginger SE. Inappropriate medication prescribing for the elderly by office-based physicians. Ann Pharmacother 1997;31:823–9.

10. Ashkenazi S, Samra Z, Konisberger H, Drucker MM, Leibovici L. Factors associated with increased risk in inappropriate empiric antibiotic treatment of childhood bacteremia. Eur J Pediatr 1996;155:545–50.
11. Ferris DG, Dekle C, Litaker MS. Women's use of over-the-counter anti-fungal medications for gynecologic symptoms. J Fam Pract 1996;42:595–600.
12. Molnar FJ, Man Son Hing M, Dalziel WB, Mitchell SL, Power BE, Byszewski AM, St John P. Assessing the quality of newspaper medical advice columns for elderly readers. Can Med Assoc J 1999;161:393–5.
13. Packer M. Use and abuse of clinical trials? Is the dose used the dose tested? Cardiology 1994; 85(Suppl 1):2–6.
14. Forman DE, Chander RB, Lapane KL, Shah P, Stoukides J. Evaluating the use of angiotensin-converting enzyme inhibitors for older nursing home residents with chronic heart failure. J Am Geriatr Soc 1998;46:1550-4.
15. Métry J-M, Meyer UA, editors. Drug regimen compliance. Chichester: John Wiley & Sons Ltd, 1999.
16. Rudd P. Clinicians and patients with hypertension: unsettled issues about compliance. Am Heart J 1995; 130: 572-9.
17. Roter DL, Hall JA, Merisca R, Nordstrom B, Cretin D, Svarstad B. Effectiveness of interventions to improve patient compliance: a meta-analysis. Med Care 1998;36:1138–61.
18. Whiting B, Goldberg A. The use of the drug disc (MEDISC): a warning system for drug interactions. In: Grahame-Smith DG, editor. Drug interactions. Baltimore: University Park Press, 1977:21–31.
19. Hartigan-Go K. Drug interaction chart. Rational Drug Use (RDU) Update Newsletter. Philippines: Department of Health, 1991:1(1).
20. Stockley IH. Drug interactions. Blackwell Scientific Publications, Oxford 1981:1–14.
21. Hansten PD. Drug Interactions. 5th edition. Philadelphia: Lea & Febiger, 1985:238–43.
22. Dufull S. Drugs and food—clinically significant interactions. Med Prog 1997;24:33-7.
23. Horn JR, Hansten PD. Drug interactions with antibacterial agents. J Fam Pract 1995;41:81–90.
24. Back DJ, Breckenridge AM, Crawford FE, MacIver M, Orme LE, Rowe PH. Interindividual variation and drug interactions with hormonal steroid contraceptives. Drugs 1981;21:46–61.
25. Janz D, Schmidt D. Anti-epileptic drugs and the failure of oral contraceptives. Lancet 1974;1:1113.
26. Levi G, O'Reilly RA, Aggeler PM, Keech GM. Pharmacokinetic analysis of the effect of barbiturate on the anticoagulant action of warfarin in man. Clin Pharmacol Ther 1970;11:372.
27. Grahame-Smith DG. 'Keep on taking the tablets': pharmacological adaptation during long-term drug therapy. Br J Clin Pharmacol 1997;44:227–38.
28. Workshop on counterfeit medicines. Geneva: World Health Organization/IFPMA, 1992.
29. Anonymous. Fatalities associated with ingestion of diethylene glycol-contaminated glycerin used to manufacture acetaminophen syrup—Haiti, Nov 1995–June 1996. Mort Morb Wkly Rep 1996;45:649–50.
30. Okuonghae HO, Ighogboja IS, Lawson JO, Nwana EJ. Diethylene glycol poisoning in Nigerian Children. Ann Trop Paediatr 1992;12:235–8.
31. Van Ginkel CJ, Rundervoort GJ. Increasing incidence of allergy to the new preservative 1,2-dibromo-2,4-dicyanobutane (methyldibromoglutaronitrile). Br J Dermatol 1995;132:918–20.
32. Reynolds RD, Smith RM. Nebulized bacteriostatic saline as a cause of bronchitis. J Fam Pract 1995;40:35–40.
33. Sweeney DF, Willcox MD, Sansey N, Leitch C, Harmis N, Wong R, Holden BA. Incidence of contamination of preserved saline solutions during normal use. CLAO J 1999;25:167–75.
34. Sulkowski SR, Haserick JR. Simulated systemic lupus erythematosus from degraded tetracycline. J Am Med Assoc 1964;189:152.
35. Gross JM. Fanconi syndrome (adult type) developing secondary to ingestion of outdated tetracycline. Ann Intern Med 1963;58:523.
36. Jim LK. Physical and chemical compatibility of intravenous ciprofloxacin with other drugs. Ann Pharmacother 1993;27:704–7.
37. Pearson SD, Trissel LA. Leaching of diethylhexyl phthalate from polyvinyl chloride containers by selected drugs and formulation components. Am J Hosp Pharm 1993;50:1405–9.
38. Trissel LA, Xu QA, Martinez JF. Compatibility and stability of aztreonam and vancomycin hydrochloride. Am J Health-Syst Pharm 1995;52:2560–4.
39. Violon D. The (in)compatibility of drugs and contrast media: a review of the literature. J Belge Radiol 1993;76:375–6.
40. Edgar TA, Lee DS, Cousins DD. Experience with a national medication error reporting program. Am J Hosp Pharm 1994;51:1335–8.

Reginald P. Sequeira

1 Central nervous system stimulants and drugs that suppress appetite

METHYLXANTHINES *(SED-13, 1; SEDA-20, 1; SEDA-21, 1; SEDA-22, 1)*

Aminophylline

Use in pregnancy In pregnant women with bronchial asthma, bronchospasm may be exacerbated during labor, necessitating infusion of aminophylline. The placental transport of aminophylline and its effects on the fetus and the neonate are poorly understood. A recent report has highlighted the potential problems (1^c).

A 26-year-old primigravida with bronchial asthma developed an acute exacerbation at 40 weeks gestation. She did not respond to salbutamol and was given hydrocortisone and aminophylline 250 mg intravenously, without improvement. She received two more doses of intravenous aminophylline, the last being 2 hours before delivery. At cesarean section she delivered a full-term female neonate weighing 3150 g with Apgar scores of 3 and 5 at 1 and 5 minutes respectively. Within 3 minutes of birth the neonate developed multifocal clonic convulsions, which failed to respond to intravenous glucose, calcium, phenobarbital, and phenytoin. She had a tachycardia, a normal blood pressure, and poor respiratory drive, and was comatose. The serum theophylline concentration was 8.6 μg/ml (47 μmol/l) at 1 hour of life. Despite ventilatory support and anticonvulsant therapy, she continued to have intermittent seizures and died 48 hours after birth. Postmortem showed normal brain structure and no evidence of hemorrhage or asphyxial brain injury.

The toxic concentrations for theophylline in neonates have not been well defined, and may vary from infant to infant. Other pharmacokinetic factors, such as low plasma protein binding and limited capacity for excretion could make neonates prone to aminophylline toxicity. Fetuses and neonates can develop theophylline toxicity even with plasma concentrations in the target range, since they can metabolize theophylline to caffeine, adding to the methylxanthine load.

Interactions *Antibiotics* Fatal aminophylline toxicity has been described, precipitated by the concomitant administration of erythromycin (2^c).

A 55-year-old man with a long history of bronchiectasis and severe obstructive pulmonary disease presented with a chest infection, having been taking oral modified-release aminophylline 450 mg bd for 4 years, with trough concentrations always in the range 6–12 mg/l (33–66 μmol/l) and no apparent toxicity. Two days before admission, his general practitioner had prescribed trimethoprim 200 mg bd for a suspected urinary tract infection. On the day of admission, he was given cefotaxime 1 g intravenously bd and erythromycin 500 mg orally qds. Other medications included captopril 25 mg tds, frusemide 80 mg bd, ranitidine 150 mg bd, protriptyline 10 mg tds, and inhaled budesonide. He was anxious and had a fine tremor, but his gas exchange was satisfactory. He had chronic renal impairment of uncertain cause and hyperkalemia (5.5 mmol/l). The possibility of aminophylline toxicity was raised, but despite this he received three doses of erythromycin. The plasma theophylline was 66 mg/l (363 μmol/l). He had an episode of ventricular tachycardia and fibrillation, was successfully resuscitated, but had a second episode of ventricular tachycardia 30 minutes later, from which he could not be resuscitated. The plasma theophylline concentration at the time of his second cardiac arrest was 58 mg/l (319 μmol/l).

Serious theophylline toxicity has also been attributed to *ciprofloxacin* (2^c).

A 79-year-old woman presented with a generalized seizure. She had long-standing asthma,

Side Effects of Drugs, Annual 23
J.K. Aronson, ed.

and her admission medication included steroid and salbutamol inhalers, oral prednisolone, and oral modified-release aminophylline 450 mg bd. Plasma theophylline concentrations over the previous 3 years had been 8–12 mg/l (44–66 μmol/l) without apparent toxicity. Seven days before presentation, she had developed a fever and cough productive of green sputum, and had been given ciprofloxacin 500 mg bd. Despite adequate gas exchange, she developed repeated episodes of self-terminating supraventricular tachycardia, associated with hypokalemia (serum potassium 3.2 mmol/l), acidosis (pH 7.05), hypotension, and difficulty in breathing. The theophylline concentration was 33 mg/l (183 μmol/l), renal function was normal, and no other causes of fits or dysrhythmias were apparent. She was unable to tolerate oral activated charcoal and hemodialysis was started. After 2 hours of dialysis, the plasma theophylline had fallen to 15 mg/l (177 μmol/l), she was in sinus rhythm, and her serum potassium was 3.8 mmol/l. She made an uneventful recovery.

These cases illustrate that serious, even fatal, adverse effects can occur when possible interactions are not considered. In both cases, experienced physicians prescribed appropriate antimicrobials, but omitted to consider the possibility of interactions with aminophylline, and failed to reduce the dose of aminophylline or to measure theophylline concentrations. In the first case the anxiety, tremor, and cardiac arrests could all have resulted from an interaction of aminophylline and erythromycin, while in the second the development of tachycardia, hypokalemia, acidosis, vomiting, and convulsions can be explained on the basis of theophylline toxicity caused by ciprofloxacin. These cases add to an extensive literature that emphasizes the potential for interaction between aminophylline and drugs metabolized by CYP1A2. Another quinolone, prulifloxacin, reduced the elimination of theophylline in healthy volunteers (3[C]), presumably by inhibiting cytochrome CYP1A2. It is unfortunate that many of the drugs commonly prescribed for respiratory infections, such as macrolides and some quinolones, are amongst those that should ideally be avoided.

Olanzapine In healthy subjects, olanzapine did not affect theophylline pharmacokinetics (4[C]). These results confirm the earlier reported in vitro findings that olanzapine is not a potent inhibitor of CYP1A2 (5).

Terbinafine In a randomized crossover study in 12 healthy volunteers terbinafine increased the AUC of theophylline by 16%, with a 14% reduction in clearance and a 24% increase in half-life (6[C]). The clinical impact of the results is difficult to define, because of the small sample size in this study and because it is not known what effect terbinafine has on steady-state theophylline concentrations. An earlier study (7[C]) showed that terbinafine reduced the clearance of caffeine, which is metabolized via similar pathways. Until more information is available, clinicians who prescribe terbinafine for patients taking chronic theophylline therapy should be cautious, and serum theophylline concentrations should be monitored.

RESPIRATORY STIMULANTS

Doxapram

Doxapram is used to treat idiopathic apnea in premature infants. *Second-degree atrioventricular heart block* developed after its administration to three neonates (78).

Thirty-six hours after an infusion of doxapram was started the first infant developed second-degree AV block, with QT interval prolongation and an increase in the QRS interval. There was no hypotension. Sinus rhythm returned 92 hours after stopping the infusion.

Doxapram was given orally, every 6 hours, to the second infant. After 43 hours second-degree AV block with a prolonged QT interval was noted. Echocardiography showed a normal heart. Doxapram was discontinued and 8 hours later sinus rhythm returned.

The third infant was given aminophylline orally and doxapram by intravenous infusion; 5 days later cisapride was added to treat suspected gastroesophageal reflux. The next day the infant had developed second-degree AV block, with a prolonged QT interval. Doxapram was withdrawn and sinus rhythm returned 36 hours later.

Cisapride can prolong the QT interval and heart block did not occur in the third case until cisapride was added.

DRUGS THAT SUPPRESS APPETITE

Fenfluramine, cardiac valvulopathies, and pulmonary hypertension

Cardiac valvulopathies *Recently concern has been expressed that dexfenfluramine may be* *associated with valvular heart disease. This resulted in its voluntary withdrawal by the manufacturers on 15 September 1997, and the US Department of Health and Human Services issued interim recommendations for people previously exposed to fenfluramine or dexfenfluramine with cardiac valvulopathies (for review see SEDA-22, 3).*

In the meantime, the protocol of a randomized, double-blind, placebo-controlled comparison of dexfenfluramine with an investigational modified-release formulation of dexfenfluramine was amended: the study medication was discontinued and echocardiographic examinations were performed on 1072 overweight patients within a median of 1 month after withdrawal of treatment (9[CR]). These patients, 80% of whom were women, had been randomly assigned to receive dexfenfluramine (366 patients), modified-release dexfenfluramine (352 patients), or placebo (354 patients). The average duration of treatment was 71–72 days in each group. Echocardiograms were assessed blind. Pooling the fenfluramine groups, there was a higher prevalence of any degree of aortic regurgitation (17 vs 12%) and mitral regurgitation (61 vs 54%) with fenfluramine. Analyses carried out using the criteria set by the FDA showed that aortic regurgitation of mild or greater severity occurred in 5% of the patients taking dexfenfluramine, 5.4% of those in the two fenfluramine groups combined, and 3.6% of those in the placebo group. Moderate or severe mitral regurgitation occurred in 1.7 and 1.8% of those taking fenfluramine and 1.2% of those taking placebo. Aortic regurgitation of mild or greater severity, mitral regurgitation of moderate or greater severity, or both occurred in 6.5, 6.9, and 4.5% respectively.

This was an unusual study, because patients enrolled for a different purpose were analyzed midway through the study in response to withdrawal of fenfluramine. In the absence of any prospective study of the association between fenfluramine and valvulopathies, the findings of this study acquire greater importance. What should not be overlooked is that exposure to fenfluramine in this study was for relatively short periods (2–3 months); whether therapy of longer duration would yield the same or different results is not known. It is also important to emphasize that the prevalences of mitral regurgitation and aortic regurgitation in this study were much lower than previously described (10[R]).

Although the findings of this study may be reassuring for patients who have taken dexfenfluramine for 2–3 months, they should not preclude the appropriate investigation of a new murmur or new symptoms in an patient with a history of exposure to dexfenfluramine, as specified in the American College of Cardiology Guidelines (11[R]).

Pretreatment echocardiography *One limitation of the study described above was that pretreatment echocardiography was not included in the original trial design, and patients with pre-existing valvular disease were therefore not excluded. According to a study of users of fenfluramine or dexfenfluramine who underwent echocardiography before taking the drug, the risk of new or prospective valvular heart disease is much lower than implied by previous prevalence studies (12[C]). In 46 patients who used fenfluramine or dexfenfluramine for 14 days or more, the primary outcome was new or worsening valvulopathy, defined as progression of either aortic regurgitation or mitral regurgitation by at least one degree of severity and disease that met FDA criteria. Two patients taking fenfluramine + phentermine developed valvular heart disease. One had mild aortic regurgitation that progressed to moderate regurgitation and the second developed new moderate aortic insufficiency. The authors argued that the referral bias in their study, which required an echocardiogram for inclusion, would have tended to result in a higher incidence of valvular disease.*

Obesity as a confounding factor *It is not clear whether valvular insufficiency is related to the use of appetite suppressants or is simply a consequence of obesity. Obese patients who took dexfenfluramine alone, dexfenfluramine in combination with phentermine, or fenfluramine in combination with phentermine, and a matched group of obese control subjects who had not taken these medications have been compared (13[CR]). A total of 1.3% of the controls (3 of 233) and 23% of the patients (53 of 233) met the case definition for cardiac valve abnormalities (OR = 22.6). The odds ratios for such cardiac valve abnormalities were 13 with dexfenfluramine alone, 25 with dexfenfluramine and phentermine, and 26 with fenfluramine and phentermine. This study has shown that the prevalence of valvular insufficiency is significantly higher among obese patients who have* *taken appetite suppressants than among subjects matched for age, sex, and body mass index who did not take such drugs. Since a higher percentage of patients than controls had trace aortic valve insufficiency, the authors questioned whether the case definition threshold for cardiac valve abnormalities in association with appetite suppressants set by the FDA and Centers for Disease Control and Prevention is perhaps too high. In this study the factors that predisposed patients to valvular insufficiency were (a) age at the start of therapy (b) use of dexfenfluramine, (c) combination of dexfenfluramine with phentermine, and (d) combination of fenfluramine with phentermine. Hence, neither the clinical significance nor the natural history of this type of valvular disease has been defined.*

Assessing risk *The risk of a subsequent clinical diagnosis of a valvular disorder of uncertain origin has been assessed in a population-based follow-up study using nested case-control analysis of 6532 subjects who took dexfenfluramine, 2371 who took fenfluramine, and 862 who took phentermine (14[CR]). The control group comprised 9281 obese subjects who did not take appetite suppressants matched with the treated subjects for age, sex, and weight. No subject had cardiovascular disease at the start of the follow-up for an average duration of 5 years. There were 11 cases of newly diagnosed idiopathic valvular disorders, five with dexfenfluramine and six with fenfluramine. There were six cases of aortic regurgitation, two of mitral regurgitation, and three of combined aortic and mitral regurgitation. There were no cases of idiopathic cardiac valve abnormalities among the controls or those who took phentermine. The 5-year cumulative incidence of idiopathic cardiac valve disorders was 0 per 10 000 among both those who had not taken appetite suppressants (95 CI = 0–15) and those who took phentermine alone (CI = 0–77), 7.1 per 10 000 among those who took either fenfluramine or dexfenfluramine for less than 4 months (CI = 3.6–18), and 35 per 10 000 among those who took either of these medications for 4 months or more (CI = 16–76). The authors concluded that the use of fenfluramine or dexfenfluramine, particularly for 4 months or longer, is associated with an increased risk of newly diagnosed cardiac valve disorders, particularly aortic regurgitation.*

The above study was based on information derived from the General Practice Research Database in the UK. Subjects who had been given at least one prescription for dexfenfluramine, fenfluramine, or phentermine after 1 January 1988, and who were 70 years or younger at the time of their first prescription were included. Subjects were considered to have a new cardiac abnormality if they had no history, on the basis of clinical records, of cardiac valvular abnormalities and if there was evidence of a new valvular disorder on the basis of echocardiography or clinical examination after exposure to appetite suppressants. All the data had been recorded before the publication of recent reports of an association between appetite suppressants and cardiac valve disorders (10[R], 15[C]–18[C]), or primary pulmonary hypertension (19[Cr]). Hence, it was possible to exclude the possibility that enhanced awareness of possible serious adverse effects of appetite suppressants had led to closer surveillance of patients who were taking these drugs. Nevertheless, the study did not provide information on the frequency of idiopathic cardiac valve disorders that are asymptomatic or otherwise not clinically diagnosed.

Echocardiography with color Doppler in 22 patients aged 25–69 years (19 women and 3 men) who had taken phen-fen for more than 3 months showed that one patient with newly discovered aortic insufficiency was asymptomatic. Some were taking several other drugs, none of which is known to precipitate valvular heart disease. Echocardiography was normal in 12 cases and abnormal in 10, including significant aortic insufficiency and significant mitral regurgitation. Ten of the patients had significant aortic insufficiency and nine had at least mild mitral insufficiency. The author inferred that fenfluramine was the likely offending agent, because (a) while it is known to cause release of serotonin, phentermine does not; carcinoid tumors, which secrete serotonin, and ergotamine, a serotonergic drug, are known to cause valvular heart disease; (b) none of the obese patients treated with phentermine and fluoxetine for more than 2 years developed pulmonary hypertension (20[C]) and the author found no valvular heart disease in this cohort either (21[C]). The recommendation that phentermine should be combined with fluoxetine, sertraline, or fluvoxamine as safer alternatives (21[C]) requires prospective studies.

Natural history *Whether cardiac valvular lesions associated with appetite suppressant* *drugs resolve, progress, or remain unchanged after withdrawal of the drugs is uncertain. In a patient who was followed for 2 years after withdrawal multivalvular regurgitation associated with fenfluramine and phentermine may have regressed (22*[C]*).*

A 44-year-old woman with morbid obesity but no history of cardiac disease developed atypical chest pain. Myocardial infarction was ruled out, and an echocardiogram showed normal chamber sizes and mildly reduced global systolic function. However, moderate to moderately severe aortic regurgitation, mild mitral regurgitation, and moderate tricuspid regurgitation were present. The estimated pulmonary artery pressure was slightly raised. Her only medications were fenfluramine 60 mg/day and phentermine 30 mg/day, which she had taken for the previous 50 weeks, during which time she had lost 40 kg. These drugs were withdrawn and 6 months later an echocardiogram showed improved left ventricular function and a reduction in the severity of all her valvular lesions, with no clinically significant change in the estimated pulmonary artery pressure. An echocardiogram obtained 2 years after the initial study showed only trace aortic and tricuspid regurgitation without mitral regurgitation.

In this case, serial echocardiography over 2 years documented regression of multivalvular regurgitation, first discovered while the patient was taking fenfluramine and phentermine. The authors argued that although she was also given lisinopril, the marked degree of improvement in all the valvular lesions after withdrawal of the appetite suppressants was unlikely to be attributable to this alone (23[C]*).*

An important area for further research is to carry out follow-up studies on larger number of patients to document the natural history of these lesions. It is somewhat reassuring, as this report suggested, that mild to moderate valvular lesions associated with fenfluramine and phentermine may be at least partially reversible on withdrawal.

Restrictive cardiomyopathy due to endocardial fibrosis occurred in a 35-year-old woman 5 months after she had started to take fenfluramine 10 mg tds and phentermine 15 mg/day (24[C]*). The endocardial findings strongly resembled the valvular lesions associated with the use of fenfluramine-phentermine. Endocardial and valvular fibrosis associated with anorectic drugs is strikingly similar to the plaque material found in patients with carcinoid syndrome and those exposed to methysergide, and all possibly arise from a common mechanism.*

Incidence *Valvular involvement has been reported in under 1% and in more than 30% of cases, but this wide range of incidences can be at least partly reconciled. The FDA surveys and the University of Minnesota study reported point prevalences and inherently overestimated the association of appetite suppressants with valvulopathy, because a certain percentage of patients will have pre-existing valvular lesions. The method of detection also plays a crucial role. Echocardiography is far more sensitive than clinical examination in detecting valvular regurgitation. The issue may also be confounded by lesion regression after withdrawal of therapy (22*[C]*). Moreover, case control studies are no substitute for objective evidence of the status of cardiac valves before drug exposure (12*[CR]*). Also the duration of exposure has varied widely in different reports.*

Why was this type of valvulopathy not recognized before? Changes in medical practice seem to have played a role as long-term and widespread use of these drugs evolved in the 1990s. Furthermore, cardiac murmurs can be more difficult to detect in obese patients (25[r]*).*

Findings in recent studies (12[CR]*–14*[CR]*) have supported earlier reports of an association between fenfluramine or its d-isomer and cardiac valvular regurgitation, but have differed with regard to the strength and clinical significance of the association (26*[C]*). Differences in design, including a lack of baseline cardiac evaluation in echocardiographic assessment (9*[CR]*, 13*[CR]*, 14*[CR]*) have precluded comparisons. Additional evidence linking the use of fenfluramine or dexfenfluramine to cardiac valvular regurgitation has reaffirmed the wisdom of the FDA's decision to withdraw them from the market. Recent epidemiological studies have ruled out the possibility that obesity itself causes a high prevalence of cardiac valvular regurgitation (27*[C]*–29*[C]*). Further studies will be necessary to clarify the need for follow-up evaluation of patients who took fenfluramine or dexfenfluramine alone or in combination with phentermine for 3 months or more or fenfluramine in high dosages (up to 120 mg/day). It is important to remember that in patients who met the FDA criteria for cardiac valvular abnormalities on echocardiography performed soon after the withdrawal of appetite suppressants, there is a possibility (ranging from as low as 5% to as high as 67%) that the abnormality is a naturally occurring* *phenomenon and not a consequence of drug use (26[C]).*

Pulmonary hypertension *Primary pulmonary hypertension associated with fenfluramine was first reported in the early 1980s. A retrospective study further established the link between pulmonary hypertension and fenfluramine (30[C]). Subsequently a multicenter case-control study in 95 patients showed a high incidence of pulmonary hypertension in patients who had used fenfluramine or dexfenfluramine (19[C]). Moreover, there was a strong suggestion of a dose-response effect, longer periods of use being associated with a progressive increase in the relative risk of pulmonary hypertension. In 1997, the first case of pulmonary hypertension in association with fenfluramine and phentermine was reported (31[C]). Eight of the 24 patients with valvular disease had newly diagnosed pulmonary hypertension, although in most cases it was attributable to valvular abnormalities (32[C]). It is not clear whether a combination of these agents poses a higher risk in predisposed individuals.*

The results of a Belgian study in 35 patients with pulmonary hypertension and 85 matched controls have been published (33[CR]). The data were collected when there was no restriction on prescribing of appetite suppressants. Of the patients, 23 had previously taken appetite suppressants, mainly fenfluramines, compared with five controls. Moreover, the patients who had been exposed to appetite suppressants tended to be on an average more severely ill and to have a shorter median delay between the onset of symptoms and diagnosis.

Incidence *The epidemiological association of pulmonary hypertension with aminorex and dexfenfluramine, both with respect to the strength of the association (estimate of relative risk) and its impact on public health, has been investigated (34[C]). Control rates of exposure were used to estimate population exposure prevalences. The estimated odds ratio for the association between pulmonary hypertension and any exposure to aminorex was 98 and for dexfenfluramine 3.7. The strong association between aminorex and pulmonary hypertension projected a 5-fold increase in the incidence of pulmonary hypertension, and thus a very noticeable epidemic. In contrast, the association with dexfenfluramine is expected to result in an incidence of only 20% and thus a repeat epidemic seems unlikely.*

Prognosis *In 62 patients (61 women) exposed to fenfluramine compared with 125 sex-matched patients with primary pulmonary hypertension, 33 patients had used dexfenfluramine alone, seven had used fenfluramine alone, and five had used both (35[C]). In 17 cases fenfluramines were taken with amphetamines. Most of the patients (81%) had used fenfluramines for at least 3 months. The interval between the start of therapy and the onset of dyspnea was 49 months (range 27 days to 23 years). The two groups differed significantly in terms of age and body mass index. Both groups had similar severe baseline hemodynamics, but the percentage of responders to an acute vasodilator was higher in patients with primary pulmonary hypertension. Hence, more patients with primary pulmonary hypertension were treated with oral vasodilators, and long-term epoprostenol infusion was more often used in fenfluramine users. Overall survival was similar in the two groups, with a 3-year survival rate of 50%.*

Mechanism *The mechanism of fenfluramine-associated pulmonary hypertension has been reviewed before (SEDA-21, 3). Since only a minority of patients exposed to fenfluramines develop pulmonary hypertension, it has been postulated that a subset may be genetically susceptible. Whether there is a related genetic abnormality in the familial PPH gene located on chromosome 2q (36[C]) or an abnormality of the angiotensin converting enzyme gene (37[C]) has yet to be explored.*

The hypothesis that nitric oxide deficiency predisposes affected individuals to anorexigen-associated pulmonary hypertension has been tested in a prospective case-control comparison with two sex-matched sets of controls: patients with primary pulmonary hypertension (n = 8) and healthy volunteers (n = 12) (38[C]). Lung production of nitric oxide and systemic plasma oxidation products of nitric oxide were measured at rest and during exercise, and were lower in patients with anorexigen-associated pulmonary hypertension than in patients with primary pulmonary hypertension. This deficiency may have resulted from increased oxidative inactivation of nitric oxide, as their oxidation product concentrations were raised in inverse proportion to nitric oxide. These findings and earlier evidence from animal studies (39) has given support to the hypothesis incriminating nitric oxide as a determinant of individual susceptibility to anorexigen-associated pulmonary hypertension.

The pressure response to endothelin-1 in the canine circulation has been investigated in isolated perfused dog lung (40). Acute treatment of the isolated lobes with fenfluramine increased pulmonary arterial pressure. Chronic treatment with fenfluramine potentiated the pulmonary vasoconstrictor response to endothelin-1. Based on these findings the authors proposed that the pulmonary vasculature becomes hyper-reactive to vasoactive substances, such as serotonin and endothelin-1, possibly leading to pulmonary hypertension.

Anorexigen-associated severe pulmonary hypertension is clinically and histopathologically indistinguishable from idiopathic or primary pulmonary hypertension. Analysis of clonality in microdissected endothelial cells of plexiform lesions in two patients with anorexigen-associated pulmonary hypertension showed a monoclonal expansion of pulmonary endothelial cells. Accelerated growth of pulmonary endothelial cells in response to anorexigens in patients with predisposition to primary pulmonary hypertension has been speculated (41).

There has been no major breakthrough in our understanding of the cellular or molecular basis of the pathophysiology of pulmonary hypertension associated with appetite suppressants.

Features *Pulmonary artery pressure and cardiac valvular status were determined in a series of 156 mostly asymptomatic patients taking fenfluramine and phentermine (42[C]). The anorexigen was withdrawn when abnormalities were noted. Pulmonary artery pressure was estimated and valvular examination was performed using Doppler echocardiography. There was borderline or mildly elevated pulmonary artery pressure in 21 patients and 31 patients had notable valvular abnormalities. It has therefore been established that asymptomatic patients may have significant echocardiographic abnormalities, representing early lesions.*

A 30-year-old woman who had taken dexfenfluramine for 7 months developed pulmonary hypertension and right heart failure during late pregnancy. She died of septicemia with multi-organ failure 4 days after a cesarean section (43[C]).

Another case of pulmonary hypertension and multi-valvular damage after prolonged use of fenfluramine with phentermine has been reported in a 70-year-old Israeli woman (44[C]).

Risk factors *Pulmonary hypertension and valvular heart disease associated with anorexigens have been described predominantly in women, which raises important questions about biological and psychological risk factors and ethical practice. Do women respond differently to these drugs because of genetic or physiological factors, or are these drugs being prescribed almost exclusively for women? Was it realistic for the regulatory authorities to believe that these drugs would be used only to treat morbid obesity? Most important, what notion of risk-benefit has allowed women and their physicians to justify the use of potentially lethal drugs to deal with concerns about body image and weight? The above poignant questions (45[r]) are pertinent to the current scenario of appetite-suppressant drug- related concerns.*

Mazindol

There have been two reports of young adult patients with a 'semen-like' urethral discharge during micturition and testicular pain attributed to mazindol (46[c]). The composition of the discharge was not identified. Voiding of the discharge did not recur after mazindol was withdrawn, and rechallenge was not performed.

Methylphenidate

Nervous system A first case of *neuroleptic malignant syndrome* probably caused by methylphenidate has been reported in a child with multicystic encephalomalacia due to severe perinatal hypoxic/ischemic encephalopathy (47[c]). At 1.5 years of age, because her circadian rhythm was irregular or reversed, methylphenidate (3 mg/day) was given for its antihypnotic effect. The diagnostic criteria of neuroleptic malignant syndrome (48[R]) were fulfilled in this case, including three major manifestations (fever, rigidity, and raised CK activity) and six minor ones (tachycardia, abnormal blood pressure, tachypnea, altered consciousness, sweating, and leukocytosis). Other predisposing factors, such as pre-existing severe brain damage suggestive of organic fragility and infection, may have contributed.

Psychiatric Methylphenidate-induced *obsessive-compulsive* symptoms are very rare (49[C]); a second case has been reported (50[c]).

An 8-year-old boy had unusual difficulties in completing a trial of methylphenidate for attention deficit hyperkinetic disorder (ADHD). Methylphenidate 10 mg/day initially improved his school performance, but by the end of the second week of treatment severe obsessive-compulsive behavior began to emerge, requiring drug withdrawal. He eventually refused to eat because he suspected that his food was being poisoned. His parents reported that he became more sensitive and easily upset, appearing increasingly tense and fearful. He continued to have intrusive distressing contamination worries. He had repetitive tic-like movements of his head and neck, frequently rubbed his face with his shirtsleeves, and avoided touching his face directly with his fingers for fear of contamination. His symptoms gradually and completely dissipated over 2–3 months without specific intervention. While very mild ADHD symptoms persisted, he remained entirely free of symptoms at 1 year. Medication was not restarted.

This case lends further support to existing anecdotal evidence associating methylphenidate with obsessive-compulsive disorder of acute onset. However, rechallenge was not attempted, and causality should be viewed as being uncertain.

Modafinil

In an open-label, randomized, crossover study in healthy men, concomitant administration of single oral doses of modafinil (200 mg) and dexamfetamine (10 mg) showed no clinically significant pharmacokinetic interaction. Each drug given separately produced a slight *increase in blood pressure* and the cardiovascular effects were more pronounced after concomitant administration. These changes were considered not to be clinically relevant and would not necessarily preclude short-term administration of the two drugs together. The most frequent adverse events with modafinil or dexamfetamine were headache, dizziness, insomnia, and dry mouth (51[c]). The importance of this study is that some patients with narcolepsy may require a change from dexamfetamine to modafinil, and arguably such a transition can be made without any washout period.

Phendimetrazine and phentermine

Despite the withdrawal of the fenfluramines, the appetite suppressants phendimetrazine and phentermine have remained in widespread use for the treatment of obesity. The list of serious complications resulting from these drugs should now be expanded to include *allergic interstitial nephritis* (52[c]).

A 47-year-old mildly obese woman began a weight reduction program that included anorectic therapy with phentermine and phendimetrazine. She had normal renal function at the start of therapy. After 3 weeks of treatment she fell ill and discontinued treatment. She was subsequently found to have leukocyturia, a rash on her face and chest, and a rise in serum creatinine from 0.8 to 2.1 mg/dl (67 to 175 μmol/l). Renal biopsy confirmed the diagnosis of acute interstitial nephritis. She was treated with corticosteroids and her renal function returned to normal.

Pseudoephedrine

Non-pigmenting fixed drug eruptions proven by oral rechallenge have been reported with pseudoephedrine; in each of these cases the erythematous lesions spontaneously remitted without residual pigmentation (53[c])–(55[c]).

OTHER CENTRALLY ACTING DRUGS *(SEDA-20, 4; SEDA-21, 6; SEDA-22, 7)*

Pemoline

Liver A 7-year-old boy with Duchenne muscular dystrophy and ADHD developed *acute hepatic failure* with features of autoimmune hepatitis (56[c]). The only medications he had taken were pemoline (56 mg/day) and cyproheptadine (2 mg/day). Pemoline was discontinued after 8 months as the presumed cause of his raised aminotransferases. Two weeks later he developed altered mental status, jaundice, and encephalopathy. The histological features of the liver and his autoimmune antibody panel were consistent with autoimmune hepatitis. He was treated with corticosteroids and azathioprine and recovered.

In another case, a 9-year-old boy with ADHD taking premoline developed signs and symptoms of liver failure requiring liver transplantation (57[c]).

During the past two decades, there have been many reports of liver failure resulting in death or transplantation in patients being treated for ADHD with pemoline. The evidence linking premoline to life-threatening liver failure has prompted the FDA to require the manufacturer to add a black box warning to package insert, whereas in the UK the Committee on Safety of Medicines withdrew marketing approval for pemoline, citing safety and a lack of adequate evidence of efficacy as the reason (58[R]).

DRUGS USED IN ALZHEIMER'S DISEASE

Donepezil

The approval of donepezil in several countries in America and Europe has been hailed as a major milestone, because it has met regulatory guidelines for the approval of a anti-dementia drugs (59[R]). Donepezil belongs to a piperidine class of reversible acetylcholinesterase inhibitors, chemically unrelated to either tacrine or physostigmine. It is highly specific for acetylcholinesterase and does not inhibit butyrylcholinesterase. The incidence of adverse effects with donezepil is comparable to that of placebo in controlled trials, and unlike tacrine liver enzyme monitoring is not required. The long-term effectiveness of donepezil in large populations is yet to be established. Moreover, while it improves cognitive symptoms it does not alter the course of the disease. Based on a limited number of studies, support for the use of donepezil in Alzheimer's disease has emerged (60[R], 61[R], 62[C], 63[C]).

Clinical trials of donepezil were funded by the manufacturer and appear to have been methodologically sound, although the absence of care-giver quality-of-life measures and outcomes related to activities of daily living is difficult to reconcile. An earlier 12-week study showed no improvement in care-giver quality of life with donepezil (62). As with most phase 3 studies, extrapolation of these results to routine practice is hampered by the fact that study populations are likely to be healthier than patients seen in routine clinical practice. Whether the results would be any different in a more heterogeneous population remains to be seen (64[r]).

In a more recent 12-week double-blind, placebo-controlled, parallel-group study, aimed at establishing the efficacy and safety of donepezil in patients with mild to moderately severe Alzheimer's disease, donepezil (5 and 10 mg od) was well tolerated and efficacious (65[C]). Adverse events significantly more common with donepezil were *nausea*, *insomnia*, and *diarrhea*, which appeared to be dose-related and did not require treatment. Seven patients treated with placebo and six in each of the donepezil groups had serious adverse events during the trial. Three had events that were considered possibly related to donepezil. These *included gastric ulceration with hemorrhage*, *syncope and a transient ischemic attack*, *nausea*, *aphakia*, *tremor*, and *sweating*. Both groups of patients treated with donepezil had falls in mean heart rate that were larger than with placebo. Two patients treated with donepezil had *electrocardiographic changes*: one developed an intraventricular conduction defect and premature ventricular extra beats, while the other had sinus dysrhythmia, left axis deviation, and increased QRS voltage, possibly secondary to left ventricular enlargement. Neither reported cardiovascular adverse events. Two patients taking placebo also had electrocardiographic abnormalities, one with bundle branch block, the other with sinus bradycardia and ventricular extra beats.

The launch of donepezil has attracted intense interest among both the scientific community and the public. The debate regarding 'lessons for healthcare policy' (66[R]) have been summarized:

1. Licensing trials in highly selected patients may provide insignificant information on which to base clinical decisions, especially when the effect sizes are small and comorbidity is common.
2. All trials evidence should be published before new drugs are marketed, and medical journals should not carry advertisements referring to unpublished data.
3. Communication of benefits and risks should emphasize clinical effect sizes rather than statistical significance.
4. Claims about effects on populations or services should be based on evidence.
5. Secrecy surrounding licensing should be ended and data from trials should be available for independent analysis.
6. Overvaluation of new technology could threaten funding for vital but more mundane care.

In response to the above publication, there has been intense debate, as reflected by several letters to the editor of the British Medical Journal (67–72).

Psychiatric *Behavioral worsening* in seven patients with Alzheimer's disease after the initiation of donepezil has been described (73[c]). Their mean age was 76 years, and their mean score on the Mini-Mental State Examination was 18. Five patients had had dementia-related delusions and irritability before taking donepezil; one had had a history of major depression and another a history of somatization disorder. At the time of donepezil initiation, four were taking sertraline, one paroxetine, one venlafaxine, and four risperidone. All took donepezil 5 mg/day, and after 4–6 weeks the dosage in five patients was increased to 10 mg/day. In the other two cases, donepezil was discontinued after 5 weeks, in one case because of gastrointestinal symptoms and in the other because of increasing agitation. After an average of 7.3 (range 1–13) weeks after starting donepezil, all seven patients had a recurrence of previous behavioral problems. Five became agitated, one became depressed, and the other became more anxious and somatically preoccupied. The pattern of behavioral change involves regression to an earlier behavioral problem.

Violent behavior has been described with donepezil (74[c]).

A 76-year-old man who was taking oxybutinin 3 mg tds for bladder instability took donepezil 5 mg/day for presumed Alzheimer's disease and 5 days later became very paranoid, believing that his wife had been stealing his money. He beat her and held her hostage in their house with a knife until their daughter intervened. He was given haloperidol 0.5 mg bd and the donepezil and oxybutinin were withdrawn. His paranoid ideation resolved within a few days and did not recur, despite withdrawal of haloperidol.

Although a causal relation between this violent incident and donepezil cannot be proved, the temporal relation was suggestive.

Hematological A *purpuric rash* associated with donepezil has been reported (75[c]).

An 82-year-old woman with hypertension taking long-term atenolol and doxazosin developed moderate cognitive impairment attributed to Alzheimer's disease. She was given donepezil 5 mg/day and after 4 days developed diarrhea, vomiting, and a purpuric rash on her trunk, arms, and legs. Platelet counts were $119–157 \times 10^9$/l. Donepezil was withdrawn, with resolution of the gastrointestinal symptoms.

Donepezil was the probable cause of this rash, because of the temporal association with treatment and its recurrence on rechallenge.

Liver Donepezil has not been associated with hepatotoxic effects, which is a distinct advantage over tacrine. Donepezil treatment benefit persisted over 98 weeks with no evidence of hepatotoxicity (76[C]).

Interactions An additive inhibitory effect of donepezil and neostigmine on acetylcholinesterase has been proposed to explain *prolonged neuromuscular blockade during anesthesia* in an 85-year-old woman taking donepezil (77[c]).

Extrapyramidal effects occurred in a patient who took donepezil and risperidone concurrently (78[c]). Although risperidone is less likely than conventional antipsychotic drugs to cause extrapyramidal effects, and is therefore particularly useful for older patients who are very susceptible to developing extrapyramidal disturbances, an increase in brain acetylcholine resulting from donepezil, along with dopamine receptor blockade by risperidone, would have led to an imbalance between cholinergic and dopaminergic systems. Although a clinically significant interaction between donepezil and risperidone seems to be rare, clinicians should be alert to such a possibility.

Metrifonate

Metrifonate has been used for the treatment of schistosomiasis for almost 40 years. Its identification as a cholinesterase inhibitor, together with recognition of the cholinergic deficit in Alzheimer's disease, has led to its use in Alzheimer's disease.

Recently two reviews (79[R], 80[R]) and two randomized, placebo-controlled, double-blind trials (81[C], 82[C]) of the use of metrifonate in Alzheimer's disease have been published. Both reviews reported a positive effect of metrifonate, with generally mild and usually transient adverse effects, consisting of gastrointestinal symptoms (such as *abdominal pain*, *diarrhea*, *flatulence*, and *nausea*, probably reflecting cholinergic overactivation) and *leg cramps*, possibly caused by the overstimulation of nicotinic receptors at the neuromuscular junction. No laboratory abnormalities were reported.

In a randomized, double-blind, placebo-controlled trial in 408 patients with Alzheimer's disease metrifonate (20 mg/kg/day for 2 weeks followed by 0.65 mg/kg/day for 24 weeks) significantly improved several mental performance scales (81[C]). Of the 273 patients treated with metrifonate 12% discontinued treatment because of adverse effects compared with 4% of the 134 patients treated with placebo. The adverse effects leading to withdrawal were mainly gastrointestinal in nature. *Diarrhea* occurred in 18% of the patients treated with metrifonate (leading to withdrawal in 3%) and in 8% of the patients treated with placebo; 2% of the patients treated with metrifonate discontinued treatment because of *nausea and vomiting* and 1% because of *dyspepsia*. Nausea occurred in 12% of the patients treated with metrifonate and in 10% of the patients treated with placebo. Vomiting occurred in 7 and 4% respectively.

In a second randomized, double-blind, placebo-controlled trial (82[C]) 480 patients were randomized to receive placebo (n = 120), a low dose of metrifonate (0.5 mg/kg/day for 2 weeks followed by 0.2 mg/kg/day for 10 weeks) (n = 121), a moderate dose of metrifonate (0.9 mg/kg/day for 2 weeks followed by 0.3 mg/kg/day for 10 weeks) (n = 121), or a high dose (2.0 mg/kg/day for 2 weeks followed by 0.65 mg/kg/day for 10 weeks) (n = 118). These doses were selected to achieve steady-state erythrocyte acetylcholinesterase inhibition of 30, 50, and 70% respectively. There was a significant dose-related improvement in several mental performance scales with metrifonate. Most of the adverse events were mild and transient. Adverse events that occurred more often in the patients treated with metrifonate were *abdominal pain* (placebo 4%, low dose 3%, moderate dose 11%, high dose 12%), *diarrhea* (8, 9, 11, 19% respectively), *flatulence* (9, 2, 8, 16%), and *leg cramps* (1, 1, 3, 8%). *Bradycardia*, presumably related to the vagotonic effect of acetylcholinesterase inhibition, led to withdrawal of treatment in three patients with asymptomatic bradycardia. All three were in the loading-dose phase of the highest metrifonate dosage regimen.

In 16 patients with Alzheimer's disease adverse effects were dose related (83[C]). In eight patients treated with 2.5 mg/kg/day for 14 days, 4 mg/kg/day for 3 days, and then 2.0 mg/kg/day for 14 days (acetylcholinesterase inhibition 88–94%) treatment had to be discontinued because of moderate to severe adverse effects in six patients on day 28 of the planned 31. In eight patients treated with 2.5 mg/kg/day for 14 days followed by 1.5 mg/kg/day for 35 days (acetylcholinesterase inhibition 89–91%) the frequency of more severe adverse effects was considerably lower despite similar acetylcholinesterase inhibition. The most frequent adverse events in the high-dose group were muscle cramps and *abdominal discomfort* during the loading-dose phase, followed by increasing *gastrointestinal symptoms* in the second loading phase, accompanied by *headache* and *muscle aches*. The adverse events profile initially improved during the maintenance phase. However, after 11 days of maintenance treatment six patients complained of generalized moderate to *severe muscle cramps, weakness, inability to resume daily activities, and difficulties with co-ordination*. The adverse events profile was much more favorable with the lower dose, with the same, but much less severe, range of adverse effects. Again the most frequent adverse effects *were gastrointestinal disturbances, muscle cramps*, and *light-headedness*. One patient had increased *sweating, dizziness*, and palpitation on day 29 and another developed severe *abdominal tenderness* on day 31, which led to the termination of treatment. No abnormalities in laboratory parameters were found. The authors proposed a maximum tolerated dose of 1.5 mg/kg/day of metrifonate for maintenance therapy in patients with Alzheimer's disease.

Patients with Alzheimer's disease taking long-term treatment with metrifonate suffered seizures after abrupt withdrawal of antimuscarinic agents (84[cr]). In one case a 58-year-old woman was given hyoscyamine for abdominal cramps by her local physician without the knowledge of her neurologists. She had a *generalized seizure* 36 hours after stopping the drug. A 66-year-old woman was treated for a skin allergy with doxepin cream in large doses. Withdrawal of this treatment led to two *complex partial seizures*. The authors speculated that the antimuscarinic drugs impaired the cholinergic receptor down-regulation that would normally occur in the presence of the increased concentrations of acetycholine caused by acetylcholinesterase inhibition. Withdrawal of the antagonist therefore abruptly exposed the receptors to high concentrations of the neurotransmitter, leading to seizures.

Tacrine *(SEDA-20, 4; SEDA-21, 6; SEDA-22, 7)*

Nervous system *Myoclonus* has been attributed to tacrine (85[c]).

A 68-year-old woman with dementia of probable Alzheimer's type for 4 years was given tacrine 40 mg/day and 24 hours later progressively developed generalized uncontrolled abnormal movements, affecting all her limbs and her mouth, suggestive of myoclonus and controlled by clonazepam. Myoclonus disappeared 24 hours after tacrine was withdrawn. Causation was established a few months later by rechallenge: myoclonus occurred during the next 48 hours.

Liver *Hepatic failure* associated with tacrine occurred outside the usual time frame of onset (within 9 months) and resulted in the death of a 75-year-old woman with Alzheimer's disease who had taken tacrine for 14 months (86[c]). Thus, the potential for delayed, life-threatening hepatotoxicity with tacrine, although unusual, should not be overlooked.

REFERENCES

1. Agarwal HS, Nanavati RN, Bhagwat MS, Kabra NS, Udani RH. Transplacental aminophylline toxicity. Indian Pediatr 1998;35:467–70.
2. Andrews PA. Interactions with ciprofloxacin and erythromycin leading to aminophylline toxicity. Nephrol Dial Transplant 1998;13:1006–8.
3. Fattore C, Cipolla G, Gatti G, Bertoli A, Orticelli G, Picollo R, Millerioux L, Ciottoli GB, Perucca E. Pharmacokinetic interactions between theophylline and prulifloxacin in healthy volunteers. Clin Drug Invest 1998;16:387–92.
4. Macias WK, Bergstrom RF, Cerimele BJ, Kassahun K, Tatum DE, Callaghan JT. Lack of effect of olanzapine on the pharmacokinetics of a single aminophylline dose in healthy men. Pharmacotherapy 1998;18:1237–48.
5. Ring BJ, Catlow J, Lindsay TJ, Gillespie T, Roskos LK, Cerimele BJ, Swanson SP, Hamman MA, Wrighton SA. Identification of the human cytochrome P450 responsible for the in vitro formation of the major oxidative metabolites of the antipsychotic agent olanzapine. J Pharmacol Exp Ther 1996;276:658–66.
6. Trepainer EF, Nafziger AN, Amsden GW. Effect of terbinafine on theophylline pharmacokinetics in healthy volunteers. Antimicrob Agents Chemother 1998;42:695–7.
7. Wahllander A, Paumgartner G. Effect of kertoconazole and terbinafine on the pharmacokinetics of caffeine in healthy volunteers. Eur J Clin Pharmacol 1989;37:279–83.
8. DeVilliers GS, Walele A, Van der Merwe PL, Kalis NN. Second-degree atrioventricular heart block after doxapram administration. J Paediatr 1998; 133:149–50.
9. Weissmann NJ, Tighe JF Jr, Gottdiender JS, Gwynne JT. An assessment of heart valve abnormalities in obese patients taking fenfluramine, sustained-release dexfenfluramine or placebo. New Engl J Med 1998;339:725–32.
10. Anonymous. Cardiac valvulopathy associated with exposure to fenfluramine or dexfenfluramine. US Department of Health and Human Services Interim Public Health Recommendations, November 1997. Morb Mortal Wkly Rep 1997;46:1061–6.
11. Anonymous. Statement of the American College of Cardiology on Recommendations for patients who have used anorectic drugs. Bethesda, MD: American College of Cardiology, 18 October 1997.
12. Wee CC, Phillips RS, Aurigemma G, Erban S, Kriegel G, Riley M, Douglas PS. Risk for valvular heart disease among users of fenfluramine and dexfenfluramine who underwent echocardiography before use of medication. Ann Intern Med 1998;129:870–4.
13. Khan MA, Herzog CA, St. Peter JV, Hartey GG, Madlon-Kay R, Dick CD, Asinger RW, Vessey JT. The prevalence of cardiac valvular insufficiency assessed by transthoracic echocardiography in obese patients treated with appetite suppressant drugs. New Engl J Med 1998;339:713–18.
14. Jick H, Vasilakis C, Weinrauch LA, Meir CR, Jick SS. A population based study of appetite-suppressant drugs and the risk of cardiac valve regurgitation. New Engl J Med 1998;339:719–24.
15. Connolly HM, Crary JL, McGoon MD, Hensrud DD, Edwards BS, Edwards WD, Schaff HV. Valvular heart disease associated with fenfluramine-phentermine. New Engl J Med 1997; 337:581–8 (erratum 1997;337:1783).
16. Graham DJ, Green L. Further cases of valvular heart disease associated with fenfluramine-phentermine. New Engl J Med 1997;337:665.
17. Kurz X, Van Ermen A. Valvular heart disease associated with fenfluramine-phentermine. New Engl J Med 1997;337:1172–3.
18. Rasmussen S, Coya BC, Glassman RD. Valvular heart disease associated with fenfluramine-phentermine. New Engl J Med 1997;337:1173.
19. Abenheim L, Moride Y, Brenot F, Rich S, Benichou J, Kurz X, Higenbottam T, Oakley C, Wouters E, Aubier M, Simonneau G, Begaud B. Appetite suppressant drugs and the risk of primary pulmonary hypertension. New Engl J Med 1996;335: 609–16.
20. Anchors JM. Fluoxetine hydrochloride is safer alternative to fenfluramine in the medical treatment of obesity. Arch Intern Med 1997;157:1270.
21. Griffen L. Asymptomatic mitral and aortic valve disease is seen in half of the patients taking 'Phen-Fen'. Arch Intern Med 1998;158:102.

22. Cannistra LB, Cannistra AJ. Regression of multivalvular regurgitation after the cessation of fenfluramine and phentermine treatment. New Engl J Med 1998;339:771.
23. Levine HJ, Gaasch WH. Vasoactive drugs in chronic regurgitant lesions in the mitral and aortic valves. J Am Coll Cardiol 1996;28:1083–91.
24. Fowles RE, Cloward TV, Yowell RL. Endocardial fibrosis associated with fenfluramine-phentermine. New Engl J Med 1998;338:1316.
25. Parisi AF. Diet-drug debate. Ann Intern Med 1998;129:903–5.
26. Devereux RB. Appetite suppressants and valvular heart disease. New Engl J Med 1998;339:765–7.
27. Singh JP, Evans JC, Levy D, Larson MG, Fried LA, Fuller DL, Lehman B, Benjamin EJ. Prevalence and clinical determinants of mitral, tricuspid, and aortic regurgitation (the Framingham Heart Study). Am J Cardiol 1999;83:897–902.
28. Klein Al, Burstow DJ, Tajik AJ, Zachariah PK, Taliercio CP, Taylor CL, Bailey KR, Seward JB. Age-related prevalence of valvular regurgitation in normal subjects: a comprehensive color flow examination of 118 volunteers. J Am Soc Echocardiogr 1990;3:54–63.
29. Bella JN, Devreux RB, Roman MJ, O'Grady MJ, Welty TK, Lee ET, Fabsitz RR, Howard BV. Relationship of left ventricular mass to fat-free and adipose body mass: the strong heart study. Circulation 1998;98:2538–44.
30. Brenot F, Herve P, Petitpretz P, Parent F, Duroux P, Simonneau G. Primary pulmonary hypertension and fenfluramine use. Br Heart J 1993;70:537–41.
31. Mark EJ, Patalas EO, Chang HT, Evans RJ, Kessler SC. Fatal pulmonary hypertension associated with short-term use of fenfluramine-phentermine. New Engl J Med 1997;337:602–6.
32. Bruce CJ, Connolly HM. Valvular heart disease, pulmonary hypertension and fenfluramine-phentermine use. Cardiol Rev 1998;15:17–19.
33. Delcroix M, Kurz X, Walckiers D, Demedts M, Naeije R. High incidence of primary pulmonary hypertension associated with appetite suppressants in Belgium. Eur Respir J 1998;12:271–6.
34. Kramer MS, Lane DA. Aminorex, dexfenfluramine, and primary pulmonary hypertension. J Clin Epidemiol 1998;51:361–4.
35. Simonneau G, Fartoukh M, Sitbon O, Humbert M, Jagot JL, Herve P. Primary pulmonary hypertension associated with the use of fenfluramine derivatives. Chest 1998;114(Suppl 3):195–9S.
36. Nichols WC, Koller DL, Slovis B, Foroud T, Terry VH, Arnold ND, Siemieniak DR, Wheeler L, Phillips III JA, Newman JH, Conneally PM, Ginsburg D, Loyd JE. Localization of the gene for familial primary pulmonary hypertension to chromosome 2q 31–32. Nat Genet 1997;15:277–80.
37. Morrell NW, Sarybaev AS, Alikhan A, Mirrakhimov MM, Aldashev AA. ACE genotype and risk of high altitude pulmonary hypertension in Kyrghyz highlanders. Lancet 1999;353:814.
38. Archer SL, Djaballah K, Humbert M, Weir EK, Fartoukh M, Ava-Santucci D, Mercier J, Simonneau G, Dinh-Xuan T. Nitric oxide deficiency in fenfluramine and dexfenfluramine-induced pulmonary hypertension. Am J Respir Crit Care Med 1998;158:1061–8.
39. Weir EK, Reeve HL, Huang J, Mitchelakis E, Nelson DP, Hampl V, Archer SL. Anorexic agents aminorex, fenfluramine and dexfenfluramine inhibit potassium current in rat pulmonary vascular smooth muscle and cause pulmonary vasoconstriction. Circulation 1996;94:2116–20.
40. Barman SA, Isales CM. Fenfluramine potentiates canine pulmonary vasoreactivity to endothelin-1. Pulm Pharmacol Ther 1998;11:183–7.
41. Tuder RM, Radisavljevic Z, Shroyer KR, Polak JM, Voelken NF. Monoclonal endothelial cells in appetite suppressant associated pulmonary hypertension. Am J Respir Crit Care Med 1998;158:1999–2001.
42. Fisher EA, Ruden R. Pulmonary artery pressures and valvular lesions in patients taking diet suppressants. Cardiovasc Rev Rep 1998;19:13–16.
43. Hellermann JP, Salomon F. Pulmonary hypertension following appetite suppressants. Ther Umsch 1998;55:548–50.
44. Goldstein SE, Levy Y, Shoenfeld Y. Pulmonary hypertension and multivalvular damage caused by anorectic drugs. Harefuah 1998;135:498–92, 568.
45. Day A. Lessons in women's health: body image and pulmonary disease. Can Med Assoc J 1998; 159:346–9.
46. Van Puijenbroek EP, Meyboom RHB. Semen-like urethral discharge during the use of Mazindol. Int J Eating Disord 1998;24:111–13.
47. Ehara HE, Maegaki Y, Takeshita K. Neuroleptic malignant syndrome and methylphenidate. Pediatr Neurol 1998;19:299–301.
48. Levenson JL. Neuroleptic malignant syndrome. Am J Psychiatry 1985;31:66–9.
49. Koizumi HM. Obsessive-compulsive symptoms following stimulants. Biol Psychiatry 1985; 20:1332–7.
50. Kouris S. Methylphenidate-induced obsessive-compulsiveness. J Am Acad Child Adolesc Psychiatry 1998;37:135.
51. Wong NY, Wang L, Hartman L, Simcoe D, Chen Y, Laughton W, Eldon R, Markland C, Grebow P. Comparison of the single-dose pharmacokinetics and tolerability of modafinil and dextroamphetamine administered alone or in combination in healthy male volunteers. J Clin Pharmacol 1998;38:971–8.
52. Markowitz GS, Tartini A, D'Agati VD. Acute interstitial nephritis following treatment with anorectic agent phentermine and phendimetrazine. Clin Nephrol 1998;50:252–4.
53. Anibarro B, Seoane FJ. Nonpigmented fixed exanthema induced by pseudoephedrine. Allergy Eur J Allergy Clin Immunol 1998;53:902–3.
54. Handioglu U, Sahin S. Nonpigmenting solitary fixed drug eruption caused by pseudoephedrine hydrochloride. J Am Acad Dermatol 1998;38:499–500.
55. Vidal C, Prieto A, Perez-Carral C, Armisen M. Nonpigmentary fixed drug eruption due to pseudo-

ephedrine. Ann Allergy Asthma Immunol 1998;80: 309–10.
56. Hochman JA, Woodard SA, Cohen MB. Exacerbation of autoimmune hepatitis: another hepatotoxic effect of pemoline therapy. Pediatrics 1998;101:106–8.
57. Adcock KG, Macelroy DE, Wolford ET, Farrington EA. Pemoline therapy resulting in transplatation. Ann Pharmacother 1998;32:422–5.
58. Anonymous. Committee on safety of medicines. Volital (Pemoline) has been withdrawn. Curr Probl Pharmacovig 1997;23:9–12.
59. Whitehouse PJ. Donepezil. Drugs Today 1998; 34:321–6.
60. Barner EL, Gray SL. Donepezil use in Alzheimer's disease. Ann Pharmacother 1998;32: 70–7.
61. Peruche B, Schulz M. Donepezil – a new agent against Alzheimer's disease. Pharm Ztg 1998;143:38–42.
62. Rogers SL, Friedhoff LT, Apter JT, Richter RW, Hartford JT, Walshe TM, Baumel B, Linden RD, Kinney FC, Doody RS, Borison RL, Ahem GL. The efficacy and safety of donepezil in patients with Alzheimer's disease: results of a US multicentre, randomized, double-blind, placebo-controlled trial. Dementia 1996;7:293–303.
63. Rogers SL, Farlow MR, Doody RS, Mohs R, Friedhoff LT, and Donepezil Study Group. A 24-week, double-blind, placebo-controlled trial of donepezil in patients with Alzheimer's disease. Neurology 1998;50:136–45.
64. Warner JP. Commentary on donepezil. Evid-Based Med 1998;3:155.
65. Rogers SL, Doody RS, Mohs RC, Friedhoff LT, the Donepezil Study Group. Donepezil improves cognition and global function in Alzheimer's disease. A 15 week, double blind, placebo-controlled study. Arch Intern Med 1998;158:1021–31.
66. Melzer D. New drug treatment for Alzheimer's disease: lessons for health care policy. Br Med J 1998;316:762–4.
67. Dening T, Lawton C. Doctors want to offer more than sympathy. Br Med J 1998;317:945.
68. Levy R. Effect of drugs can be variable. Br Med J 1998;317:945.
69. Evans M. Drugs should not need to show cost effectiveness to justify their prescription. Br Med J 1998;317:945–6.
70. Johnstone P. Information from unpublished trials should be made available. Br Med J 1998; 317:946.
71. Zamar AC, Wise MEJ, Watson JP. Treatment with metrifonate warrants multicentric trials. Br Med J 1998;317:946.
72. Baxter T, Black D, Prempeh H. SMAC's advice on use of donepezil is contradictory. Br Med J 1998;317:946.
73. Wengel SP, Roccaforte WH, Burke WJ, Bayer B, McNeilly DP, Knop D. Behavioural complication associated with donepezil. Am J Psychiatry 1998;155:1632–3.
74. Bouman WP, Pinner G. Violent behaviour associated with donepezil. Am J Psychiatry 1998; 155:1626–7.
75. Bryant CA, Ouldred E, Jackson SHD. Purpuric rash with donepezil treatment. Br Med J 1998; 317:787.
76. Rogers SL, Friedhoff LT. Long-term efficacy and safety of donepezil in the treatment of Alzheimer's disease: an interim analysis of the results of a US multicentric open label extension study. Eur Neuropsychopharmacol 1998;8:67–75.
77. Sprung J, Castellani WJ, Srinivasan V, Udayashankar S. The effects of donepezil and neostigmine in a patient with unusual pseudocholinesterase activity. Anesth Analg 1998;87:1203–5.
78. Magnuson TM, Keller BK, Burke WJ. Extrapyramidal side effects in a patient treated with risperidone plus donepezil. Am J Psychiatry 1998;155:1458–9.
79. Cummings JL. Metrifonate: overview of safety and efficacy. Pharmacotherapy 1998;18(Suppl II):43–6S.
80. Mucke HAM. Metrifonate. Treatment of Alzheimer's disease, acetylcholinesterase-inhibitor. Drugs Future 1998;23:491–7.
81. Morris JC, Cyrus PA, Orazem J, Mas J, Bieber F, Ruzicka B, Gulanski B. Metrifonate benefits cognitive, behavioral, and global function in patients with Alzheimer's disease. Neurology 1998;50:1222–30.
82. Cummings JL, Cyrus PA, Bieber F, Mas J, Orazem J, Gulanski B. Metrifonate treatment of the cognitive deficits of Alzheimer's disease. Neurology 1998;50:1214–21.
83. Cutler NR, Jhee SS, Cyrus P, Bieber F, Tan-Piengco P, Sramek JJ, Gulanski B. Safety and tolerability of metrifonate in patients with Alzheimer's disease: results of a maximum tolerated dose study. Life Sci 1998;62:1433–41.
84. Piecoro LT, Wermeling DP, Schmitt FA, Ashford JW. Seizures in patients receiving concomitant antimuscarinics and acetylcholinesterase inhibitor. Pharmacotherapy 1998;18:1129–32.
85. Abilleira S, Viguera ML, Miquel F. Myoclonus induced by tacrine. J Neurol Neurosurg Psychiatry 1998;64:281.
86. Blackart WG Jr, Sood GK, Crowe DR, Fallon MB. Tacrine: a cause of fatal hepatotoxicity? J Clin Gastroenterol 1998;26:57–9.

P.J. Cowen

2 Antidepressant drugs

MONOAMINE OXIDASE INHIBITORS (MAOIs)

Endocrine, metabolic A number of antidepressant drugs, particularly selective serotonin re-uptake inhibitors (SSRIs), can increase plasma prolactin concentrations, although galactorrhea is uncommon. A prescription event monitoring survey of about 65 000 patients (1[R]) showed that compared with SSRIs moclobemide was associated with a relative risk of *galactorrhea* of 6.7 (95% CI = 2.7–15). However, this was substantially less than the risk associated with the dopamine receptor antagonist risperidone (relative risk compared with SSRIs 32; 95% CI = 14–70). Nevertheless, the data suggest that moclobemide may be more likely to cause galactorrhea than other antidepressant drugs.

Sexual function Most conventional antidepressants lower sexual desire and performance. However, the reversible type A selective monoamine oxidase inhibitor moclobemide produced *intense pathological sexual desire* in three men with organic brain disease (two with strokes and one with idiopathic Parkinson's disease) (2[c]). In one subject the hypersexuality was associated with features of pathological jealousy in a paranoid state, but in the other two men increased sexuality was an isolated symptom. One of these patients, who had been impotent after the stroke, was not able to have sexual intercourse and resorted to telephone sex services, a most uncharacteristic behavior for him. In all cases the hypersexuality remitted when moclobemide was withdrawn. There have been two previous case reports of moclobemide-induced hypersexuality in women without organic brain disease. This must be a rare adverse effect, but it is possible that in the cases reported here the organic brain disease may have contributed to its appearance.

Interactions Four healthy volunteers treated with moclobemide (600 mg/day for 9 days) had reduced clearance of *dextrometorphan*, a marker of hepatic CYP2D6 activity (3[c]). These findings suggest that at the higher end of its therapeutic dosage range, moclobemide may inhibit the metabolism of drugs that are substrates for CYP2D6, for example antipsychotic drugs and tricyclic antidepressants (see SEDA-22, 14).

Moclobemide in conventional doses (300–600 mg/day) does not significantly potentiate the pressor effects of oral *tyramine*, and special dietary restrictions are therefore not usually necessary. However, higher doses of moclobemide are sometimes used to treat patients with resistant depression. Moclobemide 900 mg/day and 1200 mg/day have been compared with placebo in 12 healthy volunteers (4[c]). Neither dose of moclobemide significantly potentiated the pressor effect of 50 mg of tyramine, which has been estimated to be the upper limit of dietary tyramine content, even of large meals containing substantial amounts of cheese. However, one subject taking moclobemide 1200 mg/day had an increase in systolic blood pressure of over 30 mmHg. Individuals have rather different sensitivities to the pressor effects of oral tyramine challenge, and the number studied in this series was small. Accordingly, clinical extrapolation might not be straightforward. Patients taking conventional doses of moclobemide are sometimes advised to restrict their intake of cheese or other tyramine-containing foods, and this advice is clearly prudent if subjects take higher doses.

The combination of conventional MAO inhibitors with serotonin-potentiating agents, such as *SSRIs*, is contraindicated, because of the risk of the serotonin syndrome. Moclobemide may be less likely to cause this interaction, although both case reports and clinical series have suggested that some patients

Side Effects of Drugs, Annual 23
J.K. Aronson, ed.

have suffered significant adverse effects consistent with serotonin toxicity (SEDA-20, 6; SEDA-21, 10). After steady-state therapy with the SSRI fluoxetine (20–40 mg/day for 23 days), 12 subjects took fluoxetine plus moclobemide (600 mg/day) and six took fluoxetine and placebo (5[c]). There was no difference in the rates of adverse effects between the two groups and no evidence of serotonin toxicity, although fluoxetine inhibited the metabolism of moclobemide. The authors suggested that patients can be safely switched from fluoxetine to moclobemide without the need for the currently advised 5-week wash-out (which is necessary to allow the long-acting fluoxetine metabolite, norfluoxetine, to be eliminated). However, case reports have suggested that some patients can develop serotonin toxicity when moclobemide is combined with SSRIs or clomipramine (6[c]), so great caution is still needed in clinical practice.

Overdoses of moclobemide and SSRIs can cause serious and sometimes fatal serotonin toxicity (SEDA-18, 16). A similar interaction has been reported with the antidepressant venlafaxine, a potent serotonin re-uptake inhibitor (7[c]).

A 34-year-old man took 2.625 g of venlafaxine (therapeutic dose 75–375 mg/day) and 3 g of moclobemide plus an unknown amount of alcohol 1 hour before being admitted to hospital. Within 20 minutes of arrival his conscious level deteriorated and he was hypertonic, with clonus in all limbs. He was treated with intubation, paralysis, and ventilation and sedated with midazolam and morphine. He regained consciousness after 2 days.

This case report confirms the serious consequences of combined overdosage of moclobemide with drugs that potentiate brain serotonin function.

There have been previous reports of serotonin toxicity when venlafaxine was combined with therapeutic doses of conventional MAO inhibitors (SEDA 20, 21). The serotonin syndrome has been reported in four patients who were switched from the MAO inhibitor phenelzine to venlafaxine (8[c]). In two of the subjects, the 14-day wash-out period recommended when switching from phenelzine to other antidepressant drugs had elapsed.

A 25-year-old woman had been taking phenelzine (45 mg/day) for refractory migraine and tension headache, but suffered intolerable adverse effects (weight gain, edema, and insomnia). Phenelzine was withdrawn and 15 days elapsed before she took a single dose of (37.5 mg) of venlafaxine. Within 1 hour she developed agitation, twitching, shakiness, sweating, and generalized erythema with hyperthermia (38°C). Her symptoms resolved within 3 hours with no sequelae.

These cases suggest that even after the recommended 2- week wash-out from MAO inhibitors, venlafaxine can provoke serotonin toxicity in some patients.

In principle it should be possible to switch from one conventional MAO inhibitor to another without a wash-out period. However, there have been reports that patients who switched from phenelzine to tranylcypromine had hypertensive reactions, with disastrous consequences (9[c]). Whenever possible a 2-week wash-out period when switching from a conventional MAO inhibitor to tranylcypromine seems advisable.

TRICYCLIC ANTIDEPRESSANTS

Overdosage One of the major disadvantages of tricyclic antidepressants is their toxicity in overdose. A nation-wide analysis of suicide mortality in Finland has shown that between 1990 and 1995 the overall suicide mortality fell significantly from 30 per 100 000 to 27 (10[R]). However, the use of antidepressants in completed suicide showed an upward trend, while the use of more violent methods (gassing, hanging) fell. During this time prescription of moclobemide and two SSRIs (citalopram and fluoxetine) increased, while that of tricyclics (mainly doxepin and amitriptyline) remained steady. The mean annual fatal toxicity index was highest for tricyclics, such as doxepin, trimipramine, and amitripyline, and lowest for SSRIs.

Educational policies and commercial marketing of antidepressant drugs has led to an increase in the detection and treatment of depression. Conceivably this may be associated with the fall in suicide rates noted in Finland. However, overdosage of tricyclic antidepressants continues to contribute to deaths from suicide. Whether completely replacing tricyclics with less toxic compounds would lower overall suicide rate remains controversial.

SELECTIVE SEROTONIN RE-UPTAKE INHIBITORS

Nervous system SSRI-induced *movement disorders* have been comprehensively reviewed (11[R]). The use of SSRIs was associated with a range of movement disorders, including akathisia, dystonia, dyskinesia, tardive dyskinesia, Parkinsonism, and bruxism. The most frequent movement disorder was akathisia. However, clinician-based reports of adverse events solicited from SSRI manufacturers suggested that Parkinsonism might occur with an equal frequency but a later onset during treatment. As suggested before (SEDA-22, 12), concomitant treatment with antipsychotic drugs and lithium, as well as pre-existing brain damage, predisposes to the development of movement disorders with SSRIs.

Paroxetine-induced akathisia has been described in an 81-year-old man with bipolar depression. The akathisia began 1 week after paroxetine treatment (20 mg/day) and remitted within 6 days of withdrawal (12[c]). The authors pointed out that it is important to recognize SSRI-induced akathisia, because increasing agitation and restlessness early in treatment can be mistaken for worsening depression. In addition, case reports have suggested that akathisia can be associated with suicidal impulses.

It is believed that SSRIs produce movement disorders by facilitating inhibitory serotonin interactions with dopamine pathways. While all SSRIs are potent inhibitors of serotonin re-uptake, they have other pharmacological actions that might contribute to their clinical profile. Sertraline has an appreciable affinity for the dopamine re-uptake site, and for this reason might be presumed less likely to cause movement disorders than other SSRIs. However, there is little clinical evidence to support this suggestion and a case of sertraline-induced *Parkinsonism* has been reported (13[c]).

A 70-year-old woman, who had been taking sertraline 100 mg/day for seven months, gave a 6-month history of resting tremor and loss of dexterity in the right hand. She had mild bradykinesia and cogwheel rigidity in the right arm and leg. She had not taken any other medications. A brain MRI scan was normal. The sertraline was withdrawn and within a month all neurological symptoms and signs had remitted.

Psychiatric Like other antidepressants, SSRIs are occasionally associated with *manic episodes*, even in patients with no history of bipolar disorder. In this situation some argue that the affected patients may have had an underlying predisposition to bipolar illness.

In a retrospective chart review of 167 patients with a variety of anxiety disorders, excluding patients with evidence of current or previous mood disorder, manic episodes were recorded in five patients, a rate of 3% (14[c]). While this might suggest a clear effect of SSRIs to induce mania, two of the patients were taking clomipramine, a tricyclic antidepressant, albeit with potent serotonin re-uptake inhibitor properties. In addition, all the affected patients had additional diagnoses of histrionic or borderline personality disorder, known to be associated with mood instability. It is still therefore plausible that SSRIs cause mania only in patients with an underlying predisposition, although this may be more subtle that a personal or family history of bipolar illness.

Visual hallucinations are rare during antidepressant drug treatment, except after overdosage.

A 38-year-old man with a history of chronic depression developed on waking visual hallucinations of different geometric shapes after treatment with both sertraline and fluoxetine. Eventually he responded to treatment with nefazodone which did not cause hallucinations (15[c]).

Many drugs known to cause visual hallucinations (for example, lysergic acid diethylamide) have agonist activity at $5HT_2$ receptors and it is conceivable that in these patients both sertraline and fluoxetine caused sufficient activation of post-synaptic $5HT_2$ receptors to produce this visual disturbance. Interestingly although nefazodone may increase 5HT neurotransmission, it is also a $5HT_2$ receptor antagonist, so presumably could not activate $5HT_2$ receptors.

Special senses There have been previous reports of *acute angle closure glaucoma* in patients taking paroxetine (SEDA 21, 22). Paroxetine has some anticholinergic activity, and so it is uncertain whether the use of other SSRIs can also be associated with this adverse effect. In a placebo-controlled study in depressed patients a single dose of fluoxetine (20 mg) increased intraocular pressure by 4 mmHg (16[c]). This increase is within the normal diurnal range, but could be of clinical consequence in individuals predisposed to glaucoma. However, post-marketing surveillance does not currently suggest an association between the use of fluoxetine and glaucoma (17[r]).

Sexual function The adverse sexual effects of SSRIs have been reviewed (18[R]). The use of SSRIs is most frequently associated with *delayed ejaculation* and *absent* or *delayed orgasm*, but *reduced desire and arousal* have also been reported. Estimates of the prevalence of sexual dysfunction with SSRIs vary from a small percentage to over 80%. Prospective studies that enquire specifically about sexual function have reported the highest figures. Similar sexual disturbances are seen in patients taking SSRIs for the treatment of anxiety disorders (19[c]), showing that SSRI-induced sexual dysfunction is not limited to patients with depression. It is not clear whether the relative incidence of sexual dysfunction differs between the SSRIs, but it is possible that paroxetine carries the highest risk (18[R]).

Various treatments have been advocated to ameliorate sexual dysfunction in SSRI-treated patients, including $5HT_2$ receptor antagonists (cyproheptadine, mianserin, nefazodone) and $5HT_3$ receptor antagonists (granisetron) (18[c]). One of the most popular remedies is the use of dopaminergic agents, such as bupropion.

In a prospective study 47 patients who complained of SSRI-induced sexual dysfunction took bupropion 75–150 mg 1–2 hours before sexual activity (20[c]). If this was unsuccessful they were titrated to a dosage of 75 mg tds on a regular basis. Bupropion improved sexual function in 31 patients (66%). Anxiety and tremor were the most frequently reported adverse events, and seven patients discontinued for this reason. However, it should be noted that more serious adverse events (panic attacks, delirium, seizures) have been reported when bupropion and SSRIs are combined (18[R]).

The ability of SSRIs to cause *delayed ejaculation* has been used in controlled trials of men with premature ejaculation (21[c], 22[c]). Of the SSRIs, paroxetine and sertraline produced the most benefit in terms of increase in time to ejaculation, but fluvoxamine did not differ from placebo. Clomipramine was more effective than the SSRIs but caused most adverse effects. From a practical point of view many patients might prefer to take medication for sexual dysfunction when needed rather than on a regular daily basis, and it would be of interest to study the beneficial effects of SSRIs on premature ejaculation when used in this way.

Priapism is occasionally associated with the use of psychotropic drugs, such as trazodone, that are α_1-adrenoceptor antagonists. Priapism has been reported in a man taking sertarline (23[c]).

A 47-year-old man presented to the emergency room with a 4-day history of priapism and moderate pain. He reported that several brief but otherwise similar episodes had occurred during the previous month. He had a history of depression and had been taking sertraline 200 mg/day and dexamphetamine 10 mg/day. He received intracorporeal methoxamine, but when this proved ineffective was admitted and treated with intracorporeal adrenaline and a shunt procedure. However, detumesence was incomplete. At follow-up after several weeks the priapism had resolved and he had not become impotent (a significant risk in cases of prolonged priapism). He was given nefazodone with no recurrent of erectile dysfunction.

The dosage of sertraline used in this case was high and the combined use of dexamphetamine may also have been relevant.

Withdrawal effects It has been noted before that withdrawal of SSRIs, particularly those with short half-lives, can cause withdrawal symptoms (SEDA-22, 12). However, reports of such symptoms after citalopram withdrawal are rare.

A 30-year-old man with a history of major depression and panic disorder had been in remission for a year with citalopram (20 mg/day), valproate (600 mg/day), and alprazolam (3 mg/day) (24[c]). The citalopram was tapered over 3 weeks to 5 mg/day and then discontinued. The day after the last dose he experienced anxiety and irritability together with frequent short-lasting bursts of dizziness, not having previously experienced the latter. Panic and depression did not recur and after a week the symptoms resolved spontaneously.

These symptoms, particularly dizziness, are characteristic of SSRI withdrawal, and suggest that citalopram, like other SSRIs, can cause an abstinence syndrome in some patients, despite slow tapering of the dose.

Interactions The propensity of SSRIs to cause drug interactions through inhibition of CYP 450 enzymes was reviewed in SEDA-22 (p. 13). Of the various SSRIs, citalopram seems the least likely to produce this effect. The effects of citalopram on plasma concentrations of *risperidone* and *clozapine* have been prospectively studied in 15 patients with schizophrenia (25[C]). The addition of citalopram did not alter plasma concentrations of either antipsychotic drug. In contrast, in a prospective study fluvoxamine, in a low dosage of 50 mg/day, produced a 3-fold increase in plasma clozapine concentrations (n = 16), probably through inhibition of CYP1A2 (26[c]). In this study, paroxetine (20 mg/day), a potent inhibitor of CYP2D6, did not increase clozapine concentrations (n = 14), and the authors therefore suggested that CYP2D6 is not an important pathway of metabolism of clozapine. However, other studies (SEDA-21, 22) have shown that paroxetine can increase clozapine concentrations, suggesting that this combination should be used with caution.

In 10 healthy volunteers, fluvoxamine (100 mg/day for 5 days) significantly increased the peak concentrations of the anxiolytic drug *buspirone*. Concentrations of the active metabolite, 1-(2-pyrimidinyl)-piperazine, were reduced (27[c]). These effects were probably mediated through inhibition of CYP3A4 by fluvoxamine.

Fluoxetine

Cardiovascular In general, SSRIs are assumed to be safe in patients with cardiovascular disease, although there are few systematic investigations in these patients. In a prospective study of 27 depressed patients with established cardiac disease who took fluoxetine (up to 60 mg/day for 7 weeks), fluoxetine produced a statistically significant *reduction in heart rate* (6%) and *increase in supine systolic blood pressure* (2%) (28[R]). In one patient a pre-existing *dysrhythmia* worsened and this persisted after fluoxetine withdrawal. These findings suggest that, relative to tricyclic antidepressants, fluoxetine may have a relatively benign profile in patients with cardiovascular disease. However, the authors cautioned that in view of the small number of patients studied these findings cannot be widely generalized.

Interactions A problem in using fluoxetine in patients with cardiovascular disease is the risk of interactions with concomitant medications. Fluoxetine has been reported to increase serum *digoxin* concentrations (29[c]).

A 93-year-old woman with congestive cardiac failure, paroxysmal atrial fibrillation, and hypertension developed depression after the death of her daughter. For several months she had been maintained on captopril 25 mg twice daily, furosemide 40 mg/day, digoxin 0.125 mg/day, and ranitidine 150 mg bd. She was in sinus rhythm and her serum digoxin concentration was 1.0–1.4 nmol/l. She was treated with fluoxetine (10 mg/day), but a week later she developed anorexia. At the same time the serum digoxin was 4.2 nmol/l. Both digoxin and fluoxetine were discontinued and the digoxin concentration returned to the target range within 5 days, with resolution of the anorexia. Digoxin was restarted and therapeutic concentrations (0.9–1.4 nmol/l) were achieved during the next 3 weeks. Because of persisting depressive symptoms fluoxetine (10 mg/day) was given again, but the digoxin concentrations rose and after 4 days were 2.8 nmol/l. Both digoxin and fluoxetine were then withdrawn

Because digoxin has a narrow therapeutic range, this interaction, if confirmed, may be of significant clinical consequence. The mechanism is not clear, because digoxin is not a substrate for the cytochrome P450 enzymes that are inhibited by fluoxetine. The authors speculated that fluoxetine may reduce the renal clearance of digoxin; if so, it might do that by inhibiting the P glycoprotein that is responsible for the active tubular secretion of digoxin.

Paroxetine

Hematological Clozapine and SSRIs are often used together because depressive syndromes are common in patients with schizophrenia. Clozapine carries a relatively high risk of agranulocytosis, but this adverse effect is very rarely seen with SSRIs (although a case of possible fluoxetine-induced *neutropenia* was described in SEDA-22, 15). Two cases in which the addition of paroxetine to clozapine was associated with neutropenia have been reported (30[c]). The patients had been taking stable doses of clozapine for 6–12 months and had previously tolerated other SSRIs without adverse hematological consequences. In both cases the white cell count recovered when clozapine was discontinued, although paroxetine was maintained. While the apparent association of neutropenia with the combined use of clozapine and paroxetine may be spurious, these treatments are commonly used together and it will be of interest to see if other reports emerge.

There are infrequent reports that fluoxetine can be associated with abnormal bleeding, including *ecchymoses*, *melena*, and *hematuria*. Spontaneous ecchymoses have been reported in a patient taking paroxetine (31[c]).

A 47-year-old woman who had undergone bilateral mastectomies for breast cancer developed depression and was given paroxetine 20 mg/day.

After 15 days she developed widespread multiple ecchymoses over the arms, legs, and abdomen. Her platetet count, prothrombin time, partial thromboplastin time, and bleeding time were normal. Paroxetine was withdrawn and 5 days later the bruising had markedly abated and no new lesions were identified. She was subsequently treated with a tricyclic antidepressant without recurrence of the ecchymoses.

The authors noted two earlier reports of ecchymoses with paroxetine, with normal laboratory values. They speculated that an indirect effect on platelet function through inhibition of platelet 5HT uptake may be involved.

OTHER ANTIDEPRESSANTS

Bupropion

Bupropion is not marketed in the UK or Continental Europe, but has significant use as an antidepressant in the US. It is structurally and pharmacologically distinct from other antidepressants, and apparently enhances both dopamine and noradrenaline function in the brain. In some respects its adverse effects profile is similar to that of the SSRIs, *insomnia*, *agitation*, *tremor*, and *nausea* being most often reported. Unlike SSRIs, however, bupropion does not cause sexual dysfunction, which gives it an important advantage in some patients.

The main concern with the use of bupropion is that in higher dosages it is associated with a risk of *seizures* (0.4%) that is greater than that seen with SSRIs (about 0.1%). Recently a new modified-release formulation of bupropion has been marketed (32[R]). At doses of up to 300 mg the risk of seizures appears to be about 0.1%. There are insufficient data yet on the risk of seizures with higher doses of the modified-release formulation, but preliminary indications suggest that it is likely to be lower than that seen with the immediate-release formulation (32[R]).

Mirtazepine

Psychiatric Some patients appear to develop *manic symptoms* in response to some antidepressants but not others.

A 45-year-old woman had a long history of dysthymia and depression. She had taken many antidepressants, including tricyclics, SSRIs, bupropion, and venlafaxine. She had no history of mania or hypomania. She was taking setraline 250 mg/day, with only a transient response, and mirtazepine 15 mg/day was added. Within 4 days she developed clear symptoms of hypomania, with euphoric mood, mild grandiosity, pressure of speech, increased energy, and a reduced need for sleep. The mirtazepine treatment was stopped and sertraline continued; within 3 days the hypomanic symptoms had remitted. The depressive disorder then re-emerged (33[c]).

Unlike most other antidepressants, mirtazepine does not inhibit the re-uptake of monoamines, but instead blocks inhibitory α_2-adrenoceptors. It is conceivable that this pharmacological mechanism led to hypomanic symptoms in this patient.

Nefazodone

Nervous system Nefazodone is unusual amongst antidepressants in that it does not decrease and in fact may *increase rapid eye movement (REM) sleep or dream sleep*. In a controlled study treatment of depressed patients with nefazodone (400 mg/day) resulted in an increase in REM sleep, while fluoxetine (20 mg) produced the opposite effect (34[C]). In addition nefazodone increased sleep efficiency while fluoxetine reduced it. The patients' subjective assessments of sleep showed greater improvement with nefazodone than with fluoxetine. However, the overall antidepressant effects of the drugs were similar.

The function of REM sleep and its relation to depressive disorders is not clear, so it is uncertain whether the preservation of REM sleep produced by nefazodone is likely to be of clinical consequence.

Venlafaxine

Cardiovascular A meta-analysis of the effect of venlafaxine on blood pressure in patients studied in randomized placebo-controlled trials of venlafaxine, imipramine, and placebo showed that at the end of acute-phase (6 weeks) therapy the incidence of a sustained *rise in supine diastolic blood pressure* (over 90 mmHg) was significantly higher in both active treatment groups: venlafaxine 4.8% (135/2817), imipramine 4.7% (15/319), than placebo 2.1% (13/605) (35[R]). The effect of venlafaxine in causing a rise in diastolic blood pressure appeared to be dose related, with an incidence of 1.7% in patients taking less than 100 mg/day and 9.1% in those taking over 300 mg/day.

These data confirm that venlafaxine, particularly in higher dosages, can significantly increase blood pressure. At high doses venlafaxine inhibits the re-uptake of noradrenaline as well as that of serotonin, which probably accounts for the pressor effect.

Psychiatric The use of antidepressants in patients with documented bipolar illness is often associated with a risk of *manic illness*.

A 63-year-old man with a long history of bipolar illness and alcohol dependence was given nefazodone (400 mg/day) for 8 months, with no relief of a depressive episode. He was taking valproate 1500 mg/day as a mood stabilizer together with aspirin (81 mg/day), ranitidine (300 mg/day), and docusate calcium (240 mg/day). Nefazodone was tapered over 4 days and venlafaxine begun in a dosage of 37.5 mg/day. Over 3 weeks the dosage was gradually increased to 150 mg/day. Treatment with venlafaxine led to improvement in depressive symptoms, but 6 days after the dose reached 150 mg/day he became agitated, verbally and physically threatening, grandiose, and sexually disinhibited. He also had paranoid thinking and appeared to be hallucinating. The venlafaxine was discontinued but the manic symptoms persisted, and eventually required an increase in dosages of valproate and antipsychotic drugs (36[c]).

This report illustrates the difficulty of treating depressed bipolar patients with antidepressants. The presence of a mood stabilizer did not prevent the manic episode that emerged during venlafaxine treatment, and it is in any case difficult to know whether the mania was in fact due to venlafaxine or instead represented a spontaneous mood swing.

Endocrine, metabolic It is well established that SSRIs can cause hyponatremia. Similar cases have now been reported with venlafaxine.

A 90-year-old woman had a depressive disorder in addition to other medical problems, including congestive cardiac failure, seizures, dementia, and osteoporosis. She was taking phenobarbital (120 mg/day), enalapril (40 mg/day), furosemide (80 mg/day), calcium carbonate (1300 mg/day), and nortriptyline (50 mg at night). She was given additional paroxetine 20 mg, but there was no clinical response and she was changed to venlafaxine increasing to 75 mg/day. Two months later her sodium concentration had fallen to 130 mmol/l and the furosemide was withdrawn. However, 4 months later the sodium concentration had fallen to 124 mmol/l. The venlafaxine was then withdrawn and the sodium normalized within a week and remained within the reference range for the following year (37[c]).

This was complex case, because of the multiple medical problems and treatments. However, it has been reported that since the launch of venlafaxine in Australia in 1996, the Adverse Drug Reactions Advisory Committee there has received 15 reports of hyponatremia, suggesting that the association is real (38[r]).

REFERENCES

1. Dunn NR, Freemantle SN, Pearce GL, Mann RD. Galactorrhoea with moclobemide. Lancet 1998;351:802.
2. Korpelainen JT, Hiltunen P, Myllyla VV. Moclobemide-induced hypersexuality in patients with stroke and Parkinson's disease. Clin Neuropharmacol 1998;21:251–4.
3. Hartter S, Dingemanse J, Baier D, Ziegler G, Hiemke C. Inhibition of dextromethorphan metabolism by moclobemide. Psychopharmacology 1998;135:22–6.
4. Dingemanse J, Wood N, Guentert T, Oie S, Ouwerkerk M, Amrein R. Clinical pharmacology of moclobemide during chronic administration of doses to healthy subjects. Psychopharmacology 1998;140:164–72.
5. Dingemanse J, Wallnofer A, Gieschke R, Guentert T, Amrein R. Pharmacokinetic and pharmacodynamic interactions between fluoxetine and moclobemide in the investigation of development of the 'serotonin syndrome'. Clin Pharmacol Ther 1998;63:403–13.
6. Dardennes RM, Even C, Ballon N, Bange F. Serotonin syndrome caused by a clomipramine-moclobemide interaction. J Clin Psychiatry 1998;59:382–3.
7. Coorey AN, Wenck DJ. Venlafaxine overdose. Med J Aust 1998;168:523–4.
8. Diamond S, Diamond ML, Freitag FG, Urban GJ, Erdemoglu AK. Serotonin syndrome induced by transitioning from phenelzine to venlafaxine: four patient reports. Neurology 1998;51:274–6.
9. Mattes JA. Stroke resulting from a rapid switch from phenelzine to tranylcypromine. J Clin Psychiatry 1998;59:382.
10. Ohberg A, Vuori E, Klaukka T, Lonnqvist J. Antidepressants and suicide mortality. J Affect Disord 1998;50:225–33.
11. Gerber PE, Lynd LD, Leo RJ. Selective serotonin-reuptake inhibitor-induced movement disorders. Ann Pharmacother 1998;32:692–8, 712–14.
12. Bonnet-Brilhault F, Thibaut F, Leprieur A, Petit M. A case of paroxetine-induced akathisia and a

review of SSRI-induced akathisia. Eur Psychiatry 1998;13:109–11.

13. Di Rocco A, Brannan T, Prikhojan A, Yahr MD. Sertraline induced parkinsonism. A case report and an in-vivo study of effect of sertraline on dopamine metabolism. J Neural Transm 1998;105:247–51.
14. Levy D, Kimhi R, Barak Y, Aviv A, Elizur A. Antidepressant associated mania: a study of anxiety disorders patients. Psychopharmacology 1998;136:243–6.
15. Bourgeois, JA, Thomas D, Johansen T, Walker D. Visual hallucinations associated with fluoxetine and sertraline. J Clin Psychopharmacol 1998;18:482–3.
16. Costagliola C, Mastropasqua L, Steardo L. Fluoxetine oral administration increases intra-occular pressure. Br J Ophthalmol 1996;80:678.
17. Eke T, Carr S, Costagliola C, Mastropasqua L, Steardo L. Acute glaucoma, chronic glaucoma and serotoninergic drugs. Br J Ophthalmol 1998;82:976–8.
18. Rosen RC, Lane RM, Menza M. Effects of SSRIs on sexual function: a critical review. J Clin Psychopharmacol 1999;19:67–85.
19. Labbate LA, Grimes JB, Arana GW. Serotonin reuptake antidepressant effects on sexual function in patients with anxiety disorders. Biol Psychiatry 1998;43:904–7.
20. Ashton AK, Rosen RC. Buproprion as an antidote for serotonin reuptake inhibitor-induced sexual dysfunction. J Clin Psychiatry 1998;59:112–15.
21. Kim SC, Seo KK. Efficacy and safety of fluoxetine, sertraline and clomipramine in patients with premature ejaculation: a double-blind, placebo controlled study. J Urol 1998;159:425–7.
22. Waldinger MD, Hengeveld MW, Zwinderman AH, Olivier B. Effect of SSRI antidepressants on ejaculation: a double-blind, randomized, placebo-controlled study with fluoxetine, fluvoxamine, paroxetine, and sertraline. J Clin Psychopharmacol 1998;18:274–81.
23. Rand EH. Priapism in a patient taking sertraline. J Clin Psychiatry 1998;59:538.
24. Benazzi F. Citalopram withdrawal symptoms. Eur Psychiatry 1998;13:219.
25. Avenoso A, Facciola G, Scordo MG, Gitto C, Ferrante GD. No effect of citalopram on plasma levels of clozapine, risperidone and their active metabolites in patients with chronic schizophrenia. Clin Drug Invest 1998;16:393–8.
26. Wetzel H, Anghelescu I, Szegedi A, Wiesner J, Weigmann H, Hartter S, Hiemke C. Pharmacokinetic interactions of clozapine with selective serotonin reuptake inhibitors: differential effects of fluvoxamine and paroxetine in a prospective study. J Clin Psychopharmacol 1998;18:2–9.
27. Lamberg TS, Kivisto KT, Laitila J, Martensson K, Neuvonen P. The effect of fluvoxamine on the pharmacokinetics and pharmacodynamics of buspirone. Eur J Clin Pharmacol 1998;54:761–6.
28. Roose SP, Glassman AH, Attia E, Woodring S, Giardina E. Cardiovascular effects of fluoxetine in depressed patients with heart disease. Am J Psychiatry 1998;155:660–5.
29. Leibovitz A, Bilchinsky T, Gil I, Habot B. Elevated serum digoxin level associated with coadministered fluoxetine. Arch Intern Med 1998;158:1152–3.
30. George TP, Innamorato L, Sernyak MJ, Baldessarini RJ. Leukopenia associated with addition of paroxetine to clozapine. J Clin Psychiatry 1998;59:31–2.
31. Cooper TA, Valcour VG, Gibbons RB, O'Brien-Falls K. Spontaneous ecchymoses due to paroxetine administration. Am J Med 1998;104:197–8.
32. Settle EC Jr. Buproprion sustained release: side effect profile. J Clin Psychiatry 1998;59:32–6.
33. Soutullo CA, McElroy SL, Keck PE Jr. Hypomania associated with mirtazapine augmentation of sertraline. J Clin Psychiatry 1998;59:320.
34. Rush AJ, Armitage R, Gillin JC, Yonkers KA, Winokur A. Comparative effects of nefazodone and fluoxetine on sleep in outpatients with major depressive disorder. Biol Psychiatry 1998;44:3–14.
35. Thase ME. Effects of venlafaxine on blood pressure: a meta-analysis of original data from 3744 depressed patients. J Clin Psychiatry 1998;59:502–8.
36. Stoner SC, Williams RJ, Worrel J, Ramlatchman L. Possible venlafaxine-induced mania. J Clin Psychopharmacol 1999;19:184–5.
37. Masood GR, Karki SD, Patterson WR. Hyponatremia with venlafaxine. Ann Pharmacother 1998;32:49–51.
38. Boyd IW, Karki SD, Masood GR. Hyponatremia with venlafaxine. Ann Pharmacother 1998;32:981–2.

J.W. Jefferson

3 Lithium

The availability of anticonvulsant mood stabilizers has led to comparative studies with lithium. In 29 patients, the burden of taking lithium (n = 17) was compared with that of valproate (n = 12) using a visual analog scale. Adverse effects were common but not significantly different between drugs (1[C]), a finding that contrasts with the common impression that valproate is better tolerated. Indeed, a telephone interview of 11 adolescents taking lithium and 32 taking valproate found more adverse effects, poorer compliance, and greater perceived burden in the lithium group. There was a non-significant trend toward more weight gain with valproate (mean 12 kg) than with lithium (mean 9 kg) (2[C]).

Whether elderly patients taking lithium received proper monitoring was questioned in a case note audit of 91 patients, over 40% of whom had deviations from practice standards. These included absence of pretreatment laboratory tests, infrequent monitoring of serum lithium concentrations, lack of adequate adverse effects documentation, and the use of risky concomitant drugs (3[C]). In a placebo-controlled study, there was poor tolerance of lithium augmentation of antidepressants in 76% (13/17) of elderly (mean age 70 years) patients at a mean serum concentration of 0.63 mmol/l, due to *tremor and muscle twitches*, *cognitive disturbance*, *tiredness and sedation*, and *gastrointestinal upsets* (4[C]).

Despite the availability of modified-release lithium formulations for several decades, there continues to be a paucity of information about their efficacy and tolerability compared with less expensive immediate-release formulations (5[r]).

Cardiovascular *Cardiac dysrhythmias* associated with lithium intoxication in the elderly included sinus node dysfunction and junctional bradycardia (6[r]). A retrospective chart review of patients on lithium who had mild but persistent hypercalcemia (n = 12) showed a greater frequency of cardiographic conduction disturbances compared with normocalcemic patients taking lithium (n = 40) and normocalcemic bipolar patients taking anticonvulsant mood stabilizers (n = 20), although the overall frequency of cardiographic abnormalities did not differ significantly among the groups (7[C]). When 21 patients without cardiovascular disease (mean serum lithium 0.66 mmol/l) were compared with normal controls using standard electrocardiography, vector cardiography, and electrocardiographic body surface potential mapping, the only abnormality was a reduction in the initial phase of depolarization, a finding of questionable clinical significance (8[C]).

Nervous system *(see also Overdosage)* Four of 17 studies of the cognitive effects of lithium were deemed to have acceptable methods. Reported adverse effects included effects on memory, speed of information processing, and reaction time (often in the absence of subjective complaints), suggesting that *the risk of driving accidents might be increased* when patients are taking lithium (9[R], 10[R]). Interventions for lithium-induced cognitive impairment include dosage reduction, use of a modified-release formulation, treatment of thyroid dysfunction, and assessing the role of concomitant illness and medication.

Twelve cases of *status dystonicus* of varying causes included a woman with post-traumatic dystonia who was treated unsuccessfully with lithium. Despite the lack of response, her muscular spasms worsened when lithium was stopped (11[c]).

After almost a two-decade nap, interest in lithium-induced somnambulism was reawakened by a questionnaire survey of 389 clinic patients that found *sleepwalking* in 6.9% of those taking lithium alone or with other drugs compared with a 2.5% prevalence in the general population (12[C]).

Side Effects of Drugs, Annual 23
J.K. Aronson, ed.

A 52-year-old man had a 5-year history of sleepwalking 2–3 times a week beginning 3 months after starting lithium. On one occasion he was injured in a fall after *sleepwalking* through a second-story window. When lithium was stopped for 3 months, the problem resolved only to recur when it was restarted (13[c]).

Acute *delirium and confusion* have also been reported.

A 36-year-old developed a febrile confusional state in the absence of infection while taking lithium (serum concentrations 0.37 and 0.58 mmol/l) and cyamémazine, resulting in a persistent cerebellar syndrome (14[c]).

A 62-year-old woman became delirious when lithium at therapeutic concentrations was added to valproate, haloperidol, and biperidin (15[c]). The delirium resolved after all drugs were withdrawn, but 6 months later she still had choreoathetoid movements.

In a review of SSRI-induced extrapyramidal adverse effects, lithium was listed, but not discussed, as a possible risk factor (16[r]). While previous reports have suggested an association between lithium and neuroleptic malignant syndrome (NMS) (17[r]), a case-control study (n = 12 with NMS, n = 24 controls) found no such association (18[C]). Since none of the patients with neuroleptic malignant syndrome were taking lithium, little can be concluded from such a finding.

After 4 hours of mild, intermittent, hot-weather work, a 45-year-old man taking fluoxetine and lithium (serum concentration not mentioned) collapsed, became comatose, convulsed, and was febrile (42°C); consciousness returned after 6 days but cerebellar symptoms and atrophy persisted (19[c]). It was suggested that *disruption of temperature regulation* had been caused by a synergistic effect of the two drugs (although he had taken neither drug for 36 hours before the episode).

Electroneurographic studies in 34 lithium maintenance patients and controls (both healthy subjects and mood disorder patients never on lithium) showed statistically significant *reductions in sensory and motor conduction* in the lithium group (20[C]). None of the decrements was severe enough to be abnormal, and whether these findings have clinical implications is unknown.

Endocrine, metabolic *Thyroid* The many effects of lithium on thyroid physiology and on the hypothalamic/pituitary axis and their clinical impact (*goiter, hypothyroidism,* and *hyperthyroidism*) have been reviewed (21[R]). Thyroid function tests in 101 lithium maintenance patients were compared with their baseline values and with results in 82 controls without psychiatric or endocrine diagnoses. With hypothyroidism defined as a serum TSH above the reference range, eight patients were hypothyroid at baseline, and another 40 became so during treatment. Women over 60 years of age were at slightly higher risk and had higher TSH values. Patients with a positive family history of hypothyroidism had raised TSH concentrations sooner after starting lithium (3.7 vs 8.7 years). Whether any patients became clinically hypothyroid was not noted (it was stated that those with grade II hypothyroidism were almost free of symptoms) (22[CR]).

In a review of lithium-induced *subclinical hypothyroidism* (TSH over 5 mu/l, free thyroxine normal), a prevalence of up to 23% in lithium patients was contrasted with up to 10% in the general population. It was stressed that subclinical hypothyroidism from any cause can be associated with subtle neuropsychiatric symptoms, such as depression, impaired memory and concentration, and mental slowing and lethargy, as well as with other somatic symptoms. Management guidelines were discussed (23[R]).

A cross-sectional study of 121 lithium patients found no difference in thyroid function tests among those taking treatment for 0.7–6, 7–10, or 61–240 months. However, when compared with healthy volunteers (n = 24) and pre-lithium controls (n = 11), there was a significant *increase in radioiodine uptake* in all lithium groups. Serum TSH concentrations were higher in pre-lithium patients than controls and highest in those taking lithium. Being from an iodine-deficient area appeared to predispose lithium patients to abnormally high TSH values and clinical hypothyroidism (24[C]).

In a retrospective review of 201 patients taking lithium (mean duration 6.4 years), hypothyroidism requiring supplemental thyroxine developed in 10% (3.4% of men, 15% of women) after a mean duration of 56 months. Women over 50 years of age tended to have an earlier onset. Two patients developed goiter requiring surgery and two others developed thyrotoxicosis (25[C]). Despite the predominantly antithyroid effects of lithium, thyrotoxicosis continues to be described during treatment and after withdrawal (26[c], 27[c]).

Lithium has been used successfully to augment the effects of ^{131}I to treat thyrotoxicosis (28[C], 29[c], 30[c]) and metastatic thyroid carcinoma (31[CR]).

Parathyroid and calcium Evidence continues to accrue linking lithium with parathyroid/calcium abnormalities. Of 537 patients who had parathyroid glands excised for *hyperparathyroidism*, 12 (2.2%) had been taking lithium and 11 (2.0%) had been taking it long-term (mean 15.3 years, range 2–30). Manifestations included fatigue, bone pain and fracture, and abdominal pain and constipation. Six had a single adenoma and five had multigland hyperplasia. All resumed lithium, but one had a recurrence after 3 years and one had increased parathyroid hormone concentrations but a normal serum calcium. A literature review detected 27 prior reports of parathyroid adenoma and 11 of hyperplasia associated with lithium (32[CR]).

When 15 euthymic bipolar patients who had taken lithium for a mean of 49 months were compared with 10 non-lithium euthymic bipolar controls, the former had significantly *higher total serum calcium concentrations* and intact parathyroid hormone (iPTH) concentrations (33[C]). The authors advised baseline and periodic serum calcium and iPTH concentrations and bone density measurements in all lithium patients, although whether the benefit outweighs cost is open to question.

Ten patients who had taken lithium for less than 1 year and 13 who had taken it for more than 3 years were assessed for alterations in bone metabolism and parathyroid function (34[C]). There were no differences in bone mineral density, serum calcium concentration, or parathyroid hormone concentration, but both groups had increased bone turnover and the long-term group had non-significantly higher calcium and parathyroid hormone concentrations (including one hyperparathyroid patient who had an adenoma excised). The authors' conclusion that lithium therapy is not a risk factor for osteoporosis needs to be tempered by the small sample size, the case of adenoma, and the blood concentration trends.

In 53 patients studied prospectively at 1, 6, 12, and 24 months, lithium *increased serum parathyroid hormone concentrations* (apparent by 6 months) and *increased renal reabsorption of calcium* in the absence of a significant change in serum calcium (35[C]). A prospective study of 101 lithium maintenance patients and 82 healthy controls showed higher serum calcium concentrations during lithium treatment than at baseline or in the controls, and higher calcium serum concentrations in those lithium patients over 60 years of age (22[CR]).

A 51-year-old man who had taken lithium for over 10 years presented with nausea, vomiting, anorexia, hypercalcemia (3.1 mmol/l), and increased parathyroid hormone concentration (iPTH 110 ng/l). Abnormalities resolved after an oxyphilic parathyroid adenoma was excised (36[c]).

Diabetes mellitus Two patients with diabetes mellitus developed lithium toxicity (serum concentrations 3.3 and 3.0 mmol/l) in association with impaired consciousness, and hyperglycemia that resolved after intravenous insulin and fluids (37[c]). While the authors concluded that impaired glucose tolerance predisposed to lithium intoxication, the opposite is also possible.

A 45-year-old man with severe lithium-induced diabetes insipidus developed hyperosmolar, non-ketotic hyperglycemia. It was suggested that poorly controlled diabetes mellitus may have contributed to the polyuria (38[c]). Prior contact with a patient who had developed hyperosmolar coma secondary to lithium-induced diabetes insipidus (39[c]) allowed physicians 4 years later to treat her safely after a drug overdose and a surgical procedure, by avoiding intravenous replacement fluids with a high dextrose content (despite stopping lithium several years earlier, the patient continued to put out 10 l of urine daily) (40[c]).

Weight gain In a review of psychotropic drug-induced weight gain, the prevalence and magnitude of the problem with lithium was discussed together with risk factors, mechanisms, and management (41[R]). Adolescent in-patients treated with risperidone (n = 18) or conventional antipsychotic drugs (n = 19) over 6 months gained more weight than a control group but concomitant treatment with lithium was not a contributing factor (42[C]).

Prolactin Serum prolactin concentrations in long-term (n = 15) or short-term (n = 15) lithium patients did not differ from controls (43[C]).

ACTH Calcium infusion in lithium patients (n = 7) and controls (n = 7) caused similar increases in ACTH concentrations across a physiological range of calcium (44[C]).

Mineral and fluid balance Nine trace elements were measured in whole blood (oven-dried, moisture-free) from controls, pre-lithium, and lithium patients; while there were many changes related to lithium, none appeared to be clinically important (45[C]).

Effects on vitamins A cross-sectional study showed a 20% *lower serum vitamin B12* concentration in lithium patients ($n = 81$) compared with controls ($n = 14$) (serum and erythrocyte folate concentrations were normal) (46[C]).

Hematological A retrospective review of inpatients showed higher leukocyte and granulocyte counts in those taking lithium alone ($n = 38$) compared with those taking antipsychotic drugs alone ($n = 207$); lymphocyte counts were not affected. Rises in leukocyte counts above normal occurred in 18% of those taking lithium and 6% of those taking antipsychotic drugs (47[C]). The neutrophil stimulating effect of lithium was used to advantage to successfully re-treat a patient with clozapine several years after stopping it because of neutropenia (48[c]). Likewise, lithium was used to successfully stimulate neutrophil production in a patient with clozapine-induced neutropenia and in another with clozapine-induced agranulocytosis (recovery was as fast as seen with colony stimulating factor and twice as rapid as expected spontaneously) (49[c]).

In eight patients with bipolar disorder, lithium for 3–4 weeks increased neutrophil count by 88% and also caused a significant increase in CD34+ cells (although three patients had no increase in either) (50[C]).

A lithium-treated bipolar patient with acute myeloid leukemia had an unusually great increase in CD34+ cells following administration of G-CSF suggesting a boosting effect from lithium (51[c]).

After he had failed to respond to combined treatment with corticosteroids and androgens and to antilymphocyte globulin, a 16-year-old with aplastic anemia responded to lithium combined with an androgen derivative, relapsed when lithium was stopped, and responded again when it was restarted (52[c]).

When 50 bipolar lithium patients were compared with 30 healthy controls, platelet counts were similar, but the lithium group had higher concentrations of plasma β-thromboglobulin and platelet factor 4, suggesting lithium-induced *platelet activation* (53[C]).

Gastrointestinal A comprehensive review of psychoactive drug-induced hyposalivation and hypersalivation included a discussion of lithium-induced *dry mouth* (common) and *sialorrhea* (rare) (54[R]).

In an 80-year-old woman a 2-month history of *diarrhea*, *nausea*, and *abdominal distress* attributed to irritable bowel syndrome was ultimately determined to be due to early lithium intoxication (55[c]). Her lithium concentration when she was hospitalized was 1.2 mmol/l, although she had taken no lithium for the previous 10 days. Treatment with a thiazide diuretic contributed to the toxicity.

Urinary system There have been several recent reviews of the effects of lithium on the kidney (56[R], 57[R]–59[R]), and lithium received a brief mention in a review of tubulointerstitial nephritis (60[r]). Lithium can adversely alter tubular function, leading to concentration defects and polyuria, which, although initially reversible, can ultimately become permanent. There may also be a small number of patients who develop *progressive renal insufficiency* that can best be attributed to lithium (58[R]).

A 48-year-old taking lithium and chlorprothixene had a creatinine clearance of 60 ml/minute and a renal biopsy showing chronic interstitial nephritis (61[c]).

Eight years after stopping lithium because of polydipsia and polyuria, a 55-year-old woman was hospitalized with lethargy, coma, and hypernatremia (sodium concentration 156 mmol/l) after her fluid intake had been restricted (62[cR]).

While a single case is not absolute proof that lithium causes persistent polyuria, it is consistent with other observations and illustrates the risk of fluid restriction in such individuals. Studies in rats have linked lithium-induced nephrogenic diabetes insipidus to reduced the amounts of aquaporin-2, a vasopressin-regulated water channel protein (63).

Skin and appendages In a review of *lichenoid drug eruptions*, lithium was implicated in one patient with ulcerative oral lesions and in another with ulcerative genital lesions (64[r]).

Special senses The finding of reversible lithium-induced moderate *hearing loss* (especially low frequency) in guinea-pigs led to speculation that similar findings could occur in humans (although there have been no reports as yet) (65[C]).

Immunological effects In a brief report evidence has been presented that short-term exposure to lithium (less than 2 months) caused *alterations in the expression of histocompatibility antigens* (66[c]).

Use in pregnancy Pregnancy in bipolar women was found to be a 'risk-neutral' condition, in that it neither protected against nor increased episode risk in a comparison of 42 pregnant with 42 non-pregnant women who stopped lithium either rapidly (over 1–14 days) or gradually (over 15–30 days). Stopping lithium was not 'risk-neutral', and the risk was especially high in those who stopped rapidly (67[R]) (see also Withdrawal effects). These observations must be balanced against the low but real risk of *teratogenesis* from first trimester lithium exposure (68[R]).

Use in lactation Debate continues about the risks and benefits of breast-feeding when a mother is taking lithium. 'Lithium should only be used with great caution...' (69[R]); '... has been repeatedly discouraged in the literature' (70[R]); '... it also seems unwise to exposure infants unnecessarily to lithium ...' (71[R]). Given the extremely high risk of post-partum recurrence in bipolar patients, the issue is not whether the mother should take a mood stabilizer (she should), but whether the baby should be breast-fed (unresolved).

Effects on fertility Intramuscular lithium chloride produced subtherapeutic blood concentrations (by human standards) in male rose-ringed parakeets, but significantly reduced testicular weight and caused widespread degenerative changes in the testes (72). Fertility was not assessed directly.

Genetic effects In 18 patients treated with benzodiazepines and/or antipsychotic drugs there were increased chromosomal aberrations and increased sister chromatid exchange, but there were no significant differences between this group and another group of 18 patients taking lithium in addition to benzodiazepines and/or antipsychotic drugs (73[C]).

Tumor-preventing effects There was a *lower risk of cancer* in both 609 lithium patients and 2396 psychiatric controls compared with the general population, and in the lithium group there was a non-significant trend towards an even lower risk of non-epithelial tumors (74[C]).

Withdrawal effects Three issues have been addressed:

- does rapid withdrawal increase recurrence risk?
- how common is post-discontinuation refractoriness to the reinstitution of lithium?
- does withdrawal increase the risk of thyrotoxicosis?

Data from Italy have suggested that gradual withdrawal of lithium (over 15–30 days) was associated with a markedly reduced risk of early recurrence of mania and depression and a much greater likelihood of prolonged stability compared with rapid discontinuation (over 1–14 days) (75[CR]). There was a marked increase in suicidal acts during the first year after lithium discontinuation; after that the risk returned to what it had been before the start of lithium treatment. The increased risk in the first year exceeded that expected from increased affective morbidity alone. There was a 1.95-fold greater risk, during this first year in those who discontinued lithium rapidly, although this was not statistically significant (76[CR]).

In 28 patients who had responded to lithium treatment of mania or schizoaffective mania and who had recurrences after withdrawal there were equally good responses to retreatment with lithium (77[CR]). These findings add to the evidence that lithium discontinuation-induced refractoriness is the exception rather than the rule.

A 46-year-old experienced a *thyrotoxic crisis* after lithium withdrawal, adding to the case report literature that lithium withdrawal may be associated with an outpouring of thyroid hormone in predisposed individuals (27[c]).

Overdosage Reviews have addressed lithium toxicity in the elderly (6[R]) and lithium intoxication, with an emphasis on the kidney (78[R]). The 1997 Annual Report of the American Association of Poison Control Centers Toxic Exposure Surveillance System listed nine lithium-associated deaths and provided some clinical details in seven cases, including serum concentrations of 2.4–7.8 mmol/l (79[C]).

A reversible *Creutzfeldt-Jacob-like syndrome* (the 13th reportedly attributed to lithium) was described in a 65-year-old woman treated with lithium, levopromazine, and phenobarbital after she had mistakenly increased her lithium dosage (80[cr]).

Chronic neurological sequelae of intoxication included two patients with a *persistent cerebellar syndrome* and severe *cerebellar atrophy* (81[c]), one with *subcortical dementia* (82[c]), and one with a *diffuse sensorimotor peripheral neuropathy* (83[c]). This last patient also developed *rhabdomyolysis* during the acute episode in association with a serum lithium concentration of 3.1 mmol/l and a serum sodium of 163 mmol/l.

Two patients developed lithium intoxication (serum concentrations 3.3 and 3.0 mmol/l) in association with poorly controlled diabetes mellitus, suggesting that the latter is a risk factor (37[c]).

Treatment of toxicity Two patients with lithium toxicity (serum concentrations 3.5 and 4.2 mmol/l) had the well-recognized rebound increase in serum concentrations after the end of hemodialysis. Both died during hospitalization from what was cryptically described as 'unrelated events' (84[c]).

A 49-year-old with severe lithium toxicity was treated successfully with continuous veno-venous hemodiafiltration (CVVHDF); the serum lithium concentration fell from 3.0 to 0.93 mmol/l after 7 hours and there was no rebound increase after the end of the procedure (85[c]). The maximum lithium clearance was 28 ml/minute which is considerably lower than usually attained with hemodialysis.

Interactions A review of drug interactions with lithium considered both pharmacokinetic interactions (e.g. diuretics, NSAIDs) and pharmacodynamic interactions (antipsychotic drugs, SSRIs) and summarized the most important ones in tabular form (86[R]).

Antibiotics Two reviews of drug interactions with antibiotics briefly and incompletely discussed lithium (87[r], 88[r]).

Anticonvulsants The pharmacokinetics of lithium were not altered by gabapentin in 13 patients (89[C]).

Antidepressants Adverse events associated with lithium augmentation of antidepressants have been reviewed: tricyclic antidepressants and MAO inhibitors—no serious problems; *SSRIs*—a few reports of serotonin syndrome (90[R]).

Serum lithium concentrations were unchanged when breakthrough depression was treated double-blind by the addition of paroxetine (20–40 mg/day, n = 19) or amitriptyline (75–150 mg/day, n = 23) and the combinations were generally well tolerated (91[C]).

In 12 healthy volunteers, there were no clinically significant alterations in blood concentrations of lithium or nefazodone and its metabolites when the drugs were co-administered (92[C]). The addition of lithium for 6 weeks to nefazodone in 14 treatment-resistant patients produced no serious adverse effects and no drop-outs (93[C]).

A 65-year-old man who took lithium and *doxepin* for 13 years presented with a 6-month history of myoclonic jerking of both arms, which resolved when both drugs were stopped (94[c]). Whether this represented a drug interaction or a single drug effect is unclear.

Antipsychotic drugs (see also Nervous system) In a discussion of drug interactions with antipsychotic drugs, the literature on lithium was reviewed (95[R]). Caution was advised when lithium is combined with antipsychotic drugs, especially with high dosages of high-potency drugs. In a review of acute, life-threatening, drug-induced neurological syndromes, the controversy of whether lithium increases the risk of neuroleptic malignant syndrome was mentioned briefly (96[r]) (see also Nervous system).

Erythrocyte/plasma lithium concentration ratios were lower in patients taking *phenothiazines* or *haloperidol* than in those taking lithium alone (97[C], 98[C]), and the former group had a higher incidence of neurological and renal adverse effects (98[C]). *Amisulpride* In a placebo-controlled, parallel-design, double-blind study in 24 male volunteers, amisulpride 100 mg bd for 7 days did not alter lithium pharmacokinetics. *Clozapine* (see also Hematological) Five treatment-resistant patients were treated successfully with a combination of clozapine and lithium with no clinically significant adverse events (99[c]). However, a 59-year-old woman developed neurotoxic symptoms 3 days after lithium was added to clozapine; the symptoms resolved when both drugs were stopped and recurred with rechallenge (100[c]).

Calcitonin After they had received 100 units of salmon calcitonin subcutaneously for 3 days, four patients had a 30% mean reduction in serum lithium concentration, which was attributed to reduced absorption and/or increased renal excretion (101[c]).

Mazindol A woman stabilized on lithium developed toxic symptoms 3 days after starting the appetite suppressant mazindol. After 9 days her serum lithium concentration was 3.2 mmol/l (102[c]). A 58-year-old also developed lithium toxicity (serum concentration 3.2 mmol/l) after the addition of mazindol (103[c]).

Non-steroidal anti-inflammatory drugs (NSAIDs) A review of drug interactions with analgesics in the dental literature concluded that NSAIDs should be used briefly, if at all, in patients taking lithium, especially in the elderly (104[R]). In five male volunteers, ketorolac 10 mg qds for 5 days increased lithium AUC by 24% and increased the incidence and severity of lithium-related adverse effects (105[C]). There were no significant changes in serum lithium concentrations in 12 men taking over-the-counter doses of naproxen (220 mg tds) or paracetamol (650 mg qds) for 5 days (106[C]). Nevertheless, caution is still advised when combining NSAIDs with lithium.

Risperidone There were no changes in lithium pharmacokinetics when risperidone was substituted open-label for another neuroleptic drug in 13 patients (107[C]).

Sumatriptan The 1996 Canadian Product Monograph for sumatriptan apparently lists SSRIs and lithium as contraindications (such is not the case in the 1998 US package insert). However, a review of the subject found little substantiation for a severe interaction between sumatriptan and lithium (108[r]).

Interference with diagnostic routines The possibility that other substances could interfere with ion-selective electrode lithium analysis has been briefly reviewed (109[r]).

Contamination of lithium heparin blood culture bottles with Pseudomonas fluorescens led to an outbreak of *pseudobacteremia* and the unnecessary treatment of a number of children with antibiotics. Lithium had no direct role in this misadventure (110[C]).

Lithium treatment of adolescents with bipolar disorder and secondary substance abuse improved both conditions (111[C]). It was suggested, however, that lithium-induced polyuria may have diluted urine to the extent that false negative test results were obtained when screening for drugs of abuse (112). While the number of positive urine tests was actually higher (but not significantly so) in those with polyuria (113[C]), there is still a possibility that lithium-induced diabetes insipidus could increase the frequency of false negative urine drug assays, because of urine dilution.

REFERENCES

1. Levin GM. A comparison of patient-rated burden and incidence of side-effects: lithium versus valproate. Int J Psychiatry Clin Pract 1997;1:89–93.
2. McConville BJ, Sorter MT, Foster K, Barken A, Browne K, Chaney R. Lithium versus valproate side effects in adolescents with bipolar disorder. New Clinical Drug Evaluation Unit Progam. Presented at the NCDEU 38th Annual Meeting, Boca Raton, FL, 10–13 June 1998: Poster No. 74.
3. Olugbemi E, Katona C. Case note audit of lithium use in the elderly. Aging Mental Health 1998;2:151–4.
4. Stoudemire A, Hill CD, Lewison BJ, Marquardt M, Dalton S. Lithium intolerance in a medical-psychiatric population. Gen Hosp Psychiatry 1998;20:85–90.
5. Kilts CD. The ups and downs of oral lithium dosing. J Clin Psychiatry 1998;59:21–6.
6. Jefferson JW. Lithium toxicity in the elderly. In: Nelson JC, editor. Geriatric Psychopharmacology. New York: Marcel Dekker, 1998;273–83.
7. Wolf ME, Moffat M, Ranade V, Somberg JC, Lehrer E, Mosnaim AD. Lithium, hypercalcemia, and arrhythmia. J Clin Psychopharmacol 1998;18:420–3.
8. Slavicek J, Paclt I, Hamplová J, Kittnar O, Trefny Z, Horacek BM. Antidepressant drugs and heart electrical field. Physiol Res 1998;47:297–300.
9. Honig A, Arts BMG, Ponds RWHM, Riedel WJ. Lithium induced cognitive side-effects in bipolar disorder: a qualitative analysis and implications for daily practice. Int Clin Psychopharmacol 1999;14:167–71.
10. Arts BMG, Honig A, Riedel WJ, Ponds RWHM. Cognitive-side effects of lithium; a meta-

analysis and proposal for screening. Tijdschr Psychiatr 1998;40:460–8.
11. Manji H, Howard RS, Miller DH, Hirsch NP, Carr L, Bahtia K, Quinn N, Marsden CD. Status dystonicus: the syndrome and its management. Brain 1998;121:243–52.
12. Landry P, Warnes H. Nielsen T, Montplaisir J. Somnambulistic-like behavior in patients attending a lithium clinic. Int Clin Psychopharmacol 1999;14:173–5.
13. Landry P, Montplaisir J. Lithium-induced somnambulism. Can J Psychiatry 1998;43:957–8.
14. Merle C, Sotto A, Galland MC, Jourdan E, Jourdan J. Syndrome cérébelleux persistant après traitement par lithium et neuroleptique. Therapie 1998;53:511–13.
15. Normann C, Brandt C, Berger M, Walden J. Delirium and persistent dyskinesia induced by a lithium-neuroleptic interaction. Pharmacopsychiatry 1998;31:201–4.
16. Lane RM. SSRI-induced extrapyramidal side-effects and akathisia: implications for treatment. J Psychopharmacol 1998;12:192–214.
17. Pelonero AL, Levenson JL, Pandurangi AK. Neuroleptic malignant syndrome: a review. Psychiatr Serv 1998;49:1163–72.
18. Berardi D, Amore M, Keck PE, Troia M, Dell'Atti M. Clinical and pharmacologic risk factors for neuroleptic malignant syndrome: a case-control study. Biol Psychiatry 1998;44:748–54.
19. Epstein Y, Albukrek D, Kalmovitc B, Moran DS, Shapiro Y. Heat intolerance induced by antidepressants. Ann NY Acad Sci 1997;813:553–8.
20. Faravelli C, Di Bernardo M, Ricca V, Benvenuti P, Bartelli M, Ronchi O. Effects of chronic lithium treatment on the peripheral nervous system. J Clin Psychiatry 1999;60:306–10.
21. Lazarus JH. The effects of lithium therapy on thyroid and thyrotropin-releasing hormone. Thyroid 1998;8:909–13.
22. Kusalic M, Engelsmann F. Effect of lithium maintenance therapy on thyroid and parathyroid function. J Psychiatr Neurosci 1999;24:227–33.
23. Kleiner J, Altshuler L, Hendrick V, Hershman JM. Lithium-induced subclinical hypothyroidism: review of the literature and guidelines for treatment. J Clin Psychiatry 1999;60:249–55.
24. Deodhar SD, Singh B, Pathak CM, Sharan P, Kulhara P. Thyroid functions in lithium-treated psychiatric patients. Biol Trace Elem Res 1999;67:151–63.
25. Kirov G. Thyroid disorders in lithium-treated patients. J Affect Disord 1998;50:33–40.
26. Depoot I, Van Imschoot S, Lamberigts G. Lithium-geassocieerde hyperthyroïdie. Tijdschr Geneeskd 1998;54:413–16.
27. Calvo Romero JM, Puerto Pica JM. Crisis tirotóxica tras la retirada de tratamiento con litio. Rev Clin Esp 1998;198:782–3.
28. Bogazzi F, Bartalena L, Brogioni S, Scarcello G, Burelli A, Campomori A, Manetti L, Rossi G, Pinchera A, Martino E. Comparison of radioiodine with radioiodine plus lithium in the treatment of Graves' hyperthyroidism. J Clin Endocrinol Metab 1999;84:499–503.
29. Benbassat CA, Molitch ME. The use of lithium in the treatment of hyperthyroidism. Endocrinologist 1998;8:383–7.
30. Hoogenberg K, Beentjes JAM, Piers DA. Lithium as an adjunct to radioactive iodine in treatment-resistant Graves thyrotoxicosis. Ann Intern Med 1998;129:670.
31. Koong S-S, Reynolds JC, Movius EG, Keenan AM, Ain KB, Lakshmanan MC, Robbins J. Lithium as a potential adjuvant to ^{131}I therapy of metastatic, well differentiated thyroid carcinoma. J Clin Endocrinol Metab 1999;84:912–16.
32. Abdullah H., Bliss R, Guinea AI, Delbridge L. Pathology and outcome of surgical treatment for lithium-associated hyperparathyroidism. Br J Surg 1999;86:91–3.
33. Sofuoglu S, Bastürk M, Tutus A, Karaaslan F, Aslan SS, Gönül AS. Lithium-induced alterations in parathormone function in patients with bipolar affective disorder. Int J Neuropsychopharmacol 1999;2:S56.
34. Cohen O, Rais T, Lepkifker E, Vered I. Lithium carbonate therapy is not a risk factor for osteoporosis. Horm Metab Res 1998;30:594–7.
35. Mak TWL, Shek C-C, Chow C-C, Wing Y-K, Lee S. Effects of lithium therapy on bone mineral metabolism: a two-year prospective longitudinal study. J Clin Endocrinol Metab 1998;83:3857–9.
36. De Celis G, Fiter M, Latorre X, Llebaria C. Oxyphilic parathyroid adenoma and lithium therapy. Lancet 1998;352:1070.
37. Oomura S, Mukasa H, Ooji T, Mukasa H, Mukasa H, Satomura T, Tatsumoto Y. Does impaired glucose tolerance predispose to lithium intoxication in treatment of MDI? Int J Neuropsychopharmacol 1999;2:S63.
38. Azam H, Newton RW, Morris AD, Thompson CJ. Hyperosmolar nonketotic coma precipitated by lithium-induced nephrogenic diabetes insipidus. Postgrad Med J 1998;74:39–41.
39. MacGregor DA, Baker AM, Appel RG, Ober KP, Zaloga GP. Hyperosmolar coma due to lithium-induced diabetes insipidus. Lancet 1995;346:413–17.
40. MacGregor DA, Dolinski SY. Hyperosmolar coma. Lancet 1999;353:1189.
41. Ackerman S, Nolan LJ. Bodyweight gain induced by psychotropic drugs. Incidence, mechanisms and management. CNS Drugs 1998;9:135–51.
42. Kelly DL, Conley RR, Love RC, Horn SD, Ushchak CM. Weight gain in adolescents treated with risperidone and conventional antipsychotics over six months. J Child Adolesc Psychopharmacol 1998;8:151–9.
43. Sofuoglu S, Karaaslan F, Tutus A, Bastürk M, Yabanoglu I, Esel E. Effects of short and long-term lithium treatment on serum prolactin levels in patients with bipolar affective disorder. Int J Neuropsychopharmacol 1999;2:S56.
44. Haden ST, Brown EM, Stoll AL, Scott J, Fuleihan GE-H. The effect of lithium on calcium-

induced changes in adrenocorticotrophin levels. J Clin Endocrinol Metab 1999;84:198–200.
45. Singh B, Bandhu HK, Pathak CM, Garg ML, Mittal BR, Kulhara P, Singh N, Deodhar SD. Effect of lithium therapy on trace elements in blood of psychiatric patients. Trace Elem Electrolytes 1998;15:94–100.
46. Cervantes P, Ghadirian AM, Vida S. Vitamin B_{12} and folate levels and lithium administration in patients with affective disorders. Biol Psychiatry 1999;45:214–21.
47. Oyewumi LK, McKnight M, Cernovsky ZZ. Lithium dosage and leukocyte counts in psychiatric patients. J Psychiatr Neurosci 1999;24:215–21.
48. Silverston PH. Prevention of clozapine-induced neutropenia by pretreatment with lithium. J Clin Psychopharmacol 1998;18:86–8.
49. Blier P, Slater S, Measham T, Koch M, Wiviott G. Lithium and clozapine-induced neutropenia/agranulocytosis. Int Clin Psychopharmacol 1998;13:137–40.
50. Ballin A, Lehman D, Sirota P, Litvinjuk U, Meytes D. Increased number of peripheral blood CD34+ cells in lithium-treated patients. Br J Haematol 1998;100:219–21.
51. Canales MA, Arrieta R, Hernández-García C, Bustos JG, Aguado MJ, Hernández-Navarro F. A single apheresis to achieve a high number of peripheral blood CD34+ cells in a lithium-treated patient with acute myeloid leukaemia. Bone Marrow Transplant 1999;23:305.
52. Amano I, Morii T, Yamanaka T, Tsukaguchi N, Nishikawa K, Narita N, Shimoyama T. Successful lithium carbonate therapy for a patient with intractable and severe aplastic anemia. Rinsho Ketsueki 1999;40:46–50.
53. Çelik Ç, Konukoglu D, Ozmen M, Akçay T. Platelet-specific proteins in lithium carbonate treatment. Med Sci Res 1998;26:417–18.
54. Szabadi E, Tavernor S. Hypo-and hypersalivation induced by psychoactive drugs. Incidence, mechanisms and therapeutic implications. CNS Drugs 1999;11:449–66.
55. Haude V, Kretschmer H. Chronic diarrhea and increasing disability in an older woman due to an unusual cause. J Am Geriatr Soc 1999;47:261–2.
56. Batlle D, Dorhout-Mees EJ. Lithium and the kidney. In: De Broe ME, Porter GA, Bennett WM, Verpooten GA, editors. Clinical Nephrotoxins: Renal Injury from Drugs and Chemicals. Dordrecht, The Netherlands, Boston: Kluwer Academic Publishers, 1998;383–95.
57. Braden GL. Lithium-induced renal disease. In: Greenberg A, editor. Primer on Kidney Diseases. San Diego: Academic Press, 1998;332–4.
58. Gitlin M. Lithium and the kidney. An updated review. Drug Saf 1999;20:231–43.
59. Johnson G. Lithium—early development, toxicity, and renal function. Neuropsychopharmacology 1998;19:200–5.
60. Rastegar A, Kashgarian M. The clinical spectrum of tubulointerstitial nephritis. Kidney Int 1998;54:313–27.
61. Gabutti L, Gugger M, Marti H-P. Eingeschränkte Nieren-funktion bei Lithium-therapie. Ther Umsch 1998;55:562–4.
62. Stone KA. Lithium-induced nephrogenic diabetes insipidus. J Am Board Fam Pract 1999;12:43–7.
63. Frokiaer J, Marples D, Knepper MA, Nielsen S. Pathophysiology of aquaporin-2 in water balance disorders. Am J Med Sci 1998;316:291–9.
64. Ellgehausen P, Elsner P, Burg G. Drug-induced lichen planus. Clin Dermatol 1998;16:325–32.
65. Horner KC, Huang Z-WW, Higuerie D, Cazals Y. Reversible hearing impairment induced by lithium in the guinea pig. Neuroreport 1997;8:1341–5.
66. Kang BJ, Park SW, Chung TH. Can the expression of histocompatibility antigen be changed by lithium? Int J Neuropsychopharmacol 1999;2:S55.
67. Viguera AC, Cohen LS. The course and management of bipolar disorder during pregnancy. Psychopharmacol Bull 1998;34:339–46.
68. Cohen LS, Rosenbaum JF. Psychotropic drug use during pregnancy: weighing the risks. J Clin Psychiatry 1998;59:18–28.
69. Austin M-PV, Mitchell PB. Use of psychotropic medications in breast-feeding women: acute and prophylactic treatment. Aust NZ J Psychiatry 1998;32:778–84.
70. Llewellyn A, Stowe ZN. Psychotropic medications in lactation. J Clin Psychiatry 1998;59:41–52.
71. Yoshida K, Smith B, Kumar R. Psychotropic drugs in mothers' milk: a comprehensive review of assay methods, pharmacokinetics and of safety of breast-feeding. J Psychopharmacol 1999;13:64–80.
72. Banerji TK, Maitra SK, Basu A, Hawkins HK. Lithium-induced alterations in the testis of the male roseringed parakeet (*Psittacula krameri*): evidence for significant structural changes and disruption in the spermatogenetic activity. Endocr Res 1999;25:35–49.
73. Bigatti MP, Corona D, Munizza C. Increased sister chromatid exchange and chromosomal aberration frequencies in psychiatric patients receiving psychopharmacological therapy. Mutat Res Genet Toxicol Environ Mutagen 1998;413:169–75.
74. Cohen Y, Chetrit A, Cohen Y, Sirota P, Modan B. Cancer morbidity in psychiatric patients: influence of lithium carbonate treatment. Med Oncol 1998;15:32–6.
75. Baldessarini RJ, Tondo L. Recurrence risk in bipolar manic-depressive disorders after discontinuing lithium maintenance treatment: an overview. Clin Drug Invest 1998;15:337–51.
76. Baldessarini RJ, Tondo L, Hennen J. Effects of lithium treatment and its discontinuation on suicidal behavior in bipolar manic-depressive disorders. J Clin Psychiatry 1999;60:77–84.
77. Coryell W, Solomon D, Leon AC, Akiskal HS, Keller MB, Scheftner WA, Mueller T. Lithium discontinuation and subsequent effectiveness. Am J Psychiatry 1998;155:895–8.
78. Timmer RT, Sands JM. Lithium intoxication. J Am Soc Nephrol 1999;10:666–74.

79. Litovitz TL, Klein-Schwartz W, Dyer KS, Shannon M, Lee S, Powers M. 1997 Annual Report of the American Association of Poison Control Centers Toxic Exposure Surveillance System. Am J Emerg Med 1998;16:443–97.
80. Kikyo H, Furukawa T. Creutzfeldt-Jakob-like syndrome induced by lithium, levomepromazine, and phenobarbitone. J Neurol Neurosurg Psychiatry 1999;66:802–3.
81. Roy M, Stip E, Black D, Lew V, Langlois R. Dégéné rescence cérébelleuse secondaire à une intoxication aiguë au lithium. Rev Neurol (Paris) 1998;154:546–8.
82. Brumm VL, Van Gorp WG, Wirshing W. Chronic neuropsychological sequelae in a case of severe lithium intoxication. Neuropsychiatr Neuropsychology Behav Neurol 1998;11:245–9.
83. Su K-P, Lee Y-J, Lee M-B. Severe peripheral polyneuropathy and rhabdomyolysis in lithium intoxication: a case report. Gen Hosp Psychiatry 1999;21:136–7.
84. Bosinski T, Bailie GR, Eisele G. Massive and extended rebound of serum lithium concentrations following hemodialysis in two chronic overdose cases. Am J Emerg Med 1998;16:98–100.
85. Hazouard E, Ferrandière M, Rateau H, Doucet O, Perrotin D, Legras A. Continuous veno-venous haemofiltration versus continuous veno-venous haemodialysis in severe lithium self-poisoning: a toxicokinetics study in an intensive care unit. Nephrol Dial Transplant 1999;14:1605–6.
86. Müller-Oerlinghausen B. Drug interactions with lithium. A guide for clinicians. CNS Drugs 1999;11:41–8.
87. Joos AAB. Pharmakologische interaktionen von antiobiotika und psychopharmaka. Psychiatr Prax 1998;25:57–60.
88. Hersh EV. Adverse drug interactions in dental practice: interactions involving antibiotics. Part II of a series. J Am Dent Assoc 1999;130:236–51.
89. Frye MA, Kimbrell TA, Dunn RT, Piscitelli S, Grothe D, Vanderham E, Corá-Locatelli G, Post RM, Ketter TA. Gabapentin does not alter single-dose lithium pharmacokinetics. J Clin Psychopharmacol 1998;18:461–4.
90. Schweitzer I, Tuckwell V. Risk of adverse events with the use of augmentation therapy for the treatment of resistant depression. Drug Saf 1998;19:455–64.
91. Bauer M, Zaninelli R, Müller-Oerlinghausen B, Meister W. Paroxetine and amitriptyline augmentation of lithium in the treatment of major depression: a double-blind study. J Clin Psychopharmacol 1999;19:164–71.
92. Laroudie C, Salazar DE, Cosson J-P, Cheuvart B, Istin B, Girault J, Ingrand I, Decourt J-P. Pharmacokinetic evaluation of co-administration of nefazodone and lithium in healthy subjects. Eur J Clin Pharmacol 1999;54:923–8.
93. Hawley C, Sivakumaran T, Huber TJ, Ige AK. Combination therapy with nefazodone and lithium: safety and tolerability in fourteen patients. Int J Psychiatry Clin Pract 1998;2:251–4.
94. Evidente VGH, Caviness JN. Focal cortical transient preceding myoclonus during lithium and tricyclic antidepressant therapy. Neurology 1999;52:211–13.
95. ZumBrunnen TL, Jann MW. Drug interactions with antipsychotic agents. Incidence and therapeutic implications. CNS Drugs 1998;9:381–401.
96. Richard IH. Acute, drug-induced, life-threatening neurological syndromes. Neurologist 1998;4:196–210.
97. Ahmadi-Abhari SA, Dehpour AR, Emamian ES, Azizabadi-Farahani M, Farsam H, Samini M, Shokri J. The effect of concurrent administration of psychotropic drugs and lithium on lithium ratio in bipolar patients. Hum Psychopharmacol 1998;13:29–34.
98. Dehpour AR, Emamian ES, Ahmadi-Abhari SA, Azizabadi-Farahani M. The lithium ratio and the incidence of side effects. Prog Neuro-Psychopharmacol Biol Psychiatry 1998;22:959–70.
99. Moldavsky M, Stein D, Benatov R, Sirota P, Elizur A, Matzner Y, Weizman A. Combined clozapine-lithium treatment for schizophrenia and schizoaffective disorder. Eur Psychiatry 1998;13:104–6.
100. Lee S-H, Yang Y-Y. Reversible neurotoxicity induced by a combination of clozapine and lithium: a case report. Chin Med J Taipei 1999;62:184–7.
101. Passiu G, Bocchetta A, Martinelli V, Garau P, Del Zompo M, Mathieu A. Calcitonin decreases lithium plasma levels in man. Preliminary report. Int J Clin Pharmacol Res 1998;18:179–81.
102. Hendy MS, Dove AF, Arblaster PG. Mazindol-induced lithium toxicity. Br Med J 1980;280:684–5.
103. Verduijn M. Lithiumtoxiciteit door mazindol: Patiënt sprak niet te volgen taal. Pharm Weekbl 1998;133:1901.
104. Haas DA. Adverse drug interactions in dental practice: interactions associated with analgesics. Part III in a series. J Am Dent Assoc 1999;130:397–407.
105. Cold JA, ZumBrunnen TL, Simpson MA, Augustin BG, Awad E, Jann MW. Increased lithium serum and red blood cell concentrations during ketorolac coadministration. J Clin Psychopharmacol 1998;18:33–7.
106. Levin GM, Grum C, Eisele G. Effect of over-the-counter dosages of naproxen sodium and acetaminophen on plasma lithium concentrations in normal volunteers. J Clin Psychopharmacol 1998;18:237–40.
107. Demling J, Huang ML, De Smedt G. Pharmacokinetics and safety of combination therapy with lithium and risperidone in adult patients with psychosis. Int J Neuropsychopharmacol 1999;2:S63.
108. Gardner DM, Lynd LD. Sumatriptan contraindications and the serotonin syndrome. Ann Pharmacother 1998;32:33–8.
109. Linder MW, Keck PE. Standards of laboratory practice: antidepressant drug monitoring. Clin Chem 1998;44:1073–84.

110. Namnyak S, Hussain S, Davalle J, Roker K, Strickland M. Contaminated lithium heparin bottles as a source of pseudobacteraemia due to *Pseudomonas fluorescens*. J Hosp Infect 1999;41:23–8.
111. Geller B, Cooper TB, Sun K, Zimerman B, Frazier J, Willliams M, Heath J. Double-blind and placebo-controlled study of lithium for adolescent bipolar disorders with secondary substance dependency. J Am Acad Child Adolesc Psychiatry 1998;37:171–8.
112. Rohde LA, Szobot C. Lithium in bipolar adolescents with secondary substance dependency. J Am Acad Child Adolesc Psychiatry 1999; 38:4.
113. Geller B. Lithium in bipolar adolescents with secondary substance dependency (reply). J Am Acad Child Adolesc Psychiatry 1999;38:4.

Eileen Wong, Jayendra K. Patel and Alan I. Green

4 Drugs of abuse

AMPHETAMINES

Methylenedioxymethamphetamine (MDMA, Ecstasy)

The designer drug known as Ecstasy is sold on the streets as a heterogeneous substance, with enormous variations in its main active ingredients. It most often contains derivatives of methylenedioxymethamphetamine (MDMA) and 3,4-methylenedioxy-*N*-ethylamphetamine (MDE). Other amphetamine derivatives that it may contain include 3,4-methylenedioxyamphetamine (MDA), *N*-methyl-1-(1,3-benzodioxol-5-yl)-2-butanamine (MBDB), and 2,5-dimethoxy-4-bromamphetamine (DOB). The amount of active ingredient in street Ecstasy ranges from none to very high. In addition, other amphetamines or hallucinogens can be mixed in. A survey of 3021 young adults (14–24 years old) in Germany showed that regular use of Ecstasy by itself is rare (2.6%). Among lifetime users, 97% have also used cannabinoids, 59% cocaine, 48% other substances, 46% hallucinogens, and 26% opiates. The interviews revealed that the use of Ecstasy and hallucinogens is increasing, especially in young people. The authors observed that a large number of first-time users are at risk of regular use (1[C]).

As recreational use of Ecstasy has dramatically increased in recent years, further deaths related to its use have been reported. In a retrospective review of all *violent deaths* from 1992 to 1997 in South Australia, six fatalities were associated with Ecstasy abuse; all occurred after September 1995. Three victims had documented hyperthermia and there was evidence of hyperthermia in another. The authors suggested that individual susceptibility to MDMA may be caused by impaired metabolism by CYP2D6 or through genetically poor metabolism (5–9% of Caucasians). One woman, who died with a cerebral hemorrhage, had fluoxetine (a CYP2D6 inhibitor) present in her blood. Furthermore, toxicology identified para-methoxyamphetamine (PMA) in all the cases, amphetamine/methamphetamine in four cases, and MDMA in only two cases. PMA, which is sold as an MDMA substitute or is present as a contaminant, is associated with a high rate of lethal complications (2[CR]).

Another report of a death has come from Australia (3[cr]).

A 35-year-old male criminal died under suspicious circumstances. The police had seen him alive about 1.5 hours before the alleged time of death during a patrol visit to his home. Evaluation of the corpse showed an obvious head injury, and the body was in an advanced stage of rigor mortis, despite the fact that the alleged time of death had been less than 4 hours earlier. The body temperature was significantly raised, at 42°C. By witness account, the deceased had taken Ecstasy at various times during the night, after which he had been groaning before taking off his clothes and then thrashing on the floor while hitting his head and bumping into things. When resuscitation had been attempted his jaw had been locked. Toxicology detected amphetamine, metamphetamine, and PMA in the blood.

The authors suggested that in a subgroup of amphetamine abusers, a triad of amphetamine use, prolonged exertion, and hyperthermia can be potentially lethal. Any temperature above 42°C requires active cooling (until below 38.5°C) and carries a poor prognosis. In this case rigor mortis may have started almost at the time of death. An Ecstasy tablet that was allegedly from the same batch contained 50 mg of PMA.

Cardiovascular A case of transient *myocardial ischemia* associated with Ecstasy has been reported in Britain (4[cr]).

A 25-year-old man, a regular alcohol drinker with a history of asthma, had been out drinking 8 pints of lager and 4 gins. His last drink was spiked with a tablet that was presumably Ecstasy.

Side Effects of Drugs, Annual 23
J.K. Aronson, ed.

He scooped the tablet out and even though some of the tablet may have dissolved, he finished the drink. Three hours later, he awoke with restlessness, nausea, and abdominal cramps. In the emergency room, his temperature was 37.2°C and he was sweating. His heart rate was 120 and his blood pressure 130/70 mmHg. He had some abdominal discomfort. A diagnosis of Ecstasy ingestion was made, although urine MDMA concentrations were not measured. His electrocardiogram on admission showed sinus tachycardia with T-wave inversion in leads I, aVL, and V4–6, with voltage criteria for left ventricular hypertrophy. The next day the electrocardiogram had returned to normal. An echocardiogram was within normal limits. He was well on discharge.

The authors suggested that this was the first report of transient myocardial ischemia after Ecstasy. They reasoned that the myocardial ischemia did not proceed to necrosis or a dysrhythmia because the amount of drug exposure was low.

Cardiovascular autonomic functioning during MDMA use has been investigated in 12 MDMA users and a matched group of non-users (5[Cr]). Resting heart rate variability (an index of parasympathetic tone) and heart rate response to the Valsalva maneuver (Valsalva ratio, an index of overall *autonomic responsiveness*) were both reduced in the drug users. Thus, seemingly healthy users of MDMA had autonomic dysregulation, comparable to that seen in diabetes mellitus. In several users there was a total absence of post-Valsalva release bradycardia, a sign of parasympathetic dysfunction. Since no cardiac data were available for these patients before their amphetamine use and all were multidrug users, the findings must be interpreted with caution.

Respiratory Adverse effects can develop after amphetamines are abused in combination (6[cr]).

A 28-year-old healthy woman had left-sided pleuritic chest pain of 18 hours duration, having taken one tablet of Ecstasy and one tablet of Speed (metamphetamine hydrochloride) 4 hours earlier. There was surgical emphysema in her neck. On auscultation there was a crunching cardiac systolic sound. Chest X-ray showed pneumopericardium and pneumomediastinum. She was given analgesics and monitored. The chest pain subsided after 4 days.

Possible mechanisms for her respiratory problems included alveolar rupture, caused by an increase in intra-alveolar pressure, due to the exertion while she had been dancing strenuously; or it could have been secondary to her use of positive ventilatory pressure after taking the drugs; this is done by a partner, either by direct mouth-to-mouth contact or through a cardboard cylinder, to enhance the user's experience of the stimulant's effects.

Nervous system The acute and short-term effects of a recreational dose of MDMA (1.7 mg/kg) given to 13 MDMA-naive healthy volunteers in a double-blind, placebo-controlled study have been reported (7[CR]). MDMA produced a state of *enhanced mood, well-being*, and *enhanced emotional responsiveness*, with *mild depersonalization, derealization, thought disorder*, and *anxiety*. The subjects also had *changes in their sense of space and time*, *heightened sensory awareness*, and *increased psychomotor drive*. MDMA *increased blood pressure* moderately, except in one case of a transient hypertensive reaction. The most frequent somatic adverse effects were *jaw clenching*, *poor appetite*, *restlessness*, and *insomnia*. *Lack of energy, difficulty in concentrating, fatigue*, and *feelings of restlessness* during the next day were also described. The authors suggested that MDMA produces a psychological profile different from classic hallucinogens or psychostimulants. The potential risk of hypertensive effects of recreational dosages of MDMA should also be considered in the safety profile.

Using positron emission tomography (PET) with a radioligand that selectively labels the serotonin (5HT) transporter, 14 MDMA users who were currently abstaining (for 3 weeks) from use and 15 MDMA-naive controls were studied (8[C]). MDMA users showed a reduction in global and regional brain 5HT transporter binding, a measure of the number of 5HT neurons, compared with controls. Deficiency in the serotonin transporter correlated positively with the extent of previous drug use. The authors suggested that MDMA users are susceptible to MDMA-induced *serotonin neural injury*.

Psychiatric A case of MDMA-related panic disorder has been reported (9[cr]).

A 21-year-old man used increasing dosages of MDMA (7 tablets or 400–500 mg/day) over a period of 5 months. After taking six tablets one day, he developed palpitation, chest pain, sweating, vertigo, and a fear of dying. He responded well to alprazolam and was discharged. Several days later, the panic attacks recurred spontaneously. Five weeks later, he had a complete medical work-up that was unrevealing. Since his panic attacks persisted in the absence of any drugs, he was given the SSRI paroxetine 20 mg/day along with alprazolam. On this regimen his panic attacks gradually abated and stopped 3 months later. The paroxetine was gradually tapered over the next 3 months and he continued to be symptom-free at 6 months.

The authors suggested that this case may have exemplified dose-dependent serotonergic neurotoxicity from Ecstasy abuse.

Mineral and fluid balance A new case of the syndrome of inappropriate anti-diuretic hormone (SIADH) associated with MDMA has appeared (10[cr]).

A healthy 19-year-old woman complained of nausea and vomited 8 hours after taking unknown quantities of MDMA and beer; 3 hours later she suddenly clenched her jaw, had tonic contractions of all four limbs, and collapsed. She was obtunded, with occasional moaning and non-purposeful movements of the limbs. Head CT scan showed mild cerebral edema. Her serum electrolytes, including a sodium of 115 mmol/l and a corresponding urine osmolality of 522 mosm/kg, suggested SIADH. Despite treatment, the serum sodium concentration 10 hours later was 116 mmol/l, but 18 hours after treatment it rose to 125 mmol/l. She became progressively more responsive, with normalization of her sodium concentration, and after 48 hours was awake and alert, with a serum sodium concentration of 136 mmol/l.

The authors reviewed nine other reported cases of MDMA-related SIADH, all of whom were women. They concluded that MDMA-associated SIADH is multifactorial and that MDMA may stimulate vasopressin secretion in susceptible individuals. They further suggested that hyponatremia can also occur secondary to voluntary increases in fluid or water intake aimed at preventing the adverse effects of MDMA. With appropriate treatment, full recovery is possible in almost all cases of this life-threatening condition.

Liver A 27-year-old man developed *jaundice without fever* (11[c]). He regularly used Ecstasy and had recently increased his consumption. All other possible causes of acute hepatitis were ruled out. After withdrawal of Ecstasy, the condition resolved completely.

Skin and appendages Two new cases of an interesting adverse effect, *facial papules*, have been reported (12[cR]).

A 20-year-old woman was referred for diarrhea and a pruritic yellowish skin 7 days after she had taken half a tablet of Ecstasy. Her liver was enlarged and tender. Her urine was positive for MDMA. A diagnosis of acute hepatotoxicity after MDMA was made. She rapidly developed reddish papules over the face with a perioral and acne-like distribution.

A 21-year-old man developed similar skin lesions after using Ecstasy, without hepatotoxicity.

Both patients responded to a low fat diet and 1% metronidazole ointment.

The authors suggested that serotonin indirectly affects the nerve endings of the eccrine glands via other peptides, and that the interaction of MDMA with serotonin may have caused the rapid development of pimples in these abusers.

Another unusual MDMA adverse effect, *tooth wear*, has been reported (13[cr]).

A healthy 17-year-old boy, who complained of dental sensitivity that occurred only when he consumed fizzy drinks, presented with marked tooth wear. All the teeth were involved, especially the premolars and permanent molars. He ate a poorly balanced diet, with 500 ml carbonated drinks twice daily. He subsequently admitted to frequent MDMA abuse.

Current health promotions advise that Ecstasy users should frequently consume 'sports' type or fruit drinks to counteract dehydration and avoid ion imbalances. These particular drinks may be erosive to the teeth. Bruxism and trismus associated with Ecstasy use may also contribute to tooth wear.

Interactions An MDMA-related psychiatric adverse effect may have been enhanced by an SSRI (14[c]).

A 52-year-old prisoner, who was taking the SSRI citalopram 60 mg/day, suddenly became aggressive, agitated, and grandiose after Ecstasy use. He carried out peculiar compulsive movements and had extreme motor restlessness, but no fever or rigidity. He was given chlordiazepoxide and 2 days later was asymptomatic. Citalopram was reintroduced and 2 days later he reported visual hallucinations of little bugs in the cell. Promazine was substituted for citalopram and his condition improved 2 days later.

The authors suggested that SSRIs such as citalopram may potentiate the neurochemical and behavioral effects of MDMA.

COCAINE

Cardiovascular In a retrospective study of 48 men who suffered cocaine-related deaths and a control group of 51 male cocaine users who died of lethal trauma, the blood cocaine concentrations measured in the two groups were similar (15[CR]). However, concentrations of the cocaine metabolite benzoylecgonine were higher in those with cocaine-related deaths. This group also had a significantly lower body mass index, with larger hearts and heavier lungs, livers, and spleens than the control subjects. Reduced body weight, an adverse effect of long-term cocaine use, is probably related to its effects on the serotonergic system. *Cardiomegaly* is thought to result from chronic cocaine-induced excessive catecholamine stimulation, with circulatory overload, and the increased organ weight is a result of passive visceral congestion in cocaine-induced heart failure. Cardiac alterations may explain why similar blood cocaine concentrations may be lethal in some cases but benign in others. This study shows that isolated measurements of post-mortem cocaine and benzoylecgonine blood concentrations cannot be used to assess or predict cocaine toxicity.

The increasing prevalence of multisubstance abuse may influence morbidity and mortality outcomes (16[cR]).

An 18-year-old man experienced sudden and severe chest pain while drinking ethanol. He vomited, collapsed, and died. On post-mortem examination, thrombosis of the left coronary artery, dilated cardiomyopathy with congestive heart failure, and pulmonary embolism were noted. Blood analysis showed raised cocaine and marijuana concentrations and a trace of alcohol.

The author's opinion was that although multidrug use played a role, the high blood concentration of cocaine had been the main cause of death. He also noted that marijuana may interact with cocaine to produce pronounced sympathomimetic effects.

The effects of intracoronary infusion of cocaine have been studied in dogs and humans (17[CR]). The procedure can be performed safely and does not alter coronary arterial blood flow. The effects of direct intracoronary infusion of cocaine on left ventricle systolic and diastolic performance have been studied in 20 patients referred for cardiac catheterization for evaluation of chest pain. They were given saline or cocaine hydrochloride (1 mg/minute) in 15-minute intracoronary infusions, and cardiac measurements were made during the final 2–3 minutes of each infusion. The blood cocaine concentration obtained from the coronary sinus was 3.0 mg/l, which is similar in magnitude to the blood cocaine concentration reported in abusers who die of cocaine intoxication. Minimal systemic effects were produced. The overall results were that cocaine caused measurable *deterioration of left ventricular systolic and diastolic performance*.

Respiratory Two new cases of *spontaneous pneumothorax* in intranasal cocaine users have been reported from Italy (18[cr]).

A 30-year-old man, a cocaine sniffer, who had used cocaine more than five times a month for 4 years, complained of shortness of breath and acute chest pain. He had episodic cough and bloody sputum. A chest X-ray showed an 80% pneumothorax on the left side. On thoracoscopy the entire lung visceral pleura seemed to be covered by fibrinous exudate. After yttrium aluminium garnet (YAG) laser pleurodesis surgery, which abrades the pleura, he made a full recovery within 4 days.

A 24-year-old man who had been inhaling cocaine nasally 4–5 times a month for a year developed respiratory distress and chest pain 2 days after the last use, because of a right sided pneumothorax. He underwent video-assisted thoracoscopic surgery with laser pleurodesis and responded rapidly.

In both cases, pneumothorax occurred with a delay after cocaine inhalation. The authors suggested that it was therefore unlikely that these cases of pneumothorax were due to direct traumatic effects of the drug powder inhaled, to barotrauma due to exaggerated inspiration, or to a Valsalva maneuver. Histological examination in both cases showed small foreign body granulomas with polarized material in the subpleural parenchyma. The authors proposed that the pleural damage could have been directly caused by a filler substance known as mannite (a fine white powder comprised of insoluble cellulose fibers).

Nervous system In a review of *ischemic stroke* in young American adults (aged 15–44 years) admitted to 46 regional hospitals between 1988 and 1991, illicit drug use was noted in 12% and was the probable cause of stroke in 4.7% (19[C]). Multidrug use was common among users: 73% used cocaine, 29% used heroin, and 14% used phencyclidine. Drug-associated stroke in these young adults appeared to be related to vascular mechanisms (such as large and small vessel occlusive disease) rather than to hypertension or to diabetes.

Regional cerebral blood flow was assessed using single photon emission computed tomography (SPECT) and tracer HMPAO in 10 cocaine abusers within 72 hours of last cocaine use and then after 21 days of abstinence (20[CR]). Compared with controls, recent cocaine abusers had significantly reduced cerebral blood flow in 11 of 14 brain regions, with the largest reductions in the frontal cortex and parietal cortex and greater cerebral blood flow in the brain stem. These perfusion defects appeared to be primarily due to combined abuse of alcohol and cocaine. Frontal but not parietal defects appeared to resolve partially during 21 days of abstinence.

Neuropsychological performance was examined in 355 incarcerated adult male felons who were classified by DSM-IV criteria into four subgroups: alcohol dependence or abuse (n = 101), cocaine dependence or abuse (n = 60), multisubstance dependence or abuse (n = 56), and no history of drug abuse (n = 138) (21[C]). The cocaine and control groups had similar neuropsychological test scores. However, both the multisubstance and alcohol groups performed significantly worse on nearly all measures. The multisubstance group had *worse short-term memory*, *long-term memory*, and *visual motor ability*. Correlations between neuropsychological performance and length of abstinence from drug use showed that after abstinence the alcohol group had the greatest improvement on tests. Although the cocaine group had the least amount of improvement with abstinence, their overall performance was not significantly different from controls.

Assessment of smooth pursuit eye movements is valuable in the study of neurophysiological effects of a variety of clinical and subclinical disorders. In 126 patients who met DSM-IIIR criteria for dependence on alcohol, cocaine, or heroin, or dual alcohol and cocaine use, there was a significant *reduction in tracking accuracy* in the heroin-dependent and the dually-dependent subjects relative to controls (22[C]). However, the eye movement dysfunction in the drug-dependent groups was no longer detectable when the effects of antisocial personality disorder were statistically removed. The magnitude of the dysfunction correlated significantly with several antisocial personality-related features, including an increased number of criminal charges, months of incarceration, increased problems associated with drug abuse, and lower intellectual functioning. The findings suggested that there may be an association between premorbid personality traits and eye movement impairment.

Gastrointestinal *Ischemia of the small bowel and colon* after the use of cocaine has been previously reported (SEDA-22). Another case of ischemic colitis has appeared (23[cr]).

A 38-year-old man presented with a 2-day history of severe abdominal pain and bloody stools after smoking cocaine 48 hours earlier. He had abdominal pain, guarding, rebound tenderness, and high-pitched, hypoactive bowel sounds. His white blood cell count was 31×10^9/l. Radiography showed thumb-printing in the transverse colon. Endoscopy showed friable edematous mucosa with submucosal hemorrhage and patches of yellowish fibrinous material. He recovered fully with intravenous nutrition and supportive measures after 30 days.

Sexual function *Priapism* has been associated with marijuana, ethanol, and cocaine (SEDA-19, 26, 27). A new case has been reported (24[cR]).

A 44-year-old black man developed priapism 2 hours after he overdosed on 30–40 trazodone tablets 50 mg and 10 Tylenol No. 3 (paracetamol plus codeine) tablets. Toxicology analysis was positive for cocaine and opiates. The priapism required detumescence twice, on initial presentation and then 6 hours later, and 8 hours after presentation he again developed painless priapism, which resolved spontaneously after 1.5 hours.

Trazodone-induced priapism may be mediated by α-adrenoceptor antagonism. While the mechanism for cocaine-induced priapism is unclear, it may result from vasospasm, venous pooling, and sludging of blood in the penis. The authors proposed that the two drugs may act in an additive or synergistic manner and pose a greater hazard than either alone.

Use in pregnancy Among women of child-bearing age, cocaine abuse continues to be a major problem. One of the serious medical conditions linked with cocaine use during pregnancy is *premature delivery*, with an incidence in cocaine users of 17–27%. In a recent study, the mechanism of the effect of cocaine on both spontaneous and agonist-induced contractility of pregnant human myometrium has been evaluated (25[CR]). Myometrium samples from 42 women who were undergoing cesarean section at term were examined after exposure to various pharmacological probes in combination with cocaine. The results suggested that cocaine augments the contractility of uterine tissue by both adrenergic and non-adrenergic mechanisms. Cocaine increased spontaneous myometrial contractility over threefold. Prazosin, an α-adrenoceptor antagonist, blocked this effect, but only for the first 35 minutes. Cocaine increased both the sensitivity and maximal tissue response to the α-adrenoceptor agonist methoxamine. The maximal response to oxytocin, but not sensitivity, was increased by cocaine; prazosin did not inhibit this effect.

Second-generation effects The influence of exposure to cocaine in utero on the developing human nervous system, although an area of intensive research, is not yet clearly understood (SEDA-22, 21).

Prenatal cocaine exposure has been associated with neurobehavioral effects in infancy, ranging from no effect to effects on arousal and state regulation, as well as on neurophysiological and neurological functions. A recent prospective controlled study in 154 cocaine-using pregnant mothers and suitable matched controls from a rural community produced neurobehavioral effects that supported those from previous controlled studies (26[C]). The mothers underwent drug testing and medical examination during each trimester. Their infants were assessed as near to 40 weeks after conception as possible using the Brazelton Neonatal Behavioral Assessment Scale (BNBAS). When controlled for the effects of marijuana, alcohol, and tobacco use, the use of cocaine in the third trimester was negatively related to state regulation, attention, and responsiveness among the exposed infants. Twice as many cocaine-exposed infants as controls failed to come to and maintain the quiet alert state required for orientation testing.

Among the adverse outcomes of prenatal cocaine exposure, *low birth weight* and *reduced length and head circumference* have been previously reported. In a new prospective study in New York City, 386 pairs of cocaine- and crack-using mothers and their infants and 130 matched control pairs were followed during the course of pregnancy and delivery (27[C]). The neonates were assessed by physical and neurological examination, the Brazelton Neonatal Behavioral Assessment Scale (BNBAS), and the Neonatal Stress Scale during the first 48 hours of life. The results corroborated the earlier findings of *reduced fetal growth* in cocaine-exposed infants. Significantly more (17%) of the drug group had a head circumference less than the tenth percentile compared with the controls (3%). The drug group performed less well on the BNBAS and had higher measures on the Neonatal Stress Scale. They had clinically significant neurological findings, such as *jitteriness*, *increased tone*, and *an exaggerated Moro reflex*. However, some of these findings may reflect a direct neurotoxic effect of cocaine, since testing was done during the first 48 hours of life. The authors observed that crack had a more adverse outcome than cocaine. They concluded that the most important predictor of neonatal outcome may be the frequency, quantity, and type of cocaine used.

It is unclear whether abnormalities in early infancy are associated with neurodevelopmental impairment at a later age. Several studies have suggested that the findings are limited to early childhood. The possible effects of prenatal cocaine exposure on later cognitive functioning and difficulties have been reported in three studies. In the first, 236 infants at 8 and 18 months of age were evaluated; 37 had heavy exposure to cocaine in utero, 30 had light exposure, and 169 had no exposure (28[CR]). Cognitive functioning was assessed with the Bayley Scales of Infant Development. Information processing was tested with an infant-controlled habituation procedure. At 8 months, cocaine-exposed infants and controls had no differences in cognitive functioning. Their abilities to process information indexed by habituation and response to novelty were comparable. However, at 18 months the infants with high cocaine exposure performed poorly on the Mental Development Index (MDI). The 18-month MDI covers a wider range of cognitive tasks requiring integrated learning, responsiveness to environmental cues, and memory than the 8-month MDI. These results suggest that the effects of cocaine are more likely to show up when more challenging measures are used. Infants raised in environments considered high-risk, with stressors and low support, scored lower at both 8 and 18 months.

In the second study, intellectual functioning at 6–9 years was studied in 88 cocaine-exposed children and 96 unexposed children in New York City (29[C]). The participants were interviewed and underwent medical and neurological examination and psychological assessment. Child intelligence was measured with the Wechsler Intelligence Scale for Children-III (WISC-III). Intelligence quotient scores did not differ between the two groups of children, even when adjustments for co-variables were made.

The third study examined the Robert Wood Johnson database of published literature on prenatal cocaine exposure and child outcome (30[C]). Only 8 of 101 studies focused on school-age children. Intelligence quotient (IQ), receptive language, and expressive language were measured. This meta-analysis showed an average difference of 3.12 IQ points between cocaine-exposed and control groups. When the IQ distribution is shifted by this reduction, there is a 1.6-fold increase in the number of children with IQs under 70. The authors noted that the calculated *decrement in IQ* in exposed children is subtle and does not include the possible drug effect on domains of function such as language abilities.

Research on the relation between prenatal cocaine exposure and childhood behavior also continues. In a pilot study, 27 children exposed to cocaine in utero and 75 control children were assessed (31[C]). The children had a mean age of 80 months and most were first-grade students. The child's first-grade teacher (blinded to exposure status and study design) rated the children's behavior with the Conners' Teacher Rating Sales (CTRS) and the Problem Behavior Scale (PROBS 14), an investigator-developed scale that measures behaviors associated with cocaine exposure. The drug-exposed children had higher CTRS scores (i.e. more problematic behavior), but the difference was not significant. On subscales of the PROBS 14, the drug-exposed group had significantly more problematic behavior. These results appear to substantiate teachers' reports of *problematic behavior* in children with prenatal cocaine exposure.

Whether prenatal cocaine exposure causes long-term adverse effects on the developing human nervous system will continue to be investigated. The author of one review suggested that future studies on older children will be needed to answer the question about long-term consequences of exposure to cocaine; study designs should also carefully attend to methodological issues, such as the quantification of cocaine exposure and its effects (32[R]).

Overdosage Another *death* has been reported in a cocaine body packer (33[cr]).

A 49-year-old man became ill during a plane flight. He admitted to having swallowed 102 latex packages of cocaine 5 g each and 20 tablets of activated charcoal 125 mg. After stabilization in an emergency room, he suffered a seizure. After restabilization he had not defecated and was given a laxative of a mineral oil liquid paraffin. During the next 24 hours his condition worsened. His serum cocaine concentration increased from 1.95 to 2.2 mg/l. During preparation for surgery he developed an untreatable dysrhythmia and died. Autopsy showed cocaine packages in the gut, 71 ruptured and 95 intact.

The reported lethal oral dose of cocaine is 1–3 g. In this case, paraffin may have contributed to rupture of the packages by dissolving the latex.

In another cocaine body packer, non-surgical management was followed by the development of a *giant gastric ulcer* (34[cR]).

A 35-year-old man presented to the emergency room 5 days after swallowing 35 latex-wrapped packages of cocaine. He was asymptomatic but concerned that only 10 of the 35 packets had passed in his stools. He was treated with laxatives and passed only 8 packages during the next 8 days. Radiography showed that 10–15 foreign bodies remained clustered in the stomach 14 days after ingestion. Several fragments of latex wrapping were found in his stools. On exploratory laparotomy, 15 latex packages were found impacted in the antrum just proximal to the pylorus. Beneath the packages there was a giant gastric ulcer, 2.5 cm in diameter. He had an uneventful postoperative course.

Interactions *Alcohol* Cocaine abuse has a high co-morbidity with alcohol abuse. In fact, one proposal is that concurrent alcohol abuse may be an integral part of cocaine abuse. Cocaine abusers have reported that alcohol prolongs the euphoriant properties of cocaine, while ameliorating the acutely unpleasant physical and psychological sequelae, primarily paranoia and agitation. It may also lessen the dysphoria associated with acute cocaine abstinence.

In a double-blind study, subjects meeting DSM-IV criteria for cocaine dependence and alcohol abuse participated in three drug administration sessions, involving intranasal cocaine with oral alcohol, cocaine with oral placebo-alcohol, and cocaine-placebo with oral alcohol (35[C]). The cocaine-alcohol combination produced greater euphoria and an increased perception of well-being compared with cocaine alone. Heart rate was significantly higher in the cocaine-alcohol group than with either drug alone. Cocaine concentrations were greater after cocaine-alcohol than after cocaine alone. Metabolism of cocaine to form cocaethylene was observed only during cocaine-alcohol administration. The authors concluded that enhanced psychological effects during cocaine-alcohol abuse may encourage the ingestion of larger amounts of these substances, placing users at increased risk of toxicity than with either drug alone.

Anticholinergic drugs The adverse effects of heroin that had been adulterated with an anticholinergic drug were reported in SEDA-21 (p. 34). Anticholinergic poisoning involving adulterated cocaine is less common (36[cR]).

A 39-year-old man who was a recreational alcohol and cocaine user presented with agitation, hallucinations, and delirium. Physical examination was remarkable for dry flushed skin, tachycardia, dilated minimally reactive pupils, urinary retention, and an absence of bowel sounds. He was treated with intravenous fluids and a sedative. There were cocaine metabolites in the urine. Reanalysis of a urine sample by thin layer chromatography confirmed the presence of the anticholinergic drug atropine.

Neuroleptic drugs Cocaine-abusing psychiatric patients significantly more often develop neuroleptic-induced acute dystonia according to a 2-year study carried out on the island of Curacao, Antilles, where cocaine and cannabis are often abused (37[C]). The sample consisted of 29 men with neuroleptic-induced acute dystonia aged 17–45 years who had received high potency neuroleptic drugs in the month before admission; nine were cocaine users and 20 non-users. Cocaine use was a major risk factor for neuroleptic-induced acute dystonia and should be added to the list of well-known risk factors such as male sex, younger age, neuroleptic dose and potency, and a history of neuroleptic-induced acute dystonia. The authors suggested that high-risk cocaine-using psychiatric patients who start to take neuroleptic drugs should be provided with an anticholinergic drug as a prophylactic measure to prevent neuroleptic-induced acute dystonia.

HEROIN

The main life-threatening complications of heroin intoxication include acute pulmonary edema and delayed respiratory depression with coma after successful naloxone treatment. A recent prospective study has reviewed the management of 160 heroin and heroin mixture intoxication cases treated in an emergency room in Switzerland between 1991 and 1992 (38[C]). There were no rehospitalizations after discharge from the emergency room and only one death outside the hospital due to pulmonary edema, which occurred between 2.25 and 8.25 hours after intoxication. A literature review found only two reported cases of delayed pulmonary edema, which occurred 4 and 6 hours after hospitalization. The authors recommended surveillance of a heroin user for at least 8 hours after successful opiate antagonist treatment.

MARIJUANA

A recent review has summarized the evidence related to the adverse effects of acute and chronic use of cannabis (39[R]). The effects of acute usage include *anxiety*, *impaired attention*, and *increased risk of psychotic symptoms*. Probable risks of chronic cannabis consumption include *bronchitis* and *subtle impairments of attention and memory*.

Psychiatric Reports of negative outcomes associated with marijuana use continue to appear. This is despite the fact that the drug has a reputation among some in society as being generally safe. Four cases in which *psychosis* developed after relatively small amounts of marijuana were smoked for the first time have been reported (40[c]). All four patients required hospitalization and neuroleptic drug treatment. Each had a mother with manic disorder and two had psychotic features. The authors noted that marijuana is a dopamine receptor agonist, and mania may be associated with excessive dopaminergic neurotransmission. The use of marijuana may precipitate psychosis or mania in subjects who are genetically vulnerable to major mental illness.

A second study has reported the possible relation between the degree of marijuana use and the risk of associated *psychiatric disorders*. Through random urine testing of draftees to the Italian army, 133 marijuana users were identified, tested, and interviewed (41[C]). Among these marijuana users, 83% of those with cannabis dependence, 46% with cannabis abuse, and 29% of occasional users had at least one DSM-IIIR psychiatric diagnosis. With greater cannabis use, the risk of associated psychiatric disabilities tended to increase progressively.

Marijuana abuse and its possible associated risks in reinforcing further use, causing dependence, and producing *withdrawal symptoms* among adolescents with conduct symptoms and substance use disorders has been investigated in 165 men and 64 women selected and then interviewed from a group of 255 consecutive admissions to a university-based adolescent substance abuse treatment program (42[C]). All had DSM-IIIR substance dependence, 82% had conduct disorder, 18% had major depression, and 15% had attention-deficit/hyperactivity disorder. Most (79%) met the criteria for cannabis dependence. Two-thirds of the cannabis-dependent individuals admitted serious drug-related problems and reported associated drug withdrawal symptoms according to the comprehensive addiction severity index in adolescents (CASI). For the majority, progression from first to regular cannabis use was as rapid as tobacco progression and more rapid than that of alcohol.

Immunological and hypersensitivity reactions The effects of marijuana on immune function have been extensively investigated over the last two decades, and the major findings have been reviewed (43[R]). These studies suggest that marijuana *affects immune cell function of T and B lymphocytes*, *natural killer cells*, and *macrophages*. In addition, cannabis appears to *modulate host resistance*, especially the secondary immune response to various infectious agents, both viral and bacterial. Lastly, marijuana may also *affect the cytokine network*, influencing the production and function of acute-phase and immune cytokines and modulating network cells, such as macrophages and T helper cells. Under some conditions, marijuana may be immunomodulatory and promote disease.

REFERENCES

1. Schuster P, Lieb R, Lamertz C, Wittchen H-U. Is the use of ecstasy and hallucinogens increasing? Results from a community study. Eur Addict Res 1998;4:75–82.
2. Byard RW, Gilbert J, James R, Lokan RJ. Amphetamine derivative fatalities in South Australia—is 'ecstasy' the culprit? Am J Forensic Med Pathol 1998;19:261–5.
3. James RA, Dinan A. Hyperpyrexia associated with fatal paramethoxyamphetamine (PMA) abuse. Med Sci Law 1998;38:83–5.
4. D'Costa DF. Transient myocardial ischaemia associated with accidental Ecstasy ingestion. Br J Cardiol 1998;5:290–1.
5. Brody S, Krause C, Veit R, Rau H. Cardiovascular autonomic dysregulation in users of MDMA ('Ecstasy'). Psychopharmacology Berl 1998;136:390–3.
6. Ahmed JM, Salame MY, Oakley GD. Chest pain in a young girl. Postgrad Med J 1998;74:115–16.
7. Vollenweider FX, Gamma A, Liechti M, Huber T. Psychological and cardiovascular effects and short-term sequelae of MDMA ('Ecstasy') in MDMA-naive healthy volunteers. Neuropsychopharmacology 1998;19:241–51.
8. McCann UD, Szabo Z, Scheffel U, Dannals RF, Ricaurte GA. Positron emission tomographic evidence of toxic effect of MDMA ('Ecstasy') on brain serotonin neurons in human beings. Lancet 1998;352:1433–7.
9. Windhaber J, Maierhofer D, Dantendorfer K. Panic disorder induced by large doses of 3,4-methylenedioxymethamphetamine resolved by paroxetine. J Clin Psychopharmacol 1998;18: 95–6.
10. Ajaelo I, Koenig K, Snoey E. Severe hyponatremia and inappropriate antidiuretic hormone secretion following ecstasy use. Acad Emerg Med 1998;5:839–40.
11. Roques V, Perney P, Beaufort P, Hanslik B, Ramos J, Durand L, Le Bricquir Y, Blanc F. Hepatite aiguë a l'ecstasy. Presse Med 1998;27:468–70.
12. Wollina U, Kammler HJ, Hesselbarth N, Mock B, Bosseckert H. Ecstasy pimples-a new facial dermatosis. Dermatology 1998;197:171–3.
13. Murray MC, Wilson NHF. Ecstasy related tooth wear. Br Dent J 1998;185:264.
14. Lauerma H, Wuorela M, Halme M. Interaction of serotonin reuptake inhibitor and 3,4-methylenedioxymethamphetamine? Biol Psychiatry 1998;43:929.
15. Karch SB, Stephens B, Ho CH. Relating cocaine blood concentrations to toxicity-an autopsy study of 99 cases. J Forensic Sci 1998;43:41–5.
16. Daisley H, Jones Le Cointe A, Hutchinson G, Simmons V. Fatal cardiac toxicity temporally related to poly-drug abuse. Vet Hum Toxicol 1998;40: 21–2.
17. Pitts WR, Vongpatanasin W, Cigarroa JE, Hillis LD, Lange RA. Effects of the intracoronary infusion of cocaine on left ventricular systolic and diastolic function in humans. Circulation 1998;97:1270–3.

18. Torre M, Barberis M. Spontaneous pneumothorax in cocaine sniffers. Am J Emerg Med 1998;16: 546–9.
19. Sloan MA, Kittner SJ, Feeser BR, Gardner J, Epstein A, Wozniak MA, Wityk RJ, Stern BJ, Price TR, Macko RF, Johnson CJ, Earley CJ, Buchholz D. Illicit drug-associated ischemic stroke in the Baltimore-Washington Young Stroke Study. Neurology 1998;50:1688–93.
20. Kosten TR, Cheeves C, Palumbo J, Seibyl JP, Price LH, Woods SW. Regional cerebral blood flow during acute and chronic abstinence from combined cocaine-alcohol abuse. Drug Alcohol Depend 1998;50: 187–95.
21. Selby MJ, Azrin RL. Neuropsychological functioning in drug abusers. Drug Alcohol Depend 1998;50:39–45.
22. Costa L, Bauer LO. Smooth pursuit eye movement dysfunction in substance-dependent patients: mediating effects of antisocial personality disorder. Neuropsychobiology 1998;37:117–23.
23. Simmers TA, Vidakovic VM, Van Meyel JJ. Cocaine-induced ischemic colitis. Endoscopy 1998; 30:S8–9.
24. Myrick H, Markowitz JS, Henderson S. Priapism following trazodone overdose with cocaine use. Ann Clin Psychiatry 1998;10:81–3.
25. Hurd WW, Betz AL, Dombrowski MP, Fomin VP. Cocaine augments contractility of the pregnant human uterus by both adrenergic and nonadrenergic mechanisms. Am J Obstet Gynecol 1998;178:1077–81.
26. Eyler FD, Behnke M, Conlon M, Woods NS, Wobie K. Birth outcome from a prospective, matched study of prenatal crack/cocaine use. II. Interactive and dose effects on neurobehavioral assessment. Pediatrics 1998;101:237–41.
27. Datta-Bhutada S, Johnson HL, Rosen TS. Intrauterine cocaine and crack exposure: neonatal outcome. J Perinatol 1998;18:183–8.
28. Alessandri SM, Bendersky M, Lewis M. Cognitive functioning in 8- to 18-month-old drug-exposed infants. Dev Psychol 1998;34:565–73.
29. Wasserman GA, Kline JK, Bateman DA, Chiriboga C, Lumey LH, Friedlander H. Prenatal cocaine exposure and school-age intelligence. Drug Alcohol Depend 1998;50:203–10.
30. Lester BM, LaGasse LL, Seifer R. Cocaine exposure and children: the meaning of subtle effects. Science 1998;282:633–4.
31. Delaney BV, Covington C, Templin T, Ager J, Martier S. Prenatal cocaine exposure and child behavior. Pediatrics 1998;102:945–50.
32. Chiriboga CA. Neurological correlates of fetal cocaine exposure. Ann NY Acad Sci 1998;846: 109–25.
33. Visser L, Stricker B, Hoogendoorn M, Vinks A. Do not give paraffin to packers. Lancet 1998;352:1352.
34. Miller JS, Hendren SK, Liscum KR. Giant gastric ulcer in a body packer. J Trauma Inj Infect Crit Care 1998;45:617–19.
35. McCance-Katz EF, Kosten TR, Jatlow P. Concurrent use of cocaine and alcohol is more potent and potentially more toxic than use of either alone-a multiple-dose study. Biol Psychiatry 1998;44: 250–9.
36. Weiner AL, Bayer MJ, McKay CA Jr, DeMeo M, Starr E. Anticholinergic poisoning with adulterated intranasal cocaine. Am J Emerg Med 1998;16: 517–20.
37. Van Harten PN, Van Trier JCAM, Horwitz EH, Matroos GE, Hoer HW. Cocaine as a risk factor for neuroleptic-induced acute dystonia. J Clin Psychiatry 1998;59:128–30.
38. Osterwalder JJ. Patients intoxicated with heroin or heroin mixtures: how long should they be monitored? Eur J Emerg Med 1995;2:97–101.
39. Hall W, Solowij N. Adverse effects of cannabis. Lancet 1998;352:1611–16.
40. Bowers MB Jr. Family history and psychotogenic response to marijuana. J Clin Psychiatry 1998;59:198–9.
41. Troisi A, Pasini A, Saracco M, Salletta G. Psychiatric symptoms in male cannabis users not using other illicit drugs. Addiction 1998;93:487–92.
42. Crowley TJ, Macdonald MJ, Whitmore EA, Mikulich SK. Cannabis dependence, withdrawal and reinforcing effects among adolescents with conduct symptoms and substance use disorders. Drug Alcohol Depend 1998;50:27–37.
43. Klein TW, Friedman H, Specter S. Marijuana, immunity and infection. J Neuroimmunol 1998;83:102–15.

S. Curran and S. Musa

5 Hypnotics and sedatives

Hypnotics and sedatives continue to be commonly prescribed drugs, and awareness of their adverse effects is becoming more widespread. It nevertheless remains important to ensure before prescribing these drugs that patients have had a thorough assessment to exclude treatable causes for insomnia, including psychiatric drugs (1[c]), alcohol (2[R]), and physical illness (3[C]). It is also important to try other simple measures to facilitate sleep, including reducing noise, improving the sleep environment, and avoiding large meals before bed. These simple measures (sleep hygiene) are often very effective, they are sustainable, and they are not associated with any adverse effects. Hypnotics and sedatives should only be used for relatively short periods of time, if at all (4[c]).

BENZODIAZEPINES

In a prospective study of 2765 elderly subjects, the relation between benzodiazepine use and cognitive function was evaluated. The authors concluded that current benzodiazepine use, especially in recommended or higher dosages, is associated with *worse memory* among community-dwelling elderly people (5[C]).

Patients often have memory deficits after taking benzodiazepines and alcohol. In a study of hippocampal presynaptic glutamate transmission in conjunction with memory deficits induced by benzodiazepines and ethanol, reductions in hippocampal glutamate transmission closely correlated with the extent of impairment of spatial memory performance. The results strongly suggested that presynaptic dysfunction in dorsal hippocampal glutamatergic neurons would be critical for spatial memory deficits induced by benzodiazepines and ethanol (6[c]).

Side Effects of Drugs, Annual 23
J.K. Aronson, ed.

Alprazolam

Interactions Potential pharmacokinetic effects of *venlafaxine* on alprazolam have been investigated in 16 healthy volunteers. Steady-state venlafaxine 75 mg bd did not inhibit the CYP3A4 metabolism of a single dose of alprazolam 2 mg (7[c]).

Clobazam

Interactions Clobazam intoxication with *negative myoclonus* occurred 4 weeks after clobazam had been added to a stable regimen of carbamazepine and topiramate. Blood concentrations of both carbamazepine and carbamazepine epoxide were raised, and the symptoms resolved quickly when carbamazepine dosage was reduced and clobazam discontinued (8[c]).

Clonazepam

Psychiatric The addition of clonazepam to clomipramine has been reported to have caused acute *mania* (9[c]).

A 48-year-old Japanese man with a history of bipolar affective disorder, with a previous history of both depression and mania, became depressed again. He was already taking lithium carbonate 800 mg/day and carbamazepine 800 mg/day. Clomipramine was added, and the dose was increased to 225 mg/day over 2 months and then maintained for 2 months. Because clomipramine had little effect, clonazepam (3 mg/day) was added. On the first day after he took clonazepam, symptoms of hyperthymia, haughtiness, talkativeness, and flight of ideas suddenly appeared once more. Drug-induced delirium was excluded, because orientation was not disrupted and the symptoms did not fluctuate over time. Clomipramine and clonazepam were withdrawn. Because the symptoms were similar to the previous manic episode, the same prescription was reinstated, with the addition of sodium valproate 800 mg/day. After 3 months, he was discharged in remission and had no recurrence. He had not taken other benzodiazepines throughout the treatment.

This report suggests that clomipramine alone did not induce the switch to mania, and either clonazepam alone or the interaction of clomipramine and clonazepam caused maniacal change.

Diazepam

Adverse effects related with rectal diazepam are rare and mild. Animal studies and clinical experience have not shown damage to the rectal mucosa. *Respiratory difficulties* are the major potential adverse effect (10[R]).

Oxazepam

Nervous system In a study of the effects of oxazepam on implicit vs explicit memory processes, as a function of time course the effects of oxazepam (30 mg) or placebo on directly comparable tests of implicit memory and explicit memory were examined at three times in 60 healthy volunteers. Before the plasma concentration had peaked, oxazepam impaired cued recall performance relative to placebo but did not impair priming. At the time of the peak, oxazepam impaired performance in both memory tasks. After the peak, cued recall performance in the oxazepam group remained significantly impaired relative to placebo. However, oxazepam-induced impairments in priming were only marginal, suggesting that oxazepam-induced impairments in implicit memory processes begin to wane after theoretical peak drug concentrations. The results support the hypothesis that benzodiazepines cause *impaired implicit memory processes* time-dependently (11[c]).

In 30 subjects who were given an acute dose of oxazepam 30 mg, lorazepam 2 mg, or placebo, both drugs impaired explicit memory relative to placebo. Also, both oxazepam and lorazepam impaired priming performance. The results suggested that episodic memory is time-dependently impaired by both benzodiazepines (12[c]).

Temazepam

Nervous system The effects of oral temazepam 5, 10, and 30 mg on memory were studied in healthy volunteers subjected to a battery of cognitive tests and analogue mood ratings (13[c]). The lowest dose had no effect and 10 mg significantly increased only self-ratings of well-being. Temazepam 30 mg significantly improved recall of items learned before drug administration, but *impaired recall and recognition of word lists* acquired after drug administration. There was no impairment of retrieval, suggesting that automatic information processing was unaffected. Temazepam 30 mg significantly reduced self-ratings of anxiety and *increased self-ratings of sedation.* It also significantly *impaired performance in symbol copying, digit-symbol substitution, and number cancellation tasks.* It is striking that, at a dose that was sedative and impaired many aspects of performance, temazepam nevertheless improved retrieval of items learned before drug administration.

Triazolam

Nervous system The effect of triazolam on muscarinic acetylcholine receptor binding has been investigated in living brain slices by the use of a novel positron-based imaging technique (14). Stimulation of GABA/BZ receptors lowered the affinity of the muscarinic acetylcholine cholinergic receptor for its ligand, which may underlie benzodiazepine-induced *amnesia,* a serious clinical adverse effect of benzodiazepines.

Interactions In a randomized, double-blind, pharmacokinetic-pharmacodynamic study, 12 volunteers took placebo or triazolam 0.125 mg orally, together with placebo, azithromycin, erythromycin, or clarithromycin. The apparent oral clearance of triazolam was significantly reduced by *erythromycin* and *clarithromycin.* The peak plasma concentration was correspondingly increased, and the half-life was prolonged. The effects of triazolam on dynamic measures were nearly identical when triazolam was given with placebo or azithromycin, but benzodiazepine agonist effects were enhanced by erythromycin and clarithromycin (15[c]).

OTHER HYPNOTICS/ ANXIOLYTICS

Buspirone

Nervous system The efficacy and safety of buspirone have been evaluated in the management of anxiety and irritability in 22 children with pervasive developmental disorders. One child developed *abnormal involuntary movements* of the mouth, cheeks, and tongue after having taken buspirone 20 mg/day for 10 months. No other drugs were prescribed. The abnormal movements disappeared completely within 2 weeks of withdrawal of buspirone. Other adverse effects in other children were minimal and included initial sedation, slight agitation, and initial nausea (16[c]).

Interactions *Calcium antagonists* In a randomized placebo-controlled trial, the possible interactions of buspirone with verapamil and diltiazem were investigated. Both verapamil and diltiazem considerably increased plasma buspirone concentrations, probably by inhibiting its CYP3A4-mediated first-pass metabolism. Thus, enhanced effects and adverse effects of buspirone are possible when it is used with verapamil, diltiazem, or other inhibitors of CYP3A4 (17[c]).

Fluvoxamine The effects of fluvoxamine on the pharmacokinetics and pharmacodynamics of buspirone have been investigated in 10 healthy volunteers. Fluvoxamine moderately increased plasma buspirone concentrations and reduced the production of the active metabolite of buspirone. The mechanism of this interaction is probably inhibition of the CYP3A4-mediated first-pass metabolism of buspirone by fluvoxamine. However, this pharmacokinetic interaction was not associated with impaired psychomotor performance and is probably of limited clinical significance (18[c]).

Grapefruit juice In a randomized, two-phase cross-over study, the effects of grapefruit juice on the pharmacokinetics and pharmacodynamics of oral buspirone were investigated in 10 healthy volunteers. Grapefruit juice considerably increased the mean peak plasma concentration of buspirone 4.3-fold. Large amounts of grapefruit juice should be avoided in patients taking buspirone (19[c]).

Rifampicin The effects of rifampicin on the pharmacokinetics and pharmacodynamics of buspirone were investigated in 10 young healthy volunteers. There was a significant reduction in the effects of buspirone in three of the six psychomotor tests used after rifampicin pretreatment. The strong interaction between rifampicin and buspirone is probably mostly due to enhanced CYP3A4-mediated first-pass metabolism of buspirone. Buspirone will most likely have a greatly reduced anxiolytic effect when it is used together with rifampicin or other potent inducers of CYP3A4, such as phenytoin and carbamazepine (20[c]).

Chloral hydrate

Gastrointestinal A 78-year-old woman and a 45-year-old man developed *pneumatosis cystoides coli.* Both were taking chloral hydrate. It was speculated that chloral hydrate had caused the abdominal symptoms in these two patients (21[c]).

Zolpidem

Subjective responses to treatment with zolpidem were assessed in 16 944 out-patients with insomnia. *Nausea, dizziness, malaise, nightmares, agitation*, and *headache* were the most common adverse events reported. There was one serious adverse reaction in a 48-year-old woman, who developed *paranoid symptoms* during the documentation phase. There were no life-threatening adverse events (22[C]).

Interactions *Antifungal imidazoles* Potential interactions of zolpidem with three commonly-prescribed azole derivatives (ketoconazole, itraconazole, and fluconazole) have been evaluated in a controlled clinical study. Co-administration of zolpidem with ketoconazole impaired zolpidem clearance and enhanced its benzodiazepine-like agonist pharmacodynamic effects. Itraconazole and fluconazole had a small effect on zolpidem kinetics and dynamics. The findings were consistent with in vitro studies of differentially impaired zolpidem metabolism by azole derivatives (23[c]).

Fluoxetine The possible pharmacokinetic and pharmacodynamic interactions of repeated nightly zolpidem dosing with fluoxetine were evaluated in 29 healthy women. There were no clinically significant pharmacokinetic or pharmacodynamic interactions (24[c]).

REFERENCES

1. O'Keeffe ST, Lavan JN. Clinical significance of delirium subtypes in older people. Age Ageing 1999;28:115–19.
2. Curran S, Wattis JP. Alcohol abuse in older people. Geriatr Med 1996;26:45–6.
3. Koenig HG, George LK, Peterson BL, Pieper CF. Depression in medically ill hospitalised older adults: prevalence, characteristics and course of symptoms according to six diagnostic schemes. Am J Psychiatry 1997;154:1376–83.
4. Curran S. Use of sedative hypnotics in elderly psychiatric patients. Eur Neuropsychopharmacol 1997;7(Suppl 2):231.
5. Hanlon JT, Horner RD, Schmader KE, Fillenbaum GG, Lewis IK, Wall WE, Landerman LR, Pieper CF, Blazer DG, Cohen HJ. Benzodiazepine use and cognitive function among community-dwelling elderly. Clin Pharmacol Ther 1998;64:684–92.
6. Shimizu K, Matsubara K, Uezono T, Kimura K, Shiono H. Reduced dorsal hippocampal glutamate release significantly correlates with the spatial memory deficits produced by benzodiazepines and ethanol. Neuroscience 1998;83:701–6.
7. Amchin J, Zarycranski W, Taylor KP, Albano D, Klockowski PM. Effect of venlafaxine on the pharmacokinetics of alprazolam. Psychopharmacol Bull 1998;34:211–19.
8. Genton P, Nguyen VH, Mesdjian E. Carbamazepine intoxication with negative myoclonus after the addition of clobazam. Epilepsia 1998;39:115–18.
9. Ikeda M, Fujikawa T, Yanani I, Horiguchi J, Yamawaki S. Clonazepam-induced maniacal reaction in a patient with bipolar disorder. Int Clin Psychopharmacol 1998;13:189–90.
10. Dooley JM. Rectal use of benzodiazepines. Epilepsia 1998;39(Suppl 1):S24–7.
11. Buffett-Jerrott SE, Stewart SH, Bird S, Teehan, MD. An examination of differences in the time course of oxazepam's effects on implicit vs explicit memory. J Psychopharmacol 1998;12:338–47.
12. Buffett-Jerrott SE, Stewart SH, Teehan MD. A further examination of the time-dependent effects of oxazepam and lorazepam on implicit and explicit memory. Psychopharmacology 1998;138:344–53.
13. File SE, Joyce EM, Fluck E, De Bruin E, Bazari F, Nandha H, Fitton L, Adhiya S. Limited memory impairment after temazepam. Hum Psychopharmacol 1998;13:127–33.
14. Murata T, Matsumura K, Sihver S, Onoe H, Bergstrom M, Sihver W, Yonekura Y, Langstrom B, Watanabe Y. Triazolam-induced modulation of muscarinic acetylcholine receptor in living brain slices as revealed by a new positron-based imaging technique. J Neural Transm 1998;105:1117–27.
15. Greenblatt DJ, Von Moltke LL, Harmatz JS, Counihan M, Graf JA, Durol ALB, Mertzanis P, Duan SX, Wright CE, Shader RI. Inhibition of triazolam clearance by macrolide antimicrobial agents: in vitro correlates and dynamic consequences. Clin Pharmacol Ther 1998;64:278–85.
16. Buitelaar JK, Van de Gaag RJ, Van der Hoeven J. Buspirone in the management of anxiety and irritability in children with pervasive development disorders: results of an open-label study. J Clin Psychiatry 1998;59:56–9.
17. Lamberg TS, Kivisto KT, Neuvonen PJ. Effects of verapamil and diltiazem on the pharmacokinetics and pharmacodynamics of buspirone. Clin Pharmacol Ther 1998;63:640–5.
18. Lamberg TS, Kivisto KT, Laitila J, Martensson K, Neuvonen PJ. The effect of fluvoxamine on the pharmacokinetics and pharmacodynamics of buspirone. Eur J Clin Pharmacol 1998;54:761–6.
19. Lilja JJ, Kivisto KT, Backman JT, Lamberg TS, Neuvonen PJ. Grapefruit juice substantially increases plasma concentrations of buspirone. Clin Pharmacol Ther 1998;64:655–60.
20. Lamberg TS, Kivisto KT, Neuvonnen PJ. Concentrations and effects of buspirone are considerably reduced by rifampicin. Br J Clin Pharmacol 1998;45:381–5.
21. Marigold JH. Pneumatosis cystoides coli and chloral hydrate. Gut 1998;42:899–900.
22. Hajak G, Bandelow B. Safety and tolerance of zolpidem in the treatment of disturbed sleep: a post-marketing surveillance of 16,944 cases. Int Clin Psychopharmacol 1998;13:157–67.
23. Greenblatt DJ, Von Moltke LL, Harmatz JS, Mertzanis P, Graf JA, Durol ALB, Counihan M, Roth-Schechter B, Shader RI. Kinetic and dynamic interaction study of zolpidem with ketoconazole, itraconazole and fluconazole. Clin Pharmacol Ther 1998;64:661–71.
24. Allard S, Sainati S, Roth-Schechter B, Macintyre J. Minimal interaction between fluoxetine and multiple-dose zolpidem in healthy women. Drug Metab Disp 1998;26:617–22.

Alfonso Carvajal and Luis H. Martín Arias

6 Antipsychotic drugs

GENERAL

A project group at the Swedish Council on Technology Assessment in Health Care has recently analyzed more than 2000 published manuscripts on neuroleptic drugs (1[R]). The analysis concluded that neuroleptic drug therapy is often accompanied by serious, sometimes permanent, adverse effects. Hence, neuroleptic drugs should be reserved for patients with severe psychosis. Agitated and demented elderly patients should not be treated with neuroleptic drugs, unless they have pronounced psychotic symptoms. Nor should neuroleptic drugs be used in young, mentally retarded patients and other children and adolescents, except in those with severe autism, Tourette's syndrome, or schizophrenia. In fact, in schizophrenic patients there is an increased mortality and the involvement of antipsychotic drug treatment has been investigated (2[R]).

Severe adverse events associated with antipsychotic drug treatment are *epileptic seizures, QT prolongation, myocarditis* associated with clozapine, *neuroleptic malignant syndrome, hypothermia, respiratory arrest*, and *pulmonary embolism* associated with clozapine. To minimize these potential risks, practical prescribing guidelines have recently been proposed (SEDA-21, 42); they recommend careful titration of therapy, checking for a history of cardiac disorders, seizures, neuroleptic malignant syndrome, and hypotension, and regular monitoring for known adverse effects.

Further comparisons of the main features of conventional and atypical antipsychotic drugs have emerged (SEDA-22, 45; 3[R]–5[R]). The review by the Collaborative Working Group on Clinical Trial Evaluations has addressed adverse effects extensively (4[R]). The authors stressed that atypical antipsychotic drugs cause fewer extrapyramidal signs and may have a lower risk of causing tardive dyskinesia than the conventional antipsychotic drugs. The adverse effects of the atypical drugs that one should be aware of are the following (listed with the drug(s) most likely to cause them):

- *seizures* (clozapine);
- *orthostatic hypotension* (clozapine, olanzapine, quetiapine);
- *anticholinergic effects* (clozapine, olanzapine);
- *weight gain* (clozapine, olanzapine);
- *increased prolactin* (risperidone);
- *hepatic changes*(clozapine, risperidone);
- *agranulocytosis*(clozapine).

Drug interactions can be dangerous or fatal and should be avoided. Patients' individual concerns and health needs must be taken into account when selecting a drug. The atypical drugs, it is said, would be better first-line drugs for patients with specific health concerns.

The Collaborative Working Group has also drawn attention to the interpretation of certain results from clinical trials with novel antipsychotic drugs (4[R]). It has been stated, for instance, that when extrapyramidal signs are not significantly different from those with placebo, it does not necessarily mean that new antipsychotic drugs absolutely lack extrapyramidal effects. Patients who enter studies of the new antipsychotic drugs may have been previously treated with traditional neuroleptic drugs, and extrapyramidal symptoms may have persisted from this prior drug treatment.

An interesting comparison of patients' and prescribers' beliefs about the adverse effects of neuroleptic drugs has been carried out (6[C]). Psychiatrists' estimates of prevalence, but not of distress, correlated significantly with patients' reports. The authors concluded that the apparent lack of understanding of which adverse effects are most likely to cause distress to patients may adversely affect the therapeutic alliance between prescribers and patients.

Side Effects of Drugs, Annual 23
J.K. Aronson, ed.

Compliant patients have a higher incidence of adverse effects (7[C]). Logistic regression analysis identified four factors to discriminate compliant (n = 48) from non-compliant (n = 30) patients: the course of the illness, employment status of a key relative, age at the onset of the illness, and the presence or absence of adverse effects.

Cardiovascular *Conduction disturbances* are becoming a focus of increased interest (SED-13, 119; SEDA-21, 43; SEDA-22, 45). In a case-control study, haloperidol-induced QT_c prolongation was associated with *torsade de pointes* (8[C]). The odds ratio of developing *torsade de pointes* in a patient with QT_c prolongation to over 550 ms compared with those with QT_c intervals shorter than 550 ms was 33 (95% CI = 6–195). The sample was all critically ill adult patients in medical, cardiac, and surgical intensive care units at a tertiary hospital who received intravenous haloperidol and had no metabolic, pharmacological, or neurological risk factors known to cause *torsade de pointes* or if the dysrhythmia developed more than 24 hours after intravenous haloperidol. Of 223 patients who fulfilled the inclusion criteria, eight developed tardive dyskinesia. A group of 41 patients, randomly selected from the 215 without tardive dyskinesia, served as controls. The length of hospital stay after the development of haloperidol-associated tardive dyskinesia was significantly longer than that after the maximum dose of intravenous haloperidol in the control group. The overall incidence of *torsade de pointes* was 3.6 and 11% in patients who received intravenous haloperidol 35 mg or more over 24 hours.

A new case of neuroleptic drug-induced *torsade de pointes* has been published (9[c]).

A 59-year-old woman with no history of cardiac problems, except for hypertension, who was taking amlodipine 5 mg qds, cyclobenzaprine 10 mg qds, and co-triamterzide 37.5 + 25 mg qds, and who had a QT_c interval of 497 ms, was given intravenous droperidol 0.625 mg and metoclopramide 10 mg 45 minutes before surgery. About 1.75 hours after surgery she developed a polymorphic ventricular tachycardia with findings consistent with *torsade de pointes*, which resolved with defibrillation.

From time to time, cases of *sudden death* are reported (SEDA-20, 36; SEDA-22, 46), including a new case associated with thioridazine (10[c]).

A 68-year-old man with a 5-year history of Alzheimer's disease, was treated with thioridazine 25 mg tds because of violent outbursts. His other drugs, temazepam 10–30 mg at night, carbamazepine 100 mg bd for neuropathic pain, and droperidol 5–10 mg as required, were unaltered. Five days later, he was found dead, having been in his usual condition 2 hours before. Post-mortem examination showed stenosis of the coronary arteries, but no coronary thrombosis, myocardial infarction, or other significant pathology. The certified cause of death was cardiac dysrhythmia due to ischemic heart disease. Thioridazine was considered as a possible contributing factor.

QT_c prolongation has been proposed as a predictor of sudden death, and psychiatrists are encouraged to perform electrocardiograms in patients taking high-dose antipsychotic drugs to detect conduction abnormalities, especially QT_c prolongation. It has now been suggested that QT_c prolongation in itself is not necessarily an indicator of the risk of sudden death (11[r]). Instead, QT_c dispersion, the difference between the longest and the shortest QT_c interval on the 12-lead electrocardiogram, is an indication of more extreme variability in ventricular repolarization, which could be regarded as a better predictor of the risk of dysrhythmias.

Hypotension occurs with antipsychotic drugs (SEDA-22, 45). Significantly more low blood pressures were documented by 24-hour ambulatory blood pressure monitoring compared with conventional blood pressure measurement obtained an average of 3.6 times a day in patients treated with psychotropic drugs (n = 12), most of which were neuroleptic drugs (12[Cr]). This finding may be of clinical relevance, in view of the potential hemodynamic consequences of hypotension, especially in older patients taking more than one psychotropic drug.

Nervous system Different degrees of *frontal atrophy* have been observed in 31 psychotic patients who had taken neuroleptic drugs for 5 years (13[C]). All underwent computed tomography when they were drug-naive and 5 years later. Logistic regression analysis identified neuroleptic drug as having a significant impact on the development of frontal atrophy, and the estimated risk of atrophy increased by 6.4% for each additional 10 mg of chlorpromazine equivalents.

Although neuroleptic drugs are relatively effective in treating psychiatric symptoms, their mental adverse effects can impair the quality of life of some individuals. In 44 stable schizophrenic outpatients a significant proportion of the variance was explained by a combination of protracted duration of illness and dysphoric subjective responses to neuroleptic drugs (14[C]). In terms of the individual items on the Negative Subjective Response subscale, only the statement 'I feel weird, like a zombie on medication' was associated with statistically significant differences in quality of life. Patients who agreed with this statement ($n = 10$) had a significantly poorer quality of life than those who disagreed ($n = 34$). Related to this possible impairment of the quality of life is the observation, in 45 patients with chronic schizophrenia, that antipsychotic drugs played a role in the development of depressive symptoms and negative symptoms (15[C]). Duration of treatment correlated positively with the depressive and the negative symptoms.

Notwithstanding this finding, the differentiation between disease-related and neuroleptic drug-induced negative symptoms, such as *flat affect*, can be especially difficult in some patients. To investigate the interactions among psychomotor performance, negative symptoms, and neuroleptic drug effects, dopamine D_2 receptor availability (measured by the binding of ^{123}I-iodobenzamide) psychopathology, and psychomotor reaction time have been assessed in eight drug-free and eight neuroleptic drug-treated schizophrenic patients (16[C]). Negative symptoms increased in the patients taking neuroleptic drugs compared with drug-free patients and correlated positively with neuroleptic blockade of dopamine D_2/D_3 receptors. Furthermore, parkinsonism correlated with a flat affect and psychomotor retardation. There were some limitations to this observational study: the sample size was small; different neuroleptic drugs were used, including risperidone (in seven patients), which may not behave in the same way as other neuroleptic drugs, owing to its antagonistic effect on $5HT_2$ receptors, although it has been observed that dopamine D_2 receptor occupancy and extrapyramidal adverse effects with risperidone do not differ significantly from those observed with traditional neuroleptic drugs; and the duration of disease was longer in the patients who took neuroleptic drugs.

Extrapyramidal signs The antipsychotic drugs that elicit parkinsonism are those that bind with higher affinity than dopamine to D_2 receptors, while those that cause little or no parkinsonism (melperone, seroquel, clozapine) bind with lower affinity (17[R]).

Information on neurological adverse effects in particular groups of patients, such as young patients (18[C]) and those with Alzheimer's disease (19[C], 20[C]), AIDS (21[c]), or Gilles de la Tourette syndrome (22[c]), have been recently published. The use of neuroleptic drugs in patients with Alzheimer's disease is controversial because of the significant adverse effects profile associated with these drugs. Therefore, other pharmacological and psychological methods should be explored before using neuroleptic drugs in dementia. This was the conclusion of a retrospective study in which 80 patients, 40 with confirmed Alzheimer's disease and 40 with confirmed Lewy body dementia, were assessed for neuroleptic drug use and adverse effects (19[C]). Neuroleptic drugs were used in 15 of the patients with Alzheimer's disease and 21 of those with Lewy body dementia. Only six of the latter (29%) had a definite severe sensitivity reaction to neuroleptic drugs, which included cognitive impairment, parkinsonism, drowsiness, and features of the neuroleptic malignant syndrome. All the reactions occurred within 2 weeks of new neuroleptic drug prescription or a dosage change and were associated with a reduction in survival. Certain motor disturbances, measured before neuroleptic drug treatment was begun, could be used to predict the development and severity of neuroleptic drug-induced parkinsonism in patients with Alzheimer's disease treated with very low-dose neuroleptic drugs (20[C]). Parkinsonism occurred in 67% of the patients with Alzheimer's disease. Pretreatment instrumental, but not clinical, measurement of bradykinesia was a predictor of post-treatment parkinsonism.

Young schizophrenics treated with neuroleptic drugs seemed to be similarly at particular risk of extrapyramidal adverse effects (18[C]). Of 34 schizophrenic children and adolescents followed after a drug-free period that lasted up to 4 weeks at 2-year intervals, 17 had either withdrawal dyskinesia or tardive dyskinesia at some time. Patients who developed the condition had greater premorbid impairment and a greater severity of positive symptoms at baseline, and there was a trend toward more months of neuroleptic drug exposure.

Patients with AIDS are sensitive to the extrapyramidal adverse effects of neuroleptic drugs and have evidence of depletion of dopamine in the cerebrospinal fluid (SEDA-22, 52). Of 115 consecutive HIV-infected patients, six developed parkinsonism and three of the cases were precipitated by the use of neuroleptic drugs (21[c]).

Since the gamut of the clinical pharmacology of tics is broad, it is often difficult to differentiate tics from other hyperkinetic movement disorders. Of 373 cases of Giles de la Tourette syndrome, 18 had both tics and other abnormal movements; 12 were secondary to neuroleptic drug treatment (22[c]). Akathisia was the most common movement disorder.

Tremor In 15 schizophrenic in-patients aged 16–55 years, there was a 50% probability that a patient would have a tremor when the plasma concentration of chlorpromazine was 46 ng/ml or more, corresponding to the minimum that has been associated with a good clinical response (23[C]). The use of objective accelerometric recordings was said to improve the accuracy of diagnosis of neuroleptic drug-induced tremor. This conclusion was reached in a study in which repeated accelerometric recordings showed constant and regular waveforms and frequencies (4–7 Hz) in each of 14 patients treated with neuroleptic drugs and diagnosed as having neuroleptic drug-induced tremor (24[c]).

Akathisia Patients with akathisia have a subjective feeling of restless agitation, which may cause several diverse behavior patterns (SED-13, 121). It has been associated with strong effects of terror, anger, and extreme anxiety, the most serious complication being a feeling of helplessness or being out of control, which might lead to suicidal ideation or attempted suicide. Five reported cases of neuroleptic drug-induced akathisia and suicidal tendencies in psychotic patients have further emphasized these risks (25[cr]). Doctors ought to pay attention to these symptoms, as suicidal tendencies disappear when symptoms of akathisia are relieved. Patients should also be told that akathisia is a treatable adverse effect of neuroleptic drugs.

A patient whose severe akathisia was abolished by passive motion when travelling as a car passenger has been described (26[c])

A 48-year-old woman developed akathisia soon after having been treated with chlorpromazine 400 mg for a bipolar affective disorder. Although the medication was changed a number of times over the next 4 years, there was no improvement. Fluvoxamine 150 mg and fluoxetine 20 mg seemed to aggravate the movement disorder; neither orphenadrine 200 mg nor procyclidine 15 mg affected her akathisia; nor did she experience relief from propranolol up to 320 mg. Both the subjective feeling of a need to move and the fidgeting in her legs were abolished within seconds of the car's beginning to move. Other movements (e.g. rocking in a chair or using an exercise bike) were ineffective, as were relaxation techniques and hypnosis.

Since this case emphasizes the importance of sensory input in akathisia, the authors suggested that the recurrent pacing observed in akathisia may be an attempt to alleviate the condition through sensory stimulation, rather than through motor activity.

Dyskinesia Discussion about tardive dyskinesia is necessary in the process of obtaining informed consent to treatment with neuroleptic drugs (SEDA-15, 46; SEDA-21, 42, 45). The effect of education about tardive dyskinesia has been evaluated in 56 patients taking maintenance antipsychotic drugs, who completed a questionnaire assessing their knowledge of the condition (27[C]). Education made patients more knowledgeable at 6 months, but had no effect on the clinical outcome.

The hypothesis of oxidative damage to striatal neurons mediated by neuroleptic drug enhancement of glutamatergic neurotransmission has been tested in a case-control study (28[C]). Several markers of excitatory neurotransmission (*N*-acetylaspartylglutamate, *N*-acetylaspartate, aspartate, and glutamate) and of oxidative damage (superoxide dismutase, protein carbonyl content, and lipid hydroperoxides) were measured in the CSF of patients with schizophrenia who had taken neuroleptic drugs chronically, and who had (n = 11) or had not (n = 9) developed tardive dyskinesia. There was an inverse correlation between CSF concentrations of aspartate and superoxide dismutase activity in tardive dyskinesia, which suggests a causative relation between enhanced excitatory amino acid neurotransmission and the oxidative damage associated with tardive dyskinesia. Another plausible model for the development of tardive dyskinesia is that lower activity of superoxide dismutase renders the striatal neurons more vulnerable to excitatory neurotransmission that is exacerbated by neuroleptic drugs, as shown in a subgroup of patients with schizophrenia.

There are conflicting results on the possible relation between plasma iron concentrations and movement disorders (SEDA-19, 45). A significant correlation between serum ferritin concentrations and the severity of choreoathetoid movements has been recently observed (29[C]). All 30 subjects had a minimum lifetime cumulative exposure to 'classical' antipsychotic drugs of 3 years. Nevertheless, and as was stated by the authors, it is unclear whether higher body iron stores exacerbate the symptoms of tardive dyskinesia or predispose to its development.

Intermittent neuroleptic drug treatment, chronic hospitalization, and aging increase the risk of tardive dyskinesia. In a retrospective study in a psychiatric hospital in Curaçao, Netherlands Antilles 133 Afro-Caribbean in-patients (mean age, 52 years), with no organic disorders and a history of current use of neuroleptic drugs for at least 3 months, were assessed for tardive dyskinesia (30[C]). The prevalence was 36%. When the number of interruptions to neuroleptic drug therapy was split into up to two and more than two, the resulting adjusted odds ratio was 3.29 (95% CI = 1.27–8.49). Thus, the number of interruptions turned out to be the second risk factor after age. Cumulative dosages of neuroleptic or anticholinergic drugs were not risk factors.

Chronically hospitalized elderly in-patients with schizophrenia (n = 121; mean age 74 years) were rated for tardive dyskinesia and cognition (31[C]). Subjects with tardive dyskinesia (60%) were older than those without. In subjects who were taking typical neuroleptic drugs (n = 119) there was no difference in dosage between those with and without tardive dyskinesia. Cognitive scores (Mini-Mental Status Examination) were significantly lower in the subjects with tardive dyskinesia affecting the orofacial regions. This raises the question of whether neuroleptic drug-induced brain changes underlie both the dyskinesia and cognitive impairment or whether the cognitive impairment represents a degenerative process that is itself a vulnerability factor for the emergence of tardive dyskinesia.

A group of 261 neuroleptic drug-naive patients aged 55 years or over (mean 77) were identified at the time they were starting to take antipsychotic drugs (32[C]). The length of follow-up was 3–393 (mean 115) weeks; 60 developed dyskinesia. The cumulative incidences were 25, 34, and 53% after 1, 2, and 3 years respectively of cumulative antipsychotic drug treatment. A greater risk of tardive dyskinesia was associated with a history of electroconvulsive therapy (ECT), higher mean daily and cumulative antipsychotic doses, and the presence of extrapyramidal signs early in treatment. Although age was not a significant predictor of tardive dyskinesia, it is said to be more common than in younger patients. In fact, a lower incidence has been observed in a retrospective chart review in 40 adolescents taking neuroleptic drugs (33[C]). After 2 years, the figure was 18%; although comparability of those studies is far from optimal. The average daily dose, non-compliance, early age of illness, and concomitant use of antiparkinsonian drugs were associated with increased susceptibility. It must be said that abnormal involuntary movements are not always an adverse effect of neuroleptic drugs, but may be, at least partly, an inherent part of some psychotic illnesses. Five of 49 neuroleptic-naive patients with a first episode of schizophrenia had spontaneous dyskinesia (34[C]). Despite difficulties in establishing a reference figure for the incidence or prevalence of dyskinesia, Australian psychiatrists seem to underestimate the prevalence of tardive dyskinesia. According to a survey of 139 psychiatrists, 80% estimated the prevalence of 'mild reversible' tardive dyskinesia as being 5% of those treated with neuroleptic drugs (35[C]).

Multiple involuntary movements, consisting of jaw grinding, oral dyskinesias, bilateral hand rolling, vermiform tongue movements, and bilateral choreiform movements of the digits, have been described in an 11-year-old boy taking thioridazine 150 mg/day and methylphenidate 10 mg bd (36[c]). The stimulant was discontinued and within 4 weeks his movement disorder had completely disappeared. Tardive dyskinesia can affect the neural control of any voluntary muscle (SEDA-22, 50). However, smooth pursuit eye movements were not related to tardive dyskinesia in schizophrenic patients with (n = 40) and without (n = 25) the condition (37[C]).

Successful treatment of tardive dyskinesia is very difficult (SED-13, 122; SEDA-20, 40). A beneficial effect of pyridoxine has been reported (38[c]).

A 22-year-old man with chronic organic persecutory paranoid ideation and recurrent explosive attacks had been receiving neuroleptic drugs since the age of 7. While taking haloperidol, up to 25 mg/day, and trihexyphenidyl, up to 4 mg/day, he developed involuntary movements-blinking, movements of the forehead and eyebrows, tongue-thrusting, licking of the lips, smacking, and chewing-that were diagnosed as tardive dyskinesia. He scored 27 on items 1 to 7 of the Abnormal Involuntary Movement Scale (AIMS). At that time, he began to take pyridoxine, 200 mg/day. After 5 days he had a drastic reduction in severity of all movement disorders.

The uncertain cause, coupled with a high prevalence and an often disabling course have led to the testing of many other compounds in the treatment of tardive dyskinesia: hormones, electroconvulsive therapy, dietary control, antiparkinsonian drugs, benzodiazepines, and biofeedback training are among some of the approaches used in the treatment of tardive dyskinesia. Also, vitamin E has been used for its antioxidant properties (SEDA-21, 47). A meta-analysis has summarized eight double-blind placebo-controlled studies of vitamin E in the treatment of tardive dyskinesia in 221 patients (39[C]). Overall, vitamin E had a better effect than placebo; 28% of those who took vitamin E had a 33% or greater reduction in AIMS scores, compared with only 4.6% in the placebo arm. The number of patients included in any study was very small, never more than 28. The rationale for using vitamin E and for finding a better indicator of vitamin E deficiency has been explored (40[C]). Since much of the vitamin E in plasma is carried in the low-density lipoprotein fraction, relating vitamin E content to the sum of cholesterol and triglycerides in the plasma would produce the maximum specificity and sensitivity in defining vitamin E deficiency. Patients with tardive dyskinesia had lower concentrations of lipid-corrected vitamin E. However, the authors admitted that the lower concentration of vitamin E could result from, predispose to, or serve as a marker for the susceptibility to tardive dyskinesia.

Dystonia Meyge's syndrome is characterized by blepharospasm and spasm of the lower facial or oromandibular muscles (41[cr]).

A 52-year-old woman developed Meyge's syndrome 2 days after the appearance of akathisia. She had taken neuroleptic drugs for years, but her current medication had been changed to bromperidol 18 mg/day and trihexyphenidyl(benzhexol) 6 mg/day and 2 days later she developed akathisia. Oral perphenazine 12 mg and trihexyphenidyl 6 mg dose-dependently reduced the frequency of blepharospasm; the dosages of bromperidol and trihexyphenidyl were gradually reduced to 8 mg/day and 3 mg/day respectively over 3 months, by which time her symptoms had completely disappeared.

A prospective study has identified cocaine as a risk factor for neuroleptic drug-induced acute dystonia (42[C]). The study sample consisted of a high-risk group for neuroleptic-induced acute dystonia: 29 men aged 17–45 years who had used high-potency neuroleptic drugs within 24 hours of admission and had not taken neuroleptic drugs in the last month. Nine men developed acute dystonia: six of nine cocaine users and three of 20 non-users, a relative risk of 4.4 (95% CI = 1.4–13.9). Cocaine users did not differ significantly in age, mean daily neuroleptic drug dose, or peak dose.

Tardive dystonia is a late, potentially irreversible dystonic disorder caused by long-term exposure to antidopaminergic drugs; it has often been considered a subtype of tardive dyskinesia (SED-13, 123). Some features of this condition are clearly different from those of tardive dyskinesia (SEDA-20, 41). The diagnosis of tardive dystonia was first established by Burke, and it should meet the following criteria: (a) the presence of chronic dystonia; (b) a history of antipsychotic drug treatment preceding (less than 2 months) or concurrent with the onset of dystonia; and (c) exclusion of known causes of secondary dystonia (43[C]). Only a very small proportion of patients (less than 3%) receiving neuroleptic drugs develop tardive dystonia. Tardive dystonia developed at any time between 4 days and 23 years after exposure to whatever neuroleptic drug in 107 patients who fulfilled these diagnostic criteria (44[C]). Although the majority had a focal onset involving the craniocervical region, tardive dystonia tended to spread over the next 1–2 years and resulted in segmental or generalized dystonia in most cases. Once developed, it is a very persistent disorder, with a low remission rate of only 14%; withdrawal of neuroleptic drugs increases the chances of remission. Botulinum toxin injections produced symptomatic relief, but benzodiazepines were associated with a poorer outcome, probably because of reverse causality, since non-remitting patients were more likely to use benzodiazepines as a second line treatment.

A retrospective evaluation of the records of patients with idiopathic cervical dystonias (n = 82) and tardive cervical dystonias (n = 20) has been performed, in a search for clinical features that could help separate these closely related disorders (45[C]). Despite the overall similarity, the presence of a dystonic head tremor was strongly suggestive of the idiopathic form, which was present in 42% and did not occur at all in the tardive group. A family history of dystonia (10%) was also exclusive to the idiopathic group. Antecollis, a sustained contraction of the anterior neck muscles that bend the neck forwards, is a rare form of tardive dystonia that has attracted little attention. Patients with this disorder are usually quite disabled and distressed, have severe difficulties with vision, speech, and swallowing, and are unable to lie supine. In recently reported three cases (46[c]), the patients developed the symptoms after receiving a number of antipsychotic drugs for 4 months to 14 years. Neither withdrawal of antipsychotic drugs nor the administration of anticholinergic agents affected their symptoms. About 50% of patients with tardive dystonia include retrocollis; if the trunk is involved, most of the patients have back-arching opisthotonos. Five such patients experienced relief with a custom-made mechanical device that delivers constant contact to the occiput and shoulders (47[c]).

A thorough and extensive review has addressed the treatment of tardive dystonia (48[R]). For patients taking typical antipsychotic drugs, a switch to clozapine is suggested, or, if clozapine is contraindicated, to risperidone, olanzapine or sertindole. Other alternatives are anticholinergic drugs, particularly trihexyphenidyl, benzodiazepines, tetrabenazine, reserpine, tocopherol, bromocriptine, and (in children and adolescents) baclofen. Local injection of botulinum toxin, which blocks acetylcholine release at the neuromuscular junction, is very effective in the treatment of focal dystonias (SEDA-19, 45; SEDA-22, 52). The therapeutic effects of botulinum toxin last on average for 2–6 months. Surgical treatment, such as local denervation myectomy, thalamotomy, and pallidotomy, and deep brain stimulation can be considered only for patients with disabling dystonia and in those in whom medical treatment has failed to provide improvement. The successful treatment of tardive dystonia with low-dose L-dopa and benserazide, 50/12.5 mg tds, has been reported (49[c]).

Misinterpretation of symptoms has led to ineffective management of dystonia (50[c]).

A 14-year-old boy with Tourette's syndrome developed withdrawal dystonia while being treated with pimozide 12 mg/day. Increased blinking, facial pain, dystonic movements, and other facial movements at each dose reduction pointed toward withdrawal dystonia rather than toward a worsening of Tourette's syndrome.

Neuroleptic malignant syndrome Neuroleptic malignant syndrome is a rare disorder characterized by hyperthermia, raised creatine phosphokinase, extrapyramidal effects, autonomic instability, altered consciousness and leukocytosis (SEDA-20, 41). Conventional antipsychotic drugs are currently associated with the condition, although it can occur during clozapine or risperidone monotherapy. This was the conclusion of a review of neuroleptic malignant syndrome attributed to clozapine (19 cases) and risperidone (13 cases) (51[R]). Risk factors that have been proposed for the development of neuroleptic malignant syndrome include a history of prior episodes of neuroleptic malignant syndrome, the use of high potency drugs, rapid escalation in dosage or parenteral administration of neuroleptic drugs, dehydration, agitation, catatonia, and certain diagnoses, including mood disorders, schizophrenia, and mental disorders due to medical conditions (SEDA-22, 52). Acute encephalitis has now been suggested to be another risk factor (52[cr]). It has been reported in five patients who developed neuroleptic malignant syndrome after being treated with neuroleptic drugs for the psychiatric symptoms associated with encephalitis. HIV encephalitis has in particular been associated with neuroleptic malignant syndrome (SEDA-19, 47).

The occurrence of neuroleptic malignant syndrome in a patient with cancer after the use of haloperidol has given rise to some comments: (a) clinical oncologists are not familiar with the neuroleptic malignant syndrome; (b) neuroleptic malignant syndrome is difficult to diagnose, because its presentation resembles that of cancer itself, and sometimes other treatment-related complications (53[cr]).

The post-partum period is said to be a risk factor for neuroleptic malignant syndrome. During 30 months 11 cases of neuroleptic malignant syndrome were detected in a university general hospital in India (54[c]). Five patients were women and in three the onset was in the post-partum period. One patient was taking a small dose of oral chlorpromazine (20 mg). In contrast, agitation and ECT, which have been proposed as risk factors (SEDA-22, 52), have been questioned as independent risk factors in two recent letters (55[r], 56[r]). Since catatonia was mentioned without reporting the number of affected patients, the authors suggested that some of the agitated patients would actually correspond to catatonic patients. However, catatonia was present before the onset of neuroleptic malignant syndrome in only one subject from the neuroleptic malignant syndrome group (57[r]). On the other hand, ECT remains, at best, an association that possibly flags the characteristics of the primary psychiatric disorder that prompted the treatment.

Malignant catatonia associated with a low serum iron concentration carries a high risk of evolving into neuroleptic malignant syndrome. This is the main conclusion from a retrospective study in which 39 catatonic episodes in patients with low ($n = 17$) or normal ($n = 22$) serum iron concentrations were compared (58[C]). All had been exposed to neuroleptic drugs. Hypoferremia has previously been related to neuroleptic malignant syndrome (SEDA-19, 46).

New cases of neuroleptic malignant syndrome in different settings and with different features have been published (59[c]–63[c]).

A 21-year-old woman had bilateral dislocations after being struck by an automobile (59[c]). Postoperatively, she had signs of delirium and agitated behavior, and was given haloperidol 3–5 mg i.v. or i.m. and lorazepam 2 mg i.v. Her general muscular tone increased during the next several days, leading to spontaneous dislocations/subluxations of multiple joints; there was mild hyperthermia (38.4°C), a raised neutrophil count (12×10^9/l) in the absence of an identifiable source of infection, and a raised creatine phosphokinase (361 U/l; reference range 0–150). Neuroleptic malignant syndrome was diagnosed. Haloperidol and droperidol were discontinued, and she was given dantrolene sodium 1 mg/kg orally every 8 hours for 14 days. Within 24 hours her temperature had fallen and during the next week her spasticity progressively improved.

In two other cases there were features of neuroleptic malignant syndrome within 10 days of an autotransplantation with rapid improvement after withdrawal of the neuroleptic drugs (60[c]). Since neuroleptic drugs are often used during transplantation, it is important to recognize that the use of these drugs in concert with the physiological stress of the operation can result in this drug-related complication. In two new cases of neuroleptic malignant syndrome, computerized tomography showed evidence of cerebral edema, which is claimed not to have been reported before (61[c]).

A patient who developed severe hyponatremia and progressed to neuroleptic malignant syndrome, myoglobinuria, and acute renal insufficiency deserves attention (62[c]). Acute renal insufficiency has previously been reported as a severe complication (SED-13, 124; SEDA-21, 49).

A 42-year-old man with a history of paranoid schizophrenia developed confusion and emesis. His medications included buspirone and thiothixene. He also had a generalized seizure that resolved spontaneously. His serum sodium concentration was 114 mmol/l, which was thought to be secondary to psychogenic polydipsia and which was corrected. The next day his temperature rose to 40°C and the day after that he became lethargic and non-verbal and developed generalized muscle rigidity. A diagnosis of probable malignant neuroleptic syndrome was made, and he was given dantrolene sodium 1 mg/kg intravenously; neuroleptic drugs were withdrawn. The serum creatine kinase activity was over 234 500 U/l. Urinalysis showed more than 3 g/l of protein, a trace of ketones, and hemoglobin and leukocytes. By the following day, his muscle rigidity and fever had resolved and his mental status was markedly improved.

Two patients developed non-convulsive status epilepticus and neuroleptic malignant syndrome (63[c]). Whether this constitutes one syndrome or is merely the co-existence of the two is academic, because it makes no difference to therapy.

Dantrolene may be effective in reducing muscle rigidity in neuroleptic malignant syndrome (SED-13, 125; SEDA-20, 42), but according to a recent report a reliable regimen has not been established (64[c]).

A 39-year-old man receiving haloperidol 4 mg and trihexyphenidyl 2 mg for schizophrenia developed a fever of over 40°C and clouding of consciousness 19 days after the start of medication. Neuroleptic malignant syndrome was suspected and dantrolene 40–80 mg/day was given intravenously for 5 days, with no improvement; disseminated intravascular coagulation and acute renal insufficiency developed. Dantrolene 200 mg was given intravenously over 10 minutes. One hour later, his temperature fell to 38.4°C. Continuous intravenous infusion of dantrolene 400 mg/day was started in combination with oral bromocriptine 15 mg/day. Dantrolene was changed to the oral route after 14 days and medication was terminated after 28 days. He was discharged 45 days after admission.

Endocrine, metabolic There is a general belief that neuroleptic drugs cause moderate *rises in serum prolactin* of up to six times the upper limit of the reference range (SED-13, 125). In eight patients receiving neuroleptic drugs, serum prolactin concentrations were grossly raised (65[c]). The time-course of the prolactin increase has been examined in 17 subjects whose prolactin concentrations rose in the first 6–9 days of treatment with haloperidol (66[C]). The increase was followed by a plateau that persisted, with minor fluctuations, throughout the 18 days of observation. Patients whose prolactin concentrations increased above 77 ng/ml ($n = 2$) had hypothyroidism, and it is known that TRH (thyrotropin) stimulates the release of prolactin (67[C]). It was concluded that all patients should have had TSH determinations at the start of therapy with neuroleptic drugs.

The effects of neuroleptic drugs on menstrual status and the relation between menstrual status and neuroleptic efficacy and adverse effects have been explored (68[C]). In contrast to prior reports (SEDA-18, 50), there was not a high prevalence of *menstrual irregularities or amenorrhea* in 27 premenopausal women with chronic schizophrenia treated with conventional neuroleptic drugs.

Hematological In view of the association of *agranulocytosis* with clozapine and of *aplastic anemia* with remoxipride, hemopoietic disorders have been studied using information from the UK monitoring system (69[C]). The Committee on Safety of Medicines and the Medicines Control Agency in the UK received 999 reports of hemopoietic disorders related to antipsychotic drugs between 1963 and 1996; there were 65 deaths. There were 182 reports of agranulocytosis; chlorpromazine and thioridazine were associated with the highest number of deaths—27 of 56 and nine of 24 respectively. The much lower mortality with clozapine-induced agranulocytosis, two of 91 (2.2%), was explained as a function of the stringent monitoring requirements for this drug, which allows early detection and treatment.

Special senses *Pigmentary retinopathy* has occasionally been reported in patients taking neuroleptic drugs (SED-13, 127). A new case has emerged (70[c]).

A 28-year-old woman with a long history of psychiatric problems was taking fluoxetine, diazepam, methylphenidate, and thioridazine 800 mg qds. Fluorescein angiography showed confluent areas of punctate hyperfluorescence, consistent with diffuse retinal pigment epithelial alteration secondary to acute thioridazine toxic effects.

Acute toxic effects of thioridazine include nyctalopia, blurred vision, and dyschromatopsia, and typically become evident after 2–8 weeks of dosages over 800 mg/day.

Sexual function Psychotropic drug-induced *priapism* has been reviewed (71[R]). It is said that antipsychotic drugs are most commonly implicated. A prior history of prolonged erections can be identified in as many as 50% of patients presenting with priapism who are using antipsychotic drugs. According to another review, the frequency of priapism with neuroleptic drugs may be increased by the fact that schizophrenia is said to be accompanied by an increase in sexual activity (72).

In 12 men with schizophrenia (mean age 36 years) receiving neuroleptic drugs, amantadine 100 mg/day for 6 weeks improved sexual function (73[C]). All 12 patients, who had a sustained relationship with a female partner, had reported sexual dysfunction. Four areas of sexual function were assessed: desire, erection, ejaculation, and satisfaction; there was an improvement in all but ejaculation. Amantadine had no effect on the symptoms of schizophrenia.

Immunological and hypersensitivity reactions *Hypogammaglobulinemia* in a 22-year-old woman with brief psychotic disorder has been attributed to antipsychotic drug therapy (74[c]). About 4 months after she had started to receive antipsychotic drugs, her serum concentrations of total protein had fallen to 58 g/l, with an IgG concentration of 3.49 g/l, an IgA concentration of 0.54 g/l, and an IgM concentration of 0.34 g/l.

Antiphospholipid syndrome is a disorder of vascular thrombosis associated with raised concentrations of antiphospholipid antibodies. Symptomatic antiphospholipid syndrome has been described in a 42-year-old woman treated with chlorpromazine 260 mg/day (75[c]). She presented with sudden right-sided weakness, numbness, and headache. Examination confirmed upper motor neuron signs affecting the right arm, leg, and face, with hemiplegia and hemiparesthesia. Autoantibody screening showed positive antinuclear antibodies, with an IgG titer of 50 and an IgM titer of 1600. Anticardiolipin antibody was positive with a raised IgM titer of 24 (normal less than 9). The symptoms and the serological findings resolved after withdrawal of the phenothiazine.

Drug-induced *lupus erythematosus* has been reviewed (76[R], 77[R]). Neuroleptic drugs, particularly chlorpromazine and chlorprothixene, have often been associated with this autoimmune disorder. It is recommended that several diagnostic criteria for this condition should be met: (1) exposure to a drug suspected to cause lupus erythematosus; (2) no previous history of the condition; (3) detection of positive antinuclear antibodies; and (4) rapid improvement and a gradual fall in the antinuclear antibodies and other serological findings on drug withdrawal.

Risk factors The use of neuroleptic drugs in children and adolescents has been extensively reviewed (78[R]–80[R]). Typical antipsychotic drugs have been assessed in only three randomized, double-blind, placebo-controlled studies in 122 patients and atypical drugs in five (one clozapine, $n = 21$; two amisulpride, $n = 36$; and two tiapride, $n = 59$). The studies were of short durations, 4–10 weeks. Extrapyramidal signs occurred in 25–73% of those treated with the typical antipsychotic drugs. For clozapine, although the frequency of adverse effects varied, the types were similar to those reported in adults, i.e. electroencephalographic changes, fatigue, increased liver enzymes, postural hypotension, tachycardia, fever, and hypersalivation.

In a study that was claimed to be the first published placebo-controlled dose comparison of neuroleptic drugs used to treat psychoses and disruptive behavior in dementia, haloperidol 2–3 mg/day was compared with 0.50–0.75 mg/day in 71 out-patients with *Alzheimer's disease* (81[C]). After 12 weeks, there was a favorable therapeutic effect of haloperidol 2–3 mg/day, although 25% of the patients developed moderate to severe extrapyramidal signs. No patient developed tardive dyskinesia, but neuroleptic drug exposure needs to be considerably longer for that.

Tumor-inducing effects There was an *increase in markers of genotoxicity* in patients receiving long-term neuroleptic drugs in combination with other psychotropic drugs ($n = 36$) compared with controls ($n = 36$) (82[C]).

A recent study has shown an association between the frequency of *chromosomal aberrations* in lymphocytes and the probability of tumor induction (83[C]).

Second-generation effects

Use in pregnancy The risks of psychotropic drug use during pregnancy (SEDA-22, 54) have been newly reviewed (84[R], 85[R]). Although there was a small increase in the risk of organ malformations with phenothiazines, studies have failed to show an increased rate of congenital malformations with haloperidol. For the atypical antipsychotic drugs, the only data currently available come from case reports, and so far there is no evidence of teratogenicity.

Effects on fertility The effects of antipsychotic drugs on fertility are not well known (SED-13, 129). It has now been suggested that *fertility may be impaired* by neuroleptic drugs, since they increase prolactin concentrations and can cause amenorrhea (86[r]).

Overdosage Antipsychotic drugs are often taken in accidental overdosage or suicide attempts, but mortality is generally low and infrequently associated with residual impairment (SED-13, 129). Nevertheless, large differences in fatal toxicity in overdosage have been observed between different antipsychotic drugs (87[C]). Pimozide has the lowest fatal toxicity index—the number of deaths divided by the number of prescriptions—and loxapine has the highest. According to the authors, the choice of first-line antipsychotic treatment should include consideration of the possibility of fatal toxicity.

Interactions A thorough review of drug interactions with antipsychotic agents has been published (88[R]). Specific interactions with *anticholinergic drugs, antihypertensive drugs, antituberculous drugs, anxiolytic drugs, β-blockers, cimetidine, lithium, and tobacco* are addressed.

Benzodiazepines Because of the frequency of co-administration of benzodiazepines with neuroleptic drugs, it is important to consider possible adverse effects that may result from such combinations. In a brief review emphasis has been placed on pharmacokinetic interactions between neuroleptic drugs and benzodiazepines, as much information on their metabolic pathways is emerging (89[R]). Thus, the enzyme CYP3A4, which plays a dominant role in metabolism of benzodiazepines, also contributes to the metabolism of clozapine, haloperidol, and quetiapine, and neuroleptic drug plasma concentrations can rise. Intramuscular levomepromazine in combination with an intravenous benzodiazepine has been said to increase the risk of airways obstruction, on the basis of five cases of respiratory impairment in patients who received injections of psychotropic drugs (90[c]). The doses of levomepromazine were higher in the five cases that had accompanying airways obstruction than in another 95 patients who did not.

Lithium and valproate Antipsychotic drugs are often used in mood stabilizer combinations. However, there have been few controlled studies of the use of such combinations, and interactions are potentially dangerous. The advantages and disadvantages of all currently used mood stabilizer combinations have been extensively reviewed (91[R]). Some effects are well known: neurotoxicity, hypotension, somnambulistic-like events, and cardiac and respiratory arrest associated with the combination of lithium and traditional neuroleptic drugs considered as a first-line treatment for classic euphoric mania with psychotic features. Likewise, the combination of valproate and traditional neuroleptic drugs, a first-line treatment for mixed or rapid-cycling episodes or dysphoric mania with psychotic features, is associated with altered mental status and electroencephalographic abnormalities.

Selective serotonin re-uptake inhibitors Urinary retention and severe constipation occurred in a patient who started to take sertraline when already receiving haloperidol and clonazepam (92[c]). After a week, she discontinued sertraline and her symptoms disappeared in a few days.

Three adults with Giles de la Tourette syndrome had acute severe drug-induced parkinsonism when neuroleptic drugs and SSRIs were used together (93[c]). The adverse reactions were observed in three of 14 adults treated with the combination but in none of almost 75 children receiving similar treatment. The authors suggested that age-related changes in dopamine neurotransmitter systems could confer vulnerability. On the other hand, SSRIs themselves can cause parkinsonism and also inhibit P450 enzymes, leading to increases in plasma concentrations of neuroleptic drugs during combined treatment (SEDA-20, 50; SEDA-21, 51; SEDA-22, 55). Surprisingly, in a recent double-blind, randomized, placebo-controlled study there were no significant differences in plasma haloperidol or reduced haloperidol concentrations when sertraline (n = 18) or placebo (n = 18) were added at 2, 4, 6, and 8 weeks (94[C]).

INDIVIDUAL DRUGS

Amisulpride *(SEDA-22, 55)*

Amisulpride is an atypical antipsychotic drug, a benzamide derivative, which may have a low propensity to cause *extrapyramidal symptoms* (SEDA-22, 55). Its effects have recently been studied in a 4-week, double-blind, randomized trial in 319 patients with acute exacerbation of schizophrenia (95[C]). Fixed doses of amisulpride (100, 400, 800, and 1200 mg/day) and haloperidol (16 mg/day) were compared. Amisulpride 400 mg/day and 800 mg/day was effective in treating the positive symptoms of schizophrenia, with fewer extrapyramidal adverse effects than haloperidol, which was associated with the highest proportion of extrapyramidal symptoms. The incidence of extrapyramidal symptoms in patients treated with amisulpride increased with increasing dose (31, 42, 45, and 55% for 100, 400, 800, and 1200 mg/day respectively). The rate of withdrawals due to adverse events was higher with haloperidol (16%) than amisulpride (0, 5, 3, and 5% respectively).

Similarly, amisulpride 600–1200 mg/day for 3 months was effective and well tolerated in 445 schizophrenic patients aged 18–45 years (96[C]). During this time 124 patients (28%) dropped out of the study; 21% reported adverse events, neurological (35%), psychiatric (15%), or endocrine (9.1%). Seven adverse events were assessed as serious: two *suicides, two suicide attempts*, one *neuroleptic malignant syndrome*, one *somnolence*, and one *worsening of arteritis*.

In a randomized, double-blind, multicenter comparison of amisulpride 1000 mg/day (n = 70) and flupenthixol 25 mg/day (n = 62) for 6 weeks, both drugs significantly improved the acute psychotic symptoms to a similar extent (97[C]). The total numbers of drop-outs were 19 with amisulpride and 25 with flupentixol. Adverse effects accounted for 8.6 and 18% respectively of the totals. In all extrapyramidal outcome parameters, amisulpride caused significantly fewer motor adverse effects. Apart from the *extrapyramidal adverse effects*, there were treatment-emergent adverse events in 87% of the patients given amisulpride and 92% of those given flupenthixol. *Prolactin concentrations were higher* with amisulpride.

A lower dose of amisulpride (50 mg) has been tested in 20 healthy elderly volunteers (aged 65–79 years) (98[C]). There were no serious adverse events, but one subject reported a moderate *headache* for 18 hours, a second subject vomited 9 hours after dosing, and a further subject complained of mild *somnolence* for 12 hours starting 4 hours after dosing; however, there were no extrapyramidal symptoms, clinically significant hemodynamic variations, nor electrocardiographic abnormalities.

Clozapine *(SED-13, 117; SEDA-20, 46; SEDA-21, 52; SEDA-22, 56)*

There have been further attempts to establish the role of clozapine in the treatment of resistant schizophrenia. Thus, 75 schizophrenic out-patients, who met criteria for residual positive or negative symptoms after being treated for at least 6 weeks with conventional neuroleptic drugs, entered a 10-week randomized, double-blind, parallel-group comparison of clozapine (n = 38) and haloperidol (n = 37) (99[C]). There was no evidence of any superior efficacy or long-term effect of clozapine on primary or secondary negative symptoms. Long-term clozapine was associated with significant improvements in social and occupational functioning, but not in overall quality of life. There were no significant differences between the two groups in adverse effects from previous neuroleptic drug treatment, and *dizziness* (50 vs 19%), *salivation* (82 vs 19%), and *nausea* (37 vs 11%) were significantly more common in patients treated with clozapine. In contrast, *dry mouth* was significantly more common with haloperidol (62 vs 18%). Patients who completed the double-blind study (n = 58) entered a 1-year open-label clozapine study. Over the course of that year, there was a small reduction in adverse effects, apart from hypersalivation, which increased significantly. Over the first 6 months there was weight gain followed by a plateau.

In a retrospective open study of 46 patients taking clozapine for 4 years, clozapine had to be discontinued in 10 patients (21%) and serious adverse effects were rare; no patient had agranulocytosis (100[C]). The most troublesome adverse effects were *drooling, sedation*, and *weight gain*, and three patients had *seizures*.

Experiences in uncontrolled open-label studies in Chinese patients have recently been summarized (101[R]). The most common adverse effect of clozapine was *hypersalivation*, followed by *sedation*. Mandatory blood monitoring is considered an obstacle in persuading some patients to undergo a trial of clozapine, mainly for cultural reasons, summed up by the Chinese proverb that ‘a hundred grains of rice make a drop of blood’. In turn, risperidone was associated with *dizziness* and *sedation*. One patient developed *obsessive rumination* and was successfully treated with clomipramine 25 mg/day.

Some pharmacoeconomic studies have suggested that clozapine may be cost-effective in treatment-resistant schizophrenia, with savings mainly due to a fall in hospitalization expenses, including the cost of dropouts from treatment (102, 103[CR]).

It has been suggested that clozapine may be efficacious in some special group of patients (SEDA-21, 53). New information has appeared from patients with severe borderline personality disorder (104[c]), patients with aggressive schizophrenia (105[c]), and mentally retarded adults (106[cr]). Of 12 in-patients with borderline personality disorder treated with clozapine for 16 weeks, 10 developed *sedation*, which disappeared during the first month of treatment; nine had hypersialorrhea, and six had a fall in white blood cell count, which never reached values outside a clinical range of safety. Aggressive schizophrenic patients (n = 29) improved when treated with clozapine; one was withdrawn after the development of *leukopenia*. In 10 mentally retarded patients taking clozapine for 15 days to 46 months improvement was observed. Half of the patients developed *sedation* and *hypersalivation*, and one discontinued the drug after 2 weeks because of neutropenia. The putative neurotoxicity of clozapine in moderately to profoundly retarded patients (that is, those with an accentuation of cognitive deficits due to the drug's anticholinergic and sedating properties) was not observed. The small sample size, the short duration of treatment, and the lack of control groups in this study preclude definite conclusions.

Cardiovascular *Hypertension* has been reported in young men (SEDA-22, 57). Dominance of α_2 adrenoceptor blockade by clozapine has been proposed as a possible mechanism in a 52-year-old man (107[c]).

Tachycardia is a common cardiovascular adverse effect, and the prevalence of clozapine-induced electrocardiographic changes has been estimated at 10% (SEDA-20, 47; SEDA-22, 57). A new case of clozapine-induced *atrial fibrillation* in a 69-year-old man has been reported (108[c]). The correlation between plasma clozapine concentration and heart rate variability has been studied in 40 schizophrenic patients treated with clozapine 50–600 mg/day (109[C]). The patients had reduced heart rate variability parameters, which correlated negatively with plasma clozapine concentration.

Nervous system *Seizure* characteristics and *electroencephalographic abnormalities* in 12 patients taking clozapine have been identified; there was a surprisingly high incidence of focal epileptiform abnormalities (110[C]). Seizures associated with clozapine are dose-dependent (SEDA-21, 53, SEDA-22, 57). However, seizures have occasionally been reported with low doses, as in the case of a 28-year-old woman, with no history of prior seizures and not taking concomitant medication, who had seizures while taking clozapine 200 mg/day (111[c]). However, when seizures occur in patients taking low dosages of clozapine, other causes must be considered. A 75-year-old patient developed seizures while taking clozapine 12.5 mg/day, but the seizure was unlikely to have been due to clozapine, given the very low dose and non-recurrence with rechallenge at higher dosages (112[c]).

The efficacy and safety of treatment with clozapine in Parkinson's disease have previously been discussed (SEDA-22, 57). A multicenter retrospective review of the effects of clozapine in 172 patients with Parkinson's disease has been published (113[C]). The mean duration of clozapine treatment was 17 (range 1–76) months. Low-dose clozapine improved the symptoms of psychosis, anxiety, depression, hypersexuality, sleep disturbances, and akathisia. Of the 40 patients 24% withdrew as a result of adverse events, mostly sedation (n = 19). Sedation was reported in 46%, *sialorrhea* in 11%, and *postural hypotension* in 9.9%. *Neutropenia* was detected in four patients (2.3%).

It is generally believed that clozapine can improve pre-existing tardive dyskinesia (114[R], 115[cr]). Schizophrenic patients with (n = 15) and without (n = 11) tardive dyskinesia differed markedly in their dopaminergic response to haloperidol, assessed by means of plasma homovanillic acid variations, which increased, whereas this difference was not observed after clozapine (116[C]). Also, the low prevalence of akathisia in patients taking clozapine has led to the proposal that clozapine should be used to treat patients with neuroleptic-induced chronic akathisia (117[r], 118[r]).

Tardive tremor is a hyperkinetic movement disorder associated with chronic neuroleptic drug treatment, first described in 1991 as being symmetrical, of low frequency, present at rest and during voluntary movements but most prominent during posture maintenance, and often accompanied by tardive dyskinesia. Tetrabenazine is the current treatment. Sequential responsiveness to both tetrabenazine and clozapine has been reported (119[c]).

A 55-year-old man with a 15-year history of schizophrenia treated with various neuroleptic drugs developed a tremor and was given tetrabenazine 75 mg/day, with complete regression of the tremor. Three months later he developed depression, a known adverse effect of tetrabenazine, which was discontinued, with subsequent partial improvement of his depressive symptoms but reappearance of the tardive tremor. Clozapine 25 mg/day was started and increased to 75 mg/day; his tardive tremor again disappeared.

Neuroleptic malignant syndrome has been associated with clozapine (SEDA-22, 58). A new case in a 19-year-old man who developed a sudden change in level of consciousness, fever, and muscle rigidity has been reported (120[c]).

Endocrine, metabolic *Diabetic ketoacidosis and insulin-dependent hyperglycemia* has been associated with clozapine (SEDA-21, 54; SEDA-22, 58). For instance, diabetes was more common in 63 patients treated with clozapine compared with 67 treated with conventional depot antipsychotic drugs (121[C]). The percentages of type 3 diabetes mellitus were 12 and 6% respectively. Nevertheless, the mechanism by which it happens is not known. In six schizophrenic patients, clozapine increased mean concentrations of blood glucose, insulin, and C-peptide (122[C]). The authors concluded that the glucose intolerance was due to increased insulin resistance.

Weight gain is often associated with clozapine (SEDA-21, 54). In addition, in a recent study in 42 patients treated with clozapine for at least 1 year, both men and women gained weight and body mass, which is more directly related to cardiovascular morbidity (123[C]). Leptin is a hormone synthesized by adipocytes. Serum leptin concentrations correlate with body mass index. During 10 weeks *leptin concentrations increased* significantly from baseline in 12 patients treated with clozapine (124[C]).

Hematological Careful attention should be paid to possible early warnings of *agranulocytosis*, such as fever, sore throat, and lymphadenopathy. The real incidence of agranulocytosis with clozapine has been extensively discussed, since premarketing data warned that 1–2% of patients may developed this serious complication (SED-13, 126; SEDA-21, 54; SEDA-22, 59). Some of the available postmarketing data on clozapine-induced agranulocytosis are presented in Table 1 (125[CR]).

Reported cases of negative or positive rechallenge in patients with agranulocytosis have previously been collected (SEDA-20, 54; SEDA-22, 59). Now further cases have emerged. Agranulocytosis in a 58-year-old man during a second trial of clozapine, despite a successful previous trial, has been reported (126[c]). A 17-year-old boy with severe clozapine-induced neutropenia had a negative rechallenge; because he had had an unsatisfactory response to traditional antipsychotic drugs, clozapine was continued despite a fall in white blood cell count, since concomitant treatment with granulocyte colony stimulating factor was followed by rapid normalization of the white blood cell count (127[c]).

Immune-mediated mechanisms of clozapine-induced agranulocytosis have been reviewed in the context of agranulocytosis in a 46-year-old woman (128[cr]). Moreover, immune and toxic mechanisms have been explored in three patients who developed agranulocytosis and seven patients who developed neutropenia during therapy with clozapine, and in five patients who were asymptomatic while taking clozapine. There was no evidence of antineutrophil antibodies in the blood of patients shortly after an episode of clozapine-induced agranulocytosis, and an antibody mechanism seems unlikely, in view of the delay in onset of clozapine-induced agranulocytosis on reexposure to the drug (129[C]).

A case of clozapine-induced eosinophilia and subsequent neutropenia has been reported (130[c]). As the patient had a high IgE concentration, an allergic cause was proposed. In a previous study in 70 patients there was no predictive value of eosinophilia for clozapine-induced neutropenia (SEDA-21, 54).

Treatment with granulocyte colony stimulating factor and granulocyte macrophage colony stimulating factors (SEDA-20, 48) has been useful in a case of sepsis and neutropenia induced by clozapine (131[c]). Lithium may be used in combination with clozapine, and in these patients the possibility of inducing a leukocytosis and increasing the total leukocyte count and the granulocyte count has been considered (SEDA-20, 50). Lithium has even been used to prevent clozapine-induced neutropenia (SEDA-22, 59). Lithium has been used in a patient with clozapine-induced neutropenia and in another with complete agranulocytosis: in both cases lithium increased the neutrophil count to within the reference range within 6 days (132[c]). In the patient who had neutropenia, clozapine was reinstated in the presence of lithium and the neutrophil count did not fall thereafter. In addition, five patients who took combined clozapine and lithium had a significant improvement with this combination and there were no cases of agranulocytosis, neuroleptic malignant syndrome, or other adverse effects (133[c]).

Liver Hepatitis associated with clozapine has been reported (SEDA-20, 49; SEDA-22, 59). A new case of *obstructive hepatitis* has been described (134[cr]).

A 48-year-old man with schizophrenia started taking clozapine 12.5 mg/day increasing over the next 18 days to 150 mg/day. By that time he was icteric, with mild distress and fever and raised bilirubin 149 μmol/l (5.1–25.7), direct bilirubin 92 μmol/l, γ-glutamyl transpeptidase 446 IU/l (<65), AlT 100 IU/l (<40), and AsT 56 IU/l (<40). Hepatitis serology showed positive hepatitis B surface antibodies, and HBs antigen was negative, as were hepatitis A, hepatitis C, Epstein–Barr virus, and cytomegalovirus. He also had hyperglycemia, pleural effusion, eosinophilia, hematuria, and proteinuria, which also resolved on clozapine discontinuation.

Pancreas Occasional cases of *pancreatitis* have been previously related to clozapine therapy (SEDA-17, 63). A new case of this un-

Table 1. *Reported incidences of clozapine-induced agranulocytosis*

Country	Period	Number of patients	Percentage incidence (associated mortality)	Reference
Finland	1975	2260	0.70 (0.35)	SED-9, 83
USA	1990–91	11382	0.80 (0.02)	SEDA-18, 54
France	1992	2834	0.46 (ND)	SEDA-21, 54
USA	1990–94	99502	0.38 (0.01)	SEDA-22, 59
UK and Ireland	1990–94	6316	0.80 (0.03)	SEDA-22, 59
New Zealand	1988–95	693	1.15 (0.00)	SEDA-22, 59
Australia	1993–96	4061	0.90 (0.00)	124[CR]
Spain	1993–99	6354	0.16 (0.02)	Agencia Española del Medicamento (personal communication)
Total		133402	0.44 (0.018)	

common adverse effect, with a lower dose of clozapine, has been published (135[c]).

A 73-year-old woman with a 4-year history of Parkinson's disease developed hallucinations and delusions that were interpreted as secondary effects of L-dopa. She was given clozapine 25 mg/day and continued to take L-dopa. Four days later she complained of abdominal pain. She had raised serum amylase activity of 806 IU/l (reference range <220 IU/l), lipase of 2598 IU/l (<190 IU/l), creatine phosphokinase 464 IU/l (<190 IU/l), and normal concentrations of total and direct bilirubin. All others causes of pancreatitis were ruled out.

Gastrointestinal *Reflux esophagitis* has been associated with clozapine (SEDA-22, 60). It has been speculated that clozapine-reduced esophageal motility was the cause (136[r]).

Musculoskeletal *Weakness and reduced muscle tone* have previously been described in connection with clozapine (SEDA-21, 54). In a recent open study in 41 patients, strength control was evaluated before the start of clozapine titration and again at the end of the titration period (on average 9 weeks later). The results suggested that the strength deficit was primarily due to clozapine and that two distinct effects could be distinguished: an initial transient stage characterized by 'drowsiness' and a subsequent stage with dose-dependent myoclonic features (137[C]).

Rhabdomyolysis occurred in two men, aged 21 and 42 years, taking clozapine (138[c], 139[c]). The first patient had no risk factors, but calcium-dependent potassium efflux, normally responsible for membrane hyperpolarization and muscle refractoriness, was severely impaired in the patient's erythrocytes. The second patient had marked hyponatremia, due to psychogenic polydipsia, and developed a marked rise in creatine kinase activity (62 730 U/l) after correction of hyponatremia with hyperosmolar fluids.

Myokymia is characterized by undulating movements of the muscle and skin, accompanied by involuntary repetitive firing of grouped motor unit action potentials. A case associated with clozapine has been reported (140[c]).

A 33-year-old woman developed muscle twitching and spasms of the legs and back after having taken clozapine for 3 years. Neurological examination showed myokymia in both thighs, calves, and the lower lip. The myokymia disappeared 1 week after withdrawal of clozapine.

Risk factors Patients with *Lewy body dementia* may be more intolerant of neuroleptic drugs, including atypical neuroleptic drugs, than other patients with neurodegenerative dementia. However, given the symptom pattern in this dementia (because hallucinations are commonly present), it is likely that people with Lewy body dementia will be exposed to neuroleptic drugs, perhaps with dire consequences. In a recent report, two patients with Lewy body dementia taking clozapine developed confusion and behavioral symptoms (141[c]).

Age Data from an open study (n = 329) has suggested that patients between the ages of 55 and 64 years may have a better response to clozapine than those aged 65 and older, but there were no significant differences between the two age groups in the number of patients remaining on clozapine therapy and the number in whom therapy was discontinued (n = 134) (142[C]). The mean duration of clozapine therapy was 278 days. The most common adverse effects that required withdrawal were sedation (n = 12), hematological adverse effects (n = 7), and cardiovascular adverse effects (n = 6).

Genetic susceptibility Agranulocytosis due to clozapine has previously been associated with different types of human leukocyte antigen (HLA) (SEDA-20, 48; SEDA-22, 61). A further study has been performed in 61 Jewish schizophrenic patients (143[C]); in 11 of them agranulocytosis developed after clozapine treatment and in 50 controls it did not. Patients with agranulocytosis had a higher frequency of the HLA B38 antigen (8/11 or 72% vs 6/50 or 12%). The authors suggested that major histocompatibility complex gene products could be involved in clozapine-mediated hematological complications.

Withdrawal effects Psychotic decompensation has often been associated with clozapine withdrawal (SED-13, 128; SEDA-20, 55; SEDA-22, 61). In susceptible individuals, abrupt or rapid withdrawal from clozapine may be accompanied by severe psychotic decompensation, autonomic instability, symptoms of cholinergic rebound, and dystonias and dyskinesias. Four patients had severe *dystonias and dyskinesias* on abrupt withdrawal of clozapine (144[c]), and another two had *obsessive-compulsive symptoms* during withdrawal; resumption of clozapine led to the complete disappearance of the obsessive-compulsive symptoms (145[c]).

Overdosage Seven patients who took large doses of clozapine (mean 3 g, range 0.4–16 g) have been reported (146[c]). All made a full recovery and toxicokinetic modeling suggested that norclozapine was formed by a saturable process but that clozapine kinetics were linear over the estimated doses.

Interactions Both *caffeine* and clozapine are CYP1A2 substrates, and caffeine has previously been associated with changes in the metabolism of clozapine (SEDA-20, 50; SEDA-22, 61). Seven schizophrenic patients taking clozapine monotherapy participated in a study of the effects of caffeine withdrawal from the diet (147[C]). After a caffeine-free diet for 5 days, clozapine plasma concentrations fell by 50%. The authors suggested that schizophrenic patients treated with clozapine should have their caffeine intake medically supervised, and that monitoring of concentrations of clozapine and its metabolite may be warranted.

Interferon-α A synergistic effect of interferon-α and clozapine has been suggested as a cause of agranulocytosis after 7 weeks of this combined therapy in a 29-year-old patient who had been taking clozapine for more than 5 years without developing hematological abnormalities (148[c]).

Phenobarbital may stimulate the metabolism of clozapine, probably by inducing its *N*-oxidation and demethylation pathways. Seven patients taking clozapine in combination with phenobarbital had significantly lower plasma clozapine concentrations than 15 controls taking clozapine only (149[C]).

Selective serotonin re-uptake inhibitors It has previously been reported that selective serotonin re-uptake inhibitors (SSRIs) increase clozapine plasma concentrations (SEDA-20, 50; SEDA-21, 55; SEDA-22, 62). In 10 patients stabilized on clozapine (200–450 mg/day) who took fluoxetine (20 mg/day) for 8 weeks, mean plasma concentrations of clozapine, norclozapine, and clozapine *N*-oxide increased significantly by 58, 36, and 38% respectively (150[C]). The potential consequences of the interaction of SSRIs with clozapine have been illustrated by a case of fatal outcome caused by ingestion of clozapine and fluoxetine (151[c]). The blood fluoxetine concentration was 0.7 μg/ml, which would be considered a high therapeutic concentration (usual target range 0.03–0.5 μg/ml); the blood clozapine concentration was 4.9 μg/ml, which is high and lies within the lethal concentration range (1.6–7.1 μg/ml). In contrast, a recent study did not show any effect of citalopram on plasma concentrations of clozapine (n = 8), risperidone (n = 7), or their active metabolites during 8 weeks (152[C]). Dual effects were observed in a 44-year-old schizophrenic patient taking clozapine with both fluoxetine and sertraline for mood stabilization (153[c]). Clinical and motor status improved with both fluoxetine and sertraline; cognitive function improved with clozapine and fluoxetine, but was not sustained with sertraline.

Monitoring therapy Since up to 17% of patients discontinue clozapine because of adverse effects, strategies for minimizing and managing the adverse effects of clozapine have been reviewed (154[R], 155[R]). Some of the adverse effects are dose-dependent. Consequently, tailoring the dosage to the needs of each individual would be beneficial. Treatment should be begun at a low dosage, 12.5–25 mg/day. The optimal plasma concentration of clozapine is 200–350 ng/ml, which usually corresponds to a daily dose of 200–400 mg (156[R], 157[R]).

A dosing nomogram to predict clozapine steady-state plasma concentrations has been generated using data from 71 patients (158[C]). Clozapine steady-state plasma concentrations and demographic variables were obtained. The model explained 47% of the variance in clozapine concentrations. Two equations were obtained to predict steady-state plasma concentrations, one for men and one for women:

$$\text{clozapine (ng/ml)} = 0.464D + 111S + 145 \quad \text{(men)}$$

$$\text{clozapine (ng/ml)} = 1.590D + 111S - 149 \quad \text{(women)}$$

where D = dose (mg/day), S = 1 for smokers, and S = 0 for non-smokers.

A further model for optimizing individual dosage regimens using a Bayesian methodology has been proposed (159[C]).

Droperidol

Of 20 volunteers who took droperidol 5 mg orally in orange juice, none had a neutral or pleasant experience (160[C]). All reported *restlessness*; 17 felt *sedated*; 11 reported *dysphoria*, the onset being relatively immediate, and one subject broke down in tears within an hour of taking droperidol. *Suicidal feelings* emerged acutely in two subjects and were entertained in two more subjects. Among other experiences reported were *skin hypersensitivity* (five subjects), *aching in the muscles* (six subjects), *wheezing consistent with respiratory dyskinesia* (one subject), *change in voice quality* (one subject), and marked *rhinorrhea* (one subject). *Mental effort was difficult*, and all subjects reported some *problems with concentration.*

Olanzapine *(SEDA-21, 56; SEDA-22, 64)*

Several reviews have echoed olanzapine's efficacy and tolerability (161[R]–163[R]). Unlike clozapine, olanzapine has not been associated with clinically important neutropenia during premarketing. A thorough and extensive review has summarized five pivotal clinical trials comprising 3252 patients (164[R]), but the safety and the efficacy of olanzapine in long-term use has not yet been studied. Similarly, its efficacy in treatment-resistant schizophrenia has not been established. Moreover, in some recent studies olanzapine has failed to show efficacy in treatment-resistant schizophrenia (165[C], 166[C]). In one of these studies, 103 previously treatment-resistant patients with schizophrenia were given a prospective 6-week trial of 10–40 mg/day of haloperidol; 84 failed to respond and were randomly assigned to a double-blind 8-week fixed-dose trial of either olanzapine 25 mg/day alone ($n = 42$) or chlorpromazine 1200 mg/day plus benzatropine mesylate 4 mg/day ($n = 39$) (165[C]). There was no significant difference in completion rates. Neither drug produced a substantial change in the level of psychosis from pre-randomization baseline, and there were no differences between the groups in efficacy. However, olanzapine had a better adverse effects profile.

In another study, 19 patients previously treated with clozapine were switched to olanzapine (166[C]). Eight were considered to be responders and the rest decompensated, seven of them enough to require hospitalization. Nevertheless, overall Brief Psychiatric Rating Scale (BPRS) scores increased significantly from baseline to final assessment.

In a third study, supported by Eli Lilly and Company, it was concluded that olanzapine may be effective in a significant number of neuroleptic drug-resistant schizophrenic patients (167[C]). However, of 25 patients who entered an open-label trial for 6 months, 14 discontinued olanzapine, one because of an adverse effect (depression), two because of lack of compliance, and 11 because of lack of efficacy.

Even though no clear efficacy in treatment-resistant schizophrenia has been observed for olanzapine, most of the psychiatrists in an area of Northampton in the UK, who had prescribed olanzapine (nine psychiatrists, 41 patients), were happy to prescribe it when patients showed resistance to other antipsychotic drugs (168[C]).

The results of one of the clinical trials in which olanzapine (Eli Lilly) was compared with risperidone (Janssen Pharmaceutica) (see SEDA-22, 64) have given rise to a debate between researchers of the two pharmaceuticals companies on some of the possible flaws (169[r]–174[r]). Since the modal dosage over the 28-week trial was 7.2 mg/day, significantly higher than that used in actual clinical practice (average dose 4.6 mg/day), the higher incidence of risperidone-associated adverse effects could have been explained by this dosage difference.

The efficacy and safety of olanzapine in particular disorders, such as bipolar disorders (175[C], 176[C]), treatment-refractory childhood-onset schizophrenia (177[C]), or substance abuse, (178[C]) have been studied. Treatments other than lithium for the management of bipolar disorders include neuroleptic drugs. Of 14 consecutive patients with bipolar I disorder, who were inadequately responsive to standard psychotropic agents and who were given olanzapine, eight improved (175[C]). The most common adverse effects were *sedation, tremor, dry mouth,* and *increased appetite with weight gain.*

The response to olanzapine in 150 consecutive patients has been assessed by reviewing their records (176[C]). Patients with a moderate-to-marked response to olanzapine were more likely to be younger, to be female, and to have a diagnosis of bipolar disorder. No information on adverse effects was provided.

The efficacy of olanzapine in treatment-refractory childhood-onset schizophrenia has been examined in eight patients (mean age 15 years) over 8 weeks (177[C]). There was a 17% improvement in the BPRS total score. Olanzapine was moderately well tolerated. The most common adverse events were *increased appetite* (n = 6), *constipation* (n = 5), *nausea/vomiting* (n = 6), *headache* (n = 6), *somnolence* (n = 6), *insomnia* (n = 7), *difficulty in concentrating* (n = 5), *sustained tachycardia* (n = 6), *transient rises in liver transaminases* (n = 7), and *increased agitation* (n = 6).

In contrast, olanzapine was discontinued in all five preadolescent children (aged 6–11 years) within the first 6 weeks because of adverse effects or lack of therapeutic response (179[C]). The adverse effects included *sedation* (n = 3), *weight gain* (n = 3), and *akathisia* (n = 2). Furthermore, in the light of a case of intoxication in a 2.5-year-old boy who took one or two tablets of 7.5 mg and exhibited *agitation, aggressive behavior, miosis, hypersalivation, tachycardia*, and *ataxia*, it was stated that there is no recommended pediatric dose for olanzapine or any information on its effect on children (180[c]). A similar dose was well tolerated by an 8-year-old autistic boy (181[c]).

Substance abuse is a major complication in the treatment of schizophrenia. Of 60 patients with schizophrenia in an open 7-week trial of olanzapine up to 25 mg/day there was substance abuse in 23 (178[C]). There were no differences in response between the substance-abusing patients and the others. Baseline rates of extrapyramidal adverse effects did not differ between the groups. Overall the patients did not improve significantly.

Nervous system It has been suggested that in the treatment of negative symptoms of schizophrenia olanzapine may be better than haloperidol or risperidone, with fewer *extrapyramidal adverse effects* (SEDA-21, 56; SEDA-22, 64). Receptor occupancy may account for the extrapyramidal effects. To ascertain to what extent olanzapine occupies $5HT_2$ and dopamine D_2 receptors, a positron emission tomography study has been conducted in 12 patients with schizophrenia randomly assigned to 5, 10, 15, or 20 mg/day of olanzapine (182[C]). Olanzapine is a potent $5HT_2$ blocker and has higher $5HT_2$ than D_2 occupancy at all doses. Its D_2 occupancy is higher than that of clozapine and similar to that of risperidone. In the usual clinical dose range of 10–20 mg/day, D_2 occupancy is 71–80%, and this restricted range may explain its freedom from extrapyramidal adverse effects. However, doses of 30 mg/day and higher are associated with more than 80% D_2 occupancy and may have a higher likelihood of extrapyramidal adverse effects.

The relation between extrapyramidal adverse effects and the negative symptoms of schizophrenia has been studied (183[C]). Correlation analysis after 6 weeks of treatment showed that extrapyramidal symptoms correlated significantly in patients taking haloperidol (n = 10) but not in those taking olanzapine (n = 13). The results of multiple regression analysis suggested that ratings of negative signs were confounded by extrapyramidal symptoms in patients treated with haloperidol. This confusion occurred to a lesser extent with olanzapine.

Patients taking olanzapine reported a low incidence of *dystonias*, which may be about 0.3% (SEDA-22, 56). In the light of two new cases of acute dystonia associated with olanzapine in patients with previous history of dystonia or parkinsonism related to antipsychotic treatment, comparative figures have been reported. Acute dystonia occurred in 1.4% of patients who took olanzapine, compared with 5–6.3% of those taking haloperidol (184[cr]).

Whether treatment with olanzapine is useful in psychotic patients with neuroleptic-induced *parkinsonism*, or even in dopaminergic psychosis in Parkinson's disease, remains unclear. In a retrospective study of 19 patients with parkinsonism, 10 had some worsening of their parkinsonism after being treated with olanzapine, three had some motor benefit, and seven had improvement in their psychosis (185[C]). Olanzapine was also given to five patients with idiopathic Parkinson's disease and hallucinosis, and after initial treatment for 9 days, the frequency of hallucinations was significantly reduced; during this early phase of treatment, parkinsonian motor disability increased, which resulted in medication discontinuation in two of the patients (186[C]) . Worsening parkinsonism was also observed in two patients after treatment with olanzapine, 5 mg/day (187[c]). In contrast, coarse tremors induced by fluphenazine or haloperidol disappeared in three patients within days of the start of treatment with olanzapine (10 mg/day), without discontinuation or reduction in the dosage of fluphenazine or haloperidol (188[c]). Olanzapine is active at muscarinic cholinergic receptors, which may account for the observed suppression of neuroleptic-induced tremor; however, two of the three patients had been taking benzatropine, an antagonist at muscarinic acetylcholine receptors, with little tremor relief, suggesting that olanzapine could suppress tremor by means of an action other than antimuscarinic.

Akathisia has previously been reported in 16% of patients taking olanzapine (SEDA-21, 56). There has now been a report of three patients who developed severe akathisia during treatment with olanzapine (20–25 mg/day) (189[c]). In two patients the akathisia resolved after withdrawal of olanzapine; in one case, after complete remission of akathisia, olanzapine was well tolerated when reintroduced in combination with lorazepam. In the third patient, the akathisia was controlled by dosage reduction. A 33-year-old man with AIDS and a prior history of extrapyramidal symptoms with both typical antipsychotic drugs and risperidone developed dose-dependent akathisia with olanzapine 15–19 mg/day; the akathisia responded to dosage reduction and β-blockade (190[c]).

In contrast, olanzapine may sometimes improve pre-existing tardive dyskinesia (SEDA-22, 65). An elderly woman who developed moderately severe neuroleptic drug-induced dyskinetic movements responded to olanzapine 10 mg/day (191[c]).

A recent report of *neuroleptic malignant syndrome* associated with olanzapine, claimed to be the first, has been published (192[c]). The patient had all of the major manifestations of this condition and there was no other likely explanation for his illness; he had taken no other drug likely to be associated with the syndrome.

A 67-year-old man with bipolar disorder became confused, delirious, and manic. His only medications were olanzapine 10 mg/day and divalproex sodium 500 mg bd. On day 6, typical neuroleptic malignant syndrome developed. He had a fever (39.9°C), obtundation, rigidity, tremor, sweating, fluctuating pupillary diameter, labile tachycardia and hypertension, hypernatremia, and raised serum creatine kinase. Olanzapine was withdrawn and the syndrome resolved by day 12.

Another case of possible neuroleptic malignant syndrome associated with olanzapine has been reported in a patient who had taken clozapine for 3 years without incident. Symptoms suggestive of neuroleptic malignant syndrome appeared 19 days after the addition of olanzapine. This severe reaction could have resulted from clozapine alone or from an interaction of clozapine with olanzapine (193[c]).

Four patients taking olanzapine developed *speech dysfunction* (194[c]). The authors suggested that the incidence of speech abnormalities may be higher than listed in the package insert of olanzapine (impairment of articulation 2% and voice alteration less than 1%).

Psychiatric *Mania* has rarely been associated with classic neuroleptic drugs, but has been described in patients treated with new antipsychotic drugs, especially risperidone (SEDA-22, 69). Several cases of mania, presumably associated with olanzapine, have been reported (192[c], 195[c]–199[c]). The mechanism is not clear. It has been suggested that olanzapine could lead to manic symptoms in patients with schizophrenia because of its potent anti-$5HT_{2A}$ action.

Olanzapine-induced worsening of *obsessive–compulsive symptoms* has been reported (200[c]). The patient, a 35-year-old man, had had a similar response to both clozapine and risperidone in previous trials. In addition, a 35-year-old woman developed obsessive-compulsive symptoms after starting to take olanzapine (201[c]). Her symptoms remitted after withdrawal and recurred on rechallenge, which provides evidence for de novo provocation of obsessive-compulsive symptoms by olanzapine.

Paranoia and agitation occurred in two patients, a 34-year-old man and a 30-year-old woman, who had taken olanzapine for a few weeks (202[c]). Their symptoms improved when olanzapine was withdrawn.

Endocrine, metabolic Olanzapine may cause *increased serum prolactin concentrations*, but probably to a lesser extent than haloperidol does (SEDA-22, 65). Surprisingly, two women with antipsychotic-induced hyperprolactinemia, menstrual dysfunction, and galactorrhea had improvement in these adverse effects during treatment with olanzapine (203[c])

A 34-year-old woman, who developed *amenorrhea* while taking risperidone, regained her normal menstrual pattern along with a marked fall in serum prolactin concentration 8 weeks after being switched to olanzapine, whereas amantadine had failed to normalize the menses and had apparently reactivated the psychotic symptoms (204[c]). The authors suggested that olanzapine may offer advantages for selected patients in whom hyperprolactinemia occurs during treatment with other antipsychotic drugs.

Improvement in *galactorrhea* has also been observed in a case of trichotillomania refractory to a selective serotonin re-uptake inhibitor (205[c]). The patient only had a positive response with risperidone in combination with fluoxetine, but developed hyperprolactinemia and an intolerable galactorrhea. Olanzapine in combination with fluoxetine was started, with significant clinical improvement and without symptoms of galactorrhea; however, the patient had undesired weight gain of 3.6 kg after 22 weeks.

Significant *weight gain* occurs more often with olanzapine than with either haloperidol or risperidone (SEDA-22, 64). There has been a recent report of 15 patients with excessive weight gain associated with olanzapine (206[C]). The mean weight gain was 11 (range 3.6–25) kg and the mean duration of treatment was 7 (range 2–11) months.

According to the Physician's Desk Reference for 1998, *hyperglycemia* associated with olanzapine has a frequency of 1/100 to 1/1000. A recent report has drawn attention to this important reaction (207[c]).

A 32-year-old African–American man with no prior history of diabetes mellitus or glucose intolerance had a raised blood glucose concentration after 6 weeks of olanzapine therapy, and required insulin. Olanzapine was withdrawn and blood glucose concentrations returned to normal about 2 weeks later. At rechallenge hyperglycemia occurred again.

Hematological Olanzapine is relatively free of hematological adverse effects (SEDA-22, 65). Some explanations of the lower risk of *agranulocytosis* have been advanced after an in vitro cytotoxicity study (208). Like clozapine, olanzapine is oxidized to a reactive nitrenium ion by HOCl, the major oxidant produced in activated neutrophils. However, the olanzapine reactive metabolite has a lower propensity to cause toxicity to human neutrophils, monocytes, and HL-60 cells than the reactive clozapine nitrenium ion. The lower toxic potential of the olanzapine reactive metabolite, in conjunction with the lower therapeutic plasma concentrations of olanzapine compared with clozapine, may help to explain this difference between the drugs.

Seven patients, after developing *eosinophilia* (n = 1), *agranulocytosis*(n = 2), or *neutropenia* (n = 4) during neuroleptic drug therapy, were given olanzapine, with improvement and without evidence of blood dyscrasias (209[c], 210[c]). Nevertheless, a series of cases has linked early intervention with olanzapine, after discontinuation of clozapine because of agranulocytosis or neutropenia, to prolongation and worsening of agranulocytosis (SEDA-22, 65). In the light of that series, a recent review warned that this might reflect the fact that olanzapine shares many pharmacological properties with clozapine, which might make it more likely to prolong the clozapine-induced effect on white cells (211[r]).

Six cases of reduced hematological values (unspecified) associated with the use of olanzapine were reported to the Canadian Adverse Drug Reaction Monitoring Program from July 1996 to April 1998 (212[c]).

Gastrointestinal While hypersalivation is a common adverse effect of clozapine (SEDA-22, 60), dry mouth is associated with olanzapine (SEDA-21, 57; SEDA-22, 64). Drooling as an adverse effect of olanzapine has been reported in a 20-year-old woman (213[c]).

Sexual function The first two cases of *priapism* with olanzapine have been published (214[c], 215[c]). The first occurred in a 68-year-old patient taking olanzapine 5 mg at bedtime who required emergency surgery. In the second case, a 46-year-old patient taking olanzapine 15 mg/day, priapism remitted after withdrawal.

Overdosage Two deaths from overdosage of olanzapine have been described in a 59-year-old woman (216[c]) and a 43-year-old man (217[c]). In the first case, death was due to ingestion of an unknown quantity of olanzapine; however, the blood concentration (4.9 μg/ml) exceeded the usual target range of 10 ng/ml (based on the blood concentration of olanzapine administered in a repeated dosage of 10 mg/day) by nearly 500-fold. In the second case, death occurred within hours of the ingestion of as much as 600 mg of olanzapine and the drug concentration in a postmortem analysis of the blood was 1.24 μg/ml.

Interactions The pharmacokinetics of two single therapeutic doses of olanzapine have been determined in 11 healthy volunteers, before and after carbamazepine (218[C]). The dose of olanzapine given after pretreatment with carbamazepine was cleared more rapidly than olanzapine given alone. Olanzapine C_{max} and AUC were significantly lower after the second dose, the half-life was significantly shorter, and the clearance and volume of distribution were significantly increased. This interaction may be attributed to induction of CYP1A2 by carbamazepine, leading to increased first-pass and systemic metabolism of olanzapine.

Quetiapine *(SEDA-22, 65)*

The long-term efficacy and safety of quetiapine have yet to be determined. Data from short-term clinical trials (6 weeks) suggest that quetiapine may be useful for the management of psychotic disorders in patients who do not tolerate the adverse effects of the typical antipsychotic drugs or clozapine (219[R]). The most common adverse effects of quetiapine were *dizziness, hypotension, somnolence*, and *weight gain.* Dose-dependent decreases in total T_3 and T_4 and free T_4, without an increase in TSH, have been reported. Such changes have not been observed with other antipsychotic drugs. *Raised hepatic enzymes* have also been reported. In addition, two patients with idiopathic Parkinson's disease and psychosis were treated with quetiapine for 52 weeks (220[c]). Psychotic symptoms were successfully controlled without worsening of motor disability.

Risperidone *(SEDA-20, 52; SEDA-21, 57; SEDA-22, 66)*

Experience with risperidone has been reviewed with data from Canadian studies (221[R]). Furthermore, an important meta-analysis has compared risperidone with haloperidol (222[CR]). Six of the nine trials met criteria for inclusion, i.e. they were randomized and double-blind, had a duration of at least 4 weeks, and used risperidone in schizophrenic patients in a dosage range of 4–8 mg/day or in a flexible dose regimen. Risperidone was associated with higher clinical response rates (mean difference 14%; 95% CI = 5.6–22%), less prescribing of anticholinergic drugs (mean difference 18%; CI = 9.4–26%), and fewer treatment drop-outs (mean difference 13%; CI = 9.4–26%). It was concluded that risperidone was more efficacious than haloperidol, suggesting both a lower incidence of extrapyramidal symptoms and improved treatment compliance.

Similar conclusions have been reached in a Prescription Event Monitoring study of the safety of risperidone in 7684 patients treated in general practice (223[C]). Information on risperidone prescriptions issued to patients in England was gathered between July 1993 and April 1996. After 6 months, 76% of the patients for whom data were available were still taking risperidone. *Drowsiness/sedation* was the most frequent reason for stopping risperidone and the most frequently reported event (4.6 cases per 1000 patient-months). *Extrapyramidal symptoms* were rarely reported, the incidence being 3.2 per 1000 patient-months; they were more frequent in elderly patients (7.8 per 1000 patient-months). There were only four reports of *dyskinesias* and one report of *tardive dyskinesia*, which resulted in withdrawal of risperidone. Eight overdoses of risperidone alone were reported, with no serious clinical sequelae. Nine patients took risperidone during

10 pregnancies, with seven live births and three early therapeutic terminations. There were no abnormalities among the live births.

Long-term data on the efficacy and tolerability of risperidone are scant, as most of the clinical trials have been of short duration (no longer than 12 weeks). Some additional data from open studies have now emerged (224[C], 225[C]). In one of the studies, 386 patients with chronic schizophrenia took risperidone 2–16 mg/day for up 57 weeks; 247 patients were treated for at least 1 year (224[C]). All but 48 patients (88%) had been treated with antipsychotic drugs before entering the study. At the end of the study, 64% of the patients were rated as having improved on the Clinical Global Impression change scale, and extrapyramidal symptoms (scored on the Extrapyramidal Symptom Rating Scale (ESRS)) tended to be lower in severity or remained unchanged over the course of risperidone treatment; 27% of the patients required antiparkinsonian medication during the study, and 6.5% discontinued treatment prematurely because of adverse events. One or more adverse events were reported by 221 patients (57%) during risperidone treatment. *Extrapyramidal symptoms* occurred in 23%. *Insomnia and anxiety* were reported by 13 and 12% of patients. Two patients died during the 1-year study: one patient drowned and another committed suicide by hanging after 3.5 months. At the end of the study the mean *increase in body weight* was 1.8 kg.

In a retrospective study of 97patients taking risperidone under 30% of the patients were still taking risperidone after a mean period of follow-up of 102 (range 13–163) weeks (225[C]). Reasons for discontinuation included not achieving the desired therapeutic effect (n = 39), non-compliance (n = 22), adverse effects (n = 26), the patient's not liking the drug and requesting a change to a different medication (n = 17), and symptom remission (n = 6). The authors stated that in routine clinical practice the use of risperidone is plagued by many of the same problems of older antipsychotic drugs.

A randomized double-blind comparison of two dosage regimens of risperidone, 8 mg od and 4 mg bd for 6 weeks, in 211 patients has provided further information (226[C]). Neither efficacy nor ESRS scores differed significantly. At least one adverse event was reported in 72 of the patients taking once-daily therapy and 87 of the patients taking twice-daily therapy. The most frequently reported were *insomnia, anxiety, extrapyramidal symptoms, agitation*, and *headache*. The only statistically significant difference between the groups was in the incidence of anxiety, which was reported by 31% of those taking twice-daily therapy and 17% of those taking once-daily therapy.

The efficacy and safety of risperidone have been examined in special groups of patients, such as those with psychotic depression (227[C]), autistic disorders (228[C]), bipolar disorder (229[C]), mental retardation (230[C]), and children and adolescents (231[C]). For example, 62 patients with co-existing psychotic and depressive symptoms were included in a multicenter, randomized, double-blind comparison of the efficacy of risperidone (mean dose 6.9 mg/day) with that of a combination of haloperidol 9 mg/day and amitriptyline 180 mg/day (n = 61) over 6 weeks (227[C]). The results suggested that haloperidol plus amitriptyline was superior to risperidone alone. The incidence of *extrapyramidal adverse effects* was slightly higher with risperidone (37%) than haloperidol plus amitriptyline (31%); the use of concurrent anticholinergic drugs was significantly higher with risperidone (37%) than haloperidol plus amitriptyline (20%).

Adults with autistic disorder (n = 17) or pervasive developmental disorder not otherwise specified (n = 14) participated in a randomized, 12-week, double-blind, placebo-controlled trial of risperidone (228[C]). Among those who completed the study, risperidone (n = 14) was superior to placebo (n = 16) in reducing the symptoms of autism, and the most prominent adverse effect was mild transient sedation during the initial phase of drug administration. *Abnormal gait* was reported in one patient taking risperidone.

Patients with bipolar disorders may benefit from risperidone. This has been observed in an open trial of 10 patients with rapid cycling bipolar disorder who were refractory to lithium carbonate, carbamazepine, and valproate; eight improved after 6 months of treatment. One patient dropped out through non-compliance and one because of adverse effects (*agitation, anxiety, insomnia, and headache*) (229[C]). There was a similar beneficial effect in eight adults with moderate to profound mental retardation (230[C]). Risperidone was associated with a significant reduction in aggression and self injurious behavior, whereas adverse effects were primarily those of *sedation* and *restlessness*. Finally, eight of a heterogeneous group of 11 children and adolescents (mean age 9.8, range 5.5–16 years) with mood disorders and aggressive behavior, improved with a low dose of risperidone (0.75–2.5 mg/day) (231[C]). Treatment was stopped in two children because of *drowsiness*; the most bothersome adverse effect of risperidone was *weight gain* in two cases (mean increase 4 kg).

Nervous system The relation between anticholinergic effects and *cognitive adverse effects* has been studied in 22 patients (232[C]). Anticholinergic potency was indexed by a reduction in the receptor occupancy rates of quinuclidinyl benzylate. Patients who took clozapine ($n = 15$) had significantly higher anticholinergic concentrations than those who took risperidone ($n = 7$). However, they all had essentially equivalent scores on cognitive measures. These data suggest that anticholinergicity distinguishes clozapine and risperidone in vivo, but that this effect is not associated with differences in global cognitive functioning.

Risperidone produces dose-related *extrapyramidal adverse effects*, but at concentrations lower than those of conventional antipsychotic drugs (SED-13, 118; SEDA-21, 58, SEDA-22, 68). The relation between the degree of receptor occupancy and the presence of extrapyramidal symptoms is not clear, as observed in a recent SPECT study of 20 patients (233[C]). The frequency of risperidone-induced extrapyramidal signs, on the other hand, is intermediate between clozapine and conventional antipsychotic drugs, according to an open study in patients treated for at least 3 months with clozapine ($n = 41$; mean dose 426 mg/day), risperidone ($n = 23$; 4.7 mg/day), or conventional antipsychotic drugs ($n = 42$; 477 mg/day chlorpromazine equivalents) (234[C]). The point prevalence of akathisia was 7.3% in those who took clozapine, 13% in those who took risperidone, and 24% in those who took conventional antipsychotic drugs; the point prevalences of rigidity and cogwheeling were 4.9 and 2.4% respectively with clozapine, 17 and 17% with risperidone, and 36 and 26% with conventional antipsychotic drugs.

Elderly patients with dementia have been said to be at particular risk of developing extrapyramidal adverse effects, even with very low doses. In a 9-week, open-label, prospective study of risperidone for agitated behavior in 15 patients with dementia (modal dose 0.5 mg/day), extrapyramidal symptoms developed at some point during the trial in eight patients, and cognitive skills fell in three patients (235[C]). Similarly, in 22 patients with dementia and behavioral disturbances, treated with risperidone 1.5 mg/day (range 0.5 mg qds to 3 mg bd), 50% had significant improvement, but 50% had some extrapyramidal symptoms (236[C]). A further case of a severe extrapyramidal reaction in an old patient with dementia has further illustrated these risk factors (see reference 78 in Chapter 1).

Although several cases of sensitivity to risperidone with extrapyramidal signs in Lewy body dementia have previously been published (SEDA-20, 52), a case of successful treatment without extrapyramidal adverse effects has now been reported (237[c]). A 74-year-old man with Lewy body dementia treated with a combination of donezepil (5 mg in the evening) and risperidone (0.25 mg/day), had significant improvement, objectively and subjectively, within 2 weeks.

Intolerable exacerbation of *parkinsonism* with risperidone has previously been reported (SEDA-20, 52). In contrast, eight patients (five women, three men) with advanced Parkinson's disease, motor fluctuations, and levodopa-induced dyskinesia took part in an open study with a low dosage of risperidone (mean 0.187 mg/day); after an average of 11 months all the patients had moderate to pronounced reduction in levodopa-induced dyskinesia (238[C]). However, whether risperidone should be used in patients with Parkinson's disease is a subject of debate (239[r], 240[r]).

Tardive dyskinesia has occasionally been reported with risperidone (SEDA-20, 53; SEDA-21, 59; SEDA-22, 68), and several new cases have emerged (241[c]–244[c]). In two cases, advanced age and dementia may have been contributing factors.

Neuroleptic malignant syndrome has previously been associated with risperidone (SEDA-20, 52; SEDA-21, 59; SEDA-22, 68), and two new cases have been reported (245[c], 246[c]). In another case, a patient with schizoaffective disorder, who developed risperidone-related neuroleptic malignant syndrome, responded satisfactorily to supportive management and vitamin E plus vitamin B_6 (247[c]).

Psychiatric Anxiety and behavioral stimulation characterized by *anxiety, insomnia*, and *restlessness* during risperidone treatment have previously been reported (SEDA-20, 53;

SEDA-22, 69). Now, six of 13 out-patients who took part in a 10-week open trial of risperidone had an good initial response, followed by intolerable effects, including feelings of agitation and depression and periods of crying and insomnia (248[C]). The patients who developed this syndrome had a significantly higher mean baseline rating on the Brief Psychiatric Rating Scale anxiety subscale.

Obsessive-compulsive symptoms (SEDA-22, 69) developed in a 26-year-old Chinese woman taking risperidone for a chronic schizophrenic illness (249[c]). She had no history of obsessive-compulsive symptoms. Risperidone 2 mg/day, benzhexol 2 mg/day, and diazepam 10 mg at night had been prescribed after she had had adverse effects with other antipsychotic drugs.

Endocrine, metabolic *Hyperprolactinemia* and *galactorrhea* have previously been reported (SEDA-20, 53; SEDA-22, 69). Now a greater but non-significant prolactogenic effect associated with risperidone (n = 14) has been observed in an open comparison of risperidone with other neuroleptic drugs (n = 14) (250[C]).

There was a significant rise in baseline serum prolactin concentration in 10 patients after they had taken risperidone for a mean of 12 weeks (251[C]). They were compared with 10 patients who were tested after a neuroleptic drug-free wash-out period of at least 2 weeks.

Galactorrhea associated with a rise in prolactin occurred after a few weeks of treatment with risperidone in two women aged 24 and 39 (252[c]). One of them was switched to thioridazine, with an improvement in the galactorrhea, and the other continued to take risperidone owing to a robust response; her galactorrhea was partially treated with bromocriptine.

Pathological *weight gain* has been increasingly identified as a problem when atypical neuroleptic drugs are given to children (SEDA-21, 57; SEDA-22, 69). In one case unremitting weight gain, triggered by risperidone, was eventually curbed through the use of a diet containing slowly absorbed carbohydrates and a careful balance of carbohydrates, proteins, and fats (253[c]).

A 9-year-old boy with autism and overactivity was unresponsive to several drugs. Risperidone 0.5 mg bd was effective, reducing his Aberrant Behavior Checklist score from 103 to 57 by the end of the first week. Four weeks later his weight had risen from 34.6 to 37 kg. This rate of weight gain (0.6 kg/week) continued over the next 12 weeks. His weight was then contained by the use of the 'Zone' diet, with an emphasis on slowly absorbed carbohydrates (examples include apples, oatmeal, kidney beans, whole-grain pasta, and sweet potatoes) in a calorie-reduced diet containing 30% proteins and 30% fats.

Hematological Risperidone has occasionally been associated with blood dyscrasias (SEDA-21, 59; SEDA-22, 69). A 40-year-old woman developed *agranulocytosis* after taking risperidone for 2 weeks (254[c]). She had also developed agranulocytosis after treatment with several other antipsychotic drugs (chlorpromazine, haloperidol, and zuclopenthixol).

Liver There have been some published reports of *hepatotoxicity* associated with risperidone in adults (SEDA-21, 59). Two new cases, one in a 81-year-old man who took only two doses of risperidone 0.5 mg (255[c]) and the other in a 25-year-old woman (256[c]), have been reported. In the second case, liver function tests were 2.6–7.4 times higher than the upper limit of the reference range.

Risperidone has been implicated in hepatotoxicity and weight gain in boys taking long-term risperidone (SEDA-22, 69). An additional case of *liver enzyme rises and fatty liver infiltration* in the context of pre-existing obesity has been published (257[c]). The patient, a 13-year-old girl, developed the condition after taking risperidone 0.5 mg/day for 3 days.

Urinary system *Hemorrhagic cystitis* associated with risperidone has been reported, purportedly for the first time (258[c]).

An 11-year-old boy developed acute dysuria and increased frequency accompanied by gross hematuria. He was taking fluoxetine, valproic acid, benzatropine, haloperidol, clonidine, trazodone, and nasal desmopressin. One week before presentation, risperidone had been introduced instead of haloperidol to improve behavioral control. The risperidone was discontinued and haloperidol resumed, and his symptoms resolved during the following week.

Immunological and hypersensitivity reactions Risperidone has been rarely associated with allergic reactions (SEDA-22, 70). A case of *photosensitivity* has recently been reported in a 69-year-old woman (259[c]). She had an erythematous rash with areas of blistering and early desquamation. It was most pronounced in exposed areas, although there was some spread beyond.

Risk factors *Age* It has been previously stated that delirium occurs in 1.6% of elderly patients newly treated with risperidone (SEDA-22, 70). Several new cases have been reported in patients of advanced age (260[c], 261[c]). It is suggested that in these patients, treatment should begin with low dosages (0.25–0.5 mg/day) and that the dosage be gradually increased over several days with close monitoring.

A case of hypothermia associated with hypothalamic and thermoregulatory dysfunction has been reported in a patient with Prader-Willi syndrome taking risperidone and olanzapine (262[c]). Hypothermia in response to these drugs is said to result from $5HT_2$ receptor blockade and it is recommended that patients with hypothalamic dysfunction should be carefully monitored if risperidone or olanzapine are administered.

Withdrawal effects Serious withdrawal effects have occasionally been reported with risperidone (SEDA-21, 60; SEDA-22, 70). Both manic and psychotic symptoms have been described in a chronic schizophrenic patient on risperidone withdrawal (263[c]).

A 38-year-old Chinese man had responded to risperidone monotherapy for 2 weeks after 19 years of resistance to other classical agents. Three days later he lost his medicine and 2 days later his auditory hallucinations and persecutory delusions recurred. Meanwhile, vivid manic symptoms (such as heightened mood, irritability, reduced need for sleep, hyperactivity, pressured speech, flight of ideas, and grandiosity) emerged for the first time throughout the history of his illness.

Overdosage Cases of overdosage of risperidone have previously been reported (SEDA-22, 71). During 13 months a regional poisons center gathered information by telephone on 31 patients with reported risperidone overdose (264[C]). Risperidone was the sole ingestant in 15 cases (1–180 mg). The major effects in this group included lethargy (n = 7), spasm/dystonia (n = 3), hypotension (n = 2), tachycardia (n = 6), and dysrhythmias (n = 1). One patient who co-ingested imipramine died of medical complications, but symptoms resolved within 24 hours in most of the others; all patients were asymptomatic at 72 hours after ingestion.

Interactions A potential pharmacokinetic interaction between risperidone and *carbamazepine* has previously been reported (SEDA-22, 71). Carbamazepine induces CYP3A, and the metabolism of risperidone, which mainly involves CYP2D6, may also involve CYP3A. Accordingly, carbamazepine can reduce risperidone plasma concentrations. However, since carbamazepine alters the biotransformation of many agents, non-specific enzyme induction has been suggested for the risperidone and carbamazepine interaction (265[c]).

A likely pharmacokinetic interaction of risperidone with *fluoxetine* has previously been reported (SEDA-22, 71). The possibility of an added pharmacodynamic interaction between risperidone and serotonin re-uptake inhibitors has been discussed (266[r]–268[r]). Published cases of amelioration and deterioration have perpetuated the debate. Amelioration was observed in four patients with depression that had responded inadequately to selective serotonin re-uptake inhibitors by the addition of risperidone 1 mg bd (n = 2) or 0.5 mg at night (n = 2) (269[c]). Catastrophic deterioration, with the severity of obsessive-compulsive symptoms returning to pretreatment levels, was observed in a 21-year-old man when risperidone was added to fluoxetine in a dosage that was stepped up to 3 mg/day (270[c]). The different dosages used probably account for the differences in responses.

The addition of risperidone 10 mg/day over 2 months to *valproate* and *clonazepam* in a 40-year-old woman provoked marked edema in the legs and moderate edema in the arms (271[c]). The authors considered that this was a possible interaction, since edema has not been reported with either of these drug separately.

Catatonia has been reported in a 42-year-old woman taking *valproic acid*, sertraline, and risperidone (272[c]). The catatonic features evolved for the first time after a single dose of valproate and were alleviated by lorazepam; the same catatonic signs recurred after a second dose of valproate and again remitted after lorazepam. The authors considered that this was a possible interaction, since catatonia has not been reported with valproate alone. However, in contrast, a beneficial interaction has been observed when valproic acid was added to risperidone; the previous addition of valproic acid to treatment with chlorpromazine had no effect on psychotic symptoms (273[c]).

Monitoring therapy A therapeutic target range for serum risperidone concentrations has not been established, but in 20 of 22 patients taking 6 mg/day, which is considered the optimum dosage for most patients, risperidone serum concentrations were 50–150 nmol/l (274[C]). Steady-state serum concentrations of risperidone and 9-hydroxyrisperidone, the active moiety, were also measured in 42 patients; there was no correlation between the serum concentration of the active moiety and adverse effects.

Ziprasidone

Ziprasidone is a dopamine D_2 receptor antagonist with a much higher affinity for $5HT_{2A}$ receptors than for D_2 receptors. Ziprasidone 160 mg/day is as effective as haloperidol 15 mg/day, and is less likely to cause *extrapyramidal symptoms*. This has been the conclusion of a recent study in which, after a single-blind wash-out period of 4–7 days, patients were randomly assigned to one of four dosages of ziprasidone 4 mg/day (n = 19), 10 mg/day (n = 17), 40 mg/day (n = 17), or 160 mg/day (n = 20), or haloperidol 15 mg/day (n = 17) for 4 weeks (275[C]). Concomitant benzatropine use at any time during the study was less frequent with ziprasidone 160 mg/day (15%) than with haloperidol (53%). One patient taking ziprasidone 4 mg/day had *confusion and hyponatremia*, and another taking 40 mg/day had *seizures*.

Zotepine *(SEDA-22, 72)*

The use of zotepine in short-term trials (4–8 weeks) has been reviewed (276[R]). Comparisons have been carried out with haloperidol (3 trials; n = 212), chlorpromazine (two trials; n = 328), perazine (two trials; n = 81), and thiothixene (one trial; n = 94). In these double-blind trials, zotepine 150–300 mg/day was as effective as typical antipsychotic drugs in controlling the symptoms of schizophrenia. The results suggested that zotepine may be effective in the management of patients with negative symptoms and in those with treatment-resistant schizophrenia. The most common adverse effects of zotepine were *constipation, dry mouth, insomnia, sleepiness, weakness, and weight gain*. The incidence of extrapyramidal symptoms was 8–29%, significantly less than with haloperidol and chlorpromazine, but there were no differences between zotepine and some other typical antipsychotic drugs in this respect. There was an increase in the risk of generalized seizures with zotepine at dosages over 300 mg/day. No clinically relevant hematological abnormalities have been reported to date.

DEPOT FORMULATIONS

Guidelines for depot antipsychotic drug treatment in schizophrenia were developed during a consensus conference held in 1995 in Siena in Italy. A thorough review devoted to depot antipsychotic drugs has now been published (277[R]). The authors reported that depot antipsychotic drugs are associated with significantly fewer relapses and rehospitalizations than oral antipsychotic drugs. The potential disadvantages of depot drugs include patient reluctance to accept injections or a sense of being overly controlled. In addition, clinicians, and sometimes patients, fear that if adverse effects do occur they will be more difficult to manage because of an inability to withdraw treatment rapidly. In terms of adverse effects, these formulations are not associated with a significantly higher incidence of adverse effects than oral drugs. Some patients have *pain or discomfort at the injection site*. In some cases *the injection site becomes edematous and tender or pruritic*, with a palpable mass for up to 3 months. It is recommended to rotate the injection site, to limit the volume of the injection, and to assure deep intramuscular injection.

REFERENCES

1. Perry S. Report from the Swedish Council on Technology Assessment in Health Care (SBU). Treatment with neuroleptics. Int J Technol Assess Health Care 1998;14:394–400.
2. Bandelow B, Fritze J, Rüther E. Increased mortality in schizophrenia and the possible influence of antipsychotic treatment. Int J Psychiatry Clin Pract 1998;2(Suppl 2):S49–S57.

3. Jibson MD, Tandon R. New atypical antipsychotic medications. J Psychiatr Res 1998; 32:215–28.
4. Meltzer HY, Casey DE, Garver DL, Lasagna L, Marder SR, Masand PS, Miller D, Pickar D, Tandon R. Adverse effects of the atypical antipsychotics. J Clin Psychiatry 1998;59(Suppl 12):17–22.
5. Meltzer HY, Casey DE, Garver DL, Lasagna L, Marder SR, Masand PS, Miller D, Pickar D, Tandon R. Assessment of EPS and tardive dyskinesia in clinical trials. J Clin Psychiatry 1998;59(Suppl 12):23–7.
6. Day JC, Kinderman P, Bentall R. A comparison of patients' and prescribers' beliefs about neuroleptic side-effects: prevalence, distress and causation. Acta Psychiatr Scand 1998; 97:93–7.
7. Agarwal MR, Sharma VK, Kishore Kumar KV, Lowe D. Non-compliance with treatment in patients suffering from schizophrenia: a study to evaluate possible contributing factors. Int J Soc Psychiatry 1998;44: 92–106.
8. Sharma ND, Rosman HS, Padhi ID, Tisdale JE. Torsades de pointes associated with intravenous haloperidol in critically ill patients. Am J Cardiol 1998;81:238–40.
9. Michalets EL, Smith LK, Van Tassel ED. Torsade de pointes resulting from the addition of droperidol to an existing cytochrome P450 drug interaction. Ann Pharmacother 1998;32:761–5.
10. Thomas SH, Cooper PN. Sudden death in a patient taking antipsychotic drugs. Postgrad Med J 1998;74:445–6.
11. Barber JM. Risk of sudden death on high-dose antipsychotic medication: QT_c dispersion. Br J Psychiatry 1998;173:86–7.
12. Yanovski A, Kron RE, Townsend RR, Ford V. The clinical utility of ambulatory blood pressure and heart rate monitoring in psychiatric inpatients. Am J Hypertens 1998;11:309–15.
13. Madsen AL, Keidling N, Karle A, Esbjerg S, Hemmingsen R. Neuroleptics in progressive structural brain abnormalities in psychiatric illness. Lancet 1998;352:784–5.
14. Browne S, Garavan J, Gervin M, Roe M, Larkin C, O'Callaghan E. Quality of life in schizophrenia: insight and subjective response to neuroleptics. J Nerv Ment Dis 1998;186:74–8.
15. Perenyi A, Norman T, Hopwood M, Burrows G. Negative symptoms, depression, and parkinsonian symptoms in chronic, hospitalised schizophrenic patients. J Affect Disord 1998;48:163–9.
16. Heinz A, Knable MB, Coppola R, Gorey JG, Jones DW, Lee KS, Weinberger DR. Psychomotor slowing, negative symptoms and dopamine receptor availability – an IBZM SPECT study in neuroleptic-treated and drug-free schizophrenic patients. Schizophr Res 1998;31:19–26.
17. Seeman P, Tallerico T. Antipsychotic drugs which elicit little or no Parkinsonism bind more loosely than dopamine to brain D_2 receptors, yet occupy high levels of these receptors. Mol Psychiatry 1998;3:123–34.
18. Kumra S, Jacobsen LK, Lenane M, Smith A, Lee P, Malanga CJ, Karp BI, Hamburger S, Rapoport JL. Case series: spectrum of neuroleptic-induced movement disorders and extrapyramidal side effects in childhood-onset schizophrenia. J Am Acad Child Adolesc Psychiatry 1998;37:221–7
19. Ballard C, Grace J, McKeith I, Holmes C. Neuroleptic sensitivity in dementia with Lewy bodies and Alzheimer's disease. Lancet 1998;351:1032–3.
20. Caligiuri MP, Rockwell E, Jeste DV. Extrapyramidal side effects in patients with Alzheimer's disease treated with low-dose neuroleptic medication. Am J Geriatr Psychiatry 1998;6:75–82.
21. Mirsattari SM, Power C, Nath A. Parkinsonism with HIV infection. Mov Disord 1998;13:684–9.
22. Kompoliti K, Goetz CG. Hyperkinetic movement disorders misdiagnosed as tics in Gilles de la Tourette syndrome. Mov Disord 1998;13: 477–80.
23. Chetty M, Gouws E, Miller R, Moodley SV. The use of a side effect as a qualitative indicator of plasma chlorpromazine levels. Eur Neuropsychopharmacol 1999;9:77–82.
24. Rapoport A, Stein D, Shamir E, Schwartz M, Levine J, Elizur A, Weizman A. Clinico-tremorgraphic features of neuroleptic-induced tremor. Int Clin Psychopharmacol 1998;13:115–20.
25. Kasantikul D. Drug-induced akathisia and suicidal tendencies in psychotic patients. J Med Assoc Thailand 1998;81:551–4.
26. Smith M. Case report: akathisia abolished by passive movement. Acta Psychiatr Scand 1998;97:168–9.
27. Chaplin R, Kent A. Informing patients about tardive dyskinesia. Controlled trial of patient education. Br J Psychiatry 1998;172:78–81.
28. Tsai G, Goff DC, Chang RW, Flood J, Baer L, Coyle JT. Markers of glutamatergic neurotransmission and oxidative stress associated with tardive dyskinesia. Am J Psychiatry 1998;155:1207–13.
29. Wirshing DA, Bartzokis G, Pierre JM, Wirshing WC, Sun A, Tishler TA, Marder SR. Tardive dyskinesia and serum iron indices. Biol Psychiatry 1998;44:493–8.
30. Van Harten PN, Hoek HW, Matroos GE, Koeter M, Kahn RS. Intermittent neuroleptic treatment and risk for tardive dyskinesia: Curacao extrapyramidal syndromes study. Am J Psychiatry 1998;155:565–7.
31. Byne W, White L, Parella M, Adams R, Harvey PD, Davis KL. Tardive dyskinesia in a chronically institutionalized population of elderly schizophrenic patients: prevalence and association with cognitive impairment. Int J Geriatr Psychiatry 1998;13:473–9.
32. Woerner MG, Alvir JM, Saltz BL, Lieberman JA, Kane JM. Prospective study of tardive dyskinesia in the elderly: rates and risk factors. Am J Psychiatry 1998;155:1521–8.
33. McDermid SA, Hood J, Bockus S, D'Alessandro E. Adolescents on neuroleptic medication: is this population at risk for tardive dyskinesia? Can J Psychiatry 1998;43:629–31.
34. Gervin M, Browne S, Lane A, Clarke M, Waddington JL, Larkin C, O'Callaghan E. Spontaneous abnormal involuntary movements in first-

episode schizophrenia and schizophreniform disorder: baseline rate in a group of patients from an Irish catchment area. Am J Psychiatry 1998;155:1202–6.

35. Parker G, Lambert T, McGrath J, McGorry P, Tiller J. Neuroleptic management of schizophrenia: a survey and commentary on Australian psychiatric practice. Aust NZ J Psychiatry 1998;32:50–8.
36. Connor DF. Stimulants and neuroleptic withdrawal dyskinesia. J Am Acad Child Adolesc Psychiatry 1998;37:247–8.
37. Ross DE, Buchanan RW, Lahti AC, Medoff D, Bartko JJ, Compton AD, Thaker GK. The relationship between smooth pursuit eye movements and tardive dyskinesia in schizophrenia. Schizophr Res 1998;31:141–50.
38. Lerner V, Liberman M. Movement disorders and psychotic symptoms treated with pyridoxine: a case report. J Clin Psychiatry 1998;59:623–4.
39. Barak Y, Swartz M, Shamir E, Stein D, Weizman A. Vitamin E (α-tocopherol) in the treatment of tardive dyskinesia: a statistical meta-analysis. Ann Clin Psychiatry 1998;10:101–5.
40. Brown K, Reid A, White T, Henderson T, Hukin S, Johnstone C, Glen A. Vitamin E, lipids, and lipid peroxidation products in tardive dyskinesia. Biol Psychiatry 1998;43:863–7.
41. Hayashi T, Furutani M, Taniyama J, Kiyasu M, Hikasa S, Horiguchi J, Yamawaki S. Neuroleptic-induced Meige's syndrome following akathisia: pharmacologic characteristics. Psychiatry Clin Neurosci 1998;52:445–8.
42. Van Harten PN, Van Trier JC, Horwitz EH, Matroos GE, Hoek HW. Cocaine as a risk factor for neuroleptic-induced acute dystonia. J Clin Psychiatry 1998;59:128–30.
43. Burke RE, Fahn S, Jaankovic J, Marsden CD, Lang Ae, Gollomp S. Tardive dystonia: late-onset and persistent dystonia caused by antipsychotic drugs. Neurology 1982;32:1335–46.
44. Kiriakakis V, Bhatia KP, Quinn NP, Marsden CD. The natural history of tardive dystonia. A long-term follow-up study of 107 cases. Brain 1998;121:2053–66.
45. Molho ES, Feustel PJ, Factor SA. Clinical comparison of tardive and idiopathic cervical dystonia. Mov Disord 1998;13:486–9.
46. Maeda K, Ohsaki T, Kuki K, Kin K, Ikeda M, Matsumoto Y. Severe antecollis during antipsychotics treatment: a report of three cases. Prog Neuropsychopharmacol Biol Psychiatry 1998;22:749–59.
47. Krack P, Schneider S, Deuschl G. Geste device in tardive dystonia with retrocollis and opisthotonic posturing. Mov Disord 1998;13:155–7.
48. Raja M. Managing antipsychotic-induced acute and tardive dystonia. Drug Saf 1998;19:57–72.
49. Looper KJ, Chouinard G. Beneficial effects of combined L-dopa and central anticholinergic in a patient with severe drug-induced Parkinsonism and tardive dystonia. Can J Psychiatry 1998;43:646–7.
50. Mennesson M, Klink BA, Fortin AH 6th. Case study: worsening Tourette's disorder or withdrawal dystonia? J Am Acad Child Adolesc Psychiatry 1998;37:785–8.
51. Hasan S, Buckley P. Novel antipsychotics and the neuroleptic malignant syndrome: a review and critique. Am J Psychiatry 1998;155:1113–16.
52. Caroff SN, Mann SC, McCarthy M, Naser J, Rynn M, Morrison M. Acute infectious encephalitis complicated by neuroleptic malignant syndrome. J Clin Psychopharmacol 1998; 18:349–51.
53. Tanaka K, Akechi T, Yamazaki M, Hayashi R, Nishiwaki Y, Uchitomi Y. Neuroleptic malignant syndrome during haloperidol treatment in a cancer patient: a case report. Supportive Care Cancer 1998;6:536–8.
54. Alexander PJ, Thomas RM, Das A. Is risk of neuroleptic malignant syndrome increased in the postpartum period? J Clin Psychiatry 1998; 59:254–5.
55. Rasmussen KG. Risk factors for neuroleptic malignant syndrome. Am J Psychiatry 1998; 155:1639.
56. Francis A, Chandragiri S, Petrides G. Risk factors for neuroleptic malignant syndrome. Am J Psychiatry 1998;155:1639–40.
57. Sachdev P. Risk factors for neuroleptic malignant syndrome. Replies. Am J Psychiatry 1998;155:1639–40.
58. Lee JW. Serum iron in catatonia and neuroleptic malignant syndrome. Biol Psychiatry 1998; 44:499–507.
59. Cullinane CA, Brumfield C, Flint LM, Ferrara JJ. Neuroleptic malignant syndrome associated with multiple joint dislocations in a trauma patient. J Trauma Inj Infect Crit Care 1998;45:168–71.
60. Garrido SM, Chauncey TR. Neuroleptic malignant syndrome following autologous peripheral blood stem cell transplantation. Bone Marrow Transplant 1998;21:427–8.
61. Blasi C, D'Amore F, Levati M, Bandinelli MC. Sindrome maligna da neurolettici: una patologia neurologica di grande interesse per l'internista. Ann Ital Med Interna 1998;13:111–16.
62. Elizalde-Sciavolino C, Racco A, Proscia-Lieto T, Kleiner M. Severe hyponatremia, neuroleptic malignant syndrome, rhabdomyolysis and acute renal failure: a case report. Mt Sinai J Med 1998;65:284–8.
63. Yoshino A, Yoshimasu H, Tatsuzawa Y, Asakura T, Hara T. Nonconvulsive status epilepticus in two patients with neuroleptic malignant syndrome. J Clin Psychopharmacol 1998;18:347–9.
64. Tsujimoto S, Maeda K, Sugiyama T, Yokochi A, Chikusa H, Maruyama K. Efficacy of prolonged large-dose dantrolene for severe neuroleptic malignant syndrome. Anesth Analg 1998;86:1143–4.
65. Pollock A, McLaren EH. Serum prolactin concentration in patients taking neuroleptic drugs. Clin Endocrinol 1998;49:513–16.
66. Spitzer M, Sajjad R, Benjamin F. Pattern of development of hyperprolactinemia after initiation of haloperidol therapy. Obstet Gynecol 1998;91:693–5.
67. Feek CM, Sawers JS, Brown NS, Seth J, Irvine WJ, Toft AD. Influence of thyroid status on dopa-

minergic inhibition of thyrotropin and prolactin secretion: evidence for an additional feedback mechanism in the control of thyroid hormone secretion. J Clin Endocrinol Metab 1980;51:585-9.

68. Magharious W, Goff DC, Amico E. Relationship of gender and menstrual status to symptoms and medication side effects in patients with schizophrenia. Psychiatry Res 1998;77:159–66.
69. King DJ, Wager E. Haematological safety of antipsychotic drugs. J Psychopharmacol 1998;12:283–8.
70. Shah GK, Auerbach DB, Augsburger JJ, Savino PJ. Acute thioridazine retinopathy. Arch Ophthalmol 1998;116:826–7.
71. Weiner DM, Lowe FC. Psychotropic drug-induced priapism: Incidence, mechanism and management. CNS Drugs 1998;9:371–9.
72. Demyttenaere K, De Fruyt J, Sienaert P. Psychotropics and sexuality. Int Clin Psychopharmacol 1998;13(Suppl 6):S35–S41.
73. Valevski A, Modai I, Zbarski E, Zemishlany Z, Weizman A. Effect of amantadine on sexual dysfunction in neuroleptic-treated male schizophrenic patients. Clin Neuropharmacol 1998;21:355–7.
74. Abe S, Suzuki T, Hori T, Baba A, Shiraishi H. Hypogammaglobulinemia during antipsychotic therapy. Psychiatry Clin Neurosci 1998;52:115–17.
75. Lillicrap MS, Wright G, Jones AC. Symptomatic antiphospholipid syndrome induced by chlorpromazine. Br J Rheumatol 1998;37:346–7.
76. Pramatarov KD. Drug-induced lupus erythematosus. Clin Dermatol 1998;16:367–77.
77. Krohn K, Bennett R. Drug-induced autoimmune disorders. Inmunol Allergy Clin North Am 1998;18:897–911.
78. Lewis R. Typical and atypical antipsychotics in adolescent schizophrenia: efficacy, tolerability, and differential sensitivity to extrapyramidal symptoms. Can J Psychiatry 1998;43:596–604.
79. Toren P, Laor N, Weizman A. Use of atypical neuroleptics in child and adolescent psychiatry. J Clin Psychiatry 1998;59:644–56.
80. Naja WJ, Reneric JP, Bouvard MP. Neuroleptiques atypiques chez l'enfant et l'adolescent. Encephale 1998;24:378–85.
81. Devanand DP, Marder K, Michaels KS, Sackeim HA, Bell K, Sullivan MA, Cooper TB, Pelton GH, Mayeux R . A randomized, placebo-controlled dose-comparison trial of haloperidol for psychosis and disruptive behaviors in Alzheimer's disease. Am J Psychiatry 1998;155:1512–20.
82. Bigatti MP, Corona D, Munizza C. Increased sister chromatid exchange and chromosomal aberration frequencies in psychiatric patients receiving psychopharmacological therapy. Mutat Res Genet Toxicol Environ Mutagen 1998;413:169–75.
83. Bonassi S, Abbondandolo A, Camurri I, Dal Prà L, De Ferrari M, Degrassi F, Forni A, Lamberti I, Lando C, Padovani P, Sbrana I, Vecchio D, Puntoni R. Are chromosome aberrations in circulating lymphocytes predictive of future cancer onset in humans? Preliminary results of an Italian cohort study. Cancer Genet Cytogenet 1995;79:133–5.
84. Austin MP, Mitchell PB. Psychotropic medications in pregnant women: treatment dilemmas. Med J Aust 1998;169:428–31.
85. Cohen LS, Rosenbaum JF. Psychotropic drug use during pregnancy: weighing the risks. J Clin Psychiatry 1998;59(Suppl 2):18–28.
86. Currier GW, Simpson GM. Antipsychotic medications and fertility. Psychiatr Serv 1998;49:175–6.
87. Buckley N, McManus P. Fatal toxicity of drugs used in the treatment of psychotic illnesses. Br J Psychiatry 1998;172:461–4.
88. Zumbrunner TL, Jann MW. Drug interactions with antipsychotic agents. Incidence and therapeutic implications. CNS Drugs 1998;9:381–401.
89. Bourin M, Baker GB. Therapeutic and adverse effect considerations when using combinations of neuroleptics and benzidiazepines. Saudi Pharm Journal 1998;3–4:262–5.
90. Hatta K, Takahashi T, Nakamura H, Yamashiro H, Endo H, Kito K, Saeki T, Masui K, Yonezawa Y. A risk for obstruction of the airways in the parenteral use of levomepromazine with benzodiazepine. Pharmacopsychiatry 1998;31:126–30.
91. Freeman MP, Stoll AL. Mood stabilizer combinations: a review of safety and efficacy. Am J Psychiatry 1998;155:12–21.
92. Benazzi F. Urinary retention with sertraline, haloperidol, and clonazepam combination. Can J Psychiatry 1998;43:1051–2.
93. Kurlan R. Acute parkinsonism induced by the combination of a serotonin reuptake inhibitor and a neuroleptic in adults with Tourette's syndrome. Mov Disord 1998;13:178–9.
94. Lee MS, Kim YK, Lee SK, Suh KY. A double-blind study of adjunctive sertraline in haloperidol-stabilized patients with chronic schizophrenia. J Clin Psychopharmacol 1998;18:399–403.
95. Puech A, Fleurot O, Rein W. Amisulpride, and atypical antipsychotic, in the treatment of acute episodes of schizophrenia: a dose-ranging study vs haloperidol. Acta Psychiatr Scand 1998;98:65–72.
96. Wetzel H, Gründer G, Hillert A, Philipp M, Gattaz WF, Sauer H, Adler G, Schröeder J, Rein W, Benkert O. Amisulpride versus flupentixol in schizophrenia with predominantly positive symptomatology – a double-blind controlled study comparing a selective D_2-like antagonist to a mixed D_1/D_2-like antagonist. Psychopharmacology 1998;137:223–32.
97. Chabannes JP, Pelissolo A, Farah S, Gerard D. Evaluation de l'efficacité et de la tolérance de l'ámisulpride dans le traitement des psychoses schizophréniques. Encephale 1998;24:386–92.
98. Hamon-Vilcot B, Chaufour S, Deschamps C, Canal M, Zieleniuk I, Ahtoy P, Chretien P, Rosenzweig P, Nasr A, Piette F. Safety and pharmacokinetics of a single oral dose of amisulpride in healthy elderly volunteers. Eur J Clin Pharmacol 1998;54:405–9.
99. Buchanan RW, Breier A, Kirkpatrick B, Ball P, Carpenter WT Jr. Positive and negative symptom response to clozapine in schizophrenic pa-

tients with and without the deficit syndrome. Am J Psychiatry 1998;155:751–60.
100. Connelly JC, Fullick J. Experience with clozapine in a community mental health care setting. South Med J 1998;91:838–41.
101. Chong SA, Mahendran R, Wong KE. Use of atypical neuroleptics in a state mental institute. Ann Acad Med Singapore 1998;27:547–51.
102. Ghaemi SN, Ziegler DM, Peachey TJ, Goodwin FK. Cost-effectiveness of clozapine therapy for severe psychosis. Psychiatr Serv 1998;49:829–31.
103. Bret P, Jolivel C, Bret MC, Veylit S, Martin C, Garcia P. Etude médico-économique du Léponex (clozapine) au centre hospitalier Charles Perrens de Bordeaux. Encephale 1998;24:365–77.
104. Benedetti F, Sforzini L, Colombo C, Maffei C, Smeraldi E. Low-dose clozapine in acute and continuation treatment of severe borderline personality disorder. J Clin Psychiatry 1998;59:103–7.
105. Hector RI. The use of clozapine in the treatment of aggressive schizophrenia. Can J Psychiatry 1998; 43:466–72.
106. Buzan RD, Dubovsky SL, Firestone D, Dal Pozzo E. Use of clozapine in 10 mentally retarded adults. J Neuropsychiatry Clin Neurosci 1998;10: 93–5.
107. Shiwach RS. Treatment of clozapine induced hypertension and possible mechanisms. Clin Neuropharmacol 1998;21:139–40.
108. Law RA, Fuller MA, Popli A. Clozapine induced atrial fibrillation. J Clin Psychopharmacol 1998;18:170.
109. Rechlin T, Beck G, Weis M, Kaschka WP. Correlation between plasma clozapine concentration and heart rate variability in schizophrenic patients. Psychopharmacology 1998;135:338–41.
110. Silvestri RC, Bromfield EB, Khoshbin S. Clozapine-induced seizures and EEG abnormalities in ambulatory psychiatric patients. Ann Pharmacother 1998;32:1147–51.
111. Ravasia S, Dickson RA. Seizure on low-dose clozapine. Can J Psychiatry 1998;43:420.
112. Solomons K, Berman KG, Gibson BA. All that seizes is not clozapine. Can J Psychiatry 1998;43:306–7.
113. Trosch RM, Friedman JH, Lannon MC, Pahwa R, Smith D, Seeberger LC, O'Brien CF, LeWitt PA, Koller WC. Clozapine use in Parkinson's disease: a retrospective analysis of large multicentered clinical experience. Mov Disord 1998;13:377–82.
114. Casey DE. Effects of clozapine therapy in schizophrenic individuals at risk for tardive dyskinesia. J Clin Psychiatry 1998;59(Suppl 3):31–7.
115. Dalack GW, Becks L, Meador-Woodruff JH. Tardive dyskinesia, clozapine, and treatment response. Prog Neuropsychopharmacol Biol Psychiatry 1998;22:567–73.
116. Andia I, Zumarraga M, Zabalo MJ, Bulbena A, Davila R. Differential effect of haloperidol and clozapine on plasma homovanillic acid in elderly schizophrenic patients with or without tardive dyskinesia. Biol Psychiatry 1998;43:20–3.
117. Spivak B, Mester R, Abesgaus J, Wittenberg N, Adlersberg S, Gonen N, Weizman A. Clozapine treatment for neuroleptic-induced tardive dyskinesia, parkinsonism, and chronic akathisia in schizophrenic patients. J Clin Psychiatry 1997;58:318–22.
118. Levine J, Chengappa KN. Second thoughts about clozapine as a treatment for neuroleptic-induced akathisia. J Clin Psychiatry 1998;59:195.
119. Delecluse F, Elosegi JA, Gerard JM. A case of tardive tremor successfully treated with clozapine. Mov Disord 1998;13:846–7.
120. Trayer JS, Fidler DC. Neuroleptic malignant syndrome related to use of clozapine. J Am Osteopath Assoc 1998;98:168–9.
121. Hagg S, Joelsson L, Mjorndal T, Spigset O, Oja G, Dahlqvist R. Prevalence of diabetes and impaired glucose tolerance in patients treated with clozapine compared with patients treated with conventional depot neuroleptic medications. J Clin Psychiatry 1998;59:294–9.
122. Yazici KM, Erbas T, Yazici AH. The effect of clozapine on glucose metabolism. Exp Clin Endocrinol Diabetes 1998;106:475–7.
123. Frankenburg FR, Zanarini MC, Kando J, Centorrino F. Clozapine and body mass change. Biol Psychiatry 1998;43:520–4.
124. Bromel T, Blum WF, Ziegler A, Schulz E, Bender M, Fleischhaker C, Remschmidt H, Krieg JC, Hebebrand J. Serum leptin levels increase rapidly after initiation of clozapine therapy. Mol Psychiatry 1998;3:76–80.
125. Copolov DL, Bell WR, Benson WJ, Keks NA, Strazzeri DC, Johnson GF. Clozapine treatment in Australia: a review of haematological monitoring. Med J Aust 1998;168:495–7.
126. Gupta S, Noor-Khan N, Frank B. Agranulocytosis in a second clozapine trial. Psychiatr Serv 1998; 49:1094.
127. Sperner-Unterweger B, Czeipek I, Gaggl S, Geissler D, Spiel G, Fleischhacker WW. Treatment of severe clozapine-induced neutropenia with granulocyte colony-stimulating factor (G-CSF). Remission despite continuous treatment with clozapine. Br J Psychiatry 1998;172:82–4.
128. Van de Loosdrecht AA, Faber HJ, Hordijk P, Uges DR, Smit A. Clozapine-induced agranulocytosis: a case report. Immunopathophysiological considerations. Neth J Med 1998;52:26–9.
129. Guest I, Sokoluk B, MacCrimmon J, Uetrecht J. Examination of possible toxic and immune mechanisms of clozapine-induced agranulocytosis. Toxicology 1998;131:53–65.
130. Lucht MJ, Rietschel M. Clozapine-induced eosinophilia: subsequent neutropenia and corresponding allergic mechanisms. J Clin Psychiatry 1998;59:195–7.
131. Melzer M, Hassanyeh FK, Snow MH, Ong ELC. Sepsis and neutropenia induced by clozapine. Clin Microbiol Infect 1998;4:604–5.
132. Blier P, Slater S, Measham T, Koch TM, Wiviott G. Lithium and clozapine-induced neutropenia/agranulocytosis. Int Clin Psychopharmacol 1998;13:137–40.
133. Moldavsky M, Stein D, Benatov R, Sirota P, Elizur A, Matzner Y, Weizman A. Combined

clozapine-lithium treatment for schizophrenia and schizoaffective disorder. Eur Psychiatry 1998;13:104–6.
134. Thompson J, Chengappa KN, Good CB, Baker RW, Kiewe RP, Bezner J, Schooler NR. Hepatitis, hyperglycemia, pleural effusion, eosinophilia, hematuria and proteinuria occurring early in clozapine treatment. Int Clin Psychopharmacol 1998;13:95–8.
135. Gatto EM, Castronuovo AP, Uribe Roca MC. Clozapine and pancreatitis. Clin Neuropharmacol 1998;21:203.
136. Baker RW, Chengappa KN. Gastroesophageal reflux as a possible result of clozapine treatment. J Clin Psychiatry 1998;59:257.
137. Vrtunski PB, Konicki PE, Jaskiw GE, Brescan DW, Kwon KY, Jurjus G. Clozapine effects on force control in schizophrenic patients. Schizophr Res 1998;34:39–48.
138. Koren W, Koren E, Nacasch N, Ehrenfeld M, Gur H. Rhabdomyolysis associated with clozapine treatment in a patient with decreased calcium-dependent potassium permeability of cell membranes. Clin Neuropharmacol 1998;21:262–4.
139. Wicki J, Rutschmann OT, Burri H, Vecchietti G, Desmeules J. Rhabdomyolysis after correction of hyponatremia due to psychogenic polydipsia possibly complicated by clozapine. Ann Pharmacother 1998;32:892–5
140. David WS, Sharif AA. Clozapine-induced myokymia. Muscle Nerve 1998;21:827–8.
141. Burke WJ, Pfeiffer RF, McComb RD. Neuroleptic sensitivity to clozapine in dementia with Lewy bodies. J Neuropsychiatry Clin Neurosci 1998;10:227–9.
142. Sajatovic M, Ramirez LF, Garver D, Thompson P, Ripper G, Lehmann LS. Clozapine therapy for older veterans. Psychiatr Serv 1998;49:340–4.
143. Valevski A, Klein T, Gazit E, Meged S, Stein D, Elizur A, Narinsky ER, Kutzuk D, Weizman A. HLA-B38 and clozapine-induced agranulocytosis in Israeli Jewish schizophrenic patients. Eur J Immunogenet 1998;25:11–13.
144. Ahmed S, Chengappa KN, Naidu VR, Baker RW, Parepally H, Schooler NR. Clozapine withdrawal-emergent dystonias and dyskinesias: a case series. J Clin Psychiatry 1998;59:472–7.
145. Poyurovsky M, Bergman Y, Shoshani D, Schneidman M, Weizman A. Emergence of obsessive-compulsive symptoms and tics during clozapine withdrawal. Clin Neuropharmacol 1998;21:97–100.
146. Reith D, Monteleone JP, Whyte IM, Ebelling W, Holford NH, Carter GL. Features and toxicokinetics of clozapine in overdose. Ther Drug Monit 1998;20:92–7.
147. Carrillo JA, Herraiz AG, Ramos SI, Benitez J. Effects of caffeine withdrawal from the diet on the metabolism of clozapine in schizophrenic patients. J Clin Psychopharmacol 1998; 18:311–16.
148. Hoffmann RM, Ott S, Parhofer KG, Bartl R, Pape GR. Interferon-α-induced agranulocytosis in a patient on long-term clozapine therapy. J Hepatol 1998;29:170.
149. Facciola G, Avenoso A, Spina E, Perucca E. Inducing effect of phenobarbital on clozapine metabolism in patients with chronic schizophrenia. Ther Drug Monit 1998;20:628–30.
150. Spina E, Avenoso A, Facciola G, Fabrazzo M, Monteleone P, Maj M, Perucca E, Caputi AP. Effect of fluoxetine on the plasma concentrations of clozapine and its major metabolites in patients with schizophrenia. Int Clin Psychopharmacol 1998;13:141–5.
151. Ferslew KE, Hagardorn AN, Harlan GC, McCormick WF. A fatal drug interaction between clozapine and fluoxetine. J Forensic Sci 1998; 43:1082–5.
152. Avenoso A, Facciolà G, Scordo MG, Gitto C, Ferrante GD, Madia AG, Spina E. No effect of citalopram on plasma levels of clozapine, risperidone and their active metabolites in patients with chronic schizophrenia. Clin Drug Invest 1998; 16:393–8.
153. Purdon SE, Snaterse M. Selective serotonin reuptake inhibitor modulation of clozapine effects on cognition in schizophrenia. Can J Psychiatry 1998;43:84–5.
154. Young CR, Bowers MB Jr, Mazure CM. Management of the adverse effects of clozapine. Schizophr Bull 1998;24:381–90.
155. Lieberman JA. Maximizing clozapine therapy: managing side effects. J Clin Psychiatry 1998;59(Suppl 3):38–43.
156. Conley RR. Optimizing treatment with clozapine. J Clin Psychiatry 1998;59(Suppl 3):44–8.
157. Olesen OV. Therapeutic drug monitoring of clozapine treatment. Therapeutic threshold value for serum clozapine concentrations. Clin Pharmacokinet 1998;34:497–502.
158. Perry PJ, Bever KA, Arndt S, Combs MD. Relationship between patient variables and plasma clozapine concentrations: a dosing nomogram. Biol Psychiatry 1998;44:733–8.
159. Guitton C, Kinowski JM, Gomeni R, Bressolle F. A kinetic model for simultaneous fit of clozapine and norclozapine concentrations in chronic schizophrenic patients during long-term treatment. Clin Drug Invest 1998;16:35–43.
160. Healy D, Farquhar G. Inmediate effects of droperidol. Human Psychopharmacol 1998;13:113–20.
161. Wood A. Clinical experience with olanzapine, a new atypical antipsychotic. Int Clin Psychopharmacol 1998;13(Suppl 1):S59–S62.
162. Kasper S. Risperidone and olanzapine: optimal dosing for efficacy and tolerability in patients with schizophrenia. Int Clin Psychopharmacol 1998;13:253–62.
163. Gray R. Olanzapine: efficacy in treating the positive and negative symptoms of schizophrenia. Ment Health Care 1998;1:193–4.
164. Bever KA, Perry PJ. Olanzapine: a serotonin–dopamine-receptor antagonist for antipsychotic therapy. Am J Health Syst Pharm 1998;55:1003–16.

165. Conley RR, Tamminga CA, Bartko JJ, Richardson C, Peszke M, Lingle J, Hegerty J, Love R, Gounaris C, Zaremba S. Olanzapine compared with chlorpromazine in treatment-resistant schizophrenia. Am J Psychiatry 1998;155:914–20.
166. Henderson DC, Nasrallah RA, Goff DC. Switching from clozapine to olanzapine in treatment-refractory schizophrenia: safety, clinical efficacy, and predictors of response. J Clin Psychiatry 1998;59:585–8.
167. Sacristán JA, Gómez JC, Martín J, García-Bernardo E, Peralta V, Alvarez E, Gurpegui M, Mateo I, Moríñigo A, Noval D, Soler R, Palomo T, Cuesta M, Pérez-Blanco F, Massip C. Pharmacoeconomic assessment of olanzapine in the treatment of refractory schizophrenia based on a pilot clinical study. Clin Drug Invest 1998;15:29–35.
168. Baldacchino AM, Stubbs JH, Nevison-Andrews DG, Mountjoy CQ. The prescribing practices of olanzapine in a psychiatric hospital in Britain. Int J Psych Clin Pract 1998;2:203–7.
169. Schooler NR. Comments on article by Tran and colleagues, 'Double-blind comparison of olanzapine versus risperidone in treatment of schizophrenia and other psychotic disorders'. J Clin Psychopharmacol 1998;18:174–5.
170. Tollefson G, Tran PV. Reply. J Clin Psychopharmacol 1998;18:175–6.
171. Gheuens J, A Grebb J. Comments on article by Tran and colleagues, 'Double-blind comparison of olanzapine versus risperidone in treatment of schizophrenia and other psychotic disorders'. J Clin Psychopharmacol 1998;18:176–7.
172. Tollefson G, Tran PV. Reply. J Clin Psychopharmacol 1998;18:177–9.
173. Kasper S, Kufferle B. Comments on 'Double-blind comparison of olanzapine versus risperidone in the treatment of schizophrenia and other psychotic disorders', by Tran and Associates. J Clin Psychopharmacol 1998;18:353–4.
174. Tollefson G, Tran PV. Reply to Kasper and Kufferle. J Clin Psychopharmacol 1998;18:354–5.
175. McElroy SL, Frye M, Denicoff K, Altshuler L, Nolen W, Kupka R, Suppes T, Keck PE Jr, Leverich GS, Kmetz GF, Post RM. Olanzapine in treatment-resistant bipolar disorder. J Affect Disord 1998;49:119–22.
176. Zarate CA Jr, Narendran R, Tohen M, Greaney JJ, Berman A, Pike S, Madrid A. Clinical predictors of acute response with olanzapine in psychotic mood disorders. J Clin Psychiatry 1998;59:24–8.
177. Kumra S, Jacobsen LK, Lenane M, Karp BI, Frazier JA, Smith AK, Bedwell J, Lee P, Malanga CJ, Hamburger S, Rapoport JL. Childhood-onset schizophrenia: an open-label study of olanzapine in adolescents. J Am Acad Child Adolesc Psychiatry 1998;37:377–85.
178. Conley RR, Kelly DL, Gale EA. Olanzapine response in treatment-refractory schizophrenic patients with a history of substance abuse. Schizophr Res 1998;33:95–101.
179. Krishnamoorthy J, King BH. Open-label olanzapine treatment in five preadolescent children. J Child Adolesc Psychopharmacol 1998;8:107–13.
180. Yip L, Dart RC, Graham K. Olanzapine toxicity in a toddler. Pediatrics 1998;102:1494.
181. Malek-Ahmadi P, Simonds JF. Olanzapine for autistic disorder with hyperactivity. J Am Acad Child Adolesc Psychiatry 1998;37:902.
182. Kapur S, Zipursky RB, Remington G, Jones C, DaSilva J, Wilson AA, Houle S. $5HT_2$ and D_2 receptor occupancy of olanzapine in schizophrenia: a PET investigation. Am J Psychiatry 1998;155:921–8.
183. Allan ER, Sison CE, Alpert M, Connolly B, Crichton J. The relationship between negative symptoms of schizophrenia and extrapyramidal side effects with haloperidol and olanzapine. Psychopharmacol Bull 1998;34:71–4.
184. Landry P, Cournoyer J. Acute dystonia with olanzapine. J Clin Psychiatry 1998;59:384.
185. Friedman J. Olanzapine in the treatment of dopaminomimetic psychosis in patients with Parkinson's disease. Neurology 1998;50:1195–6.
186. Graham JM, Sussman JD, Ford KS, Sagar HJ. Olanzapine in the treatment of hallucinosis in idiopathic Parkinson's disease: a cautionary note. J Neurol Neurosurg Psychiatry 1998;65:774–7.
187. Jimenez-Jimenez FJ, Tallon-Barranco A, Orti-Pareja M, Zurdo M, Porta J, Molina JA. Olanzapine can worsen parkinsonism. Neurology 1998;50:1183–4.
188. Strauss AJ, Bailey RK, Dralle PW, Eschmann AJ, Wagner RB. Conventional psychotropic-induced tremor extinguished by olanzapine. Am J Psychiatry 1998;155:1132.
189. Jauss M, Schroder J, Pantel J, Bachmann S, Gerdsen I, Mundt C. Severe akathisia during olanzapine treatment of acute schizophrenia. Pharmacopsychiatry 1998;31:146–8.
190. Meyer JM, Marsh J, Simpson G. Differential sensitivities to risperidone and olanzapine in a human immunodeficiency virus patient. Biol Psychiatry 1998;44:791–4.
191. Almeida OP. Olanzapine for the treatment of tardive dyskinesia. J Clin Psychiatry 1998;59:380–1.
192. Filice GA, McDougall BC, Ercan-Fang N, Billington CJ. Neuroleptic malignant syndrome associated with olanzapine. Ann Pharmacother 1998;32:1158–9.
193. Moltz DA, Coeytaux RR. Case report: possible neuroleptic malignant syndrome associated with olanzapine. J Clin Psychopharmacol 1998;18:485–6.
194. Gaile S, Noviasky JA. Speech disturbance and marked decrease in function seen in several older patients on olanzapine. J Am Geriatr Soc 1998;46:1330–1.
195. Pozo P, Alcantara AG. Mania-like syndrome in a patient with chronic schizophrenia during olanzapine treatment. J Psychiatry Neurosci 1998;23:309–10.
196. Benazzi F, Rossi E. Mania induced by olanzapine. Hum Psychopharmacol 1998;13:585–6.
197. Reeves RR, McBride WA, Brannon GE. Olanzapine-induced mania. J Am Osteopath Assoc 1998;98:549–50.

198. London JA. Mania associated with olanzapine. J Am Acad Child Adolesc Psychiatry 1998;37:135–6.
199. Lindenmayer JP, Klebanov R. Olanzapine-induced manic-like syndrome. J Clin Psychiatry 1998;59:318–19.
200. Morrison D, Clark D, Goldfarb E, McCoy L. Worsening of obsessive-compulsive symptoms following treatment with olanzapine. Am J Psychiatry 1998;155:855.
201. Al-Mulhim A, Atwal S, Coupland NJ. Provocation of obsessive-compulsive behaviour and tremor by olanzapine. Can J Psychiatry 1998;43:645.
202. Al Jeshi A. Paranoia and agitation associated with olanzapine treatment. Can J Psychiatry 1998;43:195.
203. Canuso CM, Hanau M, Jhamb KK, Green AI. Olanzapine use in women with antipsychotic-induced hyperprolactinemia. Am J Psychiatry 1998;155:1458.
204. Gazzola LR, Opler LA. Return of menstruation after switching from risperidone to olanzapine. J Clin Psychopharmacol 1998;18:486–7.
205. Potenza MN, Wasylink S, Epperson CN, McDougle CJ. Olanzapine augmentation of fluoxetine in the treatment of trichotillomania. Am J Psychiatry 1998;155:1299–300.
206. Gupta S, Droney T, Al-Samarrai S, Keller P, Frank B. Olanzapine-induced weight gain. Ann Clin Psychiatry 1998;10:39.
207. Fertig MK, Brooks VG, Shelton PS, English CW. Hyperglycemia associated with olanzapine. J Clin Psychiatry 1998;59:687–9.
208. Gardner I, Zahid N, MacCrimmon D, Uetrecht JP. A comparison of the oxidation of clozapine and olanzapine to reactive metabolites and the toxicity of these metabolites to human leukocytes. Mol Pharmacol 1998;53:991–8.
209. Chatterton R. Experiences with clozapine and olanzapine. Aust NZ J Psychiatry 1998;32:463.
210. Finkel B, Lerner A, Oyffe I, Rudinski D, Sigal M, Weizman A. Olanzapine treatment in patients with typical and atypical neuroleptic-associated agranulocytosis. Int Clin Psychopharmacol 1998;13:133–5.
211. Lambert T. Olanzapine after clozapine: the rare case of prolongation of granulocytopenia. Aust NZ J Psychiatry 1998;32:591–2.
212. Wray CM, Sztuke-Fournier A. Olanzapine: hematological reactions. Can Med Assoc J 1998;159:81–2.
213. Perkins DO, McClure RK. Hypersalivation coincident with olanzapine treatment. Am J Psychiatry 1998;155:993–4.
214. Heckers S, Anick D, Boverman JF, Stern TA. Priapism following olanzapine administration in a patient with multiple sclerosis. Psychosomatics 1998;39:288–90.
215. Deirmenjian JM, Erhart SM, Wirshing DA, Spellberg BJ, Wirshing WC. Olanzapine-induced reversible priaprism: a case report. J Clin Psychopharmacol 1998;18:351–3.
216. Elian AA. Fatal overdose of olanzepine. Forensic Sci Int 1998;91:231–5.
217. Stephens BG, Coleman DE, Baselt RC. Olanzapine-related fatality. J Forensic Sci 1998; 43:1252–3.
218. Lucas RA, Gilfillan DJ, Bergstrom RF. A pharmacokinetic interaction between carbamazepine and olanzapine: observations on possible mechanism. Eur J Clin Pharmacol 1998;54:639–43.
219. Misra LK, Erpenbach JE, Hamlyn H, Fuller WC. Quetiapine: a new atypical antipsychotic. South Dakota J Med 1998;51:189–93.
220. Parsa MA, Bastani B. Quetiapine (Seroquel) in the treatment of psychosis in patients with Parkinson's disease. J Neuropsychiatry Clin Neurosci 1998;10:216–19.
221. Iskedjian M, Hux M, Remington GJ. The Canadian experience with risperidone for the treatment of schizophrenia: an overview. J Psychiatry Neurosci 1998;23:229–39.
222. Davies A, Adena MA, Keks NA, Catts SV, Lambert T, Schweitzer I. Risperidone versus haloperidol: I. Meta-analysis of efficacy and safety. Clin Ther 1998;20:58–71.
223. Mackay FJ, Wilton LV, Pearce GL, Freemantle SN, Mann RD. The safety of risperidone: a post-marketing study on 7,684 patients. Hum Psychopharmacol 1998;13:413–18.
224. Moller HJ, Gagiano CA, Addington DE, Von Knorring L, Torres-Plank JF, Gaussares C. Long-term treatment of chronic schizophrenia with risperidone: an open-label, multicenter study of 386 patients. Int Clin Psychopharmacol 1998;13:99–106.
225. Binder RL, McNiel DE, Sandberg DA. A naturalistic study of clinical use of risperidone. Psychiatr Serv 1998;49:524–6.
226. Nair NPV, Reiter-Schmitt B, Ronovsky K, Vyssoki D, Baeke J, Desseilles M, Kindts P, Mesotten F, Peuskens J, Addington D et al. Therapeutic equivalence of risperidone given once daily and twice daily in patients with schizophrenia. J Clin Psychopharmacol 1998;18:103–10.
227. Muller-Siecheneder F, Muller MJ, Hillert A, Szegedi A, Wetzel H, Benkert O. Risperidone versus haloperidol and amitriptyline in the treatment of patients with a combined psychotic and depressive syndrome. J Clin Psychopharmacol 1998;18:111–20.
228. McDougle CJ, Holmes JP, Carlson DC, Pelton GH, Cohen DJ, Price LH. A double-blind, placebo-controlled study of risperidone in adults with autistic disorder and other pervasive developmental disorders. Arch Gen Psychiatry 1998;55: 633–41.
229. Vieta E, Gasto C, Colom F, Martinez A, Otero A, Vallejo J. Treatment of refractory rapid cycling bipolar disorder with risperidone. J Clin Psychopharmacol 1998;18:172–4.
230. Cohen SA, Ihrig K, Lott RS, Kerrick JM. Risperidone for aggression and self-injurious behavior in adults with mental retardation. J Autism Dev Disord 1998;28:229–33.

231. Schreier HA. Risperidone for young children with mood disorders and aggressive behavior. J Child Adolesc Psychopharmacol 1998;8:49–59.
232. Tracy JI, Monaco CA, Abraham G, Josiassen RC, Pollock BG. Relation of serum anticholinergicity to cognitive status in schizophrenia patients taking clozapine or risperidone. J Clin Psychiatry 1998;59:184–8.
233. Dresel S, Tatsch K, Dahne I, Mager T, Scherer J, Hahn K. Iodine-123-iodobenzamide SPECT assessment of dopamine D_2 receptor occupancy in riperidone-treated schizophrenic patients. J Nucl Med 1998;39:1138–42.
234. Miller CH, Mohr F, Umbricht D, Woerner M, Fleischhacker WW, Lieberman JA. The prevalence of acute extrapyramidal signs and symptoms in patients treated with clozapine, risperidone, and conventional antipsychotics. J Clin Psychiatry 1998;59:69–75.
235. Lavretsky H, Sultzer D. A structured trial of risperidone for the treatment of agitation in dementia. Am J Geriatr Psychiatry 1998;6:127–35.
236. Herrmann N, Rivard MF, Flynn M, Ward C, Rabheru K, Campbell B. Risperidone for the treatment of behavioral disturbances in dementia: a case series. J Neuropsychiatry Clin Neurosci 1998;10:220–3.
237. Geizer M, Ancill RJ. Combination of risperidone and donepezil in Lewy body dementia. Can J Psychiatry 1998;43:421–2.
238. Meco G, Fabrizio E, Alessandri A, Vanacore N, Bonifati V. Risperidone in levodopa induced dyskinesiae. J Neurol Neurosurg Psychiatry 1998;64:135.
239. Friedman JH, Ott BR. Should risperidone be used in Parkinson's disease? J Neuropsychiatry Clin Neurosci 1998;10:473–4.
240. Workman RH. In Reply. J Neuropsychiatry Clin Neurosci 1998;10:474–5.
241. Silberbauer C. Risperidone-induced tardive dyskinesia. Pharmacopsychiatry 1998;31:68–9.
242. Friedman JH. Rapid onset tardive dyskinesia ('fly catcher tongue') in a neuroleptically naive patient induced by risperidone. Med Health Rhode Island 1998;81:271–2.
243. Sakkas P, Liappas J, Christodoulou GN. Tardive dyskinesia due to risperidone. Eur Psychiatry 1998;13:107–8.
244. Fischer P, Tauscher J, Kufferle B. Risperidone and tardive dyskinesia in organic psychosis. Pharmacopsychiatry 1998;31:70–1.
245. Rohrbach P, Collinot JP, Vallet G. Syndrome malin des neuroleptiques induit par la rispéridone. Ann Fr Anesth Reanim 1998;17:85–6.
246. Aguirre C, Garcia Monco JC, Mendibil B. Síndrome neuroléptico maligno asociado a risperidona. Med Clin 1998;110:239.
247. Dursun SM, Oluboka OJ, Devarajan S, Kutcher SP. High-dose vitamin E plus vitamin B_6 treatment of risperidone-related neuroleptic malignant syndrome. J Psychopharmacol 1998; 12:220–1.
248. Ashleigh EA, Larsen PD. A syndrome of increased affect in response to risperidone among patients with schizophrenia. Psychiatr Serv 1998;49:526–8.
249. Mahendran R. Obsessional symptoms associated with risperidone treatment. Aust NZ J Psychiatry 1998;32:299–301.
250. Shiwach RS, Carmody TJ. Prolactogenic effects of risperidone in male patients—a preliminary study. Acta Psychiatr Scand 1998;98:81–3.
251. Jones H, Curtis VA, Wright PA, Lucey JV. Risperidone is associated with blunting of D-fenfluramine evoked serotonergic responses in schizophrenia. Int Clin Psychopharmacol 1998; 13:199–203.
252. Popli A, Gupta S, Rangwani SR. Risperidone-induced galactorrhea associated with a prolactin elevation. Ann Clin Psychiatry 1998;10:31–3.
253. Horrigan JP, Sikich L. Diet and the atypical neuroleptics. J Am Acad Child Adolesc Psychiatry 1998;37:1126–7.
254. Finkel B, Lerner AG, Oyffe I, Sigal M. Risperidone-associated agranulocytosis. Am J Psychiatry 1998;155:855–6.
255. Phillips EJ, Liu BA, Knowles SR. Rapid onset of risperidone-induced hepatotoxicity. Ann Pharmacother 1998;32:843.
256. Benazzi F. Risperidone-induced hepatotoxicity. Pharmacopsychiatry 1998;31:241.
257. Landau J, Martin A. Is liver function monitoring warranted during risperidone treatment? J Am Acad Child Adolesc Psychiatry 1998;37: 1007–8.
258. Hudson RG, Cain MP. Risperidone associated hemorrhagic cystitis. J Urol 1998;160:159.
259. Almond DS, Rhodes LE, Pirmohamed M. Risperidone-induced photosensitivity. Postgrad Med J 1998;74:252–3.
260. Ravona-Springer R, Dolberg OT, Hirschmann S, Grunhaus L. Delirium in elderly patients treated with risperidone: a report of three cases. J Clin Psychopharmacol 1998;18:171–2.
261. Tavcar R, Dernovsek MZ. Risperidone-induced delirium. Can J Psychiatry 1998;43:194.
262. Phan TG, Yu RY, Hersch MI. Hypothermia induced by risperidone and olanzapine in a patient with Prader-Willi syndrome. Med J Aust 1998;169:230–1.
263. Lane HY, Chang WH. Manic and psychotic symptoms following risperidone withdrawal in a schizophrenic patient. J Clin Psychiatry 1998; 59:620–1.
264. Acri AA, Henretig FM. Effects of risperidone in overdose. Am J Emerg Med 1998;16:498–501.
265. Lane HY, Chang WH. Risperidone-carbamazepine interactions: is cytochrome P450 3A involved? J Clin Psychiatry 1998;59:430–1.
266. Caley CF. Extrapyramidal reactions from concurrent SSRI and atypical antipsychotic use. Can J Psychiatry 1998;43:307–8.
267. Baker RW. Possible dose-response relationship for risperidone in obsessive-compulsive disorder. J Clin Psychiatry 1998;59:134.
268. Stein DJ, Hawkridge S, Bouwer C, Emsley RA. Dr Stein and colleagues reply. J Clin Psychiatry 1998;59:134.

269. O'Connor M, Silver H. Adding risperidone to selective serotonin reuptake inhibitor improves chronic depression. J Clin Psychopharmacol 1998;18:89–91.
270. Andrade C. Risperidone may worsen fluoxetine-treated OCD. J Clin Psychiatry 1998;59:255–6.
271. Sanders RD, Lehrer DS. Edema associated with addition of risperidone to valproate treatment. J Clin Psychiatry 1998;59:689–90.
272. Lauterbach EC. Catatonia-like events after valproic acid with risperidone and sertraline. Neuropsychiatry Neuropsychol Behav Neurol 1998;11:157–63.
273. Chong SA, Tan CH, Lee EL, Liow PH. Augmentation of risperidone with valproic acid. J Clin Psychiatry 1998;59:430.
274. Olesen OV, Licht RW, Thomsen E, Bruun T, Viftrup JE, Linnet K. Serum concentrations and side effects in psychiatric patients during risperidone therapy. Ther Drug Monit 1998;20:380–4.
275. Goff DC, Posever T, Herz L, Simmons J, Kletti N, Lapierre K, Wilner KD, Law CG, Ko GN. An exploratory haloperidol-controlled dose-finding study of ziprasidone in hospitalized patients with schizophrenia or schizoaffective disorder. J Clin Psychopharmacol 1998;18:296–304.
276. Prakash A, Lamb HM. Zotepine. A review of its pharmacodynamic and pharmacokinetic properties and therapeutic efficacy in the management of schizophrenia. CNS Drugs 1998;9:153–75.
277. Kane JM, Aguglia E, Altamura AC, Ayuso Gutierrez JL, Brunello N, Fleischhacker WW, Gaebel W, Gerlach J, Guelfi JD, Kissling W, Lapierre YD, Lindstrom E, Mendlewicz J, Racagni G, Carulla LS, Schooler NR. Guidelines for depot antipsychotic treatment in schizophrenia. European neuropsychopharmacology consensus conference in Siena, Italy. Eur Neuropsychopharmacol 1998;8:55–66.

Emilio Perucca

7 Antiepileptic drugs

GENERAL TOPICS *(SED-13, 136; SEDA-20, 58; SEDA-21, 66, SEDA-22, 81)*

Efficacy and tolerability data from double-blind placebo-controlled add-on trials of new antiepileptic drugs in patients with refractory partial epilepsy have been reviewed (1[r]). Although there were differences in adverse events profiles among the various drugs, the review identified major methodological problems, which hamper comparisons across studies and drugs. These included variability in the use of COSTART terminology, marked differences in the occurrence of specific adverse events in the placebo groups (an indication of heterogeneous evaluation procedures), and the use of non-optimal dosages or non-optimal titration schedules in many trials (1[r]).

In a multicenter randomized double-blind comparison of diazepam (0.15 mg/kg followed by phenytoin 18 mg/kg), lorazepam (0.1 mg/kg), phenobarbital (15 mg/kg), and phenytoin (18 mg/kg) in 518 patients with generalized convulsive status epilepticus, lorazepam was more effective than phenytoin and at least as effective as phenobarbital or diazepam plus phenytoin (2[cr]). Drug-related adverse effects did not differ significantly among treatments and included *hypoventilation* (up to 17%), *hypotension* (up to 59%), and *cardiac rhythm disturbances* (up to 9%).

R Death associated with antiepileptic drugs

A nested case-control study showed that the risk of sudden unexpected death in epilepsy (SUDEP) increases with increasing number of seizures, increasing numbers of drugs taken (with a relative risk of 9.89 for polytherapy with three drugs compared with monotherapy), and a high frequency of dosage changes (3[Cr]). However, these data do not necessarily implicate a role of antiepileptic drugs in the pathogenesis of SUDEP: it is possible that polytherapy and frequent dosage changes are surrogate markers for the severity of the disease. On the other hand, a possible implication of carbamazepine in SUDEP was suggested in a separate survey by the observation that 11 of 14 SUDEP patients (79%) were taking carbamazepine, while only 38% of patients in the same clinic were taking it (4[Cr]). The effects of carbamazepine on heart function were discussed as a possible mechanism, but no comment was made on the possibility that the characteristics of patients taking carbamazepine may differ from those of patients taking other drugs.

Another study implicated nitrazepam as a possible cause of increased mortality (5[Cr]). Among 294 assessable children who took nitrazepam, 62 continued treatment at the last time of follow-up. There were 1.98 deaths/100 patient years during nitrazepam treatment compared with 0.58 deaths/100 patient years after nitrazepam withdrawal (RR = 3.4). The increase in risk occurred virtually entirely in younger children: among those aged under 3.4 years, the death rate per 100 patient years was 3.98 on nitrazepam compared with 0.26 off nitrazepam (RR = 15). Causes of death differed on and off nitrazepam. Of 14 deaths during nitrazepam treatment, seven were sudden, six were due to pneumonia, and one was due to cystinosis: nine patients had at least one contributing factor, such as dysphagia, gastroesophageal reflux, or recurrent aspirations. In the off nitrazepam period, there were two sudden deaths, and one death each caused by status epilepticus, head trauma, and shunt complication; only one patient had a contributing factor (gastro-esophageal reflux). These findings were interpreted as evidence that nitrazepam increases the risk of death in young children, possibly owing to its ability to increase secretions and to cause drooling, eating difficulties, and aspiration pneumonia (6[Cr], 7[Cr]). Although the data suggest a role of nitrazepam

Side Effects of Drugs, Annual 23
J.K. Aronson, ed.

in these deaths, only incomplete information was given about the distribution of other risk factors (seizure disorder, associated morbidity) in children who continued nitrazepam therapy. Nitrazepam should be used with caution in young children, especially those with difficulties in swallowing, aspiration pneumonia, or gastro-esophageal reflux.

Nervous system In a critical review it was concluded that the adverse effects of antiepileptic drugs on learning and behavior in children have been overrated (8[R]). Because of methodological flaws, many studies could not discriminate between the effects of drugs and the influence of heredity, brain damage, seizures, and psychosocial factors. Investigations using improved methods have suggested that most children taking antiepileptic drugs do not experience clinically relevant cognitive or behavioral adverse effects. In some patients, however, antiepileptic drugs do have a detrimental effect, barbiturates being among the most commonly implicated. At least with some agents, such as gabapentin, *behavioral adverse effects* occur mainly in children with pre-existing learning disability. Clinical experience may help to identify subgroups at special risk.

Endocrine, metabolic In an assessment of the effects of antiepileptic drugs on male sexual function, men taking carbamazepine had *higher plasma concentrations of sex hormone binding globulin and lower concentrations of dehydroepiandrosterone* compared with controls (9[Cr]). Patients taking phenytoin had higher total testosterone and lower dehydroepiandrosterone concentrations. Patients taking carbamazepine and phenytoin also had a *lower free androgen index*, but free testosterone, a more reliable index of active androgen concentrations, did not differ from controls. Patients taking valproate showed no differences in hormone concentrations compared with controls. Sexual experience scales showed that treated men embraced a stricter sexual morality than untreated controls, and expressed greater satisfaction with their marriages. Most of the hormonal changes could be explained by enzyme induction, and there was no evidence of hyposexuality in this population.

Compared with healthy controls, 51 patients with epilepsy taking a variety of antiepileptic drugs (mostly carbamazepine) had *higher mean plasma concentrations of homocysteine* (10[Cr]). This effect, which could be related to a reduction in the concentrations of folate and vitamin B_6, was likely to be drug-induced, but a causative role of the underlying disease could not be excluded. Although homocysteine is an experimental convulsant and a risk factor for atherosclerosis, the clinical relevance of these findings is uncertain.

Immunological and hypersensitivity reactions Within 5 days of being switched to valproate after developing a rash ascribed to carbamazepine, a 55-year-old man developed anticonvulsant *hypersensitivity syndrome* (maculopapular rash, fever, hepatitis, and eosinophilia) and ocular manifestations consistent with bilateral *anterior uveitis* (11[c]). Although mild conjunctivitis is common in the anticonvulsant hypersensitivity syndrome, uveitis has not been reported before in this context.

Risk factors Case reports have suggested that the risk of serious skin reactions to phenytoin is increased in *patients with brain tumors undergoing cranial irradiation*, but the incidence of these reactions is unknown (12[Cr]). In a retrospective study of 289 patients with brain tumors, rash occurred in 18% of exposures to antiepileptic drugs, including 22% of exposures to phenytoin, compared with an expected rate of 5–10%. Most of the rashes occurred before the start of irradiation therapy. Only one patient developed erythema multiforme. These data suggest that the risk of serious skin reactions in patients with brain tumors is actually low, even though there was an increased frequency of milder rashes. Irradiation did not appear to contribute to the risk. However, it is possible that earlier publications about the risk of serious reactions resulted in the use of lower initial dosages or earlier withdrawal of medication, before the onset of more severe manifestations. The fact that skin rashes were more common in patients with glioma than metastatic disease could be related to the effects of underlying treatments (or disease) on immune function.

INDIVIDUAL DRUGS

Benzodiazepines *(SED-13, 104; SEDA-20, 59)*

In a prospective multicenter double-blind comparison of clobazam with phenytoin or carbamazepine monotherapy in children with partial or generalized tonic-clonic seizures, the retention rate after 1 year did not differ, but exit due to inefficacy tended to be more common with clobazam (19 vs 11% for the other drugs combined), while exit due to adverse effects tended to be more common with carbamazepine or phenytoin (15 vs 4% for clobazam) (13[c]). Although all treatments were claimed to have similar efficacy, detailed descriptions of the changes in seizure frequency and the proportion of patients who gradually achieved seizure control in each treatment group were not given. *Behavioral and mood problems* tended to be more common with clobazam than with the other drugs (38/119 vs 29/116). Drooling was more common with clobazam (7/119 vs 2/116), whereas *rash or vomiting* were more common with the other treatments (9/116 vs 4/119 and 10/116 vs 4/119 respectively). *Tolerance* was reported in 7.5% of patients taking clobazam, in 4.2% of those taking carbamazepine, and in 6.7% of those taking phenytoin; however, the definition of tolerance (no seizures for 3–6 months, followed by seizures sufficiently numerous to require a switch to another drug) was questionable, and no information was given about patients with seizure relapses who required an increase in dosage. Although these results suggest that clobazam is a valuable alternative to phenytoin and carbamazepine in childhood epilepsy, more precise characterization of responses would have been desirable.

Carbamazepine *(SED-13, 145; SEDA-20, 60; SEDA-21, 69; SEDA-22, 85)*

Cardiovascular Four additional cases of carbamazepine-induced *sinus node dysfunction* ($n = 3$) and *atrioventricular block* ($n = 1$) were described in elderly Japanese women treated with 200–600 mg/day. In two of the three patients rechallenged, sinus arrest recurred within 48 hours (14[Cr]).

Hematological Serious *blood dyscrasias* from carbamazepine may be accompanied or preceded by a rash. Two additional such cases included a 66-year-old man who had severe leukopenia a few days after a generalized rash appeared on the 36th day after he started to take carbamazepine, and a 69-year-old woman who had severe leukopenia and thrombocytopenia about a month after the onset of a rash and 2 months after she started to take carbamazepine (15[Cr]). In both patients, the abnormalities resolved after withdrawal, except for the platelet count, which increased but did not fully normalize over 6 weeks. This report suggests that patients developing a rash on carbamazepine should be monitored for the possible risk of associated blood dyscrasias.

Skin and appendages A 58-year-old man developed *stomatitis and widespread edematous erythema with papules and pustules* after taking a combination of carbamazepine and paracetamol for 2 days, a most unusual treatment for headache and fever (16[cr]). The stomatitis improved but the eruption persisted for 2 months and was diagnosed as eosinophilic pustular folliculitis, a disorder that is rarely drug-induced. Recovery was achieved with steroid therapy. A role of carbamazepine was suggested by reoccurrence of eosinophilic folliculitis after patch testing and low-dose (2 mg) oral rechallenge.

Immunological and hypersensitivity reactions A 44-year-old woman allergic to phenytoin developed fever, lymphadenopathy, pneumonitis, hepatitis, and a morbilliform eruption after taking carbamazepine for 1 month (17[c]). A skin biopsy showed atypical lymphocytes in the dermis that were CD3+, CD30+, and L26−. She improved quickly after carbamazepine was withdrawn. This seems to have been the first report of carbamazepine-induced histological features of *cutaneous pseudolymphoma*, including CD30+ cells.

Cervical lymphadenopathy, fever and a maculopapular skin rash developed in a 17-year-old boy after he had taken carbamazepine for 3 weeks (up to 600 mg/day) (18[cr]). Lymph node biopsies showed features typical of *Kikuchi disease*, a rare and self-limited immune-mediated lymphadenopathy that affects mostly the cervical region. The condition cleared rapidly after withdrawal.

A 40-year-old man who had taken carbamazepine since childhood suffered for over 10 years from a *lupus-like illness* with hypocomplementemia, pancytopenia, and splenomegaly (19[c]). He later developed cryoglobulinemia with membranoproliferative glomerulonephritis and raised ANA and pANCA titers. A causative role of carbamazepine in the latter syndrome was suggested by the observation that after withdrawal the antibodies fell and cryoglobulinemia resolved.

A 54-year-old man who had been taking neuroleptic drugs for about 30 years developed *neuroleptic malignant syndrome* within 3 days of taking add-on carbamazepine (400 mg/day) (20[cr]). This syndrome does not appear to have been described with carbamazepine alone, and it was speculated that its pathogenesis could involve rebound cholinergic activity after a reduction in plasma neuroleptic drug concentrations by carbamazepine.

Risk factors The presence of a *static encephalopathy* (defined as focal or diffuse structural brain lesions associated with mild to moderately severe cognitive dysfunction) or age above 55 years were associated with a greater risk of toxicity after rapid switch-over to a carbamazepine dosage designed to yield a plasma concentration of 10 mg/l (21[c]). Moderately severe to severe adverse effects in the 11 patients in either subgroup included sedation, ataxia, and confusion.

Interactions *Clobazam* Negative myoclonus and more typical signs of carbamazepine intoxication (fatigue, ataxia, clumsiness) occurred in a 66-year-old man after he took add-on clobazam (10 mg/day) for 4 weeks (22[Cr]). Plasma concentrations of carbamazepine (58 μmol/l) and carbamazepine-10,11-epoxide (19 μmol/l) were higher than before clobazam therapy, and his symptoms resolved quickly when carbamazepine dosage was reduced and clobazam was withdrawn. The interaction was confirmed on rechallenge; however, it does not occur in most patients.

Grapefruit juice In 10 patients grapefruit juice 300 ml taken with the morning dose of carbamazepine resulted in an approximate 50% increase of plasma carbamazepine concentrations (23[C]). The interaction was ascribed to inhibition of cytochrome CYP3A4 by components of the juice.

Mianserin In 12 patients, carbamazepine (400 mg/day for 4 weeks) markedly reduced the plasma concentrations of concomitantly administered mianserin, probably due to enzyme induction (24[C]). The concentration of S-mianserin, the most potent of the enantiomers of mianserin, fell by 45%, while the plasma concentrations of desmethylmianserin changed only slightly. These data suggest that patients co-medicated with carbamazepine may require higher dosages of mianserin.

Olanzapine In 11 healthy volunteers carbamazepine (400 mg/day for 2 weeks) reduced by about 30% the AUC of olanzapine, presumably by induction of olanzapine metabolism (25[C]). Although the interaction was considered of little relevance, it cannot be excluded that some patients on carbamazepine may require higher olanzapine dosages than usual.

Felbamate *(SED-13, 153; SEDA-20, 61; SEDA-21, 70; SEDA-22, 86)*

Felbamate risk/benefit ratio

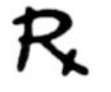

The Quality Standards Subcommittee of the American Academy of Neurology and the American Epilepsy Society (26[r]) has reviewed efficacy and safety data to establish recommendations for felbamate use in the light of the risk of aplastic anemia and liver toxicity (SEDA-22, 86). Felbamate was considered to have a favorable risk/benefit ratio in patients with Lennox-Gastaut syndrome aged over 4 years who were unresponsive to primary antiepileptic drugs, in patients over 18 years of age with intractable partial seizures that have not responded to standard antiepileptic drugs in therapeutic concentrations, and in patients who are already taking felbamate and benefit from it for more than 18 months. There are conditions in which the risk/benefit ratio is unclear, but for which use may be appropriate under certain circumstances, depending on the nature and severity of the seizure disorder; these include children with intractable partial epilepsy, patients with other generalized epilepsies unresponsive to primary agents, patients who have unacceptable sedative or cognitive effects with traditional antiepileptic drugs, and patients under 4 years with Lennox-Gastaut syndrome unresponsive to other antiepileptic drugs.

Risk/benefit assessment does not support the use of felbamate in new-onset epilepsy in children and adults, in patients who have significant prior hematological adverse events, in patients in whom follow-up and compliance will not allow careful monitoring, and in patients who are unable to discuss risk/benefits and for whom no parent or legal guardian is available to provide consent.

In patients started on felbamate, the risk/benefit ratio should be constantly assessed.

Patients should be educated about early signs of liver and bone-marrow toxicity, and about the manufacturers' recommendations. Laboratory monitoring has not been proven efficacious, but the manufacturer and the FDA suggest liver function and hematology testing at baseline and every 1–2 weeks for the first year. After that, the risk of aplastic anemia falls and the need for regular testing is less clear. A registry has been set up by the manufacturers to collect further safety data in patients started on the drug.

Gabapentin *(SED-13, 153; SEDA-20, 61; SEDA-21, 71; SEDA-22, 87)*

In an uncontrolled trial using dosages up to 6000 mg/day in 50 patients with refractory partial epilepsy, *tiredness*, *dizziness*, *headache*, and *diplopia* were the most common adverse effects (27[c]). At dosages above 3600 mg/day three patients developed *flatulence and diarrhea* and two had *myoclonic jerks*. At least in some patients, gabapentin gastrointestinal absorption did not become saturated within the explored dosage range.

Nervous system *Sensory neuropathy* occurred in a 58-year-old man who had been given up to 2400 mg/day for over 5 months for the treatment of head pain (28[c]). A mild pruritic rash had been present since starting treatment. Neuropathic symptoms included a burning sensation in the legs and hips. After withdrawal, reduced perception of tactile and noxious stimuli and neurogenic bladder dysfunction (with an associated syncopal episode) were recorded. The neuropathy improved over several months. Gabapentin is used often to treat neuropathic pain, and its role in causing the sensory neuropathy in this patient was uncertain.

Urinary system A 27-year-old man with bipolar disorder had an *increased serum creatinine concentration* (up to 1.7 mg/dl, 150 μmol/l) after taking gabapentin 2000 mg/day for several weeks, the change being reversible after drug withdrawal (29[c]). The possibility of renal dysfunction as a rare adverse effect should be considered. The patient had a history of allergic reactions to lithium, carbamazepine, clozapine, haloperidol, and lamotrigine.

Skin and appendages Serious hypersensitivity reactions to gabapentin are extremely rare. One such case may have occurred in a 32-year-old woman with HIV infection and cerebral toxoplasmosis who developed histologically confirmed *Stevens-Johnson syndrome* after taking gabapentin (300–900 mg/day) for 3 days (30[c]). Although other drugs were given, the condition resolved after withdrawal of gabapentin alone. Whether the underlying condition played a role is open to speculation.

Lamotrigine *(SED-13, 153; SEDA-20, 62; SEDA-21, 72; SEDA-22, 88)*

In a multicenter double-blind comparison of lamotrigine and phenytoin (titrated over 6 weeks from starting dosages of 100 and 200 mg/day respectively) in 181 patients with newly diagnosed epilepsy there were comparable seizure freedom rates and comparable trial discontinuation rates with the two drugs (31[cr]). *Skin rashes* leading to withdrawal occurred in 12% of patients assigned to lamotrigine and in 5% of those assigned to phenytoin, but the risk associated with lamotrigine might have been overestimated, owing to an excessively high starting dose. Central nervous system adverse effects were more common with phenytoin, the difference being statistically significant for weakness (29 vs 16%), somnolence (28 vs 7%), and ataxia (12 vs 0%).

Nervous system A multicenter study showed that lamotrigine can cause *seizure aggravation* in children with severe myoclonic epilepsy (32[C]). Of 21 patients with severe myoclonic epilepsy given lamotrigine in dosages of 2.5–12.5 mg/kg/day, seizures exacerbated in 17. The frequency of convulsive seizures increased by more than 50% in eight of 20 patients, and myoclonic seizures worsened in six out of 18. Out of five patients who improved in at least one seizure type, four had concomitant worsening of more invalidating seizures. The drug was withdrawn in 19 patients, with consequent improvement in 18. These findings suggest that lamotrigine is inappropriate in severe myoclonic epilepsy.

Insomnia is a recognized adverse effect of lamotrigine. Among 109 patients treated with lamotrigine in an adult tertiary referral center, seven had insomnia of sufficient severity to require a change of therapy (33[Cr]). The symptom occurred shortly after the start of treatment, was dose-dependent, and resolved after withdrawal or dose reduction. Unlike previous reports, in which insomnia occurred in patients with impaired cognition, no predisposing factor could be identified.

Hematological A 11-year-old girl, with congenital left renal agenesis, epilepsy from cortical dysgenesis, and chronic hepatitis B and C, developed a skin rash and *agranulocytosis* (white cell count 3.1×10^9/l, lymphocytes 92% and monocytes 8%) 15–20 days after starting to take lamotrigine (34[C]). She recovered rapidly after drug withdrawal. An inappropriately high starting dose (50 mg/day) may have contributed to the reaction.

Skin and appendages Published and unpublished cases of *Stevens-Johnson syndrome* (n = 43) and *toxic epidermal necrolysis* (n = 14) associated with lamotrigine have been reviewed (35[CR]). The patients with Stevens-Johnson syndrome were younger than those with toxic epidermal necrolysis (21 vs 31 years); the median time to onset for both reactions was 17 days; the median dosage at onset (50 mg for Stevens-Johnson syndrome, 87.5 mg for toxic epidermal necrolysis) did not differ significantly. Valproate co-medication was present in 74 and 64% of patients with Stevens-Johnson syndrome and toxic epidermal necrolysis respectively. In three patients, toxic epidermal necrolysis occurred in the context of the anticonvulsant hypersensitivity syndrome.

Sexual function A 37-year-old schizoaffective woman taking lamotrigine monotherapy developed *loss of libido* and an unpleasant feeling at touching of erogenous zones when the dosage of lamotrigine was increased from 200 to 400 mg/day (36[C]). Surprisingly, no attempt was made to determine whether the condition could be reversed by lowering the dosage. Female genital disorder is an adverse effect of selective serotonin reuptake inhibitors, and it was speculated that it could be related to the ability of lamotrigine to inhibit serotonin uptake.

Immunological and hypersensitivity reactions Twenty-six lamotrigine-associated reactions consistent with the features of the *anticonvulsant hypersensitivity syndrome* have been reviewed, including nine previously published (37[CR]). The patients were aged 3.5–74 (mean 28) years and 14 were female. Valproate was used as co-medication in 60%. Fever was present in all patients, a skin rash in 77% (with Stevens-Johnson syndrome or toxic epidermal necrolysis in five cases), hematological abnormalities in 69% (including eosinophilia in 19%), liver abnormalities in 65%, renal involvement in 23%, disseminated intravascular coagulation in 15%, and musculoskeletal disorders in 8%. Multiorgan involvement was present in 46%, and one patient died. Overall, the characteristics of the syndrome were comparable to that induced by aromatic anticonvulsants, except for a somewhat higher incidence of severe skin rashes and a lower frequency of eosinophilia and lymphadenopathy.

A 35-year-old man with Lennox-Gastaut syndrome developed *tender cervical lymphadenopathy* 14 weeks after lamotrigine was introduced, when the dosage was increased to 200 mg/day (38[c]). Frozen section examination of a biopsy specimen 10 weeks later suggested lymphoma, but further histopathological investigations documented lymphoid hyperplasia consistent with a diagnosis of pseudolymphoma, which resolved 1 month after withdrawal. This seems to be the first report of pseudolymphoma associated with lamotrigine.

A 47-year-old man developed a *rash, fever, and rigors* after taking lamotrigine (50 mg/day at maintenance) for 1 month (39[C]). The reaction subsided after withdrawal, but 3 days later he complained of left shoulder pain and numbness in the left arm. The pain worsened over the next 3 weeks and then subsided. Thereafter, he developed weakness of the left arm with muscle wasting and signs of denervation in the biceps, infraspinatus, and supraspinatus. The condition was diagnosed as neuralgic amyotrophy. Almost complete recovery occurred over 8 months. It is possible that the hypersensitivity reaction determined focal neuronal involvement at the brachial plexus.

Oxcarbazepine *(SED-12, 137; SEDA-18, 66; SEDA-19, 71; SEDA-21, 73)*

Interactions In a placebo-controlled study in healthy women, oxcarbazepine (900 mg/day) reduced the serum concentrations of *ethinylestradiol* and *levonorgestrel* by about 50% (40[Cr]). This confirms that oxcarbazepine may reduce the efficacy of the contraceptive pill, similarly to carbamazepine. Women taking oxcarbazepine should be given a contraceptive that contains 50 μg of ethinylestradiol and they should be monitored for signs of insufficient contraceptive cover, such as breakthrough bleeding.

Phenobarbital *(SED-13, 154; SEDA-20, 64; SEDA-21, 73)*

Nervous system A 12-month trial in 109 epileptic children randomized to monotherapy with phenobarbital (maintenance dose, 3.0 mg/kg/day) or phenytoin (5.0 mg/kg/day) in rural India failed to identify significant differences in either efficacy or toxicity (41[Cr]). In particular, *behavioral adverse effects* were not more common with phenobarbital. The findings suggest that phenobarbital is an acceptable first-line agent for childhood epilepsy in rural settings in developing countries.

Interactions Compared with 15 patients taking *clozapine* alone, seven patients taking similar dosages in combination with phenobarbital had significantly lower plasma clozapine concentrations (232 vs 356 ng/ml) (42[Cr]). Plasma norclozapine concentrations did not differ between the two groups, whereas clozapine *N*-oxide concentrations were significantly higher in the phenobarbital group. These findings suggest that phenobarbital stimulates the metabolism of clozapine, probably by inducing the *N*-oxidation and demethylation pathways. Although the clinical implications remain to be defined, an increase in clozapine dosage requirements may be considered in patients co-medicated with phenobarbital.

Phenytoin *(SED-13, 141; SEDA-20, 64; SEDA-21, 73; SEDA-22, 90)*

Nervous system Distal lower extremity paresthesia in stocking distribution and motor weakness with loss of the Achilles tendon reflex, associated with reduced sensory conduction velocity, occurred in an 18-year-old girl a few hours after the administration of phenytoin (7.5 mg/kg) (43[cr]). The condition regressed after phenytoin withdrawal. *Peripheral neuropathy* is a known adverse effect of phenytoin, but this is the first report of an acute neuropathy within less than a week of treatment.

Endocrine, metabolic An 18-year-old man with heterozygous point mutation in the defective allele of CYP2C9 and CYP2C19 (two enzymes involved in phenytoin metabolism) developed *gynecomastia* about 1 month after phenytoin dosage was increased from 175 to 190 mg/day, resulting in a serum phenytoin concentration of 68 μmol/l (44[cr]). Phenytoin has been rarely implicated in gynecomastia, and whether the cytochrome P450 genotype played a contributory role was unclear. The patient was co-medicated with zonisamide, which has also been rarely associated with gynecomastia.

Special senses *Ageusia* occurred in a 52-year-old man within a few hours of an intravenous infusion of phenytoin (750 mg) for the control of seizures (45[c]). The condition persisted for 2 weeks during oral phenytoin treatment and cleared in about 1 week when phenobarbital was substituted. The time course strongly suggested that phenytoin was responsible.

Immunological and hypersensitivity reactions A 32-year-old man developed *acute lung injury and renal insufficiency* after 4 days of starting phenytoin (46[c]). The symptoms mimicked a renopulmonary syndrome, and resolved completely after withdrawal of phenytoin and the addition of steroids.

Tiagabine *(SEDA-20, 65; SEDA-21, 74; SEDA-22, 91)*

Nervous system In a randomized double-blind add-on trial of tiagabine (16, 32, or 56 mg/day) in 297 patients with refractory partial seizures, adverse events significantly more common with tiagabine were *dizziness* in the 32 mg group (33 vs 15% with placebo), *tremor* in the 32 and 56 mg groups (15 and 21 vs 3%), *mental lethargy or difficulty in concentrating* in the 56 mg group (14 vs 3%), and *depressed mood* in the 16 and 56 mg groups (7% in both groups vs 0%) (47[c]). In a similar study with a dosage of 10 mg tds, the most common adverse events were *dizziness, weakness, headache, and somnolence* (48[c]), but only dizziness was significantly more common than with placebo (29 vs 10%).

Special senses Following reports of *concentric visual field defects* associated with vigabatrin (SEDA-21, 78), there has been concern that other drugs that enhance GABAergic inhibition might cause a similar disorder. Although visual field defects were detected in six of 12 patients treated with tiagabine in Australia, no details were given, and this report seems to have remained isolated (49[c]). In a controlled study, none of 15 patients treated with tiagabine monotherapy for 1.5 to 3.5 years (mean daily dose 22 mg) had evidence of a concentric visual field defect (50[c]).

Topiramate *(SEDA-20, 66; SEDA-21, 75; SEDA-22, 91)*

Nervous system *Slowed mental function* is a relatively common adverse effect of topiramate, especially at high dosages, and has been confirmed in a randomized single-blind parallel-group study in healthy volunteers. After single doses, topiramate (2.8 mg/kg) reduced performance in attention and word fluency tests, whereas lamotrigine (3.5 mg/kg) and gabapentin (17 mg/kg) had no effects (51[Cr]). After 4 weeks of multiple dosing, topiramate (5.7 mg/kg) was still associated with impairment in verbal memory and psychomotor speed, while there was no impairment with lamotrigine (7.1 mg/kg) or gabapentin (35 mg/kg). While these data suggest that topiramate can cause greater cognitive dysfunction in the short-term than lamotrigine and gabapentin, these findings should be interpreted cautiously. First, the design was less than ideal: the use of a double-blind cross-over design and inclusion of placebo would have been preferable. Second, the speed of topiramate titration was much faster than currently recommended, and it is known that neurotoxicity can be reduced by slow dose escalation. Finally, the dosage of topiramate was very high, in view of the fact that no enzyme-inducing co-medication was present.

Hemiparesis developed in a 41-year-old man and a 59-year-old woman during the first few weeks on topiramate at dosages up to 250 and 200 mg/day respectively (52[C]). The condition resolved gradually after drug withdrawal. Both patients had pre-existing cerebral damage (contralateral cerebral palsy and temporal lobe infarction respectively), which might have facilitated this hitherto unreported possible adverse effect.

Endocrine metabolic By inhibiting carbonic anhydrase, topiramate can cause *metabolic acidosis*. The first patient in whom this was described in detail was a 52-year-old man who, while taking topiramate 200 mg/day, developed a normal ion gap metabolic acidosis, which worsened during elective surgery for temporal lobectomy (53[cr]). Based on information from the manufacturers, the risk of metabolic acidosis is estimated at 1 : 100 to 1 : 1000, but the authors correctly pointed out that acidosis can become especially significant during surgery, in the elderly, or in patients on dialysis. Theoretically, there would be special concern in using topiramate in other patients at potential serious risk, such as those taking acetazolamide or those on a ketogenic diet.

Liver *Fulminant liver failure* developed in a 39-year-old woman after she had taken topiramate for about 4 months, in addition to carbamazepine. The condition occurred after she increased the dosage of topiramate to 300 mg/day, and was preceded for a few days by tiredness and somnolence (54[c]). She made an uncomplicated recovery after liver transplantation. Histological examination showed centrilobular necrosis, compatible with drug-induced fulminant liver failure. This seems to be the first report of hepatotoxicity ascribed to topiramate, but the causative role of the drug could not be determined with certainty.

Valproate sodium *(SED-13, 149; SEDA-20, 67; SEDA-21, 76; SEDA-22, 91)*

Nervous system When a 25-year-old woman with a hypothalamic hamartoma was given valproate (up to 2500 mg/day) in addition to phenytoin and phenobarbital, she became increasingly *somnolent* and *spike and wave activity in her electroencephalogram deteriorated* to the point when she appeared to be in absence status (55[c]). Her blood ammonia concentration was about three times the upper limit of the reference range. During wakefulness, electroencephalographic paroxysms increased with increasing plasma valproic acid concentrations, and resolved (together with mental status changes and hyperammonemia) when valproate was withdrawn. The data are suggestive of a paradoxical effect of valproic acid on spike and wave activity, possibly related to the underlying pathology or hyperammonemia.

A most unusual adverse effect, *uncontrollable laughter*, was reported in two men aged 17 and 20 years (56[C]). The laughter persisted for 4–6 hours after an intravenous injection of 800 mg valproate over 1 hour.

Endocrine, metabolic Women taking valproate have an increased incidence of *polycystic ovaries and hyperandrogenism* associated with weight gain and hyperinsulinemia. The reversibility of this syndrome has been documented in 16 women with valproate-related polycystic ovaries and/or hyperandrogenism who were switched to lamotrigine (57[Cr]). While taking valproate, they had centripetal obesity with associated hyperinsulinism and unfavorable serum lipid profiles. After switching to lamotrigine, in the 12 patients available for follow-up at 1 year, body-mass index and fasting serum insulin and testosterone concentrations fell, whereas HDL-cholesterol/total cholesterol ratios increased from 0.17 to 0.26. The total number of polycystic ovaries fell from 20 to 11 after 1 year of lamotrigine.

Mineral and fluid balance *Hyponatremia* (serum sodium of 128 mmol/l) was discovered accidentally in a 50-year-old man during follow-up for Henoch-Schönlein nephritis (58[c]). He was taking sodium valproate 2000 mg/day. Repeated water loads at different dosages of valproate confirmed that the ability to excrete water was dose-dependently reduced. A syndrome resembling inappropriate secretion of ADH has been described with carbamazepine and oxcarbazepine, but there have only been two other published cases implicating valproate in the pathogenesis of hyponatremia.

Hematological Valproate can cause *reduced platelet counts or function.* A recent study has shown, in addition to a reduced platelet count, impairment of procoagulatory thrombocytic functions as reflected by reduced platelet activation and an increased thrombin time (59[Cr]). Valproate-induced platelet dysfunction may be related, at least in part and in some patients, to inhibition of the arachidonic acid cascade (60[Cr]).

Sexual function A 32-year-old man developed *infertility and a low sperm count* (under 50 000/ml), with no motile sperm, less than 10% viability, and 100% with abnormal structure while taking valproate monotherapy for 5 years (61[c]). Within 4 months of switching to felbamate, he and his wife conceived twin girls, and the sperm abnormalities were largely reversed. These findings suggest that occasionally valproate can cause male infertility.

Miscellaneous In 15 patients who had a serious adverse reaction to valproate (including behavioral changes and emesis in six, raised AST in three, raised AST and pancreatitis in one, thombocytopenia in two, and unexpected death in two), erythrocyte glutathione peroxidase activity and plasma selenium and zinc concentrations were significantly reduced, whereas erythrocyte glutathione reductase activity was significantly raised relative to matched healthy controls or patients with good tolerance of valproate (62[Cr]). These findings may indicate a role for selenium-dependent antioxidant activity in individual susceptibility to the adverse effects of valproate.

Risk factors A 24-year-old man with *demyelinating disease* had fulminant progression of the disease after he experienced valproate-induced hyperammonemic encephalopathy (63[c]). Although the role of hyperammonemia is uncertain, this case raises concern for possible risks in using valproic acid in patients with fulminant demyelinating disease.

Second generation effects Three cases of *lung hypoplasia* after prenatal exposure to valproate have been reported in two female siblings and an unrelated female (64[C]). The two siblings had no other malformations, whereas the third neonate had a number of major birth defects. All three died a few hours after birth. The possibility that lung hypoplasia was caused by valproate remains speculative.

Overdosage After a valproate overdose, a 27-year-old man developed seizures, hypernatremia, respiratory failure, metabolic acidosis, liver failure, and bone marrow depression (65[C]). His plasma valproic acid concentration was 1414 mg/l. Treatment with hemodialysis was effective in enhancing valproic acid clearance, while hemoperfusion was relatively less effective, because of saturation of the column. Overall, the half-life of the drug was reduced from over 20 hours before treatment to less than 3 hours during hemodialysis/hemoperfusion; drug removal was probably favored by saturation of drug binding to plasma proteins, which resulted in a low unbound fraction (32% at the start of treatment). He was comatose for 5 days but recovered fully thereafter.

Interactions The intravenous administration of *panipenem-betamipron* in a 22-year-old man and in two young girls resulted in a marked and rapid fall in the serum concentrations of valproic acid to 0–40% of the pretreatment concentration (66[C]). In two patients, the effect was associated with epileptic seizures. Serum valproic acid began to rise again within 2 hours of stopping the antibiotic. Although the mechanism of interaction is unknown, animal studies suggest that suppression of the enterohepatic circulation of valproic acid may have been involved (67[C]).

At a concentration of 100 mg/l, valproic acid inhibits the glucuronidation of *zidovudine* in human liver microsomes by 50% (68[C]). This observation explains the previously reported effect of valproate to increase plasma zidovudine concentrations in HIV-infected patients.

Chronic valproate (600–1500 mg/day) has been associated with a slight increase in plasma *clozapine* concentrations and a slight fall in norclozapine concentrations (69[Cr]). These changes are unlikely to be clinically significant.

Vigabatrin *(SED-13, 155; SEDA-20, 70; SEDA-21, 77; SEDA-22, 92)*

In a placebo-controlled add-on comparison of three dosages of vigabatrin (1, 3, and 6 g/day) in 174 patients with partial epilepsy, *fatigue, drowsiness*, and *dizziness* were the most common treatment-related adverse events, especially at the highest dosage (70[cr]). The incidence of severe events was 2.2% in the placebo group and 8.7, 11.4, and 15.9% with 1, 3 and 6 g/day respectively. The proportion of patients who withdrew owing to adverse events was 2.2% in the placebo group and 6.5, 11.4, and 18.2% with 1, 3, and 6 g/day respectively. Four vigabatrin patients (three of whom were taking 6 g/day) had a *reduction in erythrocyte counts* to 3.4–3.5 $\times$ 10^9/l. Symptoms suggestive of retinal toxicity were not reported, but the duration of treatment was short (18 weeks) and there was no formal ophthalmological testing. Overall, efficacy and safety data from this trial suggested that 3 g/day gave optimal results. Although higher dosages may provide additional benefit in selected patients, the occurrence of retinal toxicity (see below) warrants caution about the use of high doses.

Nervous system Like other GABAergic drugs, vigabatrin may *aggravate absence seizures* and may precipitate absence status in patients with generalized epilepsies. Occasionally, absence seizures are also precipitated in patients with partial epilepsy, as in a 28-year-old man who developed de novo absence status 4 days after the dosage of vigabatrin was increased to 2 g/day (71[c]).

Special senses *Visual field defects* in patients treated with vigabatrin were discussed in SEDA-21 (p. 78) and SEDA-22 (p. 92). New evidence suggests that the prevalence of this disorder is considerable. Among 57 patients aged 19–73 years treated with vigabatrin as add-on or as monotherapy for 2–14 years, there were mildly abnormal or severely abnormal fields in 14 and 8 patients respectively (72[c]). Two patients with severe field abnormalities were symptomatic. In another study, 12 of 20 consecutive patients treated with vigabatrin had visual field constriction, severe in four and symptomatic in two (73[C]). In the latter study, visual field defects were more common in patients who were also taking valproate. Although most reports concerned adults, children may also be affected (74[C]).

Potential correlations between visual field defects and the results of ophthalmological tests are being assessed. The use of the electroretinogram as a marker for vigabatrin-induced visual field alterations has been questioned (75[c]), and the suggestion has been made that the electroretinographic changes described in some patients on vigabatrin may be due to a physiological effect of GABA not necessarily related to retinal toxicity (76[c]). Of 20 consecutive patients 14 had a reduced light/dark ratio (Arden ratio) in the standard electro-oculogram and 10 had absent oscillatory potentials in the electroretinogram (73[C]). Overall, 17 patients had abnormal electro-oculograms, electroretinograms, or both, although only 12 had constricted visual fields at perimetric testing.

The mechanism responsible for the development of the visual field defects remains elusive. Evidence for inner cone dysfunction has been presented (77[C], 78[c]), but its interpretation has been disputed (75[c], 76[c]). The possibility that retinal toxicity is due to increased GABA activity also remains to be confirmed, and vigabatrin-induced inhibition of ornithine aminotransferase has been suggested as an alternative mechanism to be considered (79[c]).

Risk factors Acute encephalopathy with stupor and generalized slow wave electroencephalographic activity developed in three men with *mild renal insufficiency* aged 24–74 years within 1–3 days of starting vigabatrin (1–2 g/day) or increasing the dosage (from 2 to 3 g/day) (80[C]). The symptoms subsided rapidly after drug withdrawal or dose reduction. Special caution is recommended when vigabatrin is used in patients with impaired renal function.

REFERENCES

1. Cramer JA, Fisher R, Ben-Menachem E, French J, Mattson RH. New antiepileptic drugs: comparison of key clinical trials. Epilepsia 1999;40:590–600.
2. Treiman DM, Meyers PD, Walton NY, Collins JF, Colling C, Rowan AJ, Handforth A, Faight E, Calabrese VP, Uthman BM, Ramsay E, Mamdani MB. A comparison of four treatments for generalized convulsive status epilepticus. New Engl J Med 1998;339:792–8.
3. Nilsson L, Farahmand BY, Persson PG, Thiblin I, Tomson T. Risk factors for sudden unexpected death in epilepsy: a case-control study. Lancet 1999;353:888–93.
4. Timmings PL. Sudden unexpected death in epilepsy: is carbamazepine implicated? Seizure 1998;7:289–91.
5. Rintahaka PJ, Nakagawa JA, Shewmon DA, Kyyronen P, Shields WD. Incidence of death in patients with intractable epilepsy during nitrazepam treatment. Epilepsia 1999;40:492–6.
6. Murphy JV, Sawasky F, Marquardt KM, Harris DJ Deaths in young children receiving nitrazepam. J Pediatr 1987;111:145–7.
7. Wyllie E, Wyllie R, Cruse RP, Rothner AD, Eremberg G. The mechanism of nitrazepam-induced drooling and aspiration. New Engl J Med 1986;314:35–8.
8. Bourgeois BFD. Antiepileptic drugs, learning and behavior in childhood epilepsy. Epilepsia 1998;39:913–21.
9. Duncan S, Blacklaw J, Beastall GH, Brodie MJ. Antiepileptic drug therapy and sexual function in men with epilepsy. Epilepsia 1999;40:197–204.
10. Schwaninger M, Ringleb P, Winter R, Kohl B, Fiehn W, Rieser PA, Walter-Sack I. Elevated plasma concentrations of homocysteine in antiepileptic drug treatment. Epilepsia 1999;40:345–50.
11. Ciernik IF, Thiel M, Widmer U. Anterior uveitis and the anticonvulsant hypersensitivity syndrome. Arch Intern Med 1998;158:192.
12. Mamon HJ, Wen PY, Burns AC, Loeffler JS. Allergic skin reactions to anticonvulsant medications in patients receiving cranial radiation therapy. Epilepsia 1999;40:341–4.
13. Canadian Study Group for Childhood Epilepsy. Clobazam has equivalent efficacy to carbamazepine and phenytoin as monotherapy for epilepsy. Epilepsia 1998;39:952–9.
14. Takayanagi K, Hisauchi I, Watanabe J-I, Maekawa Y, Fujito T, Sakai Y, Hoshi K, Kase M, Nishimura N, Inoue T, Hayashi T, Morooka S. Carbamazepine-induced sinus node dysfunction and atrioventricular block in elderly women. Jpn Heart J 1998;39:469–79.
15. Cates M, Powers R. Concomitant rash and blood dyscrasias in geriatric psychiatry patients treated with carbamazepine. Ann Pharmacother 1998;32:884–7.
16. Mizoguchi S, Setoyama M, Higashi Y, Hozumi H, Kanzaki T. Eosinophilic pustular folliculitis induced by carbamazepine. J Am Acad Dermatol 1998;38:641–3.
17. Nathan DL, Belsito DV. Carbamazepine-induced pseudolymphoma with CD-30 positive cells. J Am Acad Dermatol 1998;38:806–9.
18. Ganga A, Corda D, Gallo Carrabba G, Cossu S, Massarelli G, Rosati G. A case of carbamazepine-induced lymphadenopathy resembling Kikuchi disease. Eur Neurol 1998;39:247–8.
19. Lhotta K, Konig P. Cryoglobulinaemia, membranoproliferative glomerulonephritis and pANCA in a patient treated with carbamazepine. Nephrol Dial Transplant 1998;13:1890–1.
20. Nisijima K, Kusakabe Y, Ohtuka K, Ishiguro T. Addition of carbamazepine to long-term treatment with neuroleptics may induce neuroleptic malignant syndrome. Biol Psychiatry 1998;44:930–1.
21. Kanner AM, Bourgeois BFD, Hasegawa H, Hutson P. Rapid switchover to carbamazepine using pharmacokinetic parameters. Epilepsia 1998;39:194–200.
22. Genton P, Vi Huong N, Mesdjian E. Carbamazepine intoxication with negative myoclonus after the addition of clobazam. Epilepsia 1998;39:1115–18.
23. Garg SK, Kumar N, Bhargava VK, Prabhakar SK. Effect of grapefruit juice on carbamazepine bioavailability in patients with epilepsy. Clin Pharmacol Ther 1998;64:286–8.
24. Eap CB, Yasui N, Kaneko S, Baumann P, Powell K, Otani K. Effects of carbamazepine coadministration on plasma concentrations of the enantiomers of mianserin and its metabolites. Ther Drug Monit 1999;21:166–70.
25. Lucas RA, Gilfillan DJ, Bergstrom RF. A pharmacokinetic interaction between carbamazepine and olanzapine: observations on possible mechanism. Eur J Clin Pharmacol 1998;54:639–43.
26. French J, Smith M, Faught E, Brown L. Practice advisory: the use of felbamate in the treatment of patients with intractable epilepsy. Epilepsia 1999;40:803–8.
27. Wilson EA, Sills GJ, Forrest G, Brodie MJ. High dose gabapentin in refractory partial epilepsy: clinical observations in 50 patients. Epilepsy Res 1998;29:161–6.
28. Gould HJ. Gabapentin induced polyneuropathy. Pain 1998;74:341–3.
29. Grunze H, Dittert S, Bungert M, Erfurth A. Renal impairment as a possible side effect of gabapentin. Neuropsychobiology 1998;38:198–9.
30. Gonzalez-Sicilia L, Cano A, Serrano M, Hernandez J. Stevens-Johnson syndrome associated with gabapentin. Am J Med 1998;105:455.
31. Steiner TJ, Dellaportas CI, Findley LJ, Gross M, Gibberd FB, Perkin GD, Park DM, Abbott R. Lamotrigine monotherapy in newly diagnosed untreated epilepsy: a double-blind comparison with phenytoin. Epilepsia 1999;40:601–7.
32. Guerrini R, Dravet C, Genton P, Belmonte A, Kaminska A, Dulac O. Lamotrigine and seizure aggravation in severe myoclonic epilepsy. Epilepsia 1998;39:508–12.
33. Sadler M. Lamotrigine associated with insomnia. Epilepsia 1998;40:322–5.

34. Kraus de Camardo OA, Bode H. Agranulocytosis associated with lamotrigine. Br Med J 1999;318:1179.
35. Schlienger RG, Shapiro LE, Shear NH. Lamotrigine-induced severe cutaneous adverse reactions. Epilepsia 1998;39(Suppl 7):S22–S26.
36. Erfurth A, Amann B, Grunze H. Female genital disorder as adverse symptom of lamotrigine treatment. Neuropsychobiology 1998;38:200–1.
37. Schlienger RG, Knowles SR, Shear NH. Lamotrigine-associated anticonvulsant hypersensitivity syndrome. Neurology 1998;51:1172–5.
38. Pathak P, McLachlan RS. Drug-induced pseudolymphoma secondary to lamotrigine. Neurology 1998;50:1509–10.
39. Hennessy MJ, Koutroumanidis M, Elwes RDC. Neuralgic amyotrophy associated with hypersensitivity to lamotrigine. Neurology 1998;51:1224.
40. Fattore C. Cipolla G, Gatti G, D'Urso S, Limdo GL, Sturm Y, Bernasconi C, Perucca E. Induction of ethinylestradiol and levonorgestrel metabolism by oxcarbazepine in healthy women. Epilepsia 1999;40:783–7.
41. Pal DK, Das T, Chaudhury G, Johnson AL, Neville BGR. Randomised controlled trial to assess acceptability of phenobarbital for childhood epilepsy in rural India. Lancet 1998;351:19–23.
42. Facciola G, Avenoso A, Spina E, Perucca E. Inducing effect of phenobarbital on clozapine metabolism in patients with chronic schizophrenia. Ther Drug Monit 1998;20:628–30.
43. Yoshikawa H, Abe T, Oda Y. Extremely acute phenytoin-induced peripheral neuropathy. Epilepsia 1999;40:528–9.
44. Ikeda A, Hattori H, Odani A, Kimura J, Shibasaki H. Gynaecomastia in association with phenytoin and zonisamide in a patient having a CYP2C subfamily mutation. J Neurol Neurosurg Psychiatry 1998;65:803–4.
45. Zeller JA, Machetanz J, Kessler C. Ageusia as an adverse effect of phenytoin treatment. Lancet 1998;351:1101.
46. Polman AJ, Van der Werf TS, Tiebosch ATMC, Zijlstra JG. Early-onset phenytoin toxicity mimicking a renopulmonary syndrome. Eur Respir J 1998;11:501–3.
47. Uthman BM, Rowan AJ, Ahmann PA, Leppik IE, Schachter SC, Sommerville KW, Shu V. Tiagabine for complex partial seizures: a randomized, add-on, dose-response trial. Ann Neurol 1998;55:56–62.
48. Kalviainen R, Brodie MJ, Duncan J, Chadwick D, Edwards D, Lyby K. A double-blind, placebo-controlled trial of tiagabine given three-times daily as add-on therapy for refractory partial seizures. Epilepsy Res 1998;30:31–40.
49. Beran RG, Hung A, Plunkett M, Currie J, Sachinwalla R. Predictability of visual field defects in patients exposed to GABAergic agents, vigabatrin, or tiagabine. Neurology 1999;52(Suppl 2):A249.
50. Kalviainen R, Nousiainen I, Mantiyarvi M, Riekkinen PJ. Absence of concentric visual field defects in patients with long-term tiagabine monotherapy. Neurology 1999;52(Suppl 2):A236.
51. Martin R, Kuzniecki R, Ho S, Hetherington H, Pan J, Sinclair K, Gilliam F, Faught E. Cognitive effects of topiramate, gabapentin, and lamotrigine in healthy young volunteers. Neurology 1999;52:321–7.
52. Stephen LJ, Maxwell JE, Brodie MJ. Transient hemiparesis with topiramate. Br Med J 1999;318:845.
53. Wilner A, Raymond K, Pollard R. Topiramate and metabolic acidosis. Epilepsia 1999;40:792–5.
54. Bjoro K, Gjerstad L, Bentdal O, Osnes S, Schrumpf E. Topiramate and fulminant liver failure. Lancet 1998;352:1119.
55. Stecker MM, Kita M. Paradoxical response to valproic acid in a patient with a hypothalamic hamartoma. Ann Pharmacother 1998;332:1168–72.
56. Jacob PC, Chand RP. Pathological laughter following intravenous sodium valproate. Can J Neurol Sci 1998;25:252–3.
57. Isojarvi JIT, Rattya J, Myllyla VV, Knip M, Koivunen R, Pakarinen AJ, Tekay A, Tapanainen JS. Valproate, lamotrigine, and insulin-mediated risks in women with epilepsy. Ann Neurol 1998;43:446–51.
58. Branten AJW, Wetzels JFM, Weber AM, Koene RAP. Hyponatremia due to sodium valproate. Ann Neurol 1998;43:265–7.
59. Zeller JA, Schlesinger S, Runge U, Kessler C. Influence of valproate monotherapy on platelet activation and hematologic values. Epilepsia 1999;40:186–9.
60. Kis B, Szupera Z, Mezei Z, Gecse A, Telegdy G, Vecsei L. Valproate treatment and platelet function: the role of arachidonate metabolites. Epilepsia 1999;40:307–10.
61. Yerby MS, McCoy GB. Male infertility: possible association with valproate exposure. Epilepsia 1999;40:520–1.
62. Graf WD, Oleinik OE, Glauser TA, Maertens P, Eder DN, Pippenger C. Altered antioxidant enzyme activities in children with a serious adverse experience related to valproic acid therapy. Neuropediatrics 1998;29:195–201.
63. Blindauer KA, Harrington G, Morris GL, Ho K-C. Fulminant progression of demyelinating disease after valproate-induced encephalopathy. Neurology 1998;5:292–5.
64. Janas MS, Arroe M, Hansen SH, Graem N. Lung hypoplasia—a possible teratogenic effect of valproate. APMIS 1998;106:300–4.
65. Franssen EJF, Van Essen GG, Portman AT, De Jong A, Go G, Stegeman CA, Uges DRA. Valproic acid toxicokinetics: Serial hemodialysis and hemoperfusion. Ther Drug Monit 1999;21:289–92.
66. Yamagata T, Momoi MY, Murai K, Ikematsu K, Suwa K, Sakamoto K, Fujimura A. Panipenem-betamipron decreases in serum valproic acid concentration. Ther Drug Monit 1998;20:396–400.
67. Kojima S, Nadai M, Kitaichi K, Wang L, Nabeshima T, Hasegawa T. Possible mechanism by which the carbapenem antibiotic panipenem decreases the concentration of valproic acid in

plasma in rats. Antimicrob Agents Chemother 1998;42:3136–40.

68. Trapnell CB, Klecker RW, Jamis-Dow C, Collins JM. Glucuronidation of 3′-azido-3′-deoxythymidine (zidovudine) by human liver microsomes: Relevance to clinical pharmacokinetic interactions with atovaquone, fluconazole, methadone, and valproic acid. Antimicrob Agents Chemother 1998;42:1592–6.
69. Facciola G, Avenoso A, Scordo MG, Madia AG, Ventimiglia A, Perucca E, Spina E. Small effects of valproic acid on the plasma concentrations of clozapine and its major metabolites in patients with schizophrenic or affective disorders. Ther Drug Monit 1999;21:341–5.
70. Dean C, Mosier M, Penry K. Dose-response study of vigabatrin as add-on therapy in patients with uncontrolled partial seizures. Epilepsia 1999;40:74–82.
71. Cocito L, Primavera A, Panayiotopoulos CP, Agathonikou A, Sharoqi IA, Parker APJ. Vigabatrin aggravates absences and absence status. Neurology 1998;51:1519–20.
72. Nousiainen I, Kalviainen R, Mantiyarvi M, Riekkinen PJ. Prevalence of concentric visual field constriction in adult epilepsy patients with vigabatrin treatment. Neurology 1999;52(Suppl 2):A235–6.
73. Arndt CF, Derambure P, Defoort-Dhellemmes S, Hache JC. Outer retinal dysfunction in patients treated with vigabatrin. Neurology 1999;52:1201–5.
74. Vanhatalo S, Paakonen L. Visual field constriction in children treated with vigabatrin. Neurology 1999;52:1713–14.
75. Beck RW. Vigabatrin-associated retinal cone system dysfunction. Neurology 1998;51:1778–9.
76. Brigell MG. Vigabatrin-associated retinal cone system dysfunction. Neurology 1998;51:1779.
77. Krauss GL, Johnson MA, Miller NR. Vigabatrin-associated retinal cone system dysfunction: electroretinogram and ophthalmologic findings. Neurology 1998;50:614–18.
78. Krauss GL, Johnson MA, Miller NR. Vigabatrin-associated retinal cone system dysfunction. Neurology 1998;51:1779–81.
79. Roubertie A, Bellet H, Echenne B. Vigabatrin-associated retinal cone system dysfunction. Neurology 1998;51:1779.
80. Ifergane G, Masalha R, Zigulinski R, Merkin L, Wirguin I, Herishanu YO. Acute encephalopathy associated with vigabatrin monotherapy in patients with mild renal failure. Neurology 1998;51:314–15.

A.H. Ghodse and P.J. Bown

8 Opioid analgesics and narcotic antagonists

GENERAL

'Opioids produce analgesia but also respiratory depression, dependence and a variety of other troublesome side effects .... The clinical holy grail of analgesia without respiratory depression has yet to be attained' (1^R). This review outlines developments in opioid pharmacology that may assist in the realization of that goal. An important advance during the last decade has been the cloning of three main opioid receptor types, δ, κ, and μ, now respectively reclassified as OP, OP2, and OP3 by the International Union of Pharmacology. Structural studies from cloned μ receptors fail to support pharmacological studies proposing the existence of separate μ receptor subtypes that independently mediate analgesia and respiratory depression. However, the finding that morphine is ineffective as an analgesic in mice engineered to have no μ receptors confirms the importance of this receptor type.

The peptides endomorphin 1 and 2 have been identified in human brain and show selectivity and affinity for μ receptors. In mice, endomorphin 1 and 2 produce spinal and supraspinal analgesia. They appear to act through the regulation of calcium entry into the target cell via voltage-gated channels and also to inhibit cAMP production in μ receptor bearing cells. Clinically they mimic the action of other μ opioids. Their clinical relevance and unique adverse effects profiles await further investigation. Similarly the clinical usefulness of newly discovered receptor systems, such as the orphan opioid receptor for nociceptin (ORL1), which produces analgesia, hyperalgesia, and anti-opioid effects in animals, has yet to be defined.

Side Effects of Drugs, Annual 23
J.K. Aronson, ed.

OPIOID AGONISTS

GENERAL

Limitations to the use of opioids in cardiac surgery have been reviewed, highlighting the fact that μ receptor agonists cause dose-related *respiratory depression* through a reduction in carbon dioxide sensitivity in the respiratory centre (2^R). This depression, with a *reduced respiratory rate and hypoxia,* outlasts the analgesic effect of μ receptor agonists. Thoracic muscle rigidity on anesthetic induction with high doses of opioids has also been reported and may further compromise respiration. *Hypotension* through reduced peripheral vascular resistance occurs, while a negative inotropic effect of opioids acting directly on the heart via κ receptors is proposed, based on evidence from in vitro studies. The above effects have limited the role of opiates in patients with coronary artery disease, although they are of less importance in cardiopulmonary bypass surgery, when the heart is quiescent. In such surgery fentanyl partially blocks the expected tachycardia, hypertension, and release of inflammatory mediators that constitutes the stress response, although the block is incomplete, owing to a lack of anesthetic effect.

Biliary 'It is standard teaching that morphine should not be used to treat patients with pancreatitis because it causes a rise in biliary and pancreatic pressure' (3^R). From this starting point, this comprehensive review discusses current approaches to opioid analgesia in pancreatitis, pointing out that morphine has been reported to cause *biliary colic* in individuals without biliary tract disease and that pethidine (meperidine) has become the analgesic of choice. Direct measurement of constriction of the sphincter of Oddi is now possible using endoscopic retrograde cholangiopancreatography

(ERCP) and the basal tone of the sphincter and the frequency of phasic contractions are both observable; an increase in basal tone is believed to be the best indication of sphincter dysfunction. Morphine sulfate in intravenous doses of 2.5–5 μg/kg caused increased contractions but no change in basal pressure, while doses of 10 μg/kg plus caused in a rise in basal pressure. Pethidine increased contractions but not basal tone, while tramadol had no effect on basal pressure in a small study. Among mixed opiate agonist/antagonists, pentazocine increased basal pressure. Buprenorphine, a partial opiate agonist, resulted in no pressure changes, while the antagonist naloxone 0.4 mg intravenously had no effect alone on the sphincter basal pressure and did not stop the increase in pressure caused by morphine. However, case reports have suggested that naloxone reduces sphincter spasm in clinical situations.

The reviewers proposed that when there are concerns about the use of pethidine (in cases of renal insufficiency, allergy, reduced fit threshold, or drug seeking behaviour), buprenorphine, nalbuphine, or tramadol are the most promising opioids for analgesia, with limited adverse effects and exacerbation of the condition.

R *Opioid tolerance in neonates*

The clinical significance of opioid tolerance has been extensively reviewed (4[cR]) and the evidence for tolerance in acute and prolonged opioid administration presented. The former remains controversial while the latter has been adequately demonstrated. Different patterns of opioid use in chronic cancer-related pain are described, these being essentially escalating prescribing, steady-dose prescribing, and opioid withdrawal. The particular pattern followed by any individual is the result of the balance between physical changes in the level of nociceptive activity, psychological processes, such as increased anxiety and depression, and the degree of tolerance itself. While tolerance to an opiate reduces its clinical effectiveness, the tolerance may be beneficial if it mitigates drug adverse effects. Tolerance to respiratory depression and nausea occurs swiftly, sedation takes longer to resolve, while constipation is relatively resistant to the development of tolerance. Cross-tolerance is partial; hence switching from one opioid to another may relieve particular adverse effects without loss of clinical effect.

Physical dependence on opioids appears to occur in patients receiving opioids for long-term pain, and cases of addiction have been reported. However, rates of addiction are low and occur mainly in individuals who have a history of substance misuse. The role of long-term opioid medication in non-cancer related chronic pain remains controversial. 'Opiophobia', a fear of the legitimate use of opioid analgesics because of the potential for addiction, remains a significant issue for physicians, patients and relatives alike. The review is illustrated with a report of a 52-year-old man with multiple myeloma who displayed tolerance to oral morphine over 2 years.

Tolerance to opioids in neonates has been separately reviewed in greater detail (5[R]), and two forms of neonatal opioid exposure are considered: first, in utero exposure to opioids of neonates with opiate addicted mothers and secondly pre-term infants requiring prolonged support in intensive care when opioid administration is used to reduce the stress response. The mechanism of opioid action is also discussed. At micromolar concentrations opioids cause an increase in the cell membrane threshold, shortened action potentials, and inhibition of neurotransmitter release. At nanomolar concentrations opioid agonists are excitatory and prolong the action potential via the stimulatory G proteins (Gs) which act on the adenylate cyclase/cAMP system and on protein kinase A-dependent ion channels. Tolerance is proposed to be the result of an increase in the association of opioid receptors to Gs proteins, to an activation of N-methyl-D-aspartate receptors via protein kinase C, and calmodulin-dependent increases in cytosolic calcium, resulting in cellular hyperexcitability.

The adverse effects of opioids on neonates are similar to those described in adults (sedation, dysphoria, seizures, nausea and vomiting, urinary retention, reduced intestinal motility, biliary tract spasm, histamine release, and chest wall rigidity), but it has been proposed that differences in the densities of the different opioid receptor subtypes lead to an increased theoretical propensity for respiratory depression with given opioid doses compared with older people. However, clinical studies have not confirmed increased sensitivity to respiratory depression in neonates or young infants. Tolerance may occur more swiftly in neonates due to slower opioid metabolism and a more permeable blood brain barrier. Opioid withdrawal symptoms in neonates are similar to those for other age groups but may be mimicked by hypoxia, hypercarbia, hypoglycemia, hypocalcemia, or hypomagnesemia. Assessment of tolerance and withdrawal is made using the neonatal abstinence score rating scale and the neonatal withdrawal index.

Management of neonatal opioid withdrawal relies on gradually reducing doses of opioids to reduce the severity of withdrawal symptoms. Paregoric was formerly used as a withdrawal aid but is little used now owing to toxic effects. Tincture of opium (10% solution), consisting of 1 ml in 24 ml of sterile water, 0.05 ml/kg 4-hourly is proposed as the most suitable replacement. Speed of reduction depends on the length of neonatal exposure to opioids and a short reducing regimen (over 2–3 days) may be sufficient. A methadone replacement withdrawal regimen is also discussed, while benzodiazepines, phenobarbital, chlorpromazine, and clonidine are all reviewed as having a potential role in symptomatic relief during withdrawal; however, each has its own associated adverse effects, which limit their usefulness.

Alfentanil *(SED-13, 173; SEDA-20, 76; SEDA-21, 86; SEDA-22, 97)*

There has been a double-blind randomized control study of the effect of the antifungal drug *fluconazole* 400 mg on the pharmacokinetics and pharmacodynamics of intravenous alfentanil (6[cr]). Fluconazole given either orally or intravenously 1 hour before alfentanil 20 μg/kg iv caused a significant doubling of the half-life, through inhibition of CYP3A4, which metabolizes alfentanil. Intravenous and oral fluconazole both increased alfentanil-induced respiratory depression by reducing the respiratory rate by 10–15% compared with alfentanil alone. Alfentanil should therefore be given cautiously to patients taking fluconazole and the authors suggested that such patients require 60% less alfentanil for maintenance of analgesia, irrespective of the mode of administration of the antifungal drug.

Codeine *(SED-13, 173; SEDA-19, 82; SEDA-21, 86; SEDA-22, 98)*

In a retrospective study of patients with chronic rheumatological conditions, 290 of 644 clinic patients had received either codeine or oxycodone analgesia, of whom 137 had been given opioids for a continuous period of over 3 months (7[cr]). Adverse effects were described in 38% of both long-term and short-term opioid users, of which the most common were constipation, nausea, and sedation. *Headache, dizziness, rash or itching, confusion, insomnia, depression, diarrhea*, and *myoclonic jerking* were also reported. No significant differences in the adverse effects profile were reported between the groups and no subjects discontinued medication because of adverse effects. There were opioid abuse behaviors in 3% of the long-term users, but no association with a history of substance misuse was established.

A prospective double-blind randomized study in 184 patients with cancers involved three treatment regimens (8[c]): diclofenac alone (50 mg qds), diclofenac plus codeine (40 mg qds), or diclofenac plus imipramine (10–25 mg tds). There was no significant difference between the different treatments in terms of their analgesic effects as measured on a visual analogue scale after 4 days. However, 10 of 61 subjects taking codeine withdrew because of adverse effects compared with three taking imipramine and two taking diclofenac alone. *Gastrointestinal disturbances, dry mouth, and central nervous system disturbances* were all more frequent in those taking codeine. These results suggest that the addition of a low-potency opioid to diclofenac fails to give enhanced analgesia while the frequency of opioid-related adverse effects increases.

Nervous system Twelve cases of analgesic related headache have been reported in children aged 6–16 years, half of whom were taking paracetamol in combination with codeine (9[cr]). Headaches occurred on at least four days per week and analgesic withdrawal led to symptom resolution in 50% and some improvement in the remaining cases. This is the first report of analgesic headache in children and is consistent with the adverse effect previously described in adults.

Pancreas A second case of acute pancreatitis associated with co-codamol (paracetamol plus codeine) has been reported (10[c]).

A 20-year-old woman, who had previously taken paracetamol without adverse effects, took paracetamol 1 g and codeine 60 mg for a headache. After 3 hours she developed severe upper abdom-

inal pain radiating to the back. The abdominal pain resolved within 24 hours after phloroglucinol and tiemonium administration. Biochemical investigation showed that her serum amylase activity was raised 3-fold and the serum lipase 15-fold. Other biochemical parameters, abdominal ultrasound, and MRI were normal. Contrast enhanced computed tomography showed pancreatic edema.

The previous use of paracetamol without adverse reactions supports the theory that the reaction was linked to the addition of codeine. Drug-induced acute pancreatitis should be considered in those presenting with epigastric pain after the use of co-codamol.

Dextromethorphan *(SED-13, 174; SEDA-18, 85; SEDA-21, 87)*

Nervous system A review of *N*-methyl-D-aspartic acid (NMDA) antagonist interventions in the treatment of non-ketotic hyperglycinemia includes six cases in which dextromethorphan has been used (11[cr]). Non-ketotic hyperglycinemia is an autosomal recessive disorder in which there is failure of the glycine cleavage enzyme system, leading to impaired oxidative decarboxylation of glycine and a toxic accumulation of this amino acid. Antagonism of the NMDA receptor is hypothesized to offer partial relief to the effects of this inborn error of metabolism. Of the six cases, adverse effects were described in three. Patient 1 had profound *sedation* in response to a dose of 7.5 mg/kg of dextromethorphan administered as a single dose when the infant was 5 days old. The same daily dosage split into three doses relieved symptoms without sedation, but doses in excess of 7.5 mg/kg resulted in *somnolence, agitation*, and *involuntary movements*. Patient 4 *developed apnea, hypotonia, nystagmus, and seizures* at 38 days of age and was given dextromethorphan 1 mg/kg/day at the age of 10 months, resulting in anorexia. In patient 5 an increase in dextromethorphan dosage to 10 mg/kg/day was associated with *lethargy, apnea, and a return of seizure activity*. Further trials are required for clarification of the use of dextromethorphan in the treatment of non-ketotic hyperglycinemia.

In a trial of dextromethorphan in Parkinson's disease only one-third of the initial sample entered the double-blind placebo-controlled phase (12[cr]). One-third of the sample had a *reduction in the benefits of levodopa* when dextromethorphan 30 mg/day was given. A further one-third withdrew because of failure to gain clinical benefit from the highest tolerated dose of dextromethorphan. Adverse effects included *drowsiness, increased dystonia, increased impotence, light-headedness, sweating*, and *nausea*.

Immunological and hypersensitivity reactions Dextromethorphan-induced *anaphylactic-like symptoms* have been reported (13[c]).

A 40-year-old woman suffered repeated hives, lip swelling, and shortness of breath on taking cough suppressants containing dextromethorphan. None was sufficient to require emergency medical intervention. On challenge with dextromethorphan 1 mg mild transient pruritus occurred. After dextromethorphan 30 mg hives and nasal and conjunctival congestion occurred. Vital signs and peak flow remained stable. There was no bronchospasm or angioedema. No reaction occurred to hydrocodone and codeine.

Interactions Four subjects had markedly reduced *O*-demethylation of dextromethorphan after they had taken *moclobemide* 300 mg bd for 9 days (14[c]). *N*-demethylation was not affected. This result supports the hypothesis that moclobemide or a metabolite reduces the activity of the cytochrome enzyme CYP2D6. The clinical implications of this particular interaction remain to be clarified.

Dextropropoxyphene *(SED-13, 174; SEDA-17, 80; SEDA-18, 85)*

A systematic review of single-dose dextropropoxyphene for postoperative pain identified 130 published articles (15[R]). Of these, 11 placebo-controlled studies met the inclusion criteria for the review, six of dextropropoxyphene (65 mg) and five of the same dose of dextropropoxyphene plus paracetamol (650 mg) (co-proxamol). Pooled data from the studies showed that the incidence of nausea, drowsiness, and headache with dextropropoxyphene alone was not significantly different from placebo. Previous reports have suggested that dextropropoxyphene is significantly associated with *dizziness, sedation*, and *nausea and vomiting*. However, co-proxamol caused significantly increased dizziness (relative risk 2.2, 95% CI = 1.1–4.3) and drowsiness (2.1, 1.5–2.9). The relative risk of headache was reduced to 0.5 (0.3–0.9). Analgesic effect was greater with co-proxamol than with dextropropoxyphene alone.

Dihydrocodeine *(SED-13, 174; SEDA-17, 80; SEDA-18, 79)*

In a randomized double-blind comparison of the antitussive effect of dihydrocodeine 10 mg tds with levodropropizine 75 mg tds in 140 adults with primary lung cancer or metastatic cancer there was no significant difference between the two drugs as far as cough severity and the number of night wakings were concerned, both drugs leading to significant improvement (16[cr]). However dihydrocodeine caused significantly more *somnolence*, which was reported by 11% of this group and in some cases was continuous. Other adverse effects reported by those taking dihydrocodeine included *erythema of the abdomen* and *epigastric pain*, although constipation, a potential adverse effect of codeine derivatives, was not reported.

Fentanyl *(SED-13, 174; SEDA-20, 77; SEDA-21, 88; SEDA-22, 98)*

Fentanyl is widely used for obstetric analgesia and the dose-response relation for intrathecal fentanyl has been examined in a randomized study of 84 nulliparous full-term parturients in labor (17[c]). They received intrathecal doses of fentanyl of 5–45 μg and visual analog scales were used to measure analgesia and adverse effects. The mean duration of anesthesia increased in the dose range 5–25 μg of fentanyl and then reached a plateau. Adequate analgesia was obtained with all doses of fentanyl above 10 μg. Maternal systolic blood pressure was not significantly affected at any dose, although *diastolic blood pressure fell* significantly at 10–30 minutes after fentanyl. *Nausea and vomiting* were uncommon, but *pruritus* was common in all groups and was more severe with higher doses of fentanyl. Fetal heart rate did not change significantly with fentanyl at any dose, although the authors acknowledged that they did not undertake continuous fetal heart tracing. They concluded that there is no benefit in using doses of intrathecal fentanyl above 25 μg when fentanyl is used as the sole analgesic agent in labor.

In view of the popularity of fentanyl as an epidural analgesic in labor, its site of action is of some interest, and this has been examined in a randomized study in 55 parturients who received 0.125% bupivacaine plus one of three treatments: epidural saline plus intravenous saline; epidural fentanyl (20 μg/hour) plus intravenous saline; epidural saline plus intravenous fentanyl (20 μg/hour) (18[c]). Study treatments were continuously infused, while epidural bupivacaine was patient controlled. There was a significant reduction (28%) in bupivacaine use with epidural but not intravenous fentanyl, but there was no significant difference in the incidence of adverse effects. This result suggested that the analgesic effects of epidural fentanyl in labor are due to a spinal mechanism, rather than to systemic absorption and a supraspinal effect. However, the authors acknowledged various limitations of their study and commented that they were able to use low doses of fentanyl because of the concomitant use of bupivacaine, which acts synergistically. It is possible that this synergy allows effective analgesia of the visceral afferents at a spinal level without the need for the higher doses that are required for analgesia with fentanyl alone. Higher doses of fentanyl may mask this spinal effect.

Bupivacaine is increasingly being used in combination with fentanyl for obstetric analgesia and has been reported to reduce the incidence of pruritus. In a prospective study, 65 parturients in labor were randomly assigned to receive intrathecal fentanyl (25 μg) intrathecal bupivacaine (2.5 mg), or both as part of epidural anesthesia (19[cr]). The group that received both drugs had more prolonged analgesia and significantly less *pruritus* than those who received fentanyl alone (36 vs 95%). However, the incidence of facial pruritus was not significantly different. The type of analgesia did not affect the outcome of labor, although one patient in the combined treatment group required ephedrine for reduced blood pressure. It was proposed that pruritus is the result of stimulation of μ receptors supraspinally and in the dorsal horn of the spinal cord, and that facial itching is associated with μ receptor activation in the medullary dorsal horn, affecting the trigeminal nerve. Local anesthetics may alter this adverse effect by local neuronal blockade or by direct modulation of μ receptors. Bupivacaine also promotes opioid binding to κ receptors, which reduce pruritus. The failure to relieve facial pruritus suggests a direct effect of fentanyl in the brain stem.

The addition of bupivacaine and/or adrenaline to epidural fentanyl analgesia has also been studied in 100 women after elective cesarean section. All received fentanyl (3 μg/ml) by patient-controlled analgesia for 48 hours and were randomly assigned double-blind to receive either bupivacaine 0.01%, ephedrine 0.5 μg/ml, both, or neither (20[Cr]). Patients who received fentanyl alone made more attempts at patient-controlled analgesia than the other groups, suggesting that this regimen was less effective and the higher dose of fentanyl used perhaps contributed to a higher incidence of nausea and urinary retention and to a higher frequency of severe pruritus. The authors suggested that with lower doses of fentanyl there was less rostral spread of the drug and lower concentrations at the brain stem, thus reducing adverse effects. Breast-fed neonates were neurologically assessed at 2 and 48 hours by a pediatrician and, despite the different fentanyl requirements of mothers, neurobehavioral scores were equally high in the different groups.

Different combinations of fentanyl, bupivacaine, and clonidine were investigated in a multicenter (6 sites) trial of 78 women undergoing elective cesarean section under 'spinal block' (21[cr]). In some cases, this appeared to imply intrathecal administration, and in others combined intrathecal and epidural administration. Patients received hyperbaric bupivacaine alone, or with 75 μg of clonidine, or with 75 μg of clonidine and 12.5 μg of fentanyl. There were no reported hemodynamic differences between the groups, but sedation and pruritus were significantly more common in those who received fentanyl, occurring in 65 and 25% of subjects respectively. Apgar scores and umbilical artery blood pH were unaffected by the drug regimens.

Non-obstetric use In a prospective study of 1030 mixed surgical patients receiving patient-controlled epidural analgesia with 0.05% bupivacaine and fentanyl 4 μg/ml, the incidence of adverse effects was broadly as expected (22[CR]): *17% had pruritus, 15% nausea, 13% sedation, 6.8% hypotension, 2% motor block*, and *0.3% respiratory depression.* Two patients required naloxone for respiratory depression and sedation. Analgesia was terminated electively in 82%; 12% of cases were terminated owing to a displaced catheter, and 3% of cases required anticoagulation, while infection, adverse effects, and inadequate analgesia each accounted for termination of epidural analgesia in 1% of cases. Risk factors for adverse effects were identified as: patient age under 58 years, weight under 73 kg, being female, high fentanyl consumption (over 9 ml/hour), and lumbar placement of the epidural catheter. There was a significant association between patient age and *pruritus*, and between female sex and *nausea, hypotension*, and *sedation.*

In a randomized, double-blind, multicenter trial, 150 postoperative patients who had undergone major surgery received demand-doses of fentanyl 20, 40, or 60 μg delivered intravenously by patient-controlled analgesia (23[Cr]) and higher doses of fentanyl were associated with improved analgesic effect. Adverse effects were reported in 70 patients, and the most commonly reported were nausea and vomiting; most adverse effects were described as mild to moderate. *Bradypnea* occurred in 6% of patients who received fentanyl 60 μg, in one case sufficiently severe to warrant temporary withdrawal of treatment; *respiratory depression and moderate hypoxia* occurred in one patient on 40 μg and in one on 60 μg, again requiring withdrawal. Overall, mean respiratory rates in the 60 μg group were significantly lower than in the 20 μg group throughout the study, and at 6 hours after initiation compared with the 40 μg group. One patient developed acute *confusion and aggression* while receiving fentanyl 40 μg. The authors concluded that 40 μg of fentanyl is an appropriate dose for patient-controlled analgesia, as this balances analgesic efficacy against the incidence of adverse effects.

Mood alteration during patient-controlled epidural anesthesia with either morphine or fentanyl was compared in a randomized double-blind study of 52 patients undergoing elective hip or knee joint arthroplasty under general anesthesia (24[Cr]). Mood was assessed preoperatively and at 24, 48, and 72 hours using the bipolar version of the Profile of Mood States. Pain intensity postoperatively did not vary with morphine or fentanyl and, as expected, both fentanyl and morphine users had significant somnolence, pruritus, and nausea compared with baseline. With morphine the mean score for measures of composure/anxiety, elation/depression and clear-headedness/confusion increased, indicating a change towards the more positive pole, but there were negative changes for the fentanyl users' scores for five of the six components of the Profile of Mood States. The difference in test scores between morphine and fentanyl was significant at 48 hours of patient-controlled anesthesia and 24 hours after withdrawal. There was no correlation between mood scores and pain scores, and mood scores with fentanyl fell with increasing plasma concentrations. Previous investigations have shown transient positive feelings with intravenous fentanyl, followed by more negative feelings in the longer term. The authors suggested that the differences in mood between the two groups may have been explained by differences in the lipid solubility and pharmacokinetics of epidural morphine and fentanyl.

The interaction between propofol and fentanyl has been studied in relation to suppressing the somatic or hemodynamic responses to three types of surgical event-skin incision, peritoneum incision, and abdominal retraction (25[Cr]). Three of 99 subjects were withdrawn from the study after bradycardia of under 50 beats/minute occurred when intravenous fentanyl (dose not stated) was given to those already anesthetized with propofol. Propofol and fentanyl (concentration range 0.5–9 ng/ml maintained by computer-assisted continuous infusion for at least 30 minutes) had a predictable synergistic effect and caused a *fall in systolic blood pressure.* After stimulation, the different concentrations of fentanyl required to block somatic responses to surgery in 50% of subjects were 9.7, 15.1, and 28 ng/ml respectively for skin incision, peritoneum incision, and abdominal retraction. Concentrations required to give a 15% or less increase in post-incision systolic blood pressure were 5.3, 9.7, and 12.1 ng/ml respectively. At doses of less than 3 ng/ml of fentanyl the hemodynamic response to peritoneal incision or abdominal retraction was inadequate, even when sufficient propofol was present to suppress somatic responses. Somatic response suppression correlated with fentanyl for skin incision, fentanyl and propofol for peritoneal incision, and propofol for abdominal retraction. Prestimulation propofol reduced systolic blood pressure in a concentration-dependent fashion, while post-stimulation fentanyl significantly suppressed increases in systolic blood pressure. This difference in effect was attributed to propofol's mainly sedative and hypnotic effects, while fentanyl is primarily analgesic.

The addition of clonidine or fentanyl to local anesthetics for single shot caudal blocks has been studied in 64 children undergoing bilateral correction of vesicoureteral reflux randomized into four groups (26[CR]). The control group received a mixture of 0.25% bupivacaine with adrenaline plus 1% lidocaine; other groups received the same combination plus 1.5 μg/kg of clonidine, or the control combination plus 1 μg/kg of fentanyl, or the control combination plus 0.5 μg/kg of fentanyl plus 0.75 μg/kg of clonidine. The addition of either clonidine or fentanyl significantly prolonged anesthesia, and during recovery the groups receiving local anesthetics alone, or with the addition of fentanyl alone had significantly increased heart rates. Two of the children who received extradural fentanyl had a transient reduction in oxygen of saturation to 92% in the first hour of recovery. One of these was from the fentanyl alone group while one had received fentanyl plus clonidine. *Vomiting* occurred only in children exposed to fentanyl (nine of 29 subjects). This is the first report of *respiratory depression* in children after the caudal administration of fentanyl or clonidine, this adverse effect having been previously described with extradural opioids and clonidine in adults.

Transdermal fentanyl has been compared with modified-release oral formulations of morphine among 504 patients with advanced cancer in a multicenter, cross-sectional quality-of-life study using four widely validated scales plus original scales, generated and validated for this study (27[cr]). The authors used conversion rates 'often reported in the literature' to calculate that the fentanyl group used significantly more opiate (200–300 mg of morphine-equivalent units/day) than the oral morphine users (195 mg/day). Despite this, transdermal fentanyl patients reported fewer and less bothersome adverse effects, although these were not separately identified; 50% reported never having any adverse effects compared with 36% of morphine users without adverse effects, although measures of pain intensity showed no significant difference between the two groups. Subgroup analysis by sex showed that the difference in adverse effects between the two modes of administration was significant only in men. However, it should be noted that the mean ages of the two treatment groups were significantly different, a fact that may qualify the reported results.

Oral *itraconazole* 200 mg did not alter the pharmacokinetics of intravenous fentanyl 3 μg/kg, despite being a strong inhibitor of CYP3A4 in vitro (28[c]). In vitro research suggests that itraconazole should inhibit the elimination of fentanyl, as it been shown to do to alfentanil. This difference can be accounted for by the higher hepatic extraction ratio of fentanyl (0.8–1.0) compared with alfentanil (0.3–0.5), so that even large changes in the activity of enzymes that metabolize fentanyl significantly affect its pharmacokinetics.

Methadone *(SED-13, 176; SEDA-19, 93; SEDA-20, 79; SEDA-21, 88)*

Interactions Methadone is often used for opioid replacement therapy in intravenous drug abusers. The incidence of HIV infection is significantly higher in this population than in the general public, and interactions with drugs used for the treatment of AIDS are therefore important. The metabolism of the antiviral nucleoside *zidovudine* to the inactive glucuronide form in vitro was inhibited by atovaquone, methadone, valproic acid, and fluconazole (29[c]). The concentration of methadone required for 50% inhibition was over 8 μg/ml, a supratherapeutic concentration, thus raising questions about the clinical significance of the effect. However, in eight recently detoxified heroin addicts, acute methadone treatment increased the AUC of oral zidovudine by 41% and of intravenous zidovudine by 19%, following the start of oral methadone (50 mg/day) (30[cR]). These effects resulted primarily from inhibition of zidovudine glucuronidation, but also from reduced renal clearance of zidovudine, and methadone concentrations remained in the target range throughout. It is recommended that increased toxicity surveillance, and possibly reduction in zidovudine dose, are indicated when the two drugs are co-administered.

A similarly cautious conclusion was reached after an in vitro study of the effects of the HIV-1 protease inhibitors, *ritonavir, in dinavir*, and *saquinavir*, which are metabolized by the liver CYP3A4 (31[r]). All three protease inhibitors inhibited methadone demethylation and buprenorphine dealkylation in rank order of potency ritonavir > indinavir > saquinavir. Clinical studies are required to establish the further relevance of these observations.

A randomized, double-blind, placebo-controlled trial showed that oral *fluconazole* increased the serum methadone AUC by 35% (32[cr]). Although renal clearance was not significantly affected, mean serum methadone peak and trough concentrations rose significantly, while renal clearance was not significantly altered. This is a similar finding to that reported for alfentanil (6[cr]).

Morphine *(SED-13, 176; SEDA-19, 83; SEDA-20, 79; SEDA-21, 89; SEDA-22, 100)*

Intramuscular morphine has been compared with epidural morphine or epidural sufentanil, both with bupivacaine, in 90 patients undergoing major abdominal surgery (33[Cr]). Both epidural regimens gave significantly better postoperative analgesia at rest and during movement. The incidence of adverse effects did not differ significantly between the groups, although the intraoperative requirement for ephedrine or dopamine was higher for the epidural group. *Itching* was significantly less in the intramuscular morphine group than the epidural groups (7 vs 69%) but *nausea and vomiting* were equally common.

A prospective, randomized, double-blind study of 97 women investigated whether *droperidol* alleviated the adverse effects of epidural morphine after cesarean section (34[cr]). All groups received morphine 5 mg epidurally on delivery, accompanied by no droperidol, or droperidol 2.5 mg epidurally, or droperidol 2.5 mg intravenously. Pruritus occurred in 70% of patients, starting at 6 hours after epidural morphine, peaking at 17 hours, and with no significant difference between the different treatment regimens. Nausea and vomiting were significantly reduced by intravenous droperidol, but not by epidural droperidol. The authors concluded that droperidol acts systemically to counter the adverse effects of epidural morphine but is not entirely effective, and they suggested that its failure to alleviate pruritus may have been due to the fact that they used larger doses of morphine than some other investigators. Subhypnotic doses of propofol (20 mg) given to 120 women receiving intrathecal morphine after cesarean section also had no significant effect on pruritus (35[cr]). Higher success rates have been reported for propofol with non-obstetric patients, suggesting that labor-related factors may perpetuate this adverse effect.

Although spinal morphine provides effective analgesia, different ways of managing and minimizing its troubling adverse effects are constantly sought. *Diclofenac*, a non-steroidal anti-inflammatory drug, improves the analgesia provided by epidural morphine and may allow dosage reduction. In an investigation of this drug combination, intrathecal morphine was administered either regularly or on demand to 120 women undergoing cesarean section in doses of 0.1, 0.05, or 0.025 mg with diclofenac 75 mg intramuscularly (36[c]). Severe pruritus was significantly more common in those who received morphine 0.1 mg and there was a trend towards less vomiting with smaller doses. There was no respiratory depression. The results suggested that the adverse effects of intrathecal morphine are dose dependent and that there was no advantage in using doses of morphine larger than 0.25 mg.

Nervous system A patient with Guillain-Barré syndrome experienced *shock* with morphine sulfate (37[c]).

A 69-year-old woman developed interscapular pain after a mild respiratory infection. Non-opioid analgesics were ineffective, so she was given modified-release morphine 10 mg. On day 4 she had rapidly progressive weakness in her legs and on day 5 she was found unconscious with no detectable blood pressure. She recovered with naloxone 0.8 mg intravenously. Her paralysis persisted. Nerve conduction studies confirmed slowed neurotransmission. Further investigation excluded other potential causes and Guillain-Barré syndrome was diagnosed.

The episode of unconsciousness was attributed to opioid toxicity in a patient in whom autonomic dysfunction may already be present. It was suggested that opioid analgesics should be used with caution in patients with Guillain-Barré syndrome, because of the risk of hypotension consequent on autonomic dysfunction.

Withdrawal effects A case of acute opioid withdrawal syndrome apparently precipitated by naloxone following epidural morphine has been reported (38[c]).

A 28-year-old nulliparous woman with no history of opioid exposure underwent elective cesarean section with epidural anesthesia. On delivery she received morphine 2 mg epidurally. At 8 hours after delivery she complained of pruritus and received naloxone 0.14 mg intravenously in fractional doses. After 2 minutes she felt warm in her legs, trunk, and face. Pruritus resolved and analgesia was maintained. After 5 minutes she began to shiver in a waxing and waning pattern every 2 minutes. She was restless and agitated and had tachypnea, lacrimation, and rhinorrhea. Her symptoms resolved in 40 minutes.

Previous reports of opioid withdrawal on single exposure have been described after the administration of intramuscular morphine in healthy individuals. This case suggests that opioid dependence can occur after acute exposure to morphine by the epidural route too. An alternative explanation (39[r]) is that the stress of labor may have led to increased endogenous opioid activity, particularly β-endorphin, and that the antagonistic effect of naloxone on the endogenous opioid system contributed to the clinical effects in this patient. Moreover, the authors pointed out that many symptoms characteristic of the classic opioid withdrawal syndrome were not present in the patient.

Papaverine

The long-term outcome of penile prostheses has been compared with intracavernosal injection therapy in 115 intracavernosal injectors and 65 patients undergoing insertion of a penile prosthesis, who were followed over an average 5.4 years (40[cR]). On follow-up only 41% of the patients were still using intracavernosal injections. Of 87 injecting patients 32% reported adverse effects, including *pain* (16 cases), *prolonged erections* (5 cases), *bruising* (4), *priapism* (3), *swelling* (2), *plaque formation* (2), and *burning* (1). Unfortunately, these adverse effects are not specifically related to the various regimens for drug injection, not all of which included papaverine, which limits the value of these observations.

Liver A retrospective review of the medical records of 71 patients with erectile dysfunction examined the effect of intracavernous papaverine or a papaverine/phentolamine mixture on the liver (41[cr]). Over 18 months two of 30 of the papaverine injecting group had *changes in liver function tests*. One had transient increases in bilirubin and aspartate aminotransferase after 6 months treatment and one had a small rise in alanine aminotransferase. Both patients had a history of alcohol misuse, but neither required discontinuation of treatment. One control had a raised bilirubin. The results suggested that routine monitoring of liver function tests in all papaverine injectors may be unnecessary, but that in patients with a history of alcohol misuse or liver disease, monitoring of liver function tests before starting therapy and at 6 months is advised.

Oxycodone

Two studies of oxycodone in patients with cancer pain have been carried out. In the first, modified-release and immediate-release oxycodone were compared (42[Cr]) in a multicenter, double-blind trial involving 180 patients who were given either modified-release oxycodone, mean dose 114 mg bd, or immediate-release oxycodone 127 mg qds, four times a day for cancer-related pain. A 5-day comparison showed no significant difference in the analgesic effects of the two formulations, both of which provided effective relief of pain. However, of the 160 patients who received at least one dose of medication, 104 reported a total of 295 adverse events, significantly fewer being reported with modified-release oxycodone (109) than immediate-release oxycodone (186). Reported adverse effects included: *nausea* (18 vs 26%), *vomiting* (11 vs 23%), and *constipation* (9 vs 17%). With immediate-release oxycodone *headache* was reported by 7% and anxiety by 5%; neither was reported with modified-release oxycodone. Altogether, 7% of the modified-release group and 11% of the immediate-release group discontinued medication because of adverse effects. It is suggested that the equianalgesic effect is likely to be a factor of the rapid initial release of the modified-release formulation, allowing adequate drug concentrations to establish sufficient receptor activation, followed by a slower release of the remaining drug, which may be responsible for the reduction in adverse effects. Alternatively the peaks achieved with each administration of medication may account for the observed difference in the rates of adverse effects between the two formulations.

The second study consisted of a randomized, double-blind, cross-over comparison of the safety and efficacy of oral modified-release oxycodone with modified-release morphine in 32 patients with cancer pain, nine of whom completed the trial (43[cR]). The average dose of oxycodone was 47 mg bd compared with 73 mg bd of morphine. There were no significant differences in the degrees of sedation, nausea, or pain intensity experienced by the subjects on the different regimens and the results suggested that oxycodone may be used as an alternative to morphine.

Another randomized, double-blind, cross-over study confirmed previous findings on the adverse effects of oxycodone among sufferers of post-herpetic neuralgia (44[Cr]). Oxycodone was analgesic in this group, although 76% of the sample reported adverse effects compared with 49% of the placebo group. *Constipation*, *nausea*, and *sedation* were the most frequently reported adverse effects.

Remifentanil

Remifentanil is a pure μ receptor agonist with a very short duration of action. It therefore has to be given by continuous intravenous infusion and is used as a supplement to general anesthesia during induction and as an analgesic during maintenance of anesthesia. It has the familiar adverse effects of an opioid: *respiratory depression*, *sedation*, *nausea and vomiting*, *muscle rigidity*, *bradycardia*, and *pruritus*. These are short-lived and are antagonized by naloxone. The onset of muscle rigidity and apnea can be alarmingly rapid. Bradycardia occurred more often with remifentanil than alfentanil in patients undergoing abdominal surgery and in children undergoing strabismus surgery; the oculocardiac response was more marked with remifentanil than alfentanil (45[R]).

Sufentanil *(SED-13, 178; SEDA-20, 81; SEDA-21, 89; SEDA-22)*

Much has been published this year on various aspects of the effects of intrathecal and epidural sufentanil as an analgesic during labor in 50 nulliparous patients in a randomized double-blind study in which they received doses of 1–10 μg of sufentanil in preservative-free saline (46[cr]). The ED50 was 1.8 μg, based on numbers requesting further analgesia after 30 minutes. The incidence of adverse effects was similar in all groups (i.e. was not dose-related) and included *pruritus* of a similar intensity in all groups. There was no respiratory depression, although blood pressure and oxygen saturation fell but not in a clearly dose-related fashion. Other adverse effects included *changes in temperature sensitivity* at 30 minutes in 19 of the 50 subjects. One woman who received 5 μg of sufentanil had a *fall in oxygen saturation* to 90–92% with a respiratory rate of 16 breaths/minute 10–15 minutes after injection, but recovered spontaneously at 20 minutes. Fetal monitoring showed no significant bradycardia and there were no significant differences in 5 minutes post delivery Apgar scores. It was suggested that *hypotension* was due to the effect of intrathecal opioid rather than to an effect on the autonomic nervous system and that the temperature sensitivity changes were due to a concentration-dependent local anesthetic effect of opioids. A drop in oxygen saturation in one subject indicated the need for observation for respiratory changes when sufentanil is given intrathecally.

Combined spinal epidural analgesia has been associated with reports of increased operative deliveries, possibly due to reduced perineal sensation and motor weakness. In a comparison of combined spinal epidural analgesia (intrathecal sufentanil 10 μg followed by epidural bupivacaine and fentanyl at their next request for analgesia) with intravenous pethidine analgesia (50 mg intravenously on demand up to a maximum of 200 mg in 4 hours) in 1223 randomly assigned healthy parturients there was no significant difference in the rates of cesarean delivery for dystocia (47[Cr]). Maternal *hypotension* and *pruritus* requiring treatment occurred in 14 and 17% respectively of patients who received combined spinal epidural analgesia. *Fetal heart rate deceleration* occurred in 21% of patients who received pethidine compared with 18% of patients who received combined spinal epidural analgesia, and in each group most cases resolved spontaneously. However, profound fetal bradycardia (fetal heart rate of less than 60/minute, lasting 60 seconds or more), necessitating emergency cesarean section, occurred within 1 hour of administration of sufentanil in eight of 400 mothers, while no such events occurred with pethidine. None of the cases responded to conservative management and none was associated with maternal hypotension. Immediate postnatal neonatal outcomes were similar between the two groups, as judged by Apgar scores and umbilical artery blood gases. These findings are significant, in that an increase in cesarean deliveries due to fetal bradycardia has not previously been reported, but findings in this study must be regarded with an element of caution, as fetal monitoring was more extensive in those given combined spinal epidural analgesia. The authors suggested that fetal bradycardia might have been due to uterine hyperstimulation, associated with intrathecal opioids (although they did not consistently monitor for this), and that fetal bradycardia resulted from reduced placental perfusion secondary to uterine tetany. Alternatively, since sufentanil is highly lipid soluble, it can be detectable in plasma within 39 minutes of intrathecal administration of 15 μg. Once in the plasma, transplacental transfer can occur and the drug can have a direct vagotonic effect on the fetus. However, they believed that the most probable explanation for the bradycardia was a direct consequence of hypoperfusion of the placenta secondary to maternal hypotension, although they pointed out that none of their cases was associated with this hemodynamic change in the mother.

The absence of motor block associated with combined spinal epidural analgesia using sufentanil, noted in the previous study, has also been reported in a further investigation (48[c]) in which intrathecal sufentanil 10 μg was compared with epidural lidocaine, adrenaline, and sufentanil 40 μg in early labor. Adverse effects were not significantly different between the groups, except for more frequent and severe pruritus in the intrathecal group. Although three subjects in each group had *transient changes in fetal heart rate* within 30 minutes of medication, no intervention was necessary.

Intrathecal sufentanil and epidural bupivacaine were compared individually and in combination to establish dose-responsiveness for analgesia in labor in 100 women (49[cr]). There was no dose-responsiveness for doses of sufentanil between 2 and 10 μg. The ED50 for sufentanil was 2.3 μg alone (higher than that reported above (45[cr])) and 0.85 μg in combination with epidural bupivacaine. Adverse effects included *pruritus*(incidence 70–90%), *nausea*, and mild *somnolence* (10–30%). *Transient fetal bradycardia* was reported in two cases.

In a double-blind study of the effect of clonidine on intrathecal sufentanil 53 nulliparous women received sufentanil 5 μg intrathecally either alone or with clonidine 30 μg (50[CR]). The addition of clonidine increased the incidence of *hypotension* (12% with sufentanil alone, 63% with clonidine) and sedation (23% with sufentanil alone and 46% with clonidine). There was no significant difference in the incidence of pruritus (88%). Again, no motor blockade was observed.

The effect of sufentanil was examined in 10 healthy male volunteers to find out whether it has the same hemodynamic and sensory effects as when it is used on women in labor. Details of the method of recruitment of volunteers for this double-blind study were not provided, but they received either saline or sufentanil 10 μg intrathecally (51[cr]), and blood pressure, heart rates, oxyhemoglobin saturation, cold and pinprick sensation, motor block, and visual analog scales for sedation, pruritus, and nausea were all measured. *Pruritus* and *sensory changes to pinprick and cold* occurred only in the sufentanil group and there were no significant hemodynamic changes in either group. In view of the frequency and severity of pruritus when sufentanil is used in labor, it is interesting that all five of the male volunteers experienced this symptom, three of them severely. These findings suggested that the *hypotension* observed with the use of intrathecal sufentanil during labor and the sensory changes may not be mediated by the same pathway. The authors proposed that the hypotension observed in such studies is a direct result of pain relief, which is not an issue in the pain-free men in this investigation.

Respiratory depression has been described after sufentanil 5 μg intrathecally (52[cr]).

An 83-year-old woman scheduled for bilateral knee replacement surgery received midazolam 7.5 mg preoperatively. Continuous spinal anesthesia was planned with combined general anesthesia. Anesthesia was maintained with 0.3–0.5% of inspired isoflurane in 36% oxygen and 70% nitrous oxide while 5 mg of 0.5% bupivacaine was introduced into the subarachnoid space via an insertion at L3–4. Anesthesia extended to T11. During the procedure two top-up doses of bupivacaine 2.5 mg were administered. Postoperatively she was extubated immediately and was fully conscious on transfer to the recovery room, but 75 minutes later she had violent pain in both knees and received sufentanil 5 μg intrathecally. Analgesia was achieved in 10 minutes. At 15 minutes pruritus occurred and at 30 minutes she became unresponsive to verbal and painful stimuli and stopped breathing. Blood pressure was 120/60 mmHg, heart rate 72/minute, and oxygen saturation 97%. Ventilation with 100% oxygen via a facemask started immediately and naloxone 160 μg was injected intravenously, with full recovery of consciousness and respiration in 10 minutes.

This report is the first of respiratory depression after intrathecal sufentanil in a non-obstetric patient. Previous obstetric cases had occurred earlier and with larger doses of sufentanil. The site of action of sufentanil in this case is likely to have been supraspinal, by either direct cephalad migration in the CSF or through a systemic effect after vascular absorption.

Respiratory arrest has been reported in labor (53[c]).

A 20-year-old parturient receiving sufentanil 10 μg and bupivacaine 2.5 mg intrathecally as part of combined spinal-epidural analgesia developed pruritus 15 minutes after the injection, followed by a sleepy feeling at 20 minutes. After 25 minutes she became unresponsive and apneic; her systolic blood pressure was 130 mmHg and her heart rate 60/minute. The fetal heart rate was 86/minute. She was ventilated manually with 100% oxygen and naloxone 0.4 mg was given with prompt recovery of consciousness and respiratory effort. Drowsiness persisted, and a naloxone infusion was initiated after top-up doses of naloxone had failed to relieve it. Subsequent analgesia was with bupivacaine alone. A vacuum-assisted vaginal delivery was performed after 3 hours. The infant's Apgar score was eight at 1 minute and nine at 5 minutes. The mother and baby were subsequently well.

This case highlights the low doses at which arrest may occur.

Violent coughing in young children and adolescents exposed to small doses of sufentanil (1 μg/kg or less) has been reported (54[r]). Specific cases were not alluded to and the literature remains divided on the significance and mechanism of this age-related effect.

Tramadol *(SED-13, 76; SEDA-20, 81; SEDA-21, 90; SEDA-22, 103)*

The results of the post-marketing surveillance of modified-released tramadol in Germany have been published (55[CR]). Modified-release tramadol (mean daily dose 236 mg usually divided into two doses) was used in 3153 patients, of whom most had severe or very severe pain. During the 6-week trial, 316 adverse effects were reported by a total of 206 patients (6.5%). Adverse effects were, in decreasing order of frequency, *nausea* (3.4%), *dizziness* (1.5%), *vomiting* (1.1%), *constipation* (0.5%), *tiredness* (0.5) *sweating* (0.4%), *dry mouth* (0.3%), and *pruritus* (0.3%). *Confusion, hypotension, sleep disturbances, abdominal pain, stomach upset, gastrointestinal hemorrhage*, and *cerebral hemorrhage* were all among the less frequently reported adverse events, and 28% of events were classified as severe. Age did not affect the frequency of events, but women reported a higher frequency of adverse events than men (7.3 vs 5.7%).

In another review of tramadol, it was reported to cause less respiratory depression than morphine (45[R]). However, the authors concluded that it is less effective than morphine in the treatment of severe pain.

However, immediate postoperative pain appears to be equally well controlled by tramadol, according to a study in which tramadol and morphine were compared in 40 women undergoing hysterectomy (56[cr]). At the start of wound closure patients received either tramadol 3 mg/kg or morphine 0.2 mg/kg intravenously, which did not cause changes in arterial pressure or heart rate. There were no differences in times to spontaneous respiration, awakening, or orientation between the two groups, and ventilation frequency and pain scores were similar throughout 90 minutes. Similar numbers in each group required supplementary analgesia. Performance of the p-deletion test, a measure of psychomotor function, was more rapid in the tramadol group, but the performance of all subjects was impaired at 90 minutes compared with their pre-operative scores.

Similarly, a comparison of tramadol and morphine for subcutaneous patient-controlled analgesia after orthopedic surgery (57[cr]) showed that tramadol 40 mg subcutaneously and morphine 2 mg subcutaneously were equally effective in providing analgesia. Drug use in the first 24 hours averaged 800 mg for tramadol and 40 mg for morphine. However, *mean arterial blood pressure fell* significantly in both groups after 24 hours, with a 17% mean maximal fall from baseline concentrations for tramadol and 20% for morphine; *heart rate increased* by 17 and 15% respectively. Oxygen saturation also fell significantly in both groups, but was not associated with changes in respiratory rate. *Nausea and vomiting* were more common with tramadol (65%). In this study patients required significantly more tramadol than had been predicted, and the authors commented that at this dosage, the adverse effects profile was similar to that of morphine.

In a double-blind, randomized, cross-over study in 60 patients with osteoarthritis of the hip or knee, tramadol 50-100mg up to three times daily was compared with diclofenac (25–50 mg up to three times daily) over 4 weeks (58[cr]). Both regimens gave modest pain relief, with no significant differences between the two groups, although within individual patients there were marked differences in analgesic effectiveness. Tramadol was associated with a significantly higher rate of adverse effects (20 vs 3.3%), notably *headaches, nausea, constipation, tiredness, and vomiting*, but there was no significant difference in adverse events that required withdrawal.

A randomized double-blind comparison of the effectiveness of a single dose of tramadol 100 mg with a single dose of hydrocodone 5 mg plus paracetamol 500 mg in acute musculoskeletal pain in 68 subjects after minor trauma has been published (59[c]). Tramadol gave significantly worse analgesia. Adverse effects (*nausea and vomiting, drowsiness and dizziness, and anxiety*) were uncommon and there was no significant difference between the two drugs.

Intravenous tramadol (1.25 mg/kg), codeine (1 mg/kg), morphine (0.125 mg/kg), and saline have been compared for their effect on gastric emptying (using the paracetamol absorption test) in 10 healthy subjects in a randomized double-blind study (60[cr]). Tramadol had a measurable but statistically insignificant inhibitory effect on gastric emptying, whereas morphine and codeine significantly delayed gastric emptying. The implication of this is that the risk of regurgitation is less with tramadol than with the other opioids investigated and that tramadol is less likely to alter the pharmacokinetics of other drugs administered simultaneously.

PARTIAL OPIOID AGONISTS

Buprenorphine *(SED-13, 180; SEDA-20, 82; SEDA-21, 91; SEDA-22, 103)*

Buprenorphine is increasingly being used as a substitute for other opioids in the treatment of opioid abuse and is generally considered to be safe because of the ceiling effect. One report from Vienna described 50 opioid-dependent subjects who received gradual (10-day) detoxification with buprenorphine, contacting the out-patient clinic daily, so that buprenorphine could be administered according to their clinical need in a free dosage scheme (61). The mean daily dosage was 2.3 mg on day 1 and the highest mean daily dose was administered on day 2, followed by daily reduction over the study period. There was 70% compliance with the regimen and withdrawal symptoms during the study period were described as moderate.

Less satisfactory outcomes have been reported from France (62[c]–64[c]), where acute poisoning during buprenorphine substitution has been described in three series of patients. The first included 29 opiate addicts taking high-dosage sublingual buprenorphine with non-fatal poisoning and the second included 20 addicts who died (62[c]). Blood concentrations of buprenorphine in the first group were low (1.0–2.3 ng/ml, mean 1.4 ng/ml), but there was concomitant intake of psychotropic medication, especially benzodiazepines, in 18 cases. Blood concentrations of buprenorphine in the fatal cases were 1.1–29 (mean 8.4) ng/ml, while concentrations of its primary metabolite, norbuprenorphine, were 0.2–13 (mean 2.6) ng/ml, within or slightly over the target range. Extensive tissue distribution buprenorphine was reported (myocardium, kidney, brain, and liver) but the highest concentrations of buprenorphine and norbuprenorphine were found in the bile, and the authors suggested that this may be the sample of choice for post-mortem screening. Buprenorphine was also identified in eight of 11 hair samples assayed. Intravenous injection of crushed tablets and the concomitant use of benzodiazepines were identified as the major risk factors in the fatal cases (63[c]).

In the third report six *deaths* linked to misuse of buprenorphine-benzodiazepine combinations were described, although it is not clear whether these were different deaths, or a subset of the cases described in other papers (64[c]). Once again, the authors emphasized that blood concentrations of buprenorphine were in the target range in three subjects, although higher in three others. Exhaustive screening detected no traces of opiates in post-mortem blood, but all subjects had target range concentrations of both desmethyldiazepam and 7-aminoflunitrazepam. The risk of high-dose substitution therapy (2–8 mg) if physicians do not comply with correct practice for prescribing and using this drug were emphasized, particularly when there is a large population of patients being treated, as there was in France in 1997 (34 000 patients)

Pentazocine

The effects of pentazocine were studied in 16 non-abusing volunteers recruited via posters and local newspaper advertisements and were compared with the effects of morphine (65[CR]). Pentazocine had dose-related effects on subjective, psychomotor, and physiological variables, and the clinically relevant dose of 30 mg produced a greater magnitude of *dysphoric subjective effects* than morphine 10 mg and, unlike morphine, impaired psychomotor performance. With pentazocine, peak ratings from the adjective checklist were significantly increased for *'dry mouth'*, *'sweating'*, and *'turning of stomach'*. Compared with morphine, pentazocine led to higher ratings for *'drunk'*, *'feel bad'*, *'having pleasant bodily sensations'*, and *'having unpleasant bodily sensations'*.

Musculoskeletal There has been a further case report of *fibromyopathy* after intramuscular injection of pentazocine in a 47-year-old woman with a 4-year history of such injections into the legs (66[c]). Her thigh and buttock muscles were very hard on palpation and the overlying skin was hard, shiny, and hairless. Imaging showed fibrosis and calcification of the muscles and biopsy showed fibromyopathy. There were associated clinical and electrophysiological polyradiculopathy and multiple mononeuropathy of the lower extremities.

OPIOID ANTAGONISTS

Nalmefene *(SED-13, 179; SEDA-17, 88; SEDA-22, 104)*

The role of opioid antagonists in the treatment of pruritus in cholestatic liver disease has been reviewed (67[R]). Their use is based on the recent theory that implicates opioid neurotransmission as the cause of itching in this condition, and it has been observed that opioid antagonists, while providing relief from itching in patients with cholestasis, also cause symptoms similar to those seen in the opioid withdrawal syndrome. It has therefore been suggested that patients with cirrhosis are chronically exposed to increased concentrations of endogenous opiate receptor agonists. The review describes a study of 11 patients with cirrhosis-induced pruritus, in whom administration of nalmefene led to relief of itching within 1 month, sustained at 3 and 6 months. However, the first two patients had severe withdrawal reactions that took 3 days to subside. In the light of this experience, the trial was modified so that patients received oral nalmefene 5 mg bd with a gradual increase in dosage over 7–10 days to 20–40 mg/day, and clonidine was administered simultaneously for the first 7 days of nalmefene therapy. Despite these precautions, all patients had withdrawal reactions, including *anorexia, nausea, colicky abdominal pain, sweating, tremor*, and occasionally *visual or auditory hallucinations*. These developed within 1 hour of nalmefene therapy and diminished within 2–3 days, despite continuation of nalmefene. This review includes reports of two other studies, available in abstract form only, but which appear to have reported a lower incidence of withdrawal symptoms precipitated by nalmefene, although the dose of drug used also appeared to have been lower.

In another study in 14 patients with cholestatic liver disease, oral nalmefene was started at a dose of 2 mg bd and increased until symptomatic relief of pruritus was obtained (68[cr]). Five patients were reported to have a transient opioid withdrawal-like reaction that did not preclude continuing with treatment. Other adverse events associated with nalmefene therapy included: *perception of pins and needles* (4 cases), *anxiety and depression* (2 cases), *abdominal cramps and nausea* (2 cases), *insomnia* (3 cases), *depersonalization* (2 cases), and *changes in mood* (2 cases); *difficulties in visual focusing, dizziness, chronic goose bumps, mental 'fuzziness', anorexia, and nightmares* were each reported by one patient only. Of the cases of depersonalization, one occurred after the first dose while the other occurred in the first 2 weeks of therapy.

There were no consistent changes in biochemistry with nalmefene. Several patients had a 'breakthrough' of pruritus, which was managed by upward adjustment of dose. The authors suggested that this can be explained if nalmefene initially displaced pruritus-mediating ligands from opioid receptors, but then induced an increased density of receptors because of reduced agonist-receptor interactions, allowing further binding of pruritus-mediating ligands to receptors. In a few other patients, exacerbations of pruritus after long-term control on maintenance therapy may have been attributable to the development of tolerance towards nalmefene.

Naloxone

The review cited above (67[R]) also included a report of a randomized, double-blind, controlled trial of naloxone for the treatment of pruritus in cholestatic liver disease. Although it was effective in most patients, five had an *increase in mean scratching activity* during naloxone therapy, three patients had *anxiety*, and one developed *withdrawal symptoms*.

Naltrexone *(SED-13, 180; SEDA-20, 83; SEDA-21, 92; SEDA-22, 104)*

The use of naltrexone to relieve pruritus in cholestatic liver disease was included in the review cited earlier (67[R]). Five patients received naltrexone 50 mg/day. Pruritus scores fell, but two patients developed *severe nausea, vomiting, light-headedness*, or *tremor*, requiring withdrawal of treatment. The reviewers commented that these reactions may or may not have been related to opioid withdrawal and that the trial had had several design limitations. They pointed out that one concern relating to the chronic use of high-dose naltrexone is an asymptomatic rise in serum aminotransferases, although the doses used in this study have not been reported to produce liver function abnormalities.

A case of *panic attacks* precipitated by naltrexone has been reported (69[c]).

A 29-year woman with bulimia nervosa and a family history of anxiety was enrolled in a trial of naltrexone (100 mg/day). She had no history of opioid use. Within hours of her first dose she experienced alarm, anxiety, chest discomfort, shortness of breath, a fear of dying, sweating, nausea, and derealization. She was unable to remain at home or to go out alone. For 3 days she continued to take naltrexone, with an increasing frequency of panic attacks. On day 4 she was treated with alprazolam (0.5 mg) but relapsed after further naltrexone. Withdrawal of naltrexone lead to complete remission of symptoms.

This effect was attributed to an action of naltrexone in removing the endogenous opioid effect at μ receptors in the locus ceruleus and thus resulting in unchecked noradrenergic hyperactivity.

Interactions The effects of naltrexone on *diazepam* intoxication were investigated in 26 non-drug-abusing subjects who received either naltrexone 50 mg or placebo and 90 minutes later oral diazepam 10 mg in a double-blind crossover trial (70[cr]). Naltrexone was significantly associated with negative mood states, such as sedation, fatigue, and anxiety, compared with placebo, while positive states (friendliness, vigor, liking the effects of diazepam, feeling high from diazepam) were significantly more common with placebo. Naltrexone significantly delayed the time to peak diazepam concentrations (135 minutes) compared with placebo (75 minutes), but there were no significant differences in the concentrations of nordiazepam, the main metabolite of diazepam, at any stage in the study.

REFERENCES

1. Lambert DG. Recent advances in opioid pharmacology. Br J Anaesth 1998;81:1–2.
2. Scott BH. Opioids in cardiac surgery: cardiopulmonary bypass and inflammatory response. Int J Cardiol 1998;64(Suppl 1):S35–S41.
3. Isenhower HL, Mueller BA. Selection of narcotic analgesics for pain associated with pancreatitis. Am J Health System Pharm 1998;55:480–6.
4. Collett B-J. Opioid tolerance: The clinical perspective. Br J Anaesth 1998;81:58–68.
5. Suresh S, Anand KJS. Opioid tolerance in neonates: mechanisms, diagnosis, assessment, and management. Semin Perinatol 1998; 22:425–33.
6. Palkama VJ, Isohanni MH, Neuvonen PJ, Olkkola KT. The effect of intravenous and oral fluconazole on the pharmacokinetics and pharmacodynamics of intravenous alfentanil. Anesth Analg 1998;87:190–4.
7. Ytterberg SR, Mahowald ML, Woods SR. Codeine and oxycodone use in patients with chronic rheumatic disease pain. Arthritis Rheum 1998;41:1603–12.
8. Minotti V, De Angelis V, Righetti E, Celani MG, Rossetti R, Lupatelli M, Tonato M, Pisati R, Monza G, Fumi G, Del Favero A. Double-blind evaluation of short-term analgesic efficacy of orally administered diclofenac, diclofenac plus codeine, and diclofenac plus imipramine in chronic cancer pain. Pain 1998;74:133–7.
9. Symon DNK. Twelve cases of analgesic headache. Arch Dis Child 1998;78:555–6.
10. Renkes P, Techot P. Acetaminophen-codeine combination induced acute pancreatitis. Pancreas 1998;16:556–61.
11. Deutsch SI, Rosse RB, Mastropaolo J. Current status of NMDA antagonist interventions in the treatment of nonketotic hyperglycinemia. Clin Neuropharmacol 1998;21:71–9.
12. Metman LV, Blanchet PJ, Van Den Munckhof P, Del Dotto P, Del Dotto P, Natte R, Chase TN. A trial of dextromethorphan in parkinsonian patients with motor response complications. Mov Disord 1998;13:414–17.
13. Knowles SR, Weber E. Dextromethorphan anaphylaxis. J Allergy Clin Immunol 1998;102:316–17.
14. Hartter S, Dingemanse J, Baier D, Ziegler G, Hiemke C. Inhibition of dextromethorphan metabolism by moclobemide. Psychopharmacology 1998;135:22–6.
15. Collins SL, Edwards JE, Moore RA, McQuay HJ. Single-dose detropropoxyphene in postoperative pain: a quantitative systematic review. Eur J Clin Pharmacol 1998;54:107–12.
16. Luporini G, Barni S, March E, Daffonchio L. Efficacy and safety of levodropropizine and dihydrocodeine on nonproductive cough in primary and metastatic lung cancer. Eur Respir J 1998;12:97–101.
17. Palmer CM, Cork RC, Hays R, Van Maren G, Alves D. The dose-response relation of intrathecal fentanyl for labor analgesia. Anesthesiology 1998;88:355–61.
18. D'Angelo R, Gerancher JC, Eisenach JC, Raphael BL. Epidural fentanyl produces labor analgesia by a spinal mechanism. Anesthesiology 1998;88:1519–23.
19. Asokumar B, Newman LM, McCarthy RJ, Ivankovich AD, Tuman K. Intrathecal bupivacaine reduces pruritus and prolongs duration of fentanyl analgesia during labor: a prospective, randomised controlled trial. Anesth Analg 1998;87:1309–15.
20. Cohen S, Lowenwirt I, Pantuck CB, Amar D, E J Pantuck. Bupivacaine 0.01% and/or epinephrine 0.5 μg/ml improve epidural fentanyl analgesia after cesarean section. Anesthesiology 1998;89:1354–61.
21. Benhamou D, Thorin D, Brichant J-F, Daillant P, Milon D, Schneider M. Intrathecal clonidine and fentanyl with hyperbaric bupivacaine improves analgesia during cesarean section. Anesth Analg 1998;87:609–13.
22. Liu SS, Allen HW, Olsson GL. Patient-controlled epidural analgesia with bupivacaine and fentanyl on hospital wards. Anesthesiology 1998;88:688–95.
23. Camu F, Van Aken H, Bovill JG. Postoperative analgesic effects of three demand-dose sizes of fentanyl administered by patient-controlled analgesia. Anesth Analg 1998;87:890–5.
24. Tsueda K, Mosca PJ, Heine MF, Loyd GE, Durkis DAE, Malkani MD, Hurst HE. Mood during epidural patient-controlled analgesia with morphine or fentanyl. Anesthesiology 1998;88:885–91.
25. Kazama T, Ikeda K, Morita K. The pharmacodynamic interaction between propofol and fentanyl with respect to the suppression of somatic or hemodynamic responses to skin incision, peritoneum incision and abdominal wall retraction. Anesthesiology 1998;89:894–906.
26. Constant L, Gall O, Gouyet L, Chauvin M, Murat I. Addition of clonidine or fentanyl to local anaesthetics prolongs the duration of surgical analgesia after single shot caudal block in children. Br J Anaesth 1998;80:294–8.
27. Payne R, Mathias SD, Pasta DJ, Wanke LA, Williams R, Mahmoud R. Quality of life and cancer pain: satisfaction and side effects with transdermal fentanyl versus oral morphine. J Clin Oncol 1998;16:1588–93.
28. Palkama VJ, Neuvonen PJ, Olkkola KT. The CYP 3A4 inhibitor itraconazole has no effect on the pharmacokinetics of iv fentanyl. Br J Anaesth 1998;81:598–600.
29. Trapnell CB, Klecker RW, Jamis-Dow C, Collins JM. Glucuronidation of 3-azido-3-deoxythymidine (zidovudine) by human liver microsomes: relevance to clinical pharmacokinetic interactions with atovaquone, fluconazole, methadone and valproic acid. Antimicrob Agents Chemother 1998;42:42–7.

30. McCance-Katz EF, Rainey PM, Jatlow P, Friedland G. Methadone effects on zidovudine disposition (AIDS Clinical Trials Group 262). J Acquired Immune Defic Syndr Hum Retrovirol 1998;18:435–43.
31. Iribarne C, Berthou F, Carlhand D, Dreano Y, Picart D, Lohezic F, Riche C. Inhibition of methadone and buprenorphine *N*-dealkylations by three HIV-1 protease inhibitors. Drug Metab Disp 1998;26:257–60.
32. Cobb MN, Desai J, Brown LS Jr, Zannikos PN, Rainey PM. The effect of fluconazole on the clinical pharmacokinetics of methadone. Clin. Pharmacol Ther 1998;63:655–62.
33. Broekema AA, Veen A, Fidler V, Gielen MJM, Hennis PJ. Postoperative analgesia with intramuscular morphine at fixed rate versus epidural morphine or sufentanil and bupivacaine in patients undergoing major abdominal surgery. Anesth Analg 1998;87:1346–53.
34. Sanansilp V, Areewatana S, Tonsukchai N. Droperidol and the side effects of epidural morphine after cesarean section. Anesth Analg 1998;86:532–7.
35. Beilin Y, Bernstein HH, Zucker-Pinchoff B, Zahn J, Zenzen W. Subhypnotic doses of propofol do not relieve pruritus induced by intrathecal morphine after cesarean section. Anesth Analg 1998;86:310–13.
36. Cardoso MMSC, Carvalho JCA, Amaro AR, Prado AA, Cappel I EL. Small doses of intrathecal morphine combined with systemic diclofenac for postoperative pain control after cesarean delivery. Anesth Analg 1998;86:538–41.
37. Roca B, Mentero A, Simon E, Moulin DE, Hahn A, Hagen N. Pain and opioid analgesics in Guillain-Barré syndrome. Neurology 1998;51:924.
38. Sun HL. Naloxone-precipitated acute opioid withdrawal syndrome after epidural morphine. Anesth Analg 1998;86:544–5.
39. Eriator II, Sun HL. Naloxone, Acute opioid withdrawal syndrome or side effects? Anesth Analg 1998;87:1214.
40. Sexton WJ, Benedict JF, Jarrow JP. Comparison of long-term outcomes of penile prostheses and intracavernosal injection therapy. J Urol 1998;159:811–15.
41. Brown SL, Haas CA, Koehler M, Bodner DR, Seftel AD. Hepatotoxicity related to intracavernous pharmacotherapy with papaverine. Urology 1998;52:844–7.
42. Kaplan L, Parris WC-V, Citron ML, Khukovsky D, Reder RF, Buckley B, Kaiko R. Comparison of controlled-release and immediate-release oxycodone tablets in patients with cancer pain. J Clin Oncol 1998;16:3230–7.
43. Bruera E, Belzile M, Pituskin E, Fainsinger R, Darke E, Harsanyi Z, Babul N, Ford I. Randomised, double-blind, cross-over trial comparing safety and efficacy of oral controlled-release oxycodone with controlled release morphine in patients with cancer pain. J Clin Oncol 1998; 16:3222–9.
44. Watson CPN, Babul N. Efficacy of oxycodone in neuropathic pain. A randomised trial in postherpetic neuralgia. Neurology 1998;50;1837–41.
45. Duthie DJR. Remifentanil and tramadol. Br J Anaesth 1998;81:51–7.
46. ArkooshVA, Cooper M, Norris MC, Boxer L, Ferouz F, Silverman M, Huffnagle J, Huffnagle S, Leighton B. Intrathecal sufentanil dose response in nulliparous patients. Anesthesiology 1998;89:364–70.
47. Gambling DR, Sharma SK, Ramin SM, Lucas MJ, Leveno KJ, Wiley J, Sidawi E. A randomised study of combined spinal-epidural analgesia versus intravenous meperidine during labor. Anesthesiology 1998;89:1336–44.
48. Dunn SM, Connelly NR, Steinberg RB, Lewis TJ, Bazzell CM, Klatt J, Parker R. Intrathecal sufentanil versus epidural lidocaine with epinephrine and sufentanil for early labor analgesia. Anesth Analg 1998;87:331–5.
49. Camann W, Abouleish A, Eisenach J, Hood D, Datta S. Intrathecal sufentanil and epidural bupivacaine for labor analgesia:dose response of individual agents and in combination. Reg Anesth Pain Med 1998;23:457–62.
50. Mercier FJ, Dounas M, Bouaziz H, Des Mesnards-Smaja V, Foriet C, Veestermann MN, Fishchler M, Benhamou D. The effect of adding a minidose of clonidine to intrathecal sufentanil for labor analgesia. Anesthesiology 1998;89:594–601.
51. Riley ET, Hamilton CL, Cohen SE. Intrathecal sufentanil produces sensory changes without hypotension in male volunteers. Anesthesiology 1998;89:73–8.
52. Fournier R, Gamulin Z, Van Gessel E. Respiratory depression after 5 μg of intrathecal sufentanil. Anesth Analg 1998;87:1377–8.
53. Katsiris S, Williams S, Leighton BL, Halpern S. Respiratory arrest following intrathecal injection of sufentanil and bupivacaine in a parturient. Can J Anaesth 1998;49:880–3.
54. Yemen TA, Bennet JA, Abrams J, Van Riper DF, Horrow JC. Small doses of sufentanil will produce violent coughing in young children. Anesthesiology 1998;89:271–2.
55. Nossol S, Schwarzbold M, Stadler TH. Treatment of pain with sustained-release tramadol 100, 150, 200 mg: a post-marketing surveillance study. Int J Clin Pract 1998;52:115–21.
56. Coetzee JF, Van Loggerenberg H. Tramadol or morphine administered during operation: a study of immediate postoperative effects after abdominal hysterectomy. Br J Anaesth 1998;81:737–41.
57. Hopkins D, Shipton EA, Potgieter D, Van der Merwe CA, Boon J, De Wet C, Murphy J. Comparison of tramadol and morphine via subcutaneous PCA following major orthopaedic surgery. Can J Anaesth 1998;45:435–42.
58. Pavelka K, Peliskova Z, Stehlikova H, Ratcliffe S, Repas C. Intraindividual differences in pain relief and functional improvement in osteoarthritis with diclofenac or tramadol. Clin Drug Invest 1998;16:421–9.
59. Turturro M, Paris PM, Larkin GL. Tramadol versus hydrocodone-acetaminophen in acute musculoskeletal pain: a randomised, double-blind clinical trial. Ann Emerg Med 1998;32:139-43.

60. Crighton IM, Martin PH, Hobbs GJ, Cobby TF, Fletcher AJ, Stewart PD. A comparison of the effects of intravenous tramadol, codeine and morphine on gastric emptying in human volunteers. Anesth Analg 1998;87:445–9.
61. Diamant K, Fischer G, Schneider C, Lenzinger E, Pezawas L, Schindler S, Eder H. Outpatient detoxification with buprenorphine. Preliminary investigations. Eur Addict Res 1998, 4:198–202.
62. Tracqui A, Tournoud C, Flesch F, Kopferschmitt J, Kintz P, Devaux M, Ghysel MH, Marquet P, Pepin G, Petit G, Jaeger A, Ludes B. Intoxications aigues par traitement substitutif a base de buprenorphine haut dosage. 29 observations cliniques—20 cas mortels. Presse Med 1998;27:557–61.
63. Tracqui A, Kintz P, Ludes B. Buprenorphine-related deaths among drug addicts in France: a report on 20 fatalities. J Anal Toxicol 1998;22:430–4.
64. Reynaud M, Tracqui A, Petit G, Potard D, Courty P. Six deaths linked to misuse of buprenorphine-benzodiazepine combinations. Am J Psychiatry 1998;155:448.
65. Zacny JP, Hill JL, Black ML, Sadeghi P. Comparing the subjective, psychomotor and physiological effects of intravenous pentazocine and morphine in normal volunteers. J Pharmacol Exp Ther 1998;287:1197–207.
66. Sinsawaiwong S, Phanthumchinda K, Pentazocine-induced fibrous myopathy and localised neuropathy. J Med Assoc Thailand 1998;81:717–21.
67. Terra SG, Tsunoda SM. Opioid antagonists in the treatment of pruritus from cholestatic liver disease. Ann Pharmacother 1998;32:1228–30.
68. Begasa NV, Schmitt JM, Talbot TL, Alling DW, Swain MG, Turner ML, Jenkins JB, Jones EA. Open-label trial of oral nalmefene therapy for the pruritus of cholestasis. Hepatology 1998;27:679–84.
69. Maremmani I, Marini G, Fornai F. Naltrexone-induced panic attacks. Am J Psychiatry 1998;155:447.
70. Swift R, Davidson D, Rosen S, Fitz E, Carmar P. Naltrexone effects on diazepam intoxication and pharmacokinetics in humans. Psychopharmacology 1998;135:256–62.

Albano Del Favero

9 Anti-inflammatory and antipyretic analgesics and drugs used in gout

NON-STEROIDAL ANTI-INFLAMMATORY DRUGS (NSAIDs) AND ANTIPYRETIC ANALGESICS

℞ Analgesic-induced headaches in children

Despite widespread knowledge of analgesic-induced headache in adults who overuse analgesics (SEDA-21, 95) the condition has not been previously described in children. One report (1[C]) describes 12 children, aged 6–16 years, who gave a history of headaches on at least 4 days a week, for 3 months to 10 years. Eleven of the children had been taking paracetamol, six in combination with codeine, and one was taking ibuprofen alone. They were taking at least one dose of an analgesic for each headache and eight were taking analgesics every day.

The headaches presented with increasing frequency and were related to overuse of analgesics, a typical finding in analgesic-induced headache.

The analgesics were withdrawn; in six children the headaches resolved completely, another five children experienced a reduced frequency of headaches, and one resumed analgesic abuse.

The second report (2[C]) is a retrospective study of patients seen in a pediatric headache clinic. During 8 months 98 patients were seen for headache; 46 of them suffered from daily or near daily headache and 30 were consuming analgesics daily. Follow-up information was available in 25. The average number of weekly doses of analgesics they consumed was 26. The most commonly used medications were paracetamol and ibuprofen. In addition, a minority were taking combinations that contained aspirin, codeine, caffeine, propoxyphene, or butalbital or other NSAIDs. Abrupt discontinuation of all analgesics concomitant with initiation of 10 mg of amitriptyline (22 patients) prompted a significant reduction in the frequency and severity of headache.

The data from these studies are comparable to previous observations reported in adults (SEDA-21, 95) and suggest that daily use of analgesics can cause daily or near daily headaches in children and adolescents. However, additional controlled prospective studies are needed to address the true frequency of analgesics rebound headache among children and to evaluate possible treatments.

℞ NSAID-induced gastrointestinal bleeding: further risk factors

Cirrhosis with esophageal or cardiac varices *Aspirin can increase the risk of variceal bleeding in patients with cirrhosis. In fact, according to a case-control study (3[C]), patients with cirrhosis and esophageal or cardiac varices who take NSAIDs are three times more likely to have a first episode of variceal bleeding compared with similar patients who are not taking NSAIDs.*

In 125 patients with cirrhosis who were admitted to hospital with a first episode of bleeding related to esophageal or cardiac varices, compared with 75 patients with cirrhosis, but no previous or current history of variceal bleed-

Side Effects of Drugs, Annual 23
J.K. Aronson, ed.

ing, who were admitted to the same hospitals a questionnaire showed that more patients with a first episode of bleeding had used aspirin, either alone or in combination with other NSAIDs compared with controls (odds ratio 4.9). This increased risk of bleeding was seen only in patients with grade 2 or 3 varices.

The results of this small hospital-based study should be interpreted with caution, but as variceal bleeding is a life-threatening event and in cirrhosis other factors may also predispose to bleeding (i.e. thombocytopenia and coagulation defects) the possible benefit of therapy with aspirin or other NSAIDs should be carefully weighed against the risks of major gastrointestinal bleeding.

Cancer patients *Patients with cancer are often given an NSAID, most often to control pain that is not responding to other common analgesics (i.e. paracetamol or codeine). A retrospective study in the UK of 200 patients with advanced cancer showed that 72 (36%) were taking an NSAID, 45 were also taking a corticosteroid, and 62 had other additional risk factors for gastrointestinal toxicity (4[C]). Despite the use in 50% of patients of various 'gastroprotective' agents it was necessary to stop NSAID therapy in eight patients owing to gastrointestinal adverse effects, including three severe adverse events (two fatal perforations and one upper gastrointestinal hemorrhage).*

NSAIDs are valuable drugs in treating cancer pain, but their benefits must be weighed against the increased risk of gastrointestinal toxicity in each individual patient.

Nitrate therapy *Aspirin in low dosages (under 300 mg/day) is widely used in cardiovascular prophylaxis, but its use is accompanied by an increased risk of gastrointestinal bleeding (SEDA-21, 100). Of particular interest therefore are data from a retrospective case-control study showing that nitrate therapy may reduce the risk of aspirin-induced gastrointestinal bleeding (5[C]). As nitrates are often used in the same population of patients, such data merit further confirmation from larger prospective studies.*

Urinary system Despite the fact that a careful evaluation of all epidemiological studies on non-narcotic analgesics showed no evidence that phenacetin-free combination drugs are more nephrotoxic than simple analgesics (6[R]), the Belgian Public Health Authorities decided that combination analgesics are to become 'prescription only' (7[c]), as they have a 'devastating' effect on the kidneys. However, contrasting opinions have been published (8[R], 9[R]) and the debate is still open.

Musculoskeletal The suggestion that NSAIDs should not be used as analgesics after orthopedic surgery because they might *inhibit fracture healing* (10[C]) elicited strong disagreement (11[r], 12[C]). The belief that NSAIDs could cause more harm then benefit in patients undergoing orthopedic surgery in based on some experimental data in animals. In diverse rodent models NSAIDs inhibited bone healing, but other animal studies have shown no effect (11[r], 13, 14). In humans published evidence is almost non-existent (11[r]). In the absence of well-designed trials showing important effects on bone healing, NSAIDs should continue to be used as effective analgesics after orthopedic surgery.

Interactions *Non-steroidal anti-inflammatory drugs* There have been reports of exaggerated responses (angioedema and malaise) to bee stings in patients taking NSAIDs (SEDA-11, 88). More recently a report of resensitization to bee stings associated with diclofenac has been received by the Centre for Adverse Reactions Monitoring in New Zealand. The patient, who had been successfully desensitized to bee venom many years before, developed life-threatening anaphylaxis after a bee sting while taking diclofenac (15[c]).

Anaphylactic reactions induced by NSAIDs are associated with HLA-DRB1 genes encoding HLA-DR11 molecules, according to the results of a study in 21 patients who suffered from anaphylactic reactions to NSAIDs and 47 patients who had exclusively cutaneous reactions to these drugs (16[C]). A control group of 167 patients was studied. Patients and controls were challenged, single-blind, with aspirin, salsalate, paracetamol, piroxicam, or diclofenac. There were 88 episodes of skin reactions to NSAIDs and 26 episodes of anaphylaxis. The frequency of HLA-DR11 alleles was 59% in the anaphylaxis group compared with 16% in the control group. Neither HLA-DR and HLA-DQ alleles was associated with NSAID-induced skin reactions.

The FDA has announced its intention to require *alcohol* warnings on all over-the-counter pain medications that contain acetylsalicylic acid, salicylates, paracetamol, ibuprofen, ketoprofen, or naproxen. The proposed warnings are aimed at alerting consumers to the specific risks incurred from heavy alcohol consumption and its interaction with analgesics. For products that contain paracetamol, the warning indicates the risks of liver damage in those who drink more than three alcoholic beverages a day. For formulations that contain salicylates or the mentioned NSAIDs three or more alcoholic beverages will increase the risk of stomach bleeding (17[c]).

INDIVIDUAL DRUGS AND CLASSES

Acetylsalicylic acid (aspirin) and related compounds *(SED-13, 170; SEDA-20, 90; SEDA-21, 100; SEDA-22, 113)*

Respiratory Chronic salicylate toxicity can cause pulmonary injury, leading to respiratory distress. Lung biopsy may reveal diffuse alveolar damage and fibrosis (18[C]).

Gastrointestinal *Major hemorrhagic complications* can occur with aspirin prophylaxis, and the estimates of these complication rates are generally derived from clinical trials (SEDA-21, 100). However, the applicability of the results of such trials to the general population may be debatable, as protocols for these studies often are designed precisely to avoid enrolment of patients who are at risk of complications. Indeed differences in benefit:risk ratio have been found in trials using the same dose of aspirin (19[C], 20[C]). For this reason a recent population based historical cohort study on frequency of major complications of aspirin used for secondary stroke prevention may be of interest (21[C]). The study identified 588 patients who had a first ischemic stroke, transient ischemic attack, or amaurosis fugax during the study period. Of these, 339 patients had taken aspirin for an average of 1.7 years. The mean age of patients who had taken aspirin was 74 years. Complications occurred within 30 days of initiation of treatment in one patient, between 30 days and 6 months in 10 patients, between 6 months and 1 year in seven patients, and between 1 and 2 years in two patients. Estimated standardized morbidity ratio of gastrointestinal hemorrhage (determined on the basis of 10 observed events and 0.661 expected events, during 576 person years of observation) was 15 (95% CI = 7–28). The estimated standardized morbidity ratio of intracerebral hemorrhage (determined on the basis of only one event and 0.59 expected events) was 1.7 (CI = 0.04–9.4). One patient had a fatal gastrointestinal hemorrhage. Unfortunately these complication rates must be considered estimates, because aspirin therapy was not consistently recorded. However, the rates of complications were similar to those observed in some randomized clinical trials. On the basis of these data and of those of a meta-analysis of 16 trials involving more than 95 000 patients (21[R]), the overall benefits of aspirin, measured in terms of preventing myocardial infarction and ischemic stroke, clearly outweigh the risks.

A *gastrocolic fistula* developed in a 47-year-old woman taking aspirin and prednisone for rheumatoid arthritis (23[c]). Other similar case reports have been published (24[c], 25[c]).

Salsalate *(SEDA-21, 102)*

A 77-year-old man developed three *ulcerated lesions on his tongue* because he had difficulty in swallowing salsalate tablets. He was taught how to swallowing tablets and instructed to take tablets with water to avoid prolonged contract of salsalate with the tongue. Three weeks later, his lesions had healed and no new ones had appeared (26[C]).

ANILINE DERIVATIVES

Paracetamol *(SED-13, 199; SEDA-20, 96; SEDA-21, 103; SEDA-22, 114)*

Skin and appendages Despite its widespread use paracetamol is rarely reported to cause a *fixed drug eruption*, which has now been reported (27[C]).

A 76-year-old woman developed a bullous fixed drug eruption on her limbs after taking two paracetamol tablets for toothache. She had also fever, diarrhea, and vomiting. She had previously had two similar acute onset bullous eruptions over the same area after taking paracetamol

Overdosage A 29-year-old woman with a psychiatric disorder took an overdose of paracetamol on nine separate occasions. On the last three occasions she developed a dose-dependent, late-onset, *delayed hypersensitivity reaction*, characterized by a erythematous rash over the entire body (28[C]).

Treatment of paracetamol overdosage

Should current guidelines on the treatment of paracetamol poisoning be changed? Paracetamol is a widely used, effective, and well tolerated analgesic, but thanks also to its ready availability it is the most commonly used substance in self-poisoning (SEDA-18, 94; 29[C]) and a frequent cause of accidental overdose, especially in children (SEDA-22, 114). From recently collected prospective data (29[C], 30[C]) it has been estimated that around 58 000 people take paracetamol in overdose each year in England and Wales and that these episodes of poisoning prompted 3.3% of inquires to US regional poisons centers (31[C]), 10% of inquires to the UK National Poisons Information Service (32[C]), and up to 43% of all admissions to hospital with self-poisoning in the UK (33[C]). Despite the availability of effective antidotes for patients who seek medical intervention early after an overdose, in the US paracetamol alone accounted for 4.1% of deaths from poisoning reported to American poison centers in 1997 (31[C]). To reduce the chance of liver damage and death in cases of paracetamol overdosage, guidelines have been produced in many countries (29[C], 34[C], 35[C]) to identify patients at high risk who need to be treated soon with the antidote, N-acetylcysteine.

In general such guidelines recommend that the antidote should be given to all patients with a serum paracetamol concentration over 200 mg/l (1.32 mmol/l) 4 hours after ingestion. A nomogram, in which this value is joined to an end point of 25 mg/l (10.16 mmol/l) at 16 hours, allows identification over this period of the patients who must receive the antidote. If acetylcysteine is not administered it has been calculated that over 60% of patients with serum concentration of paracetamol above the described treatment line may develop serious liver damage and of these about 5% will die (36[C]). No deaths have been reported in any of the major treatment trials, however high the initial serum paracetamol concentrations, provided acetylcysteine was given within 10 hours of paracetamol ingestion. These data support the hypothesis that serious liver damage and death should be very uncommon if treatment guidelines are followed and if the patient presents for medical advice within the critical time of 10 hours from poisoning.

However, a recent report (36[C]) has described fatal overdose of paracetamol in four patients who presented within this time with serum paracetamol concentrations below the treatment line who, in accord with the established guidelines, were not treated with the antidote and developed fatal acute liver failure. The report has generated considerable debate by advocating changing the treatment line for the use of antidotes in patients at standard risk from paracetamol poisoning from that currently recommended, which passes through 200 mg/l at 4 hours and 25 mg/l at 16 hours, to a lower line passing through 150 mg/l at 4 hours and 30 mg/l at 12 hours.

A second 'high risk patient' line, at about half the concentration of the conventional treatment line, has been already adopted in some guidelines for patients considered at adjunctive risk of liver damage, such as those taking long-term enzyme-inducing drugs, abusing alcohol chronically, or with poor nutrition and cachexia.

However, an absolute cut-off point between a non-toxic and a toxic paracetamol overdose does not exist. Many factors should be taken into consideration in correctly interpreting the measured serum concentrations. First, the timing of the blood sample in relation to the overdose is often uncertain, and when using the treatment nomogram clinicians should assume the longest interval between poisoning and blood sampling that is consistent with the history. Second, the current treatment nomogram is useless when paracetamol overdosage has occurred over several hours or more rather than as a single episode. Third, apart from the already mentioned known risk factors, some individual differences in susceptibility to paracetamol are not well understood.

Therefore, owing to these uncertainties, it seems wise to suggest that in judging whether or not to use an antidote clinicians should always err on the side of caution: 'If there is doubt about the timing or the need of treatment, treat' (29[C]).

R

The interaction of warfarin with paracetamol

Recent reports have called attention to possible potentiation of the anticoagulant effect of warfarin by concomitant long-term paracetamol administration. In a case-control study (37[C]) on the risk factors for excessive warfarin anticoagulation the investigators studied 289 patients prospectively, 93 with an International Normalized Ratio (INR) over 6.0 and 196 with an INR of 1.7–3.3 during warfarin therapy. Paracetamol intake was independently associated with a high INR and the effect was dose-dependent. At a dosage of about 2–4 g/week the adjusted odds ratio (OR) for having an INR over 6 was 3.5 (95% CI = 1.2–10) compared with no intake of paracetamol. At an intake of 4–9 g/week the adjusted OR was 6.9 (95% CI = 2.2–22), and at an intake over 10 g/week the OR was 10 (95% CI = 2.6–38).

However, the results of this study must be interpreted with caution, for many reasons. First, despite these data and the widespread use of paracetamol as an analgesic in patients taking warfarin, only a few reports from the literature have described serious hemorrhagic complications due to potentiation of anticoagulant effect of warfarin or acenocoumarol by paracetamol (38[CR], 39[C]). Second, some pharmacological studies have failed to show such interaction (40[C]). Third, numerous factors in the Hylex study were independently associated with an increased likelihood of having an INR over 6.0 and it is therefore possible that overlap could have occurred between these factors and paracetamol intake. Fourth, the biochemical mechanism by which paracetamol may interfere with warfarin is not well understood. The normal metabolism of warfarin, which occurs via hepatic cytochrome P450, is a complex mechanism that can be competitively and non-competitively inhibited by many drugs. The normal metabolism of paracetamol, particularly when large doses of paracetamol are ingested, also involves cytochrome P450. Thus, paracetamol can exhaust the capacity of cytochrome P450 and prevent the normal metabolism of warfarin. When the normal metabolism of warfarin is prevented by paracetamol, the amount of active, non-protein bound warfarin promptly increases and may double or triple in concentration in the blood. Some pharmacological data, however, make this explanation uncertain. CYP2E1 and CYP1A2 partially metabolize paracetamol. CYP2E1 is not involved in warfarin metabolism, CYP1A2 partially metabolizes paracetamol and is responsible for metabolism of R-warfarin, the less potent anticoagulant of the two warfarin stereoisomers. While R-warfarin and paracetamol may compete for metabolism, it is unlikely that a drug that competes for or inhibits metabolism of the less potent R-warfarin would significantly increase the INR. Finally despite sporadic case reports this potential interaction is considered clinically irrelevant on the basis of a large collective experience by many clinicians in managing patients who require anticoagulation (41[c], 42[c]).

Paracetamol remains the standard analgesic in patients taking warfarin or acenocoumoral. However, the dose and duration of paracetamol therapy should be as low as possible and INR values should be monitored.

The key message from this study is that in patients on a stable warfarin regimen who begin to take repeated doses of paracetamol a possible interaction should be considered.

ANTHRANILIC ACID DERIVATIVES

Mefenamic acid *(SED-13, 241)*

Skin and appendages *Pseudoporphyria* is an infrequent adverse effect of some NSAIDs (naproxen (SEDA-12, 87), nabumetone (SEDA-16, 111), oxaprozin (SEDA-21, 106)). A 22-year-old woman developed pseudoporphyria during long-term treatment with mefenamic acid for menstrual problems. After withdrawal of mefenamic acid the skin lesions gradually disappeared, and at follow-up after 18 months she did not have any skin lesions and had minimal residual scarring (43[C]).

An unusual skin reaction characterized by widespread *pruritic papules and nodules* occurred in a 62-year-old-woman who had taken long-term mefenamic acid for arthritis. The histological findings were consistent with dermatitis herpetiformis, whereas direct immunofluorescence was suggestive of atypical bullous pemphigoid or linear IgA disease. The skin eruption responded to dapsone, but an increase in the dosage of mefenamic acid caused diarrhea and steatorrhea with IgA antigliadin antibodies. A lymphocyte stimulation test with mefenamic acid was positive. Mefenamic acid was withdrawn and all her symptoms disappeared within 2 weeks (44[C]).

Morniflumate

Immunological and hypersensitivity reactions Morniflumate is an NSAID that is widely prescribed in some countries as an antipyretic analgesic in children. A 4-year-old girl developed *angioedema* and *urticaria* 30 minutes after receiving rectal morniflumate. Her signs and symptoms resolved in 48 hours. Skin prick and intradermal tests to morniflumate were negative, but rechallenge with rectal administration caused a recurrence (45[C]).

Tolfenamic acid *(SED-13, 243)*

Hyperkalemia has been attributed to tolfenamic acid (46[c]).

A hemodialysis patient with nephrotic syndrome and diabetic end-stage renal disease developed severe hyperkalemia with muscle paresis after taking tolfenamic acid 300 mg/day for chronic headache. Five days after starting treatment he reported pain and tenderness affecting the muscles of his back and lower extremities. He had hyponatremia and severe hyperkalemia. During the following days he developed increasing weakness and became unable to move his head and limbs. Tolfenamic acid was discontinued and aggressive treatment and repeated hemodialysis started, leading to complete recovery in a few days.

In this case end-stage renal disease with nephrotic syndrome and insulin-dependent diabetes mellitus were predisposing factors to the development of hyperkalemia, but a possible role of accumulated tolfenamic acid metabolites could not be excluded. Patients with severe renal insufficiency should not receive NSAIDs.

ARYLALKANOIC ACID DERIVATIVES *(SED-13, 227; SEDA-20, 91; SEDA-21, 103; SEDA-22, 115)*

Bromfenac *(SEDA-22, 115)*

In June 1998 bromfenac was withdrawn from the market because of reports of severe *hepatic insufficiency.* Descriptions of some cases have appeared (47[C]–50[C]).

Diclofenac *(SED-13, 232; SEDA-20, 91; SEDA-21, 104; SEDA-22, 115)*

Skin and appendages *Contact dermatitis* on the eyelids developed in a 70-year-old woman after she had used eye-drops containing diclofenac. Patch tests were positive to both diclofenac and indomethacin, suggesting possible cross-reactivity between the two compounds (51[C]).

Staphylococcal scalded skin syndrome developed in a 68-year-old man after he had taken diclofenac for knee arthritis subsequently diagnosed as septic arthritis due to *Staphylococcus aureus* (52[C]). NSAIDs can predispose to severe infections (SEDA-22, 112).

Second generation effects As inhibitors of cyclo-oxygenase, NSAIDs given during pregnancy can cause adverse maternal and fetal effects (SEDA-22, 112). *Premature closure of the ductus arteriosus* occurred in a fetus who was exposed in utero to diclofenac at 34-35 weeks gestation (53[c]). Emergency cesarean section was performed and the baby girl required cardiorespiratory support and multiple medications. She gradually improved and further development was normal.

Ibuprofen *(SED-13, 228; SEDA-20, 93; SEDA-21, 105; SEDA-22, 116)*

Liver Ibuprofen has been rarely thought responsible for liver damage. A recent report has described three patients, 33–44 years old, with chronic hepatitis C infection who developed more than 5-fold increases in serum liver transaminases after taking ibuprofen for muculoskeletal pain. In all three there were no associated symptoms of hepatitis and serum transaminases normalized after ibuprofen was withdrawn (54[C]).

Urinary system High-dose ibuprofen can slow the progression of lung disease in patients with cystic fibrosis and is usually well tolerated (SEDA-20, 93). However, *transient renal insufficiency* developed in four children with cystic fibrosis who were taking maintenance ibuprofen when an intravenous aminoglycoside was added to their regimen to treat an exacerbation of lung disease (55[C]). Ibuprofen should probably be stopped during intravenous aminoglycoside therapy.

Acute deterioration in renal function can occur also in other at-risk patients, such as those with renal transplants (56[C], 57[C]).

Ketoprofen *(SED-13, 229, SEDA-20, 93; SEDA-21, 105; SEDA-22, 116)*

Skin and appendages Recent data from Sweden have confirmed the *photosensitizing potential* of topical gel formulations of ketoprofen and have included a number of reports of contact *dermatitis* (58[c]).

Overdosage A 64-year-old woman *had auditory and visual hallucinations, persecutory delusions*, and *slurred speech* after she took an overdose of ketoprofen; her psychiatric symptoms resolved within 48 hours (59[c]).

Ketorolac *(SED-13, 240; SEDA-20, 93; SEDA-21, 105; SEDA-22, 117)*

Gastrointestinal Further evidence of the unfavorable benefit:risk profile of ketorolac compared with other NSAIDs has been provided by another case-control study on first-time hospitalization for *gastroduodenal ulcer* (documented by endoscopy, radiology, surgery, or autopsy), with or without bleeding or perforation. Of all the NSAIDs used in out-patients the highest rate ratio for lesions of any degree of severity was seen with piroxicam (4.6; 95% CI = 1.4–8.3). with ketorolac ranking second highest (3.4; 95% CI = 1.4–8.3). For patients who suffered hemorrhage or perforation, the highest rate ratio observed was for ketorolac (5.9; 95% CI = 2.1–16) (60[C]).

Interactions In a pharmacokinetic study in healthy volunteers ketorolac increased the concentration of *lithium* in both serum and erythrocytes, which may reflect concentration of the drug in the CNS more accurately. Therefore ketorolac can increase the risk of adverse reactions of lithium (61[C]), as do many other NSAIDs.

Oxaprozin *(SED-13, 238; SED-20, 93; SEDA-21, 106; SEDA-22, 118)*

Toxic epidermal necrolysis occurred in a 71-year-old man after treatment with oxaprozin for shoulder pain (62[c]).

Tiaprofenic acid *(SED-13, 235; SEDA-20, 4; SEDA-21, 107)*

Tiaprofenic acid can cause a chemical interstitial cystitis, and if this complication occurs the drug should be withdrawn immediately (63[Cr]). A recent report has given some data on the frequency with which tiaprofenic acid *cystitis-related disorders* were reported to the UK Committee on Safety of Medicines. Between 1981 and 1996, 770 adverse drug reactions involving 221 patients were reported. A peak in the reporting of cystitis was noted in 1994, when tiaprofenic acid product information was changed and advice was sent to UK doctors warning about cystitis-related disorders. This peak was followed by a fall in the number of reports, but it is not clear if this was due to reduced drug usage or also to a fall in the reporting rate of such adverse reactions (64[C]).

OXICAM DERIVATIVES

(SED-13, 244; SEDA-20, 94; SEDA-21, 107; SEDA-22, 118)

Meloxicam *(SED-13, 244; SEDA-20, 94; SEDA-21, 108)*

Changes have been made to the Summary of Product Characteristics by the manufacturers of meloxicam (65[C]), in agreement with the type of adverse drug reaction reports received by the Committee on Safety of Medicine in the UK. Warnings about gastrointestinal reactions (perforation, ulceration, and/or bleeding) and skin reactions (including *erythema multiforme* and *Stevens-Johnson syndrome*) have been strengthened (66[C]).

Gastrointestinal A large prospective comparison of meloxicam 7.5 mg/day with piroxicam 20 mg/day for a median of 28 days suggested that meloxicam has a lower propensity to cause gastroduodenal adverse events. However, serious gastrointestinal events (i.e. *ulceration, perforation*, or *bleeding*), albeit rare, had similar frequencies in meloxicam and piroxicam recipients, and furthermore the difference in the incidence of adverse gastrointestinal events, although statistically significant, was clinically less relevant (67[C]). Reports received by the Swedish Adverse Drug Reaction Advisory Committee (SADRAC) have suggested that meloxicam has a similar adverse drug reactions profile to other NSAIDs (68[C]) and reports of gastrointestinal hemorrhage have started to appear (69[C]).

Piroxicam *(SED-13, 244; SEDA-20, 95)*

Piroxicam can be added to the list of NSAIDs responsible for *diaphragm-like strictures of the intestinal tract* (70[C]).

A 65 year-old woman who had taken piroxicam for the previous 3 years presented with frequent episodes of abdominal bloating and cramping, sometimes associated with nausea and vomiting, and loss of weight. Small bowel examination showed several mid-ileal strictures associated with proximal dilated bowel.

MISCELLANEOUS COMPOUNDS

Nimesulide *(SED-13, 248; SEDA-22, 119)*

Liver Recently three reports have paid attention to the possibility that *liver toxicity* may be a previously unrecognised problem with nimesulide (71[c], 72[C], 73[C]).

Fulminant hepatic failure due to massive hepatic necrosis occurred in a 58-year-old woman who took nimesulide for a few weeks for osteoarthritis. In the months before she had received a first short course of the drug, apparently without problems. When she resumed nimesulide therapy she complained of non-specific symptoms, including nausea, and appeared jaundiced. The drug was withdrawn and liver transplantation was performed, but she died of multiorgan failure. The previous exposure may have sensitized the patient with accelerated liver injury on re-exposure.

A second report described a series of five patients, two of whom died as a result of fulminant hepatic failure while taking nimesulide.

A third report referred to six cases of acute hepatitis which occurred in four patients during the first 10 weeks of treatment, and in two after 15 weeks of therapy. They were represented by jaundice (five patients), itching (2), weakness (3), and anorexia, nausea, and vomiting (2). Increases in liver enzymes varied from 1.5 to over 30 times the upper limit of the reference range. Liver biopsy showed centrilobular or panlobular bridging necrosis in the four women and intrahepatic cholestasis in the two men. Complete recovery of normal liver function tests ensued at follow-up after interruption of nimesulide therapy.

The Portuguese Pharmacy and Medicines Institute has suspended the pediatric formulation of nimesulide (74[C]). This decision has been made because of reports of serious adverse drug reactions, including liver damage, in children taking the drug. Nimesulide should be withdrawn immediately if abnormal liver-function tests develop and rechallenge must be avoided. However, it is not yet clear if the potential for hepatotoxicity of this drug is similar or greater to that found with other NSAIDs (75[R]).

Urinary system A series of 11 spontaneously reported cases in which renal impairment was associated with the use of nimesulide has been described (76[C]). The adverse events were represented by *acute renal insufficiency* (two patients) *acute deterioration of chronic renal insufficiency* (3), *fluid retention* (4), and *oliguria* and *macrohematuria* (one each). The patients had a median age of 57 (range 17-81) years and six had some predisposing condition (chronic renal insufficiency, heart failure, diabetes, use of diuretics) to NSAID-induced functional renal impairment. Apart from one patient, nimesulide was taken for a very short time (less than 8 days). A favorable outcome ensued after withdrawal of therapy in all patients. The acute deterioration of renal function described in these patients pointed to hemodynamically mediated renal impairment in all cases, with the exception of one man in whom interstitial nephritis was suspected.

This report raises doubts concerning the possibility that 'selective' COX-2 inhibitors are renal sparing.

Phenazopyridine *(SED-13, 249)*

Skin and appendages *Methemoglobinemia* is a well-known adverse effect of phenazopyridine, but yellow discoloration of the nails induced by long-term therapy has not been previously reported (77[C]).

Pyritinol *(SED-13, 249)*

Pancreas A 23-year-old student had three episodes of *acute pancreatitis* after the occasional ingestion of pyritinol for better performance in examinations. Immunological investigations pointed to a probable T cell-mediated hypersensitivity reaction (78[C]).

DRUGS USED IN THE TREATMENT OF GOUT

Allopurinol *(SED-13, 250; SEDA-21, 108)*

Immunological and hypersensitivity reactions Allopurinol-induced *hypersensitivity reactions* are characterized by a variety of manifestations (SEDA-21, 108). One report has presented evidence of a possible association between severe drug-induced erythema multiforme and reactivation of infection with human herpesvirus-6. The reactivation is thought to have contributed in some way to the development of allopurinol hypersensitivity reactions (79[C]).

A generalized *cutaneous vasculitis* has been associated with the presence in the serum of antineutrophil cytoplasmic antibodies (ANCA) with a peripheral pattern (pANCA) and antimyeloperoxidase antibodies (80[C]). A skin biopsy of a lesion showed leukocytoclastic vasculitis with eosinophilic infiltration. Allopurinol was withdrawn and the symptoms resolved completely. Allopurinol can be added to the small number of drugs that have been associated, albeit rarely, with pANCA positivity (e.g. hydralazine, propylthiouracil).

Colchicine *(SED-13, 252; SEDA-21, 109; SEDA-22, 119)*

Water and electrolytes disturbances, including inappropriate antidiuresis, can occur in patients who have taken high doses of colchicine (81[C], 82[C]), but *hypernatremia* and *polyuria* have not previously been described (83[C]).

REFERENCES

1. Symon DNK. Twelve cases of analgesics headache. Arch Dis Child 1998;78:555–6.
2. Vasconcellos E, Pina-Garza JE, Millan EJ, Warner JS. Analgesic rebound headache in children and adolescents. J Child Neurol 1998;13:443–7.
3. De Ledinghen V, Heresbach D, Fourdan O, Bernard P, Liebaert-Bories MP, Nousbaum JB, Gourlaouen A, Becker MC, Ribard D, Ingrand P, Silvain C, Beauchant M. Anti-inflammatory drugs and variceal bleeding: a case-control study. Gut 1999; 44:270–3.
4. Hawkins C. Audit and use of NSAIDs. Lancet 1998;352:658.
5. Lanas A, Bajador E, Serrano P, Arroyo M, Fuentes J, Santolaria S. Effects of nitrate and prophylactic aspirin on upper gastrointestinal bleeding: a retrospective case-control study. J Int Med Res 1998;26:120–8.
6. Delzell E, Shapiro S. A review of epidemiologic studies of nonnarcotic analgesics and chronic renal disease. Medicine 1998;77:102–21.
7. Anonymous. Analgesics combos go Rx in Belgium. Scrip 1999;2424:4.
8. De Broe ME, Elseviers WM. Analgesics nephropathy. New Engl J Med 1998;338:446–52.
9. McLaughlin JK, Lipworth L, Chow W-H, Blot WJ. Analgesic use and chronic renal failure: a critical review of the epidemiologic literature. Kidney Int 1998;54:679–86.
10. Varghese D, Kodakat S. Non-steroidal anti-inflammatories should not be used after orthopaedic surgery. Br Med J 1998;316:1390.
11. Stone GP, Richards E. NSAIDs need not usually be withheld after orthopaedic surgery. Br Med J 1998;317:1079.
12. Godden D. Effects of NSAIDs on bone healing have been widely reported in maxillofacial journals. Br Med J 1999;318:1141.
13. Dimar II JR, Ante WA, Zhang YP, Glassman SD. The effects of nonsteroidal anti-inflammatory drugs on posterior spinal fusions in the rat. Spine 1996;21:1870–6.
14. Altman RD, Latta LL, Keer R, Renfree K, Hornicek FJ, Bonavac K. Effect of nonsteroidal anti-inflammatory drugs on fracture healing: a laboratory study in rats. J Orthop Trauma 1995;9: 392–400.
15. Anonymous. Sensitisation to bee and wasp stings with NSAIDs/ACE inhibition. Reactions 1999;3:747.
16. Quiralte J, Sanchez-Garcia F, Torres M-J, Blanco C, Castello R, Ortega N, De Castro FR, Perez-Aciego P, Carrello T. Association of HLA-DR1 with the anaphylactoid reaction caused by nonsteroidal anti-inflammatory drugs. J Allergy Clin Immunol 1999;103:685–9.
17. Anonymous. Alcohol warning on over-the-counter pain medications. WHO Drug Inf 1998;12: 16.
18. Grabe DW, Manley HJ, Kim JS, McGoldrick MD, Bailie GR. Respiratory distress caused by salicylism confirmed by lung biopsy. Clin Drug Invest 1999;17:79–81.
19. Hansson L, Zanchetti A, Carruthers SG, Dahlof B, Elmfeldt D, Julius S, Menard J, Rahn KH, Wedel H, Westerling S, for the HOT Study Group. Effects of intensive blood pressure lowering and low dose aspirin in patients with hypertension: principal results of the Hypertension Optimal Treatment (HOT) randomised trial. Lancet 1998;351:1755–62.
20. Meade TW, Brennan PJ, Wilkes HC, Zuhrie SR. Thrombosis Prevention Trial. Randomised trial

of low-intensity oral anticoagulation with warfarin and low dose aspirin in the primary prevention of ischaemic heart disease in men at increased risk. Lancet 1998;351:233–41.

21. Petty GW, Brown RD Jr, Whisnant JP, Sicks JD, O'Fallon WM, Weibers DO. Frequency of major complications of aspirin, warfarin, and intravenous heparin for secondary stroke prevention. A population-based study. Ann Intern Med 1999; 130:14–22.
22. He J, Whelton PK, Vu B, Klag MJ. Aspirin and risk of hemorrhagic stroke: a meta-analysis of randomised controlled trials. J Am Med Assoc 1998; 280:1930–5.
23. Suazo-Barahona J, Gallegos J, Carmona-Sanchez R, Martinez R, Robles-Diaz G. Nonsteroidal anti-inflammatory drugs and gastrolitic fistula. J Clin Gastroenterol 1998;26:343–5.
24. Gutnik SH, Willmott D, Ziebarth J. Gastrocolic fistula—secondary to aspirin abuse. SDJ Med 1993; 46:358–60.
25. Levine MS, Kelly MR, Laufer I, Rubesin SE, Herlinger H. Gastrocolic fistulas: the increasing role of aspirin. Radiology 1993;187:359–61.
26. Ruscin JM, Astroth JD. Lingual lesions secondary to prolonged contact with salsalate tablets. Ann Pharmacother 1998;32:1248.
27. Hern S, Harman K, Clement M, Black MM. Bullous fixed drug eruption due to paracetamol with an unusual immunofluorescence pattern. Br J Dermatol 1998;139:1129–31.
28. Huitema ADR, Soesan M, Meenhorst PL, Koks CHW, Beijnen JH. A dose-dependent delayed hypersensitivity reaction to acetaminophen after repeated acetaminophen intoxications. Hum Exp Toxicol 1998;17:406–8.
29. Thomas SHL. Paracetamol (acetaminophen) poisoning. Br Med J 1998;317:1609–10.
30. Thomas SHL, Horner JE, Chew K, Connolly J, Dorani B, Bevan L, Bhattacharyya S, Bramble MG, Han KH, Rodgers A, Sen B, Tesfayohannes B, Wynne H, Bateman DN. Paracetamol poisoning in the North East of England: presentation, early management and outcome. Hum Exp Toxicol 1997; 16:495–500.
31. Litovitz TL, Klein-Schawarts W, Dyer KS, Shannon M, Lee S. 1997 Annual report of the American Association of Poison Control Centers Toxic Exposure Surveillance System. Am J Emerg Med 1998;16:443–97.
32. Vale JA, Proudfoot AT. Paracetamol (acetaminophen) poisoning. Lancet 1995;346:547-52.
33. Bialas MC, Reid PG, Beck P, Lazarus JH, Smith PNM, Scorer RC, Routledge PA. Changing patterns of self-poisoning in a UK health district. Q J Med 1996;89:893–901.
34. UK National Poisons Information Service. National guidelines: management of acute paracetamol poisoning. London: Paracetamol Information Centre in collaboration with the British Association for Accident and Emergency Medicine, 1995.
35. Bialas MC, Evans RJ, Hutchings AD, Alldridge G, Routledge PA. The impact of nationally distributed guidelines an the management of paracetamol poisoning in accident and emergency departments. J Accid Emerg Med 1998;15:13–17.
36. Bridger S, Henderson K, Glucksman E, Ellis AJ, Henry JA, Williams R. Death from low dose paracetamol poisoning. Br Med J 1998;316: 1724–5.
37. Hylek EM, Heiman H, Skates SJ, Sheehan MA, Singer DE. Acetaminophen and other risk factors for excessive warfarin anticoagulation. J Am Med Assoc 1998;279:657–72.
38. Bell WR. Acetaminophen and warfarin: undesirable synergy. J Am Med Assoc 1998;279: 702–3.
39. Bagheri H, Bachaud Bernhard N, Montastruc JL. Potentiation of the acenocoumarol anticoagulant effect by acetaminophen. Ann Pharmacother 1999;33:506.
40. Kwan D, Bartle WR, Walker SE. The effects of acetaminophen on pharmacokinetics and pharmacodynamics of warfarin. J Clin Pharmacol 1999; 39:68–75.
41. Riser J, Gilroy C, Hudson P, McCay L, Willis TA. Acetaminophen and risk factors for excess anticoagulation with warfarin. J Am Med Assoc 1998;280:696.
42. Amato MG, Bussey H, Farnett L, Lyons R. Acetaminophen and risk factors for excess anticoagulation with warfarin. J Am Med Assoc 1998; 280:695–6.
43. O'Hagan AH, Irvine AD, Allen GE, Walsh M. Pseudoporphyria induced by mefenamic acid. Br J Dermatol 1998;139:1131–2.
44. Gerbig AW, Paredes B, Hunziker T. Multiple IgA autoantibodies associated with mefenamic acid. Ann Intern Med 1998;129:588–9.
45. Matheu V, Sierra Z, Gracia MT, Caloto M, Alcazar MM, Martinez MI, Zapatero L. Morniflumate-induced urticaria-angioedema. Allergy Eur J Allergy Clin Immumol 1998;53: 812–13.
46. Nielson EH. Hyperkalaemic muscle paresis—side effect of prostaglandin inhibition in a haemodialysis patient. Nephrol Dial Transplant 1999;14: 480–2.
47. Moses PL, Schroeder B, Alkjatib O, Ferrentino N, Suppan T, Lidofsky SD. Severe hepatotoxicity associated with bromfenac sodium. Am J Gastroenterol 1999;94:1393–6.
48. Rabkin JM, Smith MJ, Orloff SL, Corless CL, Stenzel P, Olyaei AJ. Fatal fulminant hepatitis associated with bromfenac use. Ann Pharmacother 1999; 33:945–7.
49. Hunter EB, Johnston PE, Tanner G, Pinson CW, Awad JA. Bromfenac (Duract)-associated hepatic failure requiring liver transplantation. Am J Gastroenterol 1999;94:2299–301.
50. Fontana RJ, McCashland TM, Benner KG, Appelman HD, Gunartanam NT, Wisecarver JL, Rabkin JM, Lee WM et al. Acute liver failure associated with prolonged use of bromfenac leading to liver transplantation. Liver Transplant Surg 1999; 5:480–4.
51. Ueda K, Higashi N, Kume A, Ikushima-

Fujimoto M, Ogiwara S. Allergic contact dermatitis due to diclofenac and indomethacin. Contact Dermatitis 1998;39:323.

52. Oono T, Kanzaki H, Yopshioka T, Arata J. Staphylococcal scalded skin syndrome in an adult: identification of exfoliative toxin A and B genes by polymerase chain reaction. Dermatology 1997; 195:268–70.
53. Mas C, Menahem S. Premature in utero closure of the ductus arteriosus following maternal ingestion of sodium diclofenac. Aust NZ J Obstet Gynaecol 1999;39:106–7.
54. Riley TR, Smith JP. Ibuprofen induced hepatotoxicity in patients with chronic hepatitis C: a case series. Am J Gastroenterol 1998;93:1563–5.
55. Kovesi TA, Swartz R, MacDonald N. Transient renal failure due to simultaneous ibuprofen and aminoglycoside therapy in children with cystic fibrosis. New Engl J Med 1998;338:65–6.
56. Moghal NE, Hulton SA, Milford DV. Care in the use of ibuprofen as an antipyretic in children. Clin Nephrol 1998;49:293–5.
57. Stoves J, Rosenberg K, Harnden P, Turney JH. Acute interstitial nephritis due to over the counter ibuprofen in a renal transplant recipient. Nephrol Dial Transplant 1998;13:227–8.
58. Swedish adverse drug reactions advisory committee. Ketoprofen gel—contact dermatitis and photosensitivity. SADRAC Bull 1998;67:2.
59. Tavcar R, Dernovsek MZ. Ketoprofen intoxication delirium. Clin Psychopharmacol 1999;19: 95–6.
60. Menniti-Ippolito F, Maggini M, Raschetti R, Da Cas R, Traversa G, Walker AM. Ketorolac use in outpatients and gastrointestinal hospitalisation: a comparison with other non-steroidal anti-inflammatory drugs in Italy. Eur J Clin Pharmacol 1998;54:393–7.
61. Cold JA, Zumbrunnen TL, Simpson A, Augustin BG, Award E, Jann MW. Increased lithium serum and red blood cell concentration during ketorolac coadministration. J Clin Psychopharmacol 1998;18:33–7.
62. Carucci JA, Cohen DE. Toxic epidermal necrolysis following treatment with oxaprozin. Int J Dermatol 1999;38:233–4.
63. Drake MJ, Nixon PM, Crew JP. Drug-induced and urinary disorders: incidence, prevention and management. Drug Saf 1998;19:45–55.
64. Brown EG, Waller PC, Sallie BA. Tiaprofenic acid and severe cystitis. Postgrad Med J 1998;74: 443–6.
65. Anonymous. BI strengthens meloxicam warnings. Scrip 1998;31:2368.
66. Committee on Safety of Medicines/Medicines Control Agency. Meloxicam (Mobic): gastrointestinal and skin reactions. Curr Probl Pharmacovig 1998;24:13.
67. Dequere J, Hawkey C, Kahan A, Steinbruck K, Alegre C. Baum. Improvement in gastrointestinal tolerability of the selective cyclooxygenase (COX-2 inhibitor) meloxicam, compared with piroxicam: therapies (selected) trial in osteoarthritis. Br J Rheumatol 1998;37:946–51.
68. Anonymous. Meloxicam safety similar to other NSAIDs. WHO Drug Inf 1998;12:147.
69. Del Val A, llorente MJ, Y Lluch A. Upper gastrointestinal bleeding associated with meloxicam. Rev Esp Enferm Dig 1998;90:461–2.
70. Abrahamian GA, Polhamus CD, Muskat P, Karulf RE. Diaphragm-like strictures of the ileum associated with NSAID use: a rare complication. South Med J 1998;91:395–7.
71. McCormick PA, Kennedy F, Curry M, Traynor O. COX2 inhibitor and fulminant hepatic failure. Lancet 1999;353:40–1.
72. Figueras A, Estèvez F, Laporte JR. New drugs, new adverse drug reactions, and bibliographic databases. Lancet 1999;353:1447–8.
73. Van Steenbergen W, Peeters P, De Bondt J, Staessen D, Busher H. Nimesulide-induced acute hepatitis: evidence from six cases. J Hepatol 1998; 29:135–41.
74. Tolman KG. Hepatotoxicity of non-narcotic analgesics. Am J Med 1998;105:13–19.
75. Anonymous. Portugal suspends paediatric nimesulide. Scrip 1999;20:2431.
76. Leone R, Conforti A, Ghiotto E, Moretti U, Valbo E, Velo GP. Nimesulide and renal impairment. Eur J Clin Pharmacol 1999;5:151–4.
77. Amit G, Halkin A. Lemon-yellow nails and long term phenazopyridine use. Ann Intern Med 1997;127:1137.
78. Straumann A, Bauer M, Pichler WJ, Pirovino M. Acute pancreatitis due to pyritinol: an immune-mediated phenomenon. Gastroenterology 1998; 115:452–4.
79. Suzuki Y, Inagi R, Aono T, Yamanishi K, Shiohara T. Human herpesvirus 6 infection as a risk factor for the development of severe drug-induced hypersensitivity syndrome Arch Dermatol 1998; 134:1108–12.
80. Choi HK, Merkel PA, Niles JL. ANCA-positive vasculitis associated with allopurinol therapy. Clin Exp Rheumatol 1998;16:743–4.
81. Gaultier M, Bismuth C, Autret A, Pillon M. Inappropriate antidiuresis after acute colchicine poisoning. Two cases. Nouv Presse Med 1975;4: 3132–4.
82. Milne ST, Meek PD. Fatal colchicine overdose: report of a case control and review of the literature. Am J Emerg Med 1998;16:603–8.
83. Usalan C, Altun B, Ulusoy S, Erden Y, Yasavul U, Turgan C, Caglar S. Hypernatraemia and polyuria due to high-dose cochicine in a suicidal patient. Nephrol Dial Transplant 1999;14: 1556–7.

T.G. Short and C.N. Bradfield

10 General anesthetics and therapeutic gases

GENERAL TOPICS

Considerable research has been performed comparing the incidence of anesthetic drug complications and the time taken to recover from anesthesia with various anesthetic agents and techniques. In a prospective randomized study of 120 day-surgery patients desflurane and sevoflurane were associated with shorter times to awakening, extubation, and orientation than propofol infusion (1[c]). Average times to awakening at the end of anesthesia were 5, 5, and 8 minutes respectively. There were no significant differences to home readiness or actual discharge times. A review of 436 patients undergoing either sevoflurane or propofol based anesthesia showed no difference in similar recovery endpoints (2[c]). A similar review comparing sevoflurane and isoflurane anesthesia in 2008 patients found a 3–4 minute reduction in time to recovery endpoints with sevoflurane (2[c]). These differences became larger in anesthetics lasting over 3 hours and were trivial in cases less than 1 hour. Patients aged over 65 years had a 5-minute increase in recovery times after receiving isoflurane. There was no significant difference in the incidence of nausea or vomiting between isoflurane, sevoflurane, and propofol. A randomized prospective trial in 60 children undergoing out-patient anesthesia showed a 30% shorter time from discontinuation of anesthesia to eye opening and return to full wakefulness in patients receiving propofol alone compared with halothane/nitrous oxide anesthesia (3[c]). Propofol was associated with a 17% incidence of *emesis* compared with 58 and 53% for halothane/nitrous oxide and propofol/nitrous oxide anesthesia respectively.

A prospective randomized study of 185 patients compared propofol 6–8 mg/kg/h and sevoflurane 1.5% for maintenance of anesthesia (4[C]). Patients were ventilated via a laryngeal mask and no muscle relaxants were given. Both agents were suitable for this technique. Emergence was significantly faster after sevoflurane but associated with more *excitatory phenomena* and *tachycardia*.

The effects of the combination of midazolam and isoflurane on memory were studied in a randomized double blind trial of 28 volunteers (5[C]). Midazolam 0.03 mg/kg or 0.06 mg/kg combined with isoflurane 0.2% showed almost complete *abolition of explicit and implicit memory;* however, there were more variable effects on the level of sedation. The duration of deficit averaged 45 minutes. The study was remarkable for the very low doses required to abolish memory, due to synergy with the combination of midazolam and isoflurane, and abolition of memory at subhypnotic doses with this combination. However, the subjects did not undergo surgery, so caution must be exercised in extrapolating the result to surgical patients, because painful stimuli increase the dosage required to abolish memory.

Respiratory The incidence of perioperative respiratory complications has been studied prospectively in 602 children aged 1 month to 12 years undergoing elective surgery using a halothane-based anesthetic (6[C]). Exposure to environmental smoke was assessed using the history of exposure to cigarette smoke and measurement of urinary cotinine concentrations, and the respiratory complications of laryngospasm, bronchospasm, stridor, breath holding, coughing, and excessive mucus production were recorded. The incidence of respiratory complications in patients with a urinary cotinine concentration over 40 ng/ml was 42%, dropping to 24% in patients with a urinary cotinine concentration less than 10 ng/ml. Female sex and lower socioeconomic status of the

Side Effects of Drugs, Annual 23
J.K. Aronson, ed.

mother increased the incidence of respiratory complications. The study showed the importance of factors other than the anesthetic drugs and techniques used in determining complications precipitated by anesthesia.

Use in pregnancy The pharmacology and adverse effects of anesthetic drugs used for cesarean section have been reviewed (7^r).

ANESTHETIC VAPORS *(SED-13, 265; SEDA-20, 106; SEDA-21, 116; SEDA-22, 125)*

A study of single vital-capacity breath inhalational induction using either sevoflurane or isoflurane combined with 67% nitrous oxide in 67 adults showed that isoflurane was unsuitable for this technique (8^C). There was an 87% incidence of induction complications with isoflurane, *including involuntary movements, cough, laryngospasm*, and *failure of induction*.

Cardiovascular Volatile anesthetic agents *depress cardiac output*, especially in the elderly. A study of 80 patients aged over 60 years compared the effects of halothane and isoflurane with and without nitrous oxide 50% (9^C). Doses were carefully adjusted to be equipotent in all four groups. Isoflurane caused a 30% reduction in systolic and diastolic arterial pressures compared with a 17% reduction with halothane. The reductions in cardiac index were similar with the two agents, about 17%. The addition of nitrous oxide attenuated the reductions in arterial pressure. In the case of the combination of isoflurane with nitrous oxide, there was a small increase in cardiac index and a small reduction in the halothane/nitrous oxide group. Systemic vascular resistance was reduced by a greater extent with isoflurane compared with halothane and little altered by the addition of nitrous oxide. The result suggests that nitrous oxide supplementation may be advantageous in the elderly, but interpretation is limited by the fact that it does not include the effects of surgery on these important cardiac parameters.

The long QT syndrome is associated with potentially fatal ventricular dysrhythmias under anesthesia. The influence of halothane and isoflurane on the QT interval was studied in 51 healthy children (10^C). Isoflurane 2.3–3.0% *increased the average QT interval* from 425 to 475 msec at anesthesia induction. Halothane reduced the average QT interval from 428 to 407 msec. The result suggested that halothane may be the more desirable agent in children with a prolonged QT interval.

Respiratory The respiratory effects of sevoflurane and halothane have been investigated in 30 infants aged 6–24 months (11^C). Respiratory depression was greater in the sevoflurane group, with a mean minute ventilation of 4.5 compared with 5.4 l/min/m^2 and respiratory rate was lower at 38 compared with 47 breaths/min. There was a lower incidence of thoracoabdominal asynchrony with sevoflurane, but no difference in respiratory drive, as evidenced by the flow pressure generated during 100 msec of occlusion of the airway.

Gastrointestinal In a prospective study of 556 adults using isoflurane-, halothane-, and enflurane-based anesthesia for ear, nose, throat, and eye procedures the incidences of *emesis* in the various groups over the ensuing 24 hours were 36, 41, and 46% respectively (12^C). Other drugs given during anesthesia included midazolam, thiopental, morphine, and nitrous oxide. Antiemetic requirements were also less for isoflurane: 12% of patients required an antiemetic compared with 23% for halothane and enflurane. There were no differences in the overall incidence of headache or analgesic requirements in the three groups.

Another prospective study of nausea and vomiting in 50 patients undergoing arthroscopy compared sevoflurane with desflurane (13^C). Other drugs given during anesthesia included propofol and alfentanil. There was no difference in the incidence of nausea, 8 and 16% respectively, and no vomiting in either group. The desflurane group had a significantly higher incidence of sore throat (32 vs 8%). These studies have confirmed that the newer volatile anesthetics isoflurane, sevoflurane, and desflurane cause less nausea and vomiting than halothane or enflurane.

Musculoskeletal A case of *generalized muscle rigidity and hypercapnia* followed by *raised creatine kinase activity* was reported in a child undergoing general anesthesia (14^c).

A 2-year-old girl with a past history of asthma, developmental delay, short neck, and lumbar lordosis, but no known genetic defect or syndrome underwent anesthesia with midazolam and paracetamol premedication, halothane and nitrous oxide induction, and isoflurane plus nitrous oxide for maintenance of anesthesia. Difficulty with mouth opening was noted and endotracheal intubation was difficult. Limb rigidity developed rapidly. Thiopental and cisatracurium were given and the muscle rigidity abated over the next 10 minutes. The procedure was continued with a propofol infusion. No treatment for malignant hyperpyrexia was undertaken and no other markers for malignant hyperpyrexia were observed. She made a normal recovery from anesthesia. Creatine kinase activities were raised at 2370 μ/l intraoperatively and 18 046 μ/l at 20 hours postoperatively.

The case is interesting in that although episodes of masseter spasm, rigidity, rhabdomyolysis, and malignant hyperpyrexia are well known after the use of halothane and succinylcholine, they have only rarely been reported when succinylcholine was not used.

Interactions Both desflurane and sevoflurane significantly increase the neuromuscular blocking effects of *rocuronium* compared with isoflurane or propofol (15[C], 16[C]). The effective doses of rocuronium for 50% depression of single twitch height were 95, 120, 130, and 150 μg/kg for these four drugs respectively. There were no differences in recovery profiles between sevoflurane, desflurane, isoflurane, and propofol using equieffective doses. Desflurane, sevoflurane, and to a lesser extent isoflurane also potentiated the neuromuscular blocking effect of cisatracurium by 30% compared with propofol (17[C], 18[C]).

Chloroform

The very serious adverse effects of chloroform anesthesia when poorly administered have been briefly reviewed (19[R]).

Enflurane

Two patients with *hepatic failure* after enflurane anesthesia were reported from a hepatic transplant unit in France; both died while waiting for a liver transplant (20[C]). In common with halothane, hepatic failure after enflurane is thought to be caused by the metabolite trifluoroacetic acid.

Halothane

Cardiovascular In a double-blind, randomized, controlled study of 77 children undergoing halothane anesthesia for adenoidectomy the effects of atropine 0.02 mg/kg, glycopyrrolate 0.04 mg/kg, and physiological saline were compared (21[C]). There was no difference in the incidence of ventricular dysrhythmias. Atropine prevented bradycardia but was associated with sinus tachycardia in most patients. The bradycardias that occurred in the groups that received glycopyrrolate or placebo were short lived and resolved spontaneously. In a randomized, double-blind, placebo-controlled comparison of intranasal and intramuscular atropine in 80 children, the intranasal route was equally effective at preventing halothane-induced bradycardia (22[C]).

Liver *Hepatitis* after halothane anesthesia has been reviewed (23[R]). Two patterns of liver damage associated with halothane have been observed. One pattern is a mild derangement of liver enzymes, which occurs in about one in four anesthetics. The other pattern is rare but is associated with severe hepatitis, often resulting in fulminant liver failure. This severe form occurs more often in middle-aged, obese women, usually after multiple anesthetics, and is known as halothane hepatitis. It is defined as unexplained severe liver damage occurring within 28 days of halothane exposure in a person with a previously normal liver, and it occurs in 1 : 35 000 halothane exposures. With repeated exposure to halothane within 1 month the frequency of acute liver failure increases to 1 : 3700. The overall incidence of halothane hepatitis is falling, owing to reduced use of halothane. Survival after liver transplantation in patients with fulminant hepatic failure is lower than after liver transplantation for other reasons.

A case of halothane hepatitis has been reported in a child (24[c]).

A 6-year-old boy sustained pelvic injuries and a femoral fracture. The first anesthetic he received consisted of thiopental, succinylcholine, isoflurane, and nitrous oxide. He also received two units of blood. He subsequently underwent four halothane anesthetics over 6 weeks for dilatation of a urethral stricture. Two days after the last anesthetic he was noted to be jaundiced. He had a negative viral screen but was positive for antitrifluoroacetyl IgG antibodies. He developed fulminant hepatic failure with grade 2 hepatic encephalopathy and underwent an auxiliary liver transplantation 24 days after his last exposure to halothane. He died of septicemia 18 days later. Both at autopsy and on a previous hepatobiliary scan he was noted to have had extensive native liver regeneration.

Halothane hepatitis in children is rare, and occurs in 1 : 82 000 to 1 : 200 000 exposures. It has been noted that sevoflurane is not metabolized to trifluoroacetic acid and may prove to be a better alternative for repeated anesthesia in children (25[r]).

Miscellaneous Standard in vitro caffeine-halothane contracture testing was performed on 32 patients with a past history of *malignant hyperthermia* diagnosed on clinical grounds and compared to a matched control group of 120 subjects who were considered clinically to be at low risk for malignant hyperthermia (26[C]). The sensitivity of the test was 97% and the specificity 78%.

Isoflurane

Liver A case of isoflurane-induced *hepatotoxicity* has been reported in an obese 35-year-old diabetic woman (27[c]). She had had four previous halothane anesthetics, the last two of which were associated with jaundice. She made a full recovery and on a subsequent anesthetic received an infusion of propofol. Unfortunately trifluoroacetic acid antibody titers were not performed. The derangement of liver function does not appear to have been severe: peak alanine aminotransferase activity was 1410 iu/l.

Miscellaneous *Shivering* after an anesthetic develops in as many as one-half of patients recovering from isoflurane anesthesia. Most postoperative shivering appears to be thermoregulatory, although volatile anesthetics may themselves facilitate this muscular activity. In 60 adult patients the incidence of postoperative shivering was 40% in a control group, 7% after physostigmine 0.04 mg/kg, zero after meperidine 0.5 mg/kg, and zero after clonidine 1.5 μg/kg (28[C]). The centrally acting adrenoceptor agonist phenylpropylamine methylphenidate, the 5-hydroxytryptamine antagonist ketanserin, magnesium sulfate, doxapram, and hypercapnia also reduce the incidence of postoperative shivering.

Interactions In a randomized, double-blind, controlled trial in 61 patients oral *clonidine* 5 μg/kg was given 90 minutes before surgery to reduce the concentration of isoflurane at which patients wake at the end of surgery by 8% (29[C]). There was a 6–7 minute delay in waking in the clonidine group compared with the control group. Clonidine 2.5 μg/kg had no significant effect.

The effects of *alfentanil* and *esmolol* on isoflurane requirements for anesthesia have been studied in a randomized trial of 100 patients (30[C]). Alfentanil infusion to a targeted effect site concentration of 50 ng/ml, but not esmolol, reduced the minimum alveolar concentration of isoflurane required to suppress movement to surgical pain by 25%. The combination of esmolol and alfentanil caused a 74% reduction in isoflurane requirements. This study is interesting because the β-blocker esmolol had a profound effect on the isoflurane-sparing effects of alfentanil, while having little effect on its own.

Four patients with renal dysfunction in an intensive care unit received isoflurane inhalation for sedation for 8–26 days. The concentrations of isoflurane used were 20–50% of the minimum alveolar concentration. Only small increases in fluoride ion concentration, the highest being 25 μmol/l were recorded, well below the 50 μmol/l threshold associated with adverse effects on renal function (31[C]).

Sevoflurane

Cardiovascular Sevoflurane is usually well tolerated for induction of anesthesia in young children. Profound *bradycardia* was reported in four unpremedicated children aged 6 months to 2 years during anesthesia induction with sevoflurane 8% and nitrous oxide 66% (32[c]). The episodes were not associated with loss of airway or ventilation. In three of the children there was spontaneous recovery of heart rate when the sevoflurane concentration was reduced; the other child received atropine because of evidence of significantly reduced cardiac output. A previous study of sevoflurane induction of anesthesia in children with atropine premedication also had a low incidence of this complication (33[C]) which is probably due to excessive sevoflurane concentrations.

Complete atrioventricular block occurred in a 10-year-old child with a history of hypertension, severe renal dysfunction, incomplete right bundle branch block, and a ventricular septal defect that had been repaired at birth (34[c]). After slow induction with sevoflurane and nitrous oxide 66%, complete atrioventricular block occurred when the inspired sevoflurane concentration was 3% and reverted to sinus rhythm after withdrawal of the sevoflurane. The dysrhythmia recurred at the end of the procedure, possibly caused by lidocaine, which was infiltrated into the abdominal wound, and again at 24 hours in association with congestive cardiac failure following absorption of peritoneal dialysis fluid.

A case of *torsade de pointes* has been attributed to sevoflurane anesthesia (35[c]).

A 65-year-old woman, who had had normal preoperative serum electrolytes and a normal QT interval with sinus rhythm, received hydroxyzine and atropine premedication followed by thiopental and vecuronium for anesthetic induction. Endotracheal intubation was difficult and precipitated atrial fibrillation, which was refractory to disopyramide 100 mg. Anesthesia was then maintained with sevoflurane 2% and nitrous oxide 50%. Ten minutes later ventricular tachycardia ensued, refractory to intravenous lidocaine, disopyramide, and magnesium. DC cardioversion resulted in a change to a supraventricular tachycardia, which then deteriorated to torsade de pointes. External cardiac massage and further DC cardioversion were initially unsuccessful, but the cardiac rhythm reverted to atrial fibrillation 10 minutes after the sevoflurane was switched off. Two weeks later she had her operation under combined epidural and general anesthesia, with no changes in cardiac rhythm.

The role of excessive sympathetic drive as a result of the difficult intubation and the lack of opioid use during induction must be considered in this case, even if sevoflurane played a role in precipitating the dysrhythmia.

Urinary system Sevoflurane is degraded in soda lime absorbers in the anesthetic circuit to a substance called compound A, which is nephrotoxic in rats. However, there has been controversy over whether compound A causes significant renal damage in humans. The potential for renal damage using sevoflurane was investigated in 42 patients without renal disease scheduled for surgery lasting more than 4 hours (36[C]). The patients were given low-flow sevoflurane or isoflurane (fresh gas flow 1 l/min/m^2) or high-flow sevoflurane (6 l/min/m^2). None of these increased blood urea nitrogen concentrations, creatinine concentrations, or creatinine clearance. There were no significant differences in β_2-microglobulin, a marker of tubular function, or urinary glucose concentrations. However, there was an increase in the 24-hour urinary excretion of *N*-acetyl-β-glucosaminidase, a marker of *proximal tubular necrosis*, with both doses of sevoflurane but not with isoflurane. There were no significant differences in the serum and urinary fluoride concentrations between the two sevoflurane groups, despite the higher concentration of compound A (29 vs 3.9 ppm) in the expired gases of those who received low-flow sevoflurane. The maximum 24-hour protein excretion was higher with low-flow sevoflurane compared with the other two groups.

A randomized open-label study in 26 patients with renal dysfunction who received either isoflurane or sevoflurane for operations lasting up to 6 hours showed no significant differences in postoperative creatinine clearances. However, there was a significant *increase in the plasma fluoride ion concentration* with sevoflurane (37[C]). In 10 adults who were given repeat high-flow sevoflurane anesthesia there was no evidence of renal or hepatic injury and no increases in serum or urine fluoride concentrations that would indicate an increase in sevoflurane metabolism with repeated use (38[C]).

These studies have confirmed earlier findings that although there is biochemical evidence of renal damage after sevoflurane anesthesia, there are no clinically significant effects.

GASES

Nitrous oxide *(SED-13, 274; SEDA-20, 111; SEDA-21, 121; SEDA-22, 128)*

The continued use of nitrous oxide in anesthetic practice has been questioned in an editorial on the basis of its serious adverse effects and the availability of potentially safer short-acting potent analgesic drugs, such as xenon and remifentanil (39[R]).

INTRAVENOUS AGENTS

In an in vitro study of the inhibitory effects of thiopental, midazolam, and ketamine on human neutrophil function thiopental and midazolam *inhibited chemotaxis, phagocytosis, and reactive oxygen species production* at clinically relevant concentrations (40). Ketamine only impaired chemotaxis. These results may be relevant in guiding anesthetic drug therapy in septic patients.

BARBITURATE ANESTHETICS

(SED-13, 275; SEDA-20, 112; SEDA-21, 122; SEDA-22, 129)

Methohexital

The selective inhibitor of neuronal nitric oxide synthase, 7-nitroindazole prolonged the duration of methohexital-induced narcosis in rats (41). This finding is consistent with previous work showing potentiation of anesthetic agents by non-specific nitric oxide synthase inhibitors.

Thiamylyl

Severe *hypokalemia* occurred in a 14-year-old boy undergoing emergency aortic arch replacement under deep hypothermic cardiopulmonary bypass (42[c]). He was treated with thiamylal by infusion, total dose 30 mg/kg, for persistent convulsive waves on his electroencephalogram. This caused his serum potassium concentration to drop to 1.6 mmol/l. The hypokalemia was resistant to potassium chloride infusion 80 mmol/h, but responded to replacing the thiamylal infusion with midazolam. It was noted that there have also been reports of severe hypokalemia in brain-injured patients undergoing thiopental coma therapy.

MISCELLANEOUS NON-BARBITURATE ANESTHETICS

A prospective, double-blind, controlled trial in 75 patients who received low-dose opioid based anesthesia for coronary bypass grafting compared propofol, midazolam, and propofol and midazolam combined for postoperative sedation (43[C]). Mean induction doses of the single agents were 2.5 times higher than when both were used together. The single-agent groups were associated with significant *reductions in blood pressure, left atrial filling pressure, and heart rate* after induction. These hemodynamic changes returned to normal after 15 minutes with midazolam and after 30 minutes with propofol, except for the bradycardia, which remained for the duration of the sedation. The combination of propofol and midazolam had no significant hemodynamic effects, but was also associated with bradycardia lasting the duration of the sedation. There was a greater than 68% reduction in maintenance doses with the combination. The propofol and propofol-midazolam groups were associated with comparable times to awakening and extubation, while with midazolam alone recovery was slower. The study clearly showed a reduction in adverse effects from exploiting the sedative synergism between propofol and midazolam.

Etomidate *(SED-13, 276; SEDA-20, 113; SEDA-21, 124)*

A novel oral transmucosal formulation of etomidate, which is absorbed over 15 minutes was studied in 10 healthy adults at four doses: 12.5, 25, 50, and 100 mg (44[C]). Dose-related *drowsiness and light sleep* occurred 10–20 minutes after administration. Peak serum concentrations and clinical effects were noted at about 20 minutes, with no clinical effect noticeable by 60 minutes. There was no vomiting and only four patients had transient nausea. Two patients had brief episodes of involuntary tremor with the 100 mg dose. Of note was the increasingly unpleasant taste with increasing dose and the apparent reduction in absorption with higher doses.

Ketamine *(SED-13, 277; SEDA-20, 3; SEDA-21, 124)*

The pharmacology and adverse effects of ketamine have been reviewed (45[R]).

The effects of intramuscular premedication with either clonidine 2 μg/kg or midazolam 70 μg/kg on perioperative responses to ketamine anesthesia have been assessed in a placebo-controlled study in 30 patients (46[C]). Clonidine significantly reduced intraoperative oxygen consumption, mean arterial pressure, and heart rate compared with midazolam and placebo. Thus, clonidine was as effective as midazolam, the standard drug used for this purpose, in reducing the undesirable sympathetic stimulation of ketamine.

Psychiatric Ketamine is well known for producing *psychotogenic and dissociative effects* that resemble aspects of schizophrenia and dissociative states. A double-blind placebo controlled study of 23 volunteers investigated the role of lorazepam in reducing these effects after subanesthetic doses of ketamine (47[C]). Volunteers received lorazepam 2 mg or placebo 2 hours before receiving either a bolus dose of ketamine 0.26 mg/kg followed by an infusion of 0.65 mg/kg/h or a placebo infusion. The ability of lorazepam to block the undesirable effects of ketamine was limited to just some effects. It reduced the ketamine-associated emotional distress and perceptual alterations, but exacerbated the sedative, attention-impairing, and amnesic effects of ketamine. However, it failed to reduce many of the cognitive and behavioral effects of ketamine. There were no pharmacokinetic interactions between subanesthetic doses of ketamine and lorazepam.

A placebo-controlled study in 10 healthy young men showed a linear relation between ketamine plasma concentrations of 50–200 ng/ml and the severity of psychedelic effects (48[C]). The psychedelic effects were also similar to those observed in a previous study of dimethyltryptamine, an illicit LSD-25 type of drug, and were a function of plasma concentration rather than simply an emergence phenomenon. Clinically useful analgesia was obtained with plasma concentrations of 100–200 ng/ml. At plasma concentrations of 200 ng/ml all subjects had lateral nystagmus. When ketamine is given in large doses patients rapidly become unresponsive, and so the effects described in this study are usually only observed during the recovery phase. A similar placebo-controlled study of low-dose ketamine infusion in 10 volunteers also showed formal thought disorder and impairments in working and semantic memory (49[C]). The degree of thought disorder correlated with the impairment in working memory.

The use and adverse effects of S-ketamine in the intensive care unit have been reviewed (50[r]).

Midazolam and injectable benzodiazepines

(SED-13, 277; SEDA-20, 112; SEDA-21, 122; SEDA-22, 129)

The pharmacology and adverse effects of conscious sedation, with special reference to the use of benzodiazepines for conscious sedation, have been reviewed (51[R]). The pharmacology and adverse effects of midazolam in infants and children have been reviewed (52[R]).

The optimal dose of intramuscular midazolam for preoperative sedation has been studied in a double-blind prospective study of 600 patients who were age stratified (53[R]). The patients received intramuscular atropine 0.6 mg and one of five doses of midazolam 15 minutes before induction of anesthesia. For the age groups 20–39, 40–59, and 60–79 years, the optimal sedative and amnesic effects of midazolam were 0.10, 0.08, and 0.04 mg/kg respectively. The frequency with which the undesirable adverse effects of reduced blood pressure, oxygen desaturation, oversedation, loss of eyelash reflex, and tongue root depression occurred increased with age, and optimal doses for a low incidence of adverse effects were 0.08, 0.06, and 0.04 mg/kg in the same age groups respectively.

A retrospective study of diazepam infusion 0.01–0.03 mg/kg/min for the treatment of status epilepticus in 57 children resulted in control of seizures in 49 of them (54[c]). Most of the patients were seriously ill with infections; one had severe hypotension, six required ventilatory support, and seven died. Rescue thiopental infusion, when diazepam failed in nine patients, lead to a nearly universal need for mechanical ventilation and vasopressor support for hypotension.

Respiratory Intranasal midazolam is a successful route of administration for sedating children. However, it can cause *nasal burning, irritation*, and *lacrimation* (55[c]). In a study of an alternative route of administration, namely inhalation via a nebulizer, *bronchospasm* developed in two of the 10 patients studied. The formulation of midazolam has a pH of 3.0, and this was thought to be the reason it caused bronchospasm.

Nervous system A case of *opisthotonos* after flumazenil has been reported (56[c]).

A healthy 17-year-old man received an interscalene brachial plexus block using mepivacaine 600 mg and bupivacaine 150 mg. He became disorientated and showed signs of local anesthetic toxicity, for which he was given midazolam 5 mg. Flumazenil 0.5 mg was given 23 minutes after the end of the procedure, causing opisthotonos.

Similar reports have appeared in the past in patients with seizure disorders. It is recommended that flumazenil not be used in patients predisposed to seizures.

Use in pregnancy A mother with eclampsia was unsuccessfully treated with diazepam, total dose 120 mg, and phenytoin 750 mg; she received thiopental and had an emergency cesarean section at 33 weeks gestation (57[c]). The infant was *unresponsive and floppy*, requiring intubation and ventilation. At 10 hours after delivery a flumazenil infusion was begun; the baby responded with facial and limb movements within 30 seconds, resumed spontaneous ventilation, and was extubated 4 hours later. She was maintained on a slowly reducing flumazenil infusion over the next 4 days while the benzodiazepines were metabolized.

Interactions The pharmacokinetics and pharmacodynamics of midazolam are markedly affected by drugs that influence CYP3A, as shown by a study of the effects of *itraconazole*, an inhibitor of CYP3A, and *rifampicin*, an inducer of CYP3A, on oral midazolam pharmacokinetics and pharmacodynamics in nine healthy volunteers (58[C]). The half-life was prolonged from 2.7 to 7.6 hours by itraconazole and reduced to 1.0 hour by rifampicin. These effects were still present, although less marked, at 4 days after withdrawal of itraconazole and rifampicin. Similarly, after acute administration the period of drowsiness was increased from 76 to 201 minutes with itraconazole and fell to 35 minutes with rifampicin; the effects were again less marked 4 days after withdrawal.

Propofol *(SED-13, 278; SEDA-20, 114; SEDA-21, 125; SEDA-19, 130)*

Cardiovascular In a placebo-controlled study of anesthesia induction with a combination of propofol and fentanyl in 90 patients aged over 60 years, prophylactic intravenous ephedrine 0.1 or 0.2 mg/kg given 1 minute before anesthesia induction significantly attenuated the drop in blood pressure and heart rate usually observed (59[C]). Prophylactic use of ephedrine may be useful in preventing the occasional instances of cardiovascular collapse recorded after anesthesia induction using these agents in elderly people.

Nervous system Recurrent *myoclonus* due to propofol has been reported (60[c]).

An otherwise healthy 63-year-old man was anesthetized with propofol 2 mg/kg and fentanyl 1 μg/kg followed by an infusion of propofol 6 mg/kg/h. Three minutes after induction he developed myoclonus in his legs. This continued for 10 minutes and the anesthetic was abandoned. When he awoke 10 minutes later the myoclonus stopped. A repeat anesthetic with propofol soon after caused the same response. When the procedure was performed 12 days later under regional block with propofol infusion for sedation the myoclonus recurred, and lasted for 2 hours. The patient was alert after each anesthetic and did not appear to be post-ictal. An MRI scan of the spinal cord was normal.

Myoclonus after propofol has been reported before and does not appear to be associated with an adverse outcome.

Endocrine, metabolic There have been several reports of lactic acidosis with and without rhabdomyolysis.

Two fatal cases of lactic acidosis with rhabdomyolysis after propofol infusion have been reported (61[c]). Both patients were male, aged 7 and 17 years, and they presented with refractory status epilepticus. Both were treated with high-dose propofol infusions to achieve burst suppression on the electroencephalogram. During the second day of propofol infusion there was progressive severe lactic acidosis, hypoxia, pyrexia, and rhabdomyolysis, followed by hypotension, bradydysrhythmias, and renal dysfunction, leading to death. The total doses of propofol were 1275 mg/kg over 2.7 days and 482 mg/kg over 2 days.

Lactic acidosis and rhabdomyolysis have been reported in a child receiving propofol infusion for sedation in an intensive care unit (62[c]).

A previously healthy 10-month-old boy with an esophageal foreign body had endotracheal intubation to protect his airway. Midazolam and morphine did not produce satisfactory sedation and he was given propofol by infusion, increased from 3.5 to 7 mg/kg/h over 2 hours, with a total dose of about 500 mg/kg over the next 2 days. Other drugs given included cefotaxime, flucloxacillin, and ranitidine. He developed green urine, triglyceridemia of 907 mg/dl (10 mmol/l), and lactic acidosis, with a peak lactate concentration of 18 mmol/l. He also developed hypotension, with first-degree atrioventricular block and right bundle branch block, unresponsive to atropine, external cardiac pacing, or isoprenaline. Continuous veno-venous hemofiltration was instituted. He slowly improved over the next 2 days, but developed a raised CK (over 30 000 units) and myoglobinuria. A liver biopsy showed 10% necrosis of zone 3, with fatty infiltration characteristic of a toxic effect. A muscle biopsy showed large areas of muscle necrosis. Extensive investigations showed no underlying infectious or metabolic causes. He slowly recovered over 10 days and appeared to have completely recovered at 3 months.

Lactic acidosis without rhabdomyolysis has been reported in another case (63[c]).

A 61-year-old woman undergoing mitral valve surgery received fentanyl, midazolam, nitrous oxide, and propofol infusion 3 mg/kg/h during a 5 h anesthetic. She developed lactic acidosis soon after the completion of surgery and required reintubation and ventilation. The peak lactate concentration, which occurred 1 day later, was 14.3 mmol/l. There was also mild disturbance of liver function. She eventually recovered.

These cases are important because unlike previous reports of metabolic acidosis after propofol infusion, the patients had no documented infections and in at least one case received extensive investigation for other causes of the acidosis. The role of propofol in causing the metabolic problems appears to have been more likely in these than in previous reports. In the first three cases the doses of propofol used, both per hour and total, were extremely high compared with normal therapeutic practice. The subject has also been reviewed, and it was pointed out that, although suggestive, the association of fatal metabolic acidosis with propofol infusion in sick patients is as yet unproven and to date hinges on 11 case reports of patients who had multiple problems (64[r]).

An attack of *porphyria* has been reported in association with propofol (65[C]).

A 23-year-old man with a past history of Fallot's tetralogy, with repair at age 2, presented for catheter ablation of an aberrant conduction pathway causing right ventricular tachycardia, a 16-hour procedure. He was sedated with propofol at an average rate of 100 μg/kg/min, and required intubation for respiratory insufficiency half way through the procedure. He also received caffeine and isoprenaline during the procedure to induce ventricular tachycardia. After the procedure he could not be roused or extubated for a further 10 hours, and remained drowsy for a further day. He had weakness of an arm and a leg and had lancinating abdominal and shoulder pains. Urinary porphyrins, aminolevulinic acid, porphobilinogen, and coproporphyrin III were markedly raised. He made a good recovery after dextrose administration.

Propofol is regarded as being safe in patients with porphyrias. This is the first reported case in which propofol had a possible role in causing raised porphyrin concentrations perioperatively. Severe illness can also precipitate porphyria, so the association with propofol may have been incidental.

Hematological In 10 patients propofol, but not intralipos, its solvent, *inhibited platelet aggregation* both in vivo and in vitro (66[C]). This defect was not associated with a change in bleeding time, and it was assumed that the effect is not clinically significant. The cause was probably suppression of calcium influx and discharge from platelets.

Miscellaneous Propofol can cause severe *pain on injection*, especially when small distal veins are used (67[R]). A double-blind study of 25 patients showed that warming the propofol to 37°C did not reduce the incidence of injection pain when a dorsal hand vein was used (68[C]). A controlled study in 100 women showed that pretreatment with intravenous ketamine 10 mg reduced the incidence of injection pain from 84 to 26% of patients (69[C]).

Use in pregnancy In an in vitro experiment using uterine muscle strips from 10 consenting parturients undergoing cesarean section, therapeutic concentrations of propofol had no effect on isometric tension developed during contraction of the muscle (70). However, higher than therapeutic concentrations did reduce the peak muscle tension that developed. The result confirms that propofol is free of this adverse effect, which is a known cause of post-partum bleeding after the use of volatile anesthetic drugs.

REFERENCES

1. Song D, Joshi GP, White PF. Fast-track eligibility after ambulatory anesthesia: a comparison of desflurane, sevoflurane, and propofol. Anesth Analg 1998;86:267–73.
2. Ebert TJ, Robinson BJ, Uhrich TD, Mackenthun A, Pichotta P. Recovery from sevoflurane anesthesia: a comparison to isoflurane and propofol anesthesia. Anesthesiology 1998;89:1524–31.
3. Crawford MW, Lerman J, Sloan MH, Sikich N, Halpern L, Bissonnette B. Recovery characteristics of propofol anaesthesia, with and without nitrous oxide: a comparison with halothane/nitrous oxide anaesthesia in children. Paediatr Anaesth 1998; 8:49–54.
4. Keller C, Sparr HJ, Brimacombe JR. Positive pressure ventilation with the laryngeal mask airway in non-paralysed patients: comparison of sevoflurane and propofol maintenance techniques. Br J Anaesth 1998;80:332–6.
5. Ghoneim MM, Block RI, Dhanaraj VJ. Interaction of a subanaesthetic concentration of isoflurane with midazolam: effects on responsiveness, learning and memory. Br J Anaesth 1998;80:581–7.
6. Skolnick ET, Vomvolakis MA, Buck KA, Mannino SF, Sun LS. Exposure to environmental tobacco smoke and the risk of adverse respiratory events in children receiving general anesthesia. Anesthesiology 1998;88:1144–53.

7. D'Alessio JG, Ramanathan J. Effects of maternal anesthesia in the neonate. Semin Perinatol 1998;22:350–62.
8. Ti LK, Pua HL, Lee TL. Single vital capacity inhalational anesthetic induction in adults-isoflurane vs sevoflurane. Can J Anaesth 1998;45:949–53.
9. McKinney MS, Fee JPH. Cardiovascular effects of 50% nitrous oxide in older adult patients anaesthetized with isoflurane or halothane. Br J Anaesth 1998;80:169–73.
10. Michaloudis D, Fraidakis O, Petrou A, Gigourtsi C, Parthenakis F. Anaesthesia and the QT interval. Anaesthesia 1998;53:435–9.
11. Brown K, Aun C. Stocks J, Jackson E, Mackersie A, Hatch D. A comparison of the respiratory effects of sevoflurane and halothane in infants and young children. Anesthesiology 1998;89:86–92.
12. Van den Berg AA, Honjol NM, Mphanza T, Rozario CJ, Joseph D. Vomiting, retching, headache and restlessness after halothane, isoflurance and enflurane-based anaesthesia: an analysis of pooled data following nose, throat and eye surgery. Acta Anaesthesiol Scand 1998;42:658–63.
13. Naidu-Sjosvard K, Sjoberg F, Gupta A. Anaesthesia for videoarthroscopy of the knee. A comparison between desflurane and sevoflurane. Acta Anaesthesiol Scand 1998;74:464–71.
14. Medina KA, Mayhew JF. Generalised muscle rigidity and hypercarbia with halothane and isoflurane. Anesth Analg 1998;86:297–8.
15. Lowry DW, Mirakhur RK, Carrol MT. Time course of action of rocuronium during sevoflurane, isoflurane or i.v. anaesthesia. Br J Anaesth 1998; 80:544.
16. Wulf H, Ledowski T, Linstedt U, Proppe D, Sitzlack D. Neuromuscular blocking effects of rocuronium during desflurane, isoflurane, and sevoflurane anaesthesia. Can J Anaesth 1998;45: 526–32.
17. Wulf H, Kahl M, Ledowski T. Augmentation of the neuromuscular blocking effects of cisatracurium during, desflurane, sevoflurane, isoflurane or total i.v. anaesthesia. Br J Anaesth 1998;80: 308–12.
18. Tran TV, Fiset P, Varin F. Pharmacokinetics and pharmacodynamics of cisatracurium after a short infusion in patients under propofol anesthesia. Anesth Analg 1998;87:1158–63.
19. Defalque RJ, Wright AJ. An anesthetic curiosity in New York (1875–1900): a noted surgeon returns to 'open drop' chloroform. Anesthesiology 1998;88:549–51.
20. Lo SK, Wendon J, Miele-Vergani G, Williams R. Halothane-induced acute liver failure: continuing occurrence and use of liver transplantation. Eur J Gastroenterol Hepatol 1998;10:635–9.
21. Reinoso-Barbero F, Gutierrez-Marquez M, Diez-Labajo A. Prevention of halothane-induced bradycardia: is intranasal premedication indicated? Paediatr Anaesth 1998;8:195–9.
22. Annila P, Rorarius M, Reinikainen P, Oikkonen M, Baer G. Effect of pre-treatment with intravenous atropine or glycopyrrolate on cardiac arrhythmias during halothane anaesthesia for adenoidectomy in children. Br J Anaesth 1998;80: 756–60.
23. Neuberger J. Halothane hepatitis. Eur J Gastroenterol Hepatol 1998;10:631–3.
24. Munro HM, Snider SJ, Magee JC. Halothane-associated hepatitis in a 6-year-old boy: evidence for native liver regeneration following failed treatment with auxiliary liver transplantation. Anesthesiology 1998;89:524–7.
25. Murat I. There is no longer a place for halothane in paediatric anaesthesia. Paediatr Anaesth 1998;8: 184.
26. Allen GC, Larech MG, Kunselman AR. The sensitivity and specificity of the caffeine-halothane contracture test. Anesthesiology 1998;88:579–88.
27. Hasan F. Isoflurane hepatotoxicity in a patient with a previous history of halothane-induced hepatitis. Hepato-Gastroenterology. 1998;45:518–22.
28. Horne EP, Standl T, Sessler DI, Von Knobelsdorff G, Buchs C, Schulte J. Physostigmine prevents postanesthetic shivering as does meperidine or clonidine. Anesthesiology 1998;88:108–13.
29. Goyagi T, Tanaka M, Nishikawa T. Oral clonidine premedication reduces the awakening concentration of isoflurane. Anesth Analg 1998;86:410–13.
30. Johansen JW, Schneider G, Windsor AM, Sebel PS. Esmolol potentiates reduction of minimum alveolar isoflurane concentration by alfentanil. Anesth Analg 1998;87:671–6.
31. Fujino Y, Nishimura M, Nishimura S, Taenaka N, Yoshiya I. Prolonged administration of isoflurane to patients with severe renal dysfunction. Anesth Analg 1998;86:440–1.
32. Townsend P, Stokes MA. Bradycardia during rapid inhalation induction with sevoflurane in children. Br J Anaesth 1998;80:410.
33. Sigston PE, Jenkins AMC, Jackson EA, Sury MRJ, Mackersia AM, Hatch DJ. Rapid inhalation induction in children: 8% sevoflurane compared with 5% halothane. Br J Anaesth 1997;78: 62–5.
34. Maruyama K, Agata H, Ono K, Hiroki K, Fujuhara T. Slow induction with sevoflurane was associated with complete atrioventricular block in a child with hypertension, renal dysfunction and impaired cardiac conduction. Paediatr Anaesth 1998; 8:73–8.
35. Abe K, Takada K, Yoshiya I. Intraoperative torsade de pointes ventricular tachycardia and ventricular fibrillation during sevoflurane anesthesia. Anesth Analg 1998;86:701–2.
36. Higuchi H, Sumita S, Wada H, Ura T, Ikemoto T, Nakai T, Kanno M, Satoh T. Effects of sevoflurane and isoflurane on renal function and on possible markers of nephrotoxicity. Anesthesiology 1998; 89:307–22.
37. McGrath BJ, Hodgins LR, DeBree A, Frink EJ Jr, Nossaman BD, Bikhazi GB. A multicenter study evaluating the effects of sevoflurane on renal function in patients with renal insufficiency. J Cardiovasc Pharmacol Ther 1998;3:229–34.
38. Nishiyama T, Hanaoka K. Inorganic fluoride kinetics and renal and hepatic function after re-

peated sevoflurane anesthesia. Anesth Analg 1998; 87:468–73.

39. Shaw ADS, Morgan M. Nitrous oxide: time to stop laughing? Anaesthesia 1998;53;213–15.
40. Nishina K, Akamatsu H, Mikawa K, Shiga M, Maekawa N, Obara H, Niwa Y. The inhibitory effects of thiopental, midazolam, and ketamine on neutrophil functions. Anesth Analg 1998;86: 159–65.
41. Motzko D, Glade U, Tober C, Flohr H. 7-Nitro indazole enhances methohexital anesthesia. Brain Res 1998;788:353–5.
42. Irita K, Kawasaki T, Uenotsuchi T, Sakaguchi Y, Takahashi S. Does barbiturate therapy cause severe hypokalemia? Anesth Analg 1997;86:214.
43. Carrasco G, Cabre L, Sobrepere G, Costa J, Molina R, Cruspinera A, Lacasa C. Synergistic sedation with propofol and midazolam in intensive care patients after coronary artery bypass grafting. Crit Care Med 1998;26:844–51.
44. Streisand JB, Jaarsma RL, Gay MA, Badger MJ, Maland L, Nordbrock E, Stanley TH. Oral transmucosal etomidate in volunteers. Anesthesiology 1998;88:89–95.
45. Kohrs R, Durieux ME. Ketamine: teaching an old drug new tricks. Anesth Analg 1998;87:1186–93.
46. Taittonen MT, Kirvela OA, Aantaa R, Kanto JH. The effect of clonidine or midazolam premedcation on perioperative responses during ketamine anesthesia. Anesth Analg 1998;87:161–7.
47. Krystal JH, Karper LP, Bennett A, D'Souza C, Abi-Dargham A, Morrissey K, Abi-Saab D, Bremmer JD, Bowers MB, Suckow RF, Stetson P, Heninger GR, Charney DS. Interactive effects of subanesthetic ketamine and subhypnotic lorazepam in humans. Psychopharmacology 1998;135:213–29.
48. Bowdle TA, Radant AD, Cowley DS, Kharasch ED, Strassman R, Roy-Byrne PP. Psychedelic effects of ketamine in healthy volunteers: relationship to steady-state plasma concentrations. Anesthesiology 1998;88:82–8.
49. Adler CM, Goldberg TE, Malhotra AK, Pickar D, Breier A. Effects of ketamine on thought disorder, working memory, and semantic memory in healthy volunteers. Biol Psychiatry 1998;43: 811–16.
50. Adams HA. The use of (S)-ketamine in intensive care medicine. Acta Anaesthesiol Scand 1998; 42:212S–213S.
51. Minocha A, Srinivasan R. Conscious sedation: pearls and perils. Dig Dis Sci 1998;43:1835–44.
52. Blumer JL. Clinical pharmacology of midazolam in infants and children. Clin Pharmacokinet 1998;35:37–47.
53. Nishiyhama T, Matsukawa T, Hanaoka K. The effects of age and gender on the optimal premedication dose of intramuscular midazolam. Anesth Analg 1998;86:1103–8.
54. Singhi S, Banerjee S, Singhi P. Refractory status epilepticus in children: role of continuous diazepam infusion. J Child Neurol 1998;13:23–6.
55. McCormick ASM, Thomas VL, Bromley LM. Bronchospasm during inhalation of nebulized midazolam. Br J Anaesth 1998;80:564–5.
56. Watanabe S, Satumae T, Takeshima R, Taguchi N. Opisthotonos after flumazenil administered to antagonize midazolam previously administered to treat developing local anesthetic toxicity. Anesth Analg 1998;86:677–8.
57. Dixon JC, Speidel BD, Dixon JJ. Neonatal flumazenil therapy reverses maternal diazepam. Acta Paediatr Int J Paediatr 1998;87:225–6.
58. Backman JT, Kivisto KT, Olkkola KT, Neuvonen PJ. The area under the plasma concentration-time curve for oral midazolam is 400 fold larger during treatment with itraconazole than with rifampicin. Eur J Clin Pharmacol 1998; 54:53–8.
59. Michelsen I, Helbo-Hansen HS, Kohler F, Lorenzen AG, Rydlund E, Bentzon MW. Prophylactic ephedrine attenuates the hemodynamic response to propofol in elderly female patients. Anesth Analg 1998;86:477–81.
60. Kiyama S, Yoshikawa T. Persistent intraoperative myoclonus during propofol-fentanyl anaesthesia. Can J Anaesth 1998;45:283–4.
61. Hanna JP, Ramundo ML. Rhabdomyoloysis and hypoxia associated with prolonged propofol infusion in children. Neurology 1998;50:301–3.
62. Cray SH, Robinson BH, Cox PN. Lactic acidemia and bradyarrhythmia in a child sedated with propofol. Crit Care Med 1998;26:2087–92.
63. Watanabe Y. Lactic acidosis associated with propofol in an adult patient after cardiovascular surgery. J Cardiothorac Vasc Anesth 1998;12: 611–12.
64. Susla GM. Propofol toxicity in critically ill pediatric patients: show us the proof. Crit Care Med 1998;26:1959–60.
65. Asirvatham SJ, Johnson TW, Oberoi MP, Jackman WM. Prolonged loss of consciousness and elevated porphyrins following propofol administrations. Anesthesiology 1998.89:1029–31.
66. Aoki H, Mizobe T, Nozuchi S, Hiramatsu N. In vivo and in vitro studies of the inhibitory effect of propofol on platelet aggregation. Anesthesiology 1998;88:362–70.
67. Tan CH, Onsiong MK. Pain on injection of propofol. Anaesthesia 1998;53:468–76.
68. Ozturk E, Izdes S, Babacan A, Kaya K. Temperature of propofol does not reduce the incidence of injection pain. Anesthesiology 1998;89:1041.
69. Tan CH, Onsiong MK, Kua SW. The effect of ketamine pretreatment on propofol injection pain in 100 women. Anaesthesia 1998;53:296–307.
70. Shin YK, Kim YD, Collea JV. The effect of propofol on isolated human pregnant uterine muscle. Anesthesiology 1998;89:105–9.

Stephan A. Schug and Hester Cardwell

11 Local anesthetics

EFFECTS RELATED TO DIFFERENT MODES OF USE

Brachial plexus anesthesia

(SED-13, 287; SEDA-20, 123; SEDA-21, 130; SEDA-22, 134)

Neurological injury after peripheral blockade has an incidence of less than 1%. However, it has been suggested that for axillary nerve blocks, neurological damage is more likely if paresthesia is the endpoint for location of the nerve sheath, in contrast to the transarterial method. This is probably due to the increased likelihood of direct damage from a needle, intraneural injection of local anesthetic, or toxicity of the local anesthetic to the nerve (1[R]). However, published results on this issue remain contradictory (2).

A 67-year-old man had an axillary plexus block for a right palmar fasciectomy with mepivacaine 850 mg of and adrenaline 225 μg. Twenty minutes later he became *agitated* and *confused* and an electrocardiogram showed fast *atrial fibrillation.* Rapid systemic absorption of the combination of high-dose mepivacaine and adrenaline in a patient who was also taking amiodarone, sotalol, captopril, and amiloride for pre-existing cardiac disease, was felt to be responsible (3[c]).

A 59-year-old patient of grade ASA I had *psychiatric* effects associated with local anesthetic toxicity after receiving bupivacaine 50 mg and mepivacaine 75 mg for an axillary plexus block. She complained of dizziness and a 'near death experience' (4[cr]).

Side Effects of Drugs, Annual 23
J.K. Aronson, ed.

Caudal, epidural, and spinal anesthesia *(SED-13, 290; SEDA-20, 124; SEDA-21, 131; SEDA-22, 135)*

Caudal anesthesia

A study of seven children (age 36–52 weeks) given caudal anesthesia with bupivacaine 3.1 mg/kg plus adrenaline 5 μg/ml, showed significant electroencephalographic signs of central nervous system toxicity in six infants, and two children had clinical signs of possible epileptic activity. The authors stopped the study early because of the high incidence of adverse effects. They felt that these were due to the fact that no sedative or anesthetic drugs that could have masked or alleviated local anesthetic toxicity were given, and also that infants have low concentrations of α_1 acid glycoprotein, leading to increased unbound plasma concentrations (5[Cr]). However, it should be noted that 2 mg/kg is the usual upper dose limit recommended for bupivacaine. It is hardly surprising that such a high proportion of those studied showed evidence of systemic toxicity after the administration of a much higher dose of bupivacaine to such small children by a route that is known to result in rapid absorption of local anesthetic into the systemic circulation.

Epidural anesthesia

In 15 patients receiving lidocaine 300 mg plus adrenaline by cervical epidural injection, the upper cervical nerve roots C3, 4, and 5 were anesthetized. None of the patients had pre-existing pulmonary disease. Only one had symptoms of *impaired pulmonary function* at 20 minutes after epidural, and complained of dyspnea, with a reduction in maximum inspiratory pressure, FEV_1, FVC, and SpO_2. Four patients had a *bradycardia* requiring atropine, eight complained of *nausea*, and one developed *hypotension* requiring ephedrine. At 20 minutes after the epidural, all the patients had a maximum *reduction in* FEV_1 *and FVC*, ranging from 12 to 16% of preanesthetic measurements. The authors felt that as the maximum inspiratory pressure was virtually unchanged, this suggested that the motor function of the phrenic nerve was mostly intact, despite analgesia of the C3, 4, and 5 dermatomes (6[Cr]).

In a comparison of the clinical efficacy of epidural S-(–)-bupivacaine with standard racemic RS-bupivacaine in 88 patients S-(–)-bupivacaine was clinically indistinguishable from RS-bupivacaine in the three groups studied (0.75 or 0.5% S-(–)-bupivacaine and 0.5% RS-bupivacaine). *Hypotension* was distributed evenly across the groups and five patients complained of minor neurological abnormalities (*hypesthesia* and *paresthesia*), which resolved quickly after the operation (7[Cr]).

Long-term epidural catheters can be highly effective in the management of chronic pain of malignant and non-malignant origin, but they can also cause complications. *Infection* and *extravasation* of fluid to the paraspinal tissue resulting in *inadequate analgesia* have been described in a patient with non-Hodgkin's lymphoma (8[cr]).

Another patient with non-Hodgkin's lymphoma had a tunnelled thoracic epidural for analgesia and presented with *spinal cord compression.* Laminectomy showed a mass consisting of white chalk-like drug-related precipitate around the catheter tip. As the solvent for bupivacaine contains sodium hydroxide and sodium chloride, the authors assumed that the mass was a precipitate of sodium hydroxide (9[cr]).

Horner's syndrome (miosis, ptosis, anhidrosis, and vasodilatation, with increased temperature of the affected side) can result from epidural anesthesia. A case report of Horner's syndrome due to a thoracic epidural catheter has highlighted the fact that small doses of local anesthetic can block the sympathetic fibers to the face, particularly when the catheter tip is close to T_2 (10[c]). The same symptoms have been reported after obstetric epidural anesthesia (11[c]).

Drug combinations are often used in epidural anesthesia to enhance analgesic effect and minimize adverse effects. Continuous epidural analgesia (0.125% bupivacaine 12.5 mg/hour and morphine 0.25 mg/hour) has been compared with patient-controlled analgesia (morphine) in 60 patients after major abdominal surgery. Analgesia was superior in the epidural group, satisfaction and sedation scores were similar in both groups, whilst episodes of moderate nocturnal postoperative *hypoxemia* (SaO_2 85–90%) were more frequent in the epidural group (12[Cr]).

Patient-controlled epidural analgesia (0.05% bupivacaine and fentanyl 4 μg/ml) has been studied prospectively in 1030 patients requiring postoperative analgesia (13[CR]). Pruritus was the most common adverse effect, with an incidence of 17%, with risk factors of both age under 58 years and increased consumption of analgesia, over 9 ml/hour. The incidence of nausea was 15% and of sedation 13%; female sex was a slight risk factor for both. Hypotension had an incidence of 6.8% and motor block of 2%; lumbar placement of the epidural catheter was the strongest risk factor. Respiratory depression occurred in 0.3%.

Two studies have advocated the addition of opioids to local anesthetic to improve the efficacy of epidural analgesia for cesarean section (14[Cr], 15[Cr]). A test dose of lidocaine 60 mg was given to 24 patients undergoing elective cesarean section, followed by either bupivacaine 45 mg or bupivacaine 45 mg plus fentanyl 50 μg (14[Cr]). Sensory blockade to T_6 was achieved in both groups, but pain scores were significantly lower in the fentanyl group. Rescue fentanyl on uterine exteriorization was required in 40% of the control group, but in none in the fentanyl group. There were no significant differences in adverse effects, specifically pruritus, hypotension, nausea and vomiting, maternal respiratory depression, and Apgar scores.

The effects of single-dose epidural analgesia with lidocaine and morphine have been studied in 60 women undergoing elective cesarean section (15[Cr]). The patients received morphine sulfate 4 mg and 2% lidocaine 18–20 ml. Four patients proceeded to general anesthesia owing to failure of the epidural block to reach T_6, 48% of patients complained of discomfort during surgery and 23% needed supplementary analgesia. Perioperative adverse effects were hypotension 29%, bradycardia 3.6%, and shivering 5.4%. Postoperative adverse effects were pruritus 45% and nausea and vomiting 35%. Apgar scores at 1 and 5 minutes were 8 or over. At 2 and 24 hours, two babies had transient tachypnea and one had mild respiratory distress. Maternal and neonatal venous concentrations of morphine, measured at delivery, were low. The authors recommended this technique for elective cesarean section in uncomplicated obstetric patients. This study had no control group and reported a high incidence of unwanted effects and a high perioperative failure rate. Mean analgesic duration of morphine was reported as 24 hours. However, 75% of patients required additional analgesia after 12 hours. There was no record of the incidence of postoperative maternal respiratory depression.

Spinal anesthesia

Cardiovascular *Cardiovascular* complications are well recognized with spinal anesthesia. A 68-year-old was given 0.5% bupivacaine 4 ml for spinal anesthesia, and 5 minutes later complained of nausea and developed hypotension, loss of consciousness, and a tonic-clonic seizure. He had first-degree heart block 4 minutes after subarachnoid injection, followed 1 minute later by third-degree heart block, and then asystole. He was successfully resuscitated. Proposed theories included a reflex bradycardia resulting from reduced venous return and or unopposed vagal tone due to thoracic sympathectomy induced by spinal anesthesia (16[cr]).

Slow injection of hyperbaric bupivacaine 8 mg has been compared with hyperbaric bupivacaine 15 mg used to achieve bilateral block in 30 patients of ASA grades I–II (17[Cr]). There was significantly greater cardiovascular stability in the patients who had a unilateral spinal block.

Respiratory Two former preterm infants (post-conceptual age 38 weeks) both received spinal anesthetics for inguinal herniorrhaphy (block level T_4–T_6) (18[Cr]). No other medications were given. Both infants had frequent episodes of perioperative apnea and associated bradycardia. One had a 20-second bout of apnea, with an oxygen saturation of 70% and a heart rate of 80 beats/minute, the other a 30-second bout of apnea, with a saturation of 70% and a heart rate of 60 beats/minute. These episodes persisted for 8 hours into the postoperative period in one of the infants.

A patient who was receiving modified-release morphine for malignant pain suffered a respiratory arrest after intrathecal bupivacaine 12.5 mg. She recovered after treatment with naloxone. Another patient who was taking modified- release morphine was given intrathecal morphine 10 mg and bupivacaine 7.5 mg. He had respiratory distress and became comatose. Morphine-induced respiratory depression was not diagnosed and the patient subsequently died. In both cases respiratory distress and sedation was probably due to opioid action in the absence of the stimulating effect of pain on respiration, due to the intrathecal bupivacaine (19[c]).

A 20-year-old woman who received a combined spinal epidural for labor had a respiratory arrest 23 minutes after the administration of sufentanil 10 μg and bupivacaine 2.5 mg (20[cr]).

Nervous system Transient pain in the back, buttocks, and lower extremities can follow single-dose spinal anesthesia. This syndrome is currently referred to as transient radicular irritation in preference to the preceding term transient neurological symptoms, as no neurological symptoms occur. Lidocaine is still reported as the predominant culprit. However, transient radicular irritation has also been reported with bupivacaine, mepivacaine, tetracaine, and prilocaine. Osmolarity, the addition of dextrose, and speed of injection do not contribute, and even reducing the concentration of lidocaine does not alter the incidence (21[c], 22[c]). The precise cause is unclear, but three factors are strongly linked; subarachnoid lidocaine, patient positioning (with a significantly higher incidence in patients positioned for knee arthroscopy and the lithotomy position), and ambulatory surgery (21[r], 23[R]).

The interest in and controversy surrounding this syndrome continues to be high. The risk factors have been highlighted again in case reports involving lidocaine (24[cr], 25[c], 26[c]), mepivacaine (27[cr]), and bupivacaine (28[cr]).

A 50-year-old woman had a right knee arthroscopy under spinal anesthesia with 1% lidocaine 4 ml. The anesthetic and procedure were uncomplicated. At 4 hours she complained of a mild cramp in her buttocks and went home at 6 hours. By the next morning the buttock pain was severe, cramp-like in nature, and radiated down the fronts of both thighs. Walking alleviated it, simple analgesics were ineffective, and lying down made the pain worse. Neurological examination was unremarkable and the pain was gone after 36 hours.

A 74-year-old man who had a cystoscopy performed in the lithotomy position, reported dull pain in the hips, buttocks, and legs, radiating to the toes after a spinal anesthetic with 5% hyperbaric lidocaine 75 mg. The pain occurred 30 hours after the dural puncture and disappeared after 18 hours. Three months before he had had a similar anesthetic for a transurethral resection of the prostate and complained of similar but more severe symptoms of transient radicular irritation.

A 66-year-old woman with unrecognized spinal stenosis had six spinal anesthetics over 3 years. The first five were with lidocaine 2%. After 24–48 hours she developed pain in the back, hips, buttocks, and thighs, which lasted for 2–3 days. On the sixth occasion she had a spinal anesthetic with 1.5% mepivacaine 4 ml and the next day again had severe back pain radiating bilaterally to the hips and thighs.

Three patients undergoing minor surgical procedures in the lithotomy position were given a spinal anesthetic with 2% mepivacaine 3 ml. From 6 to 10 hours postoperatively they complained of burning pain in both buttocks radiating to both thighs and calves. Neurological examination in all cases was normal and all symptoms had resolved by 3–5 days postoperatively.

A 30-year-old man had a left spermatic vein ligature performed in the supine position. He had uncomplicated unilateral spinal anesthesia with 1% hyperbaric bupivacaine 8 mg. Three days later he reported an area of hypesthesia in the L3–4 dermatomes of the left leg. Sensation returned to normal after 2 weeks.

In a prospective study of 1045 patients receiving spinal anesthesia with 3% hyperbaric lidocaine for anorectal surgery in the prone position, four (0.4%) complained of aching, hypesthesia, numbness, and dull pain in both buttocks and legs on the third postoperative day. In three cases the symptoms resolved by day 5 and in one by day 7 (29[Cr]).

In a retrospective audit of 363 patients receiving spinal anesthesia, of whom 322 received hyperbaric 5% lidocaine 75–100 mg and 41 hyperbaric 0.5% bupivacaine 12.5–15 mg, six patients given lidocaine reported back pain at 24 hours; five of them had undergone arthroscopy. One patient given bupivacaine, who underwent arthroscopy, complained of backache (30[Cr]).

Over 14 months, 1863 patients received spinal anesthesia, of whom 40% were given bupivacaine, 47% lidocaine, and 13% tetracaine (31[CR]). Patients given lidocaine had a significantly higher risk of transient radicular irritation (relative risks 5.1 compared with bupivacaine and 3.2 compared with tetracaine). They were more likely to be men, have out-patient surgery, and have surgery in the lithotomy position. For those who were given lidocaine, the relative risk of transient radicular irritation was 2.6, for those in the lithotomy position 3.6, and for ambulatory surgery 1.6. Most of the patients had resolution of symptoms by 72 hours and all by 6 months

The incidence of transient radicular irritation with two different local anesthetics used for single-dose spinal anesthesia has been studied in 60 ambulatory patients given spinal anesthesia for knee arthroscopy (32[Cr]). None of those who were given 1.5% mepivacaine 45 mg developed transient radicular irritation. Six of those given 2% lidocaine 60 mg developed transient radicular irritation, but all symptoms resolved by 1–5 days. The difference between the two groups was significant.

Out of 90 patients who received intrathecal hyperbaric lidocaine 5%, mepivacaine 4%, or bupivacaine 0.5%, none in the bupivacaine group developed transient radicular irritation, but 20% in the lidocaine group and 37% in the mepivacaine group complained of a mixture of back and leg pain, classified as transient radicular irritation (33[Cr]).

When 90 patients received spinal anesthesia for gynecological procedures with 2% lidocaine, 2% prilocaine, or 0.5% bupivacaine (all 2.5 ml in 7.5% glucose), nine of the 30 patients who received lidocaine had transient radicular irritation, defined as pain or dysesthesia in the legs or buttocks, compared with none of the 30 patients who received bupivacaine (34[Cr]). The symptoms resolved within 48 hours. One of the 30 patients who received prilocaine had transient radicular irritation that lasted for 4 days.

In 200 patients given hyperbaric 5% lidocaine or hyperbaric 5% prilocaine, four developed transient radicular irritation after lidocaine (the patients were supine or prone) compared with one after prilocaine (this patient had a knee arthroscopy) (35[Cr]). There were no significant differences between the two groups.

When procaine 5% or procaine 5% with fentanyl 20 μg was given to 106 patients for spinal anesthesia, the incidence of transient radicular irritation was 0.9% (36[Cr]). There was nausea and vomiting in 17% of men and 32% of women.

Cauda equina syndrome is a rare but potentially devastating consequence of spinal or epidural anesthesia (37[c]).

A 57-year-old man with pre-existing severe vascular disease was given bupivacaine 12.5 mg with 1 : 1000 adrenaline 0.2 ml for incision and drainage of a thigh abscess. After 2–3 minutes he complained of 'severely painful warmth' on the anterior of both thighs. The pain resolved with onset of the block, but the next morning he had symptoms of cauda equina syndrome. Some perineal sensation returned over the next few days.

The authors suggested that the neurological deficit had been due to anterior spinal artery insufficiency secondary to intrathecal bupivacaine and adrenaline. They questioned the use of adrenaline in patients with multiorgan vascular disease.

Another patient with severe vascular disease was given general and epidural anesthesia with 2% isobaric lidocaine plus adrenaline for a popliteal distal vein bypass graft (38[cr]). The epidural inadvertently became a total spinal, which was discovered at the end of the operation. The patient developed cauda equina syndrome, confirmed by electromyography. He was unable to turn or sit up by himself for a month and at 12 months was walking with a cane and needed self-catheterization and medication for neuropathic pain. The cauda has a tenuous blood supply, and in this patient with pre-existing vascular disease, perioperative hypotension and the use of intrathecal adrenaline may have precipitated ischemia in an area with very poor reserve. To follow this with an accidental large dose of lidocaine, which is neurotoxic in animals when directly applied and theorized to cause interruption of nerve blood supply, would add insult to injury. The authors questioned the wisdom of performing continuous epidural anesthesia in such patients, when frequent neurological assessments cannot be performed.

Special senses When 44 patients undergoing inguinal hernia repair were given spinal anesthesia with 2% prilocaine 6 ml or 0.5% bupivacaine 3 ml, those given prilocaine had an average hearing loss of about 10 dB and 1–3 days postoperatively and those given bupivacaine had an average hearing loss of about 15 dB (39[C]). However, 10 of 22 in those given prilocaine developed hearing loss, compared with four of the 22 given bupivacaine.

Cervical plexus anesthesia

Deep cervical plexus block can cause ipsilateral phrenic nerve palsy. A patient with pre-existing respiratory disease and a contralateral raised hemidiaphragm developed hypoxia and respiratory distress when given 20 ml of plain bupivacaine 0.375% by this route for carotid endarterectomy (40[c]). Local anesthetic spread resulted in presumed stellate ganglion block, which caused nasal congestion and aggravated the respiratory distress. The symptoms resolved without intubation, but the authors advised against deep cervical plexus block in patients with diaphragmatic motion abnormalities or chronic respiratory disease.

Dental anesthesia *(SEDA-13, 288; SEDA-20, 124; SEDA-21, 131; SEDA-22, 135)*

Additives in local anesthetic solutions can cause allergic reactions (41[c]).

A 34-year-old man developed swelling and redness of the face after receiving lidocaine as Lignospan® for dental treatment. Patch testing showed *allergic contact dermatitis* due to the preservative disodium ethylenediamine tetra-acetic acid (EDTA).

Digital anesthesia

Digital block anesthesia with 1% lidocaine plus adrenaline was performed on 23 patients for surgery to finger injuries; 11 patients received adrenaline 1 : 200 000, and 12 received 1 : 100 000 (42[Cr]). A digital tourniquet was also used, but no patient developed ischemic symptoms. The authors discussed the usefulness of adrenaline as an additive to local anesthetic solutions in prolonging regional block, reducing the dose of local anesthetic required. They stated that an extensive search of the literature had revealed no sound clinical evidence to support the widely held opinion that adrenaline contributes to the risk of gangrene when it is used in digital blocks.

Glossopharyngeal nerve anesthesia

Excessive volumes of local anesthetic in a confined space can lead to life-threatening upper airway obstruction. When glossopharyngeal nerve blocks are used for tonsillectomy, children under 15 kg should be given 1 ml or less of 0.25% bupivacaine per tonsil (43[c]).

Intradermal anesthesia

Intradermal local anesthetic solutions can cause considerable *pain on injection.* Additives, such as hyaluronidase, which are used to enhance the analgesic effect of local anesthetics, can often exacerbate this (44[C]). Infiltration from the inside of a wound can be less painful than through intact skin (45[C]).

The order of injection can affect the pain of local anesthetic infiltration with buffered lidocaine; in a sequence of two injections the second injection was consistently reported to be more painful than the first. This finding has important consequences with regard to trial design in this area of research (46[C]). Buffered lidocaine warmed to 37°C was less painful than warmed plain lidocaine, plain lidocaine, and buffered lidocaine in a randomized controlled trial in 26 volunteers (47[Cr]).

Intravenous regional anesthesia

(SEDA-22, 139)

Intravenous regional anesthesia can lead to severe adverse systemic effects. Prilocaine is thought to be the safest local anesthetic for this procedure.

A 74-year-old woman was given prilocaine 400 mg for carpal tunnel surgery. Within 3 minutes she developed signs of *central nervous system toxicity, sweating, and tachycardia.* Twenty minutes later her symptoms had resolved and the cause was found to be a leak in the tourniquet.

The authors used this case to stress the importance of adequately functioning equipment and the relative safety of prilocaine (48[c]).

Chloroprocaine may also be a useful agent, but there are reports that it can cause endothelial damage, and dysrhythmias after tourniquet deflation (49[r]).

The risks of local anesthetic toxicity may be greater in pregnancy, because an increase in the unbound fraction of local anesthetic and physiological changes increase the transfer of local anesthetic into the central nervous system. The authors of a report of systemic symptoms in a pregnant patient suggested the precautionary use of a lower dose of local anesthetic than usual and a longer tourniquet time, to increase the safety of this technique during pregnancy (50[c]).

Ocular anesthesia *(SED-13, 1420; SEDA-20, 126; SEDA-21, 133; SEDA-22, 139)*

Peribulbar anesthesia Peribulbar anesthesia is generally considered safer than retrobulbar anesthesia, with a lower incidence of adverse effects. However, three reports have highlighted problems.

A 76-year-old man undergoing trabeculectomy developed *bilateral amaurosis* after a peribulbar block with 6 ml of a mixture of 2% lidocaine, 0.5% bupivacaine, and hyaluronidase (51[c]). The authors thought it unlikely that the optic nerve sheath had been penetrated and suggested that local spread to the optic nerves via the subarachnoid or subdural space had been responsible.

A 49-year-old woman had a *tonic-clonic seizure* about 15 minutes after a peribulbar block for left trabeculectomy (52[c]). She recovered and surgery continued uneventfully. However, she had severe permanent visual loss in that eye, and an MRI scan at 4 weeks showed swelling of the left optic nerve. The authors suggested that some prilocaine had been injected into the nerve sheath, causing the convulsions, local optic nerve swelling, and subsequent optic nerve atrophy.

A rare case of *hyphema* after peribulbar block with 1% lidocaine 8 ml occurred in a 38-year-old woman with a history of Fuchs' heterochromic iridocyclitis (53[c]).

Postoperative strabismus and diplopia occurred in two of 200 patients undergoing cataract extraction under peribulbar anesthesia; the symptoms resolved spontaneously by 6 months (54[C]).

Retrobulbar anesthesia Retrobulbar anesthesia can lead to serious *systemic toxicity.* However, in animal studies accidental intravitreous spread of lidocaine, bupivacaine, or a mixture of the two did not cause long-term retinal damage (55).

Topical ocular anesthesia Topical ocular anesthesia is generally well tolerated. In 14 patients 0.5% proxymetacaine had similar efficacy to 0.4% oxybuprocaine and 0.5% amethocaine but was significantly better tolerated (56[Cr]).

There has been one case report of topical anesthetic abuse (57[cr]).

A 49-year-old woman developed repeated episodes of severe keratitis after radial keratotomy for myopia. After 18 months of repeated hospital admissions, several operations, and considerably reduced visual acuity, it eventually transpired that she had been self-medicating with 1% proparacaine mixed with artificial tears to control pain after her surgery.

Non-preserved intracameral lidocaine 1% is a useful adjunct to topical anesthesia for cataract surgery. In 631 patients topical anesthesia alone was compared with combined topical and intracameral anesthesia (58[Cr]). The combination had greater efficacy – only 1% of those given combined anesthesia needing to be converted to general anesthesia compared with

40% of those given topical anesthesia alone. The authors suggest that the key difference between the two methods is reduced sensitivity to the microscope light. Another prospective study in 93 patients showed that intracameral non-preserved lidocaine was both safe and efficacious; four patients reported discomfort and none had measurable endothelial cellular changes (59[C]).

Topical anesthesia *(SEDA-20, 127; SEDA-21, 135; SEDA-22, 140)*

An 18-month-old child undergoing cardiac surgery developed *discoloration* of the hand, consistent with *severe bruising*, after application of 4% amethocaine gel, which was inadvertently left under an occlusive dressing for about 24 hours (60[c]). There were no long term sequelae and no treatment was required. The authors blamed a combination of the vasodilatory properties of amethocaine and the fact that the child was heparinized for surgery, causing capillary leak at the area of application.

In 272 children who required topical local anesthesia for venepuncture, there was no association between the duration of application of 4% amethocaine gel and the development of adverse skin reactions (61[C]). However, two reports discussed by the same authors highlighted rare adverse reactions.

A 4-year-old child with no previous exposure complained of *severe pain, erythema, and blistering* 5 minutes after the application of 4% amethocaine gel. An anesthetist who was suspected of occupational exposure developed *redness* and *blistering* after applying a test dose of amethocaine.

The authors recommended minimizing occupational contact and quickly removing the cream in patients who report pain after application of amethocaine. It is unlikely that amethocaine applied to intact skin for long periods will cause any systemic reaction, as it is rapidly metabolized by plasma cholinesterase (62[r]).

The innocuous seeming EMLA cream (Eutectic Mixture of Local Anesthetics, which contains a mixture of 2.5% prilocaine and 2.5% lidocaine) is often underestimated, and therefore carelessly used with a lack of appreciation for, or knowledge of, its adverse effects. Particular care must be taken in children.

A 5-year-old child had 35 g of EMLA applied under an occlusive dressing to eczematous skin in preparation for cryotherapy for molluscum contagiosum (63[c]). Within 1 hour the child had a generalized seizure that lasted 10 minutes. The plasma concentration of lidocaine and prilocaine 30 minutes later were 5.5 mg/l and 2.0 mg/l respectively and 6 hours later the methemoglobin concentration was 19%. The child was given vitamin C 500 mg intravenously, and 2 days later had a methemoglobin concentration of 0.3%

In 29 children with atopic dermatitis who were given EMLA cream before curettage of molluscum contagiosum there were no adverse reactions, apart from mild transient application site reactions, such as *pallor, redness, and edema.* No systemic reactions were reported, but the authors emphasized that EMLA can be rapidly absorbed through atopic skin, and they therefore recommended a maximum dose of 10 g applied under occlusive dressing for 30 minutes (64[Cr]).

Two children developed petechial eruptions after the application of EMLA for treatment curettage of molluscum contagiosum (65[cr]). Neither child became systemically unwell and subsequent reapplication of EMLA in one child did not elicit a petechial eruption.

Even topical administration of lidocaine continues to generate reports with tragic outcomes, as absorption from mucosal surfaces is underestimated. A patient due to have a bronchoscopy was given an overdose of lidocaine to anesthetize the airway by an inexperienced health worker. He was then left unobserved and subsequently developed *convulsions* and *cardiopulmonary arrest* (66[c]). He survived with *severe cerebral damage.* His lidocaine concentration was 24 μg/ml about 1 hour after initial administration (a blood concentration over 6 μg/ml is considered to be toxic).

A 19-year-old healthy volunteer undergoing bronchoscopy was given about 1200 mg of lidocaine to anesthetize the airway and was sent home after the procedure, despite complaining of chest pain. Shortly afterwards she had a *tonic-clonic seizure* and *cardiopulmonary arrest* and *died* 2 days later. The research protocol had failed to specify an upper dose limit for lidocaine (67[c]).

Local anesthetic gels and creams used liberally on traumatized epithelium can be rapidly absorbed, resulting in systemic effects, such as convulsions, particularly if excessive quantities are used. This has been highlighted in the case of a 40-year-old woman who developed *seizures* after lidocaine gel 40 ml was injected into the ureter during an attempt to remove a stone (68[c]).

INDIVIDUAL COMPOUNDS

Benzocaine *(SED-13, 293; SEDA-21, 135; SEDA-22, 141)*

Five cases of benzocaine-induced *methemoglobinemia* have been reported in 1998, following its use for transesophageal echocardiography (69[c]–72[c]). Methemoglobin concentrations >15% can lead to cyanosis, whilst concentrations over 70% lead to circulatory collapse and death (71[c], 72[c]). The degree of methemoglobinemia depends on the total dose of drug and any factors that enhance systemic absorption. The elderly and neonates are particularly susceptible to methemoglobinemia, as are those with inherited methemoglobin reductase deficiency or the abnormal hemoglobin M. Adequate monitoring and observation of patients both during and after transesophageal echocardiography is essential, as this rare complication of benzocaine and other local anesthetics, such as prilocaine, is both potentially fatal and eminently treatable.

Bupivacaine *(SED-13, 293; SEDA-20, 128; SEDA-21, 135; SEDA-22, 141)*

Cardiovascular A 13-year-old girl developed tonic-clonic *seizures* followed by *ventricular fibrillation* after subcutaneous infiltration of extensive skin abrasions with 30 mg (0.5 mg/kg) of bupivacaine over about 1 hour. She was successfully resuscitated with cardiopulmonary resuscitation and intubation, intravenous diazepam, adrenaline, and sodium bicarbonate (73[cr]). The authors noted that although the anticonvulsant effect of diazepam is significant, some animal studies have shown that diazepam can prolong the half-life of bupivacaine. They stressed the difficulty in treating bupivacaine-induced dysrhythmias and suggested the use of phenytoin as a first-line agent in their management. However, this advice is based on only two case reports.

Infusions of 0.25% bupivacaine into pig coronary arteries caused ventricular fibrillation at lower rates of infusion than 0.25% bupivacaine with 1% lidocaine (74). The lidocaine/bupivacaine mixture did not have a greater myocardial depressant effect than bupivacaine alone. The authors suggested that when regional anesthesia requires high doses of local anesthetics, bupivacaine should not be used alone, but in a mixture with lidocaine, and that lidocaine should be useful in the management of bupivacaine-induced ventricular fibrillation.

Bupivacaine *cardiotoxicity* is reduced in rats by pretreatment with low doses of calcium antagonists (75). *In vivo*, the LD50 for bupivacaine was increased from 3.08 to 3.58 mg/kg after pretreatment with verapamil 150 μg/kg, and to 3.50 mg/kg after nimodipine 200 μg/kg. Of the rats that died, only one developed cardiac arrest first, whilst the majority developed respiratory arrest. *In vitro*, bupivacaine alone dose-dependently reduced heart rate, contractile force, and coronary perfusion pressure. Dysrhythmias were also noted: bradycardias, ventricular extra beats, and ventricular tachycardia were the most common. Verapamil made no difference to these adverse effects, but nimodipine significantly reduced the negative chronotropic and dysrhythmogenic effects of bupivacaine. These results, although interesting, cannot be used to reach any clinical conclusions, particularly as the mechanism of interaction between bupivacaine and calcium antagonists has yet to be elucidated.

The reduced cardiovascular toxicity of levobupivacaine, previously demonstrated in comparison with racemic bupivacaine, has been shown again in a study in seven sheep (76). Racemic bupivacaine caused mild cardiac depression, which was superseded by central nervous system toxicity and then proceeded to severe ventricular dysrhythmias, which were fatal in three sheep, at doses of 125, 150, and 200 mg. Levobupivacaine was consistently less toxic than bupivacaine, and higher doses were needed to produce adverse effects. Convulsions were less severe and of shorter duration, and although levobupivacaine produced QRS prolongation and ventricular dysrhythmias, those that occurred were not as malignant as with bupivacaine and resulted in no deaths.

The effects of low concentrations of epidural bupivacaine on the developing neonatal brain has been studied in infant rhesus monkeys, to decide if there was a detrimental relation between perinatal analgesia with epidural bupivacaine and *later infant development* (77). The monkeys, whose mothers had been given epidurals at term (but not during labor) were subjected to a battery of neurobehavioral tests for 1 year. The authors concluded that epidural bupivacaine did not cause neonatal abnormalities or specific cognitive defects, but that it *may delay the normal course of behavioral development* It is difficult to extrapolate the results of this small study to human obstetrics.

Cetacaine

Cetacaine spray used to anesthetize the oropharynx before endoscopy led to dyspnea, central cyanosis, and an oxygen saturation of 80%; methemoglobinemia was diagnosed, and the patient recovered rapidly with methylene blue 1 mg/kg over 5 minutes (78[cr]).

Cocaine *(SED-13, 294; SEDA-20, 128; SEDA-21, 135; SEDA-22, 142)*

Cocaine is commonly used in topical anesthetics, usually in conjunction with tetracaine and adrenaline. Cocaine can cause serious adverse effects and should be used with caution, as deaths due to its use as a topical anesthetic have been reported. A 20 kg 5-year-old boy had 3 ml of adrenaline 1 : 2000 and cocaine 11.8% applied to abrasions and a laceration on his forehead. He became *tachycardic, yawned repeatedly*, and made a *repetitive verbal noise* for 2 hours. The authors attributed these symptoms to systemic cocaine toxicity, as the local anesthetic was readily absorbed from mucous membranes. They recommend a dose of cocaine plus either adrenaline or tetracaine and adrenaline of no more than 1 ml per 10 kg. However, they also pointed out that with the advent of lidocaine plus adrenaline plus tetracaine the use of cocaine should be reconsidered (79[cr]).

Dibucaine *(SED-13, 294; SEDA-21, 135)*

Low concentrations of dibucaine (0.003 and 0.03% respectively) caused irreversible *neurotoxicity* of A_β and C rabbit vagus nerve preparations (80). Dibucaine had the greatest neurotoxic effect with the lowest safety margin compared with tetracaine and bupivacaine.

Dibucaine is a common ingredient of over-the-counter topical medications, such as antihemorrhoid drugs. Two cases of contact dermatitis have been reported after the use of Proctosedyl® and *Ruscens Llorens*, both of which contain dibucaine. After patch testing, the first case was found to be *allergic* in origin and the second, photosensitive only. Neither showed cross-sensitivity to other local anesthetics (81[c], 82[c]).

Lidocaine *(SED-13, 292; SEDA-20, 128; SEDA-21, 136; SEDA-22, 142)*

Systemic toxicity Two reports have illustrated the need for particular care when using local anesthetics in neonates and small children. A 2-year-old child died from the combined effects of chloral hydrate, lidocaine, and nitrous oxide for a dental procedure (83[c]). The doses used were not clarified, but in post-mortem blood the plasma concentration of lidocaine was 12 μg/ml. It was also not clear as to the level and adequacy of perioperative monitoring. A neonate who needed a tracheostomy 10 days after a tracheo-esophageal fistula repair was given intravenous lidocaine, 1 mg/kg followed 15–20 minutes later by 0.7 mg/kg. Immediately after tonic-clonic *seizures* developed. The patient recovered, with no observable ill effects at 6 months. The authors pointed out that the dose of lidocaine used was well within recommended dose limits. However, they stressed that a more appropriate dosing schedule should be worked out for neonates. Lidocaine pharmacokinetics tend to follow a single compartment model in neonates, with an increased terminal half-life, and substantially reduced protein binding, leading to a much larger volume of distribution than in adults, but an increased proportion of unbound drug (84[cr]).

Propofol dose-dependently reduced the threshold for lidocaine- induced convulsions in rats (85). Higher doses of propofol completely abolished convulsions. However, there was no difference in the dose of lidocaine that caused cardiac arrest and death, when it was given with three different propofol infusions and placebo.

Nervous system Transient and permanent nerve damage can occur after regional anesthesia, particularly neuraxial anesthesia. The mechanism of this nerve damage is unclear. Some studies have shown an indirect effect. However, in crayfish giant axon lidocaine had a dose- and time-dependent effect on isolated nerve function *in vitro* (86). At high concentrations lidocaine caused irreversible conduction block and total loss of resting membrane potential. These results in an isolated nerve suggest a direct neurotoxic effect of lidocaine.

Immunological and hypersensitivity reactions Idiosyncratic reactions can occur with even small quantities of lidocaine, as in a 16-year-old woman, who had had an adverse reaction after administration of an unknown local anesthetic agent for a dental procedure. Patch testing elicited similar symptoms with lidocaine only, and 20 minutes after subcutaneous lidocaine 0.05 mg she developed perioral paresthesia, nausea, vomiting, vertigo, dizziness, mild agitation, drowsiness, and euphoria. Hemodynamic parameters remained stable but her symptoms were thought to be part of a genuine non-allergic, neuropsychiatric reaction, as the patch testing was double-blind and placebo-controlled (87[c]).

There have been 62 reports of *allergic contact dermatitis* to lidocaine world wide between 1972 and 1996; 49 were in Australia and several showed cross-reactivity with other amide local anesthetics, such as bupivacaine, mepivacaine, and prilocaine (88[c]).

Ropivacaine *(SED-13, 295; SEDA-20, 129; SEDA-22, 143)*

The safety, pharmacokinetics and efficacy of two doses of ropivacaine (300 and 375 mg) for wound infiltration after surgical incision have been studied in an open non-randomized study of 20 men undergoing elective hernia repair (89[C]). Efficacy was similar. There were wide variations in mean plasma concentrations of ropivacaine, the highest individual plasma concentration of total drug being 3.0 mg/ml for the 375 mg dose. One patient in the low-dose group had two episodes of bradycardia at 2 and 12 hours after drug administration. The first episode corresponded to a total plasma drug concentration of 1.3 mg/ml. Three patients in the high-dose group had several recorded episodes of sinus *bradycardia.* Two of these were within the first hour of ropivacaine administration and corresponded to plasma concentrations of 2.5 and 2.9 mg/ml. One patient in the 300 mg group complained of dizziness at 12 and 21 hours and of nausea at 12 hours. Another patient in the same group vomited 4 hours after the injection of ropivacaine. Two patients had transient hypesthesia in the leg on the operated side, thought to be due to partial block of the femoral nerve. The authors felt that systemic toxicity due to ropivacaine was unlikely to be a cause of any of these adverse effects and they concluded that high-dose ropivacaine is safe for wound infiltration.

Inadvertent intravenous injection of ropivacaine resulted in systemic toxicity in two cases (90[c], 91[c]). A 13-year-old boy weighing 44 kg was given a bolus of 20 mg of ropivacaine through an 18 gauge Tuohy needle. No CSF or blood had been aspirated. However, he immediately complained that his face '*felt different*', and within 1 minute developed a *tonic-clonic seizure* and a *tachycardia* of 160/minute. In a blood sample taken about 35 minutes later the plasma concentration of ropivacaine was 1.4 mg/ml, consistent with intravascular injection. In man symptoms of toxicity occur at plasma concentrations of 1–2 mg/ml. The authors thought that the rate of injection of epidural local anesthetic should be slower, which would give a greater safety margin between the onset of facial numbness and seizures. A ropivacaine-induced seizure also occurred in a 23-year-old woman undergoing postpartum tubal ligation. An epidural that had been inserted for labor the evening before the procedure was used to give ropivacaine 120 mg in increments over 11 minutes. She complained of nervousness and within a few seconds had a *generalized tonic-clonic seizure* and a *sinus tachycardia* of 120 beats/minute.

In both of these cases reasonable precautions had been taken to ensure correct catheter placement, but nevertheless systemic toxicity occurred. However, neither patient had any serious cardiotoxicity, reinforcing the relative safety of ropivacaine in clinical practice. However, it is worth emphasizing that large doses of local anesthetics should be given slowly and in divided doses and that lidocaine, one of the least toxic of the commonly used local anesthetics, has more obvious prodromal symptoms than ropivacaine, and could be a useful marker for intravenous injection (92[R]).

REFERENCES

1. Herman N. Neurologic complications of regional anesthesia. Semin Anesth 1998;17:64–72.
2. Gibbons JJ, Lennon RL, Rose SH, Wedel DJ, Gibson BE. Axillary block of the brachial plexus: 'You can't get there from here'. Anesthesiology 1988;68:314–15.
3. Koscielniak-Nielsen ZJ. An unusual toxic reaction to axillary block by mepivacaine with adrenaline. Acta Anaesthesiol Scand 1998;42:868–71.
4. Marsch SCU, Schaefer H-G, Castelli I. Unusual psychological manifestation of systemic local anesthetic toxicity. Anesthesiology 1998;88:531–3.
5. Breschan C, Hellstrand E, Likar R, Lonnquist P-A. Bupivacaine plasma concentrations associated with clinical and electroencephalographic signs of early central nervous system toxicity in infants during awake caudal anaesthesia. Anaesthesist 1998; 47:290–4.
6. Stevens RA, Frey K, Sheikh T, Kao TC, Mikat-Stevens M, Morales M. Time course of the effects of cervical epidural anesthesia on pulmonary function. Reg Anesth 1998;23:20–4.
7. Cox CR, Faccenda KA, Gilhooly C, Bannister J, Scott NB, Morrison LM. Extradural S(–)-bupivacaine: comparison with racemic RS-bupivacaine. Br J Anaesth 1998;80:289–93.
8. Rauck RL, Colon J, Lesser GJ, Naveira FA, Speight KL. Paraspinal fluid extravasation from long-term epidural catheter delivery system. Anesthesiology 1998;88:1672–5.
9. Johnston MKW, Harland SP. Spinal cord compression from precipitation of drug solute around an epidural catheter. Br J Neurosurg 1998;12: 445–7.
10. Liu M, Kim PS, Chen C-K, Smythe WR. Delayed Horner's syndrome as a complication of continuous thoracic epidural analgesia. J Cardiothorac Vasc Anesth 1998;12:195–6.
11. Schregel W, Brudny P. Just another explanation for: 'Horner's syndrome following low-dose epidural infusion for labour' presented by HGW Paw. Eur J Anaesthesiol 1998;15:617–18.
12. Motamed C, Spencer A, Farhat F, Bourgain JL, Lasser P, Jayr C. Postoperative hypoxaemia: continuous extradural infusion of bupivacaine and morphine vs patient-controlled analgesia with intravenous morphine. Br J Anaesth 1998;80:742–7.
13. Liu SS, Allen HW, Olsson GL. Patient- controlled epidural analgesia with bupivacaine and fentanyl on hospital wards: prospective experience with 1030 surgical patients. Anesthesiology 1998; 88:688–95.
14. Shapiro A, Fredman B, Olsfanger D, Jedeikin R. Anaesthesia for caesarean delivery: low-dose epidural bupivacaine plus fentanyl. Int J Obstet Anesth 1998;7:23–6.
15. Niruthisard S, Thaithumyanon P, Somboonviboon W, Mahutchawaroj N, Chaiyakul A. Maternal and neonatal effects of single-dose epidural anesthesia with lidocaine and morphine for cesarean delivery. J Med Assoc Thailand 1998;81: 103–9.
16. Jordi E-M, Marsch SCU, Strebel S. Third degree heart block and asystole associated with spinal anesthesia. Anesthesiology 1998;89:257–60.
17. Casati A, Fanelli G, Beccaria P, Aldegheri G, Berti M, Senatore R, Torri G. Block distribution and cardiovascular effects of unilateral spinal anaesthesia by 0.5% hyperbaric bupivacaine. A clinical comparison with bilateral spinal block. Minerva Anesthesiol 1998;64:307–12.
18. Tobias JD, Burd RS, Helikson MA. Apnea following spinal anaesthesia in two former pre-term infants. Can J Anaesth 1998;45:985–9.
19. Piquet CY, Mallaret MP, Lemoigne AH, Barjhoux CE, Danel VC, Vincent FH. Respiratory depression following administration of intrathecal bupivacaine to an opioid-dependent patient. Ann Pharmacother 1998;32:653–5.
20. Katsiris S, Williams S, Leighton BL, Halpern S. Respiratory arrest following intrathecal injection of sufentanil and bupivacaine in a parturient. Can J Anaesth 1998;45:880–3.
21. Neal JM, Pollock JE. Can scapegoats stand on shifting sands? Reg Anesth Pain Med 1998;23: 533–7.
22. DeJong RH. In my opinion: spinal lidocaine: a continuing enigma. J Clin Monit Comput 1998;14: 147–8.
23. Moore DC, Thompson GE. Commentary: neurotoxicity of local anesthetics—an issue or a scapegoat? Reg Anesth Pain Med 1998;23:605–10.
24. Henderson DJ, Faccenda KA, Morrison LMM. Transient radicular irritation with intrathecal plain lignocaine. Acta Anaesthesiol Scand 1998;42: 376–8.
25. Panadero A, Monedero P, Fernandez-Liesa JI, Percaz J, Olavide I, Iribarren MJ. Repeated transient neurological symptoms after spinal anaesthesia with hyperbaric 5% lidocaine. Br J Anaesth 1998; 81:471–2.
26. Liguori GA, Zayas VM. Repeated episodes of transient radiating back and leg pain following spinal anesthesia with 1.5% mepivacaine and 2% lidocaine. Reg Anesth Pain Med 1998;23:511– 15.
27. Sia S, Pullano C. Transient radicular irritation after spinal anaesthesia with 2% isobaric mepivacaine. Br J Anaesth 1998;81:622–4.
28. Casati A, Fanelli G, Aldegheri G, Berti M, Leoni A, Torri G. A transient neurological deficit following intrathecal injection of 1% hyperbaric bupivacaine for unilateral spinal anaesthesia. Eur J Anaesthesiol 1998;15:112–13.
29. Morisaki H, Masuda J, Kaneko S, Matsushima M, Takeda J. Transient neurologic syndrome in one thousand forty-five patients after 3% lidocaine spinal anesthesia. Anesth Analg 1998;86: 1023–6.
30. Corbey MP, Bach AB. Transient radicular irritation (TRI) after spinal anaesthesia in day-care surgery. Acta Anaesthesiol Scand 1998;42: 425–9.
31. Freedman JM, Li DK, Drasner K, Jaskela MC, Larsen B, Wi S. Transient neurologic symptoms

after spinal anesthesia: an epidemiologic study of 1,863 patients. Anesthesiology 1998;89:633–41 [Erratum in 1998;89:1614].

32. Liguori GA, Zayas VM, Chisholm MF. Transient neurologic symptoms after spinal anesthesia with mepivacaine and lidocaine. Anesthesiology 1998;88:619–23.
33. Salmela L, Aromaa U. Transient radicular irritation after spinal anesthesia induced with hyperbaric solutions of cerebrospinal fluid-diluted lidocaine 50 mg/ml or mepivacaine 40 mg/ml or bupivacaine 5 mg/ml. Acta Anaesthesiol Scand 1998; 42:765–9.
34. Hampl KF, Heinzmann-Wiedmer S, Luginbuehl I, Harms C, Seeberger M, Schneider MC, Drasner K. Transient neurologic symptoms after spinal anesthesia: a lower incidence with prilocaine and bupivacaine than with lidocaine. Anesthesiology 1998;88:629–33.
35. Martínez-Bourio R, Arzuaga M, Quintana JM, Aguilera L, Aguirre J, Sáez-Eguilaz JL, Arizaga A. Incidence of transient neurologic symptoms after hyperbaric subarachnoid anesthesia with 5% lidocaine and 5% prilocaine. Anesthesiology 1998;88: 624–8.
36. Axelrod EH, Alexander GD, Brown M, Schork MA. Procaine spinal anesthesia: a pilot study of the incidence of transient neurologic symptoms. J Clin Anesth 1998;10:404–9.
37. Tetzlaff JE, Dilger J, Yap E, Smith MP, Schoenwald PK. Cauda equina syndrome after spinal anaesthesia in a patient with severe vascular disease. Can J Anaesth 1998;45:667–9.
38. Lee DS, Bui T, Ferrarese J, Richardson PK. Cauda equina syndrome after incidental total spinal anesthesia with 2% lidocaine. J Clin Anesth 1998; 10:66–9.
39. Gultekin S, Yilmaz N, Ceyhan A, Karamustafa I, Kilic R, Unal N. The effect of different anaesthetic agents in hearing loss following spinal anaesthesia. Eur J Anaesthesiol 1998;15:61–3.
40. Stoneham MD, Wakefield TW. Acute respiratory distress after deep cervical plexus block. J Cardiothorac Vasc Anesth 1998;12:197–8.
41. Bhushan M, Beck MH. Allergic contact dermatitis from disodium ethylenediamine tetraacetic acid (EDTA) in a local anaesthetic. Contact Dermatitis 1998;38:183.
42. Wilhelmi BJ, Blackwell SJ, Miller J, Mancoll JS, Phillips LG. Epinephrine in digital blocks: revisited. Ann Plast Surg 1998;41:410–14.
43. Sher MH, Laing DI, Brands E. Life-threatening upper airway obstruction after glossopharyngeal nerve block: possibly due to an inappropriately large dose of bupivacaine? Anesth Analg 1998;86: 678.
44. Nevarre DR, Tzarnas CD. The effects of hyaluronidase on the efficacy and on the pain of administration of 1% lidocaine. Plast Reconstr Surg 1998; 101:365–9.
45. Bartfield JM, Sokaris SJ, Raccio-Robak N. Local anesthesia for lacerations: pain of infiltration inside vs outside the wound. Acad Emerg Med 1998;5:100–4.
46. Bartfield JM, Pauze D, Raccio-Robak N. The effect of order on pain of local anesthetic infiltration. Acad Emerg Med 1998;5:105– 7.
47. Colaric KB, Overton DT, Moore K. Pain reduction in lidocaine administration through buffering and warming. Am J Emerg Med 1998;16:353–6.
48. Machado HS, Bastos RS. Inadequate tourniquet inflation associated with a case of prilocaine toxicity. Eur J Anaesthesiol 1998;15:234-6.
49. Lang SA. Intravenous regional anesthesia. Anesth Analg 1998;86:1334–5.
50. Coleman M, Kelly DJ. Local anaesthetic toxicity in a pregnant patient undergoing lignocaine-induced intravenous regional anaesthesia. Acta Anaesthesiol Scand 1998;42:267–9.
51. Hamel P, Boghen D. Bilateral amaurosis following peribulbar anesthesia. Can J Ophthalmol 1998;33:216–18.
52. Dorey SE, Gillespie IH, Barton F, MacSweeney E. Magnetic resonance image changes following optic nerve trauma from peribulbar anaesthetic. Br J Ophthalmol 1998;82:586–7.
53. Belfort R Jr, Muccioli C. Hyphema after peribulbar anesthesia for cataract surgery in Fuchs' heterochromic iridocyclitis. Ocul Immunol Inflamm 1998;6:57–8.
54. Cadera W. Diplopia after peribulbar anesthesia for cataract surgery. J Pediatr Ophthalmol Strabismus 1998;35:240–1.
55. Liang C, Peyman GA, Sun G. Toxicity of intraocular lidocaine and bupivacaine. Am J Ophthalmol 1998;125:191–6.
56. Lawrenson JG, Edgar DF, Tanna GK, Gudgeon AC. Comparison of the tolerability and efficacy of unit-dose, preservative-free topical ocular anaesthetics. Ophthalmic Physiol Opt 1998;18:393–400.
57. Sugar A. Topical anesthetic abuse after radial keratotomy. J Cataract Refractive Surg 1998;24: 1535–7.
58. Masket S, Gokmen F. Efficacy and safety of intracameral lidocaine as a supplement to topical anesthesia. J Cataract Refractive Surg 1998;24: 956–60.
59. Martin RG, Miller JD, Cox CC 3rd, Ferrel SC, Raanan MG. Safety and efficacy of intracameral injections of unpreserved lidocaine to reduce intraocular sensation. J Cataract Refractive Surg 1998;24:961–3.
60. Hewitt T, Eadon H. Check long contact with Ametop. Pharm Pract 1998;8:47–8.
61. Wongprasartsuk P, Main BJ. Adverse local reactions to amethocaine cream—audit and case reports. Anaesth Intensive Care 1998;26:312–14.
62. Geraint M. Check long contact with Ametop. Pharm Pract 1998; 8:208.
63. Capron F, Perry D, Capolaghi B. Seizures and methemoglobinemia following use of prilocaine–lidocaine cream. Arch Pediatr 1998;5:812.
64. Ronnerfalt L, Fransson J, Wahlgren CF. EMLA cream provides rapid pain relief for the curettage of molluscum contagiosum in children with atopic dermatitis without causing serious application-site reactions. Pediatr Dermatol 1998;15:309–12.

65. Calobrisi SD, Drolet BA, Esterly NB. Petechial eruption after the application of EMLA cream. Pediatrics 1998;101:471–3.
66. Avery JK. Routine procedure—bad outcome. Tenn Med 1998;91:280–1.
67. Day RO, Chalmers DR, Williams KM, Campbell TJ. The death of a healthy volunteer in a human research project: implications for Australian clinical research. Med J Aust 1998;168:449–51.
68. Pantuck AJ, Goldsmith JW, Kuriyan JB, Weiss RE. Seizures after ureteral stone manipulation with lidocaine. J Urol 1997;157:2248.
69. McGrath PD, Moloney JF, Riker RR. Benzocaine- induced methemoglobinemia complicating transesophageal echocardiography: a case report. Echocardiography 1998;15:389–91.
70. Malhotra S, Kolda M, Nanda NC. Local anesthetic-induced methemoglobinemia during transesophageal echocardiography. Echocardiography 1998;15:165–7.
71. Ho RT, Nanevicz T, Yee R, Figueredo VM. Benzocaine-induced methemoglobinemia—two case reports related to transesophageal echocardiography premedication. Cardiovasc Drugs Ther 1998;12:311–12.
72. Fisher MA, Henry D, Gillam L, Chen C. Toxic methemoglobinemia: a rare but serious complication of transesophageal echocardiography. Can J Cardiol 1998;14:1157–60.
73. Yan AC, Newman RD. Bupivacaine-induced seizures and ventricular fibrillation in a 13-year-old girl undergoing wound debridement. Pediatr Emerg Care 1998;14:354–5.
74. Fujita Y, Endoh S, Yasukawa T, Sari A. Lidocaine increases the ventricular fibrillation threshold during bupivacaine-induced cardiotoxicity in pigs. Br J Anaesth 1998;80:218–22.
75. Adsan H, Tulunay M, Onaran O. The effects of verapamil and nimodipine on bupivacaine-induced cardiotoxicity in rats: an in vivo and in vitro study. Anesth Analg 1998;86:818–24.
76. Huang YF, Pryor ME, Mather LE, Veering BT. Cardiovascular and central nervous system effects of intravenous levobupivacaine and bupivacaine in sheep. Anesth Analg 1998;86:797–804.
77. Golub MS, Germann SL. Perinatal bupivacaine and infant behavior in rhesus monkeys. Neurotoxicol Teratol 1998;20:29–41.
78. Maher P. Methemoglobinemia: an unusual complication of topical anesthesia. Gastroenterol Nurs 1998;21:173–5.
79. Barnett P. Cocaine toxicity following dermal application of adrenaline-cocaine preparation. Pediatr Emerg Care 1998;14:280–1.
80. Ogawa S, Mikuni E, Nakamura T, Noda K, Ito S. Neurotoxicity of dibucaine on the isolated rabbit cervical vagus nerve. Jpn J Anesthesiol 1998;47: 439–46.
81. Lee A-Y. Allergic contact dermatitis from dibucaine in Proctosedyl ointment without cross-sensitivity. Contact Dermatitis 1998;39:261.
82. Urrutia I, Jauregui I, Gamboa P, Gonzalez G, Antepara I. Photocontact dermatitis from cinchocaine (dibucaine). Contact Dermatitis 1998;39: 139–40.
83. Engelhart DA, Lavins ES, Hazenstab CB, Sutheimer CA. Unusual death attributed to the combined effects of chloral hydrate, lidocaine, and nitrous oxide. J Anal Toxicol 1998;22:246–7.
84. Resar LM, Helfaer MA. Recurrent seizures in a neonate after lidocaine administration. J Perinatol 1998;18:193–5.
85. Lee VC, Moscicki JC, DiFazio CA. Propofol sedation produces dose-dependent suppression of lidocaine-induced seizures in rats. Anesth Analg 1998;86:652–7.
86. Kanai Y, Katsuki H, Takasaki M. Graded, irreversible changes in crayfish giant axon as manifestations of lidocaine neurotoxicity in vitro. Anesth Analg 1998;86:569–73.
87. Anibarro B, Seoane FJ. Adverse reaction to lidocaine. Allergy 1998;53:717–18.
88. Weightman W, Turner T. Allergic contact dermatitis from lignocaine: report of 29 cases and review of the literature. Contact Dermatitis 1998; 39:265–6.
89. Pettersson N, Emanuelsson BM, Reventlid H, Hahn RG. High-dose ropivacaine wound infiltration for pain relief after inguinal hernia repair: a clinical and pharmacokinetic evaluation. Reg Anesth Pain Med 1998;23:189–96.
90. Plowman AN, Bolsin S, Mather LE. Central nervous system toxicity attributable to epidural ropivacaine hydrochloride. Anaesth Intensive Care 1998;26:204–6.
91. Abouleish EI, Elias M, Nelson C. Ropivacaine-induced seizure after extradural anaesthesia. Br J Anaesth 1998;80:843–4.
92. Checketts MR, Wildsmith JA. Accidental i.v. injection of local anaesthetics: an avoidable event? Br J Anaesth 1998;80:710–11.

O. Zuzan and M. Leuwer

12 Neuromuscular blocking agents and skeletal muscle relaxants

GENERAL TOPICS

Risk factors The neuromuscular blocking effects of muscle relaxants in *patients with neuromuscular disorders* may differ significantly from those in healthy individuals. This can result in overdose and residual curarization on the one hand or in inadequate muscle relaxation on the other.

Patients with *Duchenne muscular dystrophy* often require surgery for contractures and kyphoscoliosis. The neuromuscular blocking effects of vecuronium in eight children with Duchenne muscular dystrophy (11–15 years old) have been compared with those in eight children (8–18 years old) without this disease (1[C]). After vecuronium 50 μg/kg, the median train-of-four ratio was 0.14 in the patients versus 0.86 in the controls. The median time for recovery of the train-of-four ratio from 0.1 to 0.25 was 36 minutes in the patients versus 6 minutes in the controls. The authors concluded that patients with Duchenne muscular dystrophy need smaller initial doses of vecuronium. Because of the increased recovery time, patients should be closely observed for signs of residual curarization. Monitoring of neuromuscular transmission is strongly recommended in all patients with neuromuscular disorders who are given neuromuscular blocking agents.

Use in pregnancy The pharmacokinetics of neuromuscular blocking agents in pregnancy and the impact on anesthesia for cesarean section have been reviewed (2[R]). Key statements are:

- The umbilical/maternal vein concentration ratio of non-depolarizing neuromuscular relaxants varies from 7 to 26%. Clinical doses of these drugs may induce partial curarization in neonates.
- Despite reduced plasma cholinesterase activity, the duration of the effect of succinylcholine 1 mg/kg is usually not significantly increased in pregnant women.
- At clinical doses, transplacental passage of succinylcholine is insufficient to produce paralysis of the neonate. However, inadequate muscular activity requiring ventilatory support has been reported in babies born to mothers with atypical plasma cholinesterase.

Interactions *Donepezil* has recently been approved for the treatment of Alzheimer's disease. It acts primarily as a reversible inhibitor of acetylcholinesterase with a half-life of over 70 hours. Prolonged paralysis lasting several hours and requiring postoperative mechanical ventilation in the intensive care unit has been reported after the use of succinylcholine in a patient taking long-term donepezil (3[c]).

An 85-year-old woman with a history of mild Alzheimer's disease and hypertension underwent abdominal hysterectomy. Anesthesia was induced with succinylcholine 100 mg and 40 minutes later pancuronium 2 mg. After 2 hours, when surgery was finished, train-of-four stimulation elicited three twitches, and neostigmine 5 mg plus glycopyrrolate 1 mg was given to reverse neuromuscular block. She was subsequently able to follow commands and was breathing adequately; four twitches were observed during train-of-four stimulation. Several minutes after extubation she became apneic and had to be reintubated. Further neostigmine 1 mg was given, but neuromuscular block persisted without any response to peripheral nerve stimulation. In a blood sample taken 60 minutes after the second dose

Side Effects of Drugs, Annual 23
J.K. Aronson, ed.

of neostigmine plasma cholinesterase activity was 2.1 (reference range 7.1–19 U/ml). The dibucaine number was 45 (reference range 81–87%), and the fluoride number was 84 (44–54%).

The authors of this report subsequently tested the effect of donepezil on plasma cholinesterase activity in vitro. Supratherapeutic concentrations (0.02 mg/ml) reduced plasma cholinesterase activity to 53% of the baseline. Dibucaine and fluoride numbers were not affected by neostigmine or donepezil. Others have shown previously that therapeutic doses of donepezil inhibit acetylcholinesterase by 64% (4). The authors of the present report suggested that the prolonged paralysis in this case had been due to the combined effects of atypical plasma cholinesterase and the additional inhibition of plasma cholinesterase activity by donepezil. Unfortunately, preoperative plasma cholinesterase activity was not known and low cholinesterase activity was detected under the influence of neostigmine, which inhibits both plasma cholinesterase and acetylcholinesterase. Because a very high dose of neostigmine resulted in the intensification rather than the reversal of neuromuscular block, an overdose of neostigmine may have caused the paradoxical neuromuscular block (5[R]). Hypothetically, a paradoxical block is a combination of desensitization and open channel block (SED-13, 298). So the additional dose of neostigmine should have been omitted. In addition, an excess of acetylcholine at the end- plate might have been the result of a combined inhibition of acetylcholinesterase by both donezepil and neostigmine. Until more is known, neostigmine and other cholinesterase inhibitors should be used with caution in patients taking donepezil.

DEPOLARIZING NEUROMUSCULAR BLOCKING AGENTS

Succinylcholine

Mineral and fluid balance Life-threatening *hyperkalemia* is a known adverse effect of succinylcholine in patients with severe burns.

Extrajunctional spread of acetylcholine receptors and expression of the immature type of these receptors with prolonged channel opening times have been shown after burns. This is believed to produce a massive potassium release after succinylcholine administration. As the increase in acetylcholine receptor density on the muscle surface takes some time to develop, there should be an interval after the accident during which succinylcholine can be safely given. However, the length of this interval is controversial. Referring to a lack of reports of hyperkalemic complications during the first week after the injury, it has been has suggested that succinylcholine can be given safely during the first 6–7 days after major thermal injury (6). However, based on the results of animal experiments, succinylcholine might be safe for up to 48 hours after the injury only (7). It was recommended that succinylcholine should be avoided beyond that time.

Cases of hyperkalemic cardiac arrest associated with succinylcholine in patients treated in intensive care units continue to be reported (8[c]). The exact mechanism is not known, but extrajunctional spread of acetylcholine receptors is believed to play a major role. It is strongly recommended that succinylcholine should not be given to patients who have been immobilized in the intensive care unit for more than a few days.

Special senses Succinylcholine can cause *increased intraocular pressure*. The most reliable technique to avoid this adverse effect during succinylcholine-assisted endotracheal intubation is to provide a deep level of anesthesia. Combining an intravenous anesthetic with a rapid- onset opioid, such as alfentanil, prevents increases in intraocular pressure (9[C]). This has again been demonstrated when the ultra-short acting opioid remifentanil (1 μg/kg) was given in combination with propofol (2 mg/kg) and succinylcholine (1 mg/kg) for endotracheal intubation during induction of anesthesia (10[C]). With this technique the highest intraocular pressure recorded was 18 mmHg, whereas peak values up to 35 mmHg occurred in the control group without remifentanil.

NON-DEPOLARIZING NEUROMUSCULAR BLOCKING AGENTS

Musculoskeletal Masseter muscle *rigidity is a rare but potentially dangerous adverse effect of succinylcholine* and may prevent successful airway management. Furthermore, it may be the first sign of malignant hyperthermia and rhabdomyolysis. Non-depolarizing neuromuscular blocking agents are thought to be safe with regard to masseter muscle rigidity. However, a recent report has illustrated the fact that masseter muscle rigidity not associated with the use of succinylcholine may also complicate airway management (11[c]).

A 42-year-old woman had anesthesia induced with propofol 200 mg, vecuronium 8 mg, and mask ventilation with oxygen, nitrous oxide, and 2% isoflurane. Laryngoscopy proved impossible because of spasm of the masseter muscles, and the airway was secured by blind nasal intubation. There was no evidence of rigidity of other muscle groups. Body temperature and end-tidal carbon dioxide concentration remained in the reference ranges. Masseter muscle rigidity persisted throughout the operation and resolved during recovery from anesthesia after neostigmine 2.5 mg had been given.

The authors suggested that in this case the phenomenon had been caused by vecuronium. Masseter muscle rigidity persisted during anesthesia and resolved during recovery from anesthesia after neostigmine had been given and isoflurane inhalation had been stopped. If vecuronium caused muscle rigidity in this case it was probably not mediated by effects on acetylcholine receptors, but rather by an interaction of vecuronium with ion channels (sodium, potassium and/or calcium), but it is hard to imagine how this effect could have been antagonized by a cholinesterase inhibitor. It therefore seems likely that the masseter muscle rigidity was rather caused by isoflurane, which would explain why the symptoms improved after withdrawal of isoflurane. There have been previous reports of masseter muscle rigidity associated with non-depolarizing neuromuscular blocking agents (SEDA-21, 144; 12[c], 13[c]). The mechanism is unclear. One wonders how muscle specimens from these patients might react to exposure to an inhalational anesthetic during in vitro contracture testing. Regarding the link between masseter muscle rigidity and malignant hyperthermia, muscle biopsy would not be inappropriate in patients who have masseter muscle rigidity severe enough to prevent mouth opening and conventional orotracheal intubation.

Special senses Neonates with congenital diaphragmatic hernia often develop respiratory failure. To facilitate mechanical ventilation, neuromuscular blocking agents may be used. *Sensorineural hearing loss* can occur in survivors, with a reported incidence of up to 60%. Recently, sensorineural hearing loss has been associated with the use of pancuronium. In a historical cohort study of 37 survivors of congenital diaphragmatic hernia, children with hearing loss had received significantly higher doses of pancuronium during respiratory failure than children without hearing loss (14[C]). In addition, the cumulative dose of pancuronium correlated with the intensity of hearing loss in decibels. There were no differences with regard to oxygenation and ventilation parameters or to the cumulative dose of aminoglycosides, vancomycin, or furosemide, but children with hearing loss had received a higher cumulative dose of ethacrynic acid. The authors admitted that the retrospective study design and the small sample size demanded cautious interpretation of their observations. For the time being, this report is not reason enough to avoid pancuronium if neuromuscular blockade is required. However, it should be remembered that the risk of severe neuromuscular disturbances associated with long-term administration of neuromuscular blocking agents militates against the routine use of these drugs in patients in intensive care, both children and adults. If muscle relaxants are given in this setting for more than a few hours their effect should be monitored by a peripheral nerve stimulator to avoid overdose and drug accumulation. This may prove technically difficult in neonates.

Risk factors Mivacurium has a short duration of action, because it is hydrolyzed by plasma cholinesterase. When a dose of mivacurium is injected a variable portion is inactivated before it reaches the neuromuscular junction. In *patients with very low plasma cholinesterase activity*, larger amounts of active molecules diffuse into the synaptic cleft. Consequently, the mivacurium concentration in the target compartment has a higher initial peak and takes longer to fall below a concentration that allows neuromuscular transmission. As a result, the duration of action of mivacurium is significantly prolonged in such patients. This is especially true in patients with atypical cholinesterase, who may experience profound block up to several hours duration after standard doses of mivacurium. This is a particular problem if mivacurium is used for ambulatory anesthesia, after which the patient is expected to return home, since facilities for postoperative ventilatory support may not be available. As patients with atypical cholinesterase are usually not detected by preoperative screening, it has been suggested that the patient's response to mivacurium should be tested by using a very low initial dose. However, complete paralysis for nearly 5 hours has recently been observed after a test dose of mivacurium 14 μg/kg in a patient with atypical serum cholinesterase as diagnosed by standard phenotyping and DNA sequencing (15[c]). The authors concluded that neuromuscular monitoring and facilities for long- term ventilation should always be available when mivacurium is used.

SKELETAL MUSCLE RELAXANTS

Baclofen

Musculoskeletal With regard to its effects on spinal GABA receptors, intrathecal baclofen has been compared with intrathecal fentanyl for postoperative pain treatment in six children (mean age 4.2 years) with cerebral palsy undergoing bilateral dorsal rhizotomy (16[c]). Both intrathecal baclofen and intrathecal fentanyl reduced postoperative pain. However, three of five children had severe *muscle weakness* after intrathecal baclofen 1–1.5 μg/kg, which prompted the authors to discontinue their study. An accompanying editorial dealt with the possible mechanisms of action of spinal GABA agonists on postoperative pain, suggesting that the effects on sensory processing probably cannot be separated from the changes in motor function (17[r]). Therefore, this report of muscle weakness should not prompt us to close the file on intrathecal baclofen for pain treatment. More experience is needed and different dose regimens should be tested.

Risk factors Baclofen is also used for the treatment of intractable hiccups, especially in patients with uremia. As 70% of baclofen is excreted unchanged in the urine (18), accumulation and overdosage of baclofen are a well-known problem in *patients with end-stage renal disease*. Confusion, drowsiness, and coma after standard doses have been reported (19[c]). Even very small doses can cause altered consciousness (20[c]). In addition, abdominal pain was a common adverse effect of baclofen in patients with severe renal insufficiency (20[c]). Symptoms usually resolve with dialysis (19[c], 20[c]).

Withdrawal effects Baclofen is a GABA receptor agonist used in the treatment of spinal spasticity. Like many other agents that act at the GABA receptor, abrupt termination of long-term administration can result in withdrawal symptoms. A dramatic example of life-threatening withdrawal symptoms occurred in a patient after continuous administration of intrathecal baclofen (21[c]). Another case due to intrathecal catheter malfunction showed some similarities (22[c]). As the clinical picture may resemble the neuroleptic malignant syndrome and malignant hyperthermia, the use of dantrolene has been suggested as an additional therapeutic option (22[c]), but there is only limited experience with dantrolene for the treatment of baclofen withdrawal (23[c]). A case of brain death due to baclofen withdrawal with severe hypotension and hyperthermia up to 43°C has underscored the need for immediate and aggressive treatment (24[c]). Clinicians should be suspicious of baclofen withdrawal if patients taking baclofen present with fever, muscle cramps, and hypotension. With regard to the risk of rhabdomyolysis, disseminated intravascular coagulation, acute renal insufficiency, and other organ complications, patients should be transferred to the intensive care unit and should be given parenteral baclofen.

Botulinum toxin

Musculoskeletal *Exacerbation of muscle weakness* by botulinum toxin in patients with myasthenic syndromes has been a theoretical concern. A recent example has shown that clinically relevant symptoms can occur (25[c]).

An 80-year-old woman had severe difficulty in swallowing and flaccid paralysis of her cervical muscles starting 4 days after the periocular injection of botulinum toxin (120 mouse LD50 units) for blepharospasm. She also developed bilateral facial nerve paralysis and slurred speech and could not fully close her eyes. Barium swallow and fluoroscopy showed signs of aspiration. The serum concentration of anti-acetylcholine receptor antibodies was 6.9 units (reference range 0–0.7 units). Mestinone and prednisone improved her symptoms. She had been treated with botulinum toxin on 18 occasions over the previous 13 years without any untoward effects.

While the exact cause of muscle weakness is unclear, this case militates against the use of botulinum toxin in patients with myasthenic syndromes. When the margin of safety is reduced with regard to neuromuscular transmission, botulinum toxin can result in increased morbidity or even mortality. Generalized muscle weakness after botulinum toxin has also been reported in patients with other neuromuscular disorders (26[c]). In addition, it should be remembered that both dysphagia and muscle weakness can occur after botulinum toxin injection, even in patients who do not suffer from generalized neuromuscular disorders (27[c]).

Carisoprodol

The spasmolytic effect of carisoprodol is thought to be due to interruption of neuronal communication within the reticular formation and spinal cord. Major adverse effects are *sedation* and *drowsiness*. Carisoprodol is a precursor of meprobamate, an oral anxiolytic with similarities to benzodiazepines. Consequently, *drug dependence* is a clinically relevant problem. Among patients who had taken carisoprodol for 3 months or more, up to 40% had used it in amounts larger than prescribed, and up to 30% had used it for an effect other than that for which it was prescribed (28[C]). A significant percentage of physicians were unaware of the potential of carisoprodol for abuse and of its metabolism to meprobamate. Patients with carisoprodol *withdrawal* can present with *agitation, restlessness, hallucinations, seizures, anorexia, and vomiting.*

Overdosage Carisoprodol overdose is reportedly rarely fatal. However, a review of the deaths examined at the Jefferson County Medical Examiner Office from 1986 to 1997 revealed 24 cases of carisoprodol overdosage (29[C]). In all of these 24 cases, other co-intoxicants were involved. Since the mechanism of death was *respiratory depression* in 82% of the cases, the authors suggested that carisoprodol had contributed to the fatal outcome. Carisoprodol can cause respiratory depression, and carisoprodol overdosage should be regarded as potentially fatal if other respiratory depressants add to the effect. Carisoprodol intoxication can also be associated with symptoms of CNS overactivity rather than CNS depression. *Agitation and myoclonic movement disorders* have been observed (30[cr]).

REFERENCES

1. Ririe DG, Shapiro F, Sethna NF. The response of patients with Duchenne's muscular dystrophy to neuromuscular blockade with vecuronium. Anesthesiology 1998;88:351–4.
2. Guay J, Grenier Y, Varin F. Clinical pharmacokinetics of neuromuscular relaxants in pregnancy. Clin Pharmacokinet 1998;34:483–96.
3. Sprung J, Castellani WJ, Srinivasan V, Udayashankar S. The effects of donepezil and neostigmine in a patient with unusual pseudocholinesterase activity. Anesth Analg 1998;87:1203–5.
4. Friedhoff LT, Rogers SL. Correlation between the clinical efficacy of donepezil HCl (E2020) and red-blood cell (RBC) acetylcholinesterase (ACHE) inhibition in patients with Alzheimer's disease. Clin Pharmacol Ther 1997;61:177.
5. Bevan DR, Donati F, Kopman AF. Reversal of neuromuscular blockade. Anesthesiology 1992; 77:785–805.
6. Gronert GA. Succinylcholine hyperkalemia after burns. Anesthesiology 1999;91:320–2.
7. Martyn JA. Succinylcholine hyperkalemia after burns. Anesthesiology 1999;91:321–2.
8. Biccard BM, Grant IS, Wright DJ, Nimmo SR, Hughes M. Suxamethonium and critical illness polyneuropathy. Anaesth Intensive Care 1998; 26:590–1.
9. Zimmerman AA, Funk KJ, Tidwell JL. Propofol and alfentanil prevent the increase in intraocular pressure caused by succinylcholine and endotracheal intubation during a rapid sequence induction of anesthesia. Anesth Analg 1996;83:814–17.
10. Alexander R, Hill R, Lipham WJ, Weatherwax KJ, El-Moalem HE. Remifentanil prevents an increase in intraocular pressure after succinylcholine and tracheal intubation. Br J Anaesth 1998;81:606–7.
11. Jenkins JG. Masseter muscle rigidity after vecuronium. Eur J Anaesthesiol 1999;16:137–9.
12. Polta TA, Hanisch EC Jr, Nasser JG, Ramsborg GC, Roelofs RI. Masseter spasm after pancuronium. Anesth Analg 1980;59:509–11.
13. Albrecht A, Wedel DJ, Gronert GA. Masseter muscle rigidity and nondepolarizing neuromuscular blocking agents. Mayo Clin Proc 1997;72:329–32.

14. Cheung PY, Tyebkhan JM, Peliowski A, Ainsworth W, Robertson CM. Prolonged use of pancuronium bromide and sensorineural hearing loss in childhood survivors of congenital diaphragmatic hernia. J Pediatr 1999;135:233–9.
15. Vanlinthout LE, Bartels CF, Lockridge O, Callens K, Booij LH. Prolonged paralysis after a test dose of mivacurium in a patient with atypical serum cholinesterase. Anesth Analg 1998;87:1199–202.
16. Soliman IE, Park TS, Berkelhamer MC. Transient paralysis after intrathecal bolus of baclofen for the treatment of post- selective dorsal rhizotomy pain in children. Anesth Analg 1999;89:1233–5.
17. Yaksh TL. A drug has to do what a drug has to do. Anesth Analg 1999;89:1075–7.
18. Faigle JW, Keberle H, Degen PH. Chemistry and pharmacokinetics of baclofen. In: Feldman RG, Young RR, Koella WP, editors. Spasticity: Disordered Motor Control. Chicago: Year Book, 1980:461–75.
19. Peces R, Navascues RA, Baltar J, Laures AS, Alvarez-Grande J. Baclofen neurotoxicity in chronic haemodialysis patients with hiccups. Nephrol Dial Transplant 1998;13:1896–7.
20. Chen K-S, Bullard MJ, Chien Y-Y, Lee S-Y. Baclofen toxicity in patients with severely impaired renal function. Ann Pharmacother 1997;31:1315–20.
21. Sampathkumar P, Scanlon PD, Plevak DJ. Baclofen withdrawal presenting as multiorgan system failure. Anesth Analg 1998;87:562- -3.
22. Reeves RK, Stolp-Smith KA, Christopherson MW. Hyperthermia, rhabdomyolysis, and disseminated intravascular coagulation associated with baclofen pump catheter failure. Arch Phys Med Rehabil 1998;79:353–6.
23. Khorasani A, Peruzzi WT. Dantrolene treatment for abrupt intrathecal baclofen withdrawal. Anesth Analg 1995;80:1054–6.
24. Green LB, Nelson VS. Death after acute withdrawal of intrathecal baclofen: case report and literature review. Arch Phys Med Rehabil 1999; 80:1600–4.
25. Borodic G. Myasthenic crisis after botulinum toxin. Lancet 1998;352:1832.
26. Mezaki T, Kaji R, Kohara N, Kimura J. Development of general weakness in a patient with amyotrophic lateral sclerosis after focal botulinum toxin injection. Neurology 1996;46:845–6.
27. Bakheit AMO, Ward CD, McLellan DL. Generalised botulism-like syndrome after intramuscular injections of botulinum toxin type A: a report of two cases. J Neurol Neurosurg Psychiatry 1997;62:198.
28. Reeves RR, Carter OS, Pinkofsky HB, Struve FA, Bennett DM. Carisoprodol (soma): abuse potential and physician unawareness. J Addict Dis 1999;18:51–6.
29. Davis GG, Alexander CB. A review of carisoprodol deaths in Jefferson County, Alabama. South Med J 1998;91:726–30.
30. Roth BA, Vinson DR, Kim S. Carisoprodol- induced myoclonic encephalopathy. J Toxicol Clin Toxicol 1998;36:609–12.

Michael Schachter

13 Drugs affecting autonomic functions or the extrapyramidal system

In most years there is no predominant theme as regards the adverse effects considered in this chapter. However, that is not the case this year. There has been remarkable interest in the toxicity – and of course also the efficacy – of dopamine-mimetic drugs especially in the context of Parkinson's disease. This topic forms by far the largest part of this chapter.

SYMPATHOMIMETIC DRUGS

Drugs stimulating both α- and β-adrenoceptors

Despite the very extensive non-prescribed use of ephedrine and pseudoephedrine, reports of cutaneous adverse reactions are comparatively rare. However, *fixed drug reactions* have been described and a case report from Ankara describes a solitary eruption in the groin of a 10-year-old boy given pseudoephedrine 60 mg/day; rechallenge with the drug was positive (1[c]).

Generalized skin reactions are even less frequent. A group of allergy specialists in Madrid have described two cases of *generalized dermatitis* with dissimilar histological findings in men aged 64 and 73 years (2[cr]). In one case there was severe eczema, in the other the rarer vacuolar interface dermatitis. Both patients had taken a proprietary formulation containing codeine and chlorpheniramine as well as pseudoephedrine. Oral challenges with the former two drugs was negative in both cases, but was positive for pseudoephedrine in one patient; the other was not rechallenged, because of the severity of the original reaction.

Drugs predominantly stimulating α-adrenoceptors

Phenylephrine is seldom given systemically but is still commonly used as a mydriatic for both diagnostic and therapeutic purposes. Both local and systemic adverse reactions are rare. However, a case report from Zurich has described *acute periorbital dermatitis and conjunctivitis* in a 69-year-old man given phenylephrine 5% eye-drops for ophthalmological examination (3[c]). Subsequent patch testing was strongly positive for phenylephrine eye-drops. A much more serious systemic reaction to the drops has been described in 2-month-old child given perioperative phenylephrine drops during cataract extraction (4[cr]). She developed *ventricular extra beats,* very severe *hypertension,* and *pulmonary edema* requiring intensive therapy. Extubation was possible within 3 hours and she recovered with untoward consequences. The authors commented that changes in arterial blood pressure are well described with phenylephrine eye-drops, especially in infants. Clearly precise dosage is difficult in these very young patients and they suggested that microdrops might be a safer mode of administration.

There have been responses to last year's report of *transient neurological symptoms* occurring after the addition of phenylephrine to tetracaine spinal anesthesia. It was suggested, for example, that sodium bisulfite, a preservative in the phenylephrine injection, may have been responsible for the observed toxicity (5[r]). However, the original authors rejected this, since the dose of bisulfite was small and since there is uncertain evidence whether the compound is neurotoxic in any case. Another correspondent

Side Effects of Drugs, Annual 23
J.K. Aronson, ed.

commented that tetracaine itself may be more toxic than other local anesthetics: the authors did not address this point in their reply (6[r]).

Drugs predominantly stimulating β_1-adrenoceptors

The continuing, and probably increasing, use of dobutamine stress echocardiography and perfusion scintigraphy means that the safety of this procedure attracts attention. A study from Rotterdam has examined the consequences of adding atropine to dobutamine in 200 patients with impaired left ventricular function (ejection fraction less than 35%) (7[C]). There were *cardiac dysrhythmias* in 6% of patients and significant *hypotension* in 11%, figures comparable to those in other published studies. In the 36 patients who required atropine to achieve target heart rates the incidence of adverse effects was not increased. The same group has studied over 1000 consecutive patients undergoing dobutamine stress scintigraphic imaging of the myocardium (8[C]). In these patients the incidence of dysrhythmias was about 8%, of whom about half had transient ventricular tachycardia, but only about 3% had significant hypotension (defined as a fall in systolic blood pressure of 40 mmHg). Atropine was required in nearly 40% of the patients in order to achieve target heart rates, but it is difficult to determine whether this had any influence on the occurrence of adverse effects.

A report from the Mayo Clinic has described 27 elderly patients (mean age 71 years) with aortic stenosis in whom dobutamine stress hemodynamic testing was used to assess the severity of the stenosis (9[Cr]). There were no severe adverse effects, but relatively minor problems occurred in 16 patients, *including chest pain* and *ventricular extra beats* (nine each) and *atrial dysrhythmias* (4). The authors concluded that the procedure appears to be safe in these high-risk patients, although its diagnostic value may be limited.

LEVODOPA AND DRUGS STIMULATING DOPAMINE RECEPTORS

Levodopa

Ever since the introduction of levodopa as the mainstay of antiparkinsonian therapy, there has been concern that it may be toxic, causing long-term damage to dopamine neurons. Three recent reviews have addressed this question in the light of experimental and clinical evidence over the last 30 years. One reviewer concluded that there is no evidence for irreversible levodopa-induced damage in man, only for reversible adverse effects associated with neuronal dysfunction but not neuronal death (10[R]). Others reached broadly the same conclusion, although they noted that there is in vitro evidence of damage associated with oxidative metabolism of levodopa (11[R]). They also described potential toxicity from levodopa in animals in which the nigrostriatal pathway is already damaged by other means. A third reviewer has pointed out that levodopa therapy is an entirely non-physiological means of dopamine replacement, arguing that the intermittent nature of the dopaminergic stimulus provided by most therapies, particularly levodopa, predisposes to motor complications (12[R]). He suggested that more continuous activation of dopamine receptors could minimize or eliminate these problems. The management of the complications of antiparkinsonian therapy forms a very significant focus for research. A group from the National Hospital for Neurology in London has described the use of continuous subcutaneous apomorphine infusions in 19 parkinsonian patients with severe unpredictable motor fluctuations while taking levodopa (13[Cr]). The objective was to replace levodopa during waking hours with apomorphine monotherapy. During apomorphine treatment ranging from 9 months to nearly 8 years, there was a 65% reduction in dyskinesia severity and an 85% reduction in frequency and duration, with a 70% reduction in the 'off' time. Nearly half the patients stopped taking levodopa altogether.

A less radical and much less expensive approach to the management of motor fluctuations has been described in 14 patients with advanced Parkinson's disease and levodopa-induced motor disorders (14[C]). Amantadine (mean dose 350 mg/day) reduced the severity and duration of dyskinesias by 33–75%, depending on the parameter measured. The rationale was that amantadine blocked *N*-methyl-D-aspartate receptors.

An interesting case report has drawn attention to the fact that severe response fluctuations can occur soon after the start of treatment in patients with severe disease (15[c]). Two men aged 76 and 72 years presented with advanced symptoms of Parkinson's disease and were treated with levodopa. Disabling dyskinesia occurred within days of reaching maintenance dosages of levodopa (1–1.5 g/day with benserazide). Clearly, the disease status of the patients was the determinant for this adverse reaction, not the duration of levodopa therapy.

In a review of the neuropsychiatric symptoms of Parkinson's disease and their management, it has been pointed out that nearly half of all parkinsonian patients are demented or have significant cognitive impairment (16[R]). These patients are particularly susceptible to delirium induced by levodopa and other antiparkinsonian drugs. The author recommended dosage reduction or elimination of drugs that may be responsible, starting with anticholinergic drugs but leaving levodopa unchanged if possible. He also recommended the use of the atypical neuroleptic drugs clozapine or olanzapine in severely disturbed patients in whom drug withdrawal is not feasible.

Other dopaminergic drugs

The ergot derivatives are pharmacologically interesting because of their numerous receptor interactions, but this also makes them difficult and sometimes hazardous to use. In a general review of drug-induced pleural disease it has been noted that *pleural thickening* and *effusions* may be present in up to 6% of patients treated with bromocriptine for Parkinson's disease, and that this is related to duration of exposure and cumulative dose (17[R]). The author recommended drug withdrawal in these patients. However, this does not always lead to complete resolution of the lesions (18[c]).

A 63-year-old woman with Parkinson's disease developed bilateral pleural thickening and effusions with interstitial shadowing in the lungs 4 years after starting treatment with bromocriptine. After replacement of the drug by levodopa there was gradual improvement, but some pleural thickening remained nearly 3 years later.

Other pharmacological properties of the ergot derivatives may have even more serious consequences, including *myocardial infarction* (19[c]).

A 29-year-old woman was given bromocriptine 5 mg/day postpartum to suppress lactation. Four days later she was admitted with an acute anterior myocardial infarction. Angiography showed dissection of the left main and anterior descending arteries, with occlusion of the latter. She recovered after emergency arterial grafting.

The authors speculated that bromocriptine may have caused coronary spasm. In another similar case the myocardial infarction proved fatal (20[c]).

A 30-year-old woman collapsed and died after a first dose of bromocriptine 2.5 mg. She had severe atheroma narrowing the right coronary artery proximal to the site of thrombosis. The only obvious risk factor was heavy smoking, 30 cigarettes per day.

Vasoconstriction due to ergot derivatives can also affect the cerebral circulation under similar circumstances (21[c]).

A 33-year-old woman was discharged from hospital after a normal delivery taking lisuride 0.2 mg/day for suppression of lactation. Within a day she complained of throbbing headache, which was followed by right hemiparesis and then a generalized tonic-clonic seizure starting from the right arm. She had widespread segmental vasoconstriction in the cerebral arteries and two intracerebral hemorrhages. She recovered fully within a month.

The authors commented that there have been at least seven cases in the literature of postpartum ergot-related angiopathy with bromocriptine and ergonovine. The Parkinson's Disease Research Group of the UK have reviewed their earlier report that there was excess mortality in patients with early disease treated with a combination of levodopa and the selective monoamine oxidase B inhibitor selegiline (22[Cr]). They have confirmed that there was about a 35% greater mortality in those on combined treatment compared with patients treated with levodopa alone. The excess deaths were all attributed to Parkinson's disease. The authors did not present any explanation for these findings but very reasonably suggested that the combination is inappropriate in early disease and should be used only with caution if at all in the later stages of the disease.

THE ERGOT ALKALOIDS AND RELATED DRUGS

An extraordinary report form Germany has described a 78-year-old woman who developed *gangrene* in three finger-tips on the right hand and two on the left after being given dihydroergotamine 10 mg/day as migraine prophylaxis

(23[c]). She had had Raynaud's syndrome for at least the previous 5 years and was thought to have a relatively mild from of systemic sclerosis. Comment is superfluous.

Methysergide is another drug whose use for migraine prophylaxis is declining and should soon be virtually non-existent, given its tendency to cause *retroperitoneal fibrosis* (24[R]). For any patients who still take it two hematologists have recommended a programme of 3-monthly monitoring, including clinical examination, plasma electrolytes, full blood count, and erythrocyte sedimentation rate. They have suggested that methysergide should be discontinued if any abnormalities emerge, and also concur with the widespread practice of 'drug holidays' for 3–6 months, although these are not of proven value. Despite the paper's title, the management of established fibrosis is not described, and indeed there is no treatment of proven value.

AGENTS WITH CHOLINERGIC EFFECTS

Acetylcholinesterase inhibitors

(see also Chapter 1)

A report from Madrid has described severe *urticaria* and *anaphylaxis* associated with pyridostigmine (an unspecified dose) in 54-year-old woman with myasthenia gravis (25[c]). Urticaria started almost immediately after introduction of the drug but was partially controlled by the antihistamine cetirizine. However, pyridostigmine was stopped after 2 months and the urticaria resolved completely. She was rechallenged with oral pyridostigmine, leading to an anaphylactic reaction that was treated with subcutaneous adrenaline. There were no sequelae.

AGENTS WITH ANTICHOLINERGIC EFFECTS

Reports of both new and predictable adverse effects involving anticholinergic drugs used for bladder detrusor instability continue to appear. For the first time oxybutynin, one of the most widely used of these drugs, has been described as precipitating *acute angle closure glaucoma* (26[c]). The 80-year-old woman, who was taking 2.5 mg bd, did not suffer permanent visual impairment, despite the very high intraocular pressure (56 mmHg) initially found in the affected eye.

Neuropsychiatric adverse effects seem to pose a greater problem with oxybutynin. A group of pharmacologists involved in pharmacovigilance have described five spontaneous reports of *night terrors* associated with oxybutinin (27[c]). Four were children, aged 5–8 years, being treated for enuresis, and the fifth was a 77-year-old woman with incontinence. Total daily doses were 8–12 mg in the children and 10 mg in the elderly woman: these are all towards the upper end of the recommended ranges. The efficacy and safety of oxybutynin 15 mg/day has been compared with the newer anticholinergic agent tolterodine 4 mg/day in a randomized, double-blind, placebo-controlled parallel group study in 293 patients (28[C]). The efficacies were generally similar but twice as many patients taking oxybutynin withdrew because of adverse effects (17 vs 8%). *Dry mouth* was by far the most frequent adverse effect, reported by 86% of patients taking oxybutynin and 50% of those taking tolterodine. Although there was still an excess of adverse effects after halving the dose of oxybutynin, it would not be normal practice to start treatment with this drug in a dose as high as 15 mg/day.

Jimson weed is a naturally occurring plant that is ingested to induce hallucinogenic effects. Toxicity after ingestion is due to an atropine-containing alkaloid that is present in all parts of the plant but is particularly concentrated in the seeds. Eleven patients aged 13–21 years ingested large quantities of Jimson weed pods and seeds (29). The signs and symptoms were classical of atropine poisoning. In milder cases there was asymptomatic *mydriasis* and *tachycardia* and in the more severely affected *agitation, disorientation,* and *hallucinations.* Nine of the 11 were admitted for observation. None died and none required pharmacological intervention with physostigmine to reverse the anticholinergic symptoms.

REFERENCES

1. Hindioglu U, Sahin S. Nonpigmenting solitary fixed drug eruption caused by pseudoephedrine hydrochloride. J Am Acad Dermatol 1998;38:499–500.
2. Vega F, Rosales MJ, Esteve P, Morcillo R, Panizo C, Rodriguez M. Histopathology of dermatitis due to pseudoephedrine. Allergy 1998;53:218–20.
3. Wigger-Alberti W, Elsner P, WĄthrich B. Allergic contact dermatitis to phenylephrine. Allergy 1998;53:217–18.
4. Greher M, Hartmann T, Winkler M, Zimpfer M, Crabnor CM. Hypertension and pulmonary edema associated with subconjunctival phenylephrine in a 2-month-old child during cataract extraction. Anesthesiology 1998;88:1394–6.
5. Tanaka M, Nishikawa T. Is phenylephrine or sodium bisulfite neurotoxic? Anesthesiology 1998;89:272–3.
6. Lambert DH. Transient neurologic symptoms when phenylephrine is added to tetracaine spinal anesthesia – an alternative. Anesthesiology 1998;89:273.
7. Poldermans D, Rambaldi R, Bax JJ, Cornel JH, Thomson IR, Valkema R, Boersma E, Fioretti PM, Breburda CSM, Roelandt JRTC. Safety and utility of atropine addition during dobutamine stress echocardiography for the assessment of viable myocardium in patients with severe left ventricular dysfunction. Eur Heart J 1998;19:1712–18.
8. Elhendy A, Valkema R, Van Domburg RT, Bax JJ, Nierop PR, Cornel JH, Geleijnse ML, Reijs AEM, Krenning EP, Roelandt JRTC. Safety of dobutamine-atropine stress myocardial perfusion scintigraphy. J Nucl Med 1998;39:1662–6.
9. Lin SS, Roger VL, Pascoe R, Seward JB, Pellikka PA. Dobutamine stress Doppler hemodynamics in a patients with aortic stenosis: feasibility, safety, and surgical correlations. Am Heart J 1998;136:1010–16.
10. Agid Y. Levodopa. Is toxicity a myth? Neurology 1998;50:858–63.
11. Jenner PG, Brin MF. Levodopa neurotoxicity. Experimental studies versus clinical relevance. Neurology 1998;50(Suppl 6):S39–43.
12. Chase TN. Levodopa therapy: consequences of the nonphysiologic replacement of dopamine. Neurology 1998;50(Suppl 5):S17–25.
13. Colzi A, Turner K, Lees AJ. Continuous subcutaneous waking day apomorphine in the long term treatment of levodopa induced interdose dyskinesias in Parkinson's disease. J Neurol Neurosurg Psychiatry 1998;64:573–6.
14. Metman LV, Del Sotto P, Van Den Munckhof P, Fang J, Mouradian MM, Chase TN. Amantadine as treatment for dyskinesias and motor fluctuations in Parkinson's disease. Neurology 1998;50:1323–6.
15. Onofri M, Paci C, Thomas A. Sudden appearance of invalidating dyskinesia-dystonia and off fluctuations after the introduction of levodopa in two dopaminomimetic drug naïve patients with stage IV Parkinson's disease. J Neurol Neurosurg Psychiatry 1998;65:605–6.
16. Lieberman A. Managing the neuropsychiatric complications of Parkinson's disease. Neurology 1998;50(Suppl 6):S33–9.
17. Antony VB. Drug-induced pleural disease. Clin Chest Med 1998;19:331–40.
18. Comet R, Domingo C, Such JJ, Ribera G, Sans J, Marin A. Pleuropulmonary disease as a side-effect of treatment with bromocriptine. Respir Med 1998;92:1172–4.
19. Hoppe UC, Beuckelmann DJ, Böhm M, Erdmann E. A young mother with severe chest pain. Heart 1998;79:205.
20. Dutt S, Wong F, Spurway JH. Fatal myocardial infarction associated with bromocriptine for postpartum lactation suppression. Aust NZ J Obstet Gynaecol 1998;38:116–17.
21. Roh JK, Park KS. Postpartum cerebral angiopathy with intracerebral hemorrhage in a patient receiving lisuride. Neurology 1998;50:1152–4.
22. Ben-Shlomo Y, Churchyard A, Head J, Hurwitz B, Overstall P, Ockelford J, Lees AJ. Investigation by Parkinson's Disease Research Group of United Kingdom into excess mortality seen with combined levodopa and selegiline treatment in patients with early, mild Parkinson's disease: further results of randomised trial and confidential inquiry. Br Med J 1998;316:1191–6.
23. Hahne T, Balda B-R Fingerkuppennekrosen nach Dihydroergotaminmedikation bei limitierter systemischer Sklerodermie. Hautarzt 1998;49:722–4.
24. Bucci JA, Manoharan A. The management and monitoring of methysergide-induced fibrosis. Headache Q 1998;9:321–5.
25. Castellano A, Cabrera M, Robledo T, Martinez-Cócera C, Cimarra M, Llamazares AA, Chamorro M. Anaphylaxis by pyridostigmine. Allergy 1998; 53:1108–9.
26. Sung VCT, Corridan PG. Acute angle-closure glaucoma as a side-effect of oxybutynin. Br J Urol 1998;81:634–5.
27. Valsecia ME, Malgor LA, Espindola JH, Carauni DH. New adverse effect of oxybutynin: 'night terror'. Ann Pharmacother 1998;32:506.
28. Abrams P, Freeman R, Anderström C, Mattiasson A. Tolterodine, a new antimuscarinic agent: as effective but better tolerated than oxybutynin in patients with an overactive bladder. Br J Urol 1998;81:801–10.
29. Tiongson J, Salen P. Mass ingestion of Jimson weed by eleven teenagers. Del Med J 1998;70:471–6.

Sibylle Schliemann-Willers, Andrea Bauer and Peter Elsner

14 Dermatological drugs, topical agents, and cosmetics

CONTACT ALLERGY

Recent single reports of 'new' or rare contact allergens are listed in Table 1.

Contact allergy in the anogenital region

Allergic contact dermatitis is a common anogenital disease. Predominant complaints are itching and burning. Scratching, mainly at night, and lichenification can lead to painful erosions. Topical medicaments, body-care products, popular remedies, and sanitary products are the main sources of contact allergens in the genitoanal area.

Epidemiology *During 1992–7, 1008 patients with anogenital complaints (2% of the whole test population of 54 500 patients) were patch tested in the departments of dermatology of the Information Network of Dermatological Clinics (IVDK). The standard series recommended by the German Contact Dermatitis Research Group (DKG) was tested in 978 of these patients. Other specific allergens were tested according to each patient's history. In most cases topical drugs, ointment bases, and preservatives were included, and in 466 cases patients' own products were patch tested too. In 351 patients (35%) the final diagnosis of allergic contact dermatitis was confirmed (19[CR]). Similar numbers were reported from the UK, where 201 women with anogenital dermatoses were diagnosed in a contact dermatitis clinic over 14 years. In 79 cases (39%) the diagnosis of allergic contact dermatitis was confirmed by patch tests with the European standard series, a medicament series, a corticosteroid series, and the patients' own medicaments if necessary (20[CR]). In another UK study, 39 of 135 patients tested (29%) with persisting vulval symptoms had relevant contact hypersensitivity (21[CR]). There is evidence that the vulval region and the perianal region should be considered separately, since patients with dermatoses only involving the vulva have positive patch tests less often than patients with dermatoses on the vulva and the perianal area or patients who have only perianal involvement (20[CR]).*

Relevant allergens and sources *The most frequent allergens in the study of the IVDK are listed in Table 2a, and Table 2b gives information about the patch test results obtained with topical drugs, ointment bases, and preservatives.*

Although the spectrum is comparable to that of all patients tested between 1992 and 1997, there are some allergens of pronounced significance for the anogenital region. Dibucaine HCl ranked fourth among contact allergens in this region. Furthermore, there were more positive patch test results to (chloro)methylisothiazolinone (CMI/MI) and to benzocaine among patients with anogenital complaints compared with the whole test population (19[CR]).

Topical medicaments and their ingredients, especially local anesthetics play an important role in anogenital contact allergy (19[CR]–23[CR]). Dibucaine is commonly used in topical antihemorrhoidal formulations and is a well-known sensitizer (24[CR]). Although benzocaine is not as widely used in topical anesthetic formulations in Germany, patients with anogenital dermatitis were at higher risk of sensitization. Amied-type local anaesthetics, like lidocaine HCl and tetracaine, are less potent sensitizers (25[R]). Contact allergy to local anesthetics is more often observed among patients with perianal complaints than patients with perianal and vulval or only vulval dermatitis (20[CR]).

Side Effects of Drugs, Annual 23
J.K. Aronson, ed.

Table 1. *Contact allergy to ingredients of topical drugs and cosmetics*

Ingredient	Use and vehicle	Concentration	No.	Comments	Reference
4-amino-3-nitrophenol	Hair dye	2% petrolatum	1	First report of contact allergy in a customer, 10 controls negative	(1[Cr])
Anethole	Toothpaste	5% petrolatum	1	Cheilitis, perioral eczema, stomatitis, and temporary loss of taste	(2[Cr])
Benzophenone-2	Toilet water	2% petrolatum	1	Rare contact allergen; also used as sunscreen; adequate controls: no photopatch tests	(3[Cr])
Dorzolamide	Eyedrops	0.01–10% aqua and petrolatum	1	First report of contact allergy; relatively new treatment for glaucoma; related to sulfonamides; adequate controls	(4[Cr])
Ethyl diglycol (carbitol) Chitosan gluconate	Ointment	Unknown	1	Carbitols are used in cosmetics, lacquers, varnishes, and cleaners; rare contact allergens	(5[Cr])
Krameria triandra (red rhatany)	Antihemorrhoidal gel, herbal medicine	1% petrolatum 2% ethanol	1	Contact dermatitis of the perianal region, perineum, inner buttocks and thighs; dried root of the plant is used in herbal medicine; rare contact allergen; 20 controls negative	(6[Cr])
Matricaria chamomilla (German chamomile)	Topical compress	1%	1	Allergic contact dermatitis; also positive to sesquiterpene lactone mix; no reaction to Anthemis nobilis (Roman chamomile); systemic contact dermatitis after tea ingestion	(7[Cr])
Methyl butetisalicylate	Analgesic cream	30% petrolatum	1	Contact allergy to salicylates is rare; the patient tolerated oral aspirin; 15 controls were negative	(8[Cr])
Minoxidil	Hair restorer Hydroalcoholic solution	2% ethanol	1	First report of pustular allergic contact dermatitis, confirmed by biopsy	(9[cR])
Myrrh	Essential oil used as herbal medicine for wound healing	Unknown	1	Positive patch test to myrrh solution and myrrh powder; no controls; probably unreliable report	(10[Cr])
Neo-ballistol®	Herbal remedy containing anise oil	1%	1	Generalized dermatitis after topical application	(11[Cr])
Phenylephrine	Eyedrops	1% petrolatum	1	Persistent patch test reaction for 2 months; seven controls negative	(12[Cr])
Polyoxyethylene oleylether	Non-ionic surfactant in antipruritic ointment	1% petrolatum	1	Rare allergen; positive test reactions also to cosmetic compounds and diphenhydramine (active compound of ointment)	(13[c])
PVP/hexadecene co-polymer	Skin-care product	5% petrolatum	1	First report of contact dermatitis; no controls; probably unreliable report	(14[cr])

Table 1. *Continued*

Ingredient	Use and vehicle	Concentration	No.	Comments	Reference
Prednicarbate	Topical corticosteroid in Dermatop®	10% ethanol 1% ethanol	1	Positive patch test to hydocortisone-17-butyrate and triamcinolone	(15[Cr])
Quaternium-22 Shellac	Mascara	0.1 and 0.01% aqua 20% ethanol	1	First report of contact allergy to quaternium-22; 23 controls negative	(16[Cr])
Spearmint oil	Toothpaste	5% petrolatum	1	Cheilitis; rare contact allergen; relevant ingredient seems to be carvone (SEDA-20, 156)	(17[Cr])
Spearmint oil	Toothpaste	1% petrolatum	1	Perioral contact dermatitis; positive patch test reaction to L-carvone 0.27 and 0.067%	(18[Cr])

Topical antibiotics are often used in the treatment of dermatitis with bacterial superinfection. However, in Germany sensitization to the aminoglycoside antibiotic neomycin was less frequent in patients with anogenital dermatitis (19[CR]) compared with the UK, where 15 out of 79 patients with positive patch tests and anogenital complaints were positive to neomycin (20[CR]). Framycetin contact sensitivity was frequent in the UK, partly through cross-reactivity with neomycin (21[CR]).

Another relevant substance in hemorrhoidal formulations is bufexamac, a non-steroidal anti-inflammatory drug that is a well-known sensitizer and which sometimes elicits severe dermatitis (26[CR]). Therefore, bufexamac should always be included in patch tests for anogenital dermatitis.

Corticosteroid contact allergy is well known (SEDA-21, 158–160) and has to be particularly suspected in chronic conditions affecting the perianal area (20[CR]), after long-term topical medication, and in cases of failure to ameliorate dermatitis with corticosteroids. Patch tests should then be performed both with the recommended markers budesonide (0.1% petrolatum) and tixocortol pivalate (1% petrolatum) and with the patient's own formulations.

Antifungal drugs are comparatively rare contact allergens in the anogenital region in relation to their widespread use. Clotrimazole and nystatin are preferred. In the study of the IVDK, patch tests with clotrimazole were performed in only 272 patients, leading to five positive reactions (19[CR]). In the UK study on anogenital dermatoses, five women out of 201 patients tested had positive reactions to antifungal drugs, which were unfortunately not specified in the article (20[CR]). If sensitization to nystatin is suspected, polyethylene glycol should be used as a vehicle for patch testing (27[CR]). Imidazoles may cross-react with one another (SEDA-20, 156). Most cases of contact allergy occurred with miconazole, econazole, tioconazole, and isoconazole (28[R]).

Moist toilet paper is a rare source of contact allergens. The most relevant allergens in moist toilet paper are preservatives like (chloro)methylisothiazolinone (CMI/MI) and dibromoglutaronitril + 2-phenoxyethanol (Euxyl K 400) (29[CR]–31[CR]). These substances were also relevant in the study of the IVDK (19[CR]), and are also found in bodycare products. In Germany, MCI/MI was recently replaced by iodopropyl butylcarbamate (IPBC) in moist toilet paper. A single case of contact allergy to IPBC has already been described (32[CR]). Other sources of preservatives are topical medicaments and bodycare products. Parabens, chloracetamide, and formaldehyde-releasing preservatives, like diazolidinyl urea, imidazolidinyl urea, bronopol, and quaternium 15, should also be considered (19[CR]).

Ointment bases do not seem to cause contact allergy in the anogenital region too frequently, in spite of their wide use. Wool wax alcohol and amerchol L-101 are the ones of most importance (19[CR], 20[CR]). Relevant contact sensitivity to balsam of Peru and fragrance mix is not infrequent and reflects the ubiquitous presence of these substances (21[CR]).

Topical remedies are very popular in self-treatment and patients will often not report this, since these formulations are not regarded as medicaments. Furthermore, patients often do not suspect that 'natural' remedies cause

Table 2a. *The most frequent allergens among patients with anogenital complaints*

Allergen	Number tested	Number with a a positive reaction (%)	Number with a positive reaction (% std)	IVDK total 1992–7 (% std)
Nickel sulfate	962	86 (8.9)	12.6	16–17
Balsam of Peru	962	74 (7.7)	6.6	6.5–8
Fragrance mix	960	71 (7.4)	7.2	10–13
Dibucaine HCl (cinchocaine HCl)	592	50 (8.4)	7.4	*
Thimerosal	961	48 (5.0)	5.6	5–7
Methyldibromo glutaronitrile/ 2-phenoxyethanol	958	39 (4.1)	3.1	2–3
Para-phenylenediamine	959	39 (4.1)	3.7	4–5.5
(Chloro)methyliso-thiazolinone (CMI/MI)	951	32 (3.4)	3.7	~2.5
Benzocaine	962	31 (3.2)	2.7	~1.5
Phenylmercuric acetate	736	28 (3.8)	4.0	4–8
Neomycin sulfate	962	23 (2.4)	2.1	~2.5
Wool wax alcohol	962	22 (2.3)	2.1	2.5–4
Amerchol L-101	561	21 (3.7)	2.9	*
Colophony (rosin)	961	19 (2.0)	2.3	2.5–3.5
Mercury amide chloride (ammoniated mercury)	962	19 (2.0)	1.7	~2.5
Propolis	598	17 (2.8)	2.5	*
Paraben mix	962	17 (1.8)	1.6	~1.5
Benzoylperoxide	218	15 (6.9)	7.6	*
Octylgallate	560	15 (2.7)	2.8	*
Methyldibromo-glutaronitrile	508	14 (2.8)	2.1	*
Cobalt chloride	960	13 (1.4)	2.0	4.5–5
Propylene glycol	744	12 (1.6)	1.5	*
Formaldehyde	961	12 (1.2)	1.5	~2
Hexylresorcinol	476	11 (2.3)	2.1	*
Para-tert-butylphenol formaldehyde resin (PTBP-FR)	955	11 (1.2)	1.4	~1
Thiuram mix	961	11 (1.1)	1.1	~2.5

Source: IVDK 1992–7 (n = 1008) (19[CR])
All allergens that led to positive reactions in more than 1% of the total population (i.e. 10 patients) are listed.
Column 3 shows the percentage of positive reactions.
Column 4 shows the age- and sex-standardized frequency of sensitization.
Column 5 shows the range of the age- and sex-standardized frequency of sensitization in all patients tested (n = 54.500).
std. = standardized.
* Allergens were tested in selected patients only; so a comparison in this way makes no sense.

adverse effects. Some substances lead to a considerable number of allergic reactions, for example chamomile extract and tincture of Arnica montana (19[CR]). Propolis also has pronounced sensitizing capacity (33[CR]), and sensitization to aged tee tree oil is being reported with increasing frequency (34[CR]). Contact allergy from rubber additives in condoms might be suspected in some cases, and there are anecdotal reports (35[CR]). However, in the study of the IVDK, condoms were suspected and patch tested in 17 patients without positive results (19[CR]).

Although sensitization to nickel sulfate is common in patients with anogenital contact dermatitis and in patients with dermatitis in other body sites, the relevance to anogenital complaints of sensitization to nickel sulfate should always be doubted (19[CR], 21[CR], 36[CR]). However, direct transmission of nickel between the hands and the anogenital region has to be

Table 2b. *Patch test results obtained with topical drugs, ointment bases, and preservatives*

Allergen	Test formulation	Number tested	Number with a positive reaction (%)
Bufexamac	5% petrolatum	534	9 (1.7)
Framycetin sulfate	20% petrolatum	268	7 (2.6)
Lidocaine HCl	15% petrolatum	524	6 (1.1)
Tincture of Arnica montana	20% petrolatum	241	5 (2.1)
Clotrimazole	5% petrolatum	272	5 (1.8)
Iodochlorhydroxyquin (clioquinol)	5% petrolatum	303	5 (1.7)
Chamomile extract	2.5% petrolatum	173	5 (2.9)
Tetracaine HCl (amethocaine HCl)	1% petrolatum	306	4 (1.3)
Panthenol	5% petrolatum	323	4 (1.2)
Chloramphenicol	10% petrolatum	244	3 (1.2)
Mafenide	10% petrolatum	299	3 (1.0)
Tert-butyl hydroquinone	1% petrolatum	710	8 (1.1)
Benzalkonium chloride	0.1% petrolatum	740	8 (1.1)
Bronopol	0.5% petrolatum	728	7 (1.0)
Chloroacetamide	0.2% petrolatum	743	7 (0.9)

All allergens are listed which led to positive reactions in at least 1% of the patients tested (19[CR]).

taken into account, and food may be a rare source of nickel contact in the anogenital area. In these cases relevance can be proved by oral nickel provocation and a nickel-restricted diet for a limited period may be justified (37[R]).

Conclusions *Contact allergy should always be suspected in patients with anogenital dermatitis, especially if the perianal area is involved. In patients with other chronic inflammatory diseases of the anogenital region, e.g. lichen sclerosus, contact allergy should also be excluded, since long-term use of topical medicaments on compromised skin carries an increased risk of sensitization. Patch tests in patients with anogenital eczema should include the standard series, dibucaine HCl, propolis, bufexamac, and further ingredients of topical formulations according to the patient's history. In cases of doubt, the repeated open application test (ROAT) is recommended. Patients should be advised to apply the suspected product three times a day for 3 days to an area of healthy skin on measuring 5 × 5 cm the flexural site of the forearm (38[CR]).*

Antimicrobial drugs

Antimicrobial drugs are widely used in topical medicaments, cosmetics, household products, and industrial biocides. Depending on their concentrations, they can function as disinfectants, antiseptics, or preservatives. Two recent articles have given insights into the current prevalence and rank order of sensitization to antimicrobial allergens in Europe (39[CR], 40[CR]). The most frequent antimicrobial allergens in 8521 patients who were patch tested between 1985 and 1997 in Belgium are given in Table 3 (40[CR]). In a multicenter study of the Information Network of Departments of Dermatology, sensitization rates of preservatives in the standard series were all over 1% in the test population of 11 485 patients. Thiomersal was rating highest (5.3%), chloromethyl-isothiazolinone/methyisothiazolinone, formaldehyde, and methyl-dibromo-glutaronitrile/phenoxyethanol were next at about 2%, and parabens rating lowest at 1.6%. Glutaraldehyde, a biocide mainly used as a disinfectant, showed a remarkable increase in sensitization from less than 1% in 1990 up to more than 4% at the end of 1994. Health personnel and cleaning personnel were often affected and showed a sensitization rate of 10% (39[CR], 41[CR]).

Cystamine bislactamide: a cosmetic allergen

Cystamine bislactamide is a new synthetic compound, obtained from cystamine and lactic acid molecules linked by disulfide bridges, that was for the first time incorporated into skincare products in Autumn 1996. The compound has recently been reported to be a cause of al-

Table 3. *Most frequent antimicrobial allergens in Belgium out of 8521 patients between 1985–97 (40[CR])*

Rank	Allergen	Number
1	Methyl(chloro)isothiazolinone	143*
2	Thimerosal	136
3	Merbromine	94
4	Iodine	89
5	Cetrimide	88
6	Formaldehyde	80
7	Parabens	71
8	Chloramine	43
9	Quaternium-15	32
10	Nitrofurazone	29
11	Quinoline mix	28
12	Benzyl alcohol	25
	Benzoic acid	25
	Thiocyanomethylbenzothiazole	25
	Chlorhexidine	25
13	Glutaraldehyde	22
	Methyldibromoglutaronitrile + phenoxyethanol	22
14	Chloroacetamide	20
	Diazolidinyl urea	20

* Methyl(chloro)isothiazolinone was not tested until 1987.

lergic contact dermatitis of the eyelids or face. Patch tests in 14 women with suspected contact dermatitis of the face were performed with the cosmetic product and its components; there were positive reactions to cystamine bislactamide 0.2% in water in eight of these patients, while 10 controls were negative (42[Cr]).

Formaldehyde-releasing preservatives

Formaldehyde-releasing preservatives, such as quaternium-15, diazolidinyl urea, and imidazolidinyl urea, are widely used in cosmetics and topical medications and are well-known contact sensitizers. In spite of positive patch test reactions to these preservatives in a number of patients, only some of these patients will react when they use the corresponding commercial formulations. This is because the concentrations of preservatives in the commercial products are often below the threshold necessary to produce a clinical reaction. This finding confirms the importance of using commercial formulations of topical agents in estimating the clinical relevance of patch test results (43[CR]).

The formaldehyde concentration in patch testing, which has been lowered to 1% in the standard series in recent years, has been studied in a comparison of concentrations of 1 and 2% in 3734 consecutively patch-tested patients. Since there was no significant difference between 1 and 2% formaldehyde with respect to the frequency of positive patch test reactions, while there were more irritant reactions with 2%, a 1% patch test concentration can still be recommended (44[Cr]).

Tea tree oil *(SEDA-18, 170)*

Herbal remedies, especially tea tree oil, which is extracted from *Melaleuca alternifolia*, are becoming increasingly popular. Tea tree oil is supposed to be valuable in a variety of skin conditions, including wounds, infections, eczema, and psoriasis, and has been increasingly incorporated into cosmetics for aromatherapy. Since the beginning of the 1990s, several case reports of allergic contact dermatitis have been published. Most of these adverse effects emerged after the application of aged tea tree oil. In a review on tea tree oil focussing on the allergic compounds in detail, the authors concluded that d-limonen, α-terpenes, and the aromadendrens are important allergens, whereas 1,8-cineole was not believed to be important, as has been previously stated (45[CR]). More recently it has been confirmed that tea tree oil undergoes photo-oxidation within a few days to several months, leading to degradation products, such as peroxides, epoxides and endoperoxides, which were shown to be moderate to strong sensitizers. Experimental sensitization in guinea-pigs was performed, followed by patch tests with 15 constituents of oxidized tea tree oil in 11 patients with tea tree oil contact dermatitis. The degradation products were measured by gas chromatography. All the patients reacted to α-terpinene, terpinolene, and ascaridol, the latter being a deterioration product of α-terpinene (34[CR]).

Wound dressings

Patients with chronic venous insufficiency and venous leg ulcers are at risk of sensitization to topical medications. The frequency of sensitization in these patients is up to 67% (46[CR]). In a recent study using an expanded European standard series and 20 different wound dressings for patch testing in 36 patients with chronic venous insufficiency, sensitization to modern wound dressings was found in 8.3% (three cases) and was caused by propylene glycol as an ingredient of hydrogels (47[CR]). However, it must be emphasized that positive patch test reactions to propylene glycol may indicate irritation rather than contact allergy. There were no cases of sensitization to hydrocolloids, alginates, or polyurethane foams. The rank order of allergens was headed by ointment bases (sensitization to wool wax alcohols in 33% of patients; amerchol 19%; cetearyl alcohol 14%; propylene glycol 8.3%), followed by plant resins/ ethereal oils (balsam of Peru 22%; colophony 14%; fragrance mix 8.3%; propolis 5.6%), and topical antibiotics (neomycin sulfate 17%; chloramphenicol 14%) (48[CR]).

CONTACT URTICARIA AND IMMEDIATE CONTACT REACTIONS

Chlorhexidine

Chlorhexidine is widely used as a medical disinfectant and as a preservative in various topical products, including cosmetics. Anaphylaxis is a well-known but rare event, in most cases occurring after contact to mucous membranes or wounds.

Severe *anaphylaxis* with respiratory arrest and immeasurable blood pressure has recently been reported in a man with excoriated dermatitis after he had used 0.05% chlorhexidine in a whole body bath (49[cr]). A 14-year-old girl had combined delayed and immediate types of allergy, with *urticarial* rash and *syncope*, after long-term use of an antiacne formulation containing chlorhexidine in an unknown concentration. In both cases epicutaneous tests with 1% chlorhexidine gluconate and acetate, and prick tests with 0.05 and 0.01% of the acetate solution were positive (50[Cr]).

Caution seems also to be warranted concerning polyhexanide, a chlorhexidine polymer, used in disinfectants for a relatively short time. This disinfectant was reported to have caused severe *anaphylaxis* in two young patients (51[Cr]). Both were exposed to the disinfectant Lavasept®, containing polyhexanide, on surgical wounds during orthopedic interventions. They had never been exposed to polyhexanide before, but had been exposed to chlorhexidine. However, skin prick tests were positive for polyhexanide in both cases, while chlorhexidine was negative. Negative skin prick tests to polyhexanide were obtained from controls.

Protein hydrolysates in cosmetics

Protein hydrolysates are added to hair-care products, such as shampoos and conditioners, and are supposed to 'repair' damaged hair. Hydrolysed proteins are also used in other body-care products, for example soaps, bath gels, and creams. Occasionally single reports of contact urticaria and of allergic contact dermatitis due to hair conditioner and skin cleanser have been published (SEDA-21, 166; 52[cr]). Protein hydrolysates used in hair-care products have now been tested in 11 hairdressers with hand dermatitis, in 2160 consecutive adults with suspected respiratory disease, and in 28 adults with chronic atopic dermatitis (53[CR]). The hairdressers underwent both scratch tests (1% aqueous) and patch tests (5% aqueous) with 22 protein hydrolysates (collagen, keratin, elastin, milk, wheat, almond, silk). Skin prick tests with one to three hydrolysates (1% aqueous) were conducted in the other patients. All 2199 patients were tested with hydroxypropyl trimonium hydrolized collagen (Crotein Q®). There were positive scratch/prick test reactions in 12 patients to three protein hydrolysates. Remarkably, all were women with atopic dermatitis. They reacted at least to hydroxypropyl trimonium hydrolized collagen (Crotein Q®) and 11 had positive reactions to one or more allergens in a standard prick series. In three patients clinical relevance could be confirmed by open tests with both undiluted and diluted hair conditioner containing Crotein Q® (one hairdresser with contact urticaria on the hands, two cases of contact uricaria on the head, face, and upper body). Furthermore, in seven of eight sera studied, specific IgE antibodies to Crotein Q® were detected, while 11 control sera were negative. These results show that protein hydrolysates in hair-care products may be underestimated causes of contact urticaria, particularly in patients with atopy.

Rifamycin SV

Rifamycin SV, a semisynthetic macrocyclic antibiotic derived from natural rifamycin B, has been used for years in the therapy of tuberculosis and in some European countries

Table 4. *Recent single reports of photosensitivity reactions*

Ingredient	Product/function	Test procedure	Clinical symptoms/comments	Reference
Cinchocaine (dibucaine)	Antihaemorrhoidal	Ultra Vitalux lamp with window glass to exclude UVB irradiation	Photocontact dermatitis in the perineal area, extending to the legs and arms; rare photoallergen; no controls	(56[Cr])
Diphenhydramine hydrochloride	1% diphenhydramine ointment	UVA 4.85 J/m^2	Photoallergic contact dermatitis continuing for 2 years	(57[Cr])
Fepradinol	Spray, NSAID	UVA 10 J/m^2	First report of photoallergic contact dermatitis; report probably unreliable	(58[Cr])
5-Methoxypsoralen	Bergamot aromatherapy oil	Unknown	Phototoxic eruption in a child with blistering after a body bath	(59[Cr])

as a topical antibiotic. *Anaphylaxis* has been reported after systemic administration, but it is supposed to be extremely rare after topical application. However, in Turkey two cases of severe anaphylaxis have been reported in patients with infected wounds (54[cr]). In both cases the wounds had been treated with topical rifamycin for several months before the patients experienced urticaria, angioedema, and hypotension in one case, and urticaria, wheezing, dyspnea, and hypotensive shock in the other case. In both cases prick tests with 10% rifamycin SV solution were positive, while there were no positive reactions in 20 controls.

PHOTOCONTACT DERMATITIS

Photosensitive reactions to antimicrobial drugs, including topical agents, have been reviewed (55[R]).

Recent single reports of photosensitivity due to 'new' or rare substances are listed in Table 4.

Antihistamines

Phenothiazine antihistamines can cause photoallergy followed by long-lasting photosensitivity. Recently, a photoallergic contact dermatitis followed by persistent light reaction was reported from topical dioxopromethazine hydrochloride incorporated into a gel used for the first time in a woman with periocular pruritus. Photosensitivity in sun exposed areas where she had not applied the formulation persisted for up to 500 days, with a reduced minimal erythema dose (MED) for UVA together with abnormal delayed infiltrated reactions to UVB in repeated phototests (60[cr]).

Non-steroidal anti-inflammatory drugs (NSAIDs) *(SEDA-17, 187; SEDA-18, 163; SEDA-22, 170)*

Topical NSAIDs can cause allergic, photoallergic, and phototoxic contact dermatitis. There have recently been two systematic studies of photosensitivity to these compounds and their crossreactivity (61[CR], 62[CR]). Eleven patients with confirmed photocontact dermatitis were photopatch tested with seven topical NSAIDs. Ketoprofen was the commonest cause. In five cases there was cross-sensitivity with fenofibrate, which was explained by a common benzoylketone or benzophenone molecule, and in one patient there was cross-sensitivity to tiaprofenic acid, an arylpropionic acid derivate that is not available in topical form in Europe. There was also one case of photocontact dermatitis from diclofenac, which was discovered by 1% dilution in alcohol, while 5% in petrolatum was negative in the same patient (61[CR]). In contrast to these findings, all 12 patients tested in another study reacted to both ketoprofen and tiaprofen acid, mainly after UVA irradiation, but they were negative to other arylpropionic acids (62[CR]). Furthermore, there were positive reactions to both ketoprofen and fenofibrate in eight of the 12 patients. The authors concluded that photoallergy to ketoprofen and fenofibrate is due to the molecular benzophenone structure and confirmed cross-reactivity with other benzophenones which are used as sunscreens. The cross-reactivity between ketoprofen and tiaprofenic acid was supposed to be due to the benzophenone moiety of ketoprofen, or to the very similar thiophene-phenylketone part of tiaprofenic acid, but not to their arylpropionic function.

Sunscreens *(SEDA-18, 174; SEDA-22, 170)*

A recent article has focussed on photopatch testing with sunscreens in Sweden (63[CR]). Between 1990 and 1996, 355 patients with suspected photosensitivity were photopatch tested with seven sunscreen allergens (benzophenone-3 (Eusolex 4360), isopropyldibenzoylmethane (Eusolex 8020), butylmethoydibenzoylmethane (Parsol 1789), octylmethoxycinnamate (Parsol MCX), PABA, phenylbenzimidazole sulfonic acid (Eusolex 232), 4-methylbenzylidene camphor (Eusolex 6300); 2% petrolatum). There were 42 allergic reactions in 28 patients. The most common allergen was benzophenone-3 (Eusolex 4360), with 15 photocontact and one contact allergic reaction, followed by eight photocontact and four allergic contact reactions to isopropyl dibenzoylmethane (Eusolex 8020). In six cases photocontact reactions were due to butylmethoydibenzoylmethane (Parsol 1789). Phenylbenzimidazole sulfonic acid (Eusolex 232) caused two cases of photocontact allergy, and benzophenone-3 caused contact urticaria in one patient (63[CR]). There was a similar frequency of photocontact dermatitis to Eusolex 4360, Eusolex 8020, and Parsol 1789 in an Italian study, in which nine of 36 patients had positive reactions when photopatch tested with sunscreens (UVA 10 J/m^2) (64[Cr]).

MISCELLANEOUS ADVERSE EFFECTS

Imiquimod

Imiquimod is a new addition to a class of drugs regarded as immune response modifiers. Topical formulations containing 5% of the active substance are used for the treatment of external genital and perianal warts. As imiquimod-treated warts regress, serum concentrations of interferon-α, interferon-β, interferon-γ, and tumor necrosis factor rise (65[C]). Several randomized double-blind studies on the efficacy and adverse effects of imiquimod have been published recently (66[CR], 67[CR], 68[Cr]). Local adverse effects due to irritation were common, and included *erythema*, *erosions*, *excoriation*, *flaking*, *edema*, *scabbing*, and *induration*. Mild to moderate irritation has to be expected in up to 70% of patients if a 5% imiquimod cream is applied three times per week (67[CR]).

Nitrogen mustard *(SEDA-22, 172)*

Topical nitrogen mustard (mechlorethamine) is used in the early stages of mycosis fungoides. The most common adverse reaction is allergic contact dermatitis. Furthermore, nitrogen mustard can act as a tumor promotor. In most cases squamous cell carcinomas and basal cell carcinomas were reported. Recently two cases of small malignant melanoma, 3 mm in diameter, have been reported in patients with mycosis fungoides stage 1a, with latency intervals of 18 and 10 months after cessation of local application, which had been conducted for 18 months and almost 3 years respectively (69[c]).

REFERENCES

1. Blanco R, De la Hoz B, Sanchez-Fernandez C, Sanchez-Cano M. Allergy to 4-amino-3-nitrophenol in a hair dye. Contact Dermatitis 1998;39:136.
2. Franks A. Contact allergy to anethole in toothpaste associated with loss of taste. Contact Dermatitis 1998; 38:354–5.
3. Jacobs MC. Contact allergy to benzophenone-2 in toilet water. Contact Dermatitis 1998;39:42.
4. Aalto-Korte K. Contact allergy to dorzolamide eyedrops. Contact Dermatitis 1998;39:206.
5. Pereira F, Pereira C, Lacerda MH. Contact dermatitis due to a cream containing chitin and a carbitol. Contact Dermatitis 1998;38:290–1.
6. Bujan JG, Morante J, Bayona I, Güemes M, Arechavala R. Allergic contact dermatitis from *Krameria triandra* extract. Contact Dermatitis 1998;38:120–1.
7. Rodriguez-Serna M, JM Sanchez-Motilla, Ramon R, Aliaga A. Allergic and systemic contact dermatitis from *Matricaria chamomilla* tea. Contact Dermatitis 1998;39:192–3.
8. Valsecci R, Aiolfi M, Leghissa P, Cologni L, Cortinovis R. Contact dermatitis from methyl butetisalicylate. Contact Dermatitis 1998;38:360–1.
9. Sanche-Motilla JM, Pont V, Nagore E, Rodriguez-Serna M, Sanchez JL, Aliaga A. Pustular

allergic contact dermatitis from minoxidil. Contact Dermatitis 1998;38:283–4.
10. Al-Suwaidan SN, Gad El Rab MO, Al-Fakhiry S, Al Hoqail IA, Al-Maziad A, Sherif AB. Allergic contact dermatitis from myrrh, a topical herbal medicine used to promote healing. Contact Dermatitis 1998;39: 137.
11. Sigl B. Kontaktallergie auf Neo-Ballistol. Dermatosen 1998;46:170–2.
12. Rafael M, Pereira F, Faria MA. Allergic contact blepharoconjunctivitis caused by phenylephrine, associated with persistent patch test reaction. Contact Dermatitis 1998;39:143–4.
13. Itoh M, Kantoh H, Fukuzawa M, Kurikawa Y. A case of contact dermatitis due to Restamin ointment. J Med Soc Toho Univ 1998;45:518–22.
14. Scheman A, Cummins R. Contact allergy to PVP/hexadecene copolymer. Contact Dermatitis 1998;39:201.
15. Kim HJ, Lim YS, Choi HY, K.B. M. A case of allergic contact dermatitis due to Dermatop ointment and Plancollotion. Korean J Dermatol 1998;36:460–463.
16. Scheman A. Contact allergy to quaternium-22 and shellac in mascara. Contact Dermatitis 1998;38:342–3.
17. Skrebova N, Brocks K, Karlsmark T. Allergic contact cheilitis from spearmint oil. Contact Dermatitis 1998;39:35.
18. Worm M, Jeep S, Sterry W, Zuberbier T. Perioral contact dermatitis caused by L-carvone in toothpaste. Contact Dermatitis 1998;38:338.
19. Bauer A, Geier J, Elsner P. Allergic contact dermatitis in patients with anogenital complaints. J Reprod Med 2000;45:649–54.
20. Goldsmith PC, Rycroft RJ, White IR, Ridley CM, Neill SM, McFadden JP. Contact sensitivity in women with anogenital dermatoses. Contact Dermatitis 1997;36:174–5.
21. Marren P, Wojnarowska F, Powell S. Allergic contact dermatitis and vulvar dermatoses. Br J Dermatol 1992;126:52–6.
22. Brenan JA, Dennerstein GJ, Sfameni SF, Drinkwater P, Marin G, Scurry JP. Evaluation of patch testing in patients with chronic vulvar symptoms. Australas J Dermatol 1996;37:40–3.
23. Lewis FM, Harrington CI, Gawkrodger DJ. Contact sensitivity in pruritus vulvae: a common and manageable problem. Contact Dermatitis 1994;31:264–5.
24. Wilkinson JD, Andersen KE, Lahti A, Rycroft RJ, Shaw S, White IR. Preliminary patch testing with 25% and 15% 'caine'-mixes. The EECDRG. Contact Dermatitis 1990;22:244–5.
25. Fisher A. Contact dermatitis. Third edition. Philadelphia: Lea & Febiger, 1995.
26. Bauer A, Greif C, Gebhardt M, Elsner P. A severe epicutaneous test reaction to bufexamacina hemorrhoidal therapeutic preparation. Dtsch Med Wochenschr 1999;124:1168–70.
27. De Groot A, Conemans J. Nystatin allergy. Petrolatum is not the optimal vehicle for patch testing. Clin Dermatol 1990;8:153–5.
28. Dooms-Goossens A, Matura M, Drieghe J, Degreef H. Contact allergy to imidazoles used as antimycotic agents. Contact Dermatitis 1995;33:73–7.
29. De Groot AC, Van Ginkel CJ, Weijland JW. Methyldibromoglutaronitrile (Euxyl K 400): an important 'new' allergen in cosmetics. J Am Acad Dermatol 1996;35(5 Pt 1):743–7.
30. Van Ginkel CJ, Rundervoort GJ. Increasing incidence of contact allergy to the new preservative 1,2-dibromo-2,4-dicyanobutane (methyldibromoglutaronitrile). Br J Dermatol 1995;132:918–20.
31. Blecher P, Korting HC. Tolerance to different toilet paper preparations: toxicological and allergological aspects. Dermatology 1995;191:299–304.
32. Bryld LE, Agner T, Rastogi SC, Menne T. Iodopropynyl butylcarbamate: a new contact allergen. Contact Dermatitis 1997;36:156–8.
33. Hausen B, Evers P, Stuwe H, Konig W, Wollenweber E. Propolis allergy IV. Studies with further sensitizers from propolis and constituents common to propolis, popular buds, and balsam of Peru. Contact Dermatitis 1992;26:34–44.
34. Hausen BM, Reichling J, Harkenthal M. Degradation products of monoterpenes are the sensitizing agents in tea tree oil. Am J Contact Dermatitis 1999;10:68–77.
35. Bircher AJ, Hirsbrunner P, Langauer S. Allergic contact dermatitis of the genitals from rubber additives in condoms. Contact Dermatitis 1993;28:125–6.
36. Lucke TW, Fleming CJ, McHenry P, Lever R. Patch testing in vulval dermatoses: how relevant is nickel? Contact Dermatitis 1998;38:111–12.
37. Bresser H. Oral nickel provocation and a nickel-free diet. Judications and practical implementation. Hautarzt 1992;43:610–15.
38. Johansen JD, Bruze M, Andersen KE, Frosch PJ, Dreier B, White IR, Rastogi S, Lepoittevin JP, Menne T. The repeated open application test: suggestions for a scale of evaluation. Contact Dermatitis 1998;39:95–6.
39. Schnuch A, Geier J, Uter W, Frosch PJ. Patch testing with preservatives, antimicrobials and industrial biocides. Results from a multicentre study. Br J Dermatol 1998;138:467–76.
40. Goossens A, Claes L, Drieghe J, Put E. Antimicrobials: preservatives, antiseptics and disinfectants. Contact Dermatitis 1998;39:133–4.
41. Schnuch A, Uter W, Geier J, Frosch PJ, Rustemeyer T. Contact allergies in healthcare workers. Results from the IVDK. Acta Derm Venereol 1998;78:358–63.
42. Borelli S, Piletta P, Fritz MG, Elsner P, Nestle FO. Cystamine bislactamide: a cosmetic allergen. Lancet 1998;351:1861–2.
43. Skinner SL, Marks JG. Allergic contact dermatitis to preservatives in topical medicaments. Am J Contact Dermat 1998;9:199–201.
44. Trattner A, Johansen JD, Menne T. Formaldehyde concentration in diagnostic patch testing: comparison of 1% with 2%. Contact Dermatitis 1998; 38: 9–13.
45. Beckmann B. Tea tree oil. Dermatosen 1998; 46:120–124.

46. Wilson CL, Cameron J, Powell SM, Cherry G, Ryan TJ. High incidence of contact dermatitis in leg-ulcer patients-implications for management. Clin Exp Dermatol 1991;16:250–3.
47. Aberer W, Fuchs T, Peters K, PJ F. Propylenglykol: Kutane Nebenwirkungen und Testmethodik. LiteraturĄbersicht und Ergebnisse einer Multicenterstudie der Deutschen Kontaktallergiegruppe (DKG). Dermatosen 1997;36:156–8.
48. Gallenkemper G, Rabe E, Bauer R. Contact sensitization in chronic venous insufficiency: modern wound dressings. Contact Dermatitis 1998;38: 274–8.
49. Snellman E, Rantanen T. Severe anaphylaxis after a chlorhexidine bath. J Am Acad Dermatol 1999;40(5, Pt 1):771–2.
50. Thune P. To pasienter med klorheksidinallergi-anafylaktiske reaksjoner og eksem. Tidsskr Nor Laegeforen 1998;118:3295–6.
51. Olivieri J, Eigenmann PA, Hauser C. Severe anaphylaxis to a new disinfectant: polyhexanide, a chlorhexidine polymer. Schweiz Med Wochenschr 1998;128:1508–11.
52. Van der Walle HB, Brunsveld VM. Dermatitis in hairdressers. (I). The experience of the past 4 years. Contact Dermatitis 1994;30:217–21.
53. Niinimaki A, Niinimaki M, Makinen-Kiljunen S, Hannuksela M. Contact urticaria from protein hydrolysates in hair conditioners. Allergy 1998; 53:1078–82.
54. Erel F, Karaayvaz M, Deveci M, Ozanguc N. Severe anaphylaxis from rifamycin SV. Ann Allergy Asthma Immunol 1998;81:257–60.
55. Vassileva SG, Mateev G, Parish LC. Antimicrobial photosensitive reactions. Arch Intern Med 1998;158:1993–2000.
56. Urrutia I, Jauregui I, Gamboa P, Gonzalez G, Antepara I. Photocontact dermatitis from cinchocaine (dibucaine). Contact Dermatitis 1998; 39:139–40.
57. Yamada S, Tanaka M, Kawahara Y, Inada M, Ohata Y. Photoallergic contact dermatitis due to diphenhydramine hydrochloride. Contact Dermatitis 1998;38:282.
58. Granados TR, Pinero G, Prado MC. Photoallergic contact dermatitis from fepradinol. Contact Dermatitis 1998;39:194–5.
59. Clark SM, Wilkinson SM. Phototoxic contact dermatitis from 5-methoxypsoralen in aromatherapy oil. Contact Dermatitis 1998;38:289–90.
60. Schauder S. Dioxopromethazine-induced photoallergic contact dermatitis followed by persistent light reaction. Am J Contact Dermatitis 1998;9: 82–7.
61. Adamski H, Benkalfate L, Delaval Y, Ollivier I, Le Jean S, Toubel G, Le Hir-Garreau I, Chevrant-Breton J. Photodermatitis from non-steroidal anti-inflammatory drugs. Contact Dermatitis 1998; 38:171–4.
62. Le Coz CJ, Bottlaender A, Scrivener JN, Santinelli F, Cribier BJ, Heid E, Grosshans EM. Photocontact dermatitis from ketoprofen and tiaprofenic acid: cross-reactivity study in 12 consecutive patients. Contact Dermatitis 1998;38:245–52.
63. Berne B, Ros AM. 7 years experience of photopatch testing with sunscreen allergens in Sweden. Contact Dermatitis 1998;38:61–4.
64. Ricci C, Pazzaglia M, Tosti A. Photocontact dermatitis from UV filters. Contact Dermatitis 1998; 38:343–4.
65. Tyring SK, Arany I, Stanley MA, Tomai MA, Miller RL, Smith MH, McDermott DJ, Slade HB. A randomized, controlled, molecular study of condylomata acuminata clearance during treatment with imiquimod. J Infect Dis 1998;178:551–5.
66. Beutner KR, Tyring SK, Trofatter KF, Jr., Douglas JM Jr, Spruance S, Owens ML, Fox TL, Hougham AJ, Schmitt KA. Imiquimod, a patient-applied immune-response modifier for treatment of external genital warts. Antimicrob Agents Chemother 1998; 42: 789–94.
67. Ferenczy A. Immune response modifiers: imiquimod. J Obstet Gynaecol 1998;18(Suppl 2): 76–8.
68. Syed TA, Ahmadpour OA, Ahmad SA, Ahmad SH. Management of female genital warts with an analog of imiquimod 2% in cream: a randomized, double-blind, placebo-controlled study. J Dermatol 1998;25:429–33.
69. Amichai B, Grunwald MH, Goldstein J, Finkelstein E, Halevy S. Small malignant melanoma in patients with mycosis fungoides. J Eur Acad Dermatol Venereol 1998;11:155–7.

Anthony N. Nicholson

15 Antihistamines (H_1 receptor antagonists)

Cardiovascular Although it is widely believed that cardiotoxicity of antihistamines is limited to second-generation, non-sedative compounds, both hydroxyzine and diphenhydramine can act as blockers of potassium channels. Caution should therefore be exercised in prescribing first-generation antihistamines to patients with a predisposition to cardiac dysrhythmias. For example, therapeutic doses of diphenhydramine caused *prolongation of the QT interval* in healthy volunteers and in patients undergoing angioplasty (1[C]), and it cannot be excluded that first-generation drugs that modulate potassium channels may in some circumstances cause dysrhythmias or even convulsions (2[R]). All antihistamines should be screened for cardiotoxicity, as some patients may be poor metabolizers or may be susceptible to plasma concentrations near to the usual therapeutic range. Useful information may be obtained from pharmacokinetic studies using potential inhibitors (see below under Interactions).

The single- and multiple-dose pharmacokinetics of ebastine (10 mg) have been determined in elderly and young healthy subjects using 24-hour Holter monitoring (3[C]). There were no clinically relevant effects.

Nervous system *Extrapyramidal adverse effects* Drug-induced Parkinsonism can be caused by cinnarizine and its derivative flunarizine. A retrospective study has been carried out in 74 patients with cinnarizine-induced Parkinsonism over 15 years (4[C]). Cinnarizine-induced Parkinsonism was more frequent in women, and most of the patients (66/74) recovered completely within 16 months after withdrawal. This suggests that cinnarizine-induced Parkinsonism is reversible in most cases, but there is still a question of whether it predisposes to Parkinson's disease in a few patients. Cinnarizine-induced Parkinsonism is a warning against prolonged use of an apparently harmless drug, especially in elderly people.

In a Brazilian study carried out to establish whether there are geographic differences in the cause of Parkinsonisin, the diagnosis of drug-induced Parkinsonism was made in 45 of 338 patients (5[C]). Cinnarizine and flunarizine were two of the three most commonest drugs prescribed.

Behavioural effects Children and adolescents who are given diphenhydramine as premedication, often intravenously as a bolus, to prevent the adverse effects of blood transfusion, may develop drug seeking behavior. It is recommended that in these circumstances antihistamines should be given orally or infused slowly (6[C]). Cyproheptadine (6 mg per day) was considered to be the most likely cause of aggressive behaviour in a 5 year old boy (7[c]).

Antihistamines and drowsiness

The signal characteristic of the so-called second generation of antihistamines is their freedom from sedation, and it is often claimed that such drugs may be more appropriate than those of the first generation, which cause drowsiness. However, the generality of this claim has been challenged (8[R]).

The designs of protocols used in comparisons between sedative and non-sedative compounds have been questioned. They may not accurately reflect the clinical use of each drug, and the data may be misused in advice to prescribers, even though the reason a comparator was included was merely to provide an active control. The extrapolation of the results of cognitive studies in healthy volunteers to patients may be inappropriate, as a drug that is sedating in a healthy volunteer may well not

Side Effects of Drugs, Annual 23
J.K. Aronson, ed.

be perceived to be sedating by a patient with allergic symptoms, although caution must be advised in relying on subjective assessments of performance and drowsiness. Finally, patients with mild to moderate allergic rhinitis complain of sleep difficulties and many who take a sedative may function reasonably well during the next day without further medication, especially if its activity is restricted to the sleep period. These are certainly relevant issues, and it is likely that the controversy will be settled by accepting the relative merits of each generation of drugs, and that sedative drugs will continue to be prescribed, at least for overnight ingestion and for some skin conditions.

However, there is the special case of the use of antihistamines by individuals whose work may compromise their own safety or the safety of others, e.g. transport workers. Indeed, much of the support for second-generation drugs arises from safety considerations. Nevertheless, it is sometimes suggested that recommendations for the use of antihistamines by those involved in skilled activities should be based on studies of the patients themselves carrying out their day-today work, e.g. airline pilots with allergic rhinitis operating aircraft. This is an argument that lacks careful thought. In occupational medicine it is essential that controlled studies in healthy volunteers are used to establish whether an antihistamine has sedative properties, and then to choose the drug that is least likely to impair performance or cause drowsiness.

In a comparison of the effects over 7 days of a modified-release formulation of brompheniramine (12 mg bd) and loratadine (10 mg od), physicians' and subjective assessments were better for bromopheniramine than for loratadine, but somnolence and dizziness were reported less often by those taking loratadine, although occurrences were claimed to be less frequent with bromophenirarnine as treatment continued (9[C]). The authors of a report of a comparison of the effectiveness of ebastine (10 and 20 mg) versus loratadine (10 mg) for perennial allergic rhinitis claimed that ebastine provided greater symptomatic relief than loratadine, but with a similar low incidence of central effects and headache (10[C]).

In another study, the effects of cetirizine (5, 10, and 15 mg) were studied on sleep latency, on subjective sleepiness, and on performance from 0.5–7.5 hours after ingestion (11[C]). Cetirizine produced shortened sleep latencies, increased subjective sleepiness, and impaired tracking. The authors considered that cetirizine should not be used for personnel involved in critical occupations.

The effects of fexofenadine (120, 180, and 240 mg) on performance and sleepiness have been studied in healthy volunteers. There were no changes at any time compared with placebo, and the authors suggested that fexofenadine may prove to be suitable for use by air personnel (12[C]).

Cinnarizine is used primarily in the treatment of vertigo. In a comparison of the incidence of drowsiness between cinnarizine (25 mg tds for 7 days, 25 mg bd for 15 days, and 25 mg daily for 15 days) and prochlorperazine (5 mg tds for 7 days, 5 mg bd for 15 days, and 5 mg od for 15 days), drowsiness was observed less often in those taking prochlorperazine (13[C]).

In the same way that pharmacokinetic studies have been used to ascertain whether co-administration of an inhibitor of CYP3A4 can lead to cardiotoxicity, similar studies have been carried out to indicate whether the co-administration of an inhibitor can enhance a limited sedative effect. Healthy subjects took a single dose of racemic chlorpheniramine 4 mg on two separate occasions; the second occasion coincided with the sixth day of dosing with ranitidine 75 mg bd for 8 days. Serum concentrations and urinary excretion of chlorpheniramine were not altered, and so it was considered unlikely that co-administration would enhance the potential of chlorpheniramine to cause drowsiness (14[C]).

Liver There have been reports of hepatitis induced by terfenadine, but quantitative information has been lacking on the risk of acute liver disease among users of this drug. In a population-based cohort study using general practice data in the UK carried out by the Boston Collaborative Drug Surveillance Program a causal connection to terfenadine could not be ruled out in only three cases of acute liver disease among more than 200 000 recipients (15[C]). However, the three individuals were also taking other drugs known to cause liver toxicity.

Skin and appendages A 32-year-old woman developed subacute *cutaneous lupus erythematosus* after exposure to the sun while taking cinnarizine and thiethylperazine for vertigo (16[c]). A similar eruption had occurred 10 years before, after exposure to the sun, while she was taking cinnarizine only. The problem did not occur when she was not taking the drug.

A 78-year-old woman developed generalized *lichen pemphigoides* with cinnarizine (225 mg/day) and recovered after withdrawal of the drug and anti-inflammatory drug treatment (17[c]).

A 56-year-old woman developed *itchy erythematous lesions* on the sun-exposed areas when she used diphenhydramine ointment 1% for 6 months; the condition gradually subsided with corticosteroid ointment (18[c]).

Special senses *Presbyacusis* A questionnaire showed that women taking antihistamines and/or cold formulations had a tone average 9 dB higher than those not taking such medication (19[C]). Audiography showed differences in threshold of 6.4 and 12.8 dB at 500 and 1000 Hz respectively. The medications involved were primarily meclizine for dizziness and terfenadine for allergy.

Interactions The metabolism of antihistamines is an important issue in the genesis of cardiac dysrhythmias. Co-administration of inhibitors of the enzymes that normally induce the metabolism of antihistamines has been associated with cardiac dysrhythmias, owing to raised plasma concentrations of the parent antihistamine or of a metabolite.

Astemizole Astemizole is metabolized by CYP3A4 to desmethylastemizole and norastemizole, although these metabolites may not be free of the potential to prolong the QT interval. A 77-year-old woman with QT interval prolongation and torsade de pointes had been taking astemizole 10 mg/day for 6 months (20[c]). She had markedly raised plasma concentrations of astemizole and was also taking cimetidine. However, cardiac dysrhythmias in patients taking antihistamines may be related to other factors, and in this case the patient was also taking another antihistamine and had a history of hepatitis.

Terfenadine Terfenadine is normally metabolized by CYP3A4 to fexofenadine, which has negligible cardiac effects. *Atorvastatin* is also a CYP3A4 substrate, and its effects on the pharmacokinetics of terfenadine have been studied in healthy volunteers who took atorvastatin 80 mg/day from 7 days before to 2 days after terfenadine 120 mg (21[C]). Concentrations of terfenadine and fexofenadine were measured for 72 hours. There were no alterations in the pharmacokinetics of the parent compound or of its metabolite and there were no alterations in QT_c intervals after terfenadine alone or with atorvastatin.

Drugs used in the treatment of depression and psychosis can also alter the metabolism of terfenadine. When the antidepressant *venlafaxine* was given to steady state (37.5 mg bd for 3 days and then 75 mg bd for 5 days), the pharmacokinetics of a single dose of terfenadine 120 mg were not altered and there were no changes in the electrocardiogram (22[C]). The authors concluded that cardiotoxicity is unlikely to arise with co-administration of terfenadine and venlafaxine.

Sertindole 30 mg/day, an antipsychotic drug, had no effects on the pharmacokinetics of a single dose of terfenadine (120 mg) or of its metabolite (23[C]). The authors concluded that sertindole at this dose does not inhibit the metabolism of terfenadine.

REFERENCES

1. Khalifa M, Drolet B, Dalean P, Lefez C, Gilbert M, Plante S, O'Hara GE, Gleeton O, Hmelin BA, Turgeon J. Risk of potassium currents in guinea pig ventricular myocytes and lengthening of cardiac repolarization in man by the histamine H_1 receptor antagonist diphenhydramine. J Pharmacol Exp Ther 1999;288:858–65.
2. Taglialatela M, Timmerman H, Annunsiato L. Cardiotoxic potential and CNS effects of first generation antihistamines. Trends Pharmacol Sci 2000;21:52–6.
3. Huang M-Y, Argenti D, Wilson J, Garcia J, Heald D. Pharmacokinetics and electrocardiographic effect of ebastine in young versus elderly healthy subjects. Am J Ther 1998;5:153–8.
4. Marti-Masso JF, Poza JJ. Cinnarizine-induced parkinsonism: ten years later. Mov Disord 1998; 13:453–6.
5. Cardoso F, Camargos ST, Silva GA. Etiology of parkinsonism in a Brazilian movement disorders clinic. Arg Neuropsiquiatr 1998;56:171–5.
6. Dinndorf PA, McCabe MA, Frierdich S. Risk

of abuse of diphenhydramine in children and adolescents with chronic illnesses. J Pediatr 1998;133:293–5.
7. Strayhom JM. Case study: cyproheptadine and aggression in a five year old boy. J Am Acad Child Adolesc Psychiatry 1998;37:668–70.
8. Aelony Y. First-generation vs second-generation antihistamines. Arch Intern Med 1988;158:17.
9. Druce HM, Thoden WR, Mure P, Furey A, Lockhart EA, Xic T, Galant S, Prenner M, Weinstein S, Zeiring R, Brandon ML. Brompheniramine, loratadine, and placebo in allergic rhinitis: a placebo-controlled comparative clinical trial. J Clin Pharmacol 1998;38:382–9.
10. Davies RJ. Efficacy and tolerability comparison of ebastine 10 and 20 mg with loratadine 10 mg. A double-blind, randomised study in patients with perennial allergic rhinitis. Clin Drug Invest 1998;16:413–20.
11. Nicholson AN, Turner C. Central effects of the H-1 antihistamine, cetirizine. Aviat Space Environ Med 1998;69:166–71.
12. Nicholson AN, Stone BM, Turner C, Mills SL. Antihistamines and aircrew: usefulness of fexofenadine. Aviat Space Environ Med 2000; 71:2–6.
13. Singh AK, Chattiverdi VN. Prochlorperazine versus cinnarizine in cases of vertigo. Indian J Otolaryngol Head Neck Surg 1998;50:392–7.
14. Koch KM, O'Connor-Semmes RL, Davis IM, Yin Y. Stereoselective pharmacokinetics of chlorpheniramine and the effect of ranitidine. J Pharm Sci 1998;87:1097–100.
15. Myers MW, Jick H. Terfenadine and risk of acute liver disease. Br J Clin Pharmacol 1998; 46:251–3.
16. Toll A, Campo-Pisa P, Gonzalez-Castro J, Campo-Voegeli A, Azon A, Iranso P, Lecha M, Herrero C. Subacute cutaneous lupus erythematosus associated with cinnarizine and thiethylperazine therapy. Lupus 1998;7:364–6.
17. Vlasin Z, Rulcova J, Hlubinka M. Lichenoid eruption resembling lichen pemphigoides after cinnarizine. Cesko-Slov Dermatol 1998;73:11–14.
18. Yamada S, Tanaka M, Kawahara Y, Inada M, Ohata Y. Photoallergic contact dermatitis due to diphenhydramine hydrochloride. Contact Dermatitis 1998;38:282.
19. Lee F-S, Matthews U, Mills JH, Dubno JR, Adkins WY. Gender- specific effects of medicinal drugs on hearing levels of older persons. Otolaryngol Head Neck Surg 1998;118:221–7.
20. Ikeda S, Oka H, Matunaga K, Kubo S, Asal S, Mlyahara Y, Osaka A, Kohno S. Astemizole-induced torsades de pointes in a patient with vasospastic angina. Jpn Circ J 1998;62:225–7.
21. Stem RH, Smithers JA, Olson SC. Atorvastatin does not produce a clinically significant effect on the pharmacokinetics of terfenadine. J Clin Pharmacol 199 8;38:753–7.
22. Amchin J, Zarycranski W, Taylor KP, Albano D, Klockowski PM. Effect of venlafaxine on the pharmacokinetics of terfenadine. Psychopharmacol Bull 1998;34:383–9.
23. Wong SL, Cao G, Mack R, Granneman GR. Lack of CYP3A inhibition effects of sertindole on terfenadine in healthy volunteers. Int J Clin Pharmacol Ther 1998;36:146–51.

J.W. Paterson

16 Drugs acting on the respiratory tract

INHALER PROPELLANTS

The safety of the first licensed pressurized metered dose inhaler to use a non-chlorofluorocarbon propellant, the hydrofluoroalkane 134a salbutamol sulfate inhaler, Airomir®, has been evaluated in a post-marketing surveillance study (1^{C}). A non-randomized study has been performed in 6614 patients with obstructive airways disease taking metered doses of salbutamol delivered by inhalers using either hydrofluoroalkane or chlorofluorocarbon as the propellant. There were no significant differences between the groups in the rate of hospital admissions for the condition for which salbutamol was prescribed, in visits to accident and emergency departments, or in unscheduled home visits. There were adverse events in 25% of patients in both groups. The most common adverse events were *infection, bronchospasm, and upper respiratory tract infection.* Adverse events attributed to the medication occurred in 3.1% of the patients who used the hydrofluoroalkane propellant and 0.7% of those who used the chlorofluorocarbon. This difference was significant (OR = 4.34; 95% CI = 2.22–8.52). In contrast, serious adverse events occurred more often with the chlorofluorocarbon (3.7%) than with the hydrofluoroalkane (2.7%), but this difference was not significant.

More patients using the hydrofluoroalkane (18%) withdrew from the study than patients using the chlorofluorocarbon (4.8%). Most of the withdrawals in both groups were unrelated to safety (9 and 3.2% respectively). The reasons for withdrawal included intercurrent illness, loss to follow-up, and inadvertent prescription errors. More patients using the hydrofluoroalkane withdrew because of an adverse event or because of the taste of the inhaler, 3.8 vs 0.9% and 3.1 vs 0.2% respectively. The authors concluded that the data supported the evidence already obtained in clinical trials that reformulation of salbutamol in a hydrofluoroalkane propellant does not result in changes in safety compared with a chlorofluorocarbon formulation.

Side Effects of Drugs, Annual 23
J.K. Aronson, ed.

INHALED CORTICOSTEROIDS
(SED-13, 428)

Effective dose and therapeutic ratio ℞

The concept of the L : T ratio is a useful one. L represents the local or lung availability of an inhaled drug and T the total systemic availability. This ratio will be affected by differences in first-pass metabolism. Another important variable that determines the ratio is the inhalation device. The L : T ratio for budesonide is 0.66–0.85, depending on the method of inhalation (2^{CR}).

Another way of expressing the L : T ratio concept is that of 'pulmonary targeting'. Drug properties that improve pulmonary targeting include low oral systemic availability, rapid systemic clearance, and slow absorption from the lungs. Differences in delivery devices can also produce differences in pulmonary targeting by altering the dose of drug deposited in the lungs. Allowing for both drug and inhaler differences, the relative potencies of the commonly used drugs are as follows: fluticasone propionate > budesonide = beclomethasone dipropionate > triamcinolone acetonide = flunisolide. Potency differences can be overcome by giving a larger dose of the less potent drug. However, comparisons between corticosteroids must measure the systemic effects as well as the lung effect of each dose (3^{CR}).

The importance of the inhalation device has been shown in studies of beclomethasone. Pressurized metered-dose inhalers (pMDI) containing chlorofluorocarbons produce relatively large particles that deposit less than 10% of the delivered dose in the lungs, primarily in the large airways, more than 90% being deposited in the oropharynx. A new hydrofluoroalkane beclomethasone multidose aerosol (Qvar® 3M Pharmaceuticals) delivers a smaller particle size. More than 50% is deposited in the lungs in animal and mechanical models. This has been confirmed using radio labeled Qvar® in patients with asthma and in healthy volunteers. In these subjects 50–60% of the dose is deposited throughout the airways and about 30% in the oropharynx. The breath-activated Autohaler® provides lung deposition equivalent to an optimally used Qvar® inhaler, by automatically delivering drug early in the inhalation. Neither of these devices is improved by the addition of a spacer (4[C]*).*

Measuring suppression of early morning cortisol is an indicator of the systemic activity of beclomethasone. Both inhaled and swallowed fractions cause significant systemic activity, the degree of which depends on the inhaler device used. In one study systemic activity was greater using a dry power inhaler (52%) than a pressurized metered dose inhaler with a large volume spacer (28%) (5[C]*). It was recommended that when high-dose beclomethasone is used, a pressurized metered dose inhaler with a large volume spacer would help in limiting potential adverse effects.*

The systemic availability of inhaled budesonide has been measured in 15 healthy volunteers, using an open cross-over design. Each subject was given three treatments, intravenous budesonide 0.5 mg, inhaled budesonide (from a pMDI with a Nebuhaler) 1 mg (200 µg × 5) plus oral charcoal, and inhaled budesonide 1 mg without oral charcoal. The treatment order was randomized. The mean systemic availability of inhaled compared with intravenous budesonide was 36% with charcoal and 35% without charcoal, indicating that absorption of budesonide from the gastrointestinal tract did not contribute to its systemic availability. Pulmonary deposition was 36% with charcoal and 34% without. When the inhaler was used incorrectly, i.e. the canister was shaken only before the first of the five inhalations, systemic availability fell by 50%. This shows that the performance of each inhaler is very dependent on proper use (6[C]*).*

The available studies suggest that fluticasone is more effective than beclomethasone, triamcinolone, or budesonide. However, budesonide delivered by Turbuhaler® has equivalent efficacy to fluticasone delivered by pressurized metered-dose inhaler or Diskhaler® and is more effective than beclomethasone. When comparative safety is considered, budesonide or triamcinolone delivered by pMDI has less systemic activity than fluticasone. Beclomethasone and fluticasone delivered by pMDI appear to be equivalent. Budesonide delivered by Turbuhaler® has less systemic activity than fluticasone delivered by Diskhaler® (7[CR]*).*

Endocrine, metabolic *Effects on the hypothalamic-pituitary-adrenal axis* Systemic glucocorticoids are used in the treatment of pulmonary diseases in preterm infants of very low birth-weight. This causes severe suppression of the hypothalamic-pituitary-adrenal (HPA) axis. However, the effect of inhaled corticosteroids on pituitary-adrenal function is not known. In a double-blind, randomized pilot study of the efficacy and adverse effects of inhaled fluticasone in 25 newborn preterm infants who required mechanical ventilation for treatment of respiratory distress syndrome the infants were randomized to receive inhaled fluticasone 1000 µg/day or placebo (8[C]). The HPA axis was assessed by the response to corticotropin releasing factor. All basal and post-stimulation plasma ACTH and serum cortisol concentrations were significantly less with inhaled fluticasone than placebo. Cumulative high-dose inhaled corticosteroids caused moderately severe suppression of both the pituitary and adrenal glands. This systemic activity is probably associated with pulmonary vascular absorption that avoids hepatic first-pass metabolism.

Although most patients using inhaled glucocorticosteroids have no adverse effects, systemic effects occur in a few patients. Two girls, aged 11 and 16 years, one boy aged 12 years, and one woman aged 54 years, developed hypothalamic-pituitary-adrenal axis suppression during treatment with inhaled fluticasone propionate 220–880 µg bd for long-term control of asthma; however, two of the patients also took oral prednisone or prednisolone (9[c]). In two other cases adrenal suppression occurred during treatment with low-dose inhaled fluticasone propionate for asthma (10[c]).

Because of poor growth, an 8-year-old girl's asthma medication was changed from budesonide to fluticasone propionate 250 μg/day. However, 5 months later she had developed a round face. Her early morning cortisol concentration was less than 30 nmol/l (reference range 140–720) and her growth had been no more than 0.5 cm during the past 5 months. Fluticasone propionate was discontinued. After 1 month, her Cushingoid features had resolved and her fasting morning cortisol concentration was 310 nmol/l.

A 32-year-old woman's asthma regimen was changed from budesonide to fluticasone propionate 500 μg/day and salmeterol. Eight months later, she was evaluated because of excessive bodyweight gain; her serum cortisol concentration was 16 nmol/l. Fluticasone propionate was replaced with nedocromil and 1 month later her serum cortisol concentration had normalized.

The authors commented that in the first case 250 μg of inhaled fluticasone produced greater suppression of fasting cortisol concentrations than 200 μg of budesonide.

The effect of fluticasone aqueous nasal spray on the HPA axis has been compared with that of oral prednisone and placebo, using a 6-hour co-syntropin infusion test in a 4-week, randomized, double-blind, placebo-controlled study of 105 adults with allergic rhinitis randomly assigned to receive fluticasone 200 μg od, fluticasone 400 μg bd, oral prednisone 7.5 mg od, oral prednisone 15 mg od, or placebo (11[C]). Fluticasone 400 μg bd and both doses of prednisone caused a significant reduction in the morning plasma cortisol concentration. The two fluticasone treatments produced no significant change in the HPA axis response to co-syntropin. This contrasted with oral prednisone 7.5 or 15 mg od, which significantly reduced both plasma cortisol concentrations after co-syntropin and 24-hour urinary cortisol excretion. In contrast, aqueous nasal triamcinolone spray 220 or 440 μg od for the treatment of allergic rhinitis reportedly had no measurable adverse effects on adrenocortical function in 80 children (aged 6–12 years) in a placebo-controlled, double-blind study (12[C]). Plasma triamcinolone concentrations measured over 6 hours fell rapidly and there was little or no accumulation during 6 weeks.

There has been a report of *Cushing's syndrome* after prolonged use of intranasal betamethasone 0.1% for chronic catarrh in two boys (13[c]).

Diabetes mellitus Impaired diabetic control has been reported with high doses of inhaled fluticasone (14[c]).

A 67-year-old man with asthma and non-insulin dependent diabetes mellitus, taking glibenclamide 5 mg/day and metformin 1700 mg/day had glycated hemoglobin concentrations of 7–7.3%. For asthma he used nebulized ipratropium bromide 0.5 mg and salbutamol 5 mg qds. He was given inhaled fluticasone propionate 2000 μg/day by metered dose inhaler through a Volumatic® spacer device, with beneficial effect. In the third week he developed persistent glycosuria and the dose of fluticasone was reduced stepwise to 500 μg/day. He was then rechallenged by increasing his daily dose of fluticasone from 500 to 1000 μg. Within a week he had glycosuria, which again resolved on reduction of the dose of fluticasone. His glycated hemoglobin concentration rose to 7.8% after 1000 μg/day and to 8.2% after 2000 μg/day.

Skin and appendages The effect of long-term inhaled corticosteroids (800–1000 μg/day of either budesonide or beclomethasone) on skin collagen synthesis and thickness has been prospectively investigated in 27 consecutive new asthmatic patients (15[C]). Asthma was treated with a moderate dosage of inhaled corticosteroids. Skin thickness was measured before treatment and at 3 and 6 months using ultrasound on the abdomen and the upper right arm. Suction blisters were induced on the abdominal skin using a disposable suction blister device. Blister fluid was collected and kept frozen for radioimmunoassay of PINP and PIIINP (the amino terminal propeptides of type I and type III procollagens, which reflect collagen synthesis). Skin punch biopsies were taken from the abdominal wall for determination of skin hydroxyproline. After 1–2 years 20 subjects attended for a further measurement of skin thickness. Control data were obtained in 14 healthy women who were followed for 6 months. PINP and PIIINP concentrations in blister fluid were followed in eight male volunteers for 1 year.

There was no significant change in abdominal skin thickness after 6 months of inhaled corticosteroids. In the upper arm there was a small significant reduction from 1.64 to 1.5 mm after 6 months. After 1–2 years the skin thickness in the abdomen and upper arm was unchanged in 14 subjects who had used only inhaled steroids, but in six patients who had taken supplementary oral corticosteroids for one to several weeks there was *thinning of the skin* in the upper arm but not in the abdomen. The procollagen propeptides were markedly reduced in blister fluid at 3 and 6 months. There was no significant change in skin collagen expressed as hydroxyproline. Thus, despite evidence of a reduction in collagen synthesis, skin thickness and collagen did not change, possibly because the degradation and turnover of collagen slowed down. However, in the six patients who subsequently used oral steroids skin thickness decreased.

Two cases of *perioral dermatitis* have been associated with the use of inhaled corticosteroids (16[c]).

A 38-year-old woman who had used inhaled beclomethasone daily (dosage not stated) during the winter for the past 5 years for mild asthma, developed a perioral rash with numerous small pustules and papules. She stopped using beclomethasone and was treated with oral erythromycin and topical tretinoin. Her rash resolved within 4 weeks. One year later, she restarted beclomethasone and her rash reappeared after 2 weeks. There was no recurrence of her perioral dermatitis during subsequent treatment with monthly intramuscular injections of betamethasone.

A 46-year-old woman, who had used inhaled budesonide (dosage not stated) for 8 years for vasomotor rhinitis, developed a recurrent perioral rash, which responded to treatment with oral erythromycin 1 g/day for 6 weeks. One year later, she had a recurrence, which resolved with oral erythromycin. She continued to use inhaled budesonide.

Special senses Nasal budesonide or beclomethasone 100 μg bd for 3–9 months had no effect on the eyes in 26 patients who had undergone endoscopic sinus surgery (17[C]). Ophthalmologic examination, tonometry, visual field testing, and biomicroscopic studies showed no evidence of ocular hypertension or posterior subcapsular cataract.

The use of intranasal steroids in the treatment of allergic and vasomotor rhinitis in Sweden has doubled over a period of 5 years, and the number of reported cases of *nasal septum perforation* increased over the same time (18[CR]). The most common risk factor in 32 patients with nasal septum perforation (21 women, 11 men) was steroid treatment. Information from the Swedish Drug Agency showed that 38 cases of steroid-induced perforation had been reported over 10 years. The number of adverse effects per million Defined Daily Doses averaged 0.21. The risk of perforation was greatest during the first 12 months of treatment and most cases were in young women.

Musculoskeletal *Bone mineral density in adults* Bone mineral density, bone turnover markers, and adrenal steroid hormones have been measured in 53 patients (34 women, 19 men) with chronic bronchial asthma who took either inhaled beclomethasone or budesonide in doses of at least 1500 μg/day for at least 12 months (19[C]). The patients were divided into those who had taken oral glucocorticoids for more than 1 month and those who had not. Bone mineral density was measured at the lumbar spine and the proximal femur. The values were about 1 standard deviation lower in men and women taking oral glucocorticoids or very high doses of inhaled corticosteroids. The reduction in bone mineral density was enough to a double the risk of fracture at these sites. There was suppression of both endogenous glucocorticoid and adrenal androgen production in all subjects. Adrenal androgen suppression may increase the susceptibility of postmenopausal women treated with an oral glucocorticoid to bone loss.

In a 1-year prospective, randomized, open comparison of inhaled fluticasone 500 μg bd with budesonide 800 μg bd delivered by pMDI and large volume spacer, bone mineral density was measured in 29 patients in the lumbar spine and femoral neck (20[C]). Bone mineral density in the spine increased slightly in both groups over the 12 months. Serum osteocalcin concentrations increased from baseline in both treatment groups (fluticasone +17%, budesonide +14%). The percentage change from baseline in bone mineral density of the spine correlated with the increase in serum osteocalcin. Mean serum cortisol concentrations remained in the reference range after both inhaled corticosteroids.

Bone mineral density and growth in children In 23 children, randomized to use either fluticasone 100 μg bd or beclomethasone 200 μg bd for 20 months, there was a significant increase in bone mineral density in the lumbar spine with time, following the normal growth pattern (21[C]).

Bone mineral density was measured after 7.4 months in 49 asthmatic children, 38 of whom took inhaled beclomethasone, average daily dose 276 μg, and 11 sodium cromoglycate, average daily dose 30 mg (22[C]). Children who had used beclomethasone had grown as much as those who used sodium cromoglycate. Trabecular and cortical bone mineral density in the proximal forearm and lumbar spine increased to the same extent in both groups.

The efficacy and safety of fluticasone 750 μg/day and beclomethasone 1500 μg/day delivered by a spacer device have been compared in 30 asthmatic children in a 12-week, randomized, double-blind, cross-over study (23[C]). All of the children had persistent asthma requiring 1000–2000 μg/day of inhaled corticosteroids before the trial. There was no significant difference in efficacy, as judged by daytime and night-time symptom scores and PEFR. There was a minimal reduction in serum cortisol in both groups. Both groups had identical height gain velocities. At the doses used in this trial the authors were unable to show a safety advantage of fluticasone over beclomethasone, as assessed by cortisol concentrations.

The effects of fluticasone 50 μg bd or sodium cromoglycate 20 mg qds on growth over 12 months have been studied in 122 asthmatic children aged 4–10 years (24[C]). The mean height velocity was 6 cm/year with fluticasone and 6.5 cm/year with sodium cromoglycate. There was no significant treatment difference in the mean 24-hour urinary free cortisol concentrations at 6 or 12 months. Mean predicted PEFR improved over 1 year in both groups, but to a greater extent with fluticasone. The authors concluded that growth was normal in mildly asthmatic children using fluticasone (50 μg bd) for 1 year. Fluticasone was more effective than sodium cromoglycate, with fewer withdrawals and greater improvement in lung function.

Prevention of osteoporosis with bisphosphonates The effect of high-dose inhaled corticosteroids and antiresorptive therapy with sodium etidronate has been studied for 18 months in 38 Chinese patients (24 men and 14 premenopausal women aged 30–50 years), of whom 28 were asthmatics who had already been treated for at least 12 months with high-dose inhaled corticosteroids (beclomethasone or budesonide over 1.5 mg/day), and 10 healthy controls (25[C]). The patients were randomly allocated to (1) no supplement, (2) a calcium supplement 1000 mg/day, or (3) cyclical sodium etidronate 400 mg/day for 14 days followed by calcium 1000 mg/day for 76 days. All three groups continued to take inhaled corticosteroids. Bone mineral density was measured at the lumbar spine and hip. Bone mineral density in the group 1 patients fell by about 1% over 18 months and rose by about 1.5% in the healthy controls, neither change being significant. In groups 2 and 3 bone mineral density rose significantly at 12 and 18 months by 2 and 3% respectively. Serum osteocalcin concentrations fell significantly in all three groups of asthmatic patients but not in the controls. There were no significant changes in serum alkaline phosphatase or parathyroid hormone. In the patients taking calcium, with or without etidronate, mean serum calcium increased. The authors suggested that calcium supplementation and cyclical etidronate work by reducing bone resorption, and hence reduced bone turnover, rather than by increasing bone formation. This is consistent with the fall in serum osteocalcin.

The efficacy of clodronate in treating corticosteroid-induced bone loss in asthmatic subjects has been evaluated in a double-blind study of 74 adults (41 women and 33 men, mean age 57 years) with a long history (mean 8.1 years) of oral and inhaled corticosteroid use, randomized to clodronate 800, 1600, or 2400 mg/day or placebo (26[C]). There was no increase in bone mineral density with placebo or clodronate 800 mg/day, but a significant dose-related increase with clodronate 1600 and 2400 mg/day. The most common adverse effect was gastric irritation in the patients who took the highest dose of clodronate.

Immunological and hypersensitivity reactions *Anaphylaxis* has been reported after intradermal triamcinolone (27[c]) and oral prednisolone (28[c]).

Immediately after a third series of monthly intradermal injections of triamcinolone 10 mg into the scalp an 18-year-old man became dizzy and breathless. His face and trunk became swollen and erythematous. His conjunctivae reddened and his lips became swollen. His blood pressure was 140/70 mmHg, there were widespread high-pitched wheezes in his chest, and his PEFR was 370 l/s (normal 640 l/s). After 15 minutes the skin changes resolved spontaneously and his peak flow had risen to 540 l/s. One month later he was carefully rechallenged at the same site on his scalp with triamcinolone 1 mg intradermally followed by 2.5 mg 1 hour later and 5 mg 1 hour after that. There were no adverse local or systemic reactions. A month later triamcinolone 10 mg was injected intradermally. He developed the same anaphylactic response. He had a raised total serum IgE concentration of 338 mg/l (normal 199 mg/l). Patch testing using a battery of corticosteroids including triamcinolone and its excipients were all negative. Prick tests were not performed.

A 30-year-old man with recurrent atopic eczema of the head and neck, generalized xerosis, keratosis pilaris of the arms, and a history of dyshidrosis was initially treated with prednisolone-21-acetate ointment. His skin eruption became worse. He was given oral prednisolone 25 mg, and 5 hours after the first dose developed intense generalized pruritus with erythema and swelling of the face. After 24 hours there was generalized erythema with disseminated partly follicular papules. There was an eosinophilia (1.1×10^9/l). Total IgE was not raised. Patch tests showed delayed reactions to hydrocortisone 1%, prednisolone 1%, prednisolone-21-acetate ointment, and prednisolone 2.5%. Prick and intradermal tests with methylprednisolone succinate, hydrocortisone succinate, betamethasone, and triamcinolone acetonide in concentrations up to 1 : 10 were negative at 15 minutes. However, 4 hours after intradermal testing, generalized pruritus developed and 24 hours later there was a disseminated partly follicular eczematous reaction with involvement of the flexural areas. Biopsy of the eruptions caused by prednisolone and of the positive skin reaction to methylprednisolone succinate showed superficial dermatitis with a perivascular infiltration consisting predominantly of CD4+ cells and some eosinophils. Immunofluorescence showed increased expression of HLA-DR molecules on the CD4+ and CD8+ cells. During the exanthem caused by prednisolone, interleukin-5 (14 pg/ml), interleukin-6 (38 pg/ml) and interleukin-10 (26 pg/ml) were detected in the blood; 2 months after recovery these cytokines were not detectable.

The authors of the second report commented that generalized delayed type hypersensitivity to systemic administration of a corticosteroid is rare. Despite the potent immunosuppressive effect of steroids on immunocompetent cells, the clinical features, the skin biopsy specimen, and the positive delayed skin test reactions strongly suggested an immunological mechanism: T cells were clearly involved and the high concentrations of interleukins 5, 6, and 10 were consistent with a T-helper type 2 reaction. The raised concentrations of interleukin-5 were probably responsible for the blood and tissue eosinophilia.

A 37-year-old woman who was pregnant developed *Churg-Strauss syndrome* after withdrawal of her usual high-dose inhaled corticosteroid therapy (drug not stated) that she had used for 3 years for bronchial asthma (29[c]). The authors commented that activated eosinophils and their cytotoxic products, such as eosinophil catatonic protein, may play a part in the pathogenesis of Churg-Strauss syndrome. Measuring serum concentrations of eosinophil catatonic protein may be useful in monitoring disease activity, since concentrations were increased before treatment and normalized afterwards.

INDIVIDUAL CORTICOSTEROIDS

Budesonide

Inhaled budesonide has been studied in the management of moderately severe acute asthma in children (30[C]). After treatment with nebulized terbutaline 11 children were randomly allocated to receive one dose of either budesonide 1600 μg by Turbuhaler® or prednisolone 2 mg/kg. There was no significant difference in the improvement of the pulmonary index score or PEFR. Children treated with budesonide had an earlier clinical response than those given prednisolone. Prednisolone caused a fall in serum cortisol concentration. The authors concluded that children with moderately severe asthma attacks could be effectively treated with a short-term course of inhaled budesonide, starting with a high dose and reducing over the next week.

In 81 patients with acute asthma, mean age 38 years, inhaled budesonide 1600 μg bd via Turbuhaler® was compared with oral prednisolone (40 mg on day 1 reducing to 5 mg by day 7) in a randomized, double-blind, parallel-group design (31[C]). The mean increase in FEV_1 from baseline to day 7 was 17% with budesonide and 18% with prednisolone. Mean values of morning PEFR increased from day 1 to day 7 by 67 l/s with budesonide and by 57 l/s with prednisolone. There were no statistically significant differences between the groups in either symptoms or the number of doses of rescue medication. The authors concluded that high-dose inhaled budesonide may be a substitute for oral therapy in the treatment of an acute attack of asthma.

The effect of supplementary inhaled budesonide in acute asthma has been evaluated in a randomized, double-blind comparison with standard treatment in 44 children aged 6 months to 18 years with a moderate to severe exacerbation of asthma (32[C]). Prednisone 1 mg/kg orally and nebulized salbutamol (0.15 mg/kg) every 30 minutes for three doses and then every hour for 4 hours were given to all children. In addition each child was given 2 mg of nebulized budesonide or nebulized isotonic saline. There was a more rapid discharge rate in the budesonide group. There were no adverse effects. The authors concluded that nebulized budesonide may be an effective adjunct to oral prednisone in the management of moderate to severe exacerbations of asthma.

Fluticasone propionate

Inhaled fluticasone 500 μg bd from a pressurized metered dose inhaler for 6 months has been compared with placebo in a randomized double-blind trial in 280 patients with COPD, aged 50–75 years (33[C]). There was no significant difference in the number of patients who suffered one or more exacerbations. Moderate or severe exacerbations occurred significantly more often with placebo than with fluticasone. Diary-card scores, morning PEFR, clinic FEV_1, FVC, and mid-expiratory flow all improved significantly with fluticasone. Scores for median daily cough and sputum volume were significantly lower with fluticasone than with placebo. At the end of treatment, patients using fluticasone had increased their 6 minutes walking distance significantly more than those using placebo. Fluticasone propionate was tolerated as well as placebo, with few adverse effects and no clinically important effect on mean serum cortisol concentration. The authors suggested that inhaled corticosteroids may have an important place in the long-term management of patients with COPD.

β-ADRENOCEPTOR AGONISTS

(SED-13, 427; SEDA-20, 167; SEDA-21, 181; SEDA-22, 188)

Bambuterol and cardiac failure

A retrospective study of prescriptions from three cohort studies suggested a possible adverse effect of oral bambuterol. A cohort of 12 294 patients who received at least one prescription for nedocromil acted as the control and was compared with 15 407 patients given inhaled salmeterol and 8098 patients given oral bambuterol. Questionnaires were sent to each prescriber asking for details of significant medical events after the first prescription (prescription event monitoring). From this information, rates and relative risks of non-fatal cardiac failure and ischemic heart disease were calculated. The age- and sex-adjusted relative risk of non-fatal cardiac failure associated with bambuterol was 3.41 (CI = 1.99–5.86) compared with nedocromil. When salmeterol was compared with nedocromil the relative risk for developing non-fatal cardiac failure was 1.1 (CI = 0.63–1.91). The adjusted relative risks of non-fatal ischemic heart disease with bambuterol and salmeterol compared with nedocromil were 1.23 (CI = 0.73–2.08) and 1.07 (CI = 0.69–1.66) respectively. In the month after the first prescription, the relative risk of non-fatal ischemic heart disease was 3.95 (CI = 1.38–11.31), when bambuterol was compared with nedocromil. The authors concluded that care should be exercised when prescribing long acting oral β_2 agonists for patients at risk of cardiac failure (34[C]).

This study at best generates the hypothesis that the oral use of a particular β_2 agonist is linked to an increased risk of cardiac disease. The study itself is potentially flawed, as the three cohorts of patients were not strictly comparable: they were not treated concurrently nor were they sufficiently matched for age and diagnosis before prescription of the study drugs.

The author of a discussion of this study expressed concern about aspects of the study design (35[R]). He pointed out that it took nearly 3 years to recruit the patients who preferred or needed an oral agent. A smaller proportion of patients in this cohort were treated for 'asthmatic wheeze' –57 vs 70% in the salmeterol cohort. More of the bambuterol patients were given the drug for other indications, such as dyspnea, bronchitis, cough, chest infection, emphysema, and bronchitis –15 vs 2.8%. The salmeterol cohort consisted mostly of patients who were changing to a longer acting agent and those using nedocromil were mostly changing from cromolyn. The bambuterol group was more heterogeneous. Some patients with impending or undiagnosed heart failure may have presented with dyspnea, cough, or wheeze and received bambuterol. During the first month the correct diagnosis would become evident.

Nevertheless, the reviewer also discussed a mechanism by which β_2 agonists might aggravate cardiac disease. He concluded that inhalation is the preferred method for taking β_2 agonists. For patients who cannot use an inhaler cardiac disease should be excluded before prescribing an oral β_2 agonist. The company that manufactures bambuterol has commented on the two publications, emphasizing that prescription event monitoring is not designed to study cause-and-effect relations but to generate hypotheses (36[R]). Data were missing for more than 40% of the prescriptions, and the cohorts were collected at different times. Patients in the bambuterol group were older, the prevalence of asthma was lower, and the rate of other diagnoses was higher.

A review of the pre-clinical studies, clinical studies and post-marketing surveillance data has given no support to the proposed association between bambuterol and cardiac failure. The UK Committee on Safety of Medicines has received no spontaneous reports of cardiac failure due to bambuterol. Data from the WHO database, INTDIS, show no reports of cardiac failure with bambuterol, in contrast to 10 reports for salmeterol.

So, there is no evidence that oral β_2 agonists cause cardiac failure. The epidemiological study proposing the link is inadequate, and the authors themselves have emphasized the need for prospective randomized trials.

The safety of fenoterol in severe asthma

Debate continues about the safety of fenoterol in the treatment of severe asthma. A report from the manufacturers has discussed the epidemiological data linking the use of fenoterol to asthma mortality in New Zealand. The manufacturers point out that asthma mortality started to fall in 1979 while fenoterol sales were still increasing. Sales of fenoterol in Austria, Belgium, and Germany were similar to those in New Zealand at the peak of the New Zealand asthma death epidemic, but asthma mortality in the other countries did not rise. The confounding problem that fenoterol was preferentially prescribed for the more severe cases of asthma is again mentioned. Researchers who adjust their data appropriately for asthma severity have concluded that the increased risk of death from asthma reported in patients using fenoterol is due to underlying severe disease in the patients given fenoterol (37[R]). The proponents of the hypothesis have responded by pointing out that four case-control studies all showed a significantly higher death rate in patients taking fenoterol than in patients taking other β_2 agonists. They have acknowledged that there is some evidence of selective prescribing of fenoterol in populations studied in New Zealand and Canada. However, they do not agree that the association between fenoterol and asthma deaths is due to confounding by asthma severity (38[R]). A third group has concluded that the association between fenoterol and severe life-threatening asthma is explained by the preferential prescribing of fenoterol for patients with more severe disease (39[R]). They have pointed out that doses of fenoterol (up to 3200 μg) or salbutamol (up to 1600 μg) failed to produce clinically relevant cardiac dysrhythmias in patients with acute severe asthma (40[C]). This was despite the fact that the 2-fold higher dose of fenoterol caused greater systemic β_2 effects. They have concluded that although epidemiological evidence may implicate fenoterol as a cause of asthma deaths it can only generate a hypothesis. The hypothesis is not substantiated by data from carefully controlled pharmacodynamic and pharmacoepidemiological studies. They have supported the view that excessive use of β_2 agonists, including fenoterol, in severe asthma is a marker of inadequate suppression of the underlying inflammatory process, indicating the need to introduce or optimize the dose of glucocorticoids (39[R]).

It is interesting to reflect that a similar debate followed the rise in asthma deaths in the UK in the 1960s. Most physicians now accept that excessive use of β-adrenoceptor agonists in worsening asthma indicates inadequate treatment rather than a toxic effect of the drugs.

Formoterol (eformoterol)

The pharmacokinetics and pharmacodynamics of a single oral dose of formoterol 168 μg have been studied in eight healthy men. Plasma concentrations reached a maximum of 94 pg/ml 70 minutes after administration. The biological effects peaked later, at 4 hours. Plasma potassium fell from 3.98 mmol/l to 2.33 mmol/l. There was a *fall in blood eosinophil* count from 277×10^6/l to 47×10^6/l (41[C]).

The effect of formoterol 18 μg on histamine-induced plasma exudation into sputum has been investigated in 16 healthy subjects in a double-blind, placebo-controlled, cross-over study. Plasma exudation into the airways was produced by inhalation of histamine. Sputum was induced by inhalation of hypertonic (4.5%) saline. Induced sputum was obtained at baseline and then at 30 minutes and 8 hours after histamine inhalation. Sputum concentrations of α_2-macroglobulin were measured as a marker of microvascular-epithelial exudation of bulk plasma. Histamine-induced plasma exudation 30 minutes after placebo was considerably greater than at baseline. The median difference was 11 μg/ml (95% CI = 0.9–90) expressed as α_2-macroglobulin. The effect of histamine was reduced by 5.1 (CI = 0.9–62) μg/ml 30 minutes after formoterol compared with placebo. At 8 hours histamine exudation was much less and was no longer inhibited by formoterol (42[C]).

Regular treatment with long acting β_2 agonists reduces their bronchoprotective effect against bronchoconstrictor stimuli. A randomized, double-blind, placebo-controlled, cross-over trial was designed to see whether formoterol given once daily was associated with a lesser degree of subsensitivity. Ten asthmatics using inhaled steroids were given inhaled formoterol dry powder 24 μg od or bd or identical placebo for 1 week. Bronchoprotection was estimated by measuring the PC_{20} for adenosine monophosphate (AMP) 12 hours after the first and last doses of each treatment. The PC_{20} is the concentration of AMP that causes a 20% fall in the FEV_1 and is directly proportional to the degree of bronchoprotection.

With placebo the PC_{20} values for AMP at the start and end of one week were 71 and 75 mg/l. There was a significant *loss of bronchoprotection* after 1 week of treatment with twice-daily formoterol. The PC_{20} for AMP at the start was 475 mg/l, indicating significant bronchoprotection by formoterol compared with placebo. After 1 week the PC_{20} had fallen to 127 mg/l, a near 4-fold loss of the bronchoprotective effect of formoterol. When formoterol was given od for a week the PC_{20} values were 367 and 127 mg/l, a 3-fold loss of bronchoprotection. There was no significant difference in the effects of formoterol given once or twice a day (43[C]).

A similar randomized, parallel-group, double-blind study of 67 patients with stable asthma requiring inhaled corticosteroids used the PC_{20} for inhaled metacholine as a measure of bronchoprotection. The patients were treated for 2 weeks with formoterol 12 μg od, 6 μg bd, or 24 μg bd, terbutaline 500 μg qds, or placebo. Each of the four active treatments caused a significant fall in the PC_{20} for metacholine, and there was no significant difference between them. In contrast to the reduced bronchoprotective effect the bronchodilator effect of formoterol was maintained over the 2-week treatment period (44[C]).

In a double-blind cross-over study 12 healthy subjects were randomized to receive either inhaled placebo or inhaled budesonide 1.2 mg bd for 7 days with a minimum 7-day wash out period between the two treatments. They used formoterol 24 μg bd during both treatment periods. A dose-response curve for systemic β_2 receptor responses to inhaled salbutamol (0.8–3.2 mg) was carried out before and after 7 days of each treatment. The pretreatment value of plasma cortisol averaged 407 nmol/l and fell to 22 nmol/l after 7 days of budesonide; placebo had no effect. There was a significant reduction in the peak heart rate response to salbutamol when formoterol was given with placebo. This was partially reversed when formoterol was combined with budesonide. The peak rise in heart rate with salbutamol after formoterol and placebo was 24 beats/min and increased to 35 beats/min when formoterol was given with budesonide. The peak fall in potassium with salbutamol after formoterol and placebo was 0.48 mmol/l and did not change significantly when formoterol was combined with budesonide (0.36 mmol/l) (45[C]).

The cardiovascular and metabolic responses to increasing doses of formoterol 12, 24, 48, and 96 μg administered from a dry powder inhaler have been assessed in a randomized, double-blind, cross-over study of 20 patients with mild to moderate asthma. There was no difference in the maximum effects of formoterol 12 μg and placebo. The 24 μg dose significantly *reduced plasma potassium* (average fall 0.2 mmol/l) and *increased blood glucose* (average rise 1.8 mmol/l). After formoterol 96 μg the *rise in heart rate*was 9 beats/min greater than after placebo, *systolic blood pressure rose* by an average of 4 mmHg, and *diastolic pressure fell* by an average of 3 mmHg. Plasma potassium fell by an average of 0.5 mmol/l and blood glucose rose by an average of 2.6 mmol/l. The effects on extrapulmonary parameters would only be of clinical significance at the highest dose of formoterol studied (46[C]).

The cardiac effects of formoterol and salmeterol have been studied in 12 patients with COPD, hypoxemia (P_aO_2 below 60 mmHg), and cardiac disease. Holter monitoring showed that the *heart rate was higher* after formoterol 24 μg than after either formoterol 12 μg or salmeterol 50 μg. *Supraventricular or ventricular extra beats* occurred more often after formoterol 24 μg. Formoterol 24 μg caused a significant *reduction in the plasma potassium concentration* for 9 hours after administration. The authors suggested that in patients with COPD, hypoxemia, and pre-existing cardiac dysrhythmias long-acting β_2 agonists may cause adverse cardiac effects. However, the recommended single dose of salmeterol or formoterol allows a higher safety margin than inhaled formoterol 24 μg (47[C]).

In multiple dose studies with formoterol (Oxis®, Turbuhaler®, Astra) 6, 12, and 24 μg bd, terbutaline 0.5 mg qds, or placebo in a total of 1199 patients, at least one adverse event was reported by 65% of the patients in each treatment group (48[C]). Adverse events related to the respiratory system were reported by 37% of the patients and were attributed to underlying disease. *Tremor* was reported by 2% of patients taking formoterol 6 μg bd, by 4% with 12 μg bd, and by 12% with 24 μg bd. Tremor was reported by 5% of patients taking terbutaline 0.5 mg qds. No patient reported tremor with placebo (48[C]).

In 12 stable asthmatic patients who took high doses of formoterol or terbutaline, terbutaline had significantly greater systemic effects than formoterol, as indicated by pulse, blood pressure, and heart rate. Baseline serum potassium concentrations were all within the reference range (3.7–5.3 mmol/l). There was no significant difference between the mean potassium lowering effects of formoterol 72 μg and terbutaline 6 mg. Mean maximal systolic blood pressure rose from 150 to 155 mmHg with formoterol 72 μg and from 139 to 153 mmHg with terbutaline 6 mg. The difference between treatment groups, 5 mmHg, was statistically significant. Diastolic blood pressure fell significantly with both formoterol (from 86 to 70 mmHg) and terbutaline (from 85 to 66 mmHg). Heart rate rose from 61 beats/min to 79 beats/min on day 3 in patients taking formoterol 72 μg/day compared with a rise from 63 beats/min to 86 beats/min with terbutaline 6 mg; this difference was statistically significant.

Terbutaline 10 mg/day had significantly greater effects than formoterol 120 μg on serum potassium concentrations, pulse, and heart rate. During treatment with formoterol 120 μg/day, 10 patients had *potassium concentrations below 3.7 mmol/l* on day 1, six patients on day 2, and five patients on day 3. With terbutaline 10 mg the corresponding numbers were 12, 10, and 9. However, the effect of terbutaline 10 mg was significantly greater than formoterol 120 μg over the three treatment days. Formoterol 120 μg/day caused a *rise in baseline systolic blood pressure* from 134 to 145 mmHg; terbutaline 10 mg produced a rise from 131 to 141 mmHg. The difference between the groups, 0.6 mmHg, was not statistically significant. With formoterol 120 μg/day the *heart rate rose* from 65 beats/min to 78 beats/min, and with terbutaline 10 mg/day it rose from 63 to 86 beats/min. The difference in mean heart rate rise of 8 beats/min was statistically significant. A patient taking formoterol 72 μg/day developed *atrial fibrillation* on day 1. Minor adverse events occurred in seven patients taking formoterol 72 μg/day and six patients taking terbutaline 6 mg/day. Eight patients reported adverse events when taking formoterol 120 μg/day, as did 10 patients taking terbutaline 10 mg/day. Minor adverse effects *included headache, muscle cramps, fatigue,* and *tremor* with all four treatments. Tremor was reported in 2 of 12 patients taking terbutaline 6 mg and 5 of 15 patients taking terbutaline 10 mg. The corresponding numbers for formoterol were none with formoterol 72 μg and one of 15 with formoterol 120 μg (49[C]).

A 3-month, open, uncontrolled, multicenter trial has been carried out in 1380 patients with moderate to severe persistent asthma taking inhaled corticosteroids (50[C]). Formoterol was given via a single-dose breath-activated device (Foradil®). There were significant increases in peak flow and a 3-fold reduction in the need for rescue treatment with short acting β_2 agonists. By the end of the study, 72% of the patients were taking formoterol 12 μg bd and 29% were taking 24 μg bd. Physician evaluation indicated that tolerability was very good or good in 93% of the patients. There were only minor drug-related adverse events similar to those produced by other β_2 agonists.

In 397 adults with mild to moderate asthma randomly allocated to one of three treatments for 12 weeks (formoterol 6 μg bd, terbutaline 0.5 mg qds, and placebo), formoterol was significantly more effective than either terbutaline or placebo in reducing asthma symptoms (51[C]). It also resulted in significantly higher evening peak flow readings and less use of rescue medication. The bronchodilator response to the study drugs and an additional 1.25 mg of terbutaline was similar before and at the end of the 12 weeks. This suggested that there was no loss of β-adrenoceptor mediated bronchodilatation in any of the treatment groups. No patient in any group reported a clinically relevant adverse effect.

Of 31 patients with asthma and a mean FEV_1 of 1.97 liters in a double-blind, randomized, placebo-controlled, crossover study of single inhaled doses of placebo or formoterol, 6, 12, 24, or 48 μg on five separate days, most had at least a 50% increase in specific airway conductance within 1–4 minutes (52[C]).

The maximum increase in FEV_1 was dose dependent, rising by 12% (6 μg), 18% (12 μg), 19% (24 μg), and 26% (48 μg). At 12 hours after the administration of 6, 12, 24, and 48 μg of formoterol, the mean increases in FEV_1 were still 7, 15, 18, and 27% respectively above the value seen with placebo. The most frequently reported adverse effect was headache, which occurred with all treatments, including placebo. After inhalation of formoterol 48 μg, three patients had mild *tremor* lasting for less than 1 hour. One patient had the same effect for 3 hours after placebo.

Salbutamol (albuterol)

The efficacy and safety of salbutamol inhaled using a dry powder inhaler has been compared with salbutamol inhaled using a pressurized metered-dose inhaler (pMDI) in a randomized, open, cross-over study of 12 patients with moderate to severe asthma. A total of 1600 μg of salbutamol was given on two separate days in a cumulative dose fashion in increments of 100, 100, 200, 400, and 800 μg at 3-minute intervals. FEV_1 rose progressively with each increment. The dose-response curves showed that powdered salbutamol was 3.0 times as potent (CI = 1.8–5.8) as salbutamol from the pMDI. Systolic and diastolic blood pressures did not change. Powdered salbutamol caused a greater rise in heart rate. The maximum heart rate was seen at 25–30 minutes after the last dose on each study day. The average maximum heart rate was 95 beats/min (range 78–109) for the powder and 89 beats/min (range 76–106) for the pMDI. The relative dose potency of the powder versus the pMDI was 2.0 (CI = 1.3–3.6) for lowering the serum potassium. The lowest serum potassium in an individual patient was 3.7 mmol/l after 1600 μg of the powder. No adverse events were reported on either study day. Four patients reported *tremor.* In one patient tremor was reported after each dose of powder as well as after 1600 μg inhaled from the pMDI. Cumulative doses of 800 and 1600 μg of powder caused tremor in the other three patients and two noted tremor after 1600 μg inhaled from the pMDI. Tremor was objectively measured and the dose-response curves showed a relative dose potency for the powder versus pMDI of 2.3 (CI = 1.5–4.4). Thus, salbutamol powder was more potent than salbutamol pMDI for extrapulmonary effects and even more potent as a bronchodilator. It was concluded that use of the dry powder inhaler resulted in greater lung deposition of salbutamol, causing a higher concentration not only in the airways but also in the systemic circulation (53[C]).

Salmeterol

In a randomized, double-blind, placebo-controlled, multicenter evaluation of the clinical efficacy and safety of salmeterol 42 μg bd in 538 asthmatic patients, mean peak flow rate improved significantly in the patients who used salmeterol (54[C]). The use of supplementary salbutamol, asthma symptom scores, and FEV_1 were significantly improved by salmeterol. There were no clinically significant adverse events.

In a double-blind study of 49 stable asthmatic patients who were taking inhaled corticosteroids, randomized to either salmeterol 50 μg or placebo bd for 4 weeks, the bronchodilator response to cumulative doses of inhaled salbutamol was measured before and 12 and 36 hours after the last dose (55[C]). There were no significant differences between salmeterol and placebo in maximal FEV_1 or PEFR response to inhaled salbutamol at 12 and 36 hours. Asthma control, as judged by clinic lung function and diary card parameters, was significantly better in the patients who took regular salmeterol. There were no serious adverse events. The incidence of non-serious adverse events was similar in the two groups, 56% with salmeterol and 50% with placebo. The most commonly reported adverse events were *headache* and *rhinitis.*

Inhaled salmeterol 50 μg bd has been compared with oral modified-release theophylline in 178 patients with mild to moderate chronic obstructive pulmonary disease (56[C]). Salmeterol caused a significant improvement in mean morning PEFR compared with theophylline and significantly increased the percentage of symptom-free days and nights with no additional requirement for salbutamol. Adverse events occurred in 50% of the patients who took salmeterol, and 49% of those who used theophylline. Adverse events due to the pharmacological properties of the drug were less frequent with salmeterol (4%) than theophylline (15%).

The effect of regular salbutamol 400 μg qds has been compared with that of salmeterol 50 μg bd in patients with mild to moderate bronchial asthma in a double-dummy, placebo-controlled, cross-over study of 165 patients with asthma (57[C]). Relative to placebo, mean morning PEFR increased by 30 l/min with salmeterol but did not change with salbutamol; evening PEFR increased by 25 l/min. Salmeterol improved the asthma score compared with placebo, but salbutamol produced no overall difference. Only daytime symptoms were improved by salbutamol. The asthma score fell over time with salbutamol. Both minor and major exacerbation rates were significantly less when patients used salmeterol. Major exacerbations lasted for significantly longer in patients taking salbutamol compared with those taking placebo. Tolerance did not develop to either drug; after withdrawal there was no rebound worsening of asthma control, fall in lung function, or increase in bronchial reactivity to inhaled methacholine. Although salbutamol improved daytime symptoms, there was deterioration in asthma control over time.

Formoterol dry powder 12 μg bd has been compared with salmeterol dry powder 50 μg bd in 425 asthmatic patients treated for 6 months in a randomized, open, parallel-group study (58[C]). Improvements were similar in the two groups, although evening pre-dose PEFR showed a trend in favor of formoterol, statistically significant at 2, 3, and 4 months. Both treatments were well tolerated: 190 patients taking formoterol and 193 taking salmeterol reported adverse events. This was not unexpected in a 6-month trial. The most frequent adverse events *included viral infections, asthma exacerbation, headache, rhinitis,* and *chest infections.* Exacerbation of asthma was reported as an adverse event by 41 patients (17%) taking formoterol and 54 (22%) taking salmeterol. Adverse events, assessed as possibly/probably drug related, were reported in 32 (13%) patients taking formoterol and 21 (9%) taking salmeterol. The most frequent drug-related adverse event was headache, reported by seven patients taking formoterol and 11 taking salmeterol. Other adverse events included *tremor* in five patients taking formoterol and two taking salmeterol, *exacerbation of asthma* in four patients in each group, and *palpitation* in four patients taking formoterol.

The effect of salmeterol on asthma control in 506 patients requiring inhaled corticosteroids has been evaluated in a randomized, double-blind, placebo-controlled study (59[C]). The patients received either salmeterol 42 μg bd via a metered dose inhaler or placebo for 12 weeks. Salmeterol was superior to placebo when assessed by asthma quality-of-life score, global score, asthma symptoms, and improvement in FEV_1, PEFR, and use of supplementary salbutamol to treat exacerbations. Adverse events were reported in 53% of patients taking salmeterol and 51% of patients taking placebo. Most adverse events were not related to treatment. Treatment-related adverse events occurred in 13 patients (5%) taking placebo and 11 patients (4%) taking salmeterol. Twelve patients (2%) did not complete the study because of adverse events, five taking placebo and seven taking salmeterol. In only three patients were the adverse effects considered to be potentially related to the treatment: salmeterol-*chest tightness,* placebo-shortness of breath and chest pains. *Respiratory failure* occurred in one patient taking salmeterol and was judged to be possibly related to the drug. Exacerbation of asthma occurred in 59 patients (22%) taking placebo and 53 patients (20%) taking salmeterol. The most common reason cited for exacerbation of the asthma was *respiratory infection.*

Terbutaline

Endocrine, metabolic The effects of terbutaline as a tocolytic agent on glucose metabolism has been studied in six healthy, pregnant women, with normal glucose tolerance, between the 30th and 34th weeks of pregnancy (60[C]). The women took either oral terbutaline 5 mg every 6 hours for 24 hours or no medication. The study was repeated after 1 week and each subject acted as her own control. With terbutaline fasting blood glucose increased in each subject, the mean rising from 82 to 94 mg/dl (4.6 to 5.2 mmol/l). Basal *serum insulin increased significantly,* from 18 to 27 μU/ml. *Glucagon fell* from a mean of 166 to 144 pg/ml. There was a 12% *rise in basal hepatic glucose production.* The glucose infusion rate to maintain euglycemia fell by 33% while subjects were taking oral terbutaline. Indirect calorimetry showed that terbutaline caused a significant *increase in energy expenditure.* Oxygen consumption increased by 9% (270 to 294 ml/min) and basal caloric expenditure increased by 14% (from 1.32 to 1.5 kcal/min). Thus, oral terbutaline given for 24 hours is associated with a significant reduction in peripheral insulin sensitivity and an increase in energy expenditure. Increases in basal hepatic glucose metabolism and a reduced ability of insulin to suppress hepatic glucose output are consistent with an effect of terbutaline on maternal hepatic glucose metabolism.

ANTIMUSCARINIC AGENTS
(SED-13, 425)

There is continuing discussion about the role of inhaled antimuscarinic drugs combined with β_2-adrenoceptor agonists in the treatment of acute asthma (61[C]). Five trials involving 453 patients examined the efficacy of using a single dose (250 μg) of ipratropium bromide with a β_2 agonist. There were no reductions in hospital admission rates when pooling the two trials that reported this outcome (RR = 0.93; CI = 0.65–1.32). In three trials in which pulmonary function was the major outcome measure, there was a significantly greater improvement in lung function at 60 and 120 minutes after a single inhalation of a combination of an antimuscarinic drug and a β_2 agonist. The addition of a single dose of an antimuscarinic drug was not associated with increased vomiting or tremor, but there was an apparent reduction in nausea (RR = 0.55; CI = 0.33–0.91). Five trials involving 366 children examined the effects of multiple treatments with combined ipratropium and a β_2 agonist. Pooling of four trials using hospital admission as an outcome measure showed a 30% reduction (RR = 0.72; CI = 0.53–0.99). The authors cautioned that the total number and size of studies were small and that their conclusions could be modified by results of larger trials (61[C]).

Oxitropium

Total serum IgE has been measured in 36 patients with allergic rhinitis and 11 healthy subjects given a submaximal dose of oxitropium bromide 600 μg by inhalation (62[C]). FEV_1 was greater than 80% of predicted in all subjects. Baseline FEV_1 correlated negatively with serum IgE concentration. oxitropium bromide inhalation produced an increase in FEV_1 (mean 155 ml) that was significantly greater in allergic patients with high serum IgE than in healthy subjects (64 ml) or in those with allergic rhinitis and low serum IgE (82 ml). The effect of an inhaled β_2 agonist (orciprenaline) was similar in all three groups. These findings may explain some of the variation in response to inhaled antimuscarinic drugs in patients with asthma. The data also suggested that IgE may itself modify airway tone by an increase in cholinergic responsiveness.

In a single blind, randomized, cross-over study of 12 patients the bronchodilator effects of salmeterol 50 μg and oxitropium 200 and 400 μg were compared with placebo. All treatments were taken from a metered dose inhaler. The peak effect of salmeterol was delayed but the effect was more prolonged than the effect of oxitropium. The response to salmeterol 50 μg exceeded the response to oxitropium 200 μg over 12 hours. Between 3 and 12 hours the response to salmeterol was greater than the response to oxitropium 400 μg, but the difference was not significant. There were no significant changes in pulse rate, blood pressure, or the electrocardiogram with any of the four treatments. No patients complained of adverse symptoms and none noticed any difference in the taste of the different inhalers (63[C]).

OTHER BRONCHODILATORS

Fenspiride *(SED-13, 424)*

Fenspiride is marketed as a bronchodilator with anti-inflammatory properties. Two recent in vitro studies have suggested possible mechanisms for these effects. Functional studies in human isolated bronchi showed that fenspiride causes a shift to the left of concentration effect curves for isoprenaline and sodium nitroprusside induced relaxation (64). Biochemical studies confirmed that phosphodiesterase 4 (cyclic AMP specific) and phosphodiesterase 5 (cyclic GMP specific) are the main phosphodiesterase isoforms present in human bronchi. Fenspiride inhibited both isoforms. Fenspiride facilitates relaxation of human bronchial smooth muscle in vitro, and this effect may be due to inhibition of phosphodiesterases 4 and 5.

A second study used a human lung epithelial cell line, in which histamine increased the intracellular calcium concentration and the formation of eicosanoids (65). This response was antagonized by the H_1 histamine receptor antagonist diphenhydramine but unaffected by the H_2 receptor antagonist cimetidine. Fenspiride inhibited the H_1 receptor-induced calcium increase. Histamine also caused a biphasic increase in arachidonic acid release, which was inhibited by fenspiride. This study suggests a further mechanism that would promote anti-inflammatory and antibronchoconstrictor properties.

Fenspiride has been used to treat 392 adults with an acute respiratory tract infection, most of whom were considered to have a moderate symptom score that improved with 7 days of treatment with fenspiride (66[C]). Adverse reactions were classified as only mild and tolerance was excellent, only 20 of 392 patients discontinuing the drug.

ANTIHISTAMINES USED IN ASTHMA

Ketotifen *(SED-13, 423; SEDA-22, 194)*

A further two cases of *seizures* in children induced by ketotifen have been reported (67[cr]).

A 3-month-old boy was given ketotifen (0.1 mg/kg/day) for atopic dermatitis and after 8 days developed tonic spasms of a mixed flexor extensor type, consisting of flexion of the neck and arms with extension of the legs more than 10 times a day. Each seizure lasted for 5–15 minutes. An electroencephalogram showed a hypsarrhythmic trace. Ketotifen was withdrawn and the seizures were successfully controlled with ACTH and valproic acid. An MRI scan was normal.

A 3-month-old boy was given ketotifen, 0.1 mg/kg/day, for asthmatic bronchitis. After 10 days his facial movements altered and 1 month after ketotifen was started tonic spasms began. His seizures consisted of a sudden contraction, usually bilateral and symmetrical involving the muscles of the neck, trunk, and limbs. An electroencephalogram showed a hypsarrhythmic trace. He was treated with ACTH and clonazepam without benefit. Ketotifen was withdrawn and ACTH and clonazepam were replaced with valproic acid. This resulted in seizure control, after which the electroencephalogram showed no abnormal discharges. Blood tests and an MRI scan were normal.

There is evidence that the central histaminergic neurons play an important role in inhibiting convulsions in the immature brain, where the GABA system is less effective than in the adult brain. Histamine acts via an H_1 receptor and other H_1 receptor antagonists can cause seizures. The authors proposed that ketotifen induces infantile spasms by antagonizing H_1 receptors.

DESENSITIZATION (IMMUNOTHERAPY) *(SED-13, 424)*

The incidence of adverse systemic reactions during immunotherapy for perennial allergic rhinitis using standardized extracts of *Dermatophagoides farinae* has been estimated in 386 patients who received 22 722 injections. The incidence of systemic reactions was 6.22% per patient, and 0.12% per injection. *Systemic reactions* began 3–30 minutes after an injection (average 11 minutes). Asthma, atopic dermatitis, and a high concentration of IgE (but not specific IgE) in serum were identified as important risk factors for severe systemic reactions. Systemic reactions occurred in 12 of 18 patients who had an IgE concentration over 100 IU/ml and asthma and/or atopic dermatitis. In patients who had none of these risk factors the incidence of systemic reaction was 1.64% per patient. The authors estimated that the rate of systemic reactions could be reduced by 75% if patients with identified risk factors were strictly excluded from immunotherapy for allergic rhinitis (68[C]).

Near-fatal *anaphylaxis,* a rare complication of immunotherapy, has again been reported (69[c]).

A 55-year-old man was stung by a *Polistes* wasp and had an anaphylactic reaction. Intradermal skin tests with wasp venoms were negative. Intradermal honeybee venom 1.0 μg/ml and *Polistes* wasp venom 0.1 μg/ml produced induration and erythema. Venom immunotherapy was given using the protocol of the Bayer Corporation: monthly maintenance injections of Bayer honeybee venom and *Polistes* wasp venom, 100 μg of each for 13 months without incident. Because of a national shortage of *Polistes* wasp venom manufactured by Bayer, *Polistes* wasp venom manufactured by ALK was substituted. Within minutes of receiving injections of 100 μg of Bayer honeybee venom and ALK *Polistes* wasp venom (both from new vials) he became light-headed and developed syncope. He recovered consciousness but remained hypotensive (74/0 mmHg). In a serum sample 2 hours after the start of the reaction serum tryptase was raised at 38 μg/ml (reference range 5.6–14 μg/ml) and IgE anti-honeybee venom and IgE anti-*Polistes* wasp venom concentrations were 3 and 10 ng/ml respectively.

The authors performed RAST inhibition to measure the relative potencies of the different venom extracts using the patient's serum as a source of IgE antivenom. Although they initially suspected the new source of *Polistes* wasp venom, the relative potency tests showed greater variation in the honeybee venom. The

IgG concentrations were consistent with this finding. This report emphasizes the care that must be taken with the preparation of each injection, especially when using a new batch of antigen.

A follow-up of patients for 5 years after stopping venom immunotherapy has been reported. The authors concluded that the residual risk of a systemic reaction to a sting was 5–10% in adults. No severe or life-threatening reactions occurred with 270 challenge stings in 74 patients after 1–5 years without venom immunotherapy. The authors have extended these observations to 5–10 years and attempted to identify patients at greater risk of a reaction. Patients were surveyed for 3 consecutive years to determine the frequency of systemic reactions to field stings and the course of venom sensitivity. The patients included the original 74 (group 1) and 51 other patients followed after stopping venom immunotherapy (group 2). Eleven of the 74 patients in group 1 had field stings again after 3–7 years without venom immunotherapy. One systemic reaction (dyspnea) was reported. Of the 51 patients in group 2, 15 were stung, of whom four (26%) had systemic reactions, including respiratory symptoms necessitating the use of adrenaline. Six of the 13 patients (groups 1 and 2) with a systemic reaction to a sting after stopping venom immunotherapy had had a systemic reaction during venom immunotherapy (to an injection or a sting). Only six of 76 patients who had no reaction during venom immunotherapy had a systemic reaction when stung after cessation of venom immunotherapy. Other risk factors were persistent strongly positive skin test sensitivity and the severity of the pretreatment reaction (70[C]).

MUCOLYTIC AGENTS *(SED-13, 430)*

The place of mucolytic drugs in respiratory disease has recently been reviewed (71[R]). The authors suggested that they have been inappropriately used in the past. As mucolytic agents do not improve lung function tests in COPD, the European Respiratory Society and the American Thoracic Society guidelines discourage their use in the treatment of COPD. Future trials should evaluate clinical symptoms and quality of life as well as lung function tests. Mucolytic agents should be evaluated earlier in the natural history of COPD, when mucus hypersecretion is the major feature and before lung function has deteriorated.

ANTITUSSIVES *(SED-13, 432)*

Dextromethorphan

An *anaphylactoid reaction* to dextromethorphan has been reported (72[c]).

A 40-year-old woman was seen in consultation for recurrent reactions to cough and cold formulations. She believed that all formulations she had taken had contained dextromethorphan as the active cough suppressant. She reported reactions consisting of hives, swelling of the lips, and shortness of breath. She was given 1 mg dextromethorphan mg and noted mild transient pruritus of the eyes. Hives with nasal and conjunctival congestion occurred 20 minutes after a 30 mg dose. No bronchospasm or angioedema were noted and her vital signs and peak flow remained stable. Oral diphenhydramine quickly reversed her symptoms. The patient subsequently tolerated hydrocodone and codeine without any adverse effects.

The authors noted that many opioids are potent histamine releasers and most reactions to opioids are anaphylactoid rather than IgE-mediated. It was of particular interest that the patient was able to tolerate the opioids hydrocodone and codeine.

MISCELLANEOUS DRUGS

Ambroxol

A urine sample from a patient with a severe head injury tested positive for *lysergic acid diethylamide* (LSD) (73[C]). The test was carried out using a homogeneous immunoassay CEDIA® DAU LSD (Boehringer, Mannheim). Although LSD has a half-life of 3 hours, the patient's urine tested positive for several days. Analysis of the same urine samples using high-performance liquid chromatography (HPLC) failed to detect LSD. LSD screening was then performed in urine samples obtained from 10 other patients in the same ward. All samples tested positive for LSD by the CEDIA® DAU LSD assay but negative using HPLC. All of the patients were taking ambroxol. Ambroxol was detected in the urine by HPLC. In a volunteer LSD was not detected in a fasting urine sample. After ambroxol 15 mg a urine sample obtained 90 minutes later tested positive for LSD. The addition of 50 μl of Mucosolvan juice (which contains ambroxol) to the negative fasting urine sample resulted in a positive test for LSD. The authors concluded that ambroxol should be excluded when LSD screening is performed using the CEDIA® DAU LSD test.

Dornase alfa

Dornase alfa is human recombinant deoxyribonuclease. Its role in modifying bronchial secretions in patients with cystic fibrosis has been evaluated in 54 subjects aged 5 years or over (74[C]). They were treated for 12 months with mesna by nebulizer bd and oral ambroxol (30 mg bd). Dornase alfa was then given once daily by aerosol 2.5 mg for 12 months. Mesna and ambroxol caused reductions in FEV_1 and FVC (FEV_1 fell by 11%, FVC by 13%). After 12 months of dornase alfa, FEV_1 had increased by 7.7% and FVC by 5.3%. The patients found treatment with dornase alfa more acceptable than mucolytic therapy. *Hemoptysis* was the only reported adverse effect, but it occurred frequently in only one patient.

REFERENCES

1. Ayres JG, Frost CD, Holmes WF, Williams DRR, Ward SM. Postmarketing surveillance study of a non-chlorofluorocarbon inhaler according to the safety assessment of marketed medicines guidelines. Br Med J 1998;317:926–30.
2. Borgstrom L. Local versus total systemic bioavailability as a means to compare different inhaled formulations of the same substance. J Aerosol Med Deposition Clear Eff Lung 1998; 11:55–63.
3. Kelly HW. Establishing a therapeutic index for the inhaled corticosteroids: part I. Pharmacokinetic/pharmacodynamic comparison of the inhaled corticosteroids. J Allergy Clin Immunol 1998;102:S36–51.
4. Leach C. Targeting inhaled steroids. Int J Clin Pract Suppl 1998;96:23–7.
5. Trescoli C, Ward MJ. Systemic activity of inhaled and swallowed beclomethasone dipropionate and the effect of different inhaler devices. Postgrad Med J 1998;74:675–7.
6. Thorsson L, Edsbacker S. Lung deposition of budesonide from a pressurized metered-dose inhaler attached to a spacer. Eur Respir J 1998; 12:1340–5.
7. O'Byrne PM, Pedersen S. Measuring efficacy and safety of different inhaled corticosteroid preparations. J Allergy Clin Immunol 1998;102:879–86.
8. Ng PC, Fok TF, Wong GWK, Lam CWK, Lee CH, Wong MY, Lam K, Ma KC. Pituitary-adrenal suppression in preterm, very low birth weight infants after inhaled fluticasone propionate treatment. J Clin Endocrinol Metab 1998;83:2390–3.
9. Duplantier JE, Nelson RP Jr, Morelli AR, Good RA, Kornfeld SJ. Hypothalamic-pituitary-adrenal axis suppression associated with the use of inhaled fluticasone propionate. J Allergy Clin Immunol 1998;102:699–700.
10. Zimmerman B, Gold M, Wherrett D, Hanna AK. Adrenal suppression in two patients with asthma treated with low doses of the inhaled steroid fluticasone propionate. J Allergy Clin Immunol 1998;101:425-6.
11. Vargas R, Dockhorn RJ, Findlay SR, Korenblat PE, Field EA, Kral KM. Effect of fluticasone propionate aqueous nasal spray versus oral prednisone on the hypothalamic-pituitary-adrenal axis. J Allergy Clin Immunol 1998;102:191–7.
12. Nayak AS, Ellis MH, Gross GN, Mendelson LM, Schenkel EJ, Lanier BQ, Simpson B, Mullin ME, Smith JA. The effects of triamcinolone acetonide aqueous nasal spray on adrenocortical function in children with allergic rhinitis. J Allergy Clin Immunol 1998;101:157–62.
13. Findlay CA, Macdonald JF, Wallace AM, Geddes N, Donaldson MD. Childhood Cushing's syndrome induced by betamethasone nose drops, and repeat prescriptions. Br Med J 1998;317:739–40.
14. Faul JL, Tormey W, Tormey V, Burke C. High dose inhaled corticosteroids and dose dependent loss of diabetic control. Br Med J 1998;317:1491.
15. Haapasaari K, Rossi O, Risteli J, Oikarinen A. Effects of long-term inhaled corticosteroids on skin collagen synthesis and thickness in asthmatic patients. Eur Respir J 1998;11:139–43.
16. Shiri J, Amichai B. Perioral dermatitis induced by inhaled corticosteroids. J Dermatol Treat 1998;9:259–60.
17. Ozturk F, Yuceturk AV, Kurt E, Unlu HH, Ilker SS. Evaluation of intraocular pressure and cataract formation following the long-term use of nasal corticosteroids. Ear Nose Throat J 1998;77: 846–51.
18. Cervin A, Andersson M. Intranasal steroids and septum perforation – an overlooked complication? A description of the course of events and a discussion of the causes. Rhinology 1998;36:128–32.
19. Ebeling PR, Erbas B, Hopper JL, Wark JD, Rubinfeld AR. Bone mineral density and bone turnover in asthmatics treated with long-term inhaled or oral glucocorticoids. J Bone Miner Res 1998;13:12830–9.
20. Hughes JA, Conry BG, Male SM, Eastell R. One year prospective open study of the effect of high dose inhaled steroids, fluticasone propionate

and budesonide on bone markers and bone mineral density. Thorax 1998;54:223–9.

21. Gregson RK, Rao R, Murrills AJ, Taylor PA, Warner JO. Effect of inhaled corticosteroids on bone mineral density in childhood asthma: comparison of fluticasone propionate and beclomethasone dipropionate. Osteoporosis Int 1998;8:418–22.
22. Martinati LC, Bertoldo F, Gasperi E, Fortunati P, Lo Cascio V, Boner AL. Longitudinal evaluation of bone mass in asthmatic children treated with inhaled beclomethasone dipropionate or cromolyn sodium. Allergy 1998;53(Suppl 42):705–8.
23. Fitzgerald D, Van Asperen P, Mellis C, Honner M, Smith L, Ambler G. Fluticasone propionate 750 micrograms/day versus beclomethasone dipropionate 1500 micrograms/day: comparison of efficacy and adrenal function in paediatric asthma. Thorax 1999;53:656–61.
24. Price JF, Russell G, Hindmarsh PC, Weller P, Heaf DP, Williams J. Growth during one year of treatment with fluticasone propionate and sodium cromoglycate in children with asthma. Paediatr Pulmonol 1998;24:178–86.
25. Wang WQ, Ip MS, Tsang KW, Lam KS. Antiresorptive therapy in asthmatic patients receiving high-dose inhaled steroids: a prospective study for 18 months. J Allergy Clin Immunol 1998;101:445–50.
26. Herrala J, Puolijoki H, Liippo K, Raitio M, Impivaara O, Tala E, Nieminen MM. Clodronate is effective in preventing corticosteroid-induced bone loss among asthmatic patients. Bone 1998;22:577–82.
27. Downs AM, Lear JT, Kennedy CT. Anaphylaxis to intradermal triamcinolone acetonide. Arch Dermatol 1998;134:1163–4.
28. Yawalkar N, Hari Y, Helbing A, von Greyerz S, Kappeler A, Braathen LR, Pichler WJ. Elevated serum levels of interleukins 5, 6, and 10 in a patient with drug-induced exanthem caused by systemic corticosteroids. J Am Acad Dermatol 1998;39:790–3.
29. Priori R, Tomassini M, Magrini L, Conti F, Valesini G. Churg-Strauss syndrome during pregnancy after steroid withdrawal. Lancet 1998;352:1599–600.
30. Volovitz B, Bentur L, Finkelstein Y, Mansour Y, Shalitin S, Nussinovitch M, Varsano I. Effectiveness and safety of inhaled corticosteroids in controlling acute asthma attacks in children who were treated in the emergency department: a controlled comparative study with oral prednisolone. J Allergy Clin Immunol 1998;102:605–9.
31. Nana A, Youngchaiyud P, Charoenratanakul S, Boe J, Lofdahl CG, Selroos O, Stahl E. High-dose inhaled budesonide may substitute for oral therapy after an acute asthma attack. J Asthma 1998;35:647–55.
32. Sung L, Osmond MH, Klassen TP. Randomized, controlled trial of inhaled budesonide as an adjunct to oral prednisone in acute asthma. Acad Emerg Med 1998;5:209–13.
33. Paggiaro PL, Dahle R, Bakran I, Frith L, Hollingworth K, Efthimiou J. Multicentre randomised placebo-controlled trial of inhaled fluticasone propionate in patients with chronic obstructive pulmonary disease. International COPD Study Group. Lancet 1998;351:773–80 (Erratum in 1998;351:1968).
34. Martin RM, Dunn NR, Freemantle SN, Mann RD. Risk of non-fatal cardiac failure and ischaemic heart disease with long acting beta$_2$ agonists. Thorax 1998;53:558–62.
35. Jenne JW. Can oral beta$_2$ agonists cause heart failure? Lancet 1998;352:1081–2.
36. Lindmark B, Ottosson A. Beta$_2$ agonists and heart failure. Lancet 1998;352:1709–10.
37. Kremer G, Disse B. Fenoterol and asthma mortality. Lancet 1998;352:485–6.
38. Beasley R, Nishima S, Pearce N, Crane J. Fenoterol and asthma mortality. Lancet 1998;352: 486.
39. Lipworth B, Jackson C. Fenoterol and asthma mortality. Lancet 1998;352:486–7.
40. Newhouse MT, Chapman KR, McCallum AL, Abboud RT, Bowie DM, Hodder RV, Pare PD, Mesic-Fuchs H, Molfino NA. Cardiovascular safety of high doses of inhaled fenoterol and albuterol in acute severe asthma. Chest 1996; 110:595–603.
41. Van den Berg BT, Braat MC, Van Boxtel CJ. Pharmacokinetics and effects of formoterol fumarate in healthy human subjects after oral dosing. Eur J Clin Pharmacol 1998;54:463–8.
42. Greiff L, Wollmer P, Andersson M, Svensson C, Persson CG. Effects of formoterol on histamine induced plasma exudation in induced sputum from normal subjects. Thorax 1998;53:1010–13.
43. Aziz I, Tan KS, Hall IP, Devlin MM, Lipworth BJ. Subsensitivity to bronchoprotection against adenosine monophosphate challenge following regular once-daily formoterol. Eur Respir J 1998;12:580–4.
44. Lipworth B, Tan S, Devlin M, Aiken T, Baker R, Hendrick D. Effects of treatment with formoterol on bronchoprotection against methacholine. Am J Med 1998;104:431–8.
45. Aziz I, McFarlane LC, Lipworth BJ. Concomitant inhaled corticosteroid resensitises cardiac beta$_2$-adrenoceptors in the presence of long-acting beta$_2$-agonist therapy. Eur J Clin Pharmacol 1998;54:377–81.
46 Burgess C, Ayson M, Rajasingham S, Crane J, Della CG, Till MD. The extrapulmonary effects of increasing doses of formoterol in patients with asthma. Eur J Clin Pharmacol 1998;54:141–7.
47. Cazzola M, Imperatore F, Salzillo A, Di Perna F, Calderaro F, Imperatore A, Matera MG. Cardiac effects of formoterol and salmeterol in patients suffering from COPD with preexisting cardiac arrhythmias and hypoxemia. Chest 1998;114:411–15.
48. Selroos O. The pharmacologic and clinical properties of Oxis (formoterol) Turbuhaler. Allergy 1998;53(Suppl 42):14–19.

49. Totterman KJ, Huhti L, Sutinen E, Backman R, Pietinalho A, Falck M, Larsson P, Selroos O. Tolerability to high doses of formoterol and terbutaline via Turbuhaler for 3 days in stable asthmatic patients. Eur Respir J 1998;12:573–9.
50. Clauzel A-M, Molimard M, Le Gros V, Lepere E, Febvre N, Michel F-B. Use of formoterol dry powder administered for three months via a single-dose inhaler in 1,380 asthmatic patients. J Invest Allergol Clin Immunol 1998;8:265–70.
51. Ekstrom T, Ringdal N, Sobradillo V, Runnerstrom E, Soliman S. Low-dose formoterol Turbuhaler (Oxis) b.i.d., a 3-month placebo-controlled comparison with terbutaline (q.i.d.). Respir Med 1998;92:1040–5.
52. Ringdal N, Derom E, Wahlin-Boll E, Pauwels R. Onset and duration of action of single doses of formoterol inhaled via Turbuhaler. Respir Med 1998;92:1017–21.
53. Bondesson E, Friberg K, Soliman S, Lofdahl CG. Safety and efficacy of a high cumulative dose of salbutamol inhaled via Turbuhaler or via a pressurized metered-dose aerosol in patients with asthma. Respir Med 1998;92:325–30.
54. Busse WW, Casale TB, Murray JJ, Petrocella V, Cox F, Rickard K. Efficacy, safety, and impact on quality of life of salmeterol in patients with moderate persistent asthma. Am J Managed Care 1998;4:1579–87.
55. Langley SJ, Masterson CM, Batty EP, Woodcock A. Bronchodilator response to salbutamol after chronic dosing with salmeterol and placebo. Eur Respir J 1998;11:1081–5.
56. Di Lorenzo G, Morici G, Drago A, Pellitteri ME, Mansueto P, Melluso M, Norrito F, Squassante L, Fasolo A. Efficacy, tolerability, and effects on quality of life of inhaled salmeterol and oral theophylline in patients with mild-to-moderate chronic obstructive pulmonary disease. Clin Ther 1998;20:1130–48.
57. Taylor DR, Town GI, Herbison GP, Boothman-Burrell D, Flannery EM, Hancox B, Harre B, Laubscher K, Linscott V, Ramsay CM, Richards G, Cowan J, Holbrook N, McLachlan C, Rigby S. Asthma control during long-term treatment with regular inhaled salbutamol and salmeterol. Thorax 1998;53:744–52 (Erratum in 1999;54:188).
58. Vervloet D, Ekstrom T, Pela R, Duce Gracia F, Kopp C, Silvert BD, Quebe Fehling E, Della Cioppa G, Di Benedetto G. A 6-month comparison between formoterol and salmeterol in patients with reversible obstructive airways disease. Respir Med 1998;92:836–42.
59. Kemp JP, Cook DA, Incaudo GA, Corren J, Kalberg C, Emmett A, Cox FM, Rickard K. Salmeterol improves quality of life in patients with asthma requiring inhaled corticosteroids. J Allergy Clin Immunol 1998;101:188–95.
60. Smigaj D, Roman-Drago NM, Amini SB, Caritis SN, Kalhan SC, Catalano PM. The effect of oral terbutaline on maternal glucose metabolism and energy expenditure in pregnancy. Am J Obstet Gynecol 1998;178:1041–7.
61. Plotnick LH, Ducharme FM. Should inhaled anticholinergics be added to beta$_2$ agonists for treating acute childhood and adolescent asthma? A systemic review. Br Med J 1998;317:971–7.
62. Endoh N, Ichinose M, Takahashi T, Miura M, Kageyama N, Mashito Y, Sugiura H, Ikeda K, Takasaka T, Shirato K. Relationship between cholinergic airway tone and serum immunoglobulin E in human subjects. Eur Respir J 1998;12:71–4.
63. Cazzola M, Matera MG, Di Perna F, Calderaro F, Califano C, Vinciguerra A. A comparison of bronchodilating effects of salmeterol and oxitropium bromide in stable chronic obstructive pulmonary disease. Respir Med 1998;92:354–7.
64. Cortijo J, Naline E, Ortiz JL, Berto L, Girard V, Malbezin M, Advenier C, Morcillo EJ. Effects of fenspiride on human bronchial cyclic nucleotide phosphodiesterase isoenzymes: functional and biochemical study. Eur J Pharmacol 1998;341:79–86.
65. Quartulli F, Pinelli E, Broue-Chabbert A, Gossart S, Girard V, Pipy B. Fenspiride inhibits histamine-induced responses in a lung epithelial cell line. Eur J Pharmacol 1998;348:297–304.
66. Plusa T, Nawacka D. Efficacy and tolerance of fenspiride in adult patients with acute respiratory tract infections. Pol Merkuriusz Lek 1998;5:368–71.
67. Yasuhara A, Ochi A, Harada Y, Kobayashi Y. Infantile spasms associated with a histamine H$_1$ antagonist. Neuropediatrics 1998;29:320–1.
68. Ohashi Y, Nakai Y, Tanaka A, Kakinoki Y, Washio Y, Ohno Y, Yamada K, Nasako Y. Risk factors for adverse systemic reactions occurring during immunotherapy with standardized *Dermatophagoides farinae* extracts. Acta Oto-Laryngol Suppl 1998;538:113-17.
69. Wolf BL, Hamilton RG. Near-fatal anaphylaxis after *Hymenoptera* venom immunotherapy. J Allergy Clin Immunol 1998;102:527–8.
70. Golden DB, Kwiterovich KA, Kagey-Sobotka A, Lichtenstein LM. Discontinuing venom immunotherapy: extended observations. J Allergy Clin Immunol 1998;101:298–305.
71. Del Donno M, Olivieri D. Mucoactive drugs in the management of chronic obstructive pulmonary disease. Monaldi Arch Chest Dis 1998;53:714–19.
72. Knowles SR, Weber E. Dextromethorphan anaphylaxis. J Allergy Clin Immunol 1998;102:316–17.
73. Rohrich J, Zorntlein S, Lotz J, Becker J, Kern T, Rittner C. False-positive LSD testing in urine samples from intensive care patients. J Anal Toxicol 1998;22:393–5.
74. Derelle J, Bertolo-Houriez E, Marchal F, Weber M, Virion JM, Vidailhet M. Respiratory evolution of patient with mucoviscidosis treated with mucolytic agents plus dornase alfa. Arch Pediatr 1998;5:371–7.

J.K. Aronson

17 Positive inotropic drugs and drugs used in dysrhythmias

CARDIAC GLYCOSIDES

(SED-13, 438; SEDA-20, 173; SEDA-21, 194; SEDA-22, 201)

The question of whether digoxin should be used to treat patients with mild to moderate heart failure in sinus rhythm, in the wake of recent randomized controlled trials of its efficacy, including PROVED, RADIANCE, and DIG (SEDA-18, 196; SEDA-20, 173), has been reviewed (1[R]). The authors concluded that digoxin is effective in producing symptomatic improvement in patients with mild or moderate heart failure, but that because of concerns about its safety careful consideration must be taken in each case before using it.

Of 2254 elderly patients, 724 were being treated with digoxin, of whom 187 had congestive heart failure, 90 had atrial fibrillation, and 447 were both free from heart failure and in sinus rhythm (2[Cr]). Among those who did not have heart failure or atrial fibrillation, cardiovascular and total mortality were significantly higher among those taking digoxin. Digoxin was a predictor of mortality in those subjects. In addition the incidence of non-fatal heart failure was higher among those taking digoxin. This is yet another non-randomized study purporting to show deleterious effects of digoxin during long-term use, in this case in patients in whom it was not indicated in the first place. Since similar non-randomized studies in patients with heart failure, which also showed deleterious effects (SEDA-20, 173), have since been contradicted by proper prospective randomized studies, this result should be ignored.

There has been another study of serum digoxin concentrations in patients admitted to hospital (3[C]). Of 1433 such patients, 115 had a raised concentration. Of the 82 in whom the blood sample had been taken at an appropriate time, 59 had electrocardiographic or clinical features of digoxin toxicity. The patients whose serum digoxin concentrations were over 3.2 nmol/l (2.5 ng/ml) were slightly older (78 vs 73 years) and had higher serum creatinine concentrations (273 vs 123 μmol/l) than those whose plasma concentrations were below 3.1 nmol/l. Of 47 patients with raised digoxin concentrations on admission, 21 were admitted because of digoxin toxicity, and impaired or worsening renal function contributed to high concentrations in 37 patients. A drug interaction was a contributory factor in 10 cases. These results suggest that digoxin toxicity is still very common and confirms the increased risk in elderly patients, patients with renal impairment, and patients taking drugs that may interact with digoxin. Serum potassium concentrations were not reported in this study. In another study of this sort, serum digoxin concentrations were measured in 2009 patients (4[C]). The concentration was over 2.6 nmol/l in 320 cases (9.3%) but in 51 of those the sample had been drawn too soon after the dose. When other results were omitted in cases in which the sampling time was not known, there were 138 evaluable patients, of whom 83 had clinical evidence of digoxin toxicity, an overall incidence of 4.1%. The authors concluded that digoxin toxicity was less common in their series than has previously been reported. There were no differences between the groups in serum potassium, calcium, or magnesium concentrations, but the serum creatinine concentration was significantly higher in those who had definite and possible toxicity. The mean age of the patients was 69 years. It is likely that the differences across studies of this sort are largely due to differences in renal function and age in the population being studied.

Both of these studies also underline the importance of taking blood samples for serum

Side Effects of Drugs, Annual 23
J.K. Aronson, ed.

digoxin concentration measurement at the correct time, which should be at least 6 hours after the last dose and preferably at about 11 hours.

Digoxin toxicity has been reported in two patients who took herbal remedies (5[c]). *Digitalis lanata* was found as a contaminant.

Special senses *Color vision abnormality* is a well-known adverse effect of digitalis (SEDA-20, 173), and particularly occurs in patients with digitalis toxicity. There has now been a report of two cases of digoxin-related visual disturbances in patients whose blood concentrations were in the usual target range (6[c]). A 68-year-old woman had shimmering lights in her field of vision in both eyes when in sunlight, and a 63-year-old woman complained of blurring of vision in both eyes. The serum digoxin concentrations were 2.2 and 1.3 nmol/l (1.7 and 1.0 ng/ml) respectively. Withdrawal of digoxin caused resolution of their symptoms within 1–2 weeks. Unfortunately the authors did not report serum electrolyte concentrations, and it is not clear in these cases whether digoxin toxicity was potentiated by potassium depletion.

Miscellaneous There has been a randomized, double-blind comparison of intravenous diltiazem and digoxin in 40 patients with atrial fibrillation and a ventricular rate of over 100 beats per minute (7[C]). One patient given intravenous digoxin had *a burning sensation at the site of injection,* an adverse effect that to my knowledge has not previously been reported.

Interactions The major mechanism for drug interactions with digoxin is inhibition of its renal tubular secretion by inhibition of P-glycoprotein. This mechanism has been reviewed in relation to an in vitro tissue culture model, consisting of confluent polarized renal tubular cell monolayers (8). This model has confirmed the action of several drugs that can inhibit the renal tubular secretion of digoxin in this way, including amiodarone, ciclosporin, itraconazole and ketaconazole, mifepristone, propafenone, quinidine, spironolactone, verapamil, and vinblastine and vincristine.

Amiodarone The interaction of amiodarone with digoxin is well known (SEDA-22, 201). It has also previously been reported with acetyldigoxin (SEDA-18, 198) and now more recently with digitoxin (9[c]). In two cases the half-life of digitoxin was prolonged, but there was no other information that suggested a mechanism. The author suggested that amiodarone might displace digitoxin from tissue sites, but that would have led to a shortening of the half-life rather than a prolongation. It seems more likely that amiodarone inhibits the metabolism of digitoxin.

Antifungal imidazoles Itraconazole increases steady-state serum digoxin concentrations, perhaps by inhibiting the renal tubular secretion of digoxin (SEDA-22, 202; 10[R]). An alternative proposed mechanism is inhibition of CYP3A (SEDA-21, 196), and this has been reported in rats with ketoconazole (11), although an effect on P-glycoprotein was also possible. Whatever the mechanism, ketoconazole increased the systemic availability of digoxin from 0.68 to 0.84 and reduced the mean absorption time from 1.1 to 0.3 hours. The increased systemic availability could have been explained by inhibition of CYP3A or P-glycoprotein in the gut, but the increased rate of absorption could only be explained by inhibition of the P-glycoprotein. Since the t_{max} was unaffected, the authors hypothesized that inhibition of P-glycoprotein increased the absorption rate, which would have tended to reduce the t_{max}, while inhibition of CYP3A, which would have reduced the elimination rate of digoxin, would have tended to increase the t_{max}. Thus a combination of these two effects would have had no effect on t_{max}. It should be noted that CYP3A is an important route of metabolism of digoxin in rats, but not in man.

Macrolide antibiotics Macrolide antibiotics can reduce the metabolism of digoxin in the gut before it is absorbed, by inhibiting the growth of the bacterium Eubacterium glenum, and this has been reported with clarithromycin (SEDA-22, 201). Another case of digoxin toxicity in a patient taking clarithromycin has been reported (12[c]). However, in two other cases in which clarithromycin increased serum digoxin concentrations there was an associated reduction in the rate of renal digoxin clearance, which may be another mechanism for this interaction (13[c]). The authors hypothesized that clarithromycin inhibited P-glycoprotein. This was supported by the observation of a concentration-dependent effect of clarithromycin on in vitro transcellular transport of digoxin.

Tiagabine Tiagabine, which is principally metabolized by CYP3A, had no effect on the steady-state pharmacokinetics of digoxin in 13 healthy volunteers (14[C]). This is further evidence (see above) that CYP3A is not important in the metabolism of digoxin.

Treatment of digitalis toxicity Further evidence of the efficacy of antidigoxin Fab antibody fragments in the treatment of intoxication due to oleander poisoning, previously only anecdotally reported (15[c], 16[c]) has come from a large prospective study (17[C]).

OTHER POSITIVE INOTROPIC DRUGS *(SED-13, 447; SEDA-20, 174; SEDA-21, 196; SEDA-22, 203)*

Milrinone

Milrinone, an inhibitor of phosphodiesterase type III, continues to be used intravenously in the treatment of cardiac failure (SEDA-21, 196; SEDA-22, 203). There has now been a study of the use of intermittent intravenous milrinone in 10 patients with end-stage congestive heart failure (18[C]). Some hemodynamic benefit was obtained, but this was an open uncontrolled study and firm conclusions are impossible. There was also some improvement in the quality of life. The drug was well tolerated and only one patient had an increase in *dysrhythmias* (an increased frequency of ventricular extra beats).

Cardiovascular Milrinone can cause a *tachycardia,* partly because of its vasodilatory effects and partly perhaps by a direct effect on the heart. It has recently been reported that a 74-year-old man had a tachycardia of 145 beats/min during infusion of milrinone after an operation for repair of an abdominal aortic aneurysm (19[c]). Despite the fact that milrinone does not affect β-adrenoceptors, the tachycardia was controlled by esmolol on one occasion and more impressively by metoprolol on a second occasion. However, the hemodynamic effects of milrinone were not altered by β-blockade. Presumably the beneficial effects of β-blockade were non-specific.

In the study described below (20[C]), two infants developed *junctional ectopic tachycardia* during infusion of milrinone.

Hematological Milrinone is well known to cause *thrombocytopenia* (SEDA-20, 174), and this has again been reported in a study of 19 children (12 infants and seven children aged 1–13 years) who were given either two boluses of 25 μg/kg followed by an infusion of 0.5 μg/kg/min, or a bolus of 50 μg/kg followed by a bolus of 25 μg/kg followed by an infusion of 0.75 μg/kg/min (20[C]). Of the 19 patients, 11 developed thrombocytopenia, defined as a platelet count below 100×10^{12}/l, during milrinone infusion. Of these, two infants required a platelet transfusion. By comparison in 128 patients who did not receive milrinone the incidence of thrombocytopenia was 25%, significantly lower than in those given milrinone. The occurrence of thrombocytopenia increased with increasing duration of infusion.

Vesnarinone

Vesnarinone has previously been reported to reduce mortality at low doses and to increase it at high doses (SEDA-18, 199). Now there has been another study of vesnarinone (30 or 60 mg/day) in 3833 patients with heart failure of classes III or IV and a left ventricular ejection fraction of 30% or less despite optimal treatment, followed for 286 days (21[C]). There were significantly more deaths in those given vesnarinone 60 mg/day and a shorter duration of survival. The increased death rate was due to an increase in sudden deaths, presumably because of cardiac dysrhythmias. There were similar trends in those who took 30 mg/day, but the changes were not significant. There was dose-dependent agranulocytosis, in 0.2% of those taking 30 mg/day and 1.2% of those taking 60 mg/day. This has been previously reported (SEDA-19, 189). There was also a slight increase in the risk of diarrhea, which occurred in 17% of those taking 60 mg/day compared with 12% of those taking placebo and 14.5% of those taking 30 mg/day. In contrast to the increased mortality with vesnarinone there was a short-term increase in quality of life, which occurred during the first 16 weeks but was not maintained at 6 months. Probably the increased mortality due to vesnarinone outweighs the improvement in quality of life.

DRUGS USED IN DYSRHYTHMIAS

℞ *Prodysrhythmic effects of antidysrhythmic drugs*

There have been further reviews of the prodysrhythmic effects of antidysrhythmic drugs (22[R]–25[R]).

Criteria for prodysrhythmia *The criteria that have been suggested as labelling a drug prodysrhythmic include:*

- *the new appearance of a sustained ventricular tachydysrhythmia;*
- *change from a non-sustained to a sustained tachydysrhythmia;*
- *acceleration of the rate of a tachycardia;*
- *the new appearance of a clinically significant bradydysrhythmia or conduction defect.*

Mechanisms of prodysrhythmia *Digitalis-induced dysrhythmias have been attributed to two mechanisms. First, a decrease in the automaticity of the conducting tissues mediated by delayed after-depolarization, secondary to an increase in the intracellular calcium concentration due to inhibition of the sodium/potassium pump. This mechanism leads to ventricular and supraventricular ectopic dysrhythmias. In addition, digitalis can cause atrial fibrillation by a vagotonic effect, shortening the action potential by activating an acetylcholine-sensitive potassium current; however, this is a rare effect.*

Class I antidysrhythmic drugs cause dysrhythmias principally by sodium channel blockade. Drugs that are associated with use dependence (i.e. drugs that cause sodium channel blockade at high heart rates but not at low heart rates), such as lidocaine and mexiletine, tend not to cause cardiac dysrhythmias, whereas those that block sodium channels to a greater or lesser extent at all heart rates are more likely to cause dysrhythmias. The typical varieties of dysrhythmia that can occur by this mechanism include atrial flutter with 1 : 1 atrioventricular conduction, fast monomorphic ventricular tachycardia, ventricular fibrillation, bradydysrhythmias (associated with reduced sinoatrial nodal automaticity and reduced conduction through the atrioventricular node and His–Purkinje system), and sudden death. This mechanism is also responsible for an increased threshold for pacing and defibrillation. For this reason patients with implantable cardioverter-defibrillators should not be given potent sodium channel blockers (i.e. class I antidysrhythmic drugs). Antidysrhythmic drugs can reduce the rate of a ventricular tachycardia below the detection rate of a programmed device, thereby preventing it from terminating the tachycardia. Conversely, if an antidysrhythmic drug causes incessant ventricular tachycardia, that can lead to repetitive firing of the device. If a drug increases the defibrillation threshold it may prevent an implantable defibrillator from working. In such cases the defibrillation threshold should be adjusted.

Atrial flutter with 1 : 1 atrioventricular conduction is associated with a slowing of the atrial rate, due to slowing of conduction within the atrial flutter circuit. Ventricular tachycardia is associated with slowing of conduction within a re-entrant tachycardia circuit. The increased threshold for pacing or defibrillation is due to an increased threshold for excitability of the tissues.

In ischemic heart disease there may be rate-dependent conduction blockade and preferential slowing of conduction in ischemic tissue. Slowing of the rate of conduction around a non-conducting ischemic or infarcted area may also contribute to the risk of dysrhythmias.

Both classes I and III antidysrhythmic drugs can also cause polymorphous ventricular tachycardia, particularly of the type known as torsade de pointes, due to prolongation of the QT interval and triggered by early after-depolarizations and intramural re-entry. This particularly occurs with the class IA drugs (quinidine, disopyramide, and procainamide), and with class III drugs (d-sotalol and ibutalide). The class III drug amiodarone causes torsade de pointes much less commonly than the other drugs of this class, perhaps because it tends to prolong repolarization more uniformly throughout the ventricular tissues. The mechanism whereby these antidysrhythmic drugs cause torsade de pointes may be through blockade of the activity of the delayed rectifier potassium channels or inactivation of sodium channels.

Sudden death due to antidysrhythmic drugs *Sudden death due to antidysrhythmic drugs has been reported in several trials in patients who have had ventricular dysrhythmias after myocardial infarction. The drugs that have been incriminated include disopyramide, encainide, flecainide, mexiletine, moricizine,* *procainamide, and quinidine (26[C]–32[C]). The class III drug d-sotalol has also been associated with an increased risk of mortality in such patients (33[C]). This increase in mortality is thought to be due to an increased risk of cardiac dysrhythmias, perhaps as a consequence of rate-dependent conduction block and preferential slowing of conduction in the ischemic areas. Cardiac dysrhythmias of this sort may also occur through slowing of the rate of conduction around non-conducting ischemic or infracted areas in the heart.*

Risk factors for prodysrhythmia *Several factors increase the risk of cardiac dysrhythmias in patients taking antidysrhythmic drugs. These include left ventricular hypertrophy, a low left ventricular ejection fraction, an increased frequency and repetitiveness of ventricular extra beats, an increased tendency to inducibility of ventricular tachycardia by programmed ventricular stimulation, low heart rate variability, and an abnormal signal-averaged electrocardiogram with low-amplitude fractionated electrical activity. It has been suggested that the combination of factors that best predicts a high risk of prodysrhythmia is low heart rate variability and a low left ventricular ejection fraction (23[R]).*

Management of prodysrhythmia *The management of drug-induced cardiac dysrhythmias depends on the type of dysrhythmia. In all cases the suspected drug should be withdrawn. Atrial flutter with 1 : 1 atrioventricular conduction can be treated by atrioventricular nodal blockade, using, for example, verapamil or a β-blocker. Sustained ventricular tachycardia due to rate-dependent blockade of sodium channels may respond to slowing of the heart rate with a β-blocker. In ventricular tachycardia due to overdose with tricyclic antidepressants intravenous sodium bicarbonate is the treatment of choice. Torsade de pointes should be treated by maintaining the serum potassium at over 4.5 mmol/l, the intravenous administration of magnesium sulfate (1–2 g) and if necessary shortening of the QT interval by increasing the heart rate with either isoprenaline or overdrive pacing. There is anecdotal evidence that verapamil and propranolol may also be effective.*

Adenosine *(SED-13, 450; SEDA-20, 174; SEDA-21, 197; SEDA-22, 203)*

Several studies have reported the efficacy and safety of adenosine and ATP in the treatment of tachycardias in children (34[C], 35[R], 36[C], 37[CR]).

Cardiovascular When adenosine (70 μg/kg/min) was given by intravenous infusion to 45 patients with acute myocardial infarction preceding balloon angioplasty, one patient developed persisting *hypotension* in conjunction with a large inferolateral myocardial infarction (38[C]). Transient hypotension in three other patients resolved with a reduction in the dosage. There were no cases of atrioventricular block. Symptomatic hypotension has occasionally been reported in patients with myocardial infarction who have been given adenosine (SEDA-20, 174).

Of 100 patients who received intravenous adenosine in hospital (mean dose 7.8 mg) two had a *dysrhythmia* (39[C]). One patient, a 53-year-old man with a dilated cardiomyopathy, was given adenosine 6 mg for a regular broad-complex tachycardia; the dysrhythmia resolved but was followed by prolonged asystole and cyanosis for about 15 seconds. The other patient, a 64-year-old woman with atrial fibrillation, was given adenosine 12 mg; she developed a non-sustained polymorphous ventricular tachycardia followed by sustained ventricular fibrillation requiring DC shock. In the whole series, about 40% of the patients received adenosine unnecessarily, having atrial fibrillation or atrial flutter, and the authors suggested that misuse of this sort resulted in unnecessary expense and increased risks of adverse effects. Most of this misuse was attributed to misdiagnosis by house officers who thought that rapid atrial fibrillation was a paroxysmal supraventricular tachycardia. Very few thought that adenosine would be likely to terminate atrial fibrillation.

In four out of nine patients with heart transplants, *second- or third-degree atrioventricular block* occurred during the administration of adenosine 140 μg/kg/min over 6 minutes (40[c]). In two patients the infusion had to be interrupted because of *severe discomfort and chest pain.*

Nervous system Of 12 healthy volunteers given an intrathecal injection of adenosine (500–2000 μg) one volunteer had *transient lumbar pain* lasting 30 minutes after an injection of 2000 μg (41[c]). There were no adverse effects at lower doses.

Interactions Endogenous plasma adenosine concentrations were measured in 14 kidney transplant recipients taking ciclosporin and compared with five transplant recipients not taking ciclosporin, two taking sirolimus (FK506), six patients with chronic renal insufficiency, and 10 controls (42[C]). Plasma adenosine concentrations were significantly higher in those taking *ciclosporin* and *sirolimus* and in the patients taking ciclosporin the plasma adenosine concentrations correlated with serum ciclosporin concentrations. An in vitro study showed that ciclosporin inhibited the uptake of adenosine by erythrocytes. The authors concluded that since adenosine is an immunosuppressant, the raised concentrations of adenosine in patients taking ciclosporin might contribute to the immunosuppressive action of ciclosporin. A further mechanism of the increase in adenosine concentration was possibly increased tissue release secondary to ciclosporin-induced vasoconstriction. The relevance of these results to the use of therapeutic intravenous adenosine in patients already taking ciclosporin is not clear.

Amiodarone *(SED-13, 452; SEDA-20, 175; SEDA-21, 198; SEDA-22, 204)*

There have been recent reviews of the results of major trials of amiodarone after myocardial infarction (43[R]) and in chronic heart failure (44[R]).

- In the Basel Antiarrhythmic Study of Infarct Survival (BASIS) amiodarone significantly reduced all-cause mortality from 13 to 5%, compared with no antidysrhythmic drug therapy (45[C]).
- In the Polish Arrhythmia Trial (PAT) amiodarone reduced all-cause mortality from 10.7 to 6.9% compared with placebo and cardiac mortality from 10.7 to 6.2% (46[C]).
- In the Spanish Study of Sudden Death (SSD) amiodarone reduced all-cause mortality from 15.4 to 3.5% compared with metoprolol; however, the mortality in those receiving no antidysrhythmic drugs at all was only 7.7%, and in those the effect of amiodarone was not significant (47[C]).
- In the European Myocardial Infarction Arrhythmia Trial (EMIAT) amiodarone reduced the risk of dysrhythmic deaths from 8.5 to 4.1% compared with placebo (48[C]).
- In the Canadian Amiodarone Myocardial Infarction Arrhythmia Trial (CAMIAT) amiodarone reduced dysrhythmic deaths from 6.0 to 3.3% compared with placebo; non-dysrhythmic deaths were not affected (49[C]).

In a meta-analysis of 10 studies of the use of amiodarone in patients with heart failure, the overall odds ratio for mortality with amiodarone compared with placebo was 0.79 (95% CI = 0.68–0.92). The corresponding odds ratio for adverse effects was 2.29 (1.97–2.66) (44[CR]). The benefit to risk ratio of the use of amiodarone in these patients is not yet clear. The dosage of amiodarone in these studies varied from 50 to 400 mg/day, with an average of around 250 mg/day.

The use of oral amiodarone in preventing recurrence of atrial fibrillation, for preventing recurrence after cardioversion, or for pharmacological cardioversion of atrial fibrillation has been reviewed (50[R]). There is insufficient evidence to support its use as a first-line drug for preventing recurrence of atrial fibrillation or in preventing paroxysmal atrial fibrillation.

Respiratory It has been suggested that the serum activity of lactate dehydrogenase (LDH) may be related to the occurrence of amiodarone-induced *pneumonitis,* as occurred in a 72-year-old woman in whom the serum LDH activity rose from a baseline of around 750 units/l to around 1500 units/l during acute pneumonitis and resolved with resolution of a clinical condition after withdrawal of amiodarone (51[c]). The LDH activity in bronchoalveolar lavage fluid was also increased. The proposed mechanism was leakage of lactate dehydrogenase from the pulmonary interstitial cells into the blood. Of course, a rise in the serum LDH activity is highly nonspecific, and it is not clear whether it might also rise in bronchoalveolar lavage fluid in other conditions.

Endocrine, metabolic The effects of amiodarone on thyroid function tests and in causing thyroid disease, both *hyperthyroidism* and *hypothyroidism,* have been reviewed in the context of the use of perchlorate, which acts by inhibiting iodine uptake by the thyroid gland (52[R]). Amiodarone can cause two different varieties of hyperthyroidism, one by the effects of excess iodine (so-called type 1 hyperthyroidism), the other through direct effects of the drug on the thyroid gland (so-called type 2 hyperthyroidism). The two varieties can be distinguished by differences in radio-iodine uptake by the gland: in type 1 hyperthyroidism radio-iodine uptake is normal or increased, whereas in type 2 it is reduced. In type 1 hyperthyroidism, thyroid ultrasound shows a nodular, hypoechoic gland of increased volume, whereas in type 2 the gland is normal. Hyperthyroidism due to amiodarone is very difficult to treat (SEDA-21, 199) and may not respond to carbimazole or methimazole. Corticosteroids can be added or alternatively potassium perchlorate can be used. The authors suggested that perchlorate should be used in the treatment of type 1 hyperthyroidism and corticosteroids in the treatment of type 2.

The effects of amiodarone on the thyroid gland and the management of amiodarone-induced thyroid dysfunction have been reviewed (53[R]). For amiodarone-induced hyperthyroidism amiodarone should be withdrawn and the management depends on the type of hyperthyroidism caused (see above). However, in some cases (54[C], 55[R]) worsening of thyrotoxic symptoms and heart function has been reported after withdrawal of amiodarone. When withdrawal of amiodarone is not an option, near-total thyroidectomy may be preferred. If surgery is not possible plasmapheresis may be helpful. In amiodarone-induced hypothyroidism the simplest method is to continue treatment with amiodarone and to add thyroxine as required. If amiodarone is withdrawn, restoration of the euthyroid state can be accelerated by using potassium perchlorate (see below). However, this is not recommended, because there is a high risk of recurrence after treatment and potassium perchlorate can cause serious adverse effects (SED-13, 1281).

Potassium perchlorate has also paradoxically been recommended for the treatment of amiodarone-induced hypothyroidism. Since hypothyroidism due to amiodarone tends to occur in areas in which there is sufficient iodine in the diet, it has been hypothesized that an iodinated organic inhibitor of hormone synthesis is formed and that the formation of this inhibitor is itself inhibited by perchlorate to a greater extent than thyroid hormone iodination is inhibited, since the iodinated lipids that are thought to be inhibitors require about 10 times more iodide than the hormone.

Hematological *Granulomata* have been described in the bone-marrow of two patients (56[c]). The first was a 53-year-old woman who developed leukoerythroblastosis with giant thrombocytes in the peripheral blood and was subsequently given amiodarone, and the second was a 78-year-old woman with a raised erythrocyte sedimentation rate, a mild anemia, and a polyclonal gammopathy on serum immunoelectrophoresis. In both cases the bone-marrow was hypocellular with atypical megakaryocytes and several granulomata. In the first case amiodarone was given after the onset of the peripheral blood film abnormalities and the only change in the bone-marrow was the occurrence of the granulomata. The authors proposed that the granulomata had occurred because of phospholipid accumulation.

Skin and appendages Another case of *bluish-gray discoloration of the face* after treatment with amiodarone has been reported in a 54-year-old man who took the drug for one year (57[c]). The discoloration almost completely resolved within 9 months of withdrawal.

Special senses The adverse effects of amiodarone on the eyes have been reviewed (58[R]). Amiodarone causes *lipid deposition in the cornea,* with resulting microdeposits visible on ophthalmoscopy. However, these deposits are not commonly symptomatic. The most common symptom is of seeing *blue-green rings or halos around lights,* particularly at night; other symptoms include *blurred vision, glare, dryness of the eyes, and irritation of the skin of the eyelids with chronic blepharitis.* Occasionally amiodarone may cause anterior *subcapsular deposits,* which are usually asymptomatic. Rare cases of *retinal maculopathy* have been reported, but their association with amiodarone is not clear. Amiodarone can rarely cause an *optic neuropathy* and although this is reversible on withdrawal, there may be residual field defects (SEDA-15, 171). However, there has also been a recent report of blindness attributed to bilateral optic neuropathy in a patient taking amiodarone (59[c]). Multiple *chalazia* have been reported on the eyelids, due to lipogranulomata which contained a lot of amiodarone (60[c]). *Sicca syndrome* has also occasionally been reported (61[c], 62[R], 63[C], 64[C]). *Impaired color vision* has been reported in association with *keratopathy* (SEDA-12, 153). There has been one report of *papilledema with raised intracranial* *pressure* attributed to amiodarone (SEDA-12, 153).

Interactions Various correspondents have commented on the possibility that *β-blockers* may enhance the effects of amiodarone in reducing mortality in patients who have had a myocardial infarction or are in heart failure (65[r]–67[r]).

Cibenzoline *(SED-13, 457; SEDA-17, 222; SEDA-18, 203; SEDA-20, 177)*

Cibenzoline has previously been reported to cause a *myasthenia-like syndrome* (SEDA-21, 199). Now another case has been reported (68[c]).

A 57-year-old man with chronic renal insufficiency treated by continuous and ambulatory peritoneal dialysis took cibenzoline 150 mg/day for a ventricular dysrhythmia. Four days later he developed proximal muscle weakness, progressing to generalized muscle weakness, with dysphagia and dysarthria. Hemodiafiltration on six occasions caused complete improvement and cibenzoline was withdrawn. There was no further recurrence, even when other drugs that he had been taking were restarted.

The authors suggested that cibenzoline may have inhibited ATP-dependent potassium channels in skeletal muscle. The plasma cibenzoline concentration at the height of this patient's symptoms was very high at 1890 μg/ml (usual target range 300–600) and the authors counselled caution in patients with renal insufficiency (SEDA-15, 174).

Disopyramide *(SED-13, 457; SEDA-20, 177; SEDA-21, 199; SEDA-22, 207)*

Torsade de pointes due to disopyramide is well described (SEDA-4, 180). This effect is associated with prolongation of the QT interval. Now there has been a study of the effects of disopyramide on the QT interval in patients with pre-existing QT interval prolongation (69[C]). In eight patients with QT interval prolongation during bradycardia and five patients without QT interval prolongation, disopyramide significantly prolonged the QT interval; however, the change was more pronounced in those with pre-existing bradycardia (78 vs 35 ms). The authors proposed that this difference might be due to an underlying abnormality of potassium channels in those with pre-existing bradycardia. Thus, those who are genetically predisposed to cardiac dysrhythmias may be at greater risk of the prodysrhythmic effects of antidysrhythmic drugs.

Lidocaine (lignocaine) *(SED-13, 460; SEDA-18, 205; SEDA-21, 201; SEDA-22, 208)*

The effects of *erythromycin* and *itraconazole,* which are both potent inhibitors of CYP3A4, on the pharmacokinetics of lidocaine have been studied in nine healthy volunteers. Steady-state oral erythromycin and itraconazole had no effect on the plasma concentration versus time curve of lidocaine after intravenous administration, but erythromycin increased the plasma concentrations of the major metabolite of lidocaine, monoethylglycinexylidide (MEGX) (70[C]). In contrast, itraconazole had no effect on the kinetics of MEGX. It is not clear what the interpretation of these results is, particularly since the authors did not study enough subjects to detect what might have been small but significant changes in various disposition parameters of lidocaine and did not report unbound concentrations of lidocaine or its metabolites. However, whatever the pharmacokinetic explanation, the clinical relevance is that one would expect that erythromycin would potentiate the toxic effects of lidocaine that are mediated by MEGX.

Mexiletine *(SED-13, 462; SEDA-19, 195; SEDA-21, 201; SEDA-22, 208)*

Mexiletine has been used to treat painful peripheral neuropathy in patients with HIV infection, without any evidence of efficacy (71[C], 72[C]). In one study of 22 patients, nine had adverse effects probably related to mexiletine, including *nausea* in five, *vomiting* in four, and *abdominal pain, diarrhea, dizziness, insomnia, rises in liver enzymes,* and *skin rash* in one patient each (71[C]). Adverse effects in seven patients required dosage reduction in four cases and discontinuation in three (because of a rash in one case and gastrointestinal effects in two). In the second study, in which 48 patients were treated with mexiletine, 10 had nausea and vomiting that required dosage modification; dosage modification was also occasioned by *dizziness* in one case and *urinary retention* in three cases (72[C]).

Interactions Mexiletine is metabolized mainly by CYP2D6 and CYP1A2. *Omeprazole* is an inducer of CYP1A2 and might therefore be expected to interact with mexiletine. However, in a recent study of nine healthy men there was no evidence of an effect of steady-state omeprazole 40 mg/day on the single-dose kinetics of mexiletine 200 mg (73[C]).

Procainamide *(SED-13, 463; SEDA-20, 178; SEDA-21, 202; SEDA-22, 208)*

The adverse effects of intravenous procainamide (400 mg up to three times infused over 10 minutes) have been reported in 60 adults with atrial flutter or fibrillation (74[C]). The adverse effects of procainamide were *headache* in 11%, *hypotension* in 11%, *flushing* in 3.1%, *dizziness* in 3.1%, and *hypesthesia* in 3.1%. The mean fall in systolic blood pressure was about 20 mmHg and occurred at 30–35 minutes after infusion; the corresponding fall in diastolic blood pressure was 10 mmHg. However, in seven patients there was severe hypotension, with a fall in diastolic blood pressure of up to 67 mmHg; in three cases withdrawal of the infusion was required and these patients were treated with intravenous fluids, dopamine, or both. In the severe cases the hypotension occurred during or immediately after the infusion of procainamide.

Nervous system Procainamide has been reported to cause a *chronic inflammatory demyelinating polyradiculoneuropathy* (75[c]).

A 68-year-old man took procainamide 500 mg qds for 3 years and developed distal paresthesia and dysesthesia in the legs, followed by progressive muscle weakness, mainly affecting the legs. His gait became unsteady and was wide-based. He had antinuclear antibodies directed against histones in a titer of 1 : 320, but no antibodies to double-stranded DNA. He had a circulating lupus anticoagulant. The serum procainamide concentration was 3.3 μg/l (target range 4–8). Nerve conduction studies showed a reduction in sensory nerve action potential amplitudes, a mild reduction in sensory nerve conduction velocity, prolongation of distal motor latencies, and reduced conduction velocities, but no conduction block or temporal dispersions. Electromyography was normal. A left sural nerve biopsy showed perivascular inflammation around a single vessel, without evidence of vasculitis. Myelinated nerve fibers were reduced, and scattered nerve fibers showed thin myelin sheaths. About 30% of the fibers showed randomly distributed demyelinated or remyelinated segments. Procainamide was withdrawn and prednisone was given in combination with six plasma exchanges over 2 weeks; after 1 month there was clinical improvement.

This case of polyneuropathy was attributed to a lupus-like effect of procainamide.

Lupus-like syndrome *A lupus-like syndrome with an antiphospholipid syndrome* has been attributed to procainamide in a patient with pre-existing systemic sclerosis (76[c]).

A 51-year-old Korean man with systemic sclerosis was given procainamide 2–3 g/day for suppression of ventricular dysrhythmias. About 2 years later he noticed a new skin ulcer on one of his toes. His dorsalis pedis arteries were not palpable and there was tenderness over the proximal interphalangeal and metacarpophalangeal joints. He had a pancytopenia, prolonged coagulation (with prolongation of the activated partial thromboplastin time and prothrombin time and reduced concentrations of factors XI and XII), an increase in the plasma concentration of von Willebrand factor, a raised serum creatinine concentration, a raised serum C-reactive protein concentration, hypergammaglobulinemia, and hypocomplementemia. He had positive circulating immune complexes and mixed-type cryoglobulinemia, antinuclear antibodies, anti-DNA topoisomerase I antibodies, and a positive LE cell preparation. He had anti-DNA antibodies with a high titer of antibodies to single-stranded DNA and a slightly raised titer of antibodies to double-stranded DNA. Anti-U1 ribonuclear protein, anti-Sm, and anticentromere antibodies were negative. There were high titers of β_2-glycoprotein-I-dependent IgG anticardiolipin antibodies and the lupus anticoagulant test was positive. There were antihistone antibodies. Procainamide was withdrawn and prednisolone and azathioprine given. The pancytopenia, coagulopathy, and renal dysfunction resolved, and the his general condition improved; serum concentrations of several of the antibodies returned to normal.

The authors suggested that the pre-existence of systemic sclerosis in this case and the presence of allele HIA-DQBP1* 0303 had increased the patient's susceptibility to the lupus-like syndrome and antiphospholipid syndrome.

Interactions The in vitro interaction of procainamide with *glucose* to form glucosylamines has been reported (77). The reaction was pH-dependent, with a maximum rate of association at a pH of 3.0 and a maximum rate of dissociation at a pH of 1.5. The authors suggested that the loss of procainamide in an intravenous solution of glucose could be marked.

Propafenone *(SED-13, 465; SEDA-20, 178; SEDA-21, 202; SEDA-22, 209)*

In 87 patients with atrial fibrillation who were given propafenone 2 mg/kg intravenously over 10 minutes, four had hypotension at 8–45 minutes after the start of infusion (78[C]). In two cases this was accompanied by sinus bradycardia, nausea, and slight malaise. In all cases the hypotension resolved rapidly with saline infusion; the drug was withdrawn in only one case. In two cases atrial fibrillation was transformed to asymptomatic atrial flutter with 2 : 1 atrioventricular conduction.

The adverse effects of propafenone in placebo-controlled trials in patients with atrial tachydysrhythmias have been reviewed (79[R]). The following effects were reported after single intravenous oral doses to produce conversion of atrial fibrillation to sinus rhythm. Non-cardiac adverse effects included mild *dizziness.* Mild *hypotension* was also noted, but only required withdrawal of propafenone in one of 29 patients in one study. There have been prodysrhythmic effects in several studies, including *atrial flutter with a broad QRS complex,* which can occur in up to 5% of cases; in some cases atrial flutter can have a rapid ventricular response due to 1 : 1 atrioventricular conduction, which has been attributed to slowing of atrial conduction and reduced refractoriness of the atrioventricular node. Other prodysrhythmic effects in a few patients included *sinus bradycardia with sinus pauses and effects on atrioventricular conduction.*

In patients taking long-term propafenone for supraventricular dysrhythmias adverse effects were more common and have been reported in 14–60% of cases. Cardiac adverse effects were more common in patients with structural heart disease. The non-cardiac effects were either gastrointestinal (*nausea, vomiting, taste disturbances*) or neurological (*dizziness*). Adverse effects are dose related. In one large study there was no difference between propafenone and placebo in the risk of death.

Risk factors The safety of oral propafenone in the treatment of dysrhythmias has been studied retrospectively in infants and children (80[C]). There were significant *electrophysiological adverse effects* and *prodysrhythmia* in 15 of 772 patients (1.9%). These included sinus node dysfunction in four, complete atrioventricular block in two, aggravation of supraventricular tachycardia in two, acceleration of ventricular rate during atrial flutter in one, ventricular prodysrhythmia in five, and unexplained syncope in one. Cardiac arrest or sudden death occurred in five patients (0.6%); two had a supraventricular tachycardia due to Wolff–Parkinson–White syndrome; the other three had structural heart disease. Adverse cardiac events were more common in the presence of structural heart disease and there was no difference between patients with supraventricular and ventricular dysrhythmias.

Quinidine *(SED-13, 466; SEDA-20, 179; SEDA-21, 203; SEDA-22, 209)*

Hematological In a review of all English-language reports on drug-induced *thrombocytopenia,* excluding heparin, 561 case articles reporting on 774 patients were analysed (81[C]). A definite or probable causal role for the drug used was attributed in 247 case reports, and of the 98 that were implicated quinidine was mentioned in 38 cases. The next most common drugs involved were gold salts (11 cases) and co-trimoxazole (10 cases).

Immunological and hypersensitivity reactions Life-threatening *vasculitis* has been attributed to quinidine in a healthy volunteer taking part in a clinical trial (82[c]).

A 58-year-old man took quinidine 200 mg tds for 7 days as part of an interaction study with a new α-blocker. He developed widespread maculopapular purpuric lesions on the limbs, trunk, and ears. His temperature rose to 38.4°C and some of the lesions on his fingers, toes, ears, and nose became necrotic. He had peripheral edema with a bluish purpuric discoloration of the hands and feet. There was mucous membrane involvement with purpuric, partially necrotic lesions on the tongue and palate. A skin biopsy showed necrotizing vasculitis with focal leukocytoclasia. Direct immunofluorescence showed microgranular deposits of IgA, IgM, and C3 around the superficial skin vessels. Quinidine was withdrawn and he was given intravenous methyl prednisolone followed by oral prednisone for 1 month. He recovered completely within 3 weeks.

REFERENCES

1. Soler-Soler J, Permanyer-Miralda G. Should we still prescribe digoxin in mild-to-moderate heart failure? Eur Heart J 1998;19(Suppl P):P26–31.
2. Casiglia E, Tikhonoff V, Pizziol A, Onesto C, Ginocchio G, Mazza A, Pessina AC. Should digoxin be proscribed in elderly subjects in sinus rhythm free from heart failure? A population-based study. Jpn Heart J 1998;39:639–51.
3. Marik PE, Fromm L. A case series of hospitalized patients with elevated digoxin levels. Am J Med 1998;105:110–15.
4. Williamson KM, Thrasher KA, Fulton KB, LaPointe NMA, Dunham GD, Cooper AA, Barrett PS, Patterson JH. Digoxin toxicity: an evaluation in current clinical practice. Arch Intern Med 1998;158:2444–9.
5. Slifman NR, Obermeyer WR, Aloi BK, Musser SM, Correll WA Jr, Cichowicz SM, Betz JM, Love LA. Contamination of botanical dietary supplements by Digitalis lanata. New Engl J Med 1998;339:806–11.
6. Wolin MJ. Digoxin visual toxicity with therapeutic blood levels of digoxin. Am J Ophthalmol 1998;125:406–7.
7. Tisdale JE, Padhi ID, Goldberg AD, Silverman NA, Webb CR, Higgins RSD, Paone G, Frank DM, Borzak S. A randomized, double-blind comparison of intravenous diltiazem and digoxin for atrial fibrillation after coronary artery bypass surgery. Am Heart J 1998;135:739–47.
8. Woodland C, Ito S, Koren G. A model for the prediction of digoxin-drug interactions at the renal tubular cell level. Ther Drug Monit 1998;20:134–8.
9. Laer S, Scholz H, Buschmann I, Thoenes M, Meinertz T. Digitoxin intoxication during concomitant use of amiodarone. Eur J Clin Pharmacol 1998;54:95–6.
10. Lomaestro BM, Piatek MA. Update on drug interactions with azole antifungal agents. Ann Pharmacother 1998;32:915–28.
11. Salphati L, Benet LZ. Effects of ketoconazole on digoxin absorption and disposition in rat. Pharmacology 1998;56:308–13.
12. Trivedi S, Hyman J, Lichstein E. Clarithromycin and digoxin toxicity. Ann Intern Med 1998;128:604.
13. Wakasugi H, Yano I, Ito T, Hashida T, Futami T, Nohara R, Sasayama S, Inui K-I. Effect of clarithromycin on renal excretion of digoxin: interaction with P-glycoprotein. Clin Pharmacol Ther 1998;64:123–8.
14. Snel S, Jansen JA, Pedersen PC, Jonkman JHG, Van Heiningen PNM. Tiagabine, a novel antiepileptic agent: lack of pharmacokinetic interaction with digoxin. Eur J Clin Pharmacol 1998;54:355–7.
15. Safadi R, Levy I, Amitai Y, Caraco Y. Beneficial effect of digoxin specific Fab antibody fragments in oleander intoxication. Arch Intern Med 1995;155:2121–5.
16. Shumaik GM, Wu AW, Ping AC. Oleander poisoning: treatment with digoxin specific Fab antibody fragments. Ann Emerg Med 1988;17:732–5.
17. Eddleston M, Rajapakse S, Rajakanthan, Jayalath S, Sjostrom L, Santharaj W, Thenabadu PN, Sheriff MH, Warrell DA Anti-digoxin Fab fragments in cardiotoxicity induced by ingestion of yellow oleander: a randomised controlled trial. Lancet 2000;355:967–72.
18. Cesario D, Clark J, Maisel A. Beneficial effects of intermittent home administration of the inotrope/vasodilator milrinone in patients with end-stage congestive heart failure: a preliminary study. Am Heart J 1998;135:121–9.
19. Alhashemi JA, Hooper J. Treatment of milrinone-associated tachycardia with beta-blockers. Can J Anaesth 1998; 45: 67–70.
20. Ramamoorthy C, Anderson GD, Williams GD, Lynn AM. Pharmacokinetics and side effects of milrinone in infants and children after open heart surgery. Anesth Analg 1998;86:283–9.
21. Cohn JN, Goldstein SO, Greenberg BH, Lorell BH, Bourge RC, Jaski BE, Gottlieb SO, McGrew III F, DeMets DL, White BG. A dose-dependent increase in mortality with vesnarinone among patients with severe heart failure. New Engl J Med 1998;339:1810–16.
22. Nattel S. Experimental evidence for proarrhythmic mechanisms of antiarrhythmic drugs. Cardiovasc Res 1998;37:567–77.
23. Pratt CM, Waldo AL, Camm AJ. Can antiarrhythmic drugs survive survival trials? Am J Cardiol 1998;81:24D–34D.
24. Roden DM. Mechanisms and management of proarrhythmia. Am J Cardiol 1998;82:49I–57I.
25. Friedman PL, Stevenson WG, Ferrick K, Friedman PL, Luderitz B, Waldo A, Grant AO, Pritchett E, Kaufman E, Reiffel J. Proarrhythmia. Am J Cardiol 1998;82:50N–58N.
26. The Cardiac Arrhythmia Suppression Trial (CAST) Investigators Preliminary report: effect of encainide and flecainide on mortality in a .randomized trial of arrhythmia suppression after myocardial infarction. New Engl J Med 1989;321:406–12.
27. The Cardiac Arrhythmia Suppression Trial II Investigators. Effect of the antiarrhythmic agent moricizine on survival after myocardial infarction. New Engl J Med 1992;327:227–33.
28. Impact Research Group. International mexiletine and placebo antiarrhythmic coronary trial: I. Report on arrhythmia and other findings. J Am Coll Cardiol 1984;4:1148–63.
29. Coplen SE, Antman EM, Berlin JA, Hewitt P, Chalmers TC. Efficacy and safety of quinidine therapy for maintenance of sinus rhythm after cardioversion. A meta-analysis of randomized controlled trials. Circulation 1990;82:1106–16 (Erratum 1991;83:714).
30. Flaker GC, Blackshear JL, McBride R, Kronmal RA, Halperin JL, Hart RG. Antiarrhythmic

drug therapy and cardiac mortality in atrial fibrillation. The Stroke Prevention in Atrial Fibrillation Investigators. J Am Coll Cardiol 1992;20:527–32.
31. Nattel S, Hadjis T, Talajic M. The treatment of atrial fibrillation. An evaluation of drug therapy, electrical modalities and therapeutic considerations. Drugs 1994;48:345–71.
32. Moosvi AR, Goldstein S, Van der Brug Medendorp S, Landis JR, Wolfe RA, Leighton R, Ritter G, Vasu CM, Acheson A. Effect of empiric antiarrhythmic therapy in resuscitated out of hospital cardiac arrest victims with coronary artery disease. Am J Cardiol 1990;65:1192–7.
33. Waldo AL, Camm AJ, deRuyter H, Friedman PL, MacNeil DJ, Pauls JF, Pitt B, Pratt CM, Schwartz PJ, Veltri EP. Effect of d-sotalol on mortality in patients with left ventricular dysfunction after recent and remote myocardial infarction. The SWORD Investigators. Survival With Oral d-Sotalol. Lancet 1996; 348:7–12 (Erratum 1996;348:416).
34 Dimitriu AG, Nistor N, Russu G, Cristogel F, Streanga V, Varlam L. Value of intravenous ATP in the diagnosis and treatment of tachyarrhythmias in children. Rev Med Chir Soc Med Nat Iasi 1998;102:100–2.
35. Pfammatter JP, Bauersfeld U. Safety issues in the treatment of paediatric supraventricular tachycardias. Drug Saf 1998;18:345–56.
36. Sherwood MC, Lau KC, Sholler GF. Adenosine in the management of supraventricular tachycardia in children. J Paediatr Child Health 1998;34:53–6.
37. Bakshi F, Barzilay Z, Paret G. Adenosine in the diagnosis and treatment of narrow complex tachycardia in the pediatric intensive care unit. Heart Lung 1998;27:47–50.
38. Garratt KN, Holmes DR Jr, Molina-Viamonte V, Reeder GS, Hodge DO, Bailey KR, Lobl JK, Laudon DA, Gibbons RJ. Intravenous adenosine and lidocaine in patients with acute myocardial infarction. Am Heart J 1998;136:196–204.
39. Knight BP, Zivin A, Souza J, Goyal R, Man KC, Strickberger SA, Morady F. Use of adenosine in patients hospitalized in a University Medical Center. Am J Med 1998;105:275–80.
40. Toft J, Mortensen J, Hesse B. Risk of atrioventricular block during adenosine pharmacologic stress testing in heart transplant recipients. Am J Cardiol 1998;82:696–7.
41. Rane K, Segerdahl M, Goiny M, Sollevi A. Intrathecal adenosine administration: a phase 1 clinical safety study in healthy volunteers, with additional evaluation of its influence on sensory thresholds and experimental pain. Anesthesiology 1998;89:1108–15.
42. Guieu R, Dussol B, Devaux C, Sampol J, Brunet P, Rochat H, Bechis G, Berland YF. Interactions between cyclosporine A and adenosine in kidney transplant recipients. Kidney Int 1998;53: 200–4.
43. Cairns JA. Antiarrhythmic therapy in the post-infarction setting: update from major amiodarone studies. Int J Clin Pract 1998;52:422–4.
44. Piepoli M, Villani GQ, Ponikowski P, Wright A, Flather MD, Coats AJS. Overview and meta-analysis of randomised trials of amiodarone in chronic heart failure. Int J Cardiol 1998;66:1–10.
45. Pfisterer ME, Kiowski W, Brunner H, Burckhardt D, Burkart F. Long-term benefit of 1-year amiodarone treatment for persistent complex ventricular arrhythmias after myocardial infarction. Circulation 1993;87:309–11.
46. Ceremuzynski L, Kleczar E, Krzeminska-Pakula M, Kuch J, Nartowicz E, Smielak-Korombel J, Dyduszynski A, Maciejewicz J, Zaleska T, Lazarczyk-Kedzia E, et al. Effect of amiodarone on mortality after myocardial infarction: a double-blind, placebo-controlled, pilot study. J Am Coll Cardiol 1992;20:1056–62.
47. Navarro-Lopez F, Cosin J, Marrugat J, Guindo J, Bayes de Luna A. Comparison of the effects of amiodarone versus metoprolol on the frequency of ventricular arrhythmias and on mortality after acute myocardial infarction. SSSD Investigators. Spanish Study on Sudden Death. Am J Cardiol 1993;72:1243–8.
48. Julian DG, Camm AJ, Frangin G, Janse MJ, Munoz A, Schwartz PJ, Simon P, for the European Myocardial Infarct Amiodarone Trial Investigators. Randomised trial of effect of amiodarone on mortality in patients with left-ventricular dysfunction after recent myocardial infarction: EMIAT. Lancet 1997;349:667–74.
49. Cairns JA, Connolly SJ, Roberts R, Gent M, for the Canadian Amiodarone Myocardial Infarction Arrhythmia Trial Investigators. Randomised trial of outcome after myocardial infarction in patients with repetitive ventricular premature depolarisations: CAMIAT. Lancet 1997;349:675–82.
50. Levy S. Amiodarone in atrial fibrillation. Int J Clin Pract 1998;52:429–31.
51. Drent M, Cobben NAM, Van Dieijen-Visser MP, Braat SHJ, Wouters EFM. Serum lactate dehydrogenase activity: indicator of the development of pneumonitis induced by amiodarone. Eur Heart J 1998;19:969–70.
52. Wolff J. Perchlorate and the thyroid gland. Pharmacol Rev 1998;50:89–105.
53. Newman CM, Price A, Davies DW, Gray TA, Weetman AP. Amiodarone and the thyroid: a practical guide to the management of thyroid dysfunction induced by amiodarone therapy. Heart 1998;79:121–7.
54. Leger AF, Massin JP, Laurent MF, Vincens M, Auriol M, Helal OB, Chomette G, Savoie JC. Iodine-induced thyrotoxicosis: analysis of eighty-five consecutive cases. Eur J Clin Invest 1984;14:449–55.
55. Brennan MD, Van Heerden JA, Carney JA. Amiodarone-associated thyrotoxicosis (AAT): experience with surgical management. Acta Ophthalmol Copenh 1987;65:556–64.
56. Rosenbaum H, Ben-Arie Y, Azzam ZS, Krivoy N. Amiodarone-associated granuloma in bone marrow. Ann Pharmacother 1998;32:60–2.
57. Sra J, Bremner S. Amiodarone skin toxicity. Circulation 1998;97:1105.

58. Mantyjarvi M, Tuppurainen K, Ikaheimo K. Ocular side effects of amiodarone. Surv Ophthalmol 1998;42:360–6.
59. Mindel JM. Editorial: Amiodarone and optic neuropathy – a medicolegal issue. Surv Ophthalmol 1998;42:358–9.
60. Reifler DM, Verdier DD, Davy CL, Mostow ND, Wendt VE. Multiple chalazia and rosacea in a patient treated with amiodarone. Am J Ophthalmol 1987;103:594–5.
61. Dickinson EJ, Wolman RL. Sicca syndrome associated with amiodarone therapy. Br Med J 1986;293:510.
62. Vrobel TR, Miller PE, Mostow ND, Rakita L. A general overview of amiodarone toxicity: its prevention, detection, and management. Prog Cardiovasc Dis 1989;31:393–426.
63. Greene HL, Graham EL, Werner JA, Sears GK, Gross BW, Gorham JP, Kudenchuk PJ, Trobaugh GB. Toxic and therapeutic effects of amiodarone in the treatment of cardiac arrhythmias. J Am Coll Cardiol 1983;2:1114–28.
64. Kerin NZ, Aragon E, Faitel K, Frumin H, Rubenfire M. Long-term efficacy and toxicity of high- and low-dose amiodarone regimens. J Clin Pharmacol 1989;29:418–23.
65. Collins P, Ferguson J. Narrow-band UVB (TL-01) phototherapy: an effective preventative treatment for the photodermatoses. Br J Dermatol 1995;132:956–63.
66. Landray MJ, Kendall MJ. Effect of amiodarone on mortality. Lancet 1998;351:523.
67. McCullough PA, Redle JD, Zaman AG, Archbold A, Alamgir F, Ulahannan TJ, Daoud EG, Morady F. Amiodarone prophylaxis for atrial fibrillation after cardiac surgery. New Engl J Med 1998;338:1383–4.
68. Wakutani Y, Matsushima E, Son A, Shimizu Y, Goto Y, Ishida H. Myasthenia-like syndrome due to adverse effects of cibenzoline in a patient with chronic renal failure. Muscle Nerve 1998;21:416–17.
69. Furushima H, Niwano S, Chinushi M, Ohhira K, Abe A, Aizawa Y. Relation between bradycardia dependent long QT syndrome and QT prolongation by disopyramide in humans. Heart 1998;79:56–8.
70. Isohanni MH, Neuvonen PJ, Palkama VJ, Olkkola KT. Effect of erythromycin and itraconazole on the pharmacokinetics of intravenous lignocaine. Eur J Clin Pharmacol 1998;54:561–5.
71. Kemper CA, Kent G, Burton S, Deresinski SC. Mexiletine for HIV-infected patients with painful peripheral neuropathy: a double-blind, placebo-controlled, crossover treatment trial. J Acquired Immune Defic Syndr Hum Retrovirol 1998;19:367–72.
72. Kieburtz K. Simpson D, Yiannoutsos C, Max MB, Hall CD, Ellis RJ, Marra CM, McKendall R, Singer E, Dal Pan GJ, Clifford DB, Tucker T, Cohen B, Jatlow P. Kasdan P, Shriver S, Martinez A, Millar L, Colquhoun D, Zaborski L, Dias V, Jubelt B, Noseworthy J, Barton B, Sharer L, Kerza A, Sperber K, Chusid E, Gerits P, et al. A randomized trial of amitriptyline and mexiletine for painful neuropathy in HIV infection. Neurology 1998;51:1682–8.
73. Kusumoto M, Ueno K, Tanaka K, Takeda K, Mashimo K, Kameda T, Fujimura Y, Shibakawa M, Guzman WM, Laplante S. Lack of pharmacokinetic interaction between mexiletine and omeprazole. Ann Pharmacother 1998;32:182–4.
74. Volgman AS, Carberry PA, Stambler B, Lewis WR, Dunn GH, Perry KT, Vanderlugt JT, Kowey PR. Conversion efficacy and safety of intravenous ibutilide compared with intravenous procainamide in patients with atrial flutter or fibrillation. J Am Coll CardioL 1998;31:1414–19.
75. Erdem S, Freimer ML, O'Dorisio T, Mendell JR. Procainamide-induced chronic inflammatory demyelinating polyradiculoneuropathy. Neurology 1998;50:824–5.
76. Kameda H, Mimori T, Kaburaki J, Fujil T, Takahashi T, Akaishi M, Ikeda Y. Systemic sclerosis complicated by procainamide-induced lupus and antiphospholipid syndrome. Br J Rheumatol 1998;37:1236–9.
77. Sianipar A, Parkin JE, Sunderland VB. The reaction of procainamide with glucose following admixture to glucose infusion. Int J Pharm 1998;176:55–61.
78. Bianconi L, Mennuni M. Comparison between propafenone and digoxin administered intravenously to patients with acute atrial fibrillation. Am J Cardiol 1998;82:584–8.
79. Rae AP, Camm J, Rae AP, Winters S, Page R. Placebo-controlled evaluations of propafenone for atrial tachyarrhythmias. Am J Cardiol 1998;82:59N–65N.
80. Janousek J, Paul T. Safety of oral Propafenone in the treatment of arrhythmias in infants and children (European retrospective multicenter study). Am J Cardiol 1998;81:1121–4.
81. George JN. Raskob GE, Shah SR, Rizvi MA, Hamilton SA, Osborne S, Vondracek T. Drug-induced thrombocytopenia: a systematic review of published case reports. Ann Intern Med 1998;129:886–90.
82. Lipsker D, Walther S, Schulz R, Nave S, Cribier B. Life-threatening vasculitis related to quinidine occurring in a healthy volunteer during a clinical trial. Eur J Clin Pharmacol 1998;54: 815.

A.P. Maggioni, M.G. Franzosi and R. Latini

18 β-adrenoceptor antagonists and antianginal drugs

β-ADRENOCEPTOR ANTAGONISTS *(SED-13, 488; SEDA-20, 183; SEDA-21, 207; SEDA-22, 213)*

ORGANS AND SYSTEMS

Cardiovascular Of 153 consecutive patients treated with eye-drops of timolol, three complained of unexplained *falls* and two of them had *dizziness* and *blackouts* (1^c). Two had a *cardioinhibitory carotid sinus syndrome* (a period of asystole greater than 3 seconds after carotid sinus massage) and the third a *vasodepressor carotid sinus syndrome* (a reduction in systolic blood pressure higher than 50 mmHg after carotid sinus massage). In all three cases, timolol eye-drops were discontinued. Follow-up carotid sinus massage in the two patients with a cardioinibitory carotid sinus syndrome was negative and all reported complete remission of symptoms.

Respiratory The respiratory and cardiovascular adverse effects of topical therapy with timolol or betaxolol have been studied in a randomized controlled trial in 40 elderly patients with glaucoma (2^C). Five of the 20 allocated to timolol discontinued treatment for respiratory reasons, compared with three of the 20 patients allocated to betaxolol. There were no significant differences in mean values of spirometry, pulse, or blood pressure between the groups. This study confirms that β-blockers administered as eye-drops can reach the systemic circulation and that serious adverse respiratory events can occur in elderly people, even if they are screened before treatment for cardiac and respiratory disease. These events can occur using either the selective betaxolol agent or the non-selective timolol.

Gastrointestinal *Nausea and vomiting* have been attributed to timolol eye-drops (3^c).

Severe nausea and vomiting occurred in a 77-year-old woman treated with timolol eye-drops for glaucoma. Her weight had fallen by 8 kg (13%). All physical, laboratory and instrumental examinations were negative. Gastroduodenoscopy and duodenal biopsy were unremarkable and *Helicobacter pylori* was absent. When timolol was replaced by betaxolol, her complaints disappeared and she gained 2 kg. On rechallenge 3 months later she developed severe nausea, vomiting, and anorexia after some days of treatment. She immediately stopped taking the treatment and 4 days later the symptoms disappeared.

Since timolol has been satisfactorily used by millions of patients, the incidence of serious gastrointestinal events appears to be very low. Absence of symptoms after betaxolol therapy in this patient is in agreement with its lower risk of non-cardiac adverse reactions compared with the non-selective agent timolol.

Skin and appendages β-blocker eye-drops can cause *skin rashes* (4^c).

A 70-year-old woman treated with topical timolol for glaucoma developed a papular eruption on the arms and back, consistent with prurigo. All tests were within the reference ranges. There was no improvement after 1 month of topical corticosteroids. The eruption cleared completely within 1 month of timolol withdrawal. Betaxolol eye-drops were introduced and the eruption recurred within 1 week. When β-blocker therapy was replaced by synthetic cholinergic eye-drops (drug unspecified) the eruption cleared completely without any recurrence a year later.

Although cutaneous adverse effects have been previously described after oral β-blockers, including timolol, this observation further sug-

Side Effects of Drugs, Annual 23
J.K. Aronson, ed.

gests a class effect of topical β-blockers. This case also suggests a cross-reaction between timolol and betaxolol.

Leukocytoclastic vasculitis has been reported with sotalol (5[c]).

A progressive cutaneous vasculitis occurred in a 66-year-old man treated with sotalol for the prevention of a symptomatic atrial fibrillation. After 7 days he noted a petechial eruption on his wrists and ankles. This progressed during the next days to palpable purpura on the hands, wrists, ankles, and feet. A biopsy specimen showed changes consistent with leukocytoclastic vasculitis. After withdrawal of sotalol the skin rash cleared completely without any other intervention.

Other β-blockers associated with leukocytoclastic vasculitis include propranolol, acebutolol, practolol, and alprenolol.

Use in pregnancy Two infants with features of severe β-blockade *(bradycardia, persistent hypotension), persistent hypoglycemia, pericardial effusion*, and *myocardial hypertrophy* were born before term to mothers taking long-term oral labetalol for hypertension in pregnancy. Although labetalol is considered to be generally safe in neonates, impaired urinary excretion and lower albumin binding in preterm infants may prolong the half-life of labetalol and increases its systemic availability and toxicity (6[c]).

Fetal bradycardia and pauses after each two normal beats occurred at 21 weeks gestation in a 37-year-old woman using timolol eye-drops for glaucoma; when timolol was withdrawn, the fetal heart rate recovered (7[c]). The authors concluded that when a woman taking glaucoma therapy becomes pregnant, it is usually possible to interrupt therapy during pregnancy. Treatment may be deferred until delivery of the infant.

INDIVIDUAL β-ADRENOCEPTOR ANTAGONISTS

Carvedilol

Cardiovascular In trials in patients with congestive heart failure, carvedilol was discontinued in only about 5% (8[R]). The most common adverse reactions were *edema, dizziness, bradycardia, hypotension, nausea, diarrhea*, and *blurred vision*. The rate of drug withdrawal was not different among patients under 65 years and among older ones. Renal insufficiency can occur in patients with heart failure treated with carvedilol, usually when pre-existing renal insufficiency, low blood pressure, or diffuse vascular disease were present. Patients at high risk of renal dysfunction should be carefully monitored, particularly at the beginning of treatment, and the drug should be withdrawn in case renal function worsens.

Liver *Liver function abnormalities* in trials of carvedilol occurred in 1.1% of patients taking carvdilol compared with 0.9% in patients taking placebo (8[R]). However, in all trials the patients with pre-existing liver disease were excluded, and so information on the effects of carvedilol in these patients are not available.

Overdosage Overdoses of carvedilol results mainly in *hypotension* and *bradycardia* (8[R]). For excessive bradycardia, atropine has been used successfully, while to support ventricular function intravenous glucagon, dobutamine, or isoproterenol have been recommended. For severe hypotension, adrenaline or noradrenaline can be given.

NITRATE DERIVATIVES *(SED-13, 488; SEDA-20, 184; SEDA-21, 208; SEDA-22, 218)*

Glyceryl trinitrate

Glyceryl trinitrate has been used for its relaxing action on smooth muscle during cesarean delivery, with the aim of facilitating fetal extraction. After the publication of reports, a randomized, placebo-controlled trial has been performed in 97 patients undergoing elective cesarean delivery after the 34th week of gestation (9[Cr]). Patients were randomized to receive an intravenous bolus of glyceryl trinitrate (0.25 or 0.5 mg) or placebo. Glyceryl trinitrate did not improve fetal extraction. There were no adverse reactions attributable to glyceryl trinitrate in the neonate or mother.

The safety of glyceryl trinitrate in emergency or elective cesarean delivery has been also documented in a prospective series of 23 women, who received 400–800 μg of glyceryl trinitrate spray (10[cr]). However, no conclusions about the efficacy of glyceryl trinitrate are possible, owing to the lack of a control group.

Molsidomine

A multicenter, randomized, double-blind, cross-over, placebo-controlled study has shown the efficacy of two regimens of molsidomine in 90 patients with stable angina (11[c]). Beneficial effects on exercise load did not seem to be reduced by 6 weeks of continuous therapy, suggesting lack of tolerance. The most frequently reported adverse reaction with molsidomine was *headache,* as for all other nitric oxide donors.

CALCIUM ANTAGONISTS

(SED-13, 488; SEDA-19, 203; SEDA-20, 185; SEDA-21, 208)

Amlodipine

The efficacy of amlodipine or isosorbide-5-mononitrate for 3 weeks on exercise-induced myocardial stunning have been compared in a randomized, double-blind, cross-over study in 24 patients with chronic stable angina and normal left ventricular function (12[Cr]). Amlodipine attenuated stunning, evaluated by echocardiography, significantly more than isosorbide, without difference in anti-ischemic action or hemodynamics. Amlodipine was better tolerated than isosorbide, mainly because of a lower incidence of headache (12[Cr]).

A patient presented with severe, generalized *muscle stiffness, joint pain,* and *fatigue* while taking amlodipine for hypertension and zafirlukast for asthma. Stopping zafirlukast did not change her symptoms; the dose of amlodipine was increased at different times up to 15 mg to control blood pressure better. Since the neurological symptoms worsened, in the absence of any evidence of immunological or neurological disorders, amlodipine was stopped: the symptoms disappeared within 4 days (13[cr]).

Use in pregnancy *Subcutaneous fat necrosis* in a neonate has been attributed to maternal use amlodipine during pregnancy (14[c]).

A boy weighing 4 kg was born by spontaneous normal delivery at 39 weeks to a 38-year-old Afro-Caribbean woman, whose pregnancy was complicated by essential hypertension treated with amlodipine. At 1 day the child developed firm, red, pea-sized nodular lesions on the face, buttocks, back, shoulders, and arms.

Subcutaneous fat necrosis of the newborn is relatively uncommon. It is said to be benign and painless and to resolve within a few weeks. However, in this case it was extremely painful and was relieved only by opiates. The skin changes persisted beyond the age of 6 months and remained extremely symptomatic until the age of 9 months, when the skin had become normal. Calcium abnormalities have often been reported in association with subcutaneous fat necrosis, and exposure to amlodipine during pregnancy may have resulted in impairment of enzyme systems dependent on calcium fluxes for their action; it may also have affected calcium homeostasis in the neonate. Since previous reports of teratogenicity in animals have been published, few women take calcium antagonists during pregnancy and there are no reports to date of an association between these drugs and subcutaneous fat necrosis (14[c]).

Interactions *Ciclosporin* increases the survival of allografts in man. However, it causes renal vasoconstriction and increases proximal tubular reabsorption, leading in some cases to hypertension (15[R]). The concomitant use of calcium antagonists can prevent most of these adverse effects of ciclosporin. However, some calcium antagonists (verapamil, diltiazem, nicardipine) can increase plasma concentrations of cyclosporin up to 3-fold through inhibition of cytochrome P450. Eight different studies have been performed on the combination of amlodipine and ciclosporin given for 1–6 months to kidney transplant recipients, and the results have been reviewed (16[R]). In three studies in a total of 41 patients amlodipine increased ciclosporin concentrations, while in the others, a total of 85 patients, there was no evidence of an interaction.

Diltiazem

Urinary system *Acute interstitial nephritis* has been attributed to diltiazem (17[c]).

A 53-year-old was given diltiazem for precordial pain and about 2 hours later developed an erythematous maculopapular rash mainly on the trunk and lower limbs. Four days later he developed abdominal pain radiating to both renal angles, accompanied by dysuria and tenesmus and followed 6 days later by acute renal insufficiency associated with raised liver function test results.

In this case the self-limiting resolution in 4–5 days without relapse, the presence of the skin rash, and the liver sequelae suggested a common immunoallergic mechanism. The clinical symptoms, the time relation between drug administration and the occurrence of the syndrome, the inability to explain the syndrome otherwise, and its disappearance on withdrawal of diltiazem support an association with the drug.

A retrospective analysis of postoperative renal function in patients undergoing cardiac operations has been conducted to evaluate whether the use of prophylactic intravenous diltiazem, in order to reduce the incidence of ischemia and dysrhythmias, was associated with increased renal dysfunction (18[C]). The incidence of *acute renal insufficiency* requiring dialysis was 4.4% with diltiazem versus 0.7% in the controls. Logistic regression analysis suggested that the risk of acute renal insufficiency was strongly associated with intravenous diltiazem, age, baseline serum creatinine, the presence of left main coronary disease, and the presence of cerebrovascular disease.

Skin and appendages Skin reactions ranging from exanthems to severe adverse events have been reported in association with diltiazem (SED-13, 513; SEDA-18, 215; SEDA-22, 216). Acute generalized *exanthematous pustulosis* in an 82-year-old woman was confirmed as being due to diltiazem by a positive patch test (19[c]) and three new cases of skin reactions (hypersensitivity syndrome reaction, pruritic exanthematous eruption, and acute generalized exanthematous pustulosis) possibly induced by diltiazem have been described and the literature on skin reactions associated with calcium antagonists has been reviewed (35[Cr]). The number of diltiazem-induced cutaneous events was significantly greater than those induced by either nifedipine or verapamil. However, there was no difference in the proportion of serious cutaneous adverse events due to any of these three drugs (20[Cr]).

Interactions The effects of co-administration of diltiazem, a potent inhibitor of CYP3A, on the pharmacokinetics of *lovastatin* and *pravastatin* have been evaluated in a randomized study in 10 healthy volunteers, to test the hypothesis that a substantial interaction would occur with lovastatin but not with pravastatin. Lovastatin is oxidized by CYP3A to active metabolites but pravastatin is active alone and is not so metabolized. Diltiazem significantly increased the oral AUC and maximum serum concentration of lovastatin but did not alter its half-life; it did not alter the oral AUC, maximum serum concentration, or half-life of pravastatin. The magnitude of the increase of plasma concentration of lovastatin suggested that caution is necessary when co-administering diltiazem and lovastatin (21[C]).

Many studies have shown an interaction between *ciclosporin* and diltiazem: concomitant administration allows reduction of the daily dose of ciclosporin. However, according to a study in eight renal transplant recipients, the low systemic availability and high degree of variation in diltiazem metabolism within and between patients may give unpredictable results (22[C]).

Diltiazem abolishes the acute renal hypoperfusion and vasoconstriction induced by ciclosporin in renal transplant patients. Plasma endothelin-1 may be a mediator of cyclosporin-induced renal hypoperfusion, but is not affected by diltiazem (23[C]).

Felodipine

Different skin reactions have been reported with calcium antagonists, and in particular *telangiectases* in light-exposed areas of the skin with nifedipine and amlodipine (24[R]). For the first time, telangiectases in a light-protected area, the trunk, have been described.

A 70-year-old woman took felodipine 10 mg/day and enalapril for about 1 year for hypertension. She developed telangiectatic lesions of both sides of the trunk. After excluding other causes, felodipine was withdrawn. After 2 months the lesions slightly abated, but never completely disappeared. The diagnosis was confirmed by histological evidence of enlarged capillaries parallel to the skin surface, in the absence of mast cells.

Isradipine

Interactions Studies in rodents and primates have suggested that calcium-antagonists, including darodipine, nifedipine, and verapamil, may attenuate the behavioral effects of *ethanol.* Isradipine seems to be the most effective. However, the results of published reports in man on the effects of calcium antagonists on the acute subject-rated, performance-impairing, and cardiovascular effects of ethanol, have suggested that the behavioral effects of ethanol are not attenuated by verapamil, nifedipine, or nimodipine. The same conclusions have been reached from a study in nine healthy volunteers (25[Cr]). Combined ethanol and isradipine produced increases in heart rate and reductions in blood pressure that were not observed with either drug alone. Isradipine significantly reduced peak breath alcohol concentrations, but it did not significantly alter the subject-rated performance-impairing effects of ethanol.

Adverse drug interactions with mibefradil

Mibefradil is a calcium antagonist with a novel mechanism of action: preferential block of T type calcium channels, but also to some extent of L-type calcium channels, as opposed to the other calcium antagonists, which block only L-type channels. It had a favorable pharmacokinetic profile, allowing once-a-day dosage (26[R]). It also had peculiarities, such as slight bradycardia associated with its hypotensive effect. Owing to its attractive pharmacological profile, namely an anti-ischemic action with little or no negative inotropism, mibefradil was tested in a large-scale mortality trial in heart failure (MACH-I, Mortality Assessment in Congestive Heart failure trial).

However, early in June 1998, only a few months after its launch, Roche Laboratories withdrew mibefradil from the market, after several dangerous interactions with at least 25 drugs had been reported (27[r], 28[r]). On this occasion, the FDA stated that: 'since [mibefradil] has not been shown to offer special benefits (such as treating patients who do not respond to other antihypertensive and antianginal drugs), the drug's problems are viewed as an unreasonable risk to consumers'. At the same time, no difference was found between mibefradil and placebo in an interim analysis of MACH-I data.

During development mibefradil was found to be a potent inhibitor of cytocrome P450, and in particular of its isoform CYP3A4 (26[R]). Along with its extensive use after marketing, several drug interactions attributable to mibefradil were reported. Particularly serious were interactions with tacrolimus (29[cr]), simvastatin (30[cr]), and drugs that impair sinoatrial node function (e.g. β-blockers) (31[Cr]).

Severe rhabdomyolysis has been reported in a 83-year-old woman admitted to hospital with progressive immobilizing myopathy, low back pain, and oliguria; she was taking simvastatin and mibefradil. Laboratory tests proved the existence of rhabdomyolysis, which is a known adverse effect of high doses of simvastatin. The symptoms disappeared completely after 4 weeks withdrawal. Mibefradil was probably responsible for raising plasma concentrations of simvastatin to toxic concentrations (30[cr]).

The safety and efficacy of mibefradil in association with β-blockers has been assessed in 205 patients with chronic stable angina, randomized to placebo or mibefradil 25 or 50 mg/day for 2 weeks (31[Cr]). Besides an improvement in angina with mibefradil, it dose-dependently reduced heart rate and increased the PR interval. One patient taking mibefradil had an escape junctional rhythm 26 hours after the last dose of 50 mg. The nodal rhythm disappeared on withdrawal of mibefradil, but based on the overall results it was concluded that mibefradil was safe and effective when given for a short time with β-blockers. Abrupt switch of therapy from mibefradil to other dihydropyridine calcium antagonist was reported to cause shock, fatal in one case, in four patients also taking β-blockers (32[cr]).

Nicardipine

Nicardipine has been used intravenously for hypertensive crisis in adults, although an *increase in intracranial pressure* was observed in a case series (33[Cr]). Its use in children has scarcely been documented; intravenous nicardipine proved effective in controlling blood pressure in three cases of hypertensive emergency secondary to renal disease (34[cr]). Children aged 12–14 years received intravenous infusions of 1–3 μg/kg/min for 3–27 days, which normalized blood pressure without significant adverse reactions.

Nifedipine

Cardiovascular A significant fall in pulmonary vascular resistance with high doses of oral calcium antagonists seems to be associated with an improved prognosis, and potential clinical efficacy in primary pulmonary hypertension. However, significant adverse effects have been reported during acute testing with calcium antagonists. Therefore, to identify patients who may benefit from long-term calcium antagonists therapy accurately, there is a need for a safe, potent, short-acting vasodilator. Two studies have been conducted to assess the use of inhaled nitric oxide, a selective pulmonary vasodilator, for predicting the safety of high-dose oral calcium antagonists and acute hemodynamic responses to them in primary pulmonary hypertension. In one study 17 patients with primary pulmonary hypertension undergoing a trial of nifedipine (20 mg hourly for 8 hours) were assessed for the hemodynamic response to inhaled nitric oxide, 80 parts per million for 5 minutes (35[C]). All nitric oxide responders also responded to nifedipine, and nine of the 10 nitric oxide non-responders were nifedipine non-responders. All nitric oxide responders tolerated a full trial of nifedipine without hypotension. There was a highly significant correlation between the effects of nitric oxide and nifedipine on pulmonary vascular resistance. In conclusion, the pulmonary vascular response to inhaled nitric oxide accurately predicted the acute hemodynamic response to nifedipine in primary pulmonary hypertension, and a positive response to nitric oxide was associated with a safe nifedipine trial. In patients comparable to those evaluated, a trial of nifedipine in nitric oxide non-responders appears unwarranted and potentially dangerous.

In another study the acute response to inhaled nitric oxide and high doses of oral nifedipine or verapamil was assessed in 33 consecutive patients with primary pulmonary hypertension. Ten patients responded acutely to nitric oxide, nine of whom responded acutely to calcium antagonists, without any complications. The other 23 patients failed to respond to nitric oxide and calcium antagonists. In these non-responders there were nine serious adverse effects with calcium antagonists. There was no clinical or baseline hemodynamic feature that predicted the acute vasodilator response. Long-term oral treatment with calcium antagonists was restricted to the nine acute responders, and there was a sustained clinical and hemodynamic improvement in only six patients. It was concluded that nitric oxide may be used as a screening agent for safely identifying patients with primary pulmonary hypertension who may benefit from long-term treatment with calcium antagonists (36[C]).

Hematological In a case-control surveillance of agranulocytosis and aplastic anemia conducted in the metropolitan area of Barcelona, where 178 cases of *aplastic anemia* were identified during a follow-up period of 74.5×10^6 patient years, nifedipine was associated with a significant relative risk of aplastic anemia, which translates into an absolute risk of 1.2 per patient year. Among the 178 patients, 147 were interviewed and compared with 1295 controls. Six cases (4.1%) and 11 controls (0.8%) had been exposed to nifedipine during the window period, as all of them had taken nifedipine for at least 7 months. The multivariate odds ratio was 4.6 (1.5–15). All six died within 5 months of diagnosis. The authors concluded that the risk of aplastic anemia associated with nifedipine is of a similar magnitude to that associated with chloramphenicol (1.7 per 100 000 patients) and that associated with phenylbutazone (2.2 per 100 000 patients) (37[C]).

Immunological and hypersensitivity reactions *Anaphylaxis* has been attributed to sublingual nifedipine (38[c]).

A 71-year-old man with prostatic adenocarcinoma and a pathological vertebral fracture received sublingual nifedipine for hypertension and 15 minutes later became stuporose and complained of pruritus, generalized erythema, dizziness, and nausea. His blood pressure had fallen to 60/40 mmHg, his pulse rate was 120/min, and his respiratory rate was 30/min. He had cyanosis and severe bronchospasm with no focal neurological abnormalities. After treatment with subcutaneous adrenaline, intravenous fluids, hydrocortisone, and aminophylline, his blood pressure increased to 125/70 mmHg. During the following days his neurological and pulmonary status rapidly improved.

Use in pregnancy Tocolytic therapy with nifedipine has been reported in several studies to be at least effective as ritodrine, terbutaline, or magnesium sulfate, with fewer maternal adverse effects (SEDA-18, 216; SEDA-20, 187). These observations have been confirmed by two trials in 102 and 54 pregnant women of under 34 weeks gestation, randomized to nifedipine or ritodrine. There were no differences in the time of delivery, but significantly fewer maternal adverse effects in those given nifedipine (39[C], 40[C]).

Verapamil

Interactions There have been two reports of interaction between verapamil and *macrolide antibiotics* (41[c], 42[c]).

A 53-year-old woman had periods of dizziness and episodes of fainting when she stood up 24 hours after having been given clarithromycin for an acute exacerbation of chronic obstructive pulmonary disease and verapamil for atrial fibrillation. One day later she developed severe hypotension and bradycardia. Since her symptoms matched those of severe verapamil overdosage, the drug was withdrawn and her condition improved within two days.

A 77-year-old hypertensive woman receiving both verapamil and propranolol for hypertrophic cardiomyopathy and paroxysmal atrial fibrillation, developed symptomatic bradycardia within 2–4 days of initiation of both erythromycin or clarithromycin on two separate occasions, for pneumonia and sinusitis respectively.

Verapamil is both a substrate and an inhibitor of CYP3A4, which is inhibited by clarithromycin and erythromycin. Giving these macrolide antibiotics during verapamil therapy is likely to reduce the first-pass metabolism of verapamil, increase its systemic availability, and impair its elimination. In patients taking this combination, verapamil should be started in a low dosage and its hemodynamic effects should be monitored closely.

The effects of a combination of erythromycin and verapamil on the pharmacokinetics of a single dose of *simvastatin* have been studied in a randomized, double-blind, cross-over study in 12 healthy volunteers simultaneously taking the three drugs. Both erythromycin and verapamil interacted with simvastatin, producing significant increases in the serum concentrations of simvastatin and its active metabolite simvastatin acid. The mean C_{max} of active simvastatin acid was increased about 5-fold and the $AUC_{0\rightarrow 24}$ 4-fold by erythromycin; verapamil increased the C_{max} of simvastatin acid 3.4-fold and the $AUC_{0\rightarrow 24}$ 2.8-fold. There was a substantial interindividual variation in the extent of these interactions. Concomitant use of erythromycin, verapamil, and simvastatin should be avoided (43[C]).

The interaction with *grapefruit juice* observed with several calcium antagonists, including felodipine, nifedipine, and nisoldipine, has not been confirmed with verapamil. A single dose of grapefruit juice had no effect on the pharmacokinetics of verapamil in 10 hypertensive patients taking chronic verapamil (44[C]).

REFERENCES

1. Mulcahy R, Allcock L, O'Shea D. Timolol, carotid sinus hypersensitivity, and elderly patients. Lancet 1998;352:1147–8.
2. Diggory P, Cassels-Brown A, Vail A, Hillman JS. Randomised, controlled trial of spirometric changes in elderly people receiving timolol or betaxolol as initial treatment for glaucoma. Br J Ophthalmol 1998;82:146–9.
3. Wolfhagen FHJ, Van Neerven JAFM, Groen FC, Ouwendijk RJ. Severe nausea and vomiting with timolol eye drops. Lancet 1998;352:373.
4. Girardin P, Derancourt C, Laurent R. A new cutaneous side-effect of ocular beta-blockers. Clin Exp Dermatol 1998;23:95.
5. Rustmann WC, Carpenter MT, Harmon C, Botti CF. Leukocytoclastic vasculitis associated with sotalol therapy. J Am Acad Dermatol 1998;38:111–12.
6. Crooks BNA, Deshpande SA, Hall C, Ward Platt MP, Milligan DWA. Adverse neonatal effects of maternal labetalol treatment. Arch Dis Child Fetal Neonatal Ed 1998;79:F150–1.
7. Wagenvoort AM, Van Vugt JMG, Sobotka M, Van Geijn HP. Topical timolol therapy in pregnancy: is it safe for the fetus? Teratology 1998;58: 258–62.
8. Frishman WH. Drug therapy: carvedilol. New Engl J Med 1998;339:1759–65.
9. David M, Halle H, Lichtenegger W, Sinha P, Zimmerman T. Nitroglycerin to facilitate fetal extraction during cesarean delivery. Obstet Gynecol 1998;91:119–24.
10. Craig S, Dalton R, Tuck M, Brew F. Sublingual glyceryl trinitrate for uterine relaxation at Caesarean section. A prospective trial. Aust NZ J Obstet Gynaecol 1998;38:34–9.
11. Messin R, Karpov Y, Baikova N, Bruhwyler J, Monse M-J, Guns C, Geczy J. Short- and long-term effects of molsidomine retard and molsidomine nonretard on exercise capacity and clinical status in patients with stable angina: a multicenter randomized double-blind crossover placebo-control trial. J Cardiovasc Pharmacol 1998;31: 271–6.
12. Rinaldi CA, Linka AZ, Masani ND, Avery PG, Jones E. Randomized, double-blind crossover study to investigate the effects of amlodipine and isosorbide mononitrate on the time course and severity exercise-induced myocardial stunning. Circulation 1998;98:749–56.
13. Phillips BB, Muller BA. Severe neuromuscular complications possibly associated with amlodipine. Ann Pharmacother 1998;32:1165–7.
14. Rosbotham JL, Johnson A, Haque KN, Holden CA. Painful subcutaneous fat necrosis of the newborn associated with intra-partum use of a calcium channel blocker. Clin Exp Dermatol 1998;23:19–21.
15. Curtis JJ. Hypertension following kidney transplantation. Am J Kidney Dis 1994;23:471–5.
16. Schrama YC, Koomans HA. Interactions of cyclosporin A and amlodipine: blood cyclosporin A levels, hypertension and kidney function. J Hypertens Suppl 1998;16:S33–8.

17. Abadín JA, Durán JA, Pérez de León JA. Probable diltiazem-induced acute interstitial nephritis. Ann Pharmacother 1998;32:656–8.
18. Young EW, Diab A, Kirsh MV. Intravenous diltiazem and acute renal failure after cardiac operations. Ann Thorac Surg 1998;65:1316–19.
19. Jan V, Machet L, Gironet N, Martin L, Machet MC, Lorette G, Vaillant L. Acute generalized exanthematous pustulosis induced by diltiazem: value of patch testing. Dermatology 1998;197:274–5.
20. Knowles S, Gupta AK, Shear NH. The spectrum of cutaneous reactions associated with diltiazem: three cases and a review of the literature. J Am Acad Dermatol 1998;38:201–6.
21. Azie NE, Brater DC, Becker PA, Jones DR, Hall SD. The interaction of diltiazem with lovastatin and pravastatin. Clin Pharmacol Ther 1998;64: 369–77.
22. Morris RG, Jones TE. Diltiazem disposition and metabolism in recipients of renal transplants. Ther Drug Monit 1998;20:365–70.
23. Asberg A, Christensen H, Hartmann A, Berg KJ. Diltiazem modulates cyclosporin A induced renal hemodynamic effects but not its effect on plasma endothelin-1. Clin Transplant 1998;12:363–70.
24. Karonen T, Stubb S, Keski-Oja J. Truncal telangiectases coinciding with felodipine. Dermatology 1998;196:272–3.
25. Rush CR, Pazzaglia PJ. Pretreatment with isradipine, a calcium-channel blocker, does not attenuate the acute behavioral effects of ethanol in humans. Alcohol Clin Exp Res 1998;22:539–47.
26. Billups SJ, Carter BL. Mibefradil: a new class of calcium-channel antagonists. Ann Pharmacother 1998;32:6590–71.
27. SoRelle R. Withdrawal of Posicor from market. Circulation 1998;98:831–2.
28. Li Wan Po A, Zhang WY. What lessons can be learnt from withdrawal of mibefradil from the market? Lancet 1998;351:1829–30.
29. Krahenbuhl S, Menafoglio A, Giostra E, Gallino A. Serious interaction between mibefradil and tacrolimus. Transplantation 1998;66:1113–15.
30. Schmassmann-Suhijar D, Bullingham R, Gasser R, Schmutz J. Rhabdomyolysis due to interaction of simvastatin with mibefradil. Lancet 1998;351:1929–30.
31. Alper JS, Kobrin I, DeQuattro V, Friedman R, Shepherd A, Fenster PE, Thadani U. Additional antianginal and anti-ischemic efficacy of mibefradil in patients pretreated with a beta blocker for chronic stable angina pectoris. Am J Cardiol 1997;79:1025–30.
32. Mullins ME, Horowitz Z, Linden DHJ, Smith GW, Norton RL, Stump J. Life-threatening interaction of mibefradil and β-blockers with dihydropyridine calcium channel blockers. J Am Med Assoc 1998;280:157–8.
33. Nishikawa T, Omote K, Namiki A, Takahashi T. The effects of nicardipine on cerebrospinal fluid pressure in humans. Anesth Analg 1986;65:507–10.
34. Michael J, Groshong T, Tobias JD. Nicardipine for hypertensive emergencies in children with renal disease. Pediatr Nephrol 1998;12:40–2.
35. Ricciardi MJ, Knight BP, Martinez FJ, Rubenfire M. Inhaled nitric oxide in primary pulmonary hypertension. A safe and effective agent for predicting response to nifedipine. J Am Coll Cardiol 1998;32:1068-73.
36. Sitbon O, Humbert M, Jagot JL, Taravella O, Fartoukh M, Parent F, Herve P, Simonneau G. Inhaled nitric oxide as a screening agent for safely identifying responders to oral calcium-channel blockers in primary pulmonary hypertension. Eur Respir J 1998;12:265–70.
37. Laporte JR, Ibáñez L, Ballarín E, Pérez E, Vidal X. Fatal aplastic anaemia associated with nifedipine. Lancet 1998;352:619–20.
38. Pedro-Botet J, Minguez S, Supervia A. Sublingual nifedipine-induced anaphylaxis. Arch Intern Med 1998;158:1379.
39. Koks CAM, Brölman HAM, De Kleine MJK, Manger PA. A randomized comparison of nifedipine and ritodrine for suppression of preterm labor. Eur J Obstet Gynecol Reprod Biol 1998;77:171–6.
40. García-Velasco JA, Gonzáles Gonzáles A. A prospective, randomized trial of nifedipine vs. ritodrine in threatened preterm labor. Int J Gynecol Obstet 1998;61:239–44.
41. Kaeser YA, Brunner F, Drewe J, Haefeli WE. Severe hypotension and bradycardia associated with verapamil and clarithromycin. Am J Health-Syst Pharm 1998;55:2417–18.
42. Steenbergen JA, Stauffer VL. Potential macrolide interaction with verapamil. Ann Pharmacother 1998;32:387–8.
43. Kantola T, Kivistö KT, Neuvonen PJ. Erythromycin and verapamil considerably increase serum simvastatin and simvastatin acid concentrations. Clin Pharmacol Ther 1998;64:177–82.
44. Zaidenstein R, Dishi V, Gips M, Soback S, Cohen N, Weissgarten J, Blatt A, Golik A. The effect of grapefruit juice on the pharmacokinetics of orally administered verapamil. Eur J Clin Pharmacol 1998;54:337–40.

R. Verhaeghe

19 Drugs acting on the cerebral and peripheral circulations

DRUGS USED IN THE TREATMENT OF ARTERIAL DISORDERS OF THE BRAIN AND LIMBS

Cinnarizine *(SED-13, 417; SEDA-20, 191; SEDA-22, 221)*

Liver Drug-induced *cholestasis* has only been reported once as a possible adverse effect of cinnarizine, but uncertainty remained because the patient received triazolam at the same time. A second case has been now published (1^c).

A 87-year-old man was given cinnarizine for tinnitus and developed jaundice 7 weeks later, with dark urine and pale stools. He had taken no other drugs. Bile duct obstruction was ruled out and serological tests for viral hepatitis were negative. A liver biopsy 6 weeks later showed distinct centrilobular cholestasis and a slight lymphocytic infiltrate. He recovered completely and the liver tests were normal after another 3 months without cinnarizine. No rechallenge was performed.

Immunological and hypersensitivity reactions Several drugs can cause lesions of *subacute cutaneous lupus erythematosus.*

A 32-year-old women developed an erythematous, papulosquamous, annular, polycyclic skin eruption on her neck, trunk, and lateral parts of the limbs after sunbathing while taking cinnarizine and thiethylperazine (a phenothiazine) for vertigo. She had positive antinuclear antibodies (nucleolar pattern, anti-Ro/SSA). The lesions cleared without residual scars within a few weeks after stopping both drugs and starting steroids and chloroquine.

Phenothiazines are known to induce photosensitivity, but cinnarizine is not. The authors' arguments that cinnarizine was also to blame were its structural resemblance to piperazine and a similar episode of skin eruption in the same patient after sunbathing many years ago while taking cinnarizine only, but for which she did not seek medical advice (2^c).

Ginkgo biloba *(see also Chapter 48)*

Subarachnoid hemorrhage associated with *Ginkgo biloba* (3^c) stimulated a vigorous discussion on the differences between the usual extract sold over-the-counter and a ginkgolide mixture, and their respective (absence of) effects on platelet aggregating factor and bleeding time (4, 5). The dispute points to confusion that can arise when formulations of similar origin but with variable composition are available. In general, *Ginkgo biloba* is largely considered innocuous but its efficacy has been poorly demonstrated.

DRUGS USED IN THE TREATMENT OF MIGRAINE

Ergotamine *(SED-13, 543; SEDA-20, 192; SEDA-21, 216)*

Ergotism, arterial spasm induced by ergotamine, can be due to overdose, but some patients develop an exaggerated response to a therapeutic dose. Interaction with other drugs, leading to potentiation, may be a third mechanism. Four patients developed extreme limb ischemia after a therapeutic dose of ergotamine: one even took only a single dose of 1 mg. The symptoms responded to vasodilator therapy after withdrawal of ergotamine, but one needed a minor amputation. All patients were taking antiviral treatment for HIV infection, and the authors hypothesized that ritonavir and indinavir potentiated the effect of ergotamine by inhibiting a cytochrome P450 isoenzyme responsible for its metabolism (6^c–9^c).

Side Effects of Drugs, Annual 23
J.K. Aronson, ed.

Triptans *(SEDA-20, 192; SEDA-22, 222)*

Sumatriptan is available as film-coated tablets, as prefilled syringes for self-administered subcutaneous injection, and as an intranasal spray. A fourth formulation is for rectal use. Sumatriptan suppositories appear to be well tolerated: reported adverse events were similar to those during oral or subcutaneous treatment of patients with migraine. Local events involving the anus or rectum were rarely observed (10[R], 11[C]).

A recent publication has focused on *ischemic colitis* associated with the use of sumatriptan. Retrospective review and analysis of postmarketing reports showed seven confirmed cases (colonoscopy and/or biopsy) and a new one has been added (12[r]). Seven of the patients were women. Sumatriptan was mainly given subcutaneously, the dosages were not excessive, and the median time between the last administration to the onset of symptoms was less than 24 hours in only four patients. All the patients recovered on withdrawal of sumatriptan. Although many of these patients were using other drugs, particularly β-blocking and non-steroidal anti-inflammatory drugs, confusing the analysis, the authors suggested that vasoconstrictor effects in the mesenteric circulation associated with the use of sumatriptan played a causative role in inducing the ischemia.

A long list of new triptans is appearing (almotriptan, avitriptan, eletriptan, frovatriptan, naratriptan, rizatriptan, zolmitriptan, etc.) as potential antimigraine agents, and the first are already available. They share with sumatriptan the same basic mechanism of action and profile of adverse effects. The main search is for improved lipid solubility and enhanced penetration into the brain. Further randomized comparisons should clarify whether this will result in an improved clinical balance of efficacy and tolerability. Their exact role in the treatment of migraine remains to be defined.

OTHER PERIPHERAL VASODILATORS

Sildenafil *(SEDA-22, 222)*

Cardiovascular A post-marketing survey over the first 6 months of sales of sildenafil in the US (April to the middle of November 1998) has reported details on 130 patients who died after having been given sildenafil (over 3.5 million have received a prescription for it). As expected, deaths were mostly *cardiovascular*. There was a close time relation to the administration of sildenafil (within 4–5 hours) in 44 patients, 27 of whom died during or immediately after sexual intercourse. The disturbing finding is that 16 men either took or were given glyceryl trinitrate, contrary to product labelling and to several warnings (13[R]). A survey conducted in the UK on recreational use of sildenafil among night-club customers detected combined use of sildenafil with amyl nitrate. As both drugs are vasodilators, combined use may expose users to the same risk as the combination with glyceryl trinitrate (14[c]).

Nervous system *Third nerve palsy* occurred 36 hours after a second dose of sildenafil in a 56-year-old man; the authors suggested that sildenafil caused systemic hypotension sufficient to cause neurological dysfunction, but 36 hours is a long lag time for a drug with a half-life of only a few hours (15[c]).

Special senses German researchers have clashed over the importance of reversible *changes in the electroretinogram* observed in volunteers after sildenafil 100 mg. This has been ascribed to cross-reactivity of sildenafil with phosphodiesterase type 6 in the retina, but up to now no clinically significant effects have been reported (16[c]–18[c]).

REFERENCES

1. Colle I, Reynaert H, Naegels S, Hoorens A, Urbain D. Cinnarizine-induced cholestasis. J Hepatol 1999;30:553.
2. Toll A, Campo-Pisa P, Gonzales-Castro J, Campo-Voegeli A, Azon A, Iranzo P, Lecha M, Herrero C. Subacute cutaneous lupus erythematosus with cinnarizine and thiethylperazine. Lupus 1998;7:364–6.
3. Vale S. Subarachnoid haemorrhage associated with *Gingko biloba*. Lancet 1998;352:36.
4. Skogh M. Extracts of *Gingko biloba* and bleeding or haemorrhage. Lancet 1998;352:1145–6.
5. Vale S. Reply. Lancet 1998;352:1146.
6. Caballero-Granado FJ, Viciana P, Cordero E, Gomez-Vera MJ, Del Nozal M, Lopez-Cortes LF. Ergotism related to concurrent administration of er-

gotamine tartrate and ritonavir in an AIDS patient. Antimicrob Agents Chemother 1997;41:1207.
7. Montero A, Giovannoni AG, Tyrde P. Leg ischemia in a patient receiving ritonavir and ergotamine. Ann Intern Med 1999;130:329–30.
8. Liaudet L. Severe ergotism associated with interaction between ritonavir and ergotamine. Br J Med 1999;318:771.
9. Rosenthal E, Sala F, Chichmanian RM, Batt M, Cassuto JP. Ergotism related to concurrent administration of ergotamine tartrate and indinavir. J Am Med Assoc 1999,281:987.
10. Perry CM, Markham A. Sumatriptan. An updated review of its use in migraine. Drugs 1998; 55:889–922.
11. Tepper SJ, Cochran A, Hobbs S, Woessner M, Saiers J. Sumatriptan suppositories for the acute treatment of migraine. Int J Clin Pract 1998;52:31–5.
12. Knudsen JF, Friedman B, Chen M, Goldwasser J. Ischemic colitis and sumatriptan use. Ann Intern Med 1998;158:1946–8.
13. Jackson G, Sweeney M, Osterloh IH. Sildenafil citrate (Viagra®): a cardiovascular overview. Br J Cardiol 1999;6:325–33.
14. Aldridge J, Measham F. Sidenafil (Viagra®) is used as a recreational drug in England. Br Med J 1999;318:669.
15. Donahue SP, Taylor RJ. Pupil-sparing third nerve palsy associated with sildenafil citrate (Viagra®). Am J Ophthalmol 1998;126:476–7.
16. Vobig MA, Klotz T, Stak M, Bartz-Schmidt KU, Engelmann U, Walter P. Retinal side-effects of sildenafil. Lancet 1999;353:375.
17. Zrenner E. No cause for alarm over retinal side-effects of sildenafil. Lancet 1999;353:340–1.
18. Vobig MA. Retinal side-effects of sildenafil. Lancet 1999;353:1442.

Faiez Zannad

20 Antihypertensive drugs

GENERAL

Six drug classes of antihypertensive agents are used world wide: diuretics, β-adrenoceptor antagonists, calcium antagonists, angiotensin converting enzyme (ACE) inhibitors, angiotensin II receptor antagonists, and α-adrenoceptor antagonists. Centrally-acting antihypertensive drugs are also often used, and particularly the most recently available, imidazoline receptor antagonists. In some parts of the world, reserpine and methyldopa are still in use, although less and less often, because of their poor safety record. Indeed the most prominent differences among the various classes and agents are related to their safety profiles. The emergence of ACE inhibitors, calcium antagonists, and more recently angiotensin II receptor antagonists as alternative first-line agents possibly reflects continuing concerns about adverse effects that interfere with patients quality of life, and also the possible adverse metabolic consequences of long-term treatment with the more conventional agents, such as thiazide diuretics and β-blockers. There are also important differences between classes of drugs in the amount of evidence available from randomized controlled trials on their effects on morbidity and mortality. On the one hand, the benefit of diuretics and β-blockers is well established. On the other hand, there are no reliable data about α-blockers, direct-acting vasodilators, centrally-active agents, or the most recently available angiotensin II antagonists. As for calcium antagonists and ACE inhibitors, some convincing recent data suggest that these new agents may also reduce cardiovascular mortality and morbidity (1). Some of the data relevant to the ACE inhibitor class are summarized below.

Side Effects of Drugs, Annual 23
J.K. Aronson, ed.

ANGIOTENSIN CONVERTING ENZYME INHIBITORS

(SED-13, 546; SEDA-20, 195; SEDA-21, 219; SEDA-22, 225)

In hypertension, the CAPPP trial aimed to establish ACE inhibitors as alternative first-line agents in mild to moderate hypertension. It was an open prospective study with blinded evaluation (PROBE design) comparing an antihypertensive strategy based on either captopril or conventional therapy with a β-blocker or a diuretic as first-line drugs in patients with mild to moderate hypertension. At the end of follow-up the incidence of cardiovascular events was equal with the two strategies. However, imbalances in the assignment of treatment resulted in a 2 mmHg higher average diastolic blood pressure at entry in the group assigned to captopril. This difference in blood pressure alone would be sufficient to confer an excess of cardiovascular risk within this group, could mask real differences between the regimens in their effects on coronary events, and could explain the greater risk of stroke among patients who took captopril. The authors claimed that the overall results support the position that from now on one should consider ACE inhibitors as first-line agents, equal to diuretics and β-blockers (2^C). The CAPPP study also reported a reduced risk of diabetes with captopril, which may be explained by the fact that thiazides and β-blockers cause changes in glucose metabolism and by favorable effects of ACE inhibition on insulin responsiveness.

More recently, the results of a major trial with ramipril have become available (data presented at the European Society of Cardiology Barcelona 1999 annual meeting and unpublished at the time of writing, Salim Yusuf and Peter Sleight, personal communication). The HOPE Study was a factorial design evaluation of vitamin E and/or ramipril (10 mg od), or matching placebo in order to reduce events in high-risk elderly individuals. Over 9500 patients aged over 55 years were recruited. The trial was stopped early, after a mean of 4.5 years follow-up, in March 1999 because of significant benefit in the ramipril arm. The vitamin E arm will be continued for a further 2 years. This was a well-treated population with baseline treatment: 76% aspirin, 30% lipid-lowering agents, 40% β-blockers, 47% calcium antagonists, and 15% diuretics. During the trial the use of these agents increased. The mean BP, 138/79 mmHg at baseline, was reduced only modestly (by 3.3/1.5 mmHg) by ramipril. Ramipril reduced the primary outcome, death, by 22%. The separate end-points (cardiovascular death, fatal and non-fatal myocardial infarction, fatal and non-fatal stroke, revascularization procedure, hospitalization for heart failure) were also each significantly reduced. There was no effect on unstable angina, but revascularization was reduced by 15% and heart failure hospitalization by 16%. The results were particularly impressive in the 3518 diabetics, in whom cardiovascular death was reduced by 38%, myocardial infarction by 21% stroke by 32%, and all-cause mortality by 25%. The benefit was greater in patients with higher systolic blood pressures at baseline, but benefit was apparent down to baseline systolic blood pressures of 125–130 mmHg, underlining the more recent recommendations for lower blood pressure targets in high-risk individuals, even in the so-called 'normal' range. Only about half of the stroke benefit and one-quarter of the myocardial infarction benefit could be attributed to blood pressure reduction by ramipril. Combining the primary and secondary outcomes, the number needed to treat to avoid one of these events was around six. Ramipril was well tolerated, with only about a 5% drop-out from adverse effects (mainly *cough*).

In heart failure much debate has been generated by the observation of general 'under-use' of ACE inhibitors and the use of doses smaller than have been beneficial in clinical trials. This was partly related to concern about safety with the highest doses, especially in high-risk groups, such as the elderly and patients with renal insufficiency (3[R]). Actually, outcome trials effectively excluded elderly patients (75–80 years and over), and usually patients with renal insufficiency. As elderly patients have poorer renal function, are more likely to have vascular disease in their renal and carotid arteries, and may be more prone to symptomatic hypotension, it cannot be assumed that the benefit : risk ratio observed in younger patients will be the same, at the same doses, in elderly people. The NETWORK trial, a comparison of small and large doses of enalapril in heart failure, was poorly designed and is not very conclusive. However, it suggested that apart from a trend to more fatigue with higher doses (10 mg bd), the incidence of adverse effects, including symptomatic *hypotension*, was similar across the three dosages (2.5, 5, and 10 mg bd) (4[C]). The results of the larger and better designed ATLAS trial have been presented at an international meeting and are yet to be published. They suggested that lisinopril 30 mg/day is more effective than 2.5–5 mg/day and equally well tolerated. However, amazingly, full safety data are still unavailable to the public. In the studies of left ventricular dysfunction (SOLVD) adverse effects related to the long-term use of enalapril have been thoroughly investigated in a recent paper (5[C]).

In and after myocardial infarction, more trials have been published and subjected to a meta-analysis (6[R]). This very large database has provided valuable information on the rate of the most common adverse effects. Of all trials investigated the effects of ACE inhibitors on mortality in acute myocardial infarction, only the CONSENSUS II trial did not show a positive effect. In this trial enalaprilat was infused within the 24 h after the onset of symptoms, followed by oral enalapril. The reasons for the negative result of CONSENSUS II remain unresolved, but hypotension and a *proischemic effect linked to a poorer prognosis* have been reported.

In chronic nephropathy, two trials have expanded the benefit of ACE inhibitors in slowing the progression of chronic renal insufficiency due to renal diseases other than diabetic nephropathy (7[C]–9[C]) and have provided sufficient information on the safety profile of these agents in chronic renal insufficiency. This was found to be essentially the same as in patients with normal renal function. The current practice of avoiding ACE inhibitors in severe renal insufficiency, to prevent further renal impairment and hyperkalemia, is no longer justified, although careful monitoring should still be observed.

Respiratory *Cough* is still the most commonly reported adverse effect of ACE inhibitors and limits their use in a significant number of patients. The hypothesis that this adverse effect may be genetically predetermined was recently rejected in a study in which it was shown that common genetic variants of ACE, chymase, and the B_2-bradykinin receptor did not explain the occurrence of ACE inhibitor-related cough (10[C]). The mechanism may be more complicated than just an increase in bradykinin and substance P concentrations. Increased microvasculature leakage with exaggerated kinin production and subsequent stimulation of peptide release from sensory nerves may be involved.

Urinary system *Renal insufficiency* can occur in patients taking ACE inhibitors if they have reduced glomerular filtration pressure, such as in dehydration. In a retrospective study of 64 patients, mean age 71 years, with acute renal insufficiency associated with ACE inhibitor over 85% presented with overt dehydration due to diuretics or gastrointestinal fluid loss (11[Cr]). Bilateral renal artery stenosis or stenosis in a solitary kidney was documented in 20% of cases. In seven patients dialysis was required, but none became dialysis dependent. After resolution of acute renal insufficiency, the plasma creatinine concentration returned to baseline and renal function was not significantly worsened. Two-year mortality was the highest in a subgroup of patient with pre-existing chronic renal insufficiency.

Skin and appendages *Angioedema*, a potentially fatal complication, has now been associated with several different ACE inhibitors. New cases have presented as recurrent episodes of tongue swelling with cilazapril (12[cr]) and perindopril (13[c]).

Interactions Antagonistic effects of *cyclo-oxygenase inhibitors* (indomethacin or aspirin) have been repeatedly reported, in both hypertension and heart failure, strongly suggesting that prostaglandins may participate in the clinical response to ACE inhibitors (14[C], 15[C]). There are conflicting reports on the clinical significance of this interaction. Post hoc analyses of databases derived from large clinical trials are not helpful. From the SOLVD trial, it appears that in patients with left ventricular systolic dysfunction, aspirin was associated with improved survival and reduced morbidity. In aspirin users, benefit from enalapril was retained but reduced (16[CR]). On the other hand, a similar post hoc analysis of the CATS trial database in patients with acute myocardial infarction has suggested that aspirin does not attenuate the acute and long-term effects of captopril (17[CR]). Because of the demonstrated benefits on morbidity and mortality of each agent, textbooks and official guidelines do not recommend withholding either aspirin or ACE inhibitors in patients with heart failure or myocardial infarction. Instead, with insufficient proof of lack of interaction, the use of small doses of aspirin (under 100 mg/day) is recommended. The WASH pilot study compared the effects on cardiovascular events of warfarin, aspirin, and no antithrombotic therapy in patients with heart failure, most whom were taking an ACE inhibitor. Patients taking aspirin had more events and hospitalizations related to worsening heart failure than patients in the two other groups (unpublished data, reported at the 1999 annual meeting of the European Society of Cardiology, John Cleland, personal communication). The authors speculated that this may have been related to a negative interaction between ACE inhibitor therapy and aspirin, which would counteract the beneficial effects of ACE inhibitors. A large controlled study investigating this issue (WATCH) is being planned.

Cilazapril *(SEDA-19, 213)*

Many cases of *pemphigus foliaceus* have been previously reported with ACE inhibitors, and were related to the amide group contained in these agents. A new case has been attributed to cilazapril in a 69-year-old white woman; skin lesions appeared after she had taken cilazapril for 3 months and resolved on withdrawal and the addition of prednisone and azathioprine (21[c]).

Enalapril *(SED-12, 479; SEDA-21, 221; SEDA-22, 227)*

Hematological Enalapril-induced *anemia* has been reported in a child (18[c]).

A 7-year-old girl with segmental glomerulosclerosis and nephrotic syndrome failed to respond to prednisolone and cyclophosphamide, which were discontinued. While her renal function was deteriorating she was given enalapril 2.5 mg bd. After 3 months, the enalapril was withdrawn because her hemoglobin fell from 12.7 to 6.2 g/dl. Ferritin, folate, and vitamin B_{12} were normal. Recovery was incomplete. Only 10 weeks after enalapril withdrawal her hemoglobin rose to 8.5 g/dl and remained unchanged thereafter.

The incomplete resolution of anemia in this case suggests that factors other than the speculated enalapril-related inhibition of erythropoietin may have contributed to the initial anemia (worsening renal function, frequent blood sampling, withdrawal of prednisolone). Although the hypothesized mechanism is controversial, in a prospective controlled study enalapril increased recombinant human erythropoietin requirements to maintain hemoglobin concentrations in hemodialysis patients (19[Cr]).

Skin and appendages Adult *Henoch–Schönlein purpura* has been attributed to enalapril (20[c]).

A 41-year-old man with a history of hypertension and a recent stroke was admitted 10 days after starting to take enalapril (dose not reported). He complained of severe abdominal pain, myalgia, arthralgia, paresthesia, and Raynaud's phenomenon, and had a high erythrocyte sedimentation rate, but no leukocytosis or thrombocytopenia. He developed purpura-like cutaneous lesions with acute renal insufficiency, severe hematuria, and proteinuria. Liver tests became altered. There was a polyclonal rise in IgA concentrations. Skin biopsy suggested leukocytoclastic vasculitis, with deposition of IgA and complement. Other diagnostic procedures were negative. Enalapril was withdrawn and he was given corticosteroids, after which he fully recovered (timing not reported).

Lisinopril *(SED-12, 479; SEDA-22, 228)*

Pancreas Several cases of *pancreatitis* have been reported with ACE inhibitors, including lisinopril. A 67-year-old man without other risk factors developed acute pancreatitis only 3 hours after taking lisinopril. The originality of this case resides in the fact that the patient had experienced a similar but less severe reaction to the medication 3 months before. Thus, this case probably represents the first time a patient was rechallenged with lisinopril and had a more severe adverse reaction (22[cr]).

Sexual function Lisinopril 20 mg/day has been compared with atenolol 100 mg/day in a 16-week, double-blind, randomized, controlled trial in 90 hypertensive men aged 40–49 and without a history of sexual dysfunction. The number of occasions on which they had sexual intercourse fell during the first month in both groups (23[Cr]). Subsequently, sexual activity tended to recover with lisinopril but not atenolol. The authors suggested that lisinopril may cause only a temporary *reduction in sexual function.*

Perindopril *(SED-13, 549; SEDA-21, 221; SEDA-22, 228)*

A 12-month post-marketing surveillance study has been conducted in 47 351 French patients recruited by 4788 general practitioners (24[Cr]). No new information emerged, but the frequency and distribution characteristics of the most common adverse effects were detailed.

Ramipril *(SED-13, 549; SEDA-22, 229)*

Gastrointestinal Two cases of severe *vomiting, dyspepsia, and headache* with *falls in body weight and plasma albumin* have been reported in patients on chronic peritoneal dialysis (25[c]). Both occurred a few days after they started to take ramipril (dose not reported) and totally resolved after withdrawal. Both patients subsequently took losartan, which was well tolerated. This led the authors to suggest that the mechanism was mediated by bradykinin and/or prostaglandins, through an interaction with gastrointestinal motility, which may also be affected by peritoneal dialysis.

ANGIOTENSIN II RECEPTOR ANTAGONISTS *(SED-13, 549; SEDA-20, 196; SEDA-21, 222; SEDA-22, 229)*

Angiotensin II receptor antagonists are now widely available, and significant experience of their clinical use is accruing. Beyond losartan, this class has now other agents with different receptor affinities and binding kinetics (26[R]), such as candesartan, irbesartan, telmisartan, and valsartan, and others will soon be available. Many more are undergoing clinical development. All are also being considered for the treatment of diseases other than hypertension (heart failure with or without left ventricular systolic dysfunction, during and after acute myocardial infarction, diabetic nephropathy, other forms of glomerulopathy, re-stenosis after coronary angioplasty, and atherosclerosis).

The safety profile of angiotensin II receptor antagonists is so far remarkably good. Except for *hypotension*, virtually no dose-related adverse effects have been reported. In consequence, in cases of poor blood pressure control with the first dose of an angiotensin II antagonist, one should consider increasing to the highest effective dose, rather than the more common recommendation of considering first combining another antihypertensive agent.

Respiratory *Cough* has been specifically studied, because the mechanism of action of losartan differs from the ACE inhibitor group, in that there is no accumulation of kinins, which have been implicated in the non-productive cough associated with ACE inhibitors (27[R]). Of 135 patients with ACE inhibitor-induced cough re-challenged with lisinopril, 72% developed a cough, compared with only 29 and 34% given losartan or hydrochlorothiazide respectively (28[c]). However, another study of Prescription-Event Monitoring reported observations in four cohorts of 9000 patients each exposed to losartan, enalapril, lisinopril, or perindopril. The rate of cough was high even in the losartan cohort. The authors attributed this to a carry-over effect, since presumably patients taking losartan have previously had a cough with an ACE inhibitor (29[C]). Still, the question of whether angiotensin II receptor antagonists cause cough is not settled. A compilation of three controlled trials in 1200 patients showed incidence rates of cough of 3.6% with valsartan versus 9.5% with ACE inhibitors and 0.4% with placebo (26[R]). Such preliminary concerns should perhaps give rise to a more complete account involving all angiotensin II receptor antagonists on record.

Losartan *(SEDA-20, 196; SEDA-21, 222; SEDA-22, 229)*

Hematological *Anemia* has been reported in hemodialysis patients (30[c]) and particularly in renal transplant patients (31[c]–33[c]). The suggested mechanism is similar to that of ACE inhibitors, which cause this same adverse effect. However, in a small uncontrolled but prospective study, losartan given for 3 months to 15 patients on chronic hemodialysis with anemia, neither altered plasma erythropoietin concentrations nor aggravated the anemia (34[c]). In those taking losartan there was no need for higher doses of co-administered r-Hu Epo in order to correct anemia, in contrast to controls.

Pancreas There has been a second report of *pancreatitis* with losartan (35[c]).

A 42-year-old woman with insulin-dependent diabetes and chronic renal insufficiency developed pancreatitis 5 days after taking enalapril 2.5 mg and recovered after drug withdrawal. The pancreatitis relapsed one week after her general practitioner had prescribed losartan 50 mg/day, with full recovery after withdrawal. A rechallenge test with losartan was fully positive.

The case was well documented and causality seems to have been very convincingly established. No mechanistic speculation was given by the authors.

Special senses *Dysgeusia* has been reported in several cases in which the role of losartan was not fully established. In two cases the symptom occurred some time after switching from an ACE inhibitor to losartan (1 week in one case and 3 months in the other). In both cases the dysgeusia disappeared after withdrawal of losartan (timing not reported in one case, 1 week after in the other) (36[cr]). The authors referred to previously reported cases, one with losartan (37[c]) and one with valsartan (38[c]), and to a personal communication from the manufacturer of 12 other cases within a large safety monitoring program.

Risk factors Losartan has been evaluated in 406 patients with end-stage *renal insufficiency* undergoing hemodialysis (39[C]). Only 15 discontinued the medication owing to adverse effects related to losartan. In seven the adverse reaction was hypotension. Two patients reported possible anaphylactoid reactions during treatment with AN69 dialysis membranes. Remarkably, nine patients with a history of previous anaphylactoid reaction during treatment with AN69, did not have this complication with losartan and AN69.

Interactions Because losartan is metabolized by CYP2C9 and CYP3A4 to an active metabolite, E3174, which has greater antihypertensive activity than the parent compound, the effects of co-administration of losartan 50 mg/day and *erythromycin*, a moderate inhibitor of CYP3A4, or the potent inducer *rifampicin* have been investigated in a well-designed study in healthy volunteers. There was no significant effect of erythromycin, but rifampicin produced 35 and 40% reductions in the AUCs of losartan and E3174 respectively. Losartan oral clearance increased by 44% and the half-lives of both compounds were shortened by 50% (40[C]). Given the magnitude of the effect, this interaction is likely to be of clinical relevance.

Another very similar study investigated interactions with *itraconazole*, an inhibitor of CYP3A4, and *fluconazole*, which is more specific for CYP2C9 (41[C]). Fluconazole reduced the mean peak plasma concentrations of losartan and E3174 to 30 and 47% of their control concentrations respectively. The half-life of losartan was prolonged by 67%. Itraconazole had no significant effect. The possibility of a reduced effect of losartan when co-administered with fluconazole should be expected.

DRUGS THAT ACT ON THE SYMPATHETIC NERVOUS SYSTEM *(SED-13, 550; SEDA-21, 223; SEDA-22, 230)*

IMIDAZOLINE RECEPTOR AGONISTS *(SEDA-22, 230)*

Relminidine *(SEDA-20, 215)*

Skin and appendages *A photosensitivity reaction* has been attributed to relminidine (42[c]).

A 51-year-old woman developed erythema and swelling on sun-exposed areas and complained of a local burning sensation and pruritus 10 days after she started to take relminidine 1 mg/day for mild hypertension. She recovered fully 1 week after relminidine withdrawal and treatment with prednisolone. The chronology and the results of patch and photopatch tests suggested a phototoxic reaction to relminidine.

The authors claimed that this may have been related to the double bond in the oxazoline ring of the drug.

POSTSYNAPTIC ADRENOCEPTOR ANTAGONISTS *(SED-13, 552; SEDA-21, 223; SEDA-22, 231)*

Several recent articles have reviewed the pharmacology and clinical use of α-adrenoceptor antagonists in the management of benign prostatic hyperplasia, with special focus on the recently available tamsulosin. This agent was specially designed for the treatment of benign prostatic hyperplasia, since it is highly selective for the urinary tract α_{1A}-adrenoceptors. Indeed, it produces little or no cardiovascular effects, no first dose-effect, and much less dizziness. In clinical trials, adverse effects *included dizziness, weakness, headache, and nasal congestion. Abnormal ejaculation* was the most frequent adverse effect, in 8% of the patients at 0.4 mg/day, and in 18% at 0.8 mg/day (43[R], 44[R]).

Alfuzosin

Alfuzosin is a uroselective α_1-adrenoceptor antagonist. Its safety has been investigated in a large prospective 3-year open trial in 3228 patients with benign prostatic hyperplasia. There were no unexpected adverse effects. Only 4.2% of the patients dropped out owing to adverse effects.

Immunological and hypersensitivity reactions A 75-year-old man who had taken alfuzosin for 1 year developed *muscle pain and weakness* over 4 days, accompanied by tenderness and swelling of the deltoid muscles. There was erythema, with rash, periungual purpura, and erythematous plaques over the finger joints. Serum CK, LDH, and transaminase activities were raised and ANA was positive. An MRI scan showed findings consistent with inflammation of muscle and a biopsy confirmed the diagnosis of *dermatomyosis* (45[c]). Three days after drug withdrawal there was no improvement, so prednisone was started and he recovered within a few days. The temporal relation in this case was weak.

Terazosin *(SEDA-19, 215)*

Skin and appendages Terazosin has reportedly caused a *rash* (46[c]).

A 59-year-old man developed a generalized rash 3 days after starting to take terazosin 2 mg/day for benign prostatic hyperplasia. He had mild fever, weakness, intense pruritus, and a widespread eruption of scaling erythematous plaques with a violaceous hue on the trunk and extremities. The clinical examination was otherwise unremarkable and laboratory and serological tests were negative. A skin biopsy was suggestive of a drug reaction. Terazosin was stopped, and treatment with oral prednisolone and emollients resulted in complete recovery in 2 weeks.

Sexual function *Priapism* is rare with α-blockers (47[c]).

A 20-year-old man with a cervical spinal cord injury and a neuropathic bladder was given terazosin 1 mg at night increasing 5 days later to 2 mg. He developed a full erection of his penis, which lasted 5 hours and subsided spontaneously. Terazosin was stopped and the patient experienced no further priapism.

REFERENCES

1. Guidelines Subcommittee. 1999 World Health Organization-International Society of Hypertension Guidelines for the Management of Hypertension. J Hypertens 1999;17:151–83.
2. Hansson L, Lindholm LH, Niskanen L, Lanke J, Hedner T, Niklason A, Luomanmäki K, Dahlöf B, De Faire U, Mörli C, Karlberg BE, Wester PO, Björk J-E. Effect of angiotensin-converting-enzyme inhibition compared with conventional therapy on cardiovascular morbidity and mortality in hypertension: the Captopril Prevention Project (CAPPP) randomised trial. Lancet 1999;353:611–16.
3. Cleland JGF. ACE inhibitors for the prevention and treatment of heart failure: Why are they 'under-used'? J Hum Hypertens 1995;9:435–42.
4. Poole-Wilson PA, on behalf of the NETWORK investigators. The NETWORK study. The effect of dose of an ACE inhibitor on outcome in patients with heart failure. J Am Coll Cardiol 1996;27(Suppl A):141A.
5. Kostis JB, Shelton B, Gosselin G, Goulet C, Hood WB, Kohn RM, Kubo SH Schron E, Weiss MB, Willis III PW, Young JB, Probstfield J. Adverse effects of enalapril in the Studies of Left Ventricular Dysfunction (SOLVD). Am Heart J 1996;131:350–5.
6. Latini R, Maggioni AP, Flather M, Sleight P, Tognoni G. ACE inhibitor use in patients with myocardial infarction. Summary of evidence from clinical trials. Circulation 1995;92:3132–7.
7. Ruggenenti P, Perna A, Gherardi G, Gaspari F, Benini R, Remuzzi G. Renal function and requirement for dialysis in chronic nephropathy patients on long term ramipril: REIN follow up trial. Lancet 1998;352:1252–6.
8. Ruggenenti P, Perna A, Gherardi G, Garini G, Zoccali C, Salvadori M, Scolari F, Schena FP, Remuzzi G. Renopretective properties of ACE-inhibition in non-diabetic nephropathies with non-nephrotic proteinuria. Lancet 1999;354:359–64.
9. Maschio G, Alberti D, Janin G, Locatelli F, Mann JFE, Motolese M, Ponticelli C, Ritz E, Zucchelli P, Marai P, Marcelli D, Tentori F, Oldrizzi L, Rugiu C, Salvadeo A, Villa G, Picardi L, Borghi M, Moriggi M, et al. Effect of the angiotensin-converting-enzyme inhibitor benazepril on the progression of chronic renal insufficiency. New Engl J Med 1996;334:939–45.
10. Zee RYL, Rao VS, Paster RZ, Sweet CS, Lindpaintner K. Three candidate genes and angiotensin-converting enzyme inhibitor-related cough: A pharmacogenetic analysis. Hypertension 1998;31:925–8.
11. Wynckel A, Ebikili B, Melin JP, Randoux C, Lavaud S, Chanard J. Long-term follow up of acute renal failure caused by angiotensin converting enzyme inhibitors. Am J Hypertens 1998;11: 1080–6.
12. Kyrmizakis DE, Papadakis CE, Fountoulakis EJ, Liolios AD, Skoulas JG. Tongue angioedema after long-term use of ACE inhibitors. Am J Otoryngol 1998;19:394–6.
13. Lapostolle F, Barron SW, Bekka R, Baud FJ. Lingual angioedema after perindopril use. Am J Cardiol 1998;81:523.
14. Guazzi MD, Campodonico J, Celeste F, Guazzi M, Santambrogio G, Rossi M, Trabattoni D, Alimento M. Antihypertensive efficacy of angiotensin converting enzyme inhibition and aspirin counteraction. Clin Pharmacol Ther 1998;63:79–86.
15. Spaulding C, Charbonnier B, Cohen-Solal A, Juilliere Y, Kromer EP, Benhamda K, Cador R, Weber S. Acute hemodynamic interaction of aspirin and ticlopidine with enalapril: results of a double-blind, randomized comparative trial. Circulation 1998;98:757–65.
16. Al-Khadra AS, Salem DN, Rand WM, Udelson JE, Smith JJ, Konstam MA. Antiplatelet agents and survival: a cohort analysis from the Studies of Left Ventricular Dysfunction (SOLVD) trial. J Am Coll Cardiol 1998;31:419–25.
17. Oosterga M, Anthonio RL, De Kam P-J, Kingma JH, Crijns HJGM, Van Gilst WH. Effects of aspirin on angiotensin-converting enzyme inhibition and left ventricular dilation one year after acute myocardial infarction. Am J Cardiol 1998;81:1178–81.
18. Sackey AH. Anaemia after enalapril in a child with nephrotic syndrome. Lancet 1998;352:285–6.
19. Albitar S, Genin R, Fen-Chong M, Serveaux M-O, Bourgeon B. High dose enalapril impairs the response to erythropoietin treatment in haemodialysis patients. Nephrol Dial Transplant 1998;13:1206–10.
20. Goncalves R, Cortez Pinto H, Serejo F, Ramalho F. Adult Schönlein-Henoch purpura after enalapril. J Intern Med 1998; 244: 356–7.
21. Buzon E, Perez-Bernal AM, De la Pena F, Rios JJ, Camacho F. Pemphigus foliaceus associated with cilazapril. Acta Dermatol Venereol 1998; 78:227.
22. Gershon T, Olshaker JS. Acute pancreatitis following lisinopril rechallenge. Am J Emerg Med 1998;16:523–4.
23. Fogari R, Zoppi A, Corradi L, Mugeliini A, Poletti L, Lusardi P. Sexual function in hypertensive males treated with lisinopril or atenolol: a cross-over study. Am J Hypertens 1998;11:1244–7.
24. Speirs C, Wagniart F, Poggi L. Perindopril postmarketing surveillance: a 12 month study in 47 351 hypertensive patients. Br J Clin Pharmacol 1998;46:63–70.
25. Riley S, Rutherford PA. Gastrointestinal side effects of ramipril in peritoneal dialysis patients. Peritoneal Dial Int 1998;18:83–4.
26. Birkenhäger WH, De Leeuw PW. Non-peptide angiotensin type 1 receptor antagonists in the treat-

ment of hypertension. J Hypertens 1999;17:873–81.

27. Lacourciere Y, Lefebvre J. Modulation of the renin-angiotensin-aldosterone system and cough. Can J Cardiol 1995;11(Suppl F):33F–39F.
28. Lacourciere Y, Brunner H, Irwin R, Karlberg BE, Ramsay LE, Snavely DB, Dobbins TW, Faison EP, Nelson EB. Effects of modulators of the renin angiotensin aldosterone system on cough. Losartan Cough Study Group. J Hypertens 1994;12:1387–93.
29. Mackay FJ, Pearce GL, Mann RD. Cough and angiotensin II receptor antagonists: cause or confounding. Br J Clin Pharmacol 1999;47:111–14.
30. Schwarzbeck A, Wittenmeier KW, Hallfritzsch U. Anaemia in dialysis patients as a side-effect of sartanes. Lancet 1998;352:286.
31. Ducloux D, Saint-Hillier Y, Chalopin JM. Effect of losartan on hemoglobin concentration in renal transplant recipients: a retrospective analysis. Nephrol Dial Transplant 1997;12:2683–6.
32. Brantley RP, Mrug M, Barker CV. Blockade of AT1 receptors lowers hematocrit in post-transplant erythrocytosis. J Am Soc Nephrol 1996;7:1939.
33. Horn S, Holzer H, Horina J. Losartan and renal transplantation. Lancet 1998;351:111.
34. Lang SM, Schiffl H. Losartan and anaemia of end-stage renal disease. Lancet 1998;352:1708.
35. Birck R, Keim V, Fiedler F, Van der Woude FJ, Rohmeiss P. Pancreatitis after losartan. Lancet 1998;351:1178.
36. Heeringa M, Van Puijenbroek EP. Reversible dysgeusia attributed to losartan. Ann Intern Med 1998;129:72.
37. Schlienger RG, Saxer MS, Haefeli WE. Reversible ageusia associated with losartan. Lancet 1996;347:471–2.
38. Stroeder D, Zeissing I, Heath R, Federlin K. Angiotensin-II-antagonist CGP 48933 (valsartan). Results of a double-blind, placebo-controlled multicenter study. Nieren Hochdruckkr 1994;23:217–20.
39. Saracho R, Martin-Malo A, Martinez I, Aljama P, Montenegro J. Evaluation of the losartan in hemodialysis (ELHE) study. Kidney Int Suppl 1998;54:S125–9.
40. Williamson KM, Patterson JH, McQueen RH, Adams KF Jr, Pieper JA. Effects of erythromycin or rifampin on losartan pharmacokinetics in healthy volunteers. Clin Pharmacol Ther 1998;63:316–23.
41. Kaukonen K-M, Olkkola KT, Neuvonen PJ. Fluconazole but not itraconazole decreases the metabolism of losartan to E-3174. Eur J Clin Pharmacol 1998;53:445–9.
42. Mota AV, Vasconcelos C, Correia TM, Barros MA, Mesquita-Guimaraes J. Rilmenidine-induced photosensitivity reaction. Photodermatol Photoimmunol Photomed 1998;14:132–3.
43. Narayan P, Tewari A. Overview of alpha-blocker therapy for benign prostatic hyperplasia. Urology 1998; 51(Suppl A): 38–45.
44. De Mey C. Cardiovascular effects of alpha-blockers used for the treatment of symptomatic BPH: Impact on safety and well-being. Eur Urol 1998;34(Suppl 2):18–28.
45. Vela-Casasempere P, Borras-Blasco J, Navarro-Ruiz A. Alfuzosin-associated dermatomyositis. Br J Rheumatol 1998;37:1135–6.
46. Hernandez-Cano N, Herranz P, Lazaro TE, Mayor M, Casado M. Severe cutaneous reaction due to terazosin. Lancet 1998;352:202–3.
47. Vaidyanathan S, Soni BM, Singh G, Sett P, Krishnan KR. Prolonged penile erection association with terazosin in a cervical spinal cord injury patient. Spinal Cord 1998;36:805.

Gordon T. McInnes

21 Diuretics

GENERAL CONSIDERATIONS

The recent return to popularity of diuretics in the management of hypertension reflects three major factors (1[R]):

- recognition of the effectiveness of much lower dosages than those used previously, thereby providing good antihypertensive efficacy with fewer adverse effects (SED-13, 558);
- the excellent reductions in morbidity and mortality achieved by low-dosage diuretic-based therapy in multiple randomized controlled trials (SED-13, 558);
- the increasing awareness that some diuretic-induced shrinkage of effective blood volume is essential for adequate treatment of most patients with hypertension.

Therefore, diuretics will probably continue to be the basis of antihypertensive therapy. Although some adverse events may develop with their use, most occur only with the inappropriately high dosages commonly used before 1990.

There may be theoretical advantages of certain newer agents, but data thus far have not consistently shown that these drugs are more effective in reducing morbidity and mortality compared with therapy based on diuretics or β-blockers (2[R]). The sole exception comes from a recent trial in diabetic individuals with hypertension (3[C]). This study has been criticized (4) because of failure of the randomization procedure. Since this trial had an open design, its results must be considered unsafe.

Emphasis is correctly placed on the important role of ACE inhibitors in retarding progression of renal insufficiency in diabetic and other nephropathies (5[R]). However, in these circumstances, ACE inhibitors are added to a background of other antihypertensive therapies, commonly including a diuretic. Therefore, the renal protective action of ACE inhibitors is in the context of combination regimens.

The ability of low doses of diuretics to enhance efficacy has been demonstrated for all other classes of drugs (6[R]). Moreover, the tendency for increased retention of sodium by the hypertensive kidney when non-diuretic drugs cause the blood pressure to fall has long been recognized to contribute to loss of antihypertensive efficacy, which can be restored immediately by the addition of a diuretic.

Diuretic-based antihypertensive treatment has halved the incidence of heart failure in hypertension (SED-13, 559). Furthermore, left ventricular hypertrophy is markedly reduced by diuretic therapy (SEDA-22, 234). In addition to their action in primary prevention of heart failure, loop and thiazide diuretics have been the mainstay of treatment for symptomatic heart failure (7[R]). Diuretic therapy in both acute and chronic heart failure is effective in relieving symptoms and in improving cardiovascular hemodynamics.

Despite their widespread use, diuretics have not been shown to improve survival in patients with heart failure. As it is not feasible to conduct such a trial in patients with pulmonary edema due to heart failure, the place of diuretic therapy in the management of heart failure appears secure.

Diuretics and renal cell carcinoma R

The relation between diuretic therapy and the risk of malignancies has been examined in a review of pertinent publications between 1966 and 1998 (8[C]). In nine case control studies (4185 cases), the odds ratio for renal cell carcinoma in patients treated with diuretics was 1.55 (95% CI = 1.42, 1.71; P < 0.00001) compared with non-users of diuretics. In three cohort studies of 1 226 229 patients (802 cases), patients taking diuretics had a more than 2-fold

Side Effects of Drugs, Annual 23
J.K. Aronson, ed.

risk of renal cell carcinoma compared with patients not taking diuretics. Women had an odds ratio of 2.01 (CI = 1.56, 1.67) compared with 1.96 (CI = 1.34, 2.13) in men. Thus, the cumulative evidence suggests that long-term use of diuretics may be associated with renal cell carcinoma.

One hypothetical mechanism is that hydrochlorothiazide, a cyclic imide, is converted in the stomach to a mutogenic nitroso-derivative. Rats and mice treated with diuretics have been reported to develop nephropathies and renal adenomas. Renal cell carcinoma arises in renal tubular cells, which are the principal site of action of diuretics. Contact over years or decades may have a low-grade carcinogenic effect. Most prospective randomized trials provide too short a period of observation to assess the potential for carcinogenicity unequivocally.

Although diuretics remain the best documented drug class to reduce morbidity and mortality in hypertension, these data suggest a need for continued vigilance to assess the benefit : risk ratio of all drugs used for long-term therapy of cardiovascular disorders. Given the widespread and prolonged use of diuretics and their relatively modest benefit in mild hypertension, a potential risk of malignancy most be considered carefully. Cardiovascular benefits are less in women, who are more commonly given diuretics. These considerations caution against the use of diuretic therapy in young/middle-aged women who are at low cardiovascular risk.

The findings linking diuretic therapy with renal cell carcinoma need careful scrutiny. The strength of evidence provided by observational studies is limited, and such studies have yielded contradictory and controversial results in the past. An accompanying editorial (9^R) pointed out that some of the studies reviewed appear to have been designed to evaluate predictors of renal cell carcinoma without an a priori hypothesis that diuretics might be implicated. Therefore, statistical significance (set at $P < 0.05$) may have emerged merely by chance if 20 risk factors were examined.

The findings may have been confounded by other risk factors for renal cell carcinoma. Adjustment for confounders greatly attenuated the risk (to non-significance) in one study, and in another the association with diuretic use disappeared completely. Therefore, the findings from these observational studies may have resulted from uncontrolled confounding by known or unrecognized risk factors.

Another commentary (10^R) emphasized the potential bias of observational studies and also publication bias in meta-analysis. The contemporary relevance of the findings is further reduced, since many of the studies included patients taking very high doses of thiazides. It is difficult to disentangle a drug-related effect from the association between hypertension and renal cell carcinoma.

Since renal cell carcinoma is rare, the practical importance of these observations is small-one extra case of renal cell carcinoma in 1500 patients treated for 20 years. If the hypothesis is correct, antihypertensive therapy with diuretics will prevent 20–40 strokes, 3–28 heart attacks, 3–10 cardiovascular deaths, and 4–14 deaths overall for every extra case of renal cell carcinoma. Even middle-aged women would be spared six strokes for each potential case of renal cell carcinoma. If a low grade carcinogen is involved, most patients will not live long enough for its effect to be expressed.

These data should not be disregarded, but do not contribute a sufficient body of evidence on which to judge causality. The hypothesis deserves rigorous a priori testing in further studies. Until such data become available, alarming health care providers and patients that diuretics will increase the risk of renal cell carcinoma is premature.

ORGAN AND SYSTEMS

Endocrine, metabolic *Glucose metabolism* Many of the myths concerning the effect of diuretics on carbohydrate metabolism (SED-13, 565) continue to be given prominence in apparently authoritative reviews (11^R). It is suggested that thiazides are associated with a net increased risk of death in patients with diabetes mellitus and that patients with the cardiovascular dysmetabolic syndrome may not benefit from diuretic treatment because of increased insulin resistance. Diuretic-induced hypokalemia is said to be associated with reduced insulin release and worsening of insulin resistance. It is further postulated that diuretic-induced magnesium depletion contributes to insulin resistance. It is not explained why it has been so difficult to show a real advantage of other antihypertensive agents in long-term outcome trials in such high-risk patients.

Lipid metabolism The long-term effects of antihypertensive drugs and placebo on plasma lipoproteins have been compared in a multicenter, randomized, double-blind, parallel-group study in hypertensive men (12[C]). Patients were randomized to placebo (n = 187), hydrochlorothiazide (n = 188), atenolol (n = 178), captopril (n = 188), diltiazem (n = 185), or prazosin (n = 188). After drug titration, patients who achieved a target diastolic blood pressure below 90 mmHg were followed for 1 year. At 8 weeks, hydrochlorothiazide increased total cholesterol and apolipoprotein B non-significantly compared with placebo. Patients who achieved the target blood pressure with hydrochlorothiazide (responders) showed no adverse changes in plasma lipoproteins, whereas non-responders had increases in triglycerides, total cholesterol, and LDL-cholesterol. Plasma lipids and lipoprotein profiles did not change significantly among treatment groups after 1 year, except for minor falls in HDL-lipoprotein 2 concentrations with hydrochlorothiazide, clonidine, and atenolol.

The previously reported short-term adverse lipid effects with thiazides are limited to non-responders. The forced up-titration to higher doses probably accounts for the deleterious effects on plasma lipoproteins in these patients. Therefore, low-dose thiazides can be prescribed safely for long-term therapy of hypertension in responders.

A commentary (13[R]) pointed out that even small changes in lipids might be clinically significant. The study was underpowered to show statistical significance of minor effects. Since under 50% of the patients in each group were followed for 1 year, selection bias may also have been introduced. It should be remembered that lipid changes are subsidiary to mortality. In this respect, diuretics are the best established of the antihypertensive drug classes.

Mineral and fluid balance *Hyponatremia* Treatment with thiazide diuretics is one of the most common causes of hyponatremia (14[R]). Patients with hyponatremia induced by thiazides can present with variable hypovolemia or apparent euvolemia, depending on the magnitude of sodium loss and water retention.

There is no consensus about optimal treatment of symptomatic hyponatremia. The authors of this comprehensive review recommended a targeted rate of correction that does not exceed 8 mmol/l on any day of treatment. Remaining within this target, the initial rate of correction can still be 1–2 mmol/l/h for several hours in patients with severe symptoms (SED-13, 562). They suggested the following formulae for calculating the effect of giving 1 l of infusate on serum sodium.

a. Solutions containing sodium only:
   Change in serum sodium concentration (mmol/l) =
   (infusate Na^+ − serum Na^+)/(total body water + 1)
b. Solutions containing sodium and potassium:
   Change in serum sodium concentration (mmol/l) =
   (infusate Na^+ + infusate K^+ − serum Na^+)/(total body water + 1)

Estimated total body water (in liters) is calculated as a fraction of bodyweight: 0.6 in children; 0.6 and 0.5 in non-elderly men and women respectively; 0.5 and 0.45 in elderly men and women respectively.

Loop diuretics can cause *hypernatremia* by increasing free water clearance (net water loss in the form of hypotonic fluid) (15[R]). Over-rapid correction should be avoided.

Hypokalemia A retrospective analysis of 6797 patients with ejection fractions below 0.36 enrolled in the Studies Of Left Ventricular Dysfunction (SOLVD) was conducted to assess the relation between diuretic use at baseline and the subsequent risk of dysrhythmic death (16[C]). Patients who were taking a diuretic at baseline (n = 2901) were significantly more likely to have such an event than those not taking a diuretic (n = 2896) – 3.1 vs 1.7 per 1000 person-years. On univariate analysis and after controlling for important co-variates, the relation remained significant (relative risks 1.85 and 1.37 respectively). However, the association was seen only with non-potassium-sparing diuretics (n = 2495; relative risk 1.33); for potassium-sparing diuretics, alone or in combination with a non-potassium-sparing diuretic (n = 406), the relative risk was 0.90.

These data suggest that diuretic-induced potassium disturbances may result in fatal dysrhythmias in patients with left ventricular systolic dysfunction. The authors cited much of the unreliable evidence that diuretics cause potassium depletion and that this is related to dysrhythmias (SED-13, 562). SOLVD were not randomized trials of the risk of dysrhythmic death caused by diuretics. On average, patients retaking diuretics not only had lower serum potassium concentrations, but were also older, had more severe heart failure and were more likely to be taking antidysrhythmic drugs at baseline, although they had fewer indicators of ischemic heart disease. Even controlling for bias in multivariate analysis does not exclude the influence of unrecognized confounders. It is unknown whether diuretics were continued or changed during the 3 years of the trial. Thus, it remains uncertain that diuretic therapy is related to a risk of sudden dysrhythmic death in patients with heart failure.

Diuretic-induced hypokalemia is undoubtedly associated with a risk of serious ventricular dysrhythmias if diuretics are co-administered with drugs that prolong the QT interval (SED-13, 563). Diuretics increase the risk of *torsade de pointes* during antidysrhythmic drug therapy, independent of serum potassium concentration (17[R]). The list of cardiac and non-cardiac drugs that prolong the QT interval continues to lengthen (17[R], 18[R]). Recent additions include various antidysrhythmic drugs, including ibutilide, almokalant, and dofetilide; antimicrobials, including clarithromycin, clindamycin, co-trimoxazole, pentamidine, imidazoles (ketoconazole etc), some fluoroquinolones, and antimalarials (quinine, halofantrine); histamine H_1 receptor antagonists (terfenadine and astemizole); the serotonin receptor antagonist zimeldine; antipsychotic drugs (pimozide and sertindole); tricyclic/tetracyclic antidepressants; and the cholinergic antagonist cisapride. Particular care should be taken to avoid diuretic-induced hypokalemia when any of these agents are co-prescribed.

Risk factors *Elderly people* The effects of furosemide withdrawal on postprandial blood pressure have been assessed in 20 elderly patients (mean age 73 years) with heart failure and preserved left ventricular systolic function (ejection fraction 61%) (19[C]). In 13 who were able to discontinue furosemide (mean dose 32 mg/day), maximum systolic blood pressure decline fell significantly from 25 to 11 mmHg and diastolic blood pressure from 18 to 9 mmHg over 3 months. In the continuation group (mean furosemide dose 21 mg/day), there was no change in the postprandial fall.

Postprandial hypotension is common in elderly patients with heart failure and preserved left ventricular systolic function. Withdrawal of furosemide ameliorates postprandial blood pressure changes, probably by improving left ventricular diastolic filling. Postprandial hypotension is associated with falls, syncope, and higher incidences of coronary heart disease events, stroke, and total mortality. Furosemide should be avoided in elderly patients with diastolic dysfunction.

MODERATELY POTENT DIURETICS

Chlortalidone *(SED-13, 570)*

Drug fever has been attributed to chlortalidone (20[c]).

A 58-year-old woman presented with intermittent nocturnal fever (up to 39.5°C) for 4 weeks beginning 2 weeks after the introduction of chlortalidone for hypertension. Otherwise, physical examination was normal. Investigations showed a normochromic normocytic anemia and raised erythrocyte sedimentation rate and C-reactive protein. Other biochemical tests, blood culture, and serological and immunological tests were negative. Chest radiography, lung scintigraphy, and abdominal ultrasound were unremarkable. There was no further fever after chlortalidone was withdrawn, and all biochemical tests became normal. The lymphocyte transformation test showed stimulation by chlortalidone.

Indapamide *(SED-13, 570; SEDA-21, 229)*

A case of severe acute *hepatitis* associated with indapamide has been reported (21[c]). Serum bilirubin and liver enzymes were greatly raised. All normalized over 6 months after withdrawal of indapamide.

A patient had several episodes of *fixed drug eruption* during treatment with indapamide (22[c]). The diagnosis was confirmed by positive controlled oral challenge. The possibility of cross-reactivity with other sulfonamide derivatives was investigated by controlled oral challenge tests with sulfamethoxazole, sulfadiazine, and furosemide. The tests with sulfamethoxazole and sulfadiazine were positive. This is the first report of a fixed drug eruption with indapamide.

CARBONIC ANHYDRASE INHIBITORS

Acetazolamide *(SED-13, 571; SEDA-20, 204; SEDA-21, 228; SEDA-22, 236)*

Cardiovascular A case of *anaphylactic shock* caused by a single oral dose of acetazolamide has been reported (23[c]).

A 70-year-old man was given acetazolamide 250 mg to control postoperative intraoscular pressure 5 hours after cataract removal under local anesthetic. Thirty minutes later he complained of nausea, became cyanotic, and had an acute respiratory arrest. His systolic blood pressure was 70 mmHg, his heart rate was 180/min, and there was tachypnea (40 breaths/min). Arterial gases confirmed hypoxemia (PaO_2 6.34 kPa, 47 mmHg). Pulmonary embolism and high pressure pulmonary edema were excluded by perfusion lung scanning and right-sided heart catheterization. Management was with ventilatory support, vasopressors, intravenous hydrocortisone, and diphenylhydramine. Clinical improvement occurred over 12 hours. After stabilization, sulfonamide hypersensitivity was confirmed by skin testing, suggesting cross-sensitivity with a sulfonamide derivative (acetazolamide).

Physicians should be aware of the risk of anaphylaxis to acetazolamide, particularly in patients with a history of allergy to sulfonamides.

Risk factors A *ketogenic diet* is sometimes used to control intractable seizures. Acetazolamide should be discontinued before starting the diet, because of the potential risk of severe secondary metabolic acidosis (24[r]). Acetazolamide can be reinstituted once the acid-base status of the patient has stabilized.

POTENT DIURETICS

Bumetanide *(SED-13, 574; SEDA-22, 236)*

A case of *bullous pemphigoid* induced by bumetanide has been reported (25[c]).

A 67-year-old man presented with an acute bullous eruption 6 weeks after starting bumetanide. He had numerous large tense bullae on erythematous skin, with superficial ulceration on the thighs, arms, and anterior trunk. Pruritus was severe. Routine laboratory tests were normal, except for blood eosinophilia. Biopsy of a blister showed subepidermal bullae associated with dermal infiltrates of neutrophils and eosinophils. Direct immunoflurescence showed continuous linear deposits of C3 and IgG at the basement membrane zone, confirmed by immuno-electron microscopy. Circulating IgG anti-basement membrane antibodies were localized in the roof of the blister. Compete clinical healing and normalization of immunology occurred within 2 months of withdrawal of bumetanide.

Torasemide *(SED-13, 574; SEDA-21, 229; SEDA-22, 239)*

Two cases of *vasculitis with kidney failure* related to torasemide have been reported (26[c]).

A 70-year-old man was admitted with heart failure secondary to ischemic heart disease and severe aortic stenosis. Furosemide 20 mg/day was replaced by torasemide 5 mg/day. After the second dose he developed oliguria and an erythematous morbilliform rash with palpable violet petechial lesions on the legs. Chest X-ray showed bilateral alveolar infiltrates. Serum creatinine and potassium were raised (212 μmol/l and 6.7 mmol/l respectively). Skin biopsy showed leukocytoclastic vasculitis. After withdrawal of torasemide, his renal function improved (serum creatinine 97 μmol/l) and the skin lesions resolved (leaving residual pigmented areas) within 8 days.

An 84-year-old man with ischemic heart disease and hypertension was treated with torasemide 10 mg/day for persistent edema. About 24 hours after the administration of torasemide, he developed painless, non-palpable, petechial lesions on the limbs and trunk, with oliguria. His serum creatinine was 256 μmol/l and his serum potassium 6.2 mmol/l. Skin biopsy showed non-leukocytoclastic vasculitis with a mixed inflammatory infiltrate including eosinophils. The patient was symptom free 15 days after withdrawal of torasemide.

Neither patient had a previous history of drug hypersensitivity. Torasemide has a chemical structure similar to that of sulfonamides, which are often linked to vasculitis. However, both patients had previously tolerated furosemide, another sulfonamide derivation. The temporal correlation with torasemide administration suggests a causal relation, but the mechanism is unclear.

POTASSIUM-SPARING DIURETICS

Spironolactone *(SED-13, 575; SEDA-20, 205; SEDA-21, 230; SEDA-22, 239)*

Spironolactone and its metabolite canrenone caused falsely low readings in a common assay for digoxin (AXSym MEIA) because of negative cross-reactivity (27[c]). Misleading subtarget concentrations were repeatedly reported, and falsely guided drug dosing resulted in digoxin intoxication.

Previously, only positive interference, leading to falsely high digoxin readings, have been reported with spironolactone and canrenone. Such values are unwelcome but give rise to further investigation. Negative interference is much more dangerous. Toxic concentrations may remain unidentified and intoxication can occur if therapy is based on such misleading values.

REFERENCES

1. Kaplan NM. Diuretics as a basis of antihypertensive therapy. An overview. Drugs 2000; 59(Suppl 2):21–5.
2. Moser M. National recommendations for the pharmacological treatment of hypertension: should they be revised? Arch Intern Med 1999;159:1403–6.
3. Hansson L, Lindholm LH. Niskanen L, Lanke J, Hedner T, Niklason A, Luomanmäki K, Dählöf B, De Faire U, Mörlin C, Karlberg BE, Wester PO, Bjröck J-E, for the Captopril Prevention Project (CAPPP) Study Group. Effect of angiotensin-converting-enzyme inhibition compared with conventional therapy on cardiovascular morbidity and mortality in hypertension: the Captopril Prevention Project (CAPPP) randomized trial. Lancet 1999;353:611–16.
4. Peto R. Failure of randomization by "sealed" envelopes. Lancet 1999;354:73.
5. Zanchetti A. Contribution of fixed low-dose combinations to initial therapy in hypertension. Eur Heart J 1999;1(Suppl L);L5–9.
6. Kaplan NM. Low dose combinations in the treatment of hypertension: theory and practice. J Hum Hypertens 1999;13:707–10.
7. Krämer BK, Schweda F, Riegger GAJ. Diuretic treatment and diuretic resistance in heart failure. Am J Med 1999;106:90–6.
8. Grossman E, Messerli FH, Goldbourt U. Does diuretic therapy increase the risk of renal cell carcinoma? Am J Cardiol 1999;83:1090–3.
9. Lee I-M, Hennekens CH. Diuretics and renal cell carcinoma. Am J Cardiol 1999;83:1094.
10. Lip GYH, Ferner RE. Diuretic therapy for hypertension: a cancer risk? J Hum Hypertens 1999; 13:421–3.
11. Peters AL, Hsueh W. Antihypertensive agents in diabetic patients. Great benefits, special risks. Arch Intern Med 1999;159:541–2.
12. Lakshman MR, Reda DJ, Materson BJ, Cushman WC, Freis ED, for the Department of Veterans Affairs Cooperative Study Group on Antihypertensive Agents. Diuretics and beta-blockers do not have adverse effects at 1 year on plasma lipid and lipoprotein profiles in men with hypertension. Arch Intern Med 1999;159:551–8.
13. Golomb BA, Criqui MH. Antihypertensives. Much ado about lipids. Arch Intern Med 1999;159:535–7.
14. Adrogué HJ, Madias NE. Hyponatremia. New Engl J Med 2000;342:1581–9.
15. Adrogué HJ, Madias NE. Hypernatremia. New Engl J Med 2000;342:1493–9.
16. Cooper HA, Dries DL, Davis CE, Shen YL, Domanski MJ. Diuretics and risk of arrhythmic death in patients with left ventricular dysfunction. Circulation 1999;100:1311–15.
17. Viskin S. Long QT syndromes and torsade de pointes. Lancet 1999;354:1625–33.
18. Yap YG, Camm J. Risk of torsades de pointes with non-cardiac drugs. Br Med J 2000;320:1158–9.
19. Van Kraaij DJW, Jansen RWMM, Bouwels LHR, Hoefnagels WHL. Furosemide withdrawal improves postprandial hypotension in elderly patients with heart failure and preserved left ventricular systolic function. Arch Intern Med 1999; 159:1599–605.
20. Osterwalder P, Koch J, Wüthrich B, Pichler WJ, Vetter W. Intermittent fever of unknown cause. Dtsch Med Wochenschr 1998;123:761–5.
21. Safer L, Ben Mimoun H, Brahem A, Hanza J, Harzallah S, Abdellati S, Bdioui F, Saffar H. Severe acute hepatitis induced by indapamide. Report of a case. Sem Hôp Paris 1998;74:1274.
22. De Barrio M, Tornero P, Zubeldia JM, Sierra Z, Matheu V, Herrero T. Fixed drug eruption induced by indapamide. Cross-reactivity with sulfonamides. Invest Allergol Clin Immunol 1998;8:253–5.
23. Tzanakis N, Metzidaki G, Thermos K, Spyrakich, Bouros D. Anaphylactic shock after a single oral intake of acetazolamide. Br J Ophthalmol 1998;82:588.
24. Tallian KB, Nahata MC, Tsao C-Y. Role of the ketogenic diet in children with intractable seizures. Clin Pharmacother 1998;32:349–61.
25. Boulinguez S, Bernard P, Bedanc C, Le Brun V, Bonnetblanc JM. Bullous pemphigoid induced by bumetanide. Br J Dermatol 1998;138:548–9.
26. Palop-Larrea V, Sancho-Calabuig A, Gorriz-Teruel J, Martínez-Mier I, Pollardo-Mateu LM. Vasculitis with acute kidney failure and torasemide. Lancet 1998;352:1909–10.
27. Steimer W, Müller C, Eber B, Emmanuilidis K. Intoxication due to negative canrenone interference in digoxin drug monitoring. Lancet 1999; 354:1176–7.

Gijsbert B. van der Voet and Frederik A. de Wolff

22 Metals

Aluminium *(SED-13, 583; SEDA-20, 207; SEDA-21, 232; SEDA-22, 242)*

Respiratory Specific chemical exposures and exposure assessment methods relating to studies in the alumina and primary aluminium industry have been reviewed (1[R]). In aluminium smelting, exposure to fluorides, coal tar pitch volatiles, and sulfur dioxide has tended to abate in recent years, but there is insufficient information about other exposures. Published epidemiological studies and quantitative exposure data for bauxite mining and alumina refining are virtually non-existent. Determination of possible exposure-response relations for this part of the industry through improved exposure assessment methods should be the focus of future studies.

Dental technicians are potentially exposed to various occupational dusts and chemicals and a case of *pulmonary granulomatosis* has been reported (2[c]).

A dental laboratory technician developed progressive exertional dyspnea and cough associated with pulmonary granulomatosis. Lung function studies showed a restrictive pattern with a low diffusion capacity. A high-resolution CT scan showed micronodules in both lungs, corresponding to non-caseating foreign body granulomas at histological examination. Mineralogical studies showed the presence of silica, silicates, and aluminum. The lymphocytic transformation test was positive for beryllium with the bronchoalveolar lavage.

Combined histological, mineralogical, and immunological studies led to a diagnosis of pneumoconiosis, most likely related to occupational exposure to beryllium and aluminum.

The role of aluminium in the development of *occupational asthma* has never been convincingly substantiated. Now occupational asthma has been reportedly caused by aluminium welding (3[c]).

A 32-year-old man working in a leather plant had to perform electric arc welding on mild steel, using manual metal arc and inert gas metal arc techniques. About once a month he welded aluminium pieces using a manual arc process with a flux-coated electrode. After 4 years of intermittent exposure to these various welding processes, he developed chest tightness and wheezing that occurred specifically on days when he was welding aluminium. His asthmatic symptoms started 1–4 hours after the end of exposure to aluminium and persisted for several hours. He never had myalgia, chills, or fever. He was treated with inhaled budesonide (400 μg/day) and salbutamol when necessary. Inhalation challenges combined with exposure assessment provided evidence that aluminium can cause asthmatic reactions.

Liver Histology and metal content of the liver were studied in a patient with *Wilson's disease* (4[c]). Copper and aluminium contents of the biopsied liver were measured simultaneously by neutron activation analysis. The copper content was markedly increased (814 μg/g dry weight) and there was an extremely high aluminium content (479 μg/g). On the other hand, macroscopically and histologically there was no evidence of cirrhosis, although there was mild fibrosis or inflammation of the liver. It is likely that toxic metals, such as aluminum, copper, and manganese, might be implicated in the pathogenesis of Wilson's disease.

Musculoskeletal Heavy chronic use of antacids containing aluminium and magnesium hydroxide can cause serious *skeletal impairment* (5[c]).

A 39-year-old female pharmacist who self-medicated with high doses of a potent antacid containing aluminum and magnesium hydroxide for peptic ulcer disease consumed over 18 kg of elemental aluminium and 15 kg of elemental magnesium over 8 years. This resulted in severe osteomalacia, due to profound phosphate depletion. Bone biopsy showed stainable aluminium deposits along 28% of the total bone surface, which is a unique observation in a patient with normal renal function. Treatment included withdrawing the antacid and supplementation with phosphate, calcium, and vitamin D. This produced marked subjective and objective improvement,

Side Effects of Drugs, Annual 23
J.K. Aronson, ed.

including a striking increase in her bone mineral density over the next 2 years.

Immunological and hypersensitivity reactions Aluminium salts are currently the only widely used adjuvants in human vaccines (6[R]). Recent developments in the understanding of the structure, composition, and preparation of immunostimulating complexes (ISCOMs) have been reviewed and compared.

Four cases have been reported of *persistent subcutaneous nodules* at sites of hepatitis B vaccination due to aluminium sensitization (7[c]). Symptoms included pruritic, sore, erythematous, and in two cases hyperpigmented, subcutaneous nodules, persisting for 8 months to 2 years. All the patients were positive for aluminium salts in patch tests, while immunization against hepatitis B was successful.

Interactions Aluminium toxicity is well described in patients on dialysis. Aluminium has a close chemical affinity with silicon, which may have a role in protecting against aluminium toxicity (8[C]). Serum aluminium and silicon concentrations were measured in hemodialysis patients from four different centers. Although there was no relation across all centers combined, in one center there was a reciprocal relation in patients on home hemodialysis (who did not require reverse osmosis). Median (range) aluminium concentrations were higher, 2.2 (0.4–9.6) μmol/l when serum silicon was less than 150 μmol/l, and lower, 1.1 (0.2–2.8) μmol/l when serum silicon was greater than 150 μmol/l. In patients treated by hemodialysis without reverse osmosis, high serum silicon concentrations were associated with lower serum aluminium concentrations. Further work is needed to confirm a preventive role for silicon in the accumulation and subsequent toxicity of aluminium in dialysis patients.

Arsenic *(SED-13, 585; SEDA-22, 243)*

Arsenic compounds continue to be used as therapeutic agents, being old drugs for new indications, such as various categories of leukemia (9[R]). Their use to treat acute promyelocytic leukemia is recent and is indicated when resistance develops against first line treatment with all-*trans* retinoic acid. Reports continue to be published on incidents related to the use of traditional Chinese herbal medications containing arsenic among other toxic substances (10[R]).

There is little experience with arsenic trioxide in the treatment of recurrent acute promyelocytic leukemia that is resistant to all-*trans* retinoic acid (11[c]).

A 15-year-old African American girl, with multiply recurrent acute promyelocytic leukemia that had resisted conventional chemotherapy was given arsenic trioxide (As_2O_3) 10 mg intravenously for 28 days and again for a further 28 days after a 4-week break. She had a complete remission by morphological, cytogenetic, and molecular criteria. About 6 months later she again relapsed and had another course of As_2O_3, which produced a morphological, but not a cytogenetic or molecular, remission. Arsenic trioxide was well tolerated. Skin dryness was treated with topical moisturizers. Gastrointestinal upset, including mild nausea without vomiting or cramping pain, occurred only during intravenous therapy. No other toxicity was noted.

Liver Arsenic salts can cause *liver damage* (12[c]).

A 60-year-old man, a heavy drinker, with psoriasis of the palms and soles was treated with arsenical salt derivatives from 1972 to 1982. In 1984 he had an upper gastrointestinal hemorrhage. Only hyperkeratosis and palmar erythema were observed. His liver enzymes were raised. Endoscopy showed an antral ulcer with signs of recent bleeding and grade IV esophageal varices with no evidence of bleeding. Liver biopsy showed preservation of the parenchymal architecture, fibrous expansion of the portal spaces, and minimal lymphocytic infiltration. The diagnosis was portal fibrosis compatible with idiopathic portal hypertension. When he died of multiorgan failure in 1997, autopsy showed a moderately differentiated multifocal hepatic angiosarcoma with bone, gastric, and splenic metastases.

This patient had both idiopathic portal hypertension and hepatic angiosarcoma, in which the common causative factor was the chronic use of arsenical salts for the treatment of psoriasis. In a review of the literature the authors found only five other cases in which both diseases were associated, while exposure to arsenical salts was found in only one of them.

Bismuth *(SED-13, 585; SEDA-20, 208; SEDA-21, 233; SEDA-22, 243)*

Bismuth remains a part of some regimens for the eradication of *Helicobacter pylori* in combination with antibiotics (13[R]). Bismuth salicylates are effectively used in other intestinal diseases, such as microscopic colitis (14[c]).

Biliary system *Acute cholecystitis* caused by non-O1 *Vibrio cholerae* has been described in a 55-year-old healthy traveller immediately after a vacation in Cancun, Mexico (15[cr]). During his vacation he had taken Peptobismol brand of bismuth subsalicylate 30 ml tds as prophylaxis against traveller's diarrhea. At surgery his gall bladder was acalculous, inflamed, distended, and nearly ruptured. Pathogenetic factors may have included the use of bismuth subsalicylate, distension of the gall bladder from illness-induced fasting, and bacterial toxins in the gall bladder. The authors implied that bismuth subsalicylate could have prevented the secretory diarrhea that is seen in many infections with non-O1 *Vibrio cholerae.* Diarrhea would result in evacuation of many organisms from the small bowel. Bismuth subsalicylate might have impaired this mechanism and increased the number of organisms with access to the common bile duct at the ampulla of Vater.

Chromium *(SEDA-20, 208)*

Trivalent chromium is an essential trace element. Trivalent chromium compounds are used by patients to enhance weight loss, to increase lean body mass, or to improve glycemic control. Drug histories should include attention to the use of over-the-counter nutritional supplements often regarded as harmless by the public and lay media. The recommended daily allowance of chromium picolinate is 50–200 μg, but information about its toxicity is limited.

Toxicity secondary to chronic ingestion of 6–12 times the recommended daily allowance of over-the-counter chromium picolinate has been reported (16[c]).

A 33-year-old white woman presented with weight loss, anemia, thrombocytopenia, hemolysis, liver dysfunction (aminotransferase activities 15–20 times normal, total bilirubin three times normal), and renal insufficiency. She had taken chromium picolinate 1200–2400 μg/d for the previous 4–5 months to enhance weight loss. Her plasma chromium concentrations were 2–3 times normal. After withdrawal of chromium picolinate, she was managed with supportive measures, blood transfusions, and hemodialysis. Hemolysis stabilized and her liver and renal function eventually recovered.

Endocrine, metabolic Chromium picolinate is a widely available nutritional supplement marketed for a plethora of afflictions. There is some evidence, including results from human studies, that it has a role in glucose homeostasis (17[cr]).

In a 28-year-old woman with an 18-year history of type 1 diabetes mellitus the glycosylated hemoglobin fell from 11.3 to 7.9% and her blood glucose concentration was 1.7–3.3 mmol/l lower after she had taken chromium picolinate (200 μg tds for 3 months). There were no adverse effects.

Musculoskeletal *Rhabdomyolysis* has been attributed to chromium picolinate in a 24-year-old body builder who took 1200 μg over 48 hours (18[c]).

Copper *(SED-13, 587; SEDA-20, 208; SEDA-21, 234; SEDA-22, 244)*

Hematological The effects of combined oral contraceptives, depot medroxyprogesterone acetate injections, levonorgestrel subdermal implants (Norplant), copper-containing intrauterine contraceptive devices (IUCDs), and Chinese stainless steel ring IUCDs on hemoglobin and ferritin have been studied in 2507, non-pregnant non-lactating women, aged 18–40 years, in seven countries (Bangladesh, Chile, China, the Dominican Republic, Pakistan, Thailand, and Tunisia) (19[C]). In 1295 current users of the contraceptive methods hemoglobin and ferritin concentrations were higher than in 1212 women who were starting to use contraceptives. The current users of copper IUCDs had higher hemoglobin concentrations (difference in mean concentrations of 0.3 g/dl), but lower ferritin concentrations (difference of 10 g/l) than non-users. Current use of the stainless steel ring had an adverse effect on both hemoglobin and ferritin. In 285 anemic women there were significant mean increases of hemoglobin at 12 months among the users of the hormonal contraceptives, but not among users of copper or stainless steel ring IUCDs. The authors concluded that hemoglobin and ferritin concentrations are affected by contraceptives and that the hormonal contraceptives included in the present study have a beneficial effect, while the effects of copper IUCDs should be studied further.

Gastrointestinal Two cases of *migration of IUCDs to the bowel* have been reported (20[c], 21[c]).

A 28-year-old pregnant woman developed an ileal perforation 4 weeks after the insertion of a Multiload-Cu 375 IUCD. This report documents the shortest interval between insertion and proven bowel injury by an IUCD.

A Copper-T IUCD migrated to the rectal lumen in a 36-year-old woman with menorrhagia for 3 months and a history of Copper-T insertion 6 years before.

Skin and appendages *Perimenstrual dermatitis* has been attributed to a copper-containing IUCD (22[c]).

A 41-year-old woman had a 2-year history of a recurrent, self-healing skin rash associated with abdominal pain. She had had cholinergic urticaria since 1995 and had had a copper-containing IUCD inserted 12 years before. The eruption followed a cyclical pattern, invariably appearing 3–7 days before the menses, and tending to improve spontaneously with the onset of bleeding. This non-itchy rash was associated with abdominal distension and cramps that followed a similar course. She had multiple non-itchy symmetrical erythematous papules on the upper trunk, neck, and arms. Patch testing was positive for copper sulfate. The IUCD was removed and the abdominal symptoms subsided at the following cycle. Progressive resolution of the dermatitis was observed. No cutaneous eruption was observed after 8 months and no new lesions developed after a further 5 months.

Special senses *Ocular chalcosis* has been attributed to injury with a copper-containing foreign body (23[c]).

After having suffered an open-globe injury, presumably due to a small foreign body after a grenade explosion, a 30-year-old man presented six years later with ocular chalcosis, including sunflower cataract, a multitude of tiny brownish particles in the anterior vitreous, fibrillar degeneration of the posterior vitreous and brilliant patches overriding the foveal region. The patches were measured by confocal scanning laser tomography and optical coherence tomography. Besides acquired cyandyschromatopsia, psychophysical and electrophysiological tests were unremarkable. Vision was 20/20. The central patches measured 200–700 μm in diameter and 150–200 μm in height above the inner retinal surface. With the exception of a Kayser–Fleischer ring of the cornea the patient presented all the morphological signs of ocular chalcosis. Since signs of inflammation were absent no further therapy was planned.

This man had probably suffered from a penetrating damage of the left eye caused by a copper-containing body, which had eventually dissolved. Although the observed patches on the central retina in ocular chalcosis have previously been described, their nature is not known.

Gallium *(SED-13, 588; SEDA-20, 209; SEDA-21, 235; SEDA-22, 244)*

No new adverse effects have been reported. The mechanisms of the therapeutic activity of gallium have recently been reviewed (24[R]).

Germanium *(SED-13, 588; SEDA-21, 235; SEDA-22, 245)*

Germanium compounds are at present mainly used in the semiconductor industry. They have previously been used as anticancer agents, and recently germanium oxide has been used as a supposed health-giving agent. *Nephropathy and neuropathy* have been attributed to germanium toxicity (25[c]).

A 53-year-old man developed severe general weakness, anorexia, and weight loss (16 kg in 3 months). Over the preceding 17 months he had taken a total of 400 g of lysine germanium oxide in powder form. After 15 months he developed a tingling sensation in the palms and soles and weakness of the limbs, especially the legs,. Neurological examination showed grade IV motor strength and negative deep tendon reflexes in the legs. Laboratory tests showed impaired renal function and anemia. Urinary concentration of β_2-microglobulin was raised. The blood germanium concentration was 63 μg/l and the urine concentration 2190 μg/l (normal less than 5 μg/l). Renal sonography showed no morphological abnormalities. Nerve conduction studies and needle electromyography suggested a sensorimotor polyneuropathy, predominantly involving sensory nerves. Renal biopsy showed tubulointerstitial nephritis. Abstinence from germanium and conservative management of the chronic renal insufficiency resulted in slight improvement of the weakness and renal function.

Gold *(SED-13, 588; SEDA-20, 209; SEDA-21, 236; SEDA-22, 245)*

Respiratory The pulmonary toxicity of gold salts is an uncommon cause of life-threatening *respiratory failure.* Patients who suffer from this do not usually need mechanical ventilation, and the toxicity can be difficult to diagnose when it occurs in patients with an illness with pulmonary involvement. However, severe respiratory failure requiring mechanical ventilation has been attributed to gold salt toxicity in a patient with rheumatoid arthritis (26[c]). Steroid therapy was life-saving and induced complete resolution of the lung damage.

Iron *(SED-13, 595; SEDA-20, 211; SEDA-21, 237; SEDA-22, 246)*

The toxicokinetics and toxicodynamics of iron poisoning have recently been reviewed, although no new adverse effects or toxicity were reported (27[R]). The safety and efficacy of iron dextran has recently been evaluated in patients on home renal replacement therapies, without any adverse effects (28[R]). The flow of trials on the efficacy of oral iron supplements continues without reports of any newly observed adverse effects (29[C], 30[C]).

Gastrointestinal *Gut pigmentation* has been attributed to an iron salt (31[c]).

An 80-year-old Japanese woman presented with epigastric discomfort and nausea. She had a history of hypertension, rheumatoid arthritis, iron deficiency anemia, and chronic renal insufficiency, and had taken oral ferrous sulfite for 19 months. Endoscopic examination of the duodenum showed marked pigmentation of the duodenal mucosa. Histological examination showed that the pigment had histochemical features compatible with hemosiderin and was located mainly within macrophage lysosomes in the lamina propria. Ferrous sulfite was withdrawn and the pigmentation disappeared within 7 months.

Musculoskeletal Saccharated ferric oxide, an intravenous formulation of iron that is used when oral iron is not effective in anemia, can cause *osteomalacia* during long-term use. The underlying mechanism of nephropathy leading to bone toxicity has recently been reviewed (32[R]).

Manganese *(SED-13, 1001; SEDA-20, 212; SEDA-21, 238; SEDA-22, 246)*

The neurotoxicity of manganese remains an issue, although no new aspects have been reported. The best way to monitor excessive exposure to manganese includes serum manganese concentration measurement in combination with brain MRI scanning and perhaps a battery of neurofunctional tests, as has recently been reviewed (33[R]). Studies have concentrated on manganese in patients on parenteral nutrition (34[C]) and occupational exposure (35[C]).

Mercury *(SED-13, 598; SEDA-20, 213; SEDA-21, 239; SEDA-22, 247)*

The debate on the effects of dental amalgams containing mercury on patients' health has not yet been resolved (36[R]).

Nervous system Despite their potentially disastrous adverse effects, topical mercury salts can still be found as the ingredients of some over-the-counter formulations or local remedies. *Peripheral polyneuropathy* as a result of chronic ammoniated mercury poisoning has been studied and followed over 2 years (37[c]).

A 36-year-old man developed peripheral polyneuropathy after chronic perianal use of an ammoniated mercury ointment. He had very high blood and urine mercury concentrations. Sural nerve biopsy showed mixed axonal degeneration/demyelination. His symptoms improved progressively over 2 years after withdrawal of the ointment, but neurophysiological recovery was incomplete.

The availability of safer drugs should result in a complete ban of these dangerous compounds.

Nickel *(SED-13, 599; SEDA-20, 214; SEDA-21, 240; SEDA-22, 248)*

No new adverse effects of nickel compounds have been reported. However, gold salts used in the treatment of rheumatoid arthritis may be contaminated by nickel, thus causing adverse effects not attributable to gold.

Immunological and hypersensitivity reactions Intramuscular chrysotherapy is a well established treatment for rheumatoid arthritis. Its therapeutic use has been limited by the high incidence of skin adverse effects. The pathogenic mechanisms of these are unknown, but could include allergic reactions to gold or to nickel as a contaminant. In order to investigate these mechanisms further, 15 patients who developed skin eruptions after chrysotherapy were assessed using skin biopsy and lymphocyte transformation stimulated by gold and nickel salts in vitro (38[C]). Chrysotherapy caused two main cutaneous eruptions: *lichenoid reactions* and *non-specific dermatitis*. Peripheral blood mononuclear cells from patients with lichenoid reactions proliferated in response to gold salts in vitro, while those who developed non-specific dermatitis responded mainly to nickel. Nickel was a significant contaminant of the gold formulation (sodium aurothiomalate, Myocrisin, Rhone–Poulenc Ltd), amounting to a total dose of 650 ng over 6 months. The authors suggested that a significant percentage of skin reactions during chrysotherapy are due to nickel contamination.

Platinum *(SED-13, 600; SEDA-22, 248)*

Nervous system The adverse effects of cisplatin include a *pure sensory neuropathy*, with conservation of pain and temperature sense, which is very disabling. Two more cases have been reported (39[c]).

A woman with cancer of the ovary and a man with oat cell carcinoma both developed paresthesia of all four limbs, reduced control of fine movements, and unstable gait after receiving a cumulative dose of 500 mg/m^2 of cisplatin. There was distal hypesthesia, with conservation of temperature and pain sensation, areflexia, and sensory ataxia. The woman also had continuous pseudoathetosis. Neurophysiological studies showed absence of peripheral and central sensory potentials and of H reflexes, normal electromyography, normal motor conduction, and normal mixed silent period.

The target organ in cisplatinum neurotoxicity is the dorsal root ganglion. These patients had a syndrome that clinically and neurophysiologically suggested diffuse neuropathic involvement of the dorsal ganglion, in which absence of sensory and H reflex potentials showed that the small myelinic cells were not altered, consistent with the preservation of pain and temperature sensation.

Encephalopathy has also been reported (40[c]).

A 84-year-old woman with adenocarcinoma of the ovary had two fully reversible episodes of non-convulsive encephalopathy, each following a course of cisplatin-based chemotherapy, confirming a causal relation. She developed acute confusion, a partial left homonymous hemianopia and a left extinction hemiparesthesia 7 and 10 days after treatment. Brain MRI showed long-standing cerebral microvascular changes and an electroencephalogram showed right-sided parieto-occipital periodic lateralized epileptiform discharges over a generalized background slowing of activity.

This case adds further to the clinical diversity of cisplatin toxicity and, in view of its similarity to posterior leukoencephalopathy, suggests regional endovascular injury rather than a direct cerebral toxicity as the initial event in the evolution of encephalopathy.

An *acute stroke* has been reported in a woman who had received cisplatin (41[c]).

A 21-year-old woman with a mixed germ cell tumor of the left ovary was given intravenous chemotherapy including etoposide 100 mg/m^2 on days 1–5, cisplatin 20 mg/m^2 on days 1–5, and bleomycin 30 units on days 2, 8, and 15, all of which she tolerated very well. Three weeks later she received a second cycle, which was complicated by an episode of dizziness on day 8. The following day she had an episode of transient dysphasia for 10 minutes. Her third course was uneventful until day 7, when she collapsed with a severe right-sided hemiparesis and dysphasia. Left-sided total anterior circulation infarction was confirmed on a MRI scan.

This case strongly implicated cisplatin as a potential neurotoxic agent.

Selenium *(SED-13, 600; SEDA-20, 215; SEDA-21, 240; SEDA-22, 249)*

All aspects of selenium compounds have recently been reviewed (42[R]). No new adverse effects of selenium-containing formulations have been reported.

Silver *(SED-13, 600; SEDA-20, 215; SEDA-21, 241; SEDA-22, 250)*

There is concern about the use of silver-containing formulations of uncontrolled composition (e.g. colloidal silver) with supposed activity in a host of microbial diseases. The use of silver fluoride in dental care may be contraindicated in children because of high release of fluoride (43[R]).

Skin and appendages The use of silver nitrate has been reviewed against the background of a recent case of intoxication.

A 29-year old woman complained of increasing black discoloration of the tip of her left middle finger, resembling gangrene (44[cr]). However it was established that she had been applying silver nitrate to her finger for the treatment of a small granuloma. Hence the true diagnosis was of localized tissue necrosis, secondary to application of the silver nitrate sticks. On withdrawal of the therapy, there was complete recovery.

In consequence, it is recommended that the practice of unsupervised local application of silver nitrate to the fingers should be discontinued.

Titanium *(SEDA-20, 215; SEDA-21, 241; SEDA-22, 250)*

Titanium continues to be used in medicine mainly for its mechanical benefits in surgical and dental materials, but also as a constituent of anticancer compounds.

Skin and appendages Titanium tetrachloride ($TiCl_4$) is an intermediate compound in the production of white pigment, which can cause severe *chemical burns* (45[c]). In two reported cases $TiCl_4$ caused 18–20% total body surface area burns. as a combined consequence of hydrochloric acid and the heat that was generated in areas in which this otherwise stable compound was mixed with sweat. $TiCl_4$ combined with water is extremely dangerous, and its immediate treatment (towel drying before irrigation) makes it unique among chemicals. The experience of the authors suggests that in most cases grafting will be required. These chemical burns were self-limiting and had no notable systemic sequelae. Wound biopsy specimens taken on days 3 and 6 were subjected to immunostaining, which showed that $TiCl_4$ did not retard wound healing. The exposure time to $TiCl_4$ vapor will determine the pulmonary and ophthalmological effects in each case. Clinical awareness of the propensity of $TiCl_4$ to react with water-even in the form of sweat-is vital, because prompt management can limit the extent of injury.

Zinc *(SED-13, 601; SEDA-20, 215; SEDA-21, 242; SEDA-22, 251)*

Nervous system Clioquinol (5-chloro-7-io-do-8-hydroxyquinoline) was used 30 years ago as an oral antiparasitic agent and to increase intestinal absorption of zinc in patients with acrodermatitis enteropathica, a genetic disorder of zinc absorption. However, the use of clioquinol was epidemiologically linked to *subacute myelo-optic neuropathy* (SMON), characterized by peripheral neuropathy and blindness, which affected 10 000 patients in Japan. Withdrawal of oral clioquinol led to the elimination of SMON, but the mechanism of how clioquinol induces neurotoxicity is unclear. The effect of clioquinol–metal chelates has been tested on neural crest-derived melanoma cells (46). The effect of clioquinol chelates on cells was further studied by electron microscopy and by a mitochondrial potential-sensitive fluorescent dye. Of the ions tested, only clioquinol–zinc chelate was cytotoxic. This cytotoxicity was extremely rapid, suggesting that its primary effect was on the mitochondria, and electron microscopic analysis showed that the chelate caused mitochondrial damage. This was further confirmed by the observation that the chelate reduced the mitochondrial membrane potential. The phenomenon of clioquinol–mediated toxicity appeared to be specific to zinc and was not seen with other metals tested. Since clioquinol causes increased systemic absorption of zinc, it is likely that clioquinol–zinc chelate was present in appreciable concentrations in patients with SMON and may have been the causative toxin.

Gastrointestinal Zinc chloride is a powerful corrosive agent. Reports of zinc chloride ingestion are uncommon, and there is little information about its toxicity and management. A new case of *gastric corrosion* has been reported (47[c]).

A 10-year-old girl accidentally ingested an acid soldering flux solution (pH 3.0; zinc chloride 30–60%). Systemic effects after ingestion were unremarkable, except for lethargy. Thus, chelation therapy was not considered. Severe gastric corrosion was caused by local caustic action. An antral stricture of the stomach developed about 3 weeks later, and she had a modified Heineke–Mikulicz antropyloroplasty. Postoperatively, she made an uneventful recovery. However, although she was tolerating a normal diet, a barium meal showed that her stomach was totally aperistaltic.

In this case careful long-term follow-up was considered necessary, because of the potential risk of malignancy in the damaged stomach.

REFERENCES

1. Benke G, Abramson M, Sim M. Exposures in the alumina and primary aluminium industry:an historical review. Ann Occup Hyg 1998;42:173–89.
2. Brancaleone P, Weynand B, De Vuyst P, Stanescu D, Pieters T. Lung granulomatosis in a dental technician. Am J Indust Med 1998;34:628–31.

3. Vandenplas O, Delwiche JP, Vanbilsen ML, Joly J, Roosels D. Occupational asthma caused by aluminium welding. Eur Respir J 1998;11:1182–4.
4. Yasui M, Kohmoto J, Ota K, Shinmen K, Tanaka H, Nogami H. A case of neurologic type of Wilson's disease with increased aluminum in liver comparative study with histological findings to metal contents in the liver (in Japanese). No To Shinkei-Brain Nerve 1998;50:767-72.
5. Woodson GC. An interesting case of osteomalacia due to antacid use associated with stainable bone aluminum in a patient with normal renal function. Bone 1998;22:695–8.
6. Sjolander A, Cox JC, Barr IG. ISCOMs: an adjuvant with multiple functions. J Leukocyte Biol 1998;64:713–23.
7. Skowron F, Grezard P, Berard F, Balme B, Perrot H. Persistent nodules at sites of hepatitis B vaccination due to aluminium sensitization. Contact Dermatitis 1998;39:135–6.
8. Parry R, Plowman D, Delves HT, Roberts NB, Birchall JD, Bellia JP, Davenport A, Ahmad R, Fahal I, Altmann P. Silicon and aluminium interactions in haemodialysis patients. Nephrol Dial Transplant 1998;13:1759–62.
9. Rousselot P, Dombret H, Fermand J-P. Arsenic derivatives: old drugs for new indications. Hematologie 1998;5(Suppl 2):95–7.
10. Wong ST, Chan HL, Teo SK. The spectrum of cutaneous and internal malignancies in chronic arsenic toxicities. Singapore Med J 1998;39:171–3.
11. Bergstrom SK, Gillan E, Quinn JJ, Altman AJ. Arsenic trioxide in the treatment of a patient with multiply recurrent, ATRA-resistant promyelocytic leukemia: a case report. J Pediatr Hematol Oncol 1998;20:545–7.
12. Duenas C, Perez-Alvarez JC, Busteros JL, Saez-Royuela F, Martin-Lorente JL, Yuguero L, Lopez-Morante A. Idiopathic portal hypertension and angiosarcoma associated with arsenic salt therapy. J Clin Gastroenterol 1998;26:303–5.
13. Wermeille J, Zelger G, Cunningham M. The eradication treatments of *Helicobacter pylori*. Pharm World Sci 1998;20:1–17.
14. Fine KD, Lee EL. Efficacy of open label bismuth subsalicylate for the treatment of microscopic colitis. Gastroenterology 1998;114:29–36.
15. West BC, Silberman R, Otterson WN. Acalculous cholecystitis and septicemia caused by non-O1 *Vibrio cholerae*:: first reported case and review of biliary infections with *Vibrio cholerae*. Diag Microbiol Infect Dis 1998;30:187–91.
16. Cerulli J, Grabe DW, Gauthier I, Malone M, McGoldrick MD. Chromium picolinate toxicity. Ann Pharmacother 1998;32:428–31.
17. Fox GN, Sabovic Z. Chromium picolinate supplementation for diabetes mellitus. J Fam Pract 1998;46:83–6.
18. Martin WR, Fuller RE. Suspected chromium picolinate-induced rhabdomyolysis. Pharmacotherapy 1998;18:860–2.
19. Bathija H, Lei Z-W, Cheng X-Q, Xie L, Wang Y, Rugpao S, Lipisam S, Suwanarach C, Akhter H, Ahmed Y, Islam Z, Sen A, Bahman S, Khan SA, Rabbani A, Khan T, Sued EM, Lumbiganon P, Weerawattrakul Y, Pinitsoontorn P, Bierschwale H, Silva P, Bravo C, Gajardo R, Meta N, Lavin F, Tuane R, Chong E, Hajri S, Siala N, Bessioud M, Boukhris R. Effects of contraceptives on hemoglobin and ferritin. Contraception 1998;58: 261–73.
20. Chen CP, Hsu TC, Wang W. Ileal penetration by a multiload-Cu 375 intrauterine contraceptive device. A case report with review of the literature. Contraception 1998;58:295–304.
21. Banerjee N, Kriplani A, Roy KK, Bal S, Takkar D. Retrieval of lost copper-T from the rectum. Eur J Obstet Gynecol Reprod Biol 1998;79:211–12.
22. Pujol RM, Randazzo L, Miralles J. Perimenstrual dermatitis secondary to a copper-containing intrauterine contraceptive device. Contact Dermatitis 1998;38:288.
23. Budde WM, Junemann A. Chalcosis oculi. Klin Monatsbl Augenheilkd 1998;212:184–5.
24. Bernstein LR. Mechanisms of therapeutic activity for gallium. Pharmacol Rev 1998;50:665–82.
25. Kim KM, Lim CS, Kim S, Kim SH, Park JH, Ahn C, Han JS, Lee JS. Nephropathy and neuropathy induced by a germanium-containing compound. Nephrol Dial Transplant 1998;13:3218–19.
26. Blancas R, Moreno JL, Martin F, De la Casa R, Onoro JJ, Gomez V, Prados J. Alveolar-interstitial pneumopathy after gold-salts compounds administration, requiring mechanical ventilation. Intensive Care Med 1998;24:1110–12.
27. Tenenbein M. Toxicokinetics and toxicodynamics of iron poisoning. Toxicol Lett 1998; 102/103:653–6.
28. Sloand JA, Shelly MA, Erenstone AL, Schiff MJ, Talley TE, Dhakal MP. Safety and efficacy of total dose iron dextran administration in patients on home renal replacement therapy. Peritoneal Dial Int 1998:18;522–7.
29. Harvey RSJ, Reffitt DM, Doig LA, Meenan J, Ellis RD, Thompson RP, Powell JJ. Ferric trimaltol corrects iron deficiency anaemia in patients intolerant of iron. Aliment Pharmacol Ther 1998;12:845–8.
30. Haliotis FA, Papanastasiou DA. Comparative study of tolerability and efficacy of iron protein succinylate versus iron hydroxide polymaltose complex in the treatment of iron deficiency in children. Int J Clin Pharmacol Ther 1998;36:320–5.
31. Hirasaki S, Koide N, Ogawa H, Ujike K, Okada H, Mizuno M, Ukida M, Tsuji T. A case of melanosis duodeni alleviated by the discontinuation of ferrous sulfite. Dig Endosc 1998;10:55–60.
32. Sato K, Shiraki M. Saccharated ferric oxide induced osteomalacia in Japan: iron-induced osteopathy due to nephropathy. Endocr J 1998;45:431–9.
33. Greger JL. Dietary standards for manganese: overlap between nutritional and toxicological studies. J Nutr 1998;128(Suppl 2):368S–371S.
34. Dietemann JL, Reimund JM, Diniz RLFC, Reis M Jr, Baumann R, Neugroschl C, Von Sohsten S, Warter JM. High signal in the adenohypophysis on T_1-weighted imaged presumable due to man-

ganese deposits in patients on long-term parenteral nutrition. Neuroradiology 1998;40:793–6.

35. Barrington WW, Angle CR, Willcockson NK, Padula MA, Korn T. Autonomic function in manganese alloy workers. Environ Res 1998;78:50–8.

36. Staehle HJ. Gesundheitsstörungen durch Amalgam? Med Klin 1998;93:99–106.

37. Deleu D, Hanssens Y, Al-Salmy HS, Hastie I. Peripheral polyneuropathy due to chronic use of topical ammoniated mercury. J Toxicol Clin Toxicol 1998;36:233–7.

38. Choy EH, Gambling L, Best SL, Jenkins RE, Kondeatis E, Vaughan R, Black MM, Sadler PJ, Panavi GS. Nickel contamination of gold salts: link with gold induced skin rash. Br J Rheumatol 1997;36:1054–8.

39. Cano JR, Catalan B, Jara C. Neuronopathy due to cisplatin. Rev Neurol 1998;27:606–10.

40. Lyass O, Lossos A, Hubert A, Gips M, Peretz T. Cisplatin-induced non-convulsive encephalopathy. Anti-Cancer Drugs 1998;9:100–4.

41. Gamble GE, Tyrrell P Acute stroke following cisplatin therapy. Clin Oncol 1998;10:274–5.

42. Barceloux DG. Selenium. J Toxicol Clin Toxic 1999;37:145–72.

43. Gotjamanos T, Orton V. Abnormally high fluoride levels in commercial preparations of 40 per cent silver fluoride solution: contraindication for use in children. Aust Dent J 1998;43:422–7.

44. Sankar NS, Donaldson D. Lessons to be learned: a case study approach. Finger discoloration due to silver nitrate exposure: review of uses and toxicity in clinical practice. J R Soc Promot Health 1998;118:371–4.

45. Paulsen SM, Nanney LB, Lynch JB. Titanium tetrachloride: an unusual agent with the potential to create severe burns. J Burn Care Rehabil 1998;19:377–81.

46. Arbiser JL, Kraeft SK, Van Leeuwen R, Hurwitz SJ, Selig M, Dickersin GR, Flint A, Byers HR, Chen LB. Clioquinol–zinc chelate: a candidate causative agent of subacute myelo-optic neuropathy. Mol Med 1998;4:665–70.

47. Yamataka A, Pringle KC, Wyeth J. A case of zinc chloride ingestion. J Pediatr Surg 1998; 33:660–2.

R.H.B. Meyboom

23 Metal antagonists

'Chelation therapy' is used as a non-orthodox treatment of atherosclerotic disease in many parts of the world. A postulated mechanism is the binding of calcium and other cations, causing an increase in their renal excretion. However, there is insufficient evidence of the efficacy of chelation therapy with ethylenediaminetetraacetic acid, deferoxamine, or dexrazoxane in cardiovascular disease ([1R]).

Deferiprone *(SED-13, 624; SEDA-20, 221; SEDA-21, 249; SEDA-22, 254)*

Deferiprone has been accepted in spite of serious toxicity, because of the great need for an effective iron chelator for oral use (SEDA-18, 250). In this context, two recent studies are important, because they cast doubt on the efficacy of deferiprone ([2CR], [3CR]). In the first, a long-term trial in 51 transfusion-dependent iron-overloaded patients, 19 withdrew because of adverse events: *arthropathy* (stiffness, crepitus, effusion; $n = 5$), *gastrointestinal symptoms* (severe nausea, anorexia, vomiting; $n = 5$), *granulocytopenia* ($n = 3$), *renal insufficiency* ($n = 1$), and *tachycardia* ($n = 1$) ([2CR]). In the second study, in 26 patients who continued to use the drug, there was generally no satisfactory reduction in iron stores. On the other hand, deferiprone caused fewer adverse effects and was more effective in patients who were previously well chelated and had lower initial ferritin concentrations. Also, in the long run deferiprone did not adequately control the body iron burden. In addition, in this study the alarming suspicion was raised that deferiprone may paradoxically *worsen hepatic fibrosis* in patients with thalassemia major, based on hepatic biopsies in 19 patients ([3CR]).

On the other hand, recent studies in Italy and the US reached more positive conclusions. Of 187 patients with thalassemia who were unable or unwilling to use deferoxamine, 162 completed 1 year of treatment with deferiprone (75 mg/kg/day) ([4CR]). One patient developed *agranulocytosis* and another nine had various degrees of *neutropenia* (altogether 5%). Other reasons for withdrawal were *nausea and vomiting* ($n = 4$; total frequency 24% of patients), *thrombocytopenia* below 100×10^9/l ($n = 2$), and a *fall in serum AlT* ($n = 2$). *Arthralgia* developed in 11 patients (6%). In 29 patients with poor compliance with deferoxamine treatment, who received deferiprone (70 mg/kg/day) with a minimum follow-up of 1 year, adverse effects were *pain in the knees* in three patients, reversible *neutropenia* in one, and *gastric intolerance* in one ([5CR]). A repeat liver biopsy in 20 patients showed a reduction of the grade of liver siderosis and iron content in seven. Worsening of hepatic fibrosis was not mentioned.

Liver Deferiprone paradoxically *worsened hepatic fibrosis*in patients with thalassemia major, based on hepatic biopsies in 19 patients ([3CR]). On the other hand, in another study of 20 liver biopsies worsening of hepatic fibrosis was not mentioned ([5CR]).

Deferoxamine *(SED-13, 619; SEDA-20, 221; SEDA-21, 248; SEDA-22, 254)*

Respiratory *Lung damage* has been attributed to high doses of deferoxamine in 17 patients with β-thalassemia major who were given 33 courses by continuous intravenous infusion of 10 days duration in doses up to 10 mg/kg/h ([6CR]). Respiratory dysfunction developed in two girls given the highest doses (aged 11 and 15 years). Symptoms were dyspnea, tachypnea, tachycardia, and low-grade fever. Arterial blood gas measurements showed hypoxemia and hypercapnia. Chest X-rays showed *bilateral interstitial infiltrates.* In one patient mechanical ventilation was needed for 2 weeks and it took 8 months before pulmonary function returned to normal. In both patients deferoxamine was reintroduced later on without relapse.

Side Effects of Drugs, Annual 23
J.K. Aronson, ed.

Nervous system and special senses Neurophysiological evaluation of 40 patients with β-thalassemia major showed *abnormal findings in brainstem evoked potentials*—auditory (25%), visual (15%), and somatosensory (7.5%); some had *abnormal nerve conduction velocity* (25%) and 15% had involvement of multiple neural pathways (7[CR]). Subclinical involvement of the auditory pathway was statistically associated with a higher mean daily deferoxamine dose and a longer duration of treatment. Abnormalities of the somatosensory pathways were related to old age, a long duration of deferoxamine use, and low serum copper concentrations. Multiple neural pathway involvement was related to the duration of treatment. However, deferoxamine is only partly responsible for the subclinical abnormalities of neural pathways often found in β-thalassemia major patients.

Hematological Deferoxamine increased erythroid precursors proliferation in the bone-marrow of anemic patients with chronic renal insufficiency (8[CR]). The findings in this study also suggested a synergistic effect with recombinant human erythropoietin.

℞ *Bone dysplasia with deferoxamine*

Both short stature and a short trunk are often encountered in patients with thalassemia. In a multicenter study in 476 patients 40% had a short trunk, 18% short stature, in 14% a disproportion between the upper and lower body segments (9[CR]). Spinal growth deficit starts early in infancy and is progressive. Deferoxamine-induced bone dysplasia has been identified as a contributing factor, in addition to thalassemia, hypogonadism, and siderosis. In addition to a short trunk, platyspondylosis and signs of bone dysplasia are characteristic features of bone lesions due to deferoxamine (9[CR]). The same group studied three children with β-thalassemia (one girl aged 7 and two boys aged 6 and 12) (10[CR]). The ages of first exposure to deferoxamine were 2.5, 2, and 1.5 years and the mean daily doses were 48, 49, and 55 mg/kg/day respectively (route not stated). All three had short stature, a short trunk, and reduced growth velocity. One had protrusion of the sternum, another had genu valgum. Radiographs of the spine and long bones showed various degrees of osteopenia, platyspondylosis, cupped metaphysis of the distal femur, and pseudocystic cavities with sclerotic borders at distal and proximal metaphyses of the tibia. A reduction in the dosage of deferoxamine was followed by improvement in the bone lesions and growth velocity but not height. The authors concluded that in all children receiving deferoxamine regular radiological and growth evaluation is needed, in order to limit bone dysplasia and short stature.

Another patient presented with pain and swelling at the anterior ends of the eighth and ninth ribs (11[CR]). This patient had been treated with subcutaneous deferoxamine since the age of 3 years in doses from 37 to 66 mg/kg/day, for 6 days a week. Radiologically there were rickets-like 'rosary' lesions of the costochondral junctions of the ribs. The pain disappeared within a few days after withdrawal of deferoxamine and reappeared after readministration. The mechanism underlying rickets-like changes due to deferoxamine is not known.

In a long-term evaluation of 29 patients with transfusion-dependent thalassemia major there were deferoxamine-induced skeletal changes in 15 patients: metaphyseal and spinal changes in five and spinal changes alone in 10 (12[CR]). After reduction in the dosage of deferoxamine, the metaphyseal changes regressed in two but progressed in three, whereas the spinal changes were unchanged or progressed. Two patients required surgical intervention for marked valgus knees. Of a further 21 patients with growth retardation and skeletal dysplasia, secondary to deferoxamine, four patients underwent surgery to correct genu valgum (13[Cr]). Bone histology showed abnormal chondrocytes, alteration of staining pattern of cartilage, irregular columnar cartilage, and lacunae in the cartilaginous tissue. Bone microfractures were sometimes present. Bone microstructure showed varying degrees of impaired mineralization and the hardness of bone tissue was reduced. Bone apatite was quantitatively reduced.

The mechanism underlying the effect of deferoxamine on bone formation has not been identified. In one study in 21 thalassemic patients with growth retardation and skeletal dysplasia secondary to deferoxamine, there were reduced concentrations of growth hormone in 72% of patients with bone dysplasia, compared with 41% of patients without (14[C]). Four patients with growth hormone deficiency were treated with human recombinant growth hormone. Growth velocity doubled in two patients and one patient had a partial response; the fourth patient did not respond. There was a fall in growth velocity after 1 year of treatment with growth hormone in the partial responder and in one of the responders. The following strategy may be helpful in preventing bone dysplasia during treatment with deferoxamine (12, 13):

- *Chelation therapy should be started after the age of 3 years and when iron accumulation has become established.*
- *The dosage of deferoxamine should be established on the basis of iron balance and dose response curves.*
- *Deferoxamine dosages above 50 mg/kg/day subcutaneously should be avoided.*
- *The deferoxamine dosage should be reduced if serum ferritin values are consistently below 1500–1000 ng/ml, or if the patient has reduced growth velocity.*
- *It is important to detect bone changes as early as possible, since a timely reduction in deferoxamine dosage or a switch to deferiprone may prevent serious skeletal injury.*

Risk factors In previous studies a possible relation was suggested between toxicity and the ratio of metabolite B of deferoxamine to unmetabolized deferoxamine (SEDA-18, 250). A further study has shown that there is a relation between regular deferoxamine treatment in respect to the degree of iron overload, as defined by the therapeutic index, i.e. the daily dose of deferoxamine in mg/kg/day divided by the serum ferritin concentration in ng/ml (SED-13, 621), and the ratio of metabolite B to total deferoxamine (deferoxamine plus ferrioxamine) in the plasma or urine (15[CR]). This is consistent with the hypothesis that metabolite B of deferoxamine, which is a product of the intercellular metabolism of iron-free but not iron-bound deferoxamine, inversely reflects the availability of iron in the plasma compartment. In patients who receive a high amount of chelation (measured as mean daily dose of deferoxamine in mg/kg), in relation to iron stores (as reflected by serum ferritin in μg/l), the proportion of iron-free deferoxamine that is available for metabolism is greater. Therefore, the proportion of metabolite B is higher in the urine or blood of patients who are relatively well chelated. These findings suggest that the ratio of metabolite B/ferrioxamine, expressed either as plasma AUC or urine concentration, reflects the availability of chelatable iron, and hence the risk from excess deferoxamine administration at the time the measurement is taken, but that there is unlikely to be an inherent qualitative difference in deferoxamine metabolism in at-risk patients. Further study is needed to determine whether this is of value in identifying patients with increased risk of adverse effects prospectively.

Dimercaptopropane sulfonic acid

(SED-13, 625; SEDA-20, 222; SEDA-21, 250)

In a study in the UK single oral doses of dimercaptosuccinic acid or dimercaptopropane sulfonic acid in different combinations, with or without the other chelating drugs, acetylcysteine and potassium citrate were given to 191 patients considered to have mercury toxicity from amalgam dental fillings (16[cr]). After a single administration about 5% of patients complained of *mild gastrointestinal discomfort, fatigue, mental fuzziness, headache,* and *diuresis.* These usually cleared within 6 hours of the dose and were considered to be due to heavy metal mobilization. There were no cases of hypersensitivity.

Edetic acid salts *(SED-13, 626; SEDA-20, 222; SEDA-21, 250; SEDA-22, 255)*

Respiratory Additives to drug for inhalation, such as disodium edetate or benzalkonium chloride, can cause *bronchoconstriction* (17[CR]). This may lead to reduced therapeutic effectiveness of bronchodilating drugs, for example salbutamol or ipratropium. Some products do and others don't contain these additives and, since generic prescribing is now common practice around the world, unexpected reduction in response to a bronchodilating drug may be the result of a casual change of product.

Skin and appendages Disodium edetate can cause *contact dermatitis*, for instance when used in a local anesthetic (18[CR]).

Interference with diagnostic tests A case report from Germany has underlined the clinical importance of early recognition of edetate-induced *pseudothrombocytopenia* (SEDA-21, 250; 19[CR]). In this case artefactual thrombocytopenia led to a bone-marrow puncture and treatment with high doses of corticosteroids, with severe Cushing's syndrome as a result. In such patients concomitant bleeding disorders (without true thrombocytopenia), for example menorrhagia while having an intrauterine device, may add to the confusion.

Penicillamine *(SED-13, 605; SEDA-20, 219; SEDA-21, 251; SEDA-22, 256)*

In a small trial penicillamine together with metacycline was not effective in secondary progressive multiple sclerosis (20[cr]). In an outpatient study in New Zealand, the changing patterns were studied in the use of 'slow-acting' antirheumatic drugs (21[CR]). There were increases in the use of methotrexate and of drugs in combination, whereas there was a marked reduction in the use of auranofin. Penicillamine had the highest 'average toxicity' score. However, despite the increased popularity of sulfasalazine and immunosuppressive drugs, drugs such as penicillamine continue to be used world wide. In a long-term follow-up study, the proportion of patients who continued to take their first DMARD or who were in remission at 5 years was 53% for penicillamine, compared with 34% for aurothiomalate, 31% for auranofin, and 30% for hydroxychloroquine (22[CR]). Of the 179 patients who used penicillamine, 36 discontinued the drug because of adverse effects (37 adverse effects, see Table 1). In an open randomized follow-up study of patients with rheumatoid arthritis, 98 were allocated to penicillamine (median daily dose 750 mg, range 375–1000 mg) and 102 to sulfasalazine (23[CR]). Over follow-up for 12 years as many as 95 patients (48%) died, four from peptic ulcer disease complications, illustrating the prevalence of premature mortality in patients with rheumatoid arthritis. Only four of the 98 patients continued to take penicillamine. Major reasons for discontinuation of penicillamine, other than death, were adverse effects (47 patients) and lack or loss of effect (36) (see Table 1). In neither study was any of the deaths thought to have been related to penicillamine. The picture given in Table 1 illustrates the remarkable diversity and seriousness of the adverse reactions pattern of penicillamine.

In a nested case control study in Mexican patients with rheumatoid arthritis encompassing 1274 patient years, the risk factors were determined for acquiring infectious diseases (24[CR]). In addition to the cumulative doses of methotrexate and the duration of corticosteroids use, the mean daily dose of penicillamine was a risk factor. In one patient the infection was secondary to *neutropenia.* Tests for a possible immunoglobulin deficiency were not performed.

Table 1. Adverse effects leading to the discontinuation of penicillamine in two recent studies

Reference	(23[C])	(22[C])
Total number of patients	98	179
Patients with adverse effects	47 (48%)	37 (20%)
Proteinuria	17	8
Rash, pruritus, or mouth ulcers		16
Nausea/vomiting	7	2
Rash	9	
Abdominal pain/dyspepsia	2	4
Thrombocytopenia	4	1
Leukopenia	2	2
Mouth ulcers	4	
Malaise	1	1
Exacerbation of joint pains		1
Myasthenia gravis		
Pemphigus		1
Systemic lupus erythematosus	1	

Respiratory See under Urinary system for *alveolar hemorrhage* and Skin and appendages for *dyspnea.*

Liver *Liver damage* has been attributed to penicillamine (25[cr]).

A 30-year-old Japanese man had taken sodium aurothiomalate for 3 years for polyarthritis. Lack of effectiveness led to the introduction of penicillamine, 200 mg/day. After 10 days he became febrile and two days later jaundiced. A lymphocyte stimulation test against penicillamine was positive, suggesting a type IV hypersensitivity. Later on he had a good response to tiopronin, without further adverse reactions.

Urinary system In a comprehensive study of 158 Japanese patients with rheumatoid arthritis, there was an obvious relation between exposure to disease modifying antirheumatic drugs (DMARDs) in 40 out of 49 patients with membranous nephropathy (26[CR]). In this study penicillamine (15%), bucillamine (67%), and gold compounds (17%) clearly predominated.

A patient with *nephrotic syndrome* that developed soon after the start of treatment with penicillamine has been described in detail (27[cR]).

A 12-year-old boy with a history of a generalized pruritic rash after penicillin took penicillamine up to 500 mg/day for Wilson's disease. He had a rash after using penicillamine for 1 week. The penicillamine was stopped for 3 days. He developed nephrotic syndrome 2 weeks after restarting penicillamine. On electron microscopy there was the typical picture of minimal change disease with extensive foot process effacement.

In rare cases penicillamine can cause *extracapillary glomerulonephritis* with more extensive and serious glomerular injury leading to progressive and persistent renal failure. One such patient has been described with a review of 26 similar published cases (28[cR]).

A 51-year-old woman, who used penicillamine, maximum dose 600 mg/day, for systemic sclerosis, developed microscopic hematuria after 11 months. The penicillamine was withdrawn. Three months later she had progressive renal insufficiency. A biopsy showed extracapillary glomerulonephritis, with central fibrinoid necrosis and segmentary mesangial proliferation, and marked tubulointerstitial lesions. After treatment with corticosteroids and cyclophosphamide and 12 plasma exchanges her renal function improved slightly.

In half of the 26 patients reported renal injury was associated with alveolar hemorrhage (28[cR]). In eight patients plasma exchange treatment was performed. Seven patients died, including four with alveolar hemorrhage; 12 ended up with more or less severe chronic renal insufficiency. Only seven patients regained normal renal function; five of these had had plasma exchange.

Acute renal insufficiency together with diffuse alveolar hemorrhage and bilateral pulmonary infiltrates was suspected to have been caused by penicillamine (500 mg/day for 6 months) in a 34-year-old white woman, who took penicillamine for progressive systemic sclerosis (29[cR]). Because of disseminated intravascular coagulation a biopsy was not made and the role of penicillamine remained uncertain.

Hemolytic-uremic syndrome has been described in a patient with paradoxical rapid progression of systemic sclerosis during the use of penicillamine (30[Cr]).

A 58-year-old man with a complex history of Hashimoto's thyroiditis and mixed cellularity Hodgkin's disease in complete remission developed systemic sclerosis involving the skin and the lungs but not the kidneys. He was given penicillamine 250 mg/day and prednisone 60 mg/day. After a few weeks there was rapidly progressive skin thickening, spreading from the hands to the trunk. However, his treatment was not altered, and 4 months later he developed a hemolytic uremic syndrome with microangiopathic hemolytic changes, thrombocytopenia, and acute renal insufficiency, with proteinuria, hematuria, and granular casts in the urine. The renal insufficiency persisted and he died with fulminant sepsis.

Skin and appendages Another case of the peculiar *pseudo-pseudoxanthoma elasticum* caused by the use of high doses of penicillamine has been described (31[CR]).

A 47-year-old man had been using penicillamine 1.5 mg/day for 18 years for Wilson's disease. He developed pseudo-pseudoxanthoma combined with dysphagia and dyspnea. Biopsy specimens showed systemic involvement of elastic fibers, including skin, lung, esophageal muscle, gum, and pharyngeal and cervical connective tissue. All biopsies showed abnormal elastic fibers, consisting of a central core of uneven thickness with many lateral arborizations. There were branches at right angles to the main fibers, with perpendicular lateral arborizations off these, producing a stag-horn or fractal appearance. On the other hand, the adjacent collagen fibers were normal in structure.

Penicillamine can cause a variety of bullous eruptions, such as *pemphigus foliaceus, pemphigus vulgaris,* and rarely *bullous pemphigoid.* One such case, in which the diagnosis was histologically and immunologically ascertained, has been described (32[CR]).

A 64-year-old woman, who had used penicillamine 500 mg/day for 3 years for rheumatoid arthritis, developed a bullous skin eruption affecting her neck and limbs. After treatment with prednisolone (dose not specified) she improved, but relapsed when the dose was reduced below 10 mg. Eleven months after the onset of blistering, penicillamine was discontinued and within 2 months the prednisolone was also stopped, with no recurrence of the eruption during 12 months follow-up. Direct immunofluorescence was positive for immunoglobulin G and complement component C3, and indirect immunofluorescence was positive on the roof of the NaCl split skin preparation.

A consultation of the database of the Committee on Safety of Medicines in London showed that 41 cases of bullous pemphigoid have been reported in suspected connection with penicillamine, suggesting that this adverse reaction is less rare that the published literature suggests.

Musculoskeletal The diagnostic pitfalls of penicillamine-induced *polymyositis* have been reviewed in the light of a case report (33[cR]). In this patient, postural changes were at first mistaken for possible ankylosing spondylitis. Muscular weakness and dysphagia can be mistaken for myasthenia, whereas increased 'liver enzymes' may suggest a liver reaction.

Second-generation effects The maternal use of penicillamine has in rare cases been complicated with *congenital cutis hyperelastica* (SED-13, 616). A baby with a bilateral *cleft lip* with total cleft palate was born at 41 weeks to a 22-year-old mother who had taken penicillamine (dosage not specified) throughout an uncomplicated pregnancy for Wilson's disease (34[cR]). The child did not have a lax skin. This case was found as part of a case-control study of 24 696 mothers of malformed infants. It was the only case of penicillamine exposure in the entire series. However, cleft lip has not previously been observed in association with maternal use of penicillamine, and there is little reason for suspecting the drug.

Tiopronin *(SED-13, 618)*

In a patient with a prior hypersensitivity reaction to penicillamine there was no cross-hypersensitivity to tiopronin (25[cr]).

In a comparison of tiopronin and penicillamine in the treatment of cystinuria in 15 children, *nephrotic syndrome* developed in one of the patients taking tiopronin; no further details were given (35[cr]).

REFERENCES

1. Elihu N, Anandasbapathy S, Frishman WH. Chelation therapy in cardiovascular disease: ethylenediaminetetraacetic acid, deferoxamine, and dexrazoxane. J Clin Pharmacol 1998;38:101–5.
2. Hoffbrand AV, Al-Refaie F, Davis B, Siritanakatkul N, Jackson BFA, Cochrane J, Prescott E, Wonke B. Long-term trial of deferiprone in 51 transfusion-dependent iron overloaded patients. Blood 1998;91:295–300.
3. Olivieri NF, Brittenham GM, McLaren CE, Templeton DM, Cameron RG, McClelland RA, Burt AD, Fleming KA. Long-term safety and effectiveness of iron-chelation therapy with deferiprone for thalassemia major. New Engl J Med 1998;339:417–23.
4. Cohen A, Galanello R, Piga A, Vullo C, Tricta F. A multi-center safety trial of the oral iron chelator deferiprone. Ann NY Acad Sci 1998; 850:223–6.
5. Mazza P, Amurri B, Lazzari G, Masi C, Palazzo G, Spartera MA, Guia R, Sebastio AM, Suma V, De Marco S, Semeraro F, Moscogiuri R. Oral iron chelating therapy. A single center interim report on deferiprone (L1) in thalassemia. Haematologica 1998;83:496–501.
6. Rego EM, Neto EB, Simoes BP, Zago MA. Dose-dependent pulmonary syndrome in patients with thalassemia major receiving intravenous deferoxamine. Am J Hematol 1998;58:340–1.
7. Zafeiriou DI, Kousi AA, Tsantali CT, Kontopoulos EE, Augoustidou-Savvopoulou PA, Tsoubaris PD, Athanasiou MA. Neurophysiologic evaluation of long-term desferrioxamine therapy in beta-thalassemia patients. Pediatr Neurol 1998; 18:420–4.
8. Aucella F, Scalzulli P, Musto P, Prencipe M, Valente GL, Vigilante M, Carotenuto M, Stallone C. Synergic effect of desferoxamine (DFO) and recombinant erythropoietin on erythroid precursors proliferation in chronic renal failure. G Ital Nefrol 1998;15:241–7.
9. Caruso-Nicoletti M, De Sanctis V, Capra M, Cardinale G, Cuccia L, Di Gregorio F, Filosa A, Galati MC, Lauriola A, Malizia R, Mangiagli A, Massolo F, Mastrangelo C, Meo A, Messina MF, Ponzi G, Raiola G, Ruggiero L, Tamborino G, Saviano A. Short stature and body proportion in thalassaemia. J Pediatr Endocrinol Metab 1998;11(Suppl 3):811–16.
10. Caruso-Nicoletti M, Di Bella D, Pizzarelli G, Leonardi C, Sciuto C, Coco M, Di Gregorio F. Growth failure and bone lesions due to desferrioxamine in thalassaemic patients. J Pediatr Endocrinol Metab 1998;11(Suppl 3):957–60.
11. Lauriola AL, Tangerini A, Lodi A, Gamberini MR, Testa MR, Orzincolo C, De Sanctis V, Vullo C. Rachitic rosary in a well chelated thalassaemic patient with primary amenorrhea. J Pediatr Endocrinol Metab 1998;11(Suppl 3):979–80.
12. Naselli A, Vignolo M, Di Battista E, Garzia P, Forni GL, Traverso T, Aicardi G. Long term follow-up of skeletal dysplasia in thalassaemia major. J Pediatr Endocrinol Metab 1998;11(Suppl 3):817–25.
13. De Sanctis V, Stea S, Savarino L, Scialpi V, Traina GC, Chiarelli GM, Sprocati M, Govoni R, Pezzoli D, Gamberini R, Rigolin F. Growth hormone secretion and bone histomorphometric study in thalassaemic patients with acquired skeletal dys-

plasia secondary to desferrioxamine. J Pediatr Endocrinol Metab 1998;11(Suppl 3):827–33.
14. De Sanctis V, Stea S, Savarino L, Scialpi V, Traina GC, Chiarelli GM, Sprocati M, Govoni R, Pezzoli D, Gamberini R, Rigolin F. Growth hormone secretion and bone histomorphometric study in thalassaemic patients with acquired skeletal dysplasia secondary to desferrioxamine. J Pediatr Endocrinol Metab 1998;11(Suppl 3):827–33.
15. Porter JB, Faherty A, Stallibrass L, Brookman L, Hassan I, Howes C. A trial to investigate the relationship between DFO pharmacokinetics and metabolism and DFO-related toxicity. Ann NY Acad Sci 1998;850:483–7.
16. Hibberd AR, Howard MA, Hunnisett AG. Mercury from dental amalgam fillings: Studies on oral chelating agents for assessing and reducing mercury burdens in humans. J Nutr Environ Med 1998; 8:219–31.
17. Beasley R, Fishwick D, Miles JF, Hendeles L. Preservatives in nebulizer solutions: risks without benefit. Pharmacotherapy 1998;18:130–9.
18. Bhushan M, Beck MH. Allergic contact dermatitis from disodium ethylenediamine tetraacetic acid (EDTA) in a local anaesthetic. Contact Dermatitis 1998;38:183.
19. Germing U, Glagounidis A, Sohngen D, Schneider W. EDTA-induced pseudothrombocytopenia: a case report. Z Allgmed 1998;740:891–4.
20. Dubois B, D'Hooghe MD, De Lepeleire K, Ketelaer P, Opdenakker G, Carton H. Toxicity in a double-blind, placebo-controlled pilot trial with D-penicillamine and metacycline in secondary progressive multiple sclerosis. Mult Scler 1998;4:74–8.
21. Horsfall MWJ, Shaw JP, Highton J, Cranch PJ. Changing patterns in the use of slow acting antirheumatic drugs for the treatment of rheumatoid arthritis. NZ Med J 1998;111067:200–3.
22. Jessop JD, O'Sullivan MM, Lewis PA, Williams LA, Camilleri JP, Plant MJ, Coles EC. A long-term five-year randomized controlled trial of hydroxychloroquine, sodium aurothiomalate, auranofin and penicillamine in the treatment of patients with rheumatoid arthritis. Br J Rheumatol 1998;37:992–1002.
23. Capell HA, Maiden N, Madhok R, Hampson R, Thomson EA. Intention-to-treat analysis of 200 patients with rheumatoid arthritis 12 years after random allocation to either sulfasalazine or penicillamine. J Rheumatol 1998;250:1880–5.
24. Hernandez-Cruz B, Cardiel MH, Villa AR, Alcocer-Varela J. Development, recurrence, and severity of infections in Mexican patients with rheumatoid arthritis. A nested case-control study. J Rheumatol 1998;250:1900–7.
25. Matsukawa Y, Saito N, Nishinarita S, Horie T, Ryu J. Therapeutic effect of tiopronin following D-penicillamine toxicity in a patient with rheumatoid arthritis. Clin Rheumatol 1998;17:73–4.
26. Nakano M, Ueno M, Nishi S, Shimada H, Hasegawa H, Watanabe T, Kuroda T, Sato T, Maruyama Y, Arakawa M. Analysis of renal pathology and drug history in 158 Japanese patients with rheumatoid arthritis. Clin Nephrol 1998;50:154–60.
27. Siafakas CG, Jonas MM, Alexander S, Herrin J, Furuta GT. Early onset of nephrotic syndrome after treatment with D-penicillamine in a patient with Wilson's disease. Am J Gastroenterol 1998;932:2544–6.
28. Marchand-Courville S, Dhib M, Fillastre J-P, Godin M. Extracapillary glomerulonephritis associated with D-penicillamine. Nephrologie 1998; 19:25–32.
29. Phillips D, Phillips B, Mannino D. A case study and national database report of progressive systemic sclerosis and associated conditions. J Women's Health 1998;7:1099–104.
30. Haviv YS, Safadi R. Rapid progression of scleroderma possibly associated with penicillamine therapy. Clin Drug Invest 1998;15:61–3.
31. Coatesworth AP, Darnton SJ, Green RM, Cayton RM, Antonakopoulos GN. A case of systemic pseudo-pseudoxanthoma elasticum with diverse symptomatology caused by long term penicillamine use. J Clin Pathol 1998;51:169–71.
32. Weller R, White MI. Penicillamine in the etiology of bullous pemphigoid. Ann Pharmacother 1998;322:1368.
33. Barrera P, Den Broeder AA, Van den Hoogen FHJ, Van Engelen BGM, Van de Putte LBA. Postural changes, dysphagia, and systemic sclerosis. Ann Rheum Dis 1998;57:331–8.
34. Martinez-Frias ML, Rodriguez-Pinilla E, Bermejo E, Blanco M. Prenatal exposure to penicillamine and oral clefts: case report. Am J Med Genet 1998;76:274–5.
35. Asanuma H, Nakai H, Takeda M, Shishido S, Kawamura T. Clinical study on cystinuria in children: the stone management and the prevention of calculi recurrence. Jpn J Urol 1998;89:758–65.

Pam Magee

24 Antiseptic drugs and disinfectants

ALDEHYDES *(SED-13, 644; SEDA-20, 255; SEDA-21, 254)*

Many disinfecting formulations contain aldehydes: formaldehyde, glyoxal, and glutaraldehyde. They are irritating and sensitizing and cause contact dermatitis in healthcare workers (SEDA-21, 254).

The incidence of *allergy* to aldehydes has been examined in 280 healthcare workers suffering from skin lesions (1^C). Allergy was diagnosed in 64 (23%). The majority (86%) were sensitive to only one aldehyde. Formaldehyde caused allergy slightly more often (14%) than glutaraldehyde (12%). Only five (1.9%) were sensitive to glyoxal. This hierarchy of sensitivity was also confirmed in animal testing.

BISBIGUANIDES

Chlorhexidine *(SED-13, 651; SEDA-20, 225; SEDA-21, 254; SEDA-22, 262)*

Special senses Chlorhexidine disinfectant (Hibitane) was accidentally used to irrigate the eyes of four patients; despite immediate treatment, *corneal burns* occurred in all (2^c). Chlorhexidine has also been accidentally irrigated into the anterior chamber of the eye, instead of balanced salt solution, during cataract surgery (3^c). Later in the operation, a decrease in corneal clarity was noted and an epithelial abrasion had to be performed. The inadvertent use of chlorhexidine in this patient resulted in reduced endothelial function and loss of corneal clarity.

Musculoskeletal Chlorhexidine is not normally used in arthroscopy, but it is a common irrigating fluid for surgical wounds. In three of five patients with pain, swelling, crepitus, and loss of range of movement following arthroscopy of the knee, accidental irrigation with 1% aqueous chlorhexidine was proven. Histological examination showed *partial necrosis of the cartilage*, with slight non-specific inflammation and fibrosis of synovial specimens (4^c). This shows that particular care is needed in checking irrigation fluids.

Immunological and hypersensitivity reactions Chlorhexidine is a widely used disinfectant, and anaphylaxis associated with its use is rare, although it continues to be reported with all types of use.

When chlorhexidine was used as a skin disinfectant in a 53-year-old man undergoing lung resection for adenocarcinoma, *anaphylaxis* was complicated by coronary artery spasm (5^c). He had two anaphylactic reactions accompanied by severe myocardial ischemia. Immunological testing indicated chlorhexidine as the causative substance.

Following disinfection of a drain insertion site with chlorhexidine digluconate 2% solution, a 43-year-old man had severe anaphylaxis, manifest as dyspnea, shock, and ST segment elevation (6^c). In the past he had had two episodes of contact dermatitis with chlorhexidine antiseptics.

Anaphylaxis following cystoscopy or urinary catheterization has been reported repeatedly (SEDA-18, 255; SEDA-19, 235; SEDA-20, 225), but is considered rare. In a further report of generalized urticaria after skin cleansing with and urethral instillation of chlorhexidine-containing products the authors suggest that there is under-reporting of such reactions and that alternative antiseptics should be considered in urological and gynecological procedures (7^c).

Side Effects of Drugs, Annual 23
J.K. Aronson, ed.

The use of chlorhexidine-impregnated central venous catheters is increasing. Anaphylaxis has occurred (SEDA-22, 262) with insertion of these catheters and three more cases have been reported (8[c], 9[c]). The FDA has issued a public health notice to inform health-care professionals about the potential for serious hypersensitivity reactions to medical devices impregnated with chlorhexidine. The Agency is also seeking information and reports to better evaluate the potential health hazard these products might pose, and to decide on what action, if any, should be taken. Devices that incorporate chlorhexidine that the FDA has cleared for marketing include intravenous catheters, topical antimicrobial skin dressings, and implanted antimicrobial surgical mesh.

Anaphylactoid and other reactions have been reported with chlorhexidine used topically or intraurethrally, as a lubricant on urinary catheters, and with chlorhexidine-impregnated catheters. The notice describes non-US reports of systemic reactions to chlorhexidine-impregnated gels or lubricants used during urological procedures and similarly impregnated central venous catheters. It also describes other types of reactions that have been reported in the US, including localized reactions to impregnated patches in neonates and occupational asthma in nurses exposed to chlorhexidine and alcohol aerosols (10[r]).

Polyhexanide

Polyhexanide is a polymerized form of chlorhexidine. Severe anaphylaxis occurred in a 18-year-old woman and a 15-year-old man when this new disinfectant was used to clean surgical wounds (11[c]). Immediate-type hypersensitivity to polyhexanide was suggested by positive skin prick tests. Both patients had previously been exposed to chlorhexidine, but skin tests with chlorhexidine remained negative.

ETHYLENE OXIDE *(SED-13, 649; SEDA-21, 254)*

Ethylene oxide is an alkylating agent, a directly-acting mutagen and carcinogen. Exposure to ethylene oxide has been reported predominantly in workers in sterilization units.

Monitoring of the concentration of ethylene oxide in workplace air is commonly used for exposure control. A standard of 1 ppm for workplace air is currently accepted as a threshold limit (SEDA-21, 254).

In 12 workers who were occupationally exposed to ethylene oxide during the sterilization of medical equipment, concentrations of 0.2–8.5 ppm were detected (12[C]). This study also confirmed the relation between the ethylene oxide concentration in ambient air and the amount of *N*-2-hydroxyethylvaline in human globin, which has been used as a biological marker of carcinogenicity.

ORGANIC MERCURY COMPOUNDS *(SED-13, 598; SEDA-21, 255; SEDA-22, 263)*

Thiomersal

Thiomersal, an organic mercurial, is widely used as a preservative in vaccines, in cutaneous test solutions, and in contact lens cleaners and creams.

Delayed *contact allergy* was diagnosed in a 26-year-old man who presented with a 2-year history of repeated episodes of dermatitis, swelling of the eyelids, and burning eyes (13[c]). The original diagnosis was of occupational allergy; patch tests confirmed that the conjunctivitis was due to thiomersal-containing eye drops, which had been used to treat the condition.

PHENOLIC COMPOUNDS *(SED-13, 600; SEDA-21, 255; SEDA-22, 264)*

Phenol was introduced into medicine as an antiseptic, but its use was limited by severe adverse effects. Current medical uses include cosmetic face peeling, nerve injections, and topical anesthesia. It is also an ingredient of various topical formulations, and is used as an environmental disinfectant. Systemic adverse effects appear after both oral and dermal exposure and include *central nervous stimulation followed by depression, seizures, coma, tachycardia, hypotension, dysrhythmias, pulmonary edema, metabolic acidosis*, and *hepatic* and *renal injury.* Phenol is so rapidly absorbed through the skin that severe systemic effects and even death can result within minutes to hours.

Ninety percent phenol spilled over the left sole and shoe of a 47-year-old tanker driver. He neither removed his soaked shoe nor attempted to decontaminate himself. He continued driving for 4.5 hours, after which he had vertigo and faintness. Fire fighters removed him from the vehicle, took off his shoes and clothes, and thoroughly washed his leg with copious amount of water. On admission to hospital he was alert but confused, his heart rate was 146/min, blood pressure 160/100 mmHg, and there was tense swelling and blue black discoloration of his left foot, ankle, and distal part of the leg (3% total body surface area), with hypalgesia and hypesthesia over the affected area. His leg was irrigated with large amounts of water, longitudinal incisions of his left foot were performed, and he was transferred to the intensive care unit. Shortly afterward, rapid atrial fibrillation, ventricular extra beats, reduced blood pressure (90/60 mmHg), and fever of 38.3°C developed. He was treated with intravenous crystalloids, verapamil, dopamine, and phenylephrine. All systemic symptoms resolved in 24 hours. Blood and urine cultures were negative. Over the next 3 weeks he was treated with 0.25% troclosene dressings and 1% microionized silver sulfadiazine until the swelling resolved and the wound had healed. On discharge from hospital and at a 4-month follow-up only blue-black discoloration was noted.

Although it is generally assumed that chemicals can easily be washed off the skin, in this case, despite copious amounts of irrigation with large volumes of water the patient suffered severe systemic effects (14^{c}).

REFERENCES

1. Kiec-Swierczynska M, Krecisz B, Krysiak B, Kuchowicz E, Rydzynski K. Occupational allergy to aldehydes in healthcare workers. Clinical observations, experiments. Int J Occup Med Environ Health 1998;11:349–58.
2. Nakamura Y, Inatomi T, Nishida K, Sotozono C, Kinoshita S. Four cases of chemical corneal burns by misuse of disinfectant. Jpn J Clin Ophthalmol 1998;52:786–8.
3. Klebe S, Anders N, Wollensak J. Inadvertant use of chlorhexidine as intraocular irrigation solution. J Cataract Refractive Surg 1998;24:729–30.
4. Douw CM, Bulstra SK, Vandenbroucke J, Geesink RGT, Vermeulen A. Clinical and pathological changes in the knee after accidental chlorhexidine irrigation during arthroscopy. J Bone Jt Surg Ser B 1998;80:437–40.
5. Conraads VMA, Jorens PG, Ebo DG, Claeys MJ, Bosmans JM, Vrints CJ. Coronary artery spasm complicating anaphylaxis secondary to skin disinfectant. Chest 1998;113:1417–19.
6. Ebo DG, Stevens WJ, Bridts CH, Matthieu L. Contact allergic dermatitis and life-threatening anaphylaxis to chlorhexidine. J Allergy Clin Immunol 1998;101:128–9.
7. Stables GI, Turner WH, Prescott S, Wilkinson SM. Generalised urticaria after skin cleansing and urethral instillation with chlorhexidine-containing products. Br J Urol 1998;82:756–7.
8. Nikaido S, Tanaka M, Yamoto M, Minami T, Akatsuka M, Mori H. Anaphylactoid shock caused by chlorhexidine gluconate. Jpn J Anesthesiol 1998; 47:330–4.
9. Terazawa E, Shimonaka H, Nagase K, Masue T, Dohi S. Severe anaphylactic reaction due to a chlorhexidine-impregnated central venous catheter. Anesthesiology 1998;89:1296–8.
10. Nightingale SL. Hypersensitivity to chlorhexidine-impregnated medical devices. J Am Med Assoc 1998;279:1684.
11. Olivieri J, Eigenmann PA, Hauser C. Severe anaphylaxis to a new disinfectant: polyhexanide, a chlorhexidine polymer. Schweiz Med Wochenschr 1998;128:1508–11.
12. Angerer J, Bader M, Kramer A. Ambient and biochemical effect monitoring of workers exposed to ethylene oxide. Int Arch Occup Environ Health 1998;71:14–18.
13. Iliev D, Wuthrich B. Conjunctivitis to thiomersal mistaken as hay fever. Allergy Eur J Allergy Clin Immunol 1998;53:333–4.
14. Bentur Y, Shoshan O, Tabak A, Bin-Nan A, Raman Y, Ulman Y, Berger Y, Nochlieli T, Pelad YJ. Prolonged elimination half life of phenol after dermal exposure. J Toxicol Clin Toxicol 1998; 36:707–11.

T. Midtvedt

25 Penicillins, cephalosporins, other β-lactam antibiotics, and tetracyclines

R

Antibiotic resistance—a change of strategy?

The 20th century can be characterized as the century of antibiotics. At the end of the 19th century, microbe hunters like Koch and Pasteur had named the task for the century to come: fight the germs. The development of chemotherapeutics and antibiotics that took place during the 20th century gave us excellent weapons and created dreams of therapia sterilans magna—a single-dose totally sterilizing elixir that would cause no harm to the host.

Sad to say, that dream seems still to be around. In an Editorial in the July Newsletter of the International Society of Chemotherapy it was claimed that 'the first decade of the new century is likely to be spent by clinical researchers on the evaluation and introduction of some very welcome and exciting new agents, which will continue the success of antibiotics and chemotherapy' (1[R]).

Based on our experiences during the 20th century, it has to be stressed that statements like this are no more than attempts to pull the wool over our eyes. It is easy to forecast that the new agents will very soon meet resistance. Looking back we should all admit that our strategy has been wrong—totally wrong. The 'old' and well-known microorganisms are still here, more active than ever. Tuberculosis and malaria are the two most glaring and widespread examples of our shortcomings in the proper use of antimicrobials, and several common bacterial pathogens can be added to the list. Staphylococcus aureus remains the most common pathogen in hospital-acquired infections, and multiresistance is in many places the rule rather than the exception. Vibrio cholerae continues to cause outbreaks of cholera, and Salmonella and Shigella are highly prevalent and with increasing antibiotic resistance.

Instead of dreaming of new agents capable of fighting the germs, we should try a shift in paradigm and start to look on the microbes not as enemies but as friends. And certainly they may become enemies if we treat them in an unfriendly way. Allowing myself to be personal and stating that I have worked, as a medical ecologist, with germ-free animals for more than 35 years, I have been convinced that microbes are man's best friends. From cradle to grave they follow every one of us, in a number that exceeds the number of our own cells by at least 2 log units. The normal flora on our skin and mucous membranes consists of several hundreds of bacterial strains that belong to a nearly equal number of species, together with an unknown number of other microbial species, including viruses, yeasts, and protozoans. Most of the microbes are potential pathogens, but they seldom express their pathogenicity. In fact, our own indigenous flora represent our best colonization resistance against exogenous pathogens.

Now the time has come to learn more about the basic factors involved in this resistance and the continuous cross-talk that exists on a cell-to-cell level between ourselves and our flora (2[R]). By unravelling the physiological cross-talk we should be able to create drugs that are far more specific in action than those we are currently using or are planning to use. Our new agents should be targeted at very specific goals. Today we are often shooting sparrows with guns, as we do when we use fluoroquinolones against ordinary urinary tract infections. The therapeutic outcome might be good, but we are affecting the flora in the whole gastro-

Side Effects of Drugs, Annual 23
J.K. Aronson, ed.

enterological tract as well as a down-stream area of unknown size outside the patient. Words such as 'narrow-spectrum' and 'small eco-shadow' (SEDA-19, 237) should be words of honor again. We should increase our efforts to unmask the specificity and mode of action of the antimicrobial peptides that we are producing ourselves, such as magainins, defencins, and cecropins ('autobiotics').

Steadily increasing insights into the intricate balance between types of mediators, including autobiotics and lymphokines, are also increasing the possibilities of being far more specific in our therapy. One thing I know for sure, we can not continue with our present strategy. The steadily increasing number of resistant bacterial strains has too long been a warning signal written on the wall (SEDA-22, 265).

R Antibiotics—immunological and allergic reactions

So-called hypersensitivity reactions are the most frequent adverse effects involving the immune system after exposure to therapeutic drugs or other xenobiotics. The β-lactam antibiotics are nearly always at the top of lists that record hypersensitivity reactions in postmarketing surveillance studies of drugs. It is therefore beyond doubt that hypersensitivity reactions to xenobiotics, including β-lactams, pose a significant threat to health. However, it is a sad fact that relevant predictive animals models have not been considered a key priority. One reason might be that allergic reactions, in contrast to toxic effects, have long been claimed to be unpredictable in animals. Noteworthy is a recent attempt to 'describe the current status of animal models predictive of hypersensitivity' (3[R]).

Immuno-allergy versus pseudo-allergy *The authors stated that since information about the mechanism(s) underlying a reaction might not always be known, the general term 'hypersensitivity' includes both possibly immunoallergic and pseudo-allergic reactions. The term 'immuno-allergy' should be used when highly specific mechanisms involving immunological memory and recognition are involved. The term 'pseudo-allergy' describes reactions that mimic immuno-allergy, but in which a specific immune mediated mechanism is not involved.*

Immuno-allergy *For many years, immunoallergy has been classified into four types:*

- *type I: immediate hypersensitivity or anaphylaxis;*
- *type II: antibody-mediated;*
- *type III: immune complex-mediated;*
- *type IV: delayed hypersensitivity.*

Although still often referred to, this classification is often too rigid, as it excludes simultaneous involvement of two or more mechanisms.

Pseudo-allergy *Pseudo-allergy clinically often mimics immuno-allergic reactions, although the mediators are completely different. Some major mediators were reviewed a few years ago (4[R]). The role of newer putative mechanisms, involving cytokines, kinins, and other host-derived substances, remains to be fully ascertained. Most important is the fact that that currently 'no standardized and validated animal models are available to predict pseudo-allergic reactions' (3[R]).*

Animal models *Guinea-pigs have been used for years in studies of systemic anaphylaxis. However, variations in predictability and sensitivity limit their value (5[R], 6[R]). Passive cutaneous anaphylaxis is another guinea-pig model, but it not seem to be more sensitive than systemic anaphylaxis (5[R]). Respiratory sensitization, resulting in IgE-mediated immediate hypersensitivity has been investigated in mice and guinea-pigs (7[R], 8[R]). Most often highly reactive chemicals have been used, and the models seem to be of limited value in testing antimicrobials.*

Contact sensitizers have been studied in guinea-pigs and mice, and it has been stated that 'these models can reasonably identify the majority of human contact sensitizers' (3[R]).

The best approach to induce a specific immune response against substances of low molecular weights is the use of models using hapten-carrier conjugates. These models are of value in assessing the potential for cross-reactivity between closely related compounds, such as β-lactam antibiotics (9[R]). Side-chain specific allergic reactions to β-lactams are a steadily increasing problem (SEDA-21, 260;

10[R], 11[R], 12[C]), a topic that should be more carefully evaluated.

It is obvious that in the near future the development of new animal models, e.g. transgenic and knock-out mice, will create new possibilities in predicting the sensitizing potential of new antimicrobials. The sad fact that hypersensitivity reactions are among the most commonly occurring adverse effects when antibiotics are used underlines the importance of their final conclusion that 'research efforts in academia and the industry are urgently needed' (3[R]).

PENICILLINS *(SEDA-20, 239; SEDA-21, 259; SEDA-22, 266)*

℞ *Acute desensitization*

Acute drug desensitization is commonly described as the process by which a drug-allergic individual is converted from a highly sensitive state to a state in which the drug is tolerated. The procedure involves cautious administration of incremental doses of the drug over a short period of time (hours to a few days). In the past it has mainly been considered to be of value in patients in whom IgE antibodies to a particular drug are known or assumed to exist and no alternative treatment agent is available. In clinical practice, most of the desensitization protocols have involved penicillins (13[R]). However, the principle has been applied successfully to other agents as well (14[R], 15[R]), including other antibiotics, insulin, chemotherapeutic agents, vaccines, heterologous sera, and other proteins.

Mechanism(s) responsible for acute desensitization *It has been stated (13[R]) that 'in studies of patients who were shown to have penicillin-specific IgE antibodies and who underwent successful penicillin desensitization, the data suggest that antigen-specific, mast cell desensitization is responsible for the tolerant state. Mediator depletion appears to play no role'. Additionally, the clinical observation that wheal-and-flare skin responses to penicillin often become negative with successful desensitization, while IgE responses to other antigens remain unchanged, also supports an involvement of an antigen-specific mechanism. Furthermore, both clinical reactivity and skin-test reactivity return within a few days unless a tolerant state is maintained by continued drug administration. The author stressed that these findings show 'that the desensitized state is dependent upon the continuous presence of antigen and that clinical sensitivity returns rapidly in the absence of antigen' (13[R]).*

However, the underlying mechanism(s) responsible for the antigen-specific desensitized state still remain(s) unclear. It has been hypothesized that IgE receptor aggregation may generate counter-regulatory forces that, instead of causing cell activation, actually extinguish activating signals (14[R]). The key point is that during desensitization, the drug is introduced very slowly, and the drug concentration rises gradually. The slow rate of a (possible) receptor aggregation caused by the gradual increase in drug concentration, along with suppression of cellular activation signals, may lead to antigen-specific desensitization and clinical tolerance. It has also been long thought that during desensitization, univalent drug-hapten protein conjugates are formed and may act by inhibiting the cross-linking of drug-specific IgE molecules on mast cells. It is slightly surprising that this prospect has not come into routine therapy.

Desensitization procedure *The author has given good advice about protocols to be used for desensitization (13[R]). He has underlined the importance of reminding the patient as well as health personnel that the patient has not been cured, but that his anaphylactic sensitivity will return after the drug is withdrawn. A patient who has an anaphylactic reaction to penicillin will have one at his next exposure to penicillin.*

Pancreas The list of agents associated with pancreatitis is long and diverse and is growing. Drugs such as corticosteroids, estrogens, diuretics, and chemotherapeutic agents have all been implicated. In addition, various antibiotics have been implicated, including tetracyclines, rifampicin, and isoniazid (16[R]). Recently a case of pancreatitis after administration of ampicillin has been reported (17[c]). Now a case of pancreatitis in a child due to penicillin has been reported (18[c]).

A 7-year-old boy developed epigastric pain, nausea, and vomiting, starting 10 days after a course of oral penicillin (dose and derivative not stated). He had a serum amylase activity of 1260 u/l and lipase of 528 u/l; electrolytes and liver function tests were within the reference ranges. Ultrasonography showed normal liver, spleen, and gallbladder, but his pancreas was diffusely enlarged.

Skin and appendages *Linear IgA disease* is an acquired subepidermal bullous disease characterized by linear deposits of IgA at the cutaneous basement membrane zone and by circulating IgA antibasement membrane antibodies. Although the cause(s) of linear IgA disease most often is (are) unknown, a minority of cases has been reported to follow ingestion of drugs, especially vancomycin and diclofenac. Recently a patient with penicillin-G induced linear IgA disease who had circulating IgA antibodies showing specificity against type VII collagen has been described (19[C])

A previously fit 76-year-old man developed pneumococcal pneumonia and acute confusion. He was given oxygen, digoxin, furosemide, and penicillin G 9.6 g/day. Because his symptoms of infection continued he was then given higher doses of penicillin, together with intravenous dexamethasone, and his condition slowly improved. After 10 days of treatment with penicillin (cumulative dose 125 g), he developed a maculopapular truncal eruption compatible with a drug rash. Penicillin was withdrawn and the eruption faded over several days, but 1 week later he developed a localized blistering eruption with tense clear bullae and erosions on the penis, scrotum, and inner thighs. This became generalized, affecting most of the body, and he developed large erosions over pressure-bearings sites, oral ulcers, and hemorrhagic nasal crusting. He was given oral prednisolone. His blistering abated within a month, steroid therapy was withdrawn after 3 months, and his disease remained in remission at follow-up 12 months later.

Histology of the affected skin showed subepidermal bullae and a mixed inflammatory infiltrate in the dermis. Direct immunofluorescence showed linear IgA deposition along the basement membrane. Antibasement membrane antibodies were demonstrated by indirect immunofluorescence and were identified by Western blotting to be against a 250 kDa antigen in dermal extracts. Monoclonal antibodies to collagen VII co-migrated to the same spot. Collagen VII is the major target antigen of epidermolysis bullosa acquisita (20[C]). Consequently, it is open for discussion whether such patients should be classified as having IgA epidermolysis bullosa acquisita or collagen VII linear IgA disease. The authors stated that 'our patient did not have the clinical phenotype of epidermolysis bullosa acquisita' and the diagnosis of drug induced collagen VII linear IgA disease seems well validated (16[C]).

Interactions Most β-lactams are weak organic acids that compete with the renal tubular secretion of *methotrexate* and its metabolites and reduce their clearance. Over the years, some reports have appeared describing aplastic crises in patients taking this combination (21[C], 22[c], 23[c]). The more basic interactions between piperacillin and methotrexate and its major metabolite 7-hydroxymethotrexate has recently been studied in rabbits (24). The study showed that the interaction was mainly caused by reduced renal clearance of both methotrexate and its metabolite. The authors concluded that 'renal function in patients receiving this combination should be monitored with adequate fluid intake, especially in elderly patients because dehydration might accelerate the occurrence of toxicity'.

Ampicillin

Release of prostaglandins Preterm labor and ruptures of membranes are always a matter of concern. In addition to an increased risk of intrauterine infections after preterm rupture of membranes, abnormal microbial colonization of the genitourinary tract may by itself be a factor of importance in the pathogenesis of preterm labor. Because of these possible associations between microbial flora and preterm labor, several authors have investigated the use of adjunctive antibiotic therapy in order to prolong pregnancy. Over the years, ampicillin has probably been the most commonly used antibiotic in the therapy of preterm labor. In spite of the fact that most of the trials have reported that antibiotic administration prolongs pregnancy, the mechanism(s) behind this prolongation is (are) still unclear.

However, it is well established that several antibiotics can alter intracellular calcium concentrations (25[R]–27[R]) or inhibit some enzymes, including various phospholipases (28[R]). It is also well established that bacterial products, such as phospholipases and endotoxins, can stimulate prostaglandin biosynthesis and release by the human amnion (29[R]). Therefore, because prostaglandin biosynthesis depends on the action of phospholipase A2, a calcium-dependent enzyme (28[R]), it has been hypothesized that antibiotics that interfere with phospholipase A2 might affect prostaglandin biosynthesis and release by the human amnion. The aim of a recent study was to test this hypothesis by evaluating the effect of ampicillin on the release of prostaglandin E from human amnion (30^R).

The results were very clear cut: ampicillin dose-dependently inhibited the release of prostaglandin E from human amnion in vitro. Moreover, ampicillin reversibly counteracted the rise in prostaglandin E induced by arachidonic acid or oxytocin. They concluded that 'the inhibition of prostaglandin E release from amnion, in our opinion, represents a further mechanism by which ampicillin might prevent some cases of premature delivery even in the absence of infection' (30^R).

Co-amoxiclav

Liver As mentioned before (SEDA-15, 255; SEDA-22, 266) it is well established that some penicillins, especially the penicillinase-resistant semisynthetic penicillins (oxacillin, cloxacillin, dicloxacillin, flucloxacillin) and amoxicillin/clavulanic acid, can cause liver damage. Now amoxicillin/clavulanic acid (co-amoxiclav) may have reached the top of the list. Transient rises in serum transaminases are not uncommon after the use of co-amoxiclav and hepatic dysfunction with jaundice may also occur. The following case report is a brief reminder (31^c).

A 40-year-old woman with a history of chronic sinusitis and asthma developed nausea, vomiting, abdominal pain, and diarrhea. Six weeks before she had taken a 10-day course of co-amoxiclav for acute sinusitis. Her aminotransferase activities were markedly increased, as was total bilirubin. All drugs were withdrawn, her symptoms progressively improved, and she was discharged home without a clearly identified cause of her illness. Liver function tests normalized completely within a few weeks. Two months later she had another episode of acute sinusitis and was again given co-amoxiclav. A few days later she developed nausea, vomiting, a skin rash, abdominal pain, and reduced appetite. Her AlT was 199 u/l (0–65), AsT 99 u/l (0–60), and alkaline phosphatase 362 u/l (50–180). The antibiotic was discontinued, and she completely recovered in 2 weeks and had normal liver function tests over the next several months.

The relative contributions of amoxicillin and clavulanate in co-amoxiclav-induced hepatotoxicity are incompletely understood. The previous use of amoxicillin and rechallenge with the same drug was uneventful in patients with co-amoxiclav hepatotoxicity, pointing to clavulanic acid as the more likely culprit (32^C). In a report from the UK, the incidence of liver injury with amoxicillin alone was 0.3 per 10 000 prescriptions versus 1.7 with co-amoxiclav (33^R). The risk increased after multiple use and with increasing age to 1 per 1000 prescriptions of co-amoxiclav. The main message is that the combination should be used with caution in elderly patients. A patient who has had documented hepatotoxicity related to co-amoxiclav should be well informed about this adverse drug reaction and any future use should be prohibited.

CEPHALOSPORINS *(SED-13, 711; SEDA-20, 229; SEDA-21, 260, SEDA-22, 267)*

Cefalexin

Interactions Intestinal absorption of β-lactams occurs at least in part by an active mechanism involving a dipeptide carrier, and this pathway may result in interactions with dipeptides and tripeptides (34^R, 35^R), which reduce the rate of absorption of the β-lactams. In particular, *angiotensin-converting enzyme* (ACE) *inhibitors*, which have an oligopeptide structure, are absorbed by the same carrier (36) and interact with β-lactams in isolated rat intestine (37). However, there might be a second site of interaction between ACE inhibitors and β-lactams. Both groups of substances are excreted by the renal anionic transport system, and concomitant administration of both drugs sometimes results in pronounced inhibition of the elimination of β-lactams (38). In the case of cefalexin, it may not lead to toxic effects. However, when more toxic β-lactams are used, the possibility of this interaction has to be kept in mind.

Cefixime

Hematological *Pseudolymphoma leukemia (Sezary syndrome)* has been reported to occur mainly after the use of phenytoin and other anticonvulsant drugs (39^c, 40^c), but cefixime can now be added to the list (41^c).

A 48-year-old woman developed fever and cough, for which she was given oral cefixime. After 48 hours she developed an itchy diffuse erythematous maculopapular rash all over her body. Her white blood cell count was 20×10^9/l with 8% eosinophils; 5 days later it was 12.5×10^9/l with atypical, so-called Sezary-like, cells and 64% eosinophils. A bone-marrow aspirate showed 20% atypical lymphocytes with a Sezary-like appearance, having large cerebriform nuclei. An increase in eosinophil precursors was also noted. Cefixime was withdrawn and as she continued to be febrile with a rash and her eosinophil count increased to 72% she was given corticosteroids. Her fever fell to 37.5°C, the rash improved, and her white cell count fell. At follow-up 12 months later her leukocytosis and eosinophilia had completely resolved and she did not have any other problems.

The authors stressed that, like patients with phenytoin-induced pseudolymphoma, this patient will need long-term follow-up to differentiate true pre-lymphoma. This case can be taken as a reminder that every new β-lactam coming on the market may have an adverse effects profile of its own.

Ceftriaxone

Pancreas Ceftriaxone has been reported to have caused *pancreatitis* (42[c]).

A 13-year-old boy received long-term intravenous ceftriaxone after surgical drainage of a right frontal subdural empyema secondary to sinusitis. After about 5 weeks he developed abdominal pain with profuse emesis; his serum amylase was 1133 u/l and lipase 3528 u/l. Abdominal ultrasound showed cholelithiasis and he had an uncomplicated cholecystectomy. The material in the gallbladder was 100% ceftriaxone.

The authors ended by stating that patients receiving long-term ceftriaxone may be at risk of cholelithiasis and pancreatitis. Ultrasound screening might be useful for monitoring such patients.

Hematological A case of fatal *hemolysis* after ceftriaxone has recently been reported (43[c]).

A 14-year-old girl perinatally infected with HIV, had a medical history of recurrent infections that had been treated with several antibiotics, including ceftriaxone. She was given ceftriaxone (60 mg/kg intravenously) for pneumonia and 30 minutes later complained of severe back pain, became nauseated, vomited, and collapsed. Despite intensive medical care she died within a few hours with massive intravascular hemolysis and disseminated intravascular coagulopathy. Autopsy was refused.

The authors reviewed seven other cases of hemolysis after treatment with ceftriaxone (six died) and stressed that the use of second- and third-generation cephalosporins, particularly ceftriaxone, in immunocompromised patients or those with long-standing hematological complications, should be avoided or undertaken with extreme caution.

TETRACYCLINES *(SED-13, 725; SEDA-20, 231, SEDA-21, 261, SEDA-22, 268)*

Tetracyclines in rheumatology—effects on microbes or enzymes? R

In 1942 the Swedish doctor Nana Svartz introduced sulfasalazine into clinical therapy and suggested that it might be useful in rheumatoid arthritis because of its antibacterial activity. Since then, many antimicrobial agents have been tried in the treatment of rheumatoid arthritis, based on the assumption that the disease may be due to an infectious agent. During the last few years, interest has focused on tetracyclines for the treatment of rheumatoid arthritis (44[R]), reactive arthritis (45[R]), and osteoarthritis (46[R]) and the state of the art has recently been reviewed (47[R]).

The key point is whether the tetracyclines act as antimicrobials or exert their effect through immunological or biochemical mechanisms. Several mechanisms might be involved.

Direct antimicrobial effect of tetracyclines *It is well established that a number of microorganisms found in the gastrointestinal tract are associated with reactive arthritis and that most of these organisms might be susceptible to tetracyclines. As stated in the review (47[R]), several investigations have shown clinical effects of tetracyclines in the treatment of reactive arthritis. In these cases, a more direct antibacterial effect of the triggering organism (if still present in the patient) might be the mechanism involved.*

Other effects of tetracyclines *Tetracyclines have many effects on cells involved in inflammatory reactions, including inhibition of neutrophilic functions, such as migration, phagocytosis, degranulation, and the production of free oxygen radical (48[R]). Most of these effects are supposed to be due to chelation of divalent ions and can be partly reversed by the addition of calcium ions or zinc ions. Their ability to inhibit synthesis of mitochondrial proteins may be the background for their effects on* *lymphocytes, such as inhibition of lymphocyte proliferation in response to mitogens, inhibition of interferon gamma production, and inhibition of immunoglobulin production. Enzyme inactivation caused by tetracyclines has been studied in several models. Tetracyclines inhibited gingival collagenolytic activity in diabetic mice and in humans with periodontal disease (49[C]). Subsequent studies showed that tetracyclines inactivated collagenases found in several places in the body (50[C], 51[C]). Most probably, the inhibitory effects of tetracyclines on collagenases are exerted through inactivation of metalloproteases, rather than serine proteases. As is to be expected, modified cycline molecules devoid of antibacterial effects are as effective as non-modified molecules.*

Tetracyclines have also been investigated in experimental osteoarthritis, because metalloproteases are involved in the breakdown of cartilage matrix seen in this condition. Doxycycline reduced the severity of knee osteoarthritis induced in dogs by ligamentous section (52[R]) and also reduced the degradation of type XI collagen exposed to extract of human arthritic cartilage (53[R]).

Tetracyclines are not currently first-line drugs in the treatment of rheumatoid arthritis and other forms of chronic joint diseases. The theory that rheumatoid arthritis is due to an infectious agent was recently refined to a statement that it can be a gene transfer disease in which some viruses may act as vectors (54[R]), thereby excluding a direct effect of antibacterial agents on the disease. However, this theory does not exclude use of tetracyclines in rheumatoid arthritis and other joint diseases. There is a possibility that tetracyclines with refined anti-inflammatory and enzyme inhibitory effects may be of increasing value in rheumatology. Again a potential adverse effect may turn in to be a useful one.

Respiratory Minocycline and nicotinamide therapy for bullous pemphigoid have been associated with severe *pneumonitis* (55[c]).

Liver Hepatotoxicity from tetracyclines has previously been mostly reported in patients receiving large doses intravenously, especially in pregnant women and patients with renal disease. However, a few reports have described liver reactions in previously healthy individuals with no pre-existing conditions and given 'normal' oral doses of tetracyclines (56[C], 57[C]). Recently 'a personally experienced further case of likely tetracycline-induced liver injury after low-dose tetracycline administration' has been reported (58[C]). The patient took oral doxycycline 200 mg/day for 8 days and had markedly altered liver function. The liver enzyme activities normalized only 109 days after withdrawal. The authors also reviewed all reports of liver damage to Swedish Adverse Drug Reactions Advisory Committee (SADRAC) in the period 1965–95. There were 23 liver reactions with a suspected causal relation to oral low-dose tetracycline derivatives. A causal relation was considered likely in three cases and possible in eight, giving an incidence of roughly 1 in 18 million defined daily doses. There were no deaths from these liver reactions, and liver enzyme activities normalized in all cases without any serious clinical consequences. The authors remarked that the frequency of liver reactions resulting from tetracyclines may be somewhat higher, as previous studies in Sweden suggest that only 20–50% of severe adverse reactions are reported to SADRAC (58[C]).

Gastrointestinal Thirty centers for pharmacovigilance in France have reported 81 cases of *esophageal damage* after treatment with tetracyclines collected between 1985 and 1992 (59[C]). There were 64 ulcers, eight cases of dysphagia, and nine of esophagitis. Most (96%) of the cases were caused by doxycycline and 73% of the patients were female, mean age 29 years. Prescriptions were for dermatological (54%), urogenital (23%), and ENT diseases. In a 71-year-old man, an esophagobronchial fistulation required esophagectomy. In 92% the drugs were not taken correctly, i.e. at bedtime or without a sufficient quantity of fluid. Treatment with sucralfate 1g tds did not change the outcome of tetracycline-induced esophageal ulcers (60[C]).

Tetracycline has radical-scavenging properties. This may be partly related to the ulcer-healing effect observed in a rat model of gastric mucosal injury (61).

Urinary system *Acute interstitial nephritis* leading to acute renal insufficiency has been reported after a single repeated dose of tetracycline (62[c]).

Skin and appendages The long-term esthetic results of severely tetracycline-stained teeth treated by endodontics and internal bleaching have been assessed in 20 patients and found to be excellent (63[C]). A therapeutic strategy may be bleaching after the preparation for porcelain laminate veneers or night-guard vital bleaching (64[C], 65[C]).

Minocycline

Nervous system The syndrome of *pseudotumor cerebri* consists of symptoms and signs of raised intracranial pressure in the absence of neuroimaging or cerebrospinal fluid abnormalities. Most cases are idiopathic, but several drugs have been implicated as causative or contributory.

The first description of minocycline-related pseudotumor cerebri was published in 1978 (66[C]). Further data have recently been published concerning 12 patients who developed pseudotumor cerebri after taking standard doses of minocycline for acne vulgaris (67[C]). Nine developed symptoms within 8 weeks of starting minocycline therapy. Minocycline was withdrawn, and none of the patients developed recurrences for at least 1 year afterwards. However, three patients had substantial residual visual field loss.

It seems reasonable to assume that the mechanisms may be similar to that postulated for tetracyclines, which reduce cerebrospinal fluid absorption, possibly by an effect on cyclic adenosine monophosphate at the arachnoid villi (68[r]). Minocycline crosses the blood-brain barrier more effectively than other tetracyclines, because of its greater lipid solubility. Therefore, a physician who prescribes minocycline should keep his eye on the patient's eyes.

Pancreas Minocycline has been associated with acute *pancreatitis* (69[c]).

Skin and appendages Long-term minocycline often results in *pigmentation of skin, nails, bones, thyroid, mouth*, and *eyes*. The bones of the oral cavity are probably the most frequently affected sites of pigmentation. On the skin, the blue-black pigmentation develops most frequently on the shins, ankles, and arms. Other patterns include pigmentation that is either generalized and symmetrical or develops at sites of inflammation. The pigmentation is often permanent when sites other than the skin and oral mucosa are involved (70[C], 71[c]). The pigment is a product of an oxidation reaction. In an experimental rat study, pigmentation of the thyroid gland was prevented by ascorbic acid (72). Laser treatment with was successfully used in two cases (73[c], 74[c]).

Immunological and hypersensitivity reactions Immunoallergic reactions have previously been reported with minocycline and include *lupus-like syndrome, autoimmune hepatitis, eosinophilic pneumonia, hypersensitivity syndrome, a serum sickness-like illness*, and *Sweet's syndrome* (SEDA-21, 262; SEDA-22, 271). Over 60 minocycline-induced cases of systemic lupus erythematosus and 24 cases of minocycline-induced autoimmune hepatitis were found in a review of the literature (75[R]). In 13 patients, both disorders co-existed. These patients had symmetrical polyarthralgia/polyarthritis, raised liver enzymes, and positive antinuclear antibodies; they were also generally antihistone-negative, and only two patients had p-ANCA antibodies. Minocycline-related lupus can also occur in adolescents (76[c]).

In a case-control study of young acne patients, current use of minocycline increased the risk of developing lupus-like syndrome 8.5-fold. The effect was stronger in longer-term users, but the absolute risk of developing lupus-like syndrome seemed to be relatively low (77[C]). A case of minocycline-induced hepatitis with antinuclear, antimitochondrial, and antismooth muscle antibodies has now been reported in a 19-year-old black West Indian woman who had been treated for acne for 2 years with oral minocycline (50 mg/day) and topical benzoyl peroxide (5%) (78[c]).

Seven patients (17–22 years old) developed symptoms of arthralgia and arthritis after having taken minocycline 50–100 mg bd for 6–36 months for acne vulgaris (79[C]). Increased titers of perinuclear ANCA were detected in all seven, five had fluorescent antinuclear antibodies, two had antihistone autoantibodies, and one had anticardiolipin antibodies. Symptoms resolved in five patients on withdrawal; the other two were treated with corticosteroids and also achieved remissions.

Autoimmune hepatitis has also been reported (80[C]).

Three adolescents taking therapeutic doses of minocycline for 12–20 months met the 1993 International Autoimmune Hepatitis Group criteria for autoimmune hepatitis All had hypogammaglobulinemia and positive antinuclear antibody and antismooth muscle antibody titers. Two underwent liver biopsy that showed severe chronic lymphoplasmocytic inflammation, necrosis, and fibrosis. All other causes of liver disease were excluded. One patient had resolution of symptoms after withdrawal of the drug, while two required immunosuppressive therapy.

REFERENCES

1. Anonymous. Chemotherapy for the 21st century. Antibiot Chemother 1999;3:1–3.
2. Falk PG, Hooper LV, Midtvedt T, Gordon JI. Creating and maintaining the gastrointestinal ecosystem. What we know and need to know from gnotobiology. Microbiol Mol Biol Rev 1998; 62:1157–70.
3. Choquet-Kastylevssky G, Descotes J. Value of animal models for predicting hypersensitivity reactions to medicinal products. Toxicology 1998;129:27–35.
4. Dejarnatt AC, Grant JA. Basic mechanisms of anaphylaxis and anaphylactoid reactions. Immunol Allergy Clin North Am 1992;12:33–46.
5. Chazal I, Verdier F, Virat M, Descotes J. Prediction of drug induced immediate hypersensitivity in guinea-pigs. Toxicol In Vitro 1994;8:1045–9.
6. Nagami K, Matsumoto H, Maki E. Experimental methods for immunization and challenge antigenicity studies in guinea-pigs. J Toxicol Sci 1995;20:579–90.
7. Sarlo K, Karol MH. Guinea pig predictive tests for allergy. In: Dean JH, Luster MI, Munson AE, Kiber I, editors. Immunotoxicology and Immunopharmacology, 2nd edition. New York: Raven Press, 1994;703–20.
8. Hilton J, Dearman RJ, Boylett S, Fielding I, Basketter DA, Kimber I. The mouse IgE test for the identification of potential chemical respiratory allergens: considerations of stability and controls. J Appl Toxicol 1996;16:165–70.
9. Saxon A, Swabb EA, Adkinson NF. Investigation into the immunological cross-reactivity of aztreonam with other β-lactam antibiotics. Am J Med 1985;78(Suppl 2A):19–26.
10. Adkinson NF. Beta-lactam crossreactivity. Clin Exp Allergy 1998;28:37–40.
11. Bolzacchini E, Meinhardi S, Orlandi M, Rindone B. 'In vivo' models of hapten generation. Clin Exp Allergy 1998;28(Suppl 4):83–6.
12. Pimiento AP, Martinez MG, Mena AM, Gonzalez AT, De Paz Arranz S, Rodriguez Mosquera M. Aztreonam and ceftazidime: evidence of in vivo cross-allergy. Allergy 1998;53:624–5.
13. Gruchalla RS. Acute drug desensitization. Clin Exp Allergy 1998;28(Suppl 3):63–4.
14. Sullivan TJ. Drug Allergy. In: Middleton E Jr, editor. Allergy-Principles and Practice. 4th edition. CV Mosby Co, 1993;1726.
15. Tidwell BH, Clearly JD, Lorenz KR. Antimicrobial desensitization: a review of published protocols. Hosp Pharm 1997;32:1362–70.
16. Marshall JB. Acute pancreatitis. A review with an emphasis on new developments. Arch Intern Med 1993;153:1185–98.
17. Hanline MH. Acute pancreatitis caused by ampicillin. South Med J 1987;80:1069.
18. Sammettt D, Greben C, Sayyed-Shah U. Acute pancreatitis caused by penicillin. Dig Dis Sci 1998; 43:1178–3.
19. Wakelin SH, Allen J, Zhou S, Wojnarowska F. Drug-induced linear IgA disease with antibodies to collagen VII. Br J Dermatol 1998;138:310–14.
20. Woodley DT, Burgeson RE, Lundstrom G, Bruckner-Tuderman L, Reese MJ, Briggaman RA. Epidermolysis bullosa acquisita antigen is the global carboxyl terminus of type VII procollagen. J Clin Invest 1988;81:683–7.
21. Mayall B, Poggi G, Parkin JD. Neutropenia due to low dose methotrexate therapy for psoriasis and rheumatoid arthritis may be fatal. Med J Aust 1991;155:480–4.
22. Dawson JK, Abernethy VE, Lynch MP. Methotrexate and penicillin interaction. Br J Rheumatol 1998;37:807.
23. Ronchera CL, Hernandez T, Peris JE. Pharmacokinetic interaction between high-dose methotrexate and amoxicillin. Ther Drug Monit 1993; 15:375–9.
24. Najjar TA, Abou-Auda HS, Ghilzai NM, Influence of piperacillin on the pharmacokinetics of methotrexate and 7-hydroxymethotrexate. Cancer Chemother Pharmacol 1998;45:423–8.
25. Cloutier MM, Guernsey L, Shaáfi RI. Duramycin increases intracellular calcium in airway epithelium. Membr Biochem 1993;10:107–18.
26. Burroughs SF, Johnson GJ. Beta-lactam antibiotics inhibit agonist-stimulated platelet influx. Thromb Haemost 1993;69:503–8.
27. Bird SD, Walker RJ, Hubbard MJ. Altered free calcium transients in pig kidney cells (LLC-PK-1) cultured with penicillin/streptomycin. In Vitro Cell Dev Biol Anim 1994;30A:420–4.
28. Verheij HM, Slotboom AJ, DeHaas GH. Structure and function of phospholipase A2. Rev Physiol Biochem Pharmacol 1981;91:191–203.
29. Romero R, Mazor M, Wu YK, Sirtor M, Oyarzun F, Mitchell MM. Infection in the pathogenesis of preterm labor. Semin Perinatol 1988;12:262–9.
30. Vesce F, Buzzi M, Ferretti ME, Pavan B, Bianchiotto A, Jorizzo G, Biondi C. Inhibition of amniotic prostaglandin E release by ampicillin. Am J Obstet Gynecol 1998;178:759–64.
31. Nathani MG, Mutchnik MG, Tynes DJ, Ehrinpreis MN. An unusual case of amoxicillin/clavulanic acid related hepatotoxicity. Am J Gastroenterol 1998;93:1363–5.
32. Stricker BH, Van den Broek JWG, Keuning J. Cholestatic hepatitis due to antibacterial combination of amoxicillin and clavulanic acid (Augmentin). Dig Dis Sci 1989;34:1576–80.
33. Rodriguez LG, Stricker BH, Zimmerman HJ. Risk of acute liver injury associated with the com-

bination of amoxicillin and clavulanic acid. Arch Intern Med 1996;156:1327–32.
34. Sugarwara M, Toda T, Iseki K, Miyazaki K, Shiroto H, Kondo Y, Uchino JI. Transport characteristics of cephalosporin antibiotics across intestinal brush-border membrane in man, rat and rabbit. J Pharm Pharmacol 1992;44:968–72.
35. Dantzig A, Bergin L. Uptake of cephalosporin, cephalexin, by a dipeptide transport carrier in the human intestinal cell line, Caco-2. Biochim Biophys Acta 1990;1027:211–17.
36. Friedman DI, Amidon GL. Intestinal absorption mechanism of dipeptide angiotensin converting enzyme inhibitors of the lysyl-proline type: lisinopril and SQ 29.852. J Pharm Sci 1989;78:995–8.
37. Hu M, Amidon G. Passive and carrier-mediated intestinal absorption components of captopril. J Pharm Sci 1988;77:1007–11.
38. Padoin C, Tod M, Perret G, Petitjean M. Analysis of the pharmacokinetic interaction between cephalexin and quinapril by a non-linear mixed-effect model. Antimicrob Agent Chemother 1998; 42:1463–9.
39. Rosenthal CJ, Noguera CA, Coppola A, Kapelner SN. Pseudolymphoma with mycosis fungoides manifestations, hyperresponsiveness to diphenylhydantoin, and lymphocyte dysregulation. Cancer 1982;49:2305–14.
40. Díncan H, Souteyrand P, Bignon YJ, Roger H. Hydantoin-induced cutaneous pseudolymphoma with clinical, pathologic and immunological aspects of Sezary syndrome. Arch Dermatol 1992; 128:1371–4.
41. Jabbar A, Siddique T. A case of pseudolymphoma leukemia syndrome following cefixime. Br J Haematol 1998;101:209.
42. Maranan MC, Gerber SI, Miller GG. Gallstone pancreatitis caused by cefriaxone. Pediatr Infect Dis J 1998;17:662–3.
43. Moallem HJ, Garratty G, Wakeham H, Dial S, Oligario A, Gondi A, Sreedhar PR, Fikrig S. Ceftriaxone-related fatal hemolysis in an adolescent with perinatally acquired human immunodeficiency virus infection J Pediatr 1998;133:279–81.
44. Trentham DE, Dynesius-Trentham RA. Antibiotic therapy for rheumatoid arthritis. Rheum Dis Clin North Am 1995;21:817–34.
45. Pott HG, Wittenborg A, Junge-Hulsing G. Long-term antibiotic treatment in reactive arthritis. Lancet 1988;245:146.
46. Kloppenburg M, Dijkmans BAC, Breedveld FC. Antimicrobial therapy for rheumatoid arthritis. Baillire's Clin Rheumatol 1996;9:759–69.
47. Toussirot E, Despaux J, Wendling D. Do minocycline and other tetracyclines have a place in rheumatology? Rev Rum Engl Ed 1997;64: 474–80.
48. Midtvedt T, Lingaas E, Melby K. The effect of 13 antimicrobial agents on the elimination phase of phagocytosis in human polymorphonuclear leukocytes. In: Eickenberg HU, Hahn A, Opferkuch W, editors. The Influence of Antibiotics on the Host-Parasite Relationship. Berlin: Springer Verlag, 1982;118–28.
49. Golub LM, Ramamurthy N, McNamara TF, Gomes B, Wolff M, Casino A. Tetracyclines inhibit collagenase activity. J Periodont Res 1984;19:651–5.
50. Greenwald RA, Golub LM, Laviets B, Ramamurthy NS, Gruber B, Laskin RS. Tetracyclines inhibit human synovial collagenase in vivo and in vitro. J Rheumatol 1987;14:28–32.
51. Lauhio A, Sorsa T, Lindy O, Suomalainen K, Sari H, Golub LM. The anticollagenolytic potential of lymecycline in the long-term treatment of reactive arthritis. Arthritis Rheum 1992;35:195–8.
52. Yu LP, Smith GN, Brandt KD, Meyers SL, O'Connor BL, Brandt DA. Reduction of the severity of canine osteoarthritis by prophylactic treatment with oral doxycycline. Arthritis Rheum 1992; 35:1150–9.
53. Yu LP, Smith GN, Hasty KA, Brandt KD. Doxycycline inhibits type XI collagenolytic activity of extracts from human osteoarthritic cartilage and of gelatinase. J Rheumatol 1991;18:1450–2.
54. Grubb R, Grubb A, Kjellen L, Lycke E, Åman P. Rheumatoid arthritis—a gene transfer disease. Exp Clin Immunogenet 1999;16:1–7.
55. Hara H, Fujitsuka A, Morishima C, Kurihara N, Yamaguchi Z-I, Morishima T. Severe drug-induced pneumonitis associated with minocycline and nicotinamide therapy of a bullous pemphigoid. Acta Derm Venereol 1998;78:393–4.
56. Hunt CM, Wasington K. Tetracycline-induced bile duct paucity and prolonged cholestasis. Gastroenterology 1994;107:1844–7.
57. Schrumpf E, Nordgård K, Unusual cholestatic hepatotoxicity of doxycycline in a young male. Scand J Gastroenterol 1986;21(Suppl 120):68.
58. Bjönsson E, Lindberg L, Olsson R. Liver reactions to oral low-dose tetracyclines. Scand J Gastroenterol 1997;32:390–5.
59. Champel V, Jonville-Béra A-P, Béra F, Autret E. Les tétracyclines peuvent être responsables d'ulcérations oesophagiennes si leur prise est incorrecte. Rev Prat Med Gen 1998;12:9–10.
60. Huizar JF, Podolsky I, Goldberg J. Ulceras esofagicas inducidas por doxiciclina. Rev Gastroenterol Mex 1998;63:101–5.
61. Suzuki Y, Ishihara M, Segami T, Ito M. Antiulcer effects of antioxidants, quercetin, alpha-tocopherol, nifedipine and tetracycline in rats. Jpn J Pharmacol 1998;78:435–41.
62. Bihorac A, Ozener C, Akoglu E, Kullu S. Tetracycline-induced acute interstitial nephritis as a cause of acute renal failure. Nephron 1999;81:72–5.
63. Abou Rass M. Long-term prognosis of intentional endodontics and internal bleaching of tetracycline-stained teeth. Compend Contin Educ Dent 1998;19:1034–8,1040–2, 1044.
64. Leonard RHJ. Efficacy, longevity, side effects, and patient perceptions of nightguard vital bleaching. Compend Contin Educ Dent 1998;19:766–70,772, 774.
65. Sadan A, Lemon RR. Combining treatment modalities for tetracycline-discolored teeth. Int J Periodontics Restorative Dent 1998;18:564–71.

66. Monaco F, Agnetti V, Mutani R. Benign intracranial hypertension after minocycline therapy. Eur Neurol 1978;17:48–9.
67. Chiu AM, Chuenkongkaew WL, Cornblath WT, Trobe JD. Digre KB, Dotan SA, Mussin KH, Eggenberger ER. Minocycline treatment and pseudotumor cerebri syndrome. Am J Ophthalmol 1998;126:116–21.
68. Walters B, Gubbay S. Tetracycline and benign intracranial hypertension. Br Med J 1981; 282:1240.
69. Chetaille E, Delcenserie R, Yzet T, Decocq G, Biour M, Andrejak M. Imputabilite de la minocycline dans deux observations de pancreatite aigue. Gastroenterol Clin Biol 1998;22:555–6.
70. Eisen D, Hakim MD. Minocycline-induced pigmentation. Incidence, prevention and management. Drug Saf 1998;18:431–40.
71. Cockings JM, Savage NW. Minocycline and oral pigmentation. Aust Dent J 1998;43:14–16.
72. Bowles WH. Protection against minocycline pigment formation by ascorbic acid (vitamin C). J Esthet Dent 1998;10:182–6.
73. Greve B, Schonermark MP, Raulin C. Minocycline-induced hyperpigmentation: treatment with the Q-switched Nd: YAG laser. Lasers Surg Med 1998;22:223–7.
74. Karrer S, Szeimies RM, Pfau A, Schroder J, Stolz W, Landthaler M. Minozyklin-induzierte Hyperpigmentierung. Hautarzt 1998;49:219–23.
75. Angulo JM, Sigal LH, Espinoza LR. Coexistent minocycline-induced systemic lupus erythematosus and autoimmune hepatitis. Semin Arthritis Rheum 1998;28:187–92.
76. Akin E, Miller LC, Tucker LB. Minocycline-induced lupus in adolescents. Pediatrics 1998; 101:926.
77. Sturkenboom MC, Meier CR, Jick H, Stricker BHC. Minocycline and lupus-like syndrome in acne patients. Arch Intern Med 1999;159: 493–7.
78. Pavese P, Sarrot-Reynauld F, Bonadona A, Massot C. Reaction immuno-allergique avec hepatite induite par la minocycline. Ann Med Interne 1998;149:521–3.
79. Elkayam O, Levartosky D, Brautbar C, Yaron M, Burke M, Vardinon N, Caspi D. Clinical and immunological study of 7 patients with minocycline-induced autoimmune phenomena. Am J Med 1998; 105:484–7.
80. Teitelbaum JE, Perz-Atayde AR, Cohen M, Bousvaros A, Jonas MM. Minocycline-related autoimmune hepatitis. Arch Paediatr Adolesc Med 1998;152:1132–6.

R. Walter and A. Schaffner

26 Miscellaneous antibacterial drugs

GENERAL TOPICS

Economics Pharmacoeconomic evaluations of antibacterial adverse effects are currently lacking. However, the economic impact of such adverse effects is enormous. Antibacterial drug reactions account for about 25% of adverse drug reactions. The adverse effects profile of an antimicrobial agent can contribute significantly to its overall direct costs (monitoring costs, prolonged hospitalization due to complications or treatment failures) and indirect costs (quality of life, loss of productivity, time spent by families and patients receiving medical care). In a recent study an adverse drug event in a hospitalized patient was associated on average with an excess of 1.9 days in the length of stay, extra costs of $US2262 (1990–93 values), and an almost 2-fold increase in the risk of death. In the outpatient setting, adverse drug reactions result in 2–6% of hospitalizations, and most of them were thought to be avoidable if appropriate interventions had been taken. In a review of the current literature, economic aspects of antibacterial therapy with β-lactams, aminoglycosides, vancomycin, macrolides, and fluoroquinolones have been summarized and critically evaluated (1[R]).

Computer assisted management A computerized anti-infective disease management program has been designed to provide clinicians with immediate relevant information pertaining to the treatment of infections and the use of anti-infective agents. The program incorporated expert-derived logic, patient care protocols, and patient-specific data, and presented epidemiological information, along with detailed recommendations and warnings. The authors prospectively studied the use of this program for 1 year in all 545 patients admitted to a 12-bed intensive care unit and compared the results with those of 1136 patients admitted to the same unit during the 2 years before. They found a significant reduction in orders for drugs to which the patients had reported allergies before, excessive drug dosages, antibiotic-susceptibility mismatches, and adverse effects caused by anti-infective agents. Furthermore, costs and length of hospital stay were also reduced (2[C], 3[r]).

Management of bite wounds Infected wounds of 50 patients with dog bites and 57 patients with cat bites were prospectively investigated in 18 emergency departments. These wounds had a complex microbiological mix that usually included *Pasteurella* species, but also included many other organisms not routinely identified by clinical microbiology laboratories and not previously recognized as pathogens in bite wounds. Whether antibiotics prevent infection after bites remains controversial. Currently, antibiotics are not given routinely, but they are almost always recommended for high-risk wounds. Based on the findings in this recent study, empirical therapy should include a combination of a β-lactam antibiotic and a β-lactamase inhibitor, a second-generation cephalosporin with anerobic activity, or combination therapy with either a penicillin and a first-generation cephalosporin or clindamycin and a fluoroquinolone. Azithromycin and the new ketolide antibiotics may also be useful (4[C], 5[r]).

Community-acquired bacterial meningitis In a retrospective analysis of 269 cases of microbiologically proven community-acquired bacterial meningitis between 1970 and 1995 hospital mortality was 27%. Neurological deficits developed in 21% of patients, and in 9% the deficit persisted at discharge. Three baseline clinical features (hypotension, altered mental

Side Effects of Drugs, Annual 23
J.K. Aronson, ed.

status, and seizures) were independently associated with an adverse clinical outcome. Using these variables, patients were stratified into three stages of prognostic severity. An adverse clinical outcome was associated with a delay in starting antibiotic therapy (6[C]).

Prevention of endocarditis during dentistry A new population-based, case-control study of 273 patients has confirmed that cardiac valvular abnormalities are strong risk factors for infective endocarditis (7[C]). For example, for prosthetic valves and a history of previous endocarditis the odds ratios were 75 and 37 respectively. In contrast, dental treatment did not seem to be a risk factor for infective endocarditis, even in patients with valvular abnormalities. An editorial review of the current evidence suggested that prophylaxis should be downgraded to 'not recommended' for most dental procedures, except extractions and gingival surgery (including implant placement) and for most underlying cardiac conditions, except prosthetic valves and previous endocarditis. Following this strategy, it should be possible to retain at least 80% of any putative benefits for less than 20% of the costs (8[r]).

Upper respiratory tract infections A clinical approach to antibiotic choice and dosage in the management of adult otitis media, sinusitis, and pharyngitis has been delineated (9[R]). The spectrum of activity should include coverage *of Streptococcus pneumoniae, H. influenzae*, and *M. catarrhalis.* Special attention should be paid to activity against resistant strains (penicillin-resistant *Strep. pneumoniae*, ampicillin-resistant *H. influenzae*, and β-lactamase positive *M. catarrhalis*). Favorable pharmacokinetic properties with good penetration into respiratory secretions, the achievement and maintenance of adequate concentrations at the site of infection, and a long dosing interval all contribute to successful therapy. For mild to moderate infections, the expense can be dramatically reduced by oral therapy, so that patients can be discharged earlier. Maximizing the use of out-patient oral therapy depends on the use of agents with excellent oral systemic availability in addition to the appropriate spectrum. Among the cephalosporins, cefprozil meets these criteria. The newer respiratory quinolones are also effective. Doxycycline is useful against typical pathogens, as is co-trimoxazole, although *Strep. pneumoniae* resistance is a growing problem. The macrolides should be avoided, because about 25% of intermediate penicillin-resistant strains of *Strep. pneumoniae* are naturally macrolide-resistant.

Factors that predispose to resistance include subtherapeutic antibiotic concentrations at the site of infection and prolonged treatment courses with low doses. Conversely, the best strategy for avoiding the development of resistance is to use the maximum dose and the shortest course of therapy that are consistent with eradication of the causative pathogen and to use antibiotics that are known to be associated with little or no resistance potential (10[R], 11[R]).

Treatment of severe pneumonia In an open, randomized, comparative study on the efficacy, safety, and tolerance of two different antibiotic regimens in the treatment of severe community-acquired or nosocomial pneumonia, 84 patients were analyzed (12[C]). Half were treated with piperacillin 4 g and tazobactam 500 mg every 8 hours, and half with co-amoxiclav (amoxicillin 2 g and clavulanic acid 200 mg) every 8 hours plus a single-dose of 3–6 mg/kg of an aminoglycoside (netilmicin or gentamicin). The patients were treated for between 48 hours and 21 days. Clinical cure was achieved in 81% of patients with piperacillin/tazobactam and in 65% of patients with co-amoxiclav/aminoglycoside. Cure or improvement was observed in 90% and 84% respectively. Treatment failures were recorded in 7 vs 14%. One patient in each group relapsed. There was only one fatal outcome in the piperacillin/tazobactam group compared with six in the co-amoxiclav/aminoglycoside group. The adverse event rate was non-significantly lower in the piperacillin/tazobactam group. In one patient given piperacillin/tazobactam, there were raised transaminases. In the co-amoxiclav/aminoglycoside group, acute renal insufficiency developed in two patients and possibly drug-related fever in one. Bacteriological efficacy was comparable (96 vs 92%). The authors concluded that piperacillin/tazobactam is highly efficacious in the treatment of severe pneumonia in hospitalized patients and compares favorably with the combination of co-amoxiclav/aminoglycoside.

Hematological *Thrombocytopenia* Reports of drug-induced thrombocytopenia have been systematically reviewed (13[R]). Among the

98 different drugs described in 561 articles the following antibiotics were found with level I (definite) evidence: co-trimoxazole, rifampicin, vancomycin, sulfisoxazole, cephalothin, piperacillin, methicillin, novobiocin. Drugs with level II (probable) evidence were oxytetracycline and ampicillin.

In another retrospective analysis of drug-induced thrombocytopenia reported to the Danish Committee on Adverse Drug Reactions, 192 cases caused by the most frequently reported drugs were included and analyzed (14[R]). There were pronounced drug-specific differences in the clinical appearance. Early thrombocytopenia was characteristic of cases caused by sulfonamides and co-trimoxazole. These drugs also often caused hemorrhage. Accompanying leukopenia was observed in some cases associated with co-trimoxazole. There were no patient-specific factors responsible for the heterogeneity of the clinical appearance, and factors related to the physician seemed to be of little significance.

Gastrointestinal Drug-induced *esophagitis* is rare, accounting for about 1% of all cases of esophagitis. An incidence of 3.9 in 100 000 has been reported. After the first description, there have been more than 250 observations, with more than 50 different drugs. Among those, the principal antibiotics included tetracyclines (doxycycline, metacycline, minocycline, oxytetracycline, and tetracycline), penicillins (amoxicillin, cloxacillin, penicillin V, and pivmecillinam), clindamycin, co-trimoxazole, erythromycin, lincomycin, spiramycin, and tinidazole. Doxycycline alone was involved in one-third of all cases. Risk factors included prolonged esophageal passage, due to motility disorders, stenosis, cardiomegaly, the formulation, supine position during drug ingestion, and failure to use liquid to wash down the tablet. Direct toxic effects of the drug (pH, accumulation in epithelial cells, non-uniform dispersion) also seem to contribute to the development of drug-induced esophagitis (15[R]).

Antibiotics often cause *gastrointestinal disturbances.* The intestinal flora is significantly influenced by antibiotics, resulting in a reduced barrier against opportunistic micro-organisms. Oral lincosamides and β-lactams (especially ampicillin, amoxicillin, and several cephalosporins) are most often implicated in disturbances of the intestinal flora. However, macrolides, parenteral carbapenems, and quinolones are also involved. Parenteral aminoglycosides seem to have no effect on normal intestinal flora. Risk factors for antibiotic-associated diarrhea or colitis, besides the class of drug, include combined antibiotic therapy, duration of therapy, extreme age (under 6 and over 65 years), the presence of another infection, immunodeficient state (suspected), previous diarrhea especially due to *C. difficile*, duration of hospital stay, and previous gastrointestinal interventions or enteral nutrition by feeding tubes. Among the different causes of antibiotic-associated diarrhea, strains of *C. difficile* that produce toxins are most important. A reduction of short-chain fatty acids that act like trophic factors on epithelial cells of the colon may contribute (16[r]).

Skin and appendages *Fixed drug eruptions* have been analyzed in 450 patients. The ratio of men to women was 10 : 11. The mean age of the men was 30 years, and that of the women 31 years. In 13% the fixed drug eruption occurred for the first time, 2.7% had more than 40 episodes. There was atopy in 11 and 23% had a positive family history of drug reactions. Co-trimoxazole was the most common cause of fixed drug eruptions. Other antibiotics included tetracycline, metronidazole, amoxicillin, ampicillin, erythromycin, and clindamycin (17[C]).

Special senses Drug induced *uveitis* is rare. Antibiotics that seem to be implicated include rifabutin and sulfonamides. Furthermore, nearly all antibiotics injected intracamerally have been reported to produce uveitis (18[R]). Topical administration of a corticosteroid and a cycloplegic (such as atropine) is suitable as initial treatment. Withdrawal of causative drugs is not always necessary (19[r]).

Immunological and hypersensitivity reactions The diagnosis of drug *allergy* is difficult for various reasons: the clinical manifestations are very heterogeneous, no reliable tests are available, and the pathophysiology remains unknown in most cases. Only a few drug allergies are IgE-mediated, but the involvement of drug-specific antibodies in some allergic drug disorders, such as anaphylaxis, urticaria, angioedema, and hemolytic anemia, is well known. Data indicate that T cells participate in various allergic drug reactions. Non-peptide antigens (lipids, prenylpyrophosphates, sugars, metals, or drugs) are recognized by T cells. The recognition of such non-peptide antigens may be important in the natural immune reaction to pathogens. Recently, the direct recognition of haptens by T cells has been demonstrated. Drugs are small compounds and are thought to act immunologically like haptens; their immunogenicity is therefore related to their ability to bind to proteins. Some drugs are reactive per se (for example, penicillins are recognized by T cells), and both CD4 and CD8 clones with a certain level of cross-reactivity can be generated. Other drugs are only reactive after drug metabolism, for example sulfonamides.

Based on novel findings, a new model of drug recognition by already activated T cells has been elaborated. According to this direct, metabolism-independent model of T cell stimulation, drug binding to the MHC-peptide complex, to the TCR receptor, and to other pharmacological receptors occurs without the requirement of covalent binding for presentation. It remains to be shown whether drug recognition is similar for primary sensitization, but it seems likely that drug metabolism and covalent binding are still important.

However, metabolism-independent drug presentation may serve to explain some features of drug allergies:

- that the manifestation of drug allergy is in organs without active drug metabolism such as the skin;
- that symptoms related to drug allergy often disappear rapidly after withdrawal of therapy;
- that drug allergies occur more often in association with generalized viral infections (viral-induced upregulation of MHC expression);
- that most cases of allergy are caused by only a few drugs (only those that interact with both MHC-peptide complexes and the TCR).

The functional properties of drug-specific T cells (phenotype and restriction of cell clones, oligoclonality with certain TCR Vβ families, secreted cytokines, cytotoxicity of the T cell response, superantigen-like T cell stimulation, cross-reactivity of drug-specific T cell clones) have been characterized more in detail, and some of these findings are peculiar and distinguishing from peptide-specific T cell clones (20[R]).

Risk factors for ventilator-associated pneumonia Risk factors for ventilator-associated pneumonia in 1014 critically ill patients have been investigated in a prospective cohort study (21[C]). Exposure to antibiotics was associated with low rates of early ventilator-associated pneumonia, but this effect attenuated over time. Identified risk factors were age, male sex, the primary admitting diagnosis, intensive care unit admission from the emergency department, a low Glasgow Coma Scale Score, an increased Multiple Organ Dysfunction score compared with that at admission, mechanical ventilation in the previous 24 hours, nasoenteral nutrition, enteral nutrition by any route, witnessed aspiration, and administration of paralytic agents. Stress ulcer prophylaxis was not a predictor.

AMINOGLYCOSIDE ANTIBIOTICS

Dosage regimens with aminoglycoside antibiotics R

A more complete understanding of the pharmacodynamic properties of the aminoglycosides, e.g. their concentration-dependent antimicrobial activity, the post-antibiotic effect, and the process of adaptive resistance, has established the new concept of therapy with extended dosing intervals (22[R]).

At least 27 randomized clinical trials and eight meta-analyses have compared extended-interval treatment with multiple daily dosing. In all the studies, extended-interval dosing was at least as efficacious as multiple daily dosing, and may have been slightly better; it was no more toxic, and may have been less nephrotoxic. Extended dosing is also less expensive than multiple daily dosing and markedly reduces costs. However, not all populations of patients have been included in published trials. Therefore, conventional multiple daily aminoglycoside dosing with individualized monitoring should be used in neonates and children, in patients with moderate to severe renal insufficiency (creatinine clearance below 40 ml/min), serious burns (over 20% of body surface area), ascites, severe sepsis, endocarditis, and mycobacterial disease, in pregnancy, in patients on dialysis, in invasive P. aeruginosa infection in neutropenic pa-

tients, and with concomitant administration of other nephrotoxic agents (e.g. amphotericin, cisplatin, radiocontrast agents, and NSAIDs). Extended-interval aminoglycoside dosing may be safe and efficacious in patients with mild to moderate renal insufficiency (over 40 ml/min) and febrile neutropenia, especially where the prevalence of P. aeruginosa is low. In other serious Gram-negative infections warranting aminoglycoside treatment, extended-interval dosing is strongly suggested (23[r]).

Major considerations in determining the appropriate dose of an aminoglycoside are its volume of distribution and rate of clearance. Concern has been raised regarding the use of the Cockcroft–Gault equation with either actual or ideal bodyweight, resulting in systematic errors, especially in malnourished patients (24). However, even extended-interval dosing should not obviate the need for monitoring drug concentrations. Even in patients with normal renal function in whom treatment is necessary for over 3 days, mid-interval or trough drug concentrations should be obtained once or twice a week in order to optimize the dosing regimen (23[r], 25[r]).

New studies on once-daily aminoglycoside administration continue to appear. In a randomized trial in 249 patients with suspected or proven serious infections, the safety and efficacy of gentamicin once-daily compared with three-times-a-day was assessed in 175 patients who were treated with ticarcillin–clavulanate combined with gentamicin once daily or three times daily or with ticarcillin–clavulanate alone (26[C]). The achievement of protocol-defined peak serum gentamicin concentrations was required for evaluability. There were no significant differences between treatment regimens with respect to clinical or microbiological efficacy; the incidence of nephrotoxicity was similar in the three groups. In a post-hoc analysis, renal function was better preserved in those treated with gentamicin once a day plus ticarcillin–clavulanate than with ticarcillin–clavulanate only.

In 43 patients, once-daily tobramycin (4 mg/kg/day) was at least as effective and was no more and possibly even less toxic than a twice-daily regimen (27[C]).

Once-daily amikacin was as effective and safe as twice-daily dosing in a prospective randomized study of 142 adults with systemic infections (28[C]).

The pharmacokinetics of once-daily intravenous tobramycin have been investigated in seven children with cystic fibrosis (29[c]). All responded well. There was one case of transient ototoxicity but no nephrotoxicity.

In a prospective study, only increasing duration of once-daily aminoglycoside therapy was recognized as risk factor for toxicity in 88 patients aged 70 years and over (30[C]).

Formulations The pharmacokinetics and toxicity of liposomal amikacin have been investigated in a patient treated for advanced pulmonary multidrug-resistant tuberculosis (31[c]). The serum concentrations of amikacin obtained with the liposomal formulation were considerably greater than those obtained with the conventional formulation. Liposomal amikacin was well tolerated and led to clinical improvement, but the patient's sputum remained smear- and culture-positive during the treatment period and for 9 months.

Pharmacokinetics In 25 African–American patients, aminoglycoside pharmacokinetics were consistent with the published general population values. However, there was wide interpatient pharmacokinetic variability (32[C]).

Economics of therapeutic drug monitoring Plasma concentration measurement has become routine in an effort to minimize toxicity and maximize effectiveness. The economic impact of aminoglycoside toxicity and its prevention through therapeutic drug monitoring have been investigated in a cost-effectiveness study. It was estimated that to offset the cost of providing high-level drug monitoring, i.e. serum drug concentration monitoring with assessment and consultation by trained personnel using computerized resources to determine individualized pharmacokinetic parameters, for the purpose of achieving an optimum dosage regimen, by cost saving due to reducing nephropathy, the service should reduce the risk of nephrotoxicity by 6.6%. Therefore, high-level therapeutic drug monitoring is only cost-justified in populations in which high rates of nephrotoxicity would be expected. Risk factors for a high rate of nephrotoxicity include age, duration of therapy, high drug concentrations, the presence of ascites or liver disease, and the concomitant use of nephrotoxic drugs (33[R]). The economic significance of aminoglycoside peak concentrations has been assessed in 61 febrile neutropenic patients with hematological malignancies. Since the clinical outcome and average infection-related costs depended significantly on peak aminoglycoside concentration, it was concluded that successful pharmacokinetic intervention may save money (34[C]).

Mineral and fluid balance Repeated courses of intravenous tobramycin can cause *hypomagnesemic tetany* (35[c]).

Urinary system There is an *increase in the urinary output of tubular marker proteins* after aminoglycoside administration (36[C]). Determination of *N*-acetyl-β-D-glucosaminidase activity in the urine may be used as a screening test to facilitate early detection of the nephrotoxic effect of aminoglycosides (37[C]). Urine chemiluminescence may aid in the detection of neonatal aminglycoside-induced nephropathy (38[C]).

The mechanism underlying the nephrotoxic effect of aminoglycosides is incompletely understood, but it is accompanied by a reduction in lysosomal phospholipid catabolism. A lipopeptide, daptomycin, which has bactericidal activity against Gram-positive bacteria by inhibition of the synthesis of lipoteichonic acid, prevents tobramycin-induced nephrotoxicity in rats.

Fourier transformed infrared spectroscopy has been used to monitor the hydrolysis of phosphatidylcholine phospholipase A_2 in the presence of different aminoglycosides and/or daptomycin (39[C]). Among the various aminoglycosides investigated there were major differences, directly related to chemical structure. The number of charges, the size, and the hydrophobicity of the substituents of an aminoglycoside determined the influence on the lag phase, on the maximal rate, and on the final extent of hydrolysis. Daptomycin alone eliminated the initial latency period and reduced the maximal extent of hydrolysis. When daptomycin was combined with any of the aminoglycosides, the latency period also disappeared, but the phospholipase activity was higher than with the lipopeptide alone. The strongest activation of phospholipase A_2 activation was observed when daptomycin was combined with gentamicin.

Stress proteins seem to be actively involved in aminoglycoside-induced renal damage. In a study on Wistar rats, subcutaneous gentamicin caused tubular necrosis, followed by tubular regenerative changes and interstitial fibrosis (40[C]). Both the regenerated and phenotypically altered tubulointerstitial cells were found to express heat-shock protein 47 in and around the fibrosis. Increased shedding of tubular membrane components, followed by rapid inductive repair processes with overshoot protein synthesis, can be detected by analysis of tubular marker protein in the urine of rats after administration of aminoglycosides (36[C]).

Skin and appendages Neomycin can cause *contact sensitivity*, with cross-reactivity to other aminoglycoside antibiotics (41[c]).

Special senses Hereditary *deafness* is a heterogeneous group of disorders, with different patterns of inheritance and due to a multitude of different genes (42[R], 43[R]). The first molecular defect described was the A1555G sequence change in the mitochondrial 12S ribosomal RNA gene. A description of two families from Italy and 19 families from Spain has now suggested that this mutation is not as rare as was initially thought (44[C], 45[C]). The A1555G mutation is important to diagnose, since hearing maternal relatives who are exposed to aminoglycosides may lose their hearing. This predisposition is stressed by the fact that 40 relatives in 12 Spanish families and one relative in an Italian family lost their hearing after aminoglycoside exposure. Since the mutation can easily be screened, any patient with idiopathic sensorineural hearing loss may be screened for this and possible other mutations.

Two cases of hearing loss after short-term exposure to isepamicin sulfate, a new aminoglycoside with milder adverse effects, have also been described in patients with the A1555G mutation (46[c]).

In an Italian family of whom five family members became deaf after aminoglycoside exposure, the nucleotide 961 thymidine deletion associated with a varying number of inserted cytosines in the mitochondrial 12S ribosomal RNA gene was identified as a second pathogenic mutation that could predispose to aminoglycoside ototoxicity (47[C]). Molecular analysis excluded the A1555G mutation in this family.

Profound late postoperative deafness and prolonged neuromuscular blockade with respiratory insufficiency associated with the use of an aminoglycoside developed in a patient with end-stage renal disease undergoing bilateral nephrectomy (48[c]). Concurrent end-stage renal disease, visceral inflammation from chronic dialysis and laparotomy, and the concomitant use of clonazepam and clindamycin may have contributed to these unwanted effects.

In a prospective study on the prevalence of hearing impairment in an neonatal intensive care unit population (a total of 942 neonates were screened), aminoglycoside administration did not seem to be an important risk factor for communication-related hearing impairment (49[C]). In almost all cases, another factor was the more probable cause of the hearing loss (dysmorphism, prenatal rubella or cytomegaly, a positive family history of hearing loss, and severe peri- and postnatal complications).

The risk of ototoxicity after systemic aminoglycoside administration is well known (50), but there is still uncertainty about the risk of ototoxicity after ototopical aminoglycosides when the indication was appropriate (51[r], 52[r]). Nine cases of iatrogenic topical vestibulotoxicity have been reported (53[Cr]). All had used ear drops containing gentamicin sulfate and betamethasone sodium phosphate for prolonged periods. Toxicity was primarily vestibular rather than cochlear. Although compensation occurred in unilateral cases, the disability in bilateral cases was typically severe and often resulted in litigation.

The primary target for the ototopical effects of aminoglycosides remains controversial. It was generally believed that outer hair cells are primarily affected, followed by loss of inner hair cells; that degeneration starts basally and proceeds towards the apex; and that neural fibers and ganglion cells would degenerate secondarily to loss of hair cells. However, the possibility that spiral ganglion cells may be a primary target has been raised. In a postmortem study of 10 temporal bones from 6 patients (aged 11–40 years) with cystic fibrosis, whose pulmonary infections had been treated with systemic aminoglycosides (mainly tobramycin), in most cases combined with nebulized tobramycin, cytocochleograms were analyzed for each bone (54[C]). Four bones showed typical manifestations of aminoglycoside-induced ototoxicity, with loss of hair cells in the lower turns and degeneration of ganglion cells. Six bones showed no loss or scattered loss of hair cells, but there was degeneration of the spiral ganglion cells. This study supports the hypothesis that degeneration of spiral ganglion cells may occur as a primary manifestation in some cases of aminoglycoside-induced ototoxicity.

The effects of aminoglycosides on the medial efferent system have been assessed in awake guinea-pigs (55[C], 56[C]). The ensemble background activity and its suppression by contralateral acoustic stimulation was used as a tool to study the medial efferent system. A single intramuscular dose of gentamicin 150 mg/kg reduced or abolished the suppressive effect produced by activation of the olivocochlear system by contralateral low-level broadband noise stimulation. This effect was dose dependent and could be demonstrated ipsilaterally on the compound action potential, otoacoustic emissions, and ensemble background activity of the eighth nerve. Long-term gentamicin treatment (60 mg/kg for 10 days) had no effect, at least before the development of ototoxicity. Single-dose intramuscular netilmicin 150 mg/kg displayed blocking properties similar to gentamicin, although less pronounced, while amikacin 750 mg/kg and neomycin 150 mg/kg had no effect. With tobramycin 150 mg/kg and streptomycin 400 mg/kg a decrease in suppression was usually associated with a reduction of the ensemble background activity measured without acoustic stimulation, which may be a first sign of alteration to cochlear function. There was no correlation between specificity and degree of aminoglycoside ototoxicity and their action on the medial efferent system.

Possible mechanisms and preventive strategies have also been investigated in pigmented guinea-pigs (57[C]–59[C]). Animals who received α-lipoic acid (100 mg/kg/day), a powerful free radical scavenger, in combination with amikacin (450 mg/kg/day i.m.) had a less severe rise in compound action potential threshold than animals who received amikacin alone. In a similar study on pigmented guinea-pigs, the iron chelator deferoxamine (150 mg/kg bd for 14 days) produced a significant protective effect against ototoxicity induced by neomycin (100 mg/kg/day for 14 days). The spin trap α-phenyl-tert-butyl-nitrone also protected against acute ototopical aminoglycoside ototoxicity in guinea-pigs. These studies have provided further evidence for the hypothesis that aminoglycoside ototoxicity is mediated by the formation of an aminoglycoside-iron complex and reactive oxygen species.

Six patients presented with unilateral *vestibulotoxicity* after systemic gentamicin therapy (60[C]). All had ataxia and oscillopsia, but none had a history of vertigo. The authors suggested that a subacute course of vestibulotoxicity with time for compensation or asymmetrical recovery of vestibular function after bilateral vestibular loss could have explained the lack of vertigo in these patients.

The vestibulotoxic effect of streptomycin sulfate has been successfully used in the treatment of vertigo in patients with either bilateral Menière's disease or with Menière's disease in their only hearing ear (61[C]).

Immunological and hypersensitivity reactions *Acute respiratory failure* with near-fatal *bronchoconstriction* has been reported in an adult with bronchiectasis and chronic *P. aeruginosa* airways colonization immediately after the first inhalation of a commercially available gentamicin solution (62[c]).

Miscellaneous Several patients developed severe *shaking chills*, often accompanied by fever, tachycardia, and/or a significant reduction in systolic blood pressure within 3 hours of receiving intravenous once-daily dosing regimens of gentamicin produced by Fujisawa USA, Inc. (Deerfield, Illinois). Investigations showed that gentamicin formulations that contain concentrations of endotoxin that are within the USP standards may deliver amounts of endotoxin that are above the threshold for pyrogenic reactions with once-daily dosing (63[C]).

Interactions *Loop diuretics* greatly potentiate the cochleotoxic effects of single-dose systemic aminoglycosides. In pigmented guinea-pigs the effects of high-dose topical (10 μl of a 100 mg/ml solution directly on to the round window) or single-dose systemic (100 mg/kg) gentamicin and intracardiac administration of the loop diuretic etacrynic acid (40 mg/kg) on cochlear function have been studied (64[C]). Compound action potentials were elicited at 8 kHz. All animals who received etacrynic acid had an immediate and profound rise in hearing threshold, irrespective of the method of gentamicin administration. The maximum threshold shift occurred within 30 minutes. Animals who received topical gentamicin recovered after etacrynic acid treatment; by day 20 the mean threshold shift was 7 dB. This group did not differ statistically from animals who received etacrynic acid alone. In contrast, animals who received systemic gentamicin initially recovered within 2 hours after etacrynic acid, but subsequently deteriorated over the next 24 hours. The mean threshold shift was 70 dB at day 20. Animals who received topical gentamicin had a temporary shift that resolved within 24–48 hours; by day 20, the mean threshold shift was 7 dB. Animals treated with systemic gentamicin alone did not have hearing loss. This study suggests that the potentiating effect of etacrynic acid on aminoglycoside ototoxicity is only after systematic and not topical aminoglycoside administration. This may be due to an ethacrynic acid-induced increase in leakiness of the stria vascularis, thereby facilitating diffusion of aminoglycosides from the systemic circulation into the endolymphatic fluid.

BACITRACIN

Immunological and hypersensitivity reactions *Anaphylaxis* rarely occurs after topical administration of bacitracin ointment. Two new cases have been described (65[c], 66[c]).

A 45-year-old man developed a near-fatal anaphylactic reaction after he applied bacitracin ointment to an excoriated area on his foot. He had had a similar, but less severe, episode 4 years earlier. IgE antibodies to bacitracin were positive.

A 24-year-old man injured in a motorcycle accident was treated with viscous lidocaine and bacitracin zinc ointment for extensive abrasions on the extremities. Five minutes later, he developed symptoms of severe anaphylaxis and required adrenaline, antihistamines, intravenous fluids, and corticosteroids. Two weeks later, only the prick test to bacitracin zinc ointment was positive.

CHLORAMPHENICOL AND THIAMPHENICOL

The response to chloramphenicol has been assessed in cases of bacteremia due to vancomycin-resistant enterococci, of whom 65% received chloramphenicol. Among those in whom a response could be assessed, 61% had a clinical response, and 79% had a microbiological response. Mortality was non-significantly lower in patients treated with chloramphenicol. In cases with central line-related bacteremia, there was no difference in mortality among those treated with chloramphenicol, line removal, or both. No adverse effect could be definitely attributed to chloramphenicol (67^C).

Resistance High-level chloramphenicol-resistant strains of *Neisseria meningitides* serogroup B were isolated from 11 patients in Vietnam and one patient in France. Resistance was due to the presence of the catP gene on a truncated transposon that has lost mobility because of internal deletions (68^C).

Hematological *Aplastic anemia* Controversy remains about the risk of aplastic anemia with topical chloramphenicol. In a prospective case-control surveillance of aplastic anemia in a population of patients who had taken chloramphenicol for a total of 67.2 million person years, 145 patients with aplastic anemia and 1226 controls were analyzed. Three patients and five controls had been exposed to topical chloramphenicol, but two had also been exposed to other known causes of aplastic anemia. Based on these findings, an association between ocular chloramphenicol and aplastic anemia could not be excluded, but the risk was less than one per million treatment courses (69^C). In another study, a review of the literature identified seven cases of idiosyncratic hemopoietic reactions associated with topical chloramphenicol. However, the authors failed to find an association between the epidemiology of acquired aplastic anemia and topical chloramphenicol. Furthermore, after topical therapy they failed to detect serum accumulation of chloramphenicol by high-performance liquid chromatography. They concluded that these findings support the view that topical chloramphenicol was not a risk factor for dose-related bone-marrow toxicity and that calls for abolition of treatment with topical chloramphenicol based on current data are not supported (70^C).

In a study using general practitioner-based computerized data, 442 543 patients were identified who received 674 148 prescriptions for chloramphenicol eye-drops. Among these patients, there were three with severe hematological toxicity and one with mild transient *leukopenia*. The causal link between topical chloramphenicol and hematological toxicity was not further evaluated in detail (71^c).

Acute leukaemia The occurrence of acute leukemia has been studied in relation to preceding use of drugs (before the 12 months preceding the diagnosis) in a case-control study of 202 patients aged over 15 years with a diagnosis of acute leukemia and age- and sex-matched controls (72^C). Among users of chloramphenicol or thiamphenicol the odds ratio for any use was 1.1 (0.6–2.2) whereas the odds ratio for high doses was 1.8 (0.6–5.3). Other systemic antibiotics showed no substantial relation with the occurrence of leukemia.

Skin and appendages A case of a facial *contact dermatitis* due to chloramphenicol with cross-sensitivity to thiamphenicol has been reported (73^c).

Interactions Inhibition of *tacrolimus* clearance has been observed in an adolescent renal transplant recipient who was treated with standard doses of chloramphenicol for vancomycin-resistant enterococci. Toxic concentrations of tacrolimus were observed on the second day of chloramphenicol treatment, requiring an 83% reduction in the dose of tacrolimus (74^c).

A possible interaction between *ciclosporin* and chloramphenicol has been observed in a morbidly obese 17-year-old Hispanic girl who had a cadaveric renal transplantation 5 years before and took ciclosporin and prednisone for stabilization. She was treated with chloramphenicol 875 mg qds and ceftazidime 2 g tds for vancomycin-resistant enterococcal sinusitis. There was a substantial and sustained increase in ciclosporin concentrations after chloramphenicol was added. Normalization was achieved after withdrawal of chloramphenicol (75^c).

An interaction between *warfarin* and ocular chloramphenicol (5 mg/ml; 1 drop qds in each eye), which led to an increase in INR, has been suspected in a 83-year-old white woman. The authors suggested that the effect may be due to chloramphenicol inhibition of hepatic microsomal CYP2C9, since the pharmacologically active enantiomer S-warfarin is metabolized by this enzyme) (76^c).

GLYCOPEPTIDES *(SED-13, 757; SEDA-20, 245; SEDA-21, 276; SEDA-22, 276)*

The rise in *device-related infections* associated with coagulase-negative staphylococci as well as the emergence of β-lactam antibiotic-resistant Gram-positive bacilli has resulted in an increase in the use of glycopeptide antibiotics. Glycopeptides do not show concentration-dependent killing in the therapeutic range, but they have postantibiotic and sub-MIC effects. The rate of killing is slower for teicoplanin than for vancomycin. Comparative trials of teicoplanin and vancomycin have shown either a similar incidence of adverse effects or a higher number of adverse events in patients given vancomycin. In none of the trials was vancomycin better tolerated. The most common adverse effects include hypersensitivity, fever, pruritus, rash, rigors, diarrhea, nausea/vomiting, loss of hearing/balance, abnormal liver function tests, nephrotoxicity, and hematological abnormalities.

Red man syndrome is a troublesome effect of vancomycin infusion, but is extremely uncommon with teicoplanin, despite the fact that teicoplanin has a similar structure.

Of major concern is the *nephrotoxicity* of vancomycin combined with aminoglycosides. The incidence of nephrotoxicity with teicoplanin plus an aminoglycoside is lower than that with vancomycin plus an aminoglycoside. Ototoxicity is uncommon after the administration of vancomycin, and in many case reports of hearing loss, aminoglycoside usage, or renal failure may be confounding factors. However, the risks of ototoxicity and nephrotoxicity associated with vancomycin alone are low and not clearly related to serum drug concentrations.

There are similar incidences of *rash and fever* result after vancomycin and teicoplanin, but patients who react to one glycopeptide may not react to both.

Reversible *neutropenia and thrombocytopenia* can occur after administration of vancomycin. Thrombocytopenia is more frequent with teicoplanin, but it develops mostly at higher than normal doses.

Therapeutic drug monitoring remains controversial. There is evidence that predose concentrations of teicoplanin are related to clinical outcome; the evidence is less conclusive for vancomycin. Predose concentrations can be linked to some toxic effects (nephrotoxicity for vancomycin and thrombocytopenia to teicoplanin) (77[R], 78[R]).

Teicoplanin

Overdosage A 10-day-old girl with a history of post-asphyxia acute renal failure, which recovered within 7 days, was given teicoplanin for sepsis due to *Staphylococcus hominis* (79[c]). The dosage used was erroneously high (20 mg/kg/12 hours instead of an initial dose of 16 mg/kg followed by daily doses of 6–8 mg/kg), and therapy was suspended after 5 days. She improved, and blood cultures were negative. Serum creatinine concentrations and cystatin C (as an early marker of glomerular damage) remained in the reference ranges. Urinary parameters for tubulotoxicity (*N*-acetyl-β-D-glucosaminidase, β_1-microglobulin) were higher than in the following days, but remained in the reference ranges. Urinary concentrations of epithelial growth factor were also higher during therapy than afterwards, probably indicating repair activity. Serum concentrations of teicoplanin were not determined.

Vancomycin

In a prospective, observational study of 742 consecutive patients (390 men; mean age 51 years, range 17–86), the incidence, outcomes, and predictive factors of vancomycin-associated toxic effects in general oncology practice were assessed. In all, 47% had hematological malignancies, and of the patients with solid tumors, primary urogenital (12%) and breast (10%) tumors were most common. In 72% vancomycin was given in a dosage of 2 g/day, 16% received a prophylactic dose of 1 g/day, and 12% had an other regimen not specified. *Phlebitis* occurred in 3%, predominantly those with recently inserted central venous catheters. All responded promptly to local therapy, and withdrawal of the catheter or vancomycin was never required. *Skin rashes* occurred in 11%. However, all but four patients concomitantly received a β-lactam antibiotic. None of the rashes required withdrawal, although the β-lactam antibiotic was often discontinued. There was clinical evidence of *ototoxicity* in 6% of the patients who received other ototoxic drugs and only 3% of patients who were not receiving other ototoxic drugs. There was *nephrotoxicity* in 17%. Logistic regression was used to derive a model of risk of nephrotoxicity. Factors associated with an increased risk of nephrotoxicity included administration of other mild to moderate nephrotoxic agents or (APACHE) III scores over 40. Raised serum vancomycin concentrations did not reliably predict subsequent nephrotoxicity. The derived model was prospectively tested in a validation set of 359 patients. Sensitivity of the Nephrotoxicity Risk Index for any nephrotoxicity was 71% and for serious nephrotoxicity

100%. Specificity for any nephrotoxicity was 90% and for serious nephrotoxicity 81%. A main limitation of the study was the lack of patients who received only vancomycin. The concomitant administration of other agents may therefore have confounded the results (80[C]).

Urinary system *Acute interstitial nephritis* has been reported (81[c]).

A 64-year-old white man was treated with intravenous cloxacillin 2 g/4 hours for a *S. aureus* sternal wound infection and osteomyelitis. On day 14 cloxacillin was discontinued because of a fall in renal function. Urinalysis was positive for occasional red blood cells and hyaline casts, but there were no eosinophils. He was given intravenous vancomycin 1.5 g/36 hours. Renal function gradually improved and the dosing regimen was adjusted to 1.5 g/24 hours. Pre-dose vancomycin serum concentrations were 11.0 and 6.3 mg/l on days 23 and 30. On day 32, oral ciprofloxacin 500 mg bd was added for suspected sepsis (catheter tip cultures grew *Klebsiella pneumoniae*, although blood cultures were negative). Other medications were enteric-coated aspirin, warfarin, acebutolol, and digoxin. The next day, a progressing maculopapular rash developed and the patient continued to have a fever. Acute interstitial nephritis was confirmed by kidney biopsy. Hemodialysis was required, and he was treated with prednisone and made a gradual recovery. Four months later, he was treated with vancomycin for a relapse of the sternal infection. His eosinophil count rose and peaked at 18%, and there were eosinophils in the urine.

The authors found four other published cases of vancomycin-induced acute interstitial nephritis.

Skin and appendages *Linear IgA bullous dermatosis*, an uncommon subepidermal blistering disease characterized by deposition of IgA antibodies in a linear pattern along the epidermal basement membrane zone, is rarely associated with drugs. Intravenous vancomycin has previously been implicated.

After 7 days of antibiotic therapy with intravenous vancomycin, gentamicin, and ticarcillin-clavulanate for *P. aeruginosa* and *Staphylococcus aureus* sepsis, confluent erythematous-based vesicobullae developed in a 65-year-old woman with subarachnoid hemorrhage secondary to a ruptured aneurysm. Other medications included ranitidine, glyceryl trinitrate, nimodipine, ferrous sulfate, and phenytoin.

On the tenth day of antibiotic therapy with vancomycin, imipenem, and gentamicin for an infected enterocutaneous fistula, widespread bullae developed in a 60-year-old woman.

In a 71-year-old woman with pneumonia, vesicles and bullae developed on the eighth day of antibiotic therapy that consisted of one dose of intravenous vancomycin followed by a course of nafcillin.

In all cases, the diagnosis was confirmed by direct immunofluorescence (82[c], 83[c]). In the latter two cases, the blisters resolved after treatment with oral prednisone and withdrawal of antibiotics, whereas in the first case the rash completely resolved after discontinuation of therapy only.

Vasculitis rashes have been described rarely. Two case reports have suggested that there may be cross-reactivity between vancomycin and teicoplanin with respect to biopsy-proven leukocytoclastic vasculitis (84[c]). In both cases, vancomycin-induced vasculitis improved after drug withdrawal. Teicoplanin was started and the rash reappeared several days later. In one case the rash faded after teicoplanin had been withdrawn. In the other, teicoplanin was continued, but the rash improved after prednisolone was given.

Special senses The risk of *ototoxicity* has been assessed in a prospective study of 16 patients on continuous ambulatory peritoneal dialysis treated with two infusions of vancomycin (30 mg/kg) in 2 l of peritoneal dialysate administered at 6-day intervals for episodes of peritonitis (85[C]). Patients who were too ill to respond appropriately, those with pre-existing sensorineural hearing loss, those with a narrow auditory canal, those with a discharging ear or perforated tympanic membrane, and those receiving concurrent ototoxic drugs were excluded. The authors found no evidence of ototoxicity (pure-tone audiometry, electronystagmography, and clinical assessment), even with repeated courses of vancomycin. Average serum concentrations were in the target range. No adverse effects were recorded, except for a transient generalized pruritus in one patient after the start of infusion.

Hearing loss due to vancomycin toxicity has been treated by hemoperfusion and hemodialysis (86[c]).

A 14-month-old girl with chronic renal insufficiency due to renal dysplasia was empirically treated with ceftazidime and vancomycin for fever. Her calculated creatinine clearance was 10 ml/min/1.73 m^2. She erroneously received vancomycin 1.5 g in 3 doses 6 hours apart. Her serum creatinine concentration increased and her vancomycin concentrations remained markedly high (338 mg/l 5 hours after the third dose). The half-life of vancomycin was 145 hours. Hearing loss developed. Continued charcoal hemoperfusion and hemodialysis were used to treat the disorder. Thrombocytopenia was noted as a significant consequence of hemoperfusion. The patient did not fully recovered her previous renal function and became dialysis dependent. The audiogram normalized by 6 months.

Sexual function *Priapism* has been reported in a 37-year-old man with a 30-year history of severe diabetes mellitus after two doses of vancomycin 1 g i.v. for treatment of methicillin-resistant *S. aureus* bursitis (87[c]). The authors noted that an interaction between vancomycin and other medications (cefazolin, aztreonam, cyclosporine, prednisone, mycophenolate mofetil, and co-trimoxazole) could not be ruled out.

The first case of *prostatitis* due to vancomycin-resistant enterococci has been reported in a 42-year-old liver transplant recipient (88[c]). The organism, *E. faecium*, was resistant to vancomycin, ampicillin, ciprofloxacin, and doxycycline. Treatment with a combination of rifampicin and nitrofurantoin for 6 weeks resulted in a long-lasting cure.

Immunological and hypersensitivity reactions Vancomycin can cause a chemically mediated *anaphylactoid reaction*. α-tryptase is only detected in the blood during systemic anaphylactic reactions and may be released by degranulation from activated mast cells. Plasma tryptase activities were unchanged, independent of increased histamine concentrations, antihistamine pretreatment, and clinical symptoms of anaphylactoid reaction in 40 patients receiving vancomycin (1 g over 10 minutes) before elective arthroplasty (89[C]). The authors conclude that plasma tryptase activities can be used to distinguish chemical from immunological reactions.

A 47-year-old white woman with end-stage renal disease had had anaphylactoid shock after vancomycin 1 g i.v. infused over 1.5 hours and gentamicin 90 mg 3 years before, despite premedication with diphenhydramine (90[c]). She was treated with doubling doses of vancomycin every 30 minutes for methicillin-resistant *S. epidermidis*. She had no reaction. The authors could not exclude that the previous anaphylactoid reaction had not been due to gentamicin, as no specific testing was done. Although successful vancomycin desensitization has been described, this would be the first time in a patient with a history of anaphylactoid reaction.

Miscellaneous In a prospective, randomized, double-blind, placebo-controlled study of 30 patients who required vancomycin chemoprophylaxis before elective arthroplasty, oral pretreatment with either a histamine H_1 receptor antagonist (diphenhydramine 1 mg/kg) or a histamine H_2 receptor antagonist (cimetidine 4 mg/kg) significantly reduced the histamine-related adverse effects of rapid vancomycin infusion (91[C]).

Interactions Changes in pharmacokinetics were studied in male Wistar rats when intravenous vancomycin 100 mg/kg and levofloxacin 20 mg/kg were administered together (92[C]). There was an increase in the AUC and half-life of vancomycin. There was also an increase in the AUC and a delay in the t_{max} of levofloxacin, but no effect on C_{max}; these data suggested delayed absorption of levofloxacin. Concomitant administration had no effect on the correlation between serum and hepatic tissue concentrations of levofloxacin, but it markedly reduced the correlation between the serum and renal tissue concentrations of vancomycin. Vancomycin increased serum creatinine concentrations 8 hours after administration. However, there was no difference in animals who received monotherapy compared with animals who received combined therapy. The authors suggested the cautious use of a combination of levofloxacin and vancomycin and advised monitoring blood concentrations of vancomycin in such cases.

Monitoring A total of 167 infants and children without cancer and 42 cancer patients aged 3 months to 17.5 years with normal serum creatinine concentrations and without evidence of renal dysfunction were treated with intravenous vancomycin 30–40 mg/kg/day divided every 6 hours for various infections (93[r]). In 93% of the children without cancer, the peak serum vancomycin concentrations were in an adequate target range (8–55 μg/ml). However, 10% of the children with cancers had peak serum vancomycin concentrations below 10 μg/ml, and 21% had trough concentrations less than 5 μg/ml; an increased dosage was required to achieve adequate peak concentrations. There were no treatment failures. The authors suggested the following guidelines: first, to measure the serum creatinine concentration within 24 hours of beginning therapy to verify normal renal function, and weekly thereafter to detect an eventual reduction in creatinine clearance; an increase of serum creatinine of more than 44 μmol/l (0.5 mg/dl) over baseline should be followed by monitoring serum vancomycin concentrations. Second, the peak and trough vancomycin serum concentrations measurements are not necessary in children without cancer receiving 40 mg/kg/day or less who have normal renal function and do not receive other potentially nephrotoxic drugs. This approach should be individualized, based on factors such as degree of illness, poor clinical response, or persistent positive cultures. Third, monitoring should be considered for patients with cancer, neonates, those receiving concurrent nephrotoxic drugs, patients with renal insufficiency, and for dosages over 40 mg/kg/day.

Resistance The first case of methicillin-resistant *S. aureus* (MRSA) with intermediate resistance to vancomycin was documented in May 1996. Additional cases have now been described in the US, in a 59-year-old man with diabetes mellitus and chronic renal failure suffering from peritonitis, and in a 66-year-old man with diabetes who developed a septicemia after 18 weeks of vancomycin treatment for recurrent methicillin-resistant *S. aureus* bacteremia. In a 79-year-old man with diabetes and chronic renal failure, intermediate vancomycin-resistance developed after a 6-week therapy with vancomycin for MRSA bloodstream infection; the strain was identical to eight MRSA isolates obtained from hospitals in the New York City metropolitan area. All eight isolates, but not control isolates, could be transformed in vitro to develop intermediate resistance to vancomycin. Both the presence of glycopeptides and environmental factors, as demonstrated by increased resistance of *S. aureus* to antibiotics in the presence of prosthetic material in animals, can exert selective pressure to develop new resistance mechanisms (94[C], 95[C], 96[r]).

Reports of vancomycin-dependent enterococci that grow only in the presence of vancomycin and are best treated by discontinuation of the compound continue to appear (97[c]).

LINCOSAMIDES

Clindamycin

New indication Long-term oral clindamycin therapy has been successfully used in a 36-year-old woman in late-stage AIDS who presented with disseminated, nodular cutaneous lesions and underlying osteomyelitis due to a microsporidial infection with an Encephalitozoon-like species (98[c]).

In a multicenter, double-blind, randomized trial in 87 patients, clindamycin + primaquine was compared with co-trimoxazole as therapy for AIDS-related *Pneumocystis carinii* pneumonia; efficacy was similar. In patients with PaO_2 under 70 mmHg, clindamycin + primaquine was associated with fewer adverse events and less steroid use, but more rashes (99[C]).

Cardiovascular Clindamycin may prolong the QT interval and cause *ventricular fibrillation* (100[c]).

Gastrointestinal In a 1-year retrospective study at a tertiary hospital in Spain, 17% of 148 episodes of *diarrhea* associated with *Clostridium difficile* developed after therapy with clindamycin (101[C]). The possible association of toxin-positive *C. difficile*-induced colitis and the use of clindamycin phosphate vaginal cream for bacterial vaginosis has been reported in a 25-year-old white woman postpartum (102[c]).

Skin and appendages A first report of clindamycin-induced *fixed drug eruption* has been published (100[C]).

MACROLIDES

In 169 patients with acute infective rhinitis, azithromycin (500 mg/day for 3 days) resulted in a better cure rate after 11 days than placebo; however, after 25 days the results for both improvement and cure were equal (103[C]). Clarithromycin (250 mg bd for 10 days) was as effective as cefuroxime axetil (250 mg bd for 10 days) in the treatment of acute maxillary sinusitis in a randomized, double-blind, multicenter study of 370 patients; 10% of patients in each group had adverse events (104[C]). In a multicenter, parallel group, double-blind trial in 420 evaluable patients aged 6 months to 16 years with community-acquired pneumonia, the therapeutic effect of azithromycin (once daily for 5 days) was similar to that of co-amoxiclav in children under 5 years and to that of erythromycin tds for 10 days. Treatment-related adverse events occurred in 11% of those given azithromycin and 31% in the comparator group (105[C]). In a double-blind, randomized, multicenter trial in 302 children, a 10-day course of erythromycin estolate (40 mg/kg/day in two doses) was as safe and effective as amoxicillin (50 mg/kg/day in two doses) in acute otitis media. Treatment-related adverse events occurred in 5.3% of patients given erythromycin and in 7.3% of patients given amoxicillin (106[C]).

Azithromycin (500 mg/day for 3 days) has been used to treat acute periapical abscesses (107[C]). Of 150 patients treated with azithromycin 18 reported a total of 26 adverse events. Slightly more (24 out of 153) treated with co-amoxiclav reported 34 adverse events, but this difference did not reach statistical significance. Most of the adverse events (44/60) were gastrointestinal, mostly diarrhea or abdominal pain. There were no significant differences between the two groups in the severity of adverse events or in the number of withdrawals because of adverse events.

Treatment of facial comedonic and papulopustular acne with azithromycin (500 mg/day for 4 days in four cycles every 10 days) may be at least as effective as minocycline (100 mg/day for 6 weeks). Both were well tolerated and mild adverse effects were reported in 10% of patients given azithromycin and 12% of those given minocycline (108[C]).

In an uncontrolled study of 24 HIV-infected patients, roxithromycin (300 mg bd for 4 weeks) was effective against cryptosporidial diarrhea (109[C]). The most limiting adverse effects were *abdominal pain* (two patients), *raised hepatic enzymes* (two patients), and abdominal pain with raised hepatic enzymes (one patient). Minor symptoms occurred in nine patients.

In combination with proton pump inhibitors and other antibiotics, macrolides are still successfully used for the eradication of *Helicobacter pylori* infection (110[C], 111[C]). However, resistance of *H. pylori* to macrolides has emerged in a number of countries. The first case of *H. pylori* resistance to clarithromycin has now also been documented in Denmark and follows increased used of this macrolide in eradication regimens (112[c]). In a double-blind, multicenter trial in 328 patients with *H. pylori* infection and non-ulcer dyspepsia, omeprazole 20 mg bd, amoxicillin 1 g bd, and clarithromycin 500 mg bd was compared with omeprazole alone. The rate of success and quality of life were similar in both groups. There were no serious adverse events. However, there were 12 withdrawals in the group given omeprazole and antibiotics and two in the group given omeprazole alone. Diarrhea occurred in 63 patients in those given omeprazole and antibiotics and in 10 patients given omeprazole alone (113[C]). In another double-blind placebo-controlled trial eradication of *H. pylori* (omeprazole 20 mg, amoxicillin 1 g, and clarithromycin 500 mg bd) in long-term users of NSAIDs with past or current peptic ulcer or troublesome dyspepsia led to impaired healing of gastric ulcers and did not affect the rate of peptic ulcers or dyspepsia over 6 months (114[C]).

Azithromycin may be useful in reducing ciclosporin-induced gingival hyperplasia in renal transplant recipients (115[C]).

In a murine model of virus-induced lung injury, erythromycin significantly improved survival rate. This may be explained by inhibition of inflammatory-cell responses and suppression of nitric oxide overproduction in the lungs of the virus-infected mice (116[C]).

Mycobacterium avium complex (MAC) infection The incidence of disseminated MAC infection has increased dramatically with the AIDS epidemic. Treatment regimens for patients with a positive culture for MAC from a sterile site should include two or more drugs, including clarithromycin. Prophylaxis against disseminated MAC should be considered for patients with a CD4 cell count of less than 50 $\times 10^6$/l (117[R]). In a randomized, open-label trial in 37 patients with HIV-associated disseminated MAC infection, treatment with clarithromycin + ethambutol produced more rapid resolution of bacteremia, and was more effective at sterilization of blood cultures after 16 weeks than azithromycin + ethambutol (118[C]). However, in a randomized, double-blind, placebo-controlled multicenter trial in 174 HIV-infected patients with CD4 cell counts of under 100 $\times$ 10^6/l, azithromycin (1200 mg once a week) was safe and effective in preventing disseminated MAC infection, death due to MAC infection, and respiratory tract infections (119[C]).

Clarithromycin (0.75–2 g/day), minocycline (200 mg/day), and clofazimine (100 mg/day) for 15 months was investigated as treatment of MAC lung disease in 30 HIV-negative patients. Eight patients did not complete the study owing to deviations from protocol or adverse effects. Persistently negative cultures were found in 14 of the other patients. There were three cases of *hepatic disturbances* and three of ototoxicity, which required a reduction in clarithromycin dosage after a short interruption of treatment (120[C]).

Prophylaxis before insertion of intrauterine contraceptive devices (IUCDs) In a triple-masked, randomized, placebo-controlled study of 1867 women, prophylaxis with azithromycin 500 mg 1 hour before IUCD insertion did not affect the rate of IUCD removal, the frequency of postinsertion medical attention, or the risk of upper genital tract infection at 90 days. Women were at low risk of sexually transmitted disease according to self-reported medical history. Gastrointestinal adverse effects were infrequent (3% azithromycin; 2% placebo). Fewer women taking azithromycin (0.7%) than taking placebo (1.3%) were treated with antibiotics for pelvic tenderness; however, this difference was not statistically significant (121[C]). Since cervical infections increase the risk of pelvic infection in women who use IUCDs, generalization of these results may be difficult (122[r]).

Cystic fibrosis and the multidrug resistant protein In an open study, children with end-stage lung disease or chronic airflow limitation unresponsive to conventional therapy were treated with long-term azithromycin. Seven children (mean age 12 years), all of whom were colonized with *P. aeruginosa* and who took azithromycin for more than 3 months, were studied. There was a significant improvement in FVC and FEV_1 (123[c]). The mechanism whereby azithromycin works is unknown, but it may be other than antibacterial. It has been hypothesized that the effect may be due to upregulation of a P-glycoprotein, a member of the family of multidrug resistant proteins, since erythromycin upregulates P-glycoprotein expression in a monkey model. Multidrug resistance (MDR) is homologous to CFTR, and previous in vitro experiments have shown that the MDR and CFTR genes can complement each other (124[r]). However, direct proof of this hypothesis is lacking at the moment.

Cardiovascular In an FDA database analysis, 346 cases of *cardiac dysrhythmias* associated with erythromycin were identified. There was a preponderance of women, as there was among those with life-threatening ventricular dysrhythmias and deaths after intravenous erythromycin lactobionate. A sex difference in cardiac repolarization response to erythromycin is a potential contributing factor, since in an in vitro experiment on rabbit hearts, erythromycin caused significantly greater *QT prolongation* in female than in male hearts (125[C]).

Nervous system Clarithromycin may be associated with *delirium* (126[c]).

Skin and appendages Allergic reactions to macrolides seem to be very rare. Cross-reaction between different macrolides has not been previously described. Roxithromycin-induced generalized *urticaria* and tachycardia with a positive prick-test and a cross-reaction to erythromycin and clarithromycin has now been reported in a 31-year-old woman (127[c]). Other case reports have associated the use of clarithromycin with fixed drug eruptions and hypersensitivity reactions (128[c], 129[c]). The second possible case of *leukocytoclastic vasculitis* associated with clarithromycin has been reported in an 83-year-old woman who was treated for pneumonia. All her symptoms resolved after withdrawal and a short course of corticosteroids (130[c]).

Special senses Bilateral *ischemic optic neuropathy* may develop secondary to acute ergotism after administration of ergotamine tartrate and macrolides (131[c]).

Immunological and hypersensitivity reactions A 46-year-old man with asthma was treated with oral roxithromycin 300 mg/day for 5 days for purulent rhinitis and 2 weeks later developed arthritis, mononeuritis multiplex, eosinophilia (64%), eosinophilic infiltrations in the bone-marrow, raised IgE concentrations, and transient pulmonary infiltrates. *Churg–Strauss syndrome* was diagnosed. Retrospectively, a similar course of disease was observed 1 year before, after the administration of azithromycin (132[c]).

Interactions Erythromycin interacts with *simvastatin*, probably by inhibiting its metabolism by CYP3A4. In a randomized, double-blind cross-over study of 12 healthy volunteers, erythromycin significantly increased mean peak serum concentration and AUC for both unchanged simvastatin and its active metabolite simvastatin acid. However, there was extensive interindividual variability in the extent of this interaction (133[C]). Rhabdomyolysis, acute renal insufficiency, pancreatitis, ileus, livedo reticularis, and raised aminotransferase activities developed in a patient who had taken *lovastatin* for 7 years and took erythromycin before a dental procedure. In a review of the literature, three other reported instances of erythromycin and lovastatin interaction presenting with rhabdomyolysis, raised aminotransferase activities, and acute renal insufficiency were identified (134[c]).

A phase I clinical trial in 30 healthy men examined possible pharmacokinetic interactions between *rifabutin* and two macrolide antibiotics (azithromycin and clarithromycin), but was terminated because of adverse events. Neutropenia developed in 14 participants who took rifabutin, including all 12 subjects who also took azithromycin or clarithromycin. There was no pharmacokinetic interaction between azithromycin and rifabutin. However, the mean concentrations of rifabutin and 25-*O*-desacetylrifabutin (an active metabolite) in participants who took clarithromycin and rifabutin were respectively more than 400 and 3700% of concentrations in those who took rifabutin alone (135[C]).

The effect of macrolides on serum *theophylline* concentration and clearance has been investigated in 53 patients with moderate asthma treated with theophylline (400 mg/day) in a randomized trial. Erythromycin (500 mg bd) and roxithromycin (150 mg bd), but not clarithromycin (250 mg bd) or azithromycin (250 mg bd) caused increased serum theophylline concentrations and reduced clearance.

A 77-year-old woman taking *verapamil* and propranolol for hypertrophic cardiomyopathy and paroxysmal atrial fibrillation developed symptomatic bradycardia on two separate occasions within days of taking either erythromycin or clarithromycin. The proposed mechanism of the interaction was inhibition of cytochrome P450, since verapamil is a substrate of an isoenzyme that is inhibited by some macrolides (136[c], 137[c]). Severe hypotension and bradycardia after combined therapy with verapamil and clarithromycin has been reported in another case (138[c]).

Azithromycin may increase the anticoagulation effect of *warfarin* (139), and an abdominal hematoma has been reported after combined acenocoumarol and roxithromycin treatment (140[c]).

The association of frank psychosis due to combined therapy with *prednisone* and clarithromycin has been reported (141[c]).

Both *tiagabine* and erythromycin are metabolized by cytochrome P450. In an open-label, cross-over study of 13 healthy volunteers, tiagabine (4 mg bd) and erythromycin (500 mg bd) were co-administered for 4 days. Maximum plasma concentration, AUC, and half-life of tiagabine were comparable when tiagabine was administered alone or in combination with erythromycin. The t_{max} was prolonged after administration with erythromycin in women; this effect may be due to a differential effect of erythromycin on gastric emptying (142[C]). The interpretation of these findings may be limited by the rather low doses of tiagabine used in the study and the short time of co-administration.

Clarithromycin (500 mg bd for 10 days) significantly increased the steady-state maximum plasma concentration and the steady-state AUC of loratadine (10 mg/day for 10 days) (143[C]). In contrast, the addition of loratadine did not affect the steady-state pharmacokinetics of clarithromycin or its active metabolite, 14(R)-hydroxyclarithromycin. No QT_c interval exceeded 439 ms in any subject.

Erythromycin (333 mg tds for 10 days) had no effect on the pharmacokinetics of *felbamate* (3.0 or 3.6 g/d) used as monotherapy in epilepsy (144[C]).

In vitro testing systems for prediction of drug interactions in vivo Some macrolides form a complex with human CYP3A, leading to inactivation of the enzyme. A large number of pharmacokinetic drug interactions with macrolides can be explained by this metabolic inhibition. The interaction of common macrolides with triazolam, a substrate that is almost entirely metabolized by CYP3A, has been investigated in vitro using human liver microsomes. The results were verified in a controlled clinical trial in vivo in 12 healthy volunteers. The in vitro model identified macrolides that may impair triazolam clearance. The authors noted that in vitro models may be of value in providing a prospective estimate of the probability of a specific drug interaction. Such systems may allow cost-effective targeting of clinical drug interaction studies (145[C]).

QUINOLONES

Ciprofloxacin

In a multicenter, double-blind study 234 patients with acute bacterial exacerbations of chronic bronchitis, ciprofloxacin (500 mg bd) was associated with a trend toward a longer infection-free interval and a significantly higher bacteriological eradication rate compared with clarithromycin (500 mg bd) after 14 days (146[C]). In a similar study, ciprofloxacin (500 mg bd) was associated with an infection-free interval and clinical response that were similar to those achieved with cefuroxime axetil (500 mg bd), but the bacteriological eradication rate associated with ciprofloxacin was significantly higher (147[C]).

Nervous system The administration of ciprofloxacin may be associated with *confusion and general seizures* (148[c]) or *psychosis* (149[c], 150[c]).

Gastrointestinal Ciprofloxacin has been associated with *pseudomembranous colitis* (151[c]).

Urinary system A ciprofloxacin-associated *acute renal insufficiency* in cancer patients has previously been reported. Two cases of suggested ciprofloxacin-induced acute renal insufficiency in cancer patients undergoing high-dose chemotherapy and autologous stem cell rescue have now been added (152[c]). A case report has suggested that ciprofloxacin overdose may lead to acute renal insufficiency characterized by acute tubular necrosis with distal nephron apoptosis (153[c]).

Skin and appendages Ciprofloxacin can cause a *fixed drug eruption* (154[c]).

Special senses Topical 0.2% ciprofloxacin (0.2 ml od for 7 days) did not significantly affect the auditory brainstem response thresholds of guinea-pigs, whereas 4% gentamicin (0.2 ml od for 7 days) resulted in *total hearing loss* (155[C]).

Musculoskeletal An acute reversible *arthropathy* has been described in a child with cancer treated with a short course of ciprofloxacin for febrile neutropenia (156[c]).

Tendinopathy and *tendon rupture* as adverse events of fluoroquinolones have been reported before, and reports continue to appear (157[c], 158[c]). Another study has reported tendinitis and tendon rupture in six patients taking fluoroquinolones. Identified risk factors included renal insufficiency, glucocorticoid therapy, secondary hyperparathyroidism, advanced age, and diabetes mellitus (159[c]). A case of Achilles tendon rupture without any sudden pain has been reported in a 45-year-old female runner who developed bilateral tendinopathy of the Achilles tendon after repeated treatment with ciprofloxacin; histological analysis showed cystic changes with focal necrosis (160[c]).

Use in pregnancy Treatment with fluoroquinolones during embryogenesis was not associated with an increased risk of major malformations in a multicenter, prospective, controlled trial in 400 women. A higher rate of therapeutic abortions has been observed in quinolone-exposed women. This may be explained by the misperception of a major risk related to quinolones during pregnancy (161[C]).

Interactions Ciprofloxacin may alter plasma *clozapine* concentrations, which may be mediated by inhibition of cytochrome P450 enzymes (162[R]).

Ciprofloxacin may interact with *phenytoin* reducing phenytoin concentrations (163[c]). Besides this kinetic interaction, the possible epileptogenic potential of ciprofloxacin itself may contribute to the development of seizure activity.

A lower than expected phenytoin serum concentration has been measured in a 78-year-old white woman with a grade III astrocytoma of the right parieto-occipital region treated with ciprofloxacin (500 mg bd). Increased renal excretion has been suggested to be at least partly responsible for the increased clearance (164[c]).

Ciprofloxacin (500 mg bd) did not interfere with the ovarian suppression produced by the *oral contraceptive* Marvelon (30 μg of ethinylestradiol plus 150 μg of desogestrel) in 24 healthy women in a randomized, double-blind, placebo-controlled, cross-over trial (165[C]).

Fleroxacin

Encephalopathy with unconsciousness has been reported in a 48-year-old woman with Machado–Joseph disease after the administration of fleroxacin (200 mg/day) for 3 days. She recovered after withdrawal. The serum and cerebrospinal fluid concentrations of fleroxacin were within normal limits (166[c]).

Gatifloxacin

To study the impact on the normal intestinal microflora, the new broad-spectrum fluoroquinolone gatifloxacin was given to 18 healthy volunteers (400 mg/day orally). In the aerobic intestinal microflora *E. coli* strains were eliminated or strongly suppressed and the number of enterococci fell significantly, while the number of staphylococci increased. In the anerobic microflora the numbers of *Clostridia* and fusobacteria fell significantly. The microflora normalized 40 days after the gatifloxacin withdrawal. No selection or overgrowth of resistant bacterial strains or yeasts occurred (167[C]).

Grepafloxacin

Grepafloxacin is a new fluoroquinolone for the treatment of community-acquired respiratory tract infections. Its toxicological profile is similar to that of other fluoroquinolones. Its phototoxic potential is comparable to that of ciprofloxacin, but its effect on the QT interval is much less pronounced. In phase II and III trials in a total of more than 3000 patients, the most common adverse events with grepafloxacin 400 or 600 mg were gastrointestinal, such as *nausea, vomiting*, and *diarrhea.* Significantly more patients reported a mild unpleasant metallic taste with grepafloxacin than with ciprofloxacin, but under 1% of patients withdrew because of this. *Headache* occurred significantly more often with ciprofloxacin than grepafloxacin. In a study of more than 9000 patients, only 2.3% reported adverse events (*nausea* 0.8%; *gastrointestinal symptoms* 0.4%; *dizziness* 0.3%; *photosensitization* 0.04%). Rarely, an unpleasant taste has been reported as an adverse event in spontaneous reports (168[C]).

Levofloxacin

Levofloxacin has an improved pharmacokinetic profile that allows convenient once-daily dosing in either an oral or parenteral formulation. Levofloxacin has enhanced activity against Gram-positive aerobic organisms, including penicillin-resistant pneumococci. In comparative trials involving commonly used regimens, levofloxacin had equivalent if not greater activity in the treatment of community-acquired pneumonia, acute bacterial exacerbations of chronic bronchitis, acute bacterial sinusitis, acute pyelonephritis, and complicated urinary tract infection (169[R]).

In a prospective, multicenter open-label trial, 313 patients with clinical signs and symptoms of bacterial infections of the respiratory tract, skin, or urinary tract were treated with levofloxacin. Of these, 134 patients had a pathogen recovered from the primary infection site and had an MIC of the pathogen to levofloxacin determined. Levofloxacin generated clinical and microbiological response rates of about 95%. These response rates included pathogens such as *Strep. pneumoniae* and *S. aureus.* In a logistic regression analysis, the clinical outcome was predicted by the ratio of peak plasma concentration to MIC and site of infection. Microbiological eradication was predicted by the peak concentration/MIC ratio. Both clinical and microbiological outcomes were most likely to be favorable if the peak concentration/MIC ratio was at least 12 (170[C]).

Lomefloxacin

Photosensitivity was found in 44 (1.03%) of 4276 patients treated with lomefloxacin in Japan. Most cases were not severe and improved after withdrawal. Risk factors for a sensitivity reaction were age over 60 years with concomitant diseases and complications, total amount of lomefloxacin over 20 g, treatment for longer than 30 days, and previous treatment with a quinolone (171[C]).

Moxifloxacin

Moxifloxacin is a new 8-methoxyquinolone that has potent antimicrobial activity against both Gram-negative and Gram-positive bacteria and anerobes. In vitro it is highly effective against a wide spectrum of respiratory tract pathogens, has excellent efficacy against pneumococcal strains resistant to β-lactam and macrolide antibiotics, and has good activity against atypical respiratory tract pathogens. It does not seem to have phototoxic potential.

In a phase I trial, single-dose pharmacokinetics have been reported after oral administration of 50–800 mg in 45 healthy Caucasian men. Moxifloxacin was well tolerated. There were no serious adverse events, dropouts, or deaths. Only *weakness* was reported more often in the active treatment group. Other adverse events in subjects taking the active treatment included *Herpes simplex* labialis and *an ear disorder.* There were no changes in laboratory parameters, electrocardiograms, electroencephalograms, or findings on physical examination. Mean maximum concentrations of moxifloxacin in plasma ranged from 0.29 mg/l (50 mg dose) to 4.73 mg/l (800 mg dose) and were reached 0.4–4 hours after drug administration (MICs at which 90% of isolates of penicillin-resistant *Strep. pneumoniae* were inhibited were below 0.125 mg/l). Plasma concentrations fell in a biphasic manner: within 4–5 hours, they fell to 30–55% of the C_{max}. A terminal half-life of 11–14 hours accounted for most of the AUC. Protein binding was about 48%. There was partial tubular reabsorption. No major active metabolites were detected. Concentrations in saliva were higher than in the plasma during the absorption phase, whereas in the terminal phase there was a constant saliva : plasma concentration ratio of 0.5–1 (172[C]).

In an open-label, randomized, cross-over study, the absolute systemic availability of a single 100 mg dose of moxifloxacin was 0.92 in 10 healthy men (mean age 29 years). There was no evidence of active tubular secretion. Both the oral and intravenous formulations were well tolerated, with five reported possible or probable drug-related adverse events, including *headache, nausea*, and localized *urticaria* (173[C]).

In contrast to some other fluoroquinolones, moxifloxacin appears to have a low propensity for causing CNS excitatory effects. The most common adverse events are *gastrointestinal disturbances.* The systemic availability of moxifloxacin is substantially reduced by coadministration with an *antacid* or *iron*. However, it does not interact with theophylline or warfarin (174[R]).

Norfloxacin

Special senses *A corneal ulcer* associated with deposits of norfloxacin in the right eye has been reported in a 40-year-old man with right trigeminal and facial nerve palsies and reduced tear secretion. The patient stopped using norfloxacin ophthalmic solution and recovered (175[c]).

Ofloxacin

The safety and efficacy of topical ofloxacin ear drops 0.3% (0.25 ml bd) has been compared with that of co-amoxiclav oral suspension (40 mg/kg/day) for acute otitis media in 286 children aged 1–12 years with tympanostomy tubes in place. Topical ofloxacin was as effective as and better tolerated than systemic therapy with co-amoxiclav. Treatment-related adverse event rates were 31% for co-amoxiclav and 6% for ofloxacin (176[C]).

Sparfloxacin

An analysis of phase III trials showed that 401 of 1585 patients treated with sparfloxacin reported at least one adverse event related to the study medication. Adverse events that were reported more often with sparfloxacin than with comparator drugs include *photosensitivity reactions* and *prolongation of the QT_c interval.* Gastrointestinal symptoms (*diarrhea, nausea, dyspepsia, abdominal pain, vomiting*, and *flatulence*), *insomnia*, and *taste disturbances* were also more common in patients taking comparator drugs. Sparfloxacin was discontinued in 6.6% of patients, whereas 8.9% of patients taking other drugs stopped therapy owing to adverse events (177[C]).

Interactions Concurrent treatment with *antacids* reduces the oral absorption of many quinolones. In an open-label, single-dose (400 mg), randomized, four-way cross-over study of 20 male volunteers (aged 18–38 years), Maalox (30 ml) given 4 hours after sparfloxacin did not cause a statistically significant reduction in the rate and extent of sparfloxacin absorption. In contrast, Maalox given 2 hours before or 2 hours after sparfloxacin did reduce its absorption: AUC fell by 23% and 17% respectively and mean C_{max} by 29 and 13% (178[C]).

Trovafloxacin

Trovafloxacin is a new fluoroquinolone with enhanced activity against Gram-positive and anerobic micro-organisms that can be given once a day. It is effective in the treatment of nosocomial or community-acquired respiratory tract infections, meningococcal meningitis in children, and urinary tract infections. Common adverse events included *dizziness, headache*, and *gastrointestinal intolerance* (179[R]). However, in 1999, trovafloxacin was withdrawn from the market owing to *hepatotoxicity.*

SULFONAMIDES, TRIMETHOPRIM, AND CO-TRIMOXAZOLE

The broad-spectrum bacteriostatic sulfonamides remain among the most widely used antibiotics, owing to their low cost, low toxicity, and excellent activity against common bacterial diseases. They interfere with bacterial synthesis of folic acid by inhibiting dihydropteroate synthetase. The synergistic action with trimethoprim, an inhibitor of dihydrofolate reductase, has brought about an enormous resurgence in sulfonamide use. Adverse reactions are uncommon and include *nausea, vomiting, diarrhea, anorexia*, and *hypersensitivity reactions.* Severe adverse events are rare, but cases of *erythema multiforme, Stevens–Johnson syndrome, Lyell's syndrome*, and *exfoliative dermatitis* have been described (180[R]).

Sulfonamides

Skin and appendages A case of *linear IgA dermatosis* with erythema multiforme-like clinical features has been reported in a 19-year-old man several days after completion of a 5-day course of treatment with sulfadimethoxynum (500 mg bd) for a flu-like syndrome. Treatment with methylprednisolone (150 mg) with gradual dosage reduction was started. Slow improvement was followed by a flare-up after reduction to 80 mg/day. Therapy was changed to dapsone 100 mg/day, and there was a dramatic improvement (181[c]). Fixed drug eruption has been described in a patient treated with the non-thiazide sulfonamide diuretic indapamide; an oral challenge test showed cross-reactivity to sulfamethoxazole and sulfadiazine (182[c]).

A mechanism for generalized drug-induced delayed skin reactions to sulfamethoxazole may be perforin-mediated killing of keratinocytes by drug-specific CD4+ lymphocytes. The requirement of interferon-γ pretreatment of keratinocytes for efficient specific killing might explain the increased frequency of drug allergies in generalized viral infections such as HIV, when interferon-γ concentrations are raised (183[C]).

Trimethoprim

Skin and appendages At least eight cases of skin eruptions associated with trimethoprim (*fixed drug eruptions, toxic epidermal necrolysis, phototoxic eruption*, and *erythema multiforme*) have been previously reported. Generalized erythematous skin eruptions have now been reported in a 20-year-old Japanese woman and a 70-year-old Japanese man (184[c]). Patch tests showed that trimethoprim alone was responsible for the erythematous papular type skin eruption in the young woman. The old man's skin responded to both trimethoprim and sulfamethoxazole.

Topical provocation of fixed drug eruption and positive reactions with co-trimoxazole are extremely rare and have never been seen on unaffected skin. In a 42-year-old Caucasian woman with histopathologically confirmed fixed drug eruption induced by co-trimoxazole, positive topical provocation by trimethoprim was obtained on both involved and uninvolved skin (185[c]).

Amino acids A median *increase in serum homocysteine* of 50% (range 27–333%) was found in seven healthy male volunteers after a 2-week course of trimethoprim 300 mg bd. Concomitantly, serum folate concentrations fell significantly. By day 50, baseline values of homocysteine and folate were regained. Since tetrahydrofolate serves as a methyl group carrier in the remethylation of homocysteine to methionine, the inhibitory effect of trimethoprim on dihydrofolate reductase may be most important, but other mechanisms could not be excluded (186[c]).

Immunological and hypersensitivity reactions The case histories of 13 patients (12 women and one man, aged 22–68 years) with *anaphylactic reactions* to trimethoprim alone that were reported to a national drug safety unit have been analyzed. Nine were classified as probable anaphylaxis. The casual relation between exposure to trimethoprim and anaphylaxis was classified as definite in three reports, possible in four, and probable in six. In one patient, IgE antibodies against trimethoprim were demonstrated (187[C]).

Interactions Fatal bone-marrow suppression has been reported in an 82-year-old woman who took *methotrexate* 7.5 mg/week for 1 year for rheumatoid arthritis without hematological problems. She was given trimethoprim 100 mg/day at first and later 200 mg/day. One week later, she developed severe pancytopenia. The bone-marrow failed to recover despite treatment with folinic acid and G-CSF, and she died of bronchopneumonia. In a literature review, the authors found two other cases of bone-marrow suppression after treatment with methotrexate and trimethoprim with full recovery of both. This interaction is also listed in the *British National Formulary* 1997 (188[c], 189[c]).

Miscellaneous *Culture-negative arthritis, bilateral uveitis, mucocutaneous Stevens–Johnson syndrome, and eosinophilia* developed in a 31-year-old woman after 3 days of therapy with oral trimethoprim 160 mg bd for a lower urinary tract infection. At the start of antibiotic therapy, corticosteroids and local anesthetics were injected into the lateral aspect of the right knee. Recovery was rapid after trimethoprim was withdrawn. Two months later she developed headache, nausea, malaise, and bilateral uveitis after taking trimethoprim again (136[c]).

Co-trimoxazole

Respiratory *Pneumonitis* developed after the administration of co-trimoxazole in a patient with intractable ulcerative colitis complicated by *Pneumocystis carinii* pneumonia. This patient had also previously had sulfasalazine-induced pneumonitis (190[c]).

Mineral and fluid balance A 41-year-old black man with AIDS and sickle cell anemia was treated on two separate occasions with co-trimoxazole and prednisone 40 mg/day for *Pneumocystis carinii* pneumonia. On both occasions he developed a hyperkalemic metabolic acidosis together with renal tubular acidosis after several days of therapy. Hyperkalemia due to co-trimoxazole has been repeatedly reported. This may be due to the trimethoprim component, which bears structural homology to the potassium-sparing diuretic amiloride. However, there are only a few reports on concurrent acidosis. This could be explained if the action of trimethoprim, like that of amiloride, is limited to the cortical collecting tubule but does not affect the medullary collecting tubule, which has a large capacity to secrete hydrogen ions and may therefore prevent the development of acidosis. Predisposing factors for the rare adverse effect of renal tubular acidosis in this case may have been aldosterone deficiency or resistance, medullary dysfunction of sickle cell anemia, and renal insufficiency. All these factors could contribute to impaired renal handling of secretion of hydrogen ions (191[c]). According to studies on animals, tetroxoprim, which is structurally similar to trimethoprim, has stronger antikaliuretic effects than trimethoprim. Tetroxoprim-induced hyperkalemia has not been described yet. However, it is only rarely used and dosages are low (192[R]).

Immunological and hypersensitivity reactions The incidence of adverse reactions to co-trimoxazole in HIV-infected patients is high. Several reports have shown that a incremental increase in drug dosage may allow a significant proportion of patients to tolerate prophylactic dosages of co-trimoxazole. In a new study, eight of 14 selected HIV-infected patients (13 men, 1 woman; patients who experienced severe reactions such as anaphylaxis or Stevens–Johnson syndrome were excluded) were successfully desensitized and after a regimen of gradual incremented exposure over 11 days as an outpatient procedure could continue to take co-trimoxazole (193[C]). *N*-acetylcysteine (3 g of a 20% liquid solution bd) did not prevent hypersensitivity reactions to co-trimoxazole in HIV-infected patients (194[C]). Although cross-reactivity can occur, dapsone may be used for patients with mild hypersensitivity reactions to co-trimoxazole for prophylaxis of *Pneumocystis carinii* pneumonia (195[C]).

REFERENCES

1. Beringer PM, Wong-Beringer A, Rho JP. Economic aspects of antibacterial adverse effects. Pharmacoeconomics 1998;13:35–49.
2. Evans RS, Pestotnik SL, Classen DC, Clemmer TP, Weaver LK, Orme JF Jr, Lloyd JF, Burke JP. A computer-assisted management program for antibiotics and other antiinfective agents. New Engl J Med 1998;338:232–8.
3. Garibaldi RA. Computers and the quality of care—a clinician's perspective. New Engl J Med 1998;338:259–60.
4. Talan DA, Citron DM, Abrahamian FM, Morgan GJ, Goldstein EJC. Bacteriologic analysis of infected dog and cat bites. New Engl J Med 1999;340:85–92.
5. Fleisher GR. The management of bite wounds. New Engl J Med 1999;340:138–40.
6. Aronin SI, Peduzzi P, Quagliarello VJ. Community-acquired bacterial meningitis: risk stratification for adverse clinical outcome and effect of antibiotic timing. Ann Intern Med 1998; 129:862–9.
7. Strom BL, Abrutyn E, Berlin JA, Kinman JL, Feldman RS, Stolley PD, Levison ME, Korzeniowski OM, Kaye D. Dental and cardiac risk factors for infective endocarditis. A population-based, case-control study. Ann Intern Med 1998; 129:761–9.
8. Durack DT. Antibiotics for prevention of endocarditis during dentistry: time to scale back? Ann Intern Med 1998;129:829–31.
9. Cunha BA. Antibiotic selection for the treatment of sinusitis, otitis media, and pharyngitis. Infect Dis Clin Pract 1998;7(Suppl 5):S324–6.
10. Cunha BA, Shea KW. Emergence of antimicrobial resistance in community-acquired pulmonary pathogens. Semin Respir Infect 1998;13:43–53.
11. Cunha BA. Antibiotic resistance. Control strategies. Crit Care Clin 1998;14:309–27.
12. Speich R, Imhof E, Vogt M, Grossenbacher M, Zimmerli W. Efficacy, safety, and tolerance of piperacillin/tazobactam compared to co-amoxiclav plus an aminoglycoside in the treatment of severe pneumonia. Eur J Clin Microbiol Infect Dis 1998;17:313–17.
13. George JN, Raskob GE, Shah SR, Rizvi MA, Hamilton SA, Osborne S, Vondracek T. Drug-induced thrombocytopenia: a systematic review of published case reports. Ann Intern Med 1998;129:886–90.
14. Pedersen BU, Andersen M, Hansen PB. Drug-specific characteristics of thrombocytopenia caused by non-cytotoxic drugs. Eur J Clin Pharmacol 1998;54:701–6.
15. Zerbib F. Les oesophagites médicamenteuses. Hepato-Gastro 1998;5:115–20.
16. Nord CE, Bergogne-Berezin E, McFarland LV, Breves G. Impact des antibiotiques sur le tube digestif. Presse Med 1998;27:2004–5.
17. Mahboob A, Haroon TS. Drugs causing fixed eruptions: a study of 450 cases. Int J Dermatol 1998;37:833–8.
18. Moorthy RS, Valluri S, Jampol LM. Drug-induced uveitis. Surv Ophthalmol 1998;42: 557–70.
19. Anonymous. Drug-induced uveitis can usually be easily managed. Drugs Ther Perspect 1998; 11:11–14.
20. Pichler WJ, Schnyder B, Zanni MP, Hari Y, Von Greyers S. Role of T cells in drug allergies. Allergy 1998;53:225–32.
21. Cook DJ, Walter SD, Cook RJ, Griffith LE, Guyatt GH, Leasa D, Jaeschke RZ, Brun-Buisson C. Incidence of and risk factors for ventilator-associated pneumonia in critically ill patients. Ann Intern Med 1998;129:433–40.
22. Lacy MK, Nicolau DP, Nightingale CH, Quintiliani R. The pharmacodynamics of aminoglycosides. Clin Infect Dis 1998;27:23–7.
23. Gerberding JL. Aminoglycoside dosing: timing is of the essence. Am J Med 1998;105:256–8.
24. Kotler DP, Sordillo EM. Nutritional status and aminoglycoside dosing. Clin Infect Dis 1998; 26:249–50.
25. Bailey TC, Reichley RM. Nutritional status and aminoglycoside dosing. Clin Infect Dis 1998; 26:251–2.
26. Gilbert DN, Lee BL, Dworkin RJ, Legget JL, Chambers HF, Modin G, Tauber MG, Sande MA. A randomized comparison of the safety and efficacy of once-daily gentamicin or thrice-daily gentamicin in combination with ticarcillin–clavulanate. Am J Med 1998;105:182–91.
27. Sanchez-Alcaraz A, Vargas A, Quintana MB, Rocher A, Querol JM, Poveda JL, Hermenegildo M. Therapeutic drug monitoring of tobramycin: once-daily versus twice-daily dosage schedules. J Clin Pharm Ther 1998;23:367–73.
28. Karachalios GN, Houpas P, Tziviskou E, Papalimneou V, Georgiou A, Karachaliou I, Halkiadaki D. Prospective randomized study of once-daily versus twice-daily amikacin regimens in patients with systemic infections. Int J Clin Pharmacol Ther 1998;36:561–4.
29. Bragonier R, Brown NM. The pharmacokinetics and toxicity of once-daily tobramycin therapy in children with cystic fibrosis. J Antimicrob Chemother 1998;42:103–6.
30. Paterson DL, Robson JM, Wagener MM. Risk factors for toxicity in elderly patients given aminoglycosides once daily. J Gen Intern Med 1998;13:735–9.
31. Whitehead TC, Lovering AM, Cropley IM, Wade P, Davidson RN. Kinetics and toxicity of liposomal and conventional amikacin in a patient with multidrug-resistant tuberculosis. Eur J Clin Microbiol Infect Dis 1998;17:794–7.
32. Oparaoji EC, Siram S, Elemihe U, Mezghebe HM, Cho T, Bashiri M, Piedrahita K, Pipalla RS. Aminoglycoside pharmacokinetics in African-Americans with normal renal function. J Clin Pharmacol Ther 1998;23:191–7.
33. Slaughter RL, Cappelletty DM. Economic impact of aminoglycoside toxicity and its prevention

through therapeutic drug monitoring. Pharmacoeconomics 1998;14:385–94.

34. Binder L, Schiel X, Binder C, Menke CFA, Schuttrumpf S, Armstrong VW, Unterhalt M, Erichsen N, Hiddemann W, Ollerich M. Clinical outcome and economic impact of aminoglycoside peak concentrations in febrile immunocompromised patients with hematologic malignancies. Clin Chem 1998;44:408–14.
35. Adams JP, Conway SP, Wilson C. Hypomagnesaemic tetany associated with repeated courses of intravenous tobramycin in a patient with cystic fibrosis. Respir Med 1998;92:602–4.
36. Scherberich JE, Mondorf WA. Nephrotoxic potential of antiinfective drugs as assessed by tissue-specific proteinuria of renal antigens. Int J Clin Pharmacol Ther 1998;36:152–8.
37. Marchewka Z, Dlugosz A. Enzymes in urine as markers of nephrotoxicity of cytostatic agents and aminoglycoside antibiotics. Int Urol Nephrol 1998;30:339–48.
38. Panova LD, Farkhutdinov RR, Akhmadeeva EN. [Urine chemiluminescence in preclinical diagnosis of neonatal drug-induced nephropathy]. Urol Nefrol Mosk 1998;4:25–9.
39. Carrier D, Bou KM, Kealey A. Modulation of phospholipase A-2 activity by aminoglycosides and daptomycin: a Fourier transform infrared spectroscopic study. Biochemistry 1998;37:7589–97.
40. Cheng M, Razzaque MS, Nazneen A, Taguchi T. Expression of the heat shock protein 47 in gentamicin-treated rat kidneys. Int J Exp Pathol 1998;79:125–32.
41. Kimura M, Kawada A. Contact sensitivity induced by neomycin with cross-sensitivity to other aminoglycoside antibiotics. Contact Dermatitis 1998; 39:148–50.
42. Hardisty RE, Fleming J, Steel KP. The molecular genetics of inherited deafness—current knowledge and recent advances. J Laryngol Otol 1998; 112:432–7.
43. Steel KP. Progress in progressive hearing loss. Science 1998;279:1870–1.
44. Casano RAMS, Bykhovskaya Y, Johnson DF, Hamon M, Torricelli F, Bigozzi M, Fischel-Ghodsian N. Hearing loss due to the mitochondrial A1555G mutation in Italian families. Am J Med Genet 1998;79:388–91.
45. Estivill X, Govea N, Barcelo A, Perello E, Badenas C, Romero E, Moral L, Scozzari R, D'Urbano L, Zeviani M, Torroni A. Familial progressive sensorineural deafness is mainly due to the mtDNA A1555G mutation and is enhanced by treatment of aminoglycosides. Am J Hum Genet 1998;62:27–35.
46. Usami S-I, Abe S, Tono T, Komune S, Kimberling WJ, Shinkawa H. Isepamicin sulfate-induced sensorineural hearing loss in patients with the 1555 A $\rightarrow$ G mitochondrial mutation. ORL J Otorhinolaryngol Relat Spec 1998;60:164–9.
47. Casano RA, Johnson DF, Bykhovskaya Y, Torricelli F, Bigozzi M, Fischel-Ghodsian N. Inherited susceptibility to aminoglycoside ototoxicity: genetic heterogeneity and clinical implications. Am J Otolaryngol 1999;20:151–6.
48. Gilbert TB, Jacobs SC, Quaddoura AA. Deafness and prolonged neuromuscular blockade following single-dose peritoneal neomycin irrigation. Can J Anaesth 1998;45:568–70.
49. Hess M, Finckh-Kramer U, Bartsch M, Kewitz G, Versmold H, Gross M. Hearing screening in at-risk neonate cohort. Int J Pediatr Otorhinolaryngol 1998;46:81–9.
50. Tange RA. Ototoxicity. Adv Drug React Toxicol Rev 1998;17:75–89.
51. Indudharan R. Ototopic aminoglycosides and ototoxicity. J Otolaryngol 1998;27:182.
52. Walby P, Stewart R, Kerr AG. Aminoglycoside ear drop ototoxicity: a topical dilemma? Clin Otolaryngol 1998;23:289–90.
53. Marais J, Rutka JA. Ototoxicity and topical eardrops. Clin Otolaryngol 1998;23:360–7.
54. Sone M, Schachern PA, Paparella MM. Loss of spiral ganglion cells as primary manifestation of aminoglycoside ototoxicity. Hear Res 1998; 115:217–23.
55. Lima da Costa D, Erre J-P, Pehourq F, Aran J-M. Aminoglycoside ototoxicity and the medial efferent system: II. Comparison of acute effects of different antibiotics. Audiology 1998;37:162–73.
56. Lima da Costa D, Erre J-P, Aran J-M. Aminoglycoside ototoxicity and the medial efferent system: I. Comparison of acute and chronic gentamicin treatments. Audiology 1998;37:151–61.
57. Conlon BJ, Perry BP, Smith DW. Attenuation of neomycin ototoxicity by iron chelation. Laryngoscope 1998;108:284–7.
58. Conlon BJ, Aran J-M, Erre J-P, Smith DW. Attenuation of aminoglycoside-induced cochlear damage with the metabolic antioxidant alpha-lipoic acid. Hear Res 1999;128:40–4.
59. Hester TO, Jones RO, Clerici WJ. Protection against aminoglycoside otic drop-induced ototoxicity by a spin trap: I. Acute effects. Otolaryngol Head Neck Surg 1998;119:581–7.
60. Waterston JA, Halmagyi GM. Unilateral vestibulotoxicity due to systemic gentamicin therapy. Acta Oto Laryngol 1998;118:474–8.
61. Balyan FR, Taibah A, De Donato G, Aslan A, Falcioni M, Russo A, Sanna M. Titration streptomycin therapy in Menière's disease: long-term results. Otolaryngol Head Neck Surg 1998; 118:261–6.
62. Melani AS, Di Gregorio A. Acute respiratory failure due to gentamicin aerosolization. Monaldi Arch Chest Dis 1998;53:274–6.
63. Anonymous. Endotoxin-like reactions associated with intravenous gentamicin—California, 1998. Morb Mortal Wkly Rep 1998;47:877–80.
64. Conlon BJ, McSwain SD, Smith DW. Topical gentamicin and ethacrynic acid: effects on cochlear function. Laryngoscope 1998;108:1087–9.
65. Lin FL, Woodmansee D, Patterson R. Near-fatal anaphylaxis to topical bacitracin ointment. J Allergy Clin Immunol 1998;101:136–7.

66. Saryan JA, Dammin TC, Bouras AE. Anaphylaxis to topical bacitracin zinc ointment. Am J Emerg Med 1998;16:512–13.
67. Lautenbach E, Schuster MG, Bilker WB, Brennan PJ. The role of chloramphenicol in the treatment of bloodstream infection due to vancomycin-resistant *Enterococcus*. Clin Infect Dis 1998;27:1259–65.
68. Galimand M, Gerbaud G, Guibourdenche M, Riou J-Y, Courvalin P. High-level chloramphenicol resistance in *Neisseria meningitidis*. New Engl J Med 1998;339:868–74.
69. Laporte JR, Vidal X, Ballarin E, Ibanez L. Possible association between ocular chloramphenicol and aplastic anaemia—the absolute risk is very low. Br J Clin Pharmacol 1998;46:181–4.
70. Walker S, Diaper CJ, Bowman R, Bowman R, Sweeney G, Seal DV, Kirkness CM. Lack of evidence for systemic toxicity following topical chloramphenicol use. Eye 1998;12:875–9.
71. Lancaster T, Swart AM, Jick H. Risk of serious haematological toxicity with use of chloramphenicol eye drops in a British general practice database. Br Med J 1998;316:667.
72. Traversa G, Menniti-Ippolito F, Da Cas R, Mele A, Pulsoni A, Mandelli F. Drug use and acute leukemia. Pharmacoepidemiol Drug Saf 1998;7:113–23.
73. Le CC, Santinelli F. Facial contact dermatitis from chloramphenicol with cross-sensitivity to thiamphenicol. Contact Dermatitis 1998;38:108–9.
74. Schulman SL, Shaw LM, Jabs K, Leonard MB, Brayman KL. Interaction between tacrolimus and chloramphenicol in a renal transplant recipient. Transplantation 1998;65:1397–8.
75. Bui L, Huang DD. Possible interaction between cyclosporine and chloramphenicol. Ann Pharmacother 1999;33:252–3.
76. Leone R, Ghiotto E, Conforti A, Velo G. Potential interaction between warfarin and ocular chloramphenicol. Ann Pharmacother 1999;33:114.
77. Wilson AP. Comparative safety of teicoplanin and vancomycin. Int J Antimicrob Agents 1998;10:143–52.
78. MacGowan AP. Pharmacodynamics, pharmacokinetics, and therapeutic drug monitoring of glycopeptides. Ther Drug Monit 1998;20:473–7.
79. Fanos V, Mussap M, Khoory BJ, Vecchini S, Plebani M, Benini D. Renal tolerability of teicoplanin in a case of neonatal overdose. J Chemother 1998;10:381–4.
80. Elting LS, Rubenstein EB, Kurtin D, Rolston KVI, Fangtang J, Martin CG, Raad II, Whimbey EE, Manzullo E, Bodey GP. Mississippi mud in the 1990s: risks and outcomes of vancomycin-associated toxicity in general oncology practice. Cancer 1998;83:2597–607.
81. Wai AO, Lo AMS, Abdo A, Marra F. Vancomycin-induced acute interstitial nephritis. Ann Pharmacother 1998;32:1160–4.
82. Nousari HC, Costarangos C, Anhalt GJ. Vancomycin-associated linear IgA bullous dermatosis. Ann Intern Med 1998;129:507–8.
83. Bernstein EF, Schuster M. Linear IgA bullous dermatosis associated with vancomycin. Ann Intern Med 1998;129:508–9.
84. Marshall C, Street A, Galbraith K. Glycopeptide-induced vasculitis-cross-reactivity between vancomycin and teicoplanin. J Infect 1998;37:82–3.
85. Gendeh BS, Gibb AG, Aziz NS, Kong N, Zahir ZM. Vancomycin administration in continuous ambulatory peritoneal dialysis: the risk of ototoxicity. Otolaryngol Head Neck Surg 1998;118:551–8.
86. Panzarino VM, Feldstein TJ, Kashtan CE. Charcoal hemoperfusion in a child with vancomycin overdose and chronic renal failure. Pediatr Nephrol 1998;12:63–4.
87. Czachor JS, Garzaro P, Miller JR. Vancomycin and priapism. New Engl J Med 1998;338:1701.
88. Taylor SE, Paterson DL, Yu VL. Treatment options for chronic prostatitis due to vancomycin-resistant *Enterococcus faecium*. Eur J Clin Microbiol Infect Dis 1998;17:798–800.
89. Renz CL, Laroche D, Thurn JD, Finn HA, Lynch JP, Thisted R, Moss J. Tryptase levels are not increased during vancomycin-induced anaphylactoid reactions. Anesthesiology 1998;89:620–5.
90. Sorensen SJ, Wise SL, Al Tawfig JA, Robb JL, Cushing HE. Successful vancomycin desensitization in a patient with end-stage renal disease and anaphylactic shock to vancomycin. Ann Pharmacother 1998;32:1020–3.
91. Renz CL, Thurn JD, Finn HA, Lynch JP, Moss J. Oral antihistamines reduce the side effects from rapid vancomycin infusion. Anesth Analg 1998;87:681–5.
92. Mori H, Nakajima T, Nakayama A, Yamori M, Izushi F, Gomita Y. Interaction between levofloxacin and vancomycin in rats—study of serum and organ levels. Chemotherapy 1998;44:181–9.
93. Thomas MP, Steele RW. Monitoring serum vancomycin concentrations in children: is it necessary? Pediatr Infect Dis J 1998;17:351–3.
94. Smith TL, Pearson ML, Wilcox KR, Cruz C, Lancaster MV, Robinson-Dunn B, Tenover FC, Zervos MJ, Band JD, White E, Jarvis WR, Arduino MJ, Carr JH, Clark N, Hill B, McAllister S, Miller JM, Jennings G. Emergence of vancomycin resistance in *Staphylococcus aureus*. New Engl J Med 1999;340:493–501.
95. Sieradzki K, Roberts RB, Haber SW, Tomasz A. The development of vancomycin resistance in a patient with methicillin-resistant *Staphylococcus aureus* infection. New Engl J Med 1999;340:517-23.
96. Waldvogel FA. New resistance in *Staphylococcus aureus*. New Engl J Med 1999;340:556–7.
97. Majumdar A, Lipkin GW, Eliott TSJ, Wheeler DC. Vancomycin-dependent enterococci in a uraemic patient with sclerosing peritonitis. Nephrol Dial Transplant 1999;14:765–7.
98. Kester KE, Turiansky GW, McEvoy PL. Nodular cutaneous microsporidiosis in a patient with AIDS and successful treatment with long-term oral clindamycin therapy. Ann Intern Med 1998;128:911–14.

99. Toma E, Thorne A, Singer J, Raboud J, Lemieux C, Trottier S,Bergeron MG, Tsoukas C, Falutz J, Lalonde R, Gaudreau C, Therrien R, Dascal A, Smail F, Senay H, Shafran S, Taylor G, Aoki F, Gill J, Sinave C, Johnston L, Cameron W. Clindamycin with primaquine vs. trimethoprim–sulfamethoxazole therapy for mild and moderately severe *Pneumocystis carinii* pneumonia in patients with AIDS: a multicenter, double-blind, randomized trial (CTN 004). Clin Infect Dis 1998;27:524–30.

100. Gabel A, Schymik G, Mehmel HC. Ventricular fibrillation due to long QT syndrome probably caused by clindamycin. Am J Cardiol 1999; 83:813–15.

101. Barreiro PM, Pintor E, Buron MR, Diaz B, Valverde J, De la Torre F. Diarrea asociada a *Clostridium difficile*. Estudio retrospectivo a un ano en un hospital terciario. Enferm Infecc Microbiol Clin 1998;16:359–63.

102. Meadowcroft AM, Diaz PR, Latham GS. *Clostridium difficile* toxin-induced colitis after use of clindamycin phosphate vaginal cream. Ann Pharmacother 1998;32:309–11.

103. Haye R, Lingaas E, Hoivik HO, Odegard T. Azithromycin versus placebo in acute infectious rhinitis with clinical symptoms but without radiological signs of maxillary sinusitis. Eur J Clin Microbiol Infect Dis 1998;17:309–12.

104. Stefansson P, Jacovides A, Jablonicky P, Sedani S, Staley H. Cefuroxime axetil versus clarithromycin in the treatment of acute maxillary sinusitis. Rhinology 1998;36:173–8.

105. Harris J-AS, Kolokathis A, Campbell M, Cassell GH, Hammerschlag MR. Safety and efficacy of azithromycin in the treatment of community-acquired pneumonia in children. Pediatr Infect Dis J 1998;17:865–71.

106. Scholz H, Noack R. Multicenter, randomized, double-blind comparison of erythromycin estolate versus amoxicillin for the treatment of acute otitis media in children. AOM Study Group. Eur J Clin Microbiol Infect Dis 1998;17:470–8.

107. Adriaenssen CF. Comparison of the efficacy, safety and tolerability of azithromycin and co-amoxiclav in the treatment of acute periapical abscesses. J Int Med Res 1998;26:257–65.

108. Gruber F, Grubisic GH, Kastelan M, Brajac I, Lenkovic M, Zamolo G. Azithromycin compared with minocycline in the treatment of acne comedonica and papulo–pustulosa. J Chemother 1998;10:469–73.

109. Sprinz E, Mallman R, Barcellos S, Silbert S, Schestatsky G, Bem-David D. AIDS-related cryptosporidial diarrhoea: an open study with roxithromycin. J Antimicrob Chemother 1998;41(Suppl B):85–91.

110. Pohle T, Stoll R, Kirchner T, Heep M, Lehn N, Bock H, Domschke W. Eradication of Helicobacter pylori with lansoprazole, roxithromycin and metronidazole—an open pilot study. Aliment Pharmacol Ther 1998;12:1273–8.

111. Laine L, Suchower L, Frantz J, Connors A, Nell G. Twice-daily, 10-day triple therapy with omeprazole, amoxicillin, and clarithromycin for *Helicobacter pylori* eradication in duodenal ulcer disease: results of three multicenter, double-blind, United States trials. Am J Gastroenterol 1998;93:2106–12.

112. Petersen AM, Schradieck W, Krogfelt KA. *Helicobacter pylori*-resistens over for clarithromycin. Ugeskr Laeg 1998;160:3412-13.

113. Blum AL, Talley NJ, O'Morain C, Van Zanten SV, Labenz J, Stolte M, Louw JA, Stubberod A, Theodors A, Sundin M, Bolling-Sternevald E, Junghard O. Lack of effect of treating *Helicobacter pylori* infection in patients with nonulcer dyspepsia. Omeprazole plus clarithromycin and amoxicillin. New Engl J Med 1998;339:1875–81.

114. Hawkey CJ, Tulassay Z, Szczepanski L, Van Rensberg CJ, Filipowicz-Sosnowsks A, Lanas A, Wason CM, Peacock RA, Gillon KRW. Randomised controlled trial of *Helicobacter pylori* eradication in patients on non-steroidal anti-inflammatory drugs: HELP NSAIDs study. Helicobacter Eradication for Lesion Prevention. Lancet 1998;352:1016–21.

115. Nash MM, Zaltzman JS. Efficacy of azithromycin in the treatment of cyclosporine-induced gingival hyperplasia in renal transplant recipients. Transplantation 1998;65:1611–15.

116. Sato K, Suga M, Akaike T, Fujii-S, Muranaka H, Doi T, Maeda H, Ando M. Therapeutic effect of erythromycin on influenza virus-induced lung injury in mice. Am J Respir Crit Care Med 1998;157:853–7.

117. Faris MA, Raasch RH, Hopfer RL, Butts JD. Treatment and prophylaxis of disseminated *Mycobacterium avium* complex in HIV-infected individuals. Ann Pharmacother 1998;32:564–73.

118. Ward TT, Rimland D, Kauffman C, Huycke M, Evans TG, Heifets L. Randomized, open-label trial of azithromycin plus ethambutol vs. clarithromycin plus ethambutol as therapy for *Mycobacterium avium* complex bacteremia in patients with human immunodeficiency virus infection. Clin Infect Dis 1998;27:1278–85.

119. Oldfield III EC, Fessel WJ, Dunne MW, Dickinson G, Wallace MR, Byrne W, Chung R, Wagner KF, Paparello SF, Craig DB, Melcher G, Zajdowicz M, Williams RF, Kelly JW, Zelasky M, Heifets LB, Berman JD. Once weekly azithromycin therapy for prevention of *Mycobacterium avium* complex infection in patients with AIDS: a randomized, double-blind, placebo-controlled multicenter trial. Clin Infect Dis 1998;26: 611–19.

120. Roussel G, Igual J. Clarithromycin with minocycline and clofazimine for *Mycobacterium avium intracellulare*complex lung disease in patients without the acquired immune deficiency syndrome. Int J Tuberc Lung Dis 1998;2:462–70.

121. Walsh T, Grimes D, Frezieres R, Nelson A, Bernstein L, Coulson A, Bernstein G. Randomised controlled trial of prophylactic antibiotics before insertion of intrauterine devices. Lancet 1998; 351:1005–8.

122. Coggins C, Sloan NL. Prophylactic antibiotics before insertion of intrauterine devices. Lancet 1998;351:1962–3.
123. Jaffe A, Francis J, Rosenthal M, Bush A. Long-term azithromycin may improve lung function in children with cystic fibrosis. Lancet 1998; 351:420.
124. Altschuler EL. Azithromycin, the multidrug-resistant protein, and cystic fibrosis. Lancet 1998; 351:1286.
125. Drici MD, Knollmann BC, Wang WX, Woosley RL. Cardiac actions of erythromycin: influence of female sex. J Am Med Assoc 1998;280:1774–6.
126. Mermelstein HT. Clarithromycin-induced delirium in a general hospital. Psychosomatics 1998; 39:540–2.
127. Kruppa A, Scharffetter Kochanek K, Krieg T, Hunzelmann N. Immediate reaction to roxithromycin and prick test cross-sensitization to erythromycin and clarithromycin. Dermatology 1998; 196:335–6.
128. Rosina P, Chieregato C, Schena D. Fixed drug eruption from clarithromycin. Contact Dermatitis 1998;38:105.
129. Igea JM, Lazaro M. Hypersensitivity reaction to clarithromycin. Allergy 1998;53:107–9.
130. Gavura SR, Nusinowitz S. Leukocytoclastic vasculitis associated with clarithromycin. Ann Pharmacother 1998;32:543–5.
131. Sommer S, Delemazure B, Wagner M, Xenard L, Rozot P. Neuropathie optique ischemique bilateral secondaire a un ergotisme aigu. J Fr Ophtalmol 1998;21:123–5.
132. Dietz A, Hubner C, Andrassy K. Makrolid-Antibiotika induzierte Vaskulitis (Churg–Strauss Syndrom). Laryngorhinootologie 1998;77:111–14.
133. Kantola T, Kivisto KT, Neuvonen PJ. Erythromycin and verapamil considerably increase serum simvastatin and simvastatin acid concentrations. Clin Pharmacol Ther 1998;64:177–82.
134. Wong PW, Dillard TA, Kroenke K. Multiple organ toxicity from addition of erythromycin to long-term lovastatin therapy. South Med J 1998;91:202–5.
135. Apseloff G, Foulds G, LaBoy GL, Willavize S, Vincent J. Comparison of azithromycin and clarithromycin in their interactions with rifabutin in healthy volunteers. J Clin Pharmacol 1998;38:830–5.
136. Arola O, Peltonen R, Rossi T. Arthritis, uveitis, and Stevens–Johnson syndrome induced by trimethoprim. Lancet 1998;351:1102.
137. Steenbergen JA, Stauffer VL. Potential macrolide interaction with verapamil. Ann Pharmacother 1998;32:387–8.
138. Kaeser YA, Brunner F, Drewe J, Haefeli WE, Jolley MR, Bess DT. Severe hypotension and bradycardia associated with verapamil and clarithromycin. Am J Health Syst Pharm 1998;55: 2417–18.
139. Woldtvedt BR, Cahoon CL, Bradley LA, Miller SJ. Possible increased anticoagulation effect of warfarin induced by azithromycin. Ann Pharmacother 1998;32:269–70.
140. Chassany O, Logeart I, Choulika S, Caulin C. Hematome parietal abdominal lors d'un traitement associant acenocoumarol et roxithromycine. Presse Med 1998;27:1103.
141. Finkenbine RD, Frye MD. Case of psychosis due to prednisone–clarithromycin interaction. Gen Hosp Psychiatry 1998;20:325–6.
142. Thomsen MS, Groes L, Agerso H, Kruse T. Lack of pharmacokinetic interaction between tiagabine and erythromycin. J Clin Pharmacol 1998;38:1051–6.
143. Carr RA, Edmonds A, Shi H, Locke CS, Gustavson LE, Craft JC, Harris SI, Palmer R. Steady-state pharmacokinetics and electrocardiographic pharmacodynamics of clarithromycin and loratadine after individual or concomitant administration. Antimicrob Agents Chemother 1998; 42:1176–80.
144. Sachdeo BC, Narang-Sachdeo S, Montgomery PA, Shumaker RC, Perhach JL, Lyness WH, Rosenberg A. Evaluation of the potential interaction between felbamate and erythromycin in patients with epilepsy. J Clin Pharmacol 1998; 38:184–90.
145. Greenblatt DJ, Von Moltke LL, Harmatz JS, Counihan M, Graf JA, Durol ALB, Mertzanis P, Su Xiang Duan, Wright CE, Shader RI. Inhibition of triazolam clearance by macrolide antimicrobial agents: in vitro correlates and dynamic consequences. Clin Pharmacol Ther 1998;64:278–85.
146. Chodosh S, Schreurs A, Siami G, et al. (37 authors). Efficacy of oral ciprofloxacin vs. clarithromycin for treatment of acute bacterial exacerbations of chronic bronchitis. The Bronchitis Study Group. Clin Infect Dis 1998;27:730–8.
147. Chodosh S, McCarty J, Farkas S, et al. (40 authors). Randomized, double-blind study of ciprofloxacin and cefuroxime axetil for treatment of acute bacterial exacerbations of chronic bronchitis. The Bronchitis Study Group. Clin Infect Dis 1998; 27:722–9.
148. Tattevin P, Messiaen T, Pras V, Ronco P, Biour M. Confusion and general seizures following ciprofloxacin administration. Nephrol Dial Transplant 1998;13:2712–13.
149. Zabala S, Gascon A, Bartolome C, Castieila J, Juyol M. Ciprofloxacino y psicosis aguda. Enferm Infecc Microbiol Clin 1998;16:42.
150. James EA, Demian AZ. Acute psychosis in a trauma patient due to ciprofloxacin. Postgrad Med J 1998;74:189–90.
151. De la Puebla Gimenez RAF, Varano MTL, Sanchez EG. Colitis seudomembranosa por ciprofloxacino. Med Clin (Barc) 1998;111:278–9.
152. Raja N, Miller WE, McMillan R, Mason JR. Ciprofloxacin-associated acute renal failure in patients undergoing high-dose chemotherapy and autologous stem cell rescue. Bone Marrow Transplant 1998;21:1283–4.
153. Dharnidharka VR, Nadeau K, Cannon CL, Harris HW, Rosen S. Ciprofloxacin overdose: acute renal failure with prominent apoptotic changes. Am J Kidney Dis 1998;31:710–12.

154. Maquirriain Gorriz M, Merino Munoz F, Tres Belzunegui JC, Sangros Gonzales FJ. Erupcion fija por farmacos inducida por ciprofloxacino. Aten Primaria 1998;21:585–6.
155. Ikiz AO, Serbetcioglu B, Guneri EA, Sutay S, Ceryan K. Investigation of topical ciprofloxacin ototoxicity in guinea pigs. Acta Otolaryngol Stockh 1998;118:808–12.
156. Mullen CA, Petropoulos D, Rytting M, Jeha S, Zipf T, Roberts WM, Rolston KV. Acute reversible arthropathy in a pediatric patient with cancer treated with a short course of ciprofloxacin for febrile neutropenia. J Pediatr Hematol Oncol 1998; 20: 516–17.
157. Blanco AC, Bravo TR. Tendinitis bilateral secundaria a ciprofloxacino. Aten Primaria 1998; 21:184–5.
158. West MB, Gow P. Ciprofloxacin, bilateral Achilles tendonitis and unilateral tendon rupture—a case report. NZ Med J 1998;111:18–19.
159. Gabutti L, Stoller R, Marti H-P. Fluoroquinolone als Ursache von Tendinopathien. Ther Umsch 1998;55:558–61.
160. Petersen W, Laprell H. Die 'schleichende' Ruptur der Achillessehne nach Ciprofloxacin induzierter Tendopathie. Ein Fallbericht. Unfallchirurg 1998;101:731–4.
161. Loebstein R, Addis A, Ho E, Andreou R, Sage S, Donnenfeld AE, Schick B, Bonati M, Moretti M, Lalkin A, Pastuszak A, Koren G. Pregnancy outcome following gestational exposure to fluoroquinolones: a multicenter prospective controlled study. Antimicrob Agents Chemother 1998;42:1336–9.
162. Joos AA. Pharmakologische Interaktionen von Antibiotika und Psychopharmaka. Psychiatr Prax.1998;25:57–60.
163. Otero MJ, Moran D, Valverde MP. Interaction between phenytoin and ciprofloxacin. Ann Pharmacother 1999;33:251–2.
164. McLeod R, Trinkle R. Comment: unexpectedly low phenytoin concentration in a patient receiving ciprofloxacin. Ann Pharmacother 1998;32:1110–11.
165. Scholten PC, Droppert RM, Zwinkels MGJ, Moesker HL, Nauta JJP, Hoepelman IM. No interaction between ciprofloxacin and an oral contraceptive. Antimicrob Agents Chemother 1998; 42:3266–8.
166. Kimura M, Fujiyama J, Nagai A, Hirayama M, Kuriyama M. [Encephalopathy induced by fleroxacin in a patient with Machado–Joseph disease]. Rinsho Shinkeigaku 1998;38:846–8.
167. Edlund C, Nord CE. Ecological effect of gatifloxacin on the normal human intestinal microflora. J Chemother 1999;11:50–3.
168. Lode H, Vogel F, Elies W. Grepofloxacin: a review of its safety profile based on clinical trials and postmarketing surveillance. Clin Ther 1999; 21:61–74.
169. Wimer SM, Schoonover L, Garrison MW. Levofloxacin: a therapeutic review. Clin Ther 1998; 20:1049–70.
170. Preston SL, Drusano GL, Berman AL, Fowler CL, Chow AT, Dornseif B, Reichl V, Natarajan J, Corrado M. Pharmacodynamics of levofloxacin: a new paradigm for early clinical trials. J Am Med Assoc 1998;279:125–9.
171. Arata J, Horio T, Soejima R, Ohara K. Photosensitivity reactions caused by lomefloxacin hydrochloride: a multicenter survey. Antimicrob Agents Chemother 1998;42:3141–5.
172. Stass H, Dalhoff A, Kubitza D, Schuhly U. Pharmacokinetics, safety, and tolerability of ascending single doses of moxifloxacin, a new 8-methoxy quinolone, administered to healthy subjects. Antimicrob Agents Chemother 1998;42: 2060–5.
173. Ballow C, Lettieri J, Agarwal V, Liu P, Stass H, Sullivan JT. Absolute bioavailability of moxifloxacin. Clin Ther 1999;21:513–22.
174. Balfour JA, Wiseman LR. Moxifloxacin. Drugs 1999;57:363–73.
175. Konishi M, Yamada M, Mashima Y. Corneal ulcer associated with deposits of norfloxacin. Am J Ophthalmol 1998;125:258–60.
176. Goldblatt EL, Dohar J, Nozza RJ, Nielsen RW, Goldberg T, Sidman JD, Seidlin M. Topical ofloxacin versus systemic amoxicillin/clavulanate in purulent otorrhea in children with tympanostomy tubes. Int J Pediatr Otorhinolaryngol 1998;46:91–101.
177. Lipsky BA, Dorr MB, Magner DJ, Talbot GH. Safety profile of sparfloxacin, a new fluoroquinolone antibiotic. Clin Ther 1999;21:148–59.
178. Johnson RD, Dorr MB, Talbot GH, Caille G. Effect of Maalox on the oral absorption of sparfloxacin. Clin Ther 1998;20:1149–58.
179. Alghasham AA, Nahata MC. Trovafloxacin: a new fluoroquinolone. Ann Pharmacother 1999;33:48–60.
180. Connor EE. Sulfonamide antibiotics. Prim Care Update Ob Gyns 1998;5:32–5.
181. Tonev S, Vasileva S, Kadurina M. Depot sulfonamide associated linear IgA bullous dermatosis with erythema multiforme-like clinical features. J Eur Acad Dermatol Venereol 1998;11:165–8.
182. De Barrio M, Tornero P, Zubeldia JM, Sierra Z, Matheu V, Herrero T. Fixed drug eruption induced by indapamide. Cross-reactivity with sulfonamides. J Invest Allergol Clin Immunol 1998; 8:253–5.
183. Schnyder B, Frutig K, Mauri Hellweg D, Limat A, Yawalkar N, Pichler WJ. T-cell-mediated cytotoxicity against keratinocytes in sulfamethoxazole-induced skin reaction. Clin Exp Allergy 1998;28:1412–17.
184. Hattori N, Hino H. Generalized erythematous skin eruptions due to trimethoprim itself and co-trimoxazole. J Dermatol 1998;25:269–71.
185. Ozkaya BE, Gungor H. Trimethoprim-induced fixed drug eruption: positive topical provocation on previously involved and uninvolved skin. Contact Dermatitis 1998;39:87–8.
186. Smulders YM, De Man AME, Stehouwer CD, Slaats-EH. Trimethoprim and fasting plasma homocysteine. Lancet 1998;352:1827–8.

187. Bijl AMH, Van der Klauw MM, Van Vliet ACM, Stricker BHC. Anaphylactic reactions associated with trimethoprim. Clin Exp Allergy 1998; 28:510–12.
188. Steuer A, Gumpel JM. Methotrexate and trimethoprim: a fatal interaction. Br J Rheumatol 1998;37:105–6.
189. Richards AJ. Re: Interaction between methotrexate and trimethoprim. Br J Rheumatol 1998; 37:806.
190. Oshitani N, Matsumoto T, Moriyama Y, Kudoh S, Hirata K, Kuroki T. Drug-induced pneumonitis caused by sulfamethoxazole, trimethoprim during treatment of *Pneumocystis carinii* pneumonia in a patient with refractory ulcerative colitis. J Gastroenterol 1998;33:578–1.
191. Sheehan MT, Wen SF. Hyperkalemic renal tubular acidosis induced by trimethoprim/sulfamethoxazole in an AIDS patient. Clin Nephrol 1998;50:188–93.
192. Gabriels G, Stockem E, Greven J. Hyperkaliämie nach Trimethoprim oder Pentamidin. Eine bisher wenig beachtete Nebenwirkung antimikrobieller Therapiemassnahmen bei AIDS-Patienten. Dtsch Med Wochenschr 1998;123:1351–5.
193. Theodore CM, Holmes D, Rodgers M, McLean KA. Co-trimoxazole desensitization in HIV-seropositive patients. Int J STD AIDS 1998; 9:158–61.
194. Walmsley SL, Khorasheh S, Singer J, Djurdjev O, Schlech W, Thompson W, Duperval R, Toma E, Tsoukas C, Senay H, Wells P, Uetrecht J, Shear N, Rachlis A, Fong B, McGreer A, Smaill F, Cohen J, Ford P, Gilmour J, Mackie I, Williams K, Montaner J, Zarowny D. A randomized trial of *N*-acetylcysteine for prevention of trimethoprim–sulfamethoxazole hypersensitivity reactions in *Pneumocystis carinii* pneumonia prophylaxis (CTN 057). J Acquired Immune Defic Syndr Hum Retrovirol 1998;19: 498–505.
195. Holtzer CD, Flaherty JF Jr, Coleman RL. Cross-reactivity in HIV-infected patients switched from trimethoprim–sulfamethoxazole to dapsone. Pharmacotherapy 1998;18:831–5.

Christine Chiou, Andreas H. Groll and Thomas J. Walsh

27 Antifungal drugs

AMPHOTERICIN B FORMULATIONS *(SED-13, 774; SEDA-20, 250; SEDA-21, 282; SEDA-22, 285)*

Owing to its broad-spectrum fungicidal activity, amphotericin remains the mainstay of treatment of most invasive fungal infections. Compared with conventional amphotericin B deoxycholate, the recently approved lipid formulations of amphotericin facilitate treatment in patients with suspected and proven invasive mycoses, who are intolerant of or refractory to conventional amphotericin.

Amphotericin B deoxycholate (D-AmB)

There has been an open, randomized comparison of D-AmB 0.5 mg/kg/day intravenously versus fluconazole 400 mg/day orally for empirical antifungal therapy in neutropenic patients with cancer and fever refractory to broad-spectrum antibiotics (1^C). Patients with abnormal hepatic or renal function were excluded, as were those with proven or suspected invasive fungal infection. The mean duration of therapy was 8.3 days with D-AmB and 7.9 days with fluconazole. Altogether, 32/48 patients randomized to receive D-AmB and 19/52 randomized to receive fluconazole had adverse affects (67 vs 36%). Two patients developed immediate *hypersensitivity reactions* (flushing, hypotension, bronchospasm) to D-AmB and had to be withdrawn. *Hypokalemia* was noted in 25 patients (52%), and *nephrotoxicity*, defined as a rise in serum creatinine of 0.5 mg/dl (44 μmol/l) or more compared with the baseline value, in nine patients (19%). The corresponding frequencies with fluconazole were 23 and 6% respectively. Treatment success rates and mortality were similar (46 vs 56% and 33 vs 27% respectively).

Side Effects of Drugs, Annual 23
J.K. Aronson, ed.

The adverse effects of D-AmB have been reviewed in a retrospective analysis of 102 adult patients (median age, 61 years) with a variety of underlying conditions who were admitted to a small community hospital in Honolulu and who received the drug for treatment of presumed or proven fungal infections that were mostly due to *Candida* spp. (2^C). The average total dose of D-AmB was comparatively low (162 mg; range 10–840 mg). The initial dose averaged 16 mg (range 1–50 mg) and the total duration of therapy was 8.3 days (range 1–46 days). Chills, fever, and/or nausea were noted in 25% of the patients. *Hypokalemia* (a serum potassium concentration below 3.5 mmol/l) occurred in 19%, and *nephrotoxicity* (defined as a serum creatinine concentration of at least 1.6 mg/dl (141 μmol/l) with an increase of at least 0.5 mg/dl (44 μmol/l) during D-AmB therapy) in 15% of patients. Nephrotoxicity increased with increasing total dose of amphotericin, while infusion-associated toxicity decreased with advancing age. The overall response rate to therapy with D-AmB was 83%.

Mineral and fluid balance In dialyzed patients receiving amphotericin it may be necessary to give it during dialysis in order to avoid *hyperkalemia.* Serum potassium concentrations were determined at the end of a 2-hour infusion of D-AmB (1 mg/kg/day) in a 2-year-old girl with systemic candidiasis receiving long-term hemodialysis for renal dysplasia (3^r). The potassium concentration was 6.7 mmol/l, despite dialysis against a 1.5 mmol/l potassium bath just before the infusion. The next dose was given during dialysis, and the serum potassium concentration was 2.6 mmol/l after the infusion.

Urinary system It has been suggested that amphotericin-induced *nephrotoxicity* may be mitigated by increasing renal blood flow and glomerular filtration rate with low-dose dopamine (1–3 μg/kg/min). The efficacy of low-dose dopamine in preventing nephrotoxicity associated with D-AmB has been evaluated in a prospective randomized study of 71 patients after antineoplastic chemotherapy for autologous bone-marrow transplantation or acute leukemia (4[C]). The patients were randomly assigned to receive low-dose dopamine by continuous infusion (3 μg/kg/min) or no dopamine. D-AmB 0.5 or 1.0 mg/kg/day was given for 8 and 13 days on average respectively. Nephrotoxicity, defined as a 1.5-fold or greater increase in baseline serum creatinine concentration, was slightly less common, but not significantly so, in those given dopamine (67 vs 80%). The grade of nephrotoxicity was the same. Ten patients developed grade IV nephrotoxicity and were withdrawn from the study. The authors concluded that dopamine offers little benefit in preventing D-AmB associated nephrotoxicity.

Immunological and hypersensitivity reactions A literature review found no support for the routine use of a test dose of amphotericin before the first therapeutic dose of D-AmB, as is still recommended by the manufacturer (5[r]). The mechanism of common infusion-related adverse effects does not appear to be allergic in nature, and true allergic reactions are rare. Moreover, the absence of a reaction to the test dose does not necessarily indicate that patients will not have a severe infusion-related reaction later in the course of therapy, and the procedure of administering a test dose may lead to a detrimental delay in adequate antifungal therapy. The authors recommended starting therapy with D-AmB at the full therapeutic target dose with careful bedside monitoring for infusion-related adverse events throughout therapy.

Amphotericin B deoxycholate formulated in parenteral lipid emulsions

The safety of two formulation of intravenous D-AmB has been investigated in a randomized, open comparison in neutropenic patients with refractory fever of unknown origin or pulmonary infiltrates (6[C]). D-AmB was given in a dose of 0.75 mg/kg/day either in 250 ml of a 5% glucose solution or mixed with 250 ml of a 20% lipid emulsion (IlD-AmB; Intralipid 20%, Kabi-Pharmacia, Erlangen, Germany) on eight consecutive days and then on alternate days as a 1-hour to 4-hour infusion. The mean number of days of treatment was 11.3 vs 9.9 days. There were no statistically significant differences between the two cohorts with respect to the incidence of infusion-related adverse events, such as fever and chills, renal impairment, or treatment failure. However, grade 3–4 acute *dyspnea* occurred slightly more often with the lipid emulsion formulation, and there were significantly more other severe respiratory events in patients receiving lipid emulsion, raising the possibility of a causal relation via fat overload or incompatibility between D-AmB and the lipid emulsion.

The efficacy and tolerability of amphotericin prepared in a 20% lipid emulsion (Intralipid 20%, Pharmacia–Upjohn, Milan, Italy) have been evaluated in 16 patients with HIV infection and esophageal candidiasis or cryptococcosis and compared with standard amphotericin in a matched group of 24 patients (7[c]). While both formulations had apparently similar clinical and microbiological efficacy, fewer patients receiving the lipid emulsion formulation required premedication or symptomatic therapy for infusion-associated adverse events, and fewer patients were withdrawn because of adverse effects. Renal adverse effects (*a rise in serum creatinine and/or electrolyte loss*) were more common in patients who received the conventional formulation.

The efficacy and safety of amphotericin in Intralipid 20 or 5% glucose has been evaluated in a retrospective case analysis in 30 patients with AIDS and cryptococcal meningitis who received either formulation 1 mg/kg/day for 20 days with or without flucytosine (n = 20) or fluconazole (n = 4), followed by maintenance therapy with fluconazole 400 mg/day (8[C]). Twenty patients received D-AmB in 500 ml 5% glucose over 5 hours, and 10 received D-AmB in 100 ml of 20% Intralipid given over 2 hours. Complete clinical resolution was obtained in 55 and 60% of the patients respectively. There were no differences regarding infusion-related adverse effects, nephrotoxicity, or anemia.

Amphotericin B Colloidal Dispersion (ABCD)

ABCD has been compared with D-AmB in a prospective, randomized, double-blind study of the empirical treatment of fever and neutropenia in 213 patients (9[C]). Patients were stratified by age and concomitant use of ciclosporin or tacrolimus and then randomized to receive ABCD (4 mg/kg/day) or D-AmB (0.8 mg/kg/day) for 14 days. Renal dysfunction was less likely to develop and occurred later with

ABCD than D-AmB. Likewise, the absolute and percentage fall in the serum potassium concentration from baseline to the end of therapy was greater with D-AmB than ABCD. However, probable or possible infusion-related *hypoxia* and *chills* were more common with ABCD than D-AmB. There was a therapeutic response in 50% of the patients who received ABCD and 43% of those who received D-AmB. Thus, ABCD was of comparable efficacy and less nephrotoxic than D-AmB, but infusion-related events were more common with ABCD.

The safety and efficacy of ABCD have been evaluated in 148 immunocompromised patients with candidemia (10[C]). ABCD was given intravenously in a median daily dose of 3.9 (range 0.1–9.1) mg/kg for a median of 12 (range 1–72) days. In the safety analysis (n = 148 patients), *nephrotoxicity* occurred in 16% of the patients, with either doubling of the baseline serum creatinine concentration or an increase of 1.0 mg/dl (88 μmol/l) or a 50% fall in calculated creatinine clearance. Severe adverse events were believed to be probably or possibly related to ABCD in 36 patients (24%), including *chills* and *fever* (9.5%), *hypotension* and *abnormal kidney function* (4%), *tachycardia, asthma, hypotension* (3%), and *dyspnea* (2%). ABCD was withdrawn in 12% because of toxicity. The overall response rate in 89 evaluable patients was 66% with candidemia alone and 14% with disseminated candidiasis.

The safety and efficacy of ABCD has been studied in 133 patients with invasive fungal infections and renal impairment due to either D-AmB or pre-existing renal disease (11[C]). The mean daily dose of ABCD was 3.4 (range 0.1–5.5) mg/kg, and the mean duration of therapy was 21 (range 1–207) days. Although individual patients had increases in serum creatinine concentrations, ABCD did not have an adverse effect on renal function: the mean serum creatinine concentration tended to fall slightly with days on therapy and increases were not dose-related. Six patients discontinued ABCD therapy because of *nephrotoxicity*. Infusion-related adverse events occurred at least once in 74 patients (56%); however, while 43% of patients had infusion-related toxic effects on day 1, only 18% reported these events by day 7. There were complete or partial responses in 50% of the intention-to-treat population and in 67% of the 58 evaluable patients.

Immunological and hypersensitivity reactions *Anaphylaxis* is rare with amphotericin (12[R]). It is important to note that a patient may tolerate one formulation and respond with anaphylaxis to another. Anaphylaxis after ABCD occurred in a patient who had previously been treated with both D-AmB and amphotericin B lipid complex (ABLC) without infusion-related adverse effects (13[c]). During the first infusion of ABCD he developed spontaneously reversible severe back pain and then swelling of his lips, respiratory distress, and left sided hemiparesis, which resolved after 24 hours. An MRI scan suggested an ischemic event in the right putamen, lending support to the hypothesis that he had had an anaphylactic reaction to ABCD, hypoperfusion, and a subsequent stroke.

In another notable report, serious adverse events (fever, severe rigors, a fall in blood pressure, *worsening mental status, increasing creatinine concentration*, and *leukocytosis*) occurred after unrecognized substitution of one amphotericin formulation (ABLC) by another (ABCD) (14[c]). After discovery of the switch, ABLC therapy was reinstituted and tolerated without incident.

These cases underscore the need to monitor patients closely when infusing the first dose of a different formulation of amphotericin.

Amphotericin B Lipid Complex (ABLC)

The safety and efficacy of amphotericin B Lipid Complex (ABLC) have been evaluated in 556 cases of proven or presumptive invasive fungal infection treated in an open-label, single-patient, US emergency-use study of patients who were refractory to or intolerant of conventional antifungal therapy (15[C]). Treatment was with a daily dosage of either 5 mg/kg (87%) or 3 mg/kg. The investigators had the option of reducing the daily dosage as clinically warranted. Treatment was for 7 days in 540 patients (97%). During the course of ABLC therapy, serum creatinine concentrations in all patients fell significantly from baseline. In 162 patients with serum creatinine concentrations of at least 2.5 mg/dl (221 μmol/l) at baseline, the mean serum creatinine concentration fell significantly from the first week to the sixth week. The serum creatinine concentration increased from baseline to the end of therapy in 132 patients (24%). *Hypokalemia* (serum potassium concentration of less than 3 mmol/l) developed in 4.6%, and *hypomagnesemia* (serum magnesium concentration of less than 0.75 mmol/l) in 18%. There was a rise in serum bilirubin in 142/284 patients (33%); the overall increase was from 4.66 to 6.59 mg/dl (79 to 112 μmol/l) at the end of therapy. The mean *alkaline phosphatase activity rose* from 273 to 320 iu/l. There was no significant change overall in alanine aminotransferase activity, but the activity increased by the end of treatment in 16% of patients with initially normal values. There were complete or partial responses to therapy with ABLC in 167 of 291 mycologically confirmed cases evaluable for therapeutic response (57%).

The safety and efficacy of ABLC 5 mg/kg/day in patients with neutropenia and intolerance or refractoriness to D-AmB have been reported in two smaller series of 25 treatment courses from the UK. In one (16[c]), the mean serum creatinine at the start of therapy was 139 μmol/l and at the end of therapy 132 μmol/l; there were no infusion-related adverse events. There was an *increase in alanine aminotransferase activity* in 12 of the 22 analyzed treatment courses. In the other series (17[c]), there was an increase in serum creatinine in five of 18 courses (28%), and *hypokalemia* (less than 2.5 mmol/l) in two courses (11%); premedication for infusion-associated reactions was required in three courses (17%). There were modest increases in serum alanine transaminase activities in five patients (30%).

In contrast to these reports, there was a frequent prevalence of adverse events with ABLC in the treatment of suspected or documented invasive fungal infections in 19 Scandinavian patients with mostly hematological malignancies (18[c]). The mean starting dose of ABLC was 4.1 mg/kg/day, given for a median of 3 (range 1–19) days. ABLC was withdrawn because of adverse events in 14/19 patients (74%). These included *rising creatinine concentrations* (n = 12), *increased serum bilirubin* (n = 7), *erythema* (n = 6), *increased alanine aminotransferase* (n = 6), *fever and chills* (n = 5), *hypoxemia* (n = 3), *hemolysis* (n = 2), and *back pain* and *increased serum alkaline phosphatase activity* (n = 1 each). In patients with renal adverse effects, there were significantly *increased serum creatinine concentration* (from 85 mmol/l to 199 mmol/l) and *increased bilirubin concentration* (from 17 to 77 μmol/l) in seven patients. The authors stated that while all the patients were very ill at the time of the start of ABLC therapy, in all cases the adverse effects had a direct and obvious correlation with the administration of ABLC. However, the reason for this unusual high rate of adverse events remains unclear.

Nervous system Reversible *parkinsonism* has been attributed to ABLC (19[c]).

A 10-year-old bone-marrow recipient was given ABLC 7 mg/kg/day for prolonged periods of time. Ablation therapy before transplantation included cytosine arabinoside, cyclophosphamide, and total body irradiation. The patient developed progressive parkinsonian features; an MRI scan showed non-specific frontal cortex white matter abnormalities, and brain MR spectroscopy was consistent with significant neuronal loss in the left insular cortex, left basal ganglia, and left frontal white matter. He was given co-careldopa (carbidopa + levodopa) and made a slow recovery within 4 months. A follow-up MRI scan again showed frontal white matter changes, but repeat MR spectroscopy showed marked improvement in the areas previously examined.

In contrast to its renal toxicity, the neurological adverse effects of amphotericin are less well known. However, several reports have described a clinical syndrome of *akinetic mutism, incontinence*, and *parkinsonism* in patients who had received large doses of D-AmB given in association with central nervous system irradiation or infection (12[R]). The reported case shows that, regardless of the formulation of amphotericin, severe neurological adverse effects can occur, in particular in patients receiving large dosages of amphotericin after cranial irradiation.

Mineral and fluid balance Rapid infusion of D-AmB can cause *hyperkalemia*, in particular in the setting of renal insufficiency (12[R]). Fatal cardiopulmonary arrest has been reported in a 4-year-old boy with acute leukemia and disseminated invasive candidiasis after the third infusion of ABLC 5 mg/kg/day, infused over 1 hour (3[c]). During resuscitation he had a serum potassium concentration of 16 mmol/l; there was no evidence of hemolysis or rhabdomyolysis and serum creatinine and potassium concentrations had been within the reference ranges earlier in the day. Autopsy showed numerous fungal abscesses, including several in the myocardium.

Urinary system There has been a retrospective comparison of the renal effects of

ABLC with D-AmB in the treatment of invasive candidiasis and cryptococcosis in dosages of 0.6–5 mg/kg/day; most patients received 5 mg/kg/day (20[c]). *Changes in serum creatinine* were evaluated in three ways: doubling of the baseline value, an increase from below 1.5 mg/dl (132 μmol/l) at baseline to over 1.5 mg/dl, and an increase from below 1.5 mg/dl at baseline to at least 2.0 mg/dl (177 μmol/l). These endpoints were achieved significantly more often with D-AmB than with ABLC, and the time needed to reach each of the endpoints was significantly shorter with D-AmB. An increased serum creatinine concentration was reported as an adverse event more often in patients receiving D-AmB than in patients receiving ABLC (24 vs 43%).

Immunological and hypersensitivity reactions A life-threatening event has been reported after the use of ABLC in a patient previously treated with D-AmB (21[c]). Ninety minutes after the start of the first dose of ABLC, the patient developed *tachycardia, tachypnea, dyspnea*, and severe *hypoxemia* with radiological evidence of *bilateral interstitial infiltrates*, and required transient mechanical ventilation. After the event, treatment was continued with D-AmB without undesirable effects.

Liposomal amphotericin B (L-AmB)

The safety, tolerance, and pharmacokinetics of liposomal amphotericin B (L-AmB; AmBisomer) have been evaluated in an open-label, sequential-dose-escalation, multiple-dose phase I/II study of 36 patients with neutropenia and persistent fever requiring empirical antifungal therapy (22[C]). The patients received doses of 1, 2.5, 5.0, or 7.5 mg/kg/day of L-AmB for a mean of 9.2 days. L-AmB was well tolerated: infusion-related adverse effects (fever, chills, rigor) occurred in 15 (5%) of all 331 infusions, and only two patients (5%) required premedication (*dyspnea and generalized flushing; facial urticaria*). *Hypotension* (one infusion) and *hypertension* (three infusions) were infrequent. One patient each had *sharp flank pain* and *dyspnea* during one infusion; these symptoms did not recur during subsequent infusions. Serum creatinine, potassium, and magnesium concentrations were not significantly changed from baseline, and there were no net increases in serum transaminases. There was, however, a significant *increase in serum alkaline phosphatase activity* and *increase in bilirubin concentration* in the overall population as well as in individual dosage groups. One patient who received concomitant L-asparaginase had *increases in serum lipase and amylase activities* in association with symptoms of *pancreatitis* while receiving L-AmB; however, as he continued to receive the drug, the serum lipase and amylase returned to baseline. L-AmB had non-linear pharmacokinetics consistent with reticuloendothelial uptake and redistribution. There were no breakthrough fungal infections during therapy.

L-AmB 5 mg/kg/day and D-AmB 1 mg/kg/day have been compared in the treatment of proven or suspected invasive fungal infections in neutropenic patients in a randomized multicenter study (23[C]). Significantly more patients given D-AmB had a greater than 100% increase in baseline serum creatinine. Treatment was temporarily discontinued or the dosage reduced because of an increase in serum creatinine in 18/54 (33%) patients treated with D-AmB vs 2/51 (4%) treated with L-AmB. There was no statistically significant difference in the number of patients with infusion-related toxicity (fever/chills), hypokalemia, or increases in serum transaminases, alkaline phosphatase, or serum bilirubin. In 66 patients eligible for analysis of efficacy there was a trend to an improved overall response rate and a significant difference in the rate of complete responses in favor of L-AmB; death rates were also lower in patients treated with L-AmB.

The efficacy of two dosages of L-AmB in the treatment of proven or probable invasive aspergillosis in neutropenic patients with cancer or those undergoing bone marrow transplantation has been studied in a prospective, randomized, open, multicenter trial in 120 patients randomized to receive either 1 or 4 mg/kg/day of L-AmB; 87 patients were available for evaluation (24[C]). There was at least one toxic event during treatment in 15 of 41 patients given 1 mg/kg/day and 25 of 46 given 4 mg/kg/day, but the numbers of events per patient were similar. These events included *headache, nausea, diarrhea, rash, liver toxicity, myalgia, dyspnea, fever, chills*, and *back pain*. Renal toxicity definitely related to L-AmB therapy occurred in 1/41 patients treated with 1 mg/kg/day and 5/46 patients treated with 4 mg/kg/day. Only in one case was treatment permanently discontinued because of toxicity related to L-AmB (4 mg/kg/day). No patient died as a result of L-AmB toxicity. Overall, L-AmB was effective in 50–60% of patients; however, the number of cases with proven invasive aspergillosis was too small to allow a meaningful comparison of the two dosages regarding efficacy in this life-threatening disease.

The safety and efficacy of L-AmB have been compared with that of ABLC in a retrospective analysis of 59 adult patients with hematological malignancies who received 68 courses of either L-AmB (n = 32) or ABLC (n = 36) for a variety of presumed or confirmed invasive fungal infections (25[c]). The median daily dosages were 1.9 (range 0.7–4.0) mg/kg for L-AmB and 4.8 (range 1.9–5.8) mg/kg for ABLC. There was no statistically significant difference in the overall outcome; *febrile reactions* were significantly more common with ABLC (36 vs 6%), but there were no significant differences in the median creatinine concentrations at baseline and at the end of therapy or in the number of patients with urinary loss of potassium or magnesium.

In an open-label, sequential phase II clinical study of three different regimens of L-AmB for visceral leishmaniasis (2 mg/kg on days 1–6 and on day 10; 2 mg/kg on days 1–4 and on day 10; 2 mg/kg on days 1, 5, and 10) in Indian and Kenyan patients in three developing countries there were few infusion-associated adverse effects (26[C]). Of 32 Brazilian patients (15 of whom received 2 mg/kg on days 1–10 because of poor responses to regimen 1) 37% had a *fever* with one or more infusions, 9% had *chills*, and 6% had *back pain;* in addition, three patients had respiratory distress and/or *cardiac dysrhythmias*. There were different response rates to the three regimens in the different countries, leading to the recommendation of 2 mg/kg on days 1–4 and day 10 in India and Kenya, and 2 mg/kg on days 1–10 in Brazil.

Urinary system L-AmB has been given to an immunosuppressed renal transplant patient with cerebral aspergillosis for almost 10 months at a cumulative dose of 42 g with no apparent changes in the function of the renal allograft, as measured by serum creatinine, creatinine clearance, and potassium concentrations (27[c]). Therapy was ultimately successful and discontinued after surgical resection of a residual sclerotic lesion.

Amphotericin can cause *hyposthenuria*, although this rarely becomes clinically important (12[R]). A 43-year-old HIV-infected patient presented with *nephrogenic diabetes insipidus* associated with D-AmB therapy for ocular candidiasis; rechallenge was positive (28[r]).

Miscellaneous Three cases of *chest discomfort* associated with infusion of L-AmB at a dosage of 3 mg/kg/hour for 1 hour have been reported (29[cr]).

The first patient had chest tightness and difficulty in breathing and the second had dyspnea and acute hypoxia (PaO_2 55 mmHg; 7.3 kPa), both within 10 minutes of the start of the infusion. The third complained of chest pain 5 minutes after the start of two infusions. In all cases the symptoms resolved on terminating therapy. Two patients were later rechallenged with slower infusions and tolerated the drug well.

A review of the literature showed that similar reactions had been reported anecdotally in several clinical trials of L-AmB, with all other formulations, and with liposomal daunorubicin and doxorubicin. While the pathophysiology of such reactions is yet unclear, the authors recommended infusing L-AmB over at least 2 hours with careful monitoring of adverse events.

Risk factors *Neonates* The safety and efficacy of liposomal amphotericin in 40 preterm and four full-term infants with invasive yeast infections have been studied retrospectively (30[C]). The initial dosage was 1 mg/kg/day, and was increased stepwise by 1 mg/kg to a maximum of 5 mg/kg depending on the clinical condition. There were no infusion-associated reactions. Blood pressure, hepatic, renal, and hematological indices were not altered. Hypokalemia was noted in 16 infants but was always transient and responsive to potassium supplementation. Treatment with liposomal amphotericin was successful in 72% of the children. However, 12 of the 40 preterm infants succumbed to the fungal infection; all had a birth weight of less than 1.5 kg.

Changes in serum creatinine and serum potassium have been measured in 21 infants of very low birth weight who received amphotericin for presumed or documented yeast infections (31[c]). The median dosage was 2.6 (range 1–5) mg/kg/day, and the median duration of therapy was 28 (11–79) days. Hypokalemia (below 3 mmol/l) was observed in 30% before treatment and in 15% during treatment. However, 21 days after the end of therapy, hypokalemia was not present in any patient. The maximum creatinine concentration fell from 121 (71–221) μmol/l to 68 (31–171) μmol/l during treatment and 46 (26–62) μmol/l at 21 days after the end of therapy. However, creatinine concentrations were available for only 10, 18, and 15 of the 21 patients respectively, and no information was provided on the number of patients who had an increase in serum creatinine during therapy. All patients responded to therapy with liposomal amphotericin, although the number of proven invasive fungal infections was small (7/21).

PYRIMIDINE ANALOGUES

Flucytosine (5-fluorocytosine)

(SED-13, 779)

Experience with flucytosine monotherapy of cryptococcosis has been reviewed in 27 patients treated between 1968 and 1973 who were selected for this form of therapy on the basis of criteria associated with good prognosis (32[c]). Flucytosine was given as primary therapy to 18 patients and as secondary therapy (following failure of D-AmB) to nine patients in dosages of 4–10 g/day in four divided doses for 8 weeks. Toxicity associated with flucytosine was uncommon and mild. Mild *leukopenia* (nadir 3–4 $\times 10^9$/l) developed in three patients, and mild *thrombocytopenia* (101 $\times 10^9$/l) and worsening *anemia* occurred in one patient each. Therapy was stopped early or changed in two patients. In the first, therapy was stopped after 31 days because of a white cell count of 4.1 $\times 10^9$/l; despite the shortened course of therapy, the patient achieved a long-term cure, and the leukopenia was ultimately believed to be secondary to sarcoidosis. There was bone-marrow suppression in the second patient shortly after the withdrawal of flucytosine (because of failure to respond); later resumption of flucytosine during AmB therapy for this critically ill patient was associated with severe bone-marrow suppression and death.

Combination therapy with fluconazole (200 mg/day for 2 months) and flucytosine (150 mg/kg/day for the first 2 weeks; n = 30) has been compared with fluconazole monotherapy (200 mg/day for 2 months; n = 28) in a randomized open trial in Ugandan patients with AIDS-associated cryptococcal meningitis (33[C]). Patients in both groups who survived for 2 months received maintenance therapy with fluconazole (200 mg three times per week for 4 months). There were no serious adverse events in any of the patients. The combination therapy prevented death within 2 weeks and significantly increased the survival rate at 6 months (32 vs 12%). However, the rate of positive cryptococcal antigen titers remained high at 2 months after treatment in both groups.

AZOLE DERIVATIVES *(SED-13, 782; SEDA-20, 252; SEDA-21, 282; SEDA-22, 293)*

Fluconazole

The use of fluconazole in 726 children under 1 year of age, reported in 78 publications, has been reviewed (34[R]). The patients received a wide range of dosages for up to 162 days. Fluconazole was well tolerated and efficacious in the therapy of systemic candidiasis and candidemia in children under 1 year of age, including neonates and very low birth-weight infants. The daily dosage recommended by the manufacturers is 6 mg/kg, to be reduced in patients with impaired renal function in accordance with the guidelines given for adults.

The efficacy and safety of fluconazole in neonates with *Candida* fungemia has been evaluated in a multicenter prospective study (35[c]). Fluconazole was safe and effective even in complicated cases of *Candida* fungemia, including infants of very low birth weights. Two of 50 neonates developed *raised liver enzymes* during fluconazole therapy and two others had raised serum creatinine concentrations. In none of them did these abnormalities necessitate discontinuation of antifungal therapy.

Skin and appendages A patient developed a longitudinal band of *pigmentation in the diseased nail* after fluconazole therapy for onychomycosis at a dosage of 150 mg once a week for 4 weeks (36[c]).

Interactions Fluconazole and related azoles are potent inhibitors of CYP3A4, which metabolizes many drugs.

Zidovudine glucuronidation in human hepatic microsomes in vitro was inhibited more by the combination of fluconazole with valproic acid than with other drugs, such as atovaquone and methadone (37[c]).

The pharmacokinetic interaction of fluconazole 400 mg od and indinavir 1000 mg tds has been evaluated in a placebo-controlled, cross-over study for 8 days; there was no significant interaction (38[c]).

In a randomized, double-blind, placebo-controlled, cross-over study of nine subjects fluconazole 400 mg reduced the clearance of *alfentanil* 20 μg/kg by 55% and increased alfentanil-induced subjective effects (39[c]).

In a randomized, double-blinded, placebo-controlled study of 25 patients fluconazole 200 mg/day increased *methadone* concentrations, but patients treated with fluconazole did not have signs or symptoms of significant narcotic overdose (40[c]).

In an open cross-over study of 10 young healthy subjects fluconazole 150 mg increased the serum concentrations of *ethinylestradiol* 30–35 μg/day (41[c]). These findings suggest that there is a potential for a clinically significant interaction between fluconazole and ethinylestradiol in oral contraceptives.

Itraconazole

The systemic availability of itraconazole and the bioequivalence of single 200 mg doses of itraconazole solution and two capsule formulations have been evaluated in a cross-over study of 30 male volunteers (42[c]). Itraconazole and hydroxyitraconazole were 30–37% more available from the solution than from either capsule formulation. However, the values of C_{max}, t_{max}, and half-lives were comparable. There were no differences in safety and tolerance.

In a double-blind comparison in oropharyngeal candidiasis in 244 patients with AIDS, itraconazole oral solution and fluconazole capsules (each 100 mg/day for 14 days) were equally efficacious; there were no significant differences in adverse effects (43[C]).

Itraconazole oral solution and fluconazole tablets have been compared in oropharyngeal candidiasis in HIV/AIDS patients in a prospective randomized, blind, multicenter trial (44[C]). Both regimens of itraconazole oral solution (100 mg bd for 7 days or 100 mg od for 14 days) were equivalent to fluconazole (100 mg od for 14 days). Itraconazole oral solution was well tolerated.

The efficacy and safety of intermittent itraconazole therapy have been investigated in 635 patients with onychomycosis (45[C]). Intermittent itraconazole (400 mg/day for 1 week per month for 2 months) was effective and safe. Most adverse events were minor and occurred infrequently; there were no major changes in liver function tests.

Two dosages of itraconazole have been compared in the treatment of tinea corporis or tinea cruris in a multicenter, randomized, double-blind, parallel-group study, which showed that itraconazole 200 mg for 1 week (54 patients) is similarly effective, equally well tolerated, and at least as safe as the established regimen of itraconazole 100 mg for 2 weeks (60 patients) (46[C]). In a similar study of tinea pedis or tinea manum, itraconazole 400 mg once a week (66 patients) and itraconazole 100 mg once every 4 weeks (69 patients) were both effective; the two schedules were equally well tolerated and safe (47[C]).

In a double-blind, randomized, placebo-controlled, multicenter trial in plantar or moccasin-type tinea pedis in 72 patients, itraconazole 200 mg bd was significantly more effective than placebo; its safety and tolerability were comparable with placebo (48[C]).

Itraconazole (28 patients) and terbinafine (27 patients) have been compared in a double-blind, randomized study of tinea capitis (49[c]). The cure rates at week 12 were 86 and 78% respectively. Adverse events were mild and did not warrant discontinuation of therapy.

Immunological and hypersensitivity reactions Itraconazole 200 mg bd for 2 weeks caused a *serum sickness-like reaction* in a 53-year-old woman with Menière's disease (50[c]).

Risk factors *Children* The safety, tolerability, and pharmacokinetics of itraconazole and its active metabolite hydroxyitraconazole after administration of itraconazole solution in hydroxypropyl-β-cyclodextrin have been investigated in a multicenter study of 26 infants and children aged 6 months to 12 years with mucosal candidiasis or at risk of invasive fungal disease (51[C]). There was a trend to lower minimum plasma concentrations in children aged 6 months to 2 years. The systemic absorption of the solubilizer hydroxypropyl-β-cyclodextrin was less than 1%. Given at 5 mg/kg/day, this new formulation provided potentially therapeutic concentrations in plasma, somewhat lower than those attained in adults, and it was well tolerated and safe.

Itraconazole 100 mg/day has been studied in 24 children with *Trichophyton tonsurans* tinea capitis (52). Itraconazole was well tolerated, but 15 children required re-treatment due to persistent infection.

Interactions Itraconazole increases the risk of skeletal muscle toxicity of some *HMG-CoA reductase inhibitors* (statins) by increasing their serum concentrations, but not all statins are equally affected. The increase in serum concentrations of atorvastatin is by inhibition of CYP3A4. In a randomized, double-blind, cross-over study of 10 healthy volunteers itraconazole 200 mg increased the AUC and half-life of atorvastatin 40 mg about 3-fold, with a change in C_{max} (53[c]). The concomitant use of itraconazole and other potent inhibitors of CYP3A4 with atorvastatin should therefore be avoided, or the dose of atorvastatin should be reduced accordingly.

Itraconazole 100 mg/day, greatly increased plasma concentrations of lovastatin 40 mg and its active metabolite, lovastatin acid in 10 healthy volunteers; in contrast, fluvastatin concentrations were not significantly increased by itraconazole (54[c]). In two other studies in 10 healthy volunteers. itraconazole 200 mg greatly increased serum concentrations of simvastatin 40 mg and simvastatin acid, but had only minor effects on pravastatin 40 mg (55[c]).

An interaction between itraconazole 600 mg bd and *tacrolimus* in organ transplant has been reported in a 17-year-old man with cystic fibrosis who received a hepato-pulmonary transplant (56[c]). High trough concentrations of tacrolimus were noted, despite the relatively low dosage (0.1–0.3 mg/kg/day). Another patient also experienced an interaction of tacrolimus 0.085 mg/kg bd with itraconazole 200–400 mg per day, with resulting ketoacidosis, neutropenia, and thrombocytopenia, requiring the withdrawal of both drugs (57[c]).

In a study of the effects of itraconazole (200 mg daily) and rifampicin 600 mg/day on the pharmacokinetics and pharmacodynamics of oral *midazolam* 7.5–15 mg during and 4 days after the end of the treatment, switching from inhibition to induction of metabolism caused an up to 400-fold change in the AUC of oral midazolam (58[c]).

Rifampicin 600 mg/day for 14 days had a very strong inducing effect on the metabolism of a single dose of itraconazole 200 mg, indicating that these two drugs should not be used concomitantly (59[c]).

Grapefruit juice did not affect the pharmacokinetics of itraconazole in 22 healthy men while orange juice reduced the C_{max}, T_{max}, and AUC (60[C]).

Famotidine, a histamine H_2 receptor antagonist (40 mg/kg/day) reduced the peak and trough concentrations of itraconazole 200 mg/kg/day by about 35% in 18 patients undergoing chemotherapy for hematological malignancies (61[C]).

In 11 healthy volunteers *omeprazole* 40 mg reduced the systemic availability of itraconazole 200 mg; these two drugs should therefore not be used together (62[C]).

Zolpidem is a short-acting imidazole-pyridine hypnotic which is mainly transformed by CYP3A4. However, itraconazole 200 mg did not alter the pharmacokinetics and pharmacodynamics of zolpidem 10 mg in 10 healthy volunteers (63[c]). Therefore, unlike triazolam, zolpidem may be used in normal or nearly normal doses together with itraconazole.

Itraconazole 200 mg had no significant effect on serum concentrations of *clozapine* (200–550 mg/day) or desmethylclozapine in 7 schizophrenic patients (64[C]).

Fentanyl is metabolized by CYP3A4. However, although itraconazole is a strong inhibitor of CYP3A enzymes, the pharmacokinetics and pharmacodynamics of fentanyl 3 μg/kg were similar after both itraconazole 200 mg and placebo in 10 healthy volunteers (65[C]).

The interaction of itraconazole with oral *methylprednisolone* has been examined in a randomized, double-blind, cross-over study of 10 healthy volunteers taking either oral itraconazole 200 mg od or placebo for 4 days (66[c]). On day 4 each subject took methylprednisolone 16 mg. Itraconazole increased the total AUC of methylprednisolone 3.9-fold compared with placebo, the peak plasma methylprednisolone concentration 1.9-fold, and the half-life 2.4-fold. This effect was probably through inhibition of CYP3A4.

Two adults with acute lymphoblastic leukemia developed unusually severe neurotoxicity caused by *vincristine*, which was probably the result of an interaction with itraconazole suspension (67[c]).

Ketoconazole

Interactions *Zolpidem*, an imidazopyridine hypnotic, is metabolized by CYP3A. Ketoconazole 200 mg bd impaired the clearance of zolpidem 5 mg and enhanced its benzodiazepine-like pharmacodynamic effects. In contrast, itraconazole 100 mg bd and fluconazole 100 mg bd had small effects on zolpidem kinetics and dynamics (68[c]).

In a double-blind, cross-over kinetic and dynamic study of the interaction of ketoconazole with *alprazolam* and *triazolam*, two CYP3A4 substrate drugs with different kinetic profiles, impaired clearance by ketoconazole had more profound clinical consequences for triazolam than for alprazolam (69[C]).

Ketoconazole 400 mg caused a minor reduction in the clearance of *ropivacaine*, a local anesthetic, which is mostly metabolized by CYP1A2 (70[c]).

Donepezil 5 mg produced no change in plasma concentrations of ketoconazole 200 mg (71[c]).

Halofantrine, a highly lipophilic antimalarial drug with poor and erratic absorption, is metabolized to its equipotent metabolite, desbutylhalofantrine, and this is inhibited by oral ketoconazole (72[c]).

ALLYLAMINES *(SED-13, 793; SEDA-21, 288; SEDA-22, 290)*

Terbinafine

The safety and efficacy of terbinafine 250 mg/day and itraconazole 200 mg/day given for 12 weeks for toenail onychomycosis have been compared in a randomized, double-blind study of 372 patients (73[C]). Adverse events were reported in 39% of the terbinafine-treated patients and in 35% of the itraconazole-treated patients. The mean values of biochemical parameters of liver and kidney function did not change significantly. Terbinafine produced higher rates of clinical cure (76 vs 58%) and mycological cure (73 vs 46%) than itraconazole.

Hematological With increasing use of terbinafine worldwide, anecdotal cases of hematological toxicity are being reported. The projected rate of all *blood dyscrasias* associated with terbinafine has been estimated to be 32 per million patient years (74[r]).

Severe reversible *agranulocytosis* associated with oral terbinafine has been reported (74[c], 75[c]).

A 55-year-old woman who was taking concurrent paroxetine and who presented with fever, diarrhea, and vomiting. A bone-marrow biopsy showed overall reduced cellularity, and the aspirate showed a profound shift toward the production of immature myeloid cells, consistent with maturation arrest. Treatment consisted of withdrawal of all out-patient medications, hydration, intravenous fluids, broad-spectrum antibiotics and G-CSF 5 μg/kg for 5 days. Mature granulocytes appeared in the peripheral blood on the fifth day in hospital, and the patient was discharged on the seventh hospital day with an absolute neutrophil count of 6.2×10^9/l. Paroxetine was resumed weeks after discharge from hospital without hematological toxicity over 6 months.

A 60-year-old man presented with fever, oral mucositis, pedal cellulitis, and bacteremia after a 6-week course of terbinafine 250 mg. He was taking concurrent yohimbine for impotence. Bone-marrow examination showed a hypocellular marrow with myeloid maturation arrest. Treatment consisted of withdrawal of out-patient medications, broad-spectrum antibiotics, hydration, and G-CSF, and was ultimately successful. Yohimbine was resumed later without any adverse effects.

Thrombocytopenia with epistaxis has been reported in a 25-year-old Yemeni woman with familial-ethnic leukopenia after treatment with terbinafine 250 mg for 4 weeks (76[c]). The platelet count recovered from a nadir of 63×10^{12}/l to 314×10^{12}/l after drug withdrawal.

Liver Hepatotoxicity of terbinafine is probably idiosyncratic and most likely a hypersensitivity reaction. Four further cases of *cholestatic hepatitis* associated with the administration of terbinafine have been reported (77[c], 78[c]). All the patients presented with jaundice and direct hyperbilirubinemia, various other clinical signs of hepatitis, and mild to moderate rises in alkaline phosphatase and hepatic transaminase activities. Biopsies in two patients showed cellular infiltrates in the portal tracts and hepatocellular and canalicular cholestasis (n = 1) and hepatocyte degeneration (n = 1). In the two cases with long-term follow-up, hepatitis was reversible after withdrawal of terbinafine and liver tests normalized within 6 months.

Skin and appendages Ten cases of severe skin reactions probably associated with terbinafine requiring drug withdrawal have been reported: *erythema multiforme* (five patients), *erythroderma* (one), severe *urticaria* (one), *iipityriasis rosea* (one), and worsening of pre-existing *psoriasis* (two) (79[c]). All the patients made an uneventful recovery with appropriate therapy. The authors pointed out that patients should be counselled about discontinuing terbinafine at the onset of a skin eruption and about seeking medical advice about further management.

Acute generalized exanthematous pustulosis associated with terbinafine has been described in two more patients (80[c], 81[c]). Both presented within 7–10 days after starting to take terbinafine with generalized pustular dermatosis and leukocytosis; fever was a presenting symptom in one patient. Treatment with systemic corticosteroids was successful in both cases.

A further case of *severe pustular psoriasis* provoked de novo by oral terbinafine has been reported in a 65-year-old man 2 weeks after the start of therapy for onychomycosis (82[c]). Treatment of psoriasis was complicated and ultimately required continuous systemic and topical antipsoriatic therapy.

Cutaneous lupus erythematosus attributed to terbinafine has been reported in two previously healthy women (83[c], 84[c]). In the first patient the lesions improved but did not resolve completely; in the second the symptoms resolved completely with appropriate therapy and the patient remained disease-free after withdrawal of all medication. Another woman with a previous history suggestive of lupus erythematosus developed a widespread flare in her skin 1 week after starting oral terbinafine (85[c]). The eruption ultimately responded to systemic treatment with corticosteroids.

Special senses *Taste disturbance* is a rare adverse effect of terbinafine. It is usually reversible, with a median time to recovery of 42 days. However, a 46-year-old woman had complete loss of taste after taking oral terbinafine, with persistent taste disturbances for 3 years after stopping the drug (86[c]).

A 38-year-old man presented with acute right otitis media and unrelated *painless bilateral enlargement of the parotid glands* 15 days after taking oral terbinafine for tinea cruris (87[c]). He stopped taking terbinafine and 12 days later the swelling had significantly abated and completely disappeared 4 weeks later.

Immunological and hypersensitivity reactions A 66-year-old man with temporal arteritis and hypertension developed a *hypersensitivity reaction* 4.5 weeks after starting to take terbinafine, with a skin eruption, fever, lymphadenopathy, and hepatic dysfunction (88[c]). Concomitant medications included prednisone, doxazosin, and aspirin. His symptoms and signs resolved within 6 weeks after withdrawal of terbinafine and continuation of all the other medications. The hypersensitivity syndrome reaction in this case was idiosyncratic, with no apparent predisposing factors.

Risk factors *Children* The plasma pharmacokinetics of terbinafine and five known metabolites have been investigated in 12 children mean age 8 (range 5–11) years who took a 125 mg capsule od for 6-8 weeks for tinea capitis (89[C]). The metabolism of terbinafine was similar to that observed in adults, and comparable steady-state plasma concentrations were measured after administration of the same oral dose in milligrams. Steady-state was reached by day 21 with no further accumulation up to day 56. Terbinafine was effective in all patients and safe and well tolerated over 56 days.

In a randomized double-blind comparison of terbinafine ($n = 27$) with itraconazole ($n = 28$) for 2 weeks for tinea capitis in Pakistani children, mean age 8 years, fever, body ache, and vertigo were seen with terbinafine in one patient each, and urticaria with itraconazole in two patients (90[C]). There were no significant changes in hematological and biochemical profiles.

In an open assessment of the efficacy, safety, and tolerability of oral terbinafine 125–250 mg/day for 1, 2, and 4 weeks for tinea capitis in 132 Brazilian children aged 1–14 years, adverse events were reported in 10 patients (91[C]). The drug was prematurely discontinued in one patient. In the post-treatment evaluation, two patients had abnormal bilirubin concentrations and eight patients abnormal alkaline phosphatase activities; none was considered clinically relevant.

Interactions Terbinafine is metabolized extensively by various pathways, including *N*-demethylation and *N*-oxidation. However, terbinafine metabolism uses only a small fraction of the total hepatic cytochrome P450 capacity. The propensity of terbinafine for drug interactions is therefore thought to be small.

Theophylline is largely metabolized by CYP1A2. In a randomized, cross-over study of 12 healthy volunteers, terbinafine increased theophylline exposure by 16%, with a 14% reduction in clearance and a 24% increase in half-life (92[C]). These pharmacokinetic changes may predispose individuals to accumulation of theophylline and unwanted toxicity. Caution should be taken in prescribing terbinafine for patients taking long-term theophylline.

Contradictory interactions of terbinafine with *warfarin* have been reported (93[c], 94[c]).

A 71-year-old woman taking a stable dose of warfarin and cimetidine was treated with terbinafine, and 32 days later developed profuse intestinal bleeding associated with a prothrombin time of 120 minutes, suggestive of an interaction between warfarin and terbinafine, either directly or through the mediation of cimetidine (which can reduce terbinafine clearance by 33%)

A 68-year-old woman taking warfarin, glibenclamide, metformin, furosemide, and spironolactone was given terbinafine 250 mg/day and 4 weeks later required progressive increases in the warfarin dosage to maintain a therapeutic INR; after withdrawal of terbinafine, her warfarin requirements returned to baseline over 4 weeks, supporting enzyme induction with gradual onset and offset.

Since a pharmacokinetic study of a single dose of warfarin in 26 healthy volunteers treated with terbinafine showed no significant interaction, and since a large post-marketing study of terbinafine did not find any cases of interaction of warfarin with terbinafine, the manufacturers (95[c]) and others (96[c]) have cautioned about any generalization regarding a interaction between terbinafine and warfarin.

An interaction of terbinafine with *nortriptyline* has been reported (97[c]).

A 74-year-old man taking a stable dose of nortriptyline for depression developed signs of nortriptyline intoxication 14 days after starting to take terbinafine. Nortriptyline serum concentrations were several times higher than the usual target range and fell to baseline after withdrawal of terbinafine. Rechallenge led to the same clinical and laboratory findings.

REFERENCES

1. Malik IA, Moid I, Aziz Z, Khan S, Suleman M. A randomized comparison of fluconazole with amphotericin B as empiric anti-fungal agents in cancer patients with prolonged fever and neutropenia. Am J Med 1998;105:478–83.
2. Pathak A, Pien FD, Carvalho L. Amphotericin B use in a community hospital, with special emphasis on side effects. Clin Infect Dis 1998;26:334–8.
3. Barcia JP. Hyperkalemia associated with rapid infusion of conventional and lipid complex formulations of amphotericin B. Pharmacotherapy 1998;18:874–6.
4. Camp MJ, Wingard JR, Gilmore CE, Lin LS, Dix SP, Davidson TG, Geller RB. Efficacy of low-dose dopamine in preventing amphotericin B nephrotoxicity in bone marrow transplant patients and leukemia patients. Antimicrob Agents Chemother 1998;42:3103–6.
5. Griswold MW, Briceland LL, Stein DS. Is amphotericin B test dosing needed? Ann Pharmacother 1998;32:475–7.
6. Schoffski P, Freund M, Wunder R, Petersen D, Kohne CH, Hecker H, Schubert U, Ganser A. Safety and toxicity of amphotericin B in glucose 5% or intralipid 20% in neutropenic patients with pneumonia or fever of unknown origin: randomised study. Br Med J 1998;317:379–84.
7. Manfredi R, Chiodo F. Case-control study of amphotericin B in a triglyceride fat emulsion versus conventional amphotericin B in patients with AIDS. Pharmacotherapy 1998;18:1087–92.
8. Torre D, Banfi G, Tambini R, Speranza F, Zeroli C, Martegani R, Airoldi M, Fiori G. A retrospective study on the efficacy and safety of amphotericin B in a lipid emulsion for the treatment of cryptococcal meningitis in AIDS patients. J Infect 1998;37:36–8.
9. White MH, Bowden RA, Sandler ES, Graham ML, Noskin GA, Wingard JR, Goldman M, Van Burik JA, McCabe A, Lin JS, Gurwith M, Miller CB. Randomized, double-blind clinical trial of amphotericin B colloidal dispersion vs amphotericin B in the empirical treatment of fever and neutropenia. Clin Infect Dis 1998;27:296–302.
10. Noskin GA, Pietrelli L, Coffey G, Gurwith M, Liang LJ. Amphotericin B colloidal dispersion for treatment of candidemia in immunocompromised patients. Clin Infect Dis 1998;26:461–7.
11. Anaissie EJ, Mattiuzzi GN, Miller CB, Noskin GA, Gurwith MJ, Mamelok RD, Pietrelli LA. Treatment of invasive fungal infections in renally impaired patients with amphotericin B colloidal dispersion. Antimicrob Agents Chemother 1998;42:606–11.
12. Groll AH, Piscitelli SC, Walsh TJ. Clinical pharmacology of systemic antifungal agents: a comprehensive review of agents in clinical use, current investigational compounds, and putative targets for antifungal drug development. Adv Pharmacol 1998;44:343–500.
13. Kauffman CA, Wiseman SW. Anaphylaxis upon switching lipid-containing amphotericin B formulations. Clin Infect Dis 1998;26:1237–8.

14. Johnson JR, Kangas PJ, West M. Serious adverse event after unrecognized substitution of one amphotericin B lipid preparation for another. Clin Infect Dis 1998;27:1342–3.
15. Walsh TJ, Hiemenz JW, Seibel NL, Perfect JR, Horwith G, Lee L, Silber JL, DiNubile MJ, Reboli A, Bow E, Lister J, Anaissie EJ. Amphotericin B lipid complex for invasive fungal infections: analysis of safety and efficacy in 556 cases. Clin Infect Dis 1998;26:1383–96.
16. Allsup D, Chu P. The use of amphotericin B lipid complex in 15 patients with presumed or proven fungal infection. Br J Haematol 1998;102:1109–10.
17. Myint H, Kyi AA, Winn RM. An open, noncomparative evaluation of the efficacy and safety of amphotericin B lipid complex as treatment of neutropenic patients with presumed or confirmed pulmonary fungal infections. J Antimicrob Chemother 1998;41:424–6.
18. Ringden O, Jonsson V, Hansen M, Tollemar J, Jacobsen N. Severe and common side-effects of amphotericin B lipid complex. Bone Marrow Transplant 1998;22:733–4.
19. Manley TJ, Chusid MJ, Rand SD, Wells D, Margolis DA. Reversible parkinsonism in a child after bone marrow transplantation and lipid-based amphotericin B therapy. Pediatr Infect Dis J 1998;17:433–4.
20. Luke RG, Boyle JA. Renal effects of amphotericin B lipid complex. Am J Kidney Dis 1998;31:780–5.
21. Garnacho-Montero J, Ortiz-Leyba C, Garcia Garmendia JL, Jimenez F. Life-threatening adverse event after amphotericin B lipid complex treatment in a patient treated previously with amphotericin B deoxycholate. Clin Infect Dis 1998;26:1016.
22. Walsh TJ, Yeldandi V, McEvoy M, Gonzalez C, Chanock S, Freifeld A, Seibel NI, Whitcomb PO, Jarosinski P, Boswell G, Bekersky I, Alak A, Buell D, Barret J, Wilson W. Safety, tolerance, and pharmacokinetics of a small unilamellar liposomal formulation of amphotericin B (AmBisome) in neutropenic patients. Antimicrob Agents Chemother 1998;42:2391–8.
23. Leenders AC, Daenen S, Jansen RL, Hop WC, Lowenberg B, Wijermans PW, Cornelissen J, Herbrecht R, Van der Lelie H, Hoogsteden HC, Verbrugh HA, De Marie S. Liposomal amphotericin B compared with amphotericin B deoxycholate in the treatment of documented and suspected neutropenia-associated invasive fungal infections. Br J Haematol 1998;103:205–12.
24. Ellis M, Spence D, De Pauw B, Meunier F, Marinus A, Collette L, Sylvester R, Meis J, Boogaerts M, Selleslag D, Krcmery V, Von Sinner W, MacDonald P, Doyen C, Vandercam B. An EORTC international multicenter randomized trial (EORTC number 19923) comparing two dosages of liposomal amphotericin B for treatment of invasive aspergillosis. Clin Infect Dis 1998;27:1406–12.
25. Clark AD, McKendrick S, Tansey PJ, Franklin IM, Chopra R. A comparative analysis of lipid-complexed and liposomal amphotericin B preparations in haematological oncology. Br J Haematol 1998;103:198–204.
26. Berman JD, Badaro R, Thakur CP, Wasunna KM, Behbehani K, Davidson R, Kuzoe F, Pang L, Weerasuriya K, Bryceson AD. Efficacy and safety of liposomal amphotericin B (AmBisome) for visceral leishmaniasis in endemic developing countries. Bull WHO 1998;76:25–32.
27. Carlini A, Angelini D, Burrows L, De Quirico G, Antonelli A. Cerebral aspergillosis: long term efficacy and safety of liposomal amphotericin B in kidney transplant. Nephrol Dial Transplant 1998;13:2659–61.
28. Araujo JJ, Dominguez A, Bueno C, Rodriguez J, Rios MJ, Muniain MA, Perez R. Nephrogenous diabetes insipidus secondary to the administration of amphotericin B and liposomal amphotericin B. Enferm Infecc Microbiol Clin 1998;16:204–5.
29. Johnson MD, Drew RH, Perfect JR. Chest discomfort associated with liposomal amphotericin B: report of three cases and review of the literature. Pharmacotherapy 1998;8:1053–61.
30. Scarcella A, Pasquariello MB, Giugliano B, Vendemmia M, De Lucia A. Liposomal amphotericin B treatment for neonatal fungal infections. Pediatr Infect Dis J 1998;17:146–8.
31. Weitkamp JH, Poets CF, Sievers R, Musswessels E, Groneck P, Thomas P, Bartmann P. Candida infection in very low birth-weight infants: outcome and nephrotoxicity of treatment with liposomal amphotericin B (AmBisome). Infection 1998;26:11–15.
32. Hospenthal DR, Bennett JE. Flucytosine monotherapy for cryptococcosis. Clin Infect Dis 1998;27:260–4.
33. Mayanja-Kizza H, Oishi K, Mitarai S, Yamashita H, Nalongo K, Watanabe K, Izumi T, Ococi-Jungala, Augustine K, Mugerwa R, Nagatake T, Matsumoto K. Combination therapy with fluconazole and flucytosine for cryptococcal meningitis in Ugandan patients with AIDS. Clin Infect Dis 1998;26:1362–6.
34. Schwarze R, Penk A, Pittrow L. Administration of fluconazole in children below 1 year of age: review. Mycoses 1998;41(Suppl 1):61–70.
35. Huttova M, Hartmanova I, Kralinsky K; Filka J, Uher J, Kurak J, Krizan S, Krcmery V Jr. Candida fungemia in neonates treated with fluconazole: report of forty cases, including eight with meningitis. Pediatr Infect Dis J 1998;17:1012–15.
36. Kar HK. Longitudinal melanonychia associated with fluconazole therapy. Int J Dermatol 1998;37:719–20.
37. Trapnell CB, Klecker RW, Jamis-Dow C, Collins JM. Glucuronidation of 3′-azido-3′-deoxythymidine (zidovudine) by human liver microsomes: relevance to clinical pharmacokinetic interactions with atovaquone, fluconazole, methadone, and valproic acid. Antimicrob Agents Chemother 1998;2:1592–6.
38. De Wit S, Debier M, De Smet M, McCrea J, Stone J, Carides A, Matthews C, Deutsch P, Clumeck N. Effect of fluconazole on indinavir pharmacokinetics in human immunodefi-

ciency virus-infected patients. Antimicrob Agents Chemother 1998;42:223–7.
39. Palkama VJ, Isohanni MH, Neuvonen PJ, Olkkola KT. The effect of intravenous and oral fluconazole on the pharmacokinetics and pharmacodynamics of intravenous alfentanil. Anesth Analg 1998;87:190–4.
40. Cobb MN, Desai J, Brown LS Jr, Zannikos PN, Rainey PM. The effect of fluconazole on the clinical pharmacokinetics of methadone. Clin Pharmacol Ther 1998;63:655–62.
41. Sinofsky FE, Pasquale SA. The effect of fluconazole on circulating ethinyl estradiol levels in women taking oral contraceptives. Am J Obstet Gynecol 1998;178:300–4.
42. Barone JA, Moskovitz BL, Guarnieri J, Hassell AE, Colaizzi JL, Bierman RH, Jessen L. Enhanced bioavailability of itraconazole in hydroxypropyl-beta-cyclodextrin solution versus capsules in healthy volunteers. Antimicrob Agents Chemother 1998;42:1862–5.
43. Phillips P, De Beule K, Frechette G, Tchamouroff S, Vandercam B, Weitner L, Hoepelman A, Stingi G, Clotet B. A double-blind comparison of itraconazole oral solution and fluconazole capsules for the treatment of oropharyngeal candidiasis in patients with AIDS. Clin Infect Dis 1998;26:1368–73.
44. Graybill JR, Vazquez J, Darouiche RO, Morhart R, Greenspan D, Tuazon C, Wheat LJ, Carey J, Leviton I, Hewitt RG, Macgregor RR, Valenti W, Restrepo M, Moskovitz BL. Randomized trial of itraconazole oral solution for oropharyngeal candidiasis in HIV/AIDS patients. Am J Med 1998;104:33–9.
45. Haneke E, Abeck D, Ring J. Safety and efficacy of intermittent therapy with itraconazole in finger- and toenail onychomycosis: a multicentre trial. Mycoses 1998;11:521–7.
46. Boonk W, De Geer D, De Kreek E, Remme J, Van Huystee B. Itraconazole in the treatment of tinea corporis and tinea cruris: comparison of two treatment schedules. Mycoses 1998;41:509–14.
47. Schuller J, Remme JJ, Rampen FH, Van Neer FC. Itraconazole in the treatment of tinea pedis and tinea manuum: comparison of two treatment schedules. Mycoses 1998;41:515–20.
48. Svejgaard E, Avnstorp C, Wanscher B, Nilsson J, Heremans A. Efficacy and safety of short-term itraconazole in tinea pedis: a double-blind, randomized, placebo-controlled trial. Dermatology 1998;197:368–72.
49. Jahangir M, Hussain I, Ul Hasan M, Haroon TS. A double-blind, randomized, comparative trial of itraconazole versus terbinafine for 2 weeks in tinea capitis. Br J Dermatol 1998;139:672–4.
50. Park H, Knowles S, Shear NH. Serum sickness-like reaction to itraconazole. Ann Pharmacother 1998;32:1249.
51. De Repentigny L, Ratelle J, Leclerc JM, Cornu G, Sokal EM, Jacqmin P, De Beule K. Repeated-dose pharmacokinetics of an oral solution of itraconazole in infants and children. Antimicrob Agents Chemother 1998;42:404–8.
52. Abdel-Rahman SM, Powell DA, Nahata MC. Efficacy of itraconazole in children with *Trichophyton tonsurans* tinea capitis. J Am Acad Dermatol 1998;38:443–6.
53. Kantola T, Kivisto KT, Neuvonen PJ. Effect of itraconazole on the pharmacokinetics of atorvastatin. Clin Pharmacol Ther 1998;64:58–65.
54. Kivisto KT, Kantola T, Neuvonen PJ. Different effects of itraconazole on the pharmacokinetics of fluvastatin and lovastatin. Br J Clin Pharmacol 1998;46:49–53.
55. Neuvonen PJ, Kantola T, Kivisto KT. Simvastatin but not pravastatin is very susceptible to interaction with the CYP3A4 inhibitor itraconazole. Clin Pharmacol Ther 1998;63:332–41.
56. Billaud EM, Guillemain R, Tacco F, Chevalier P. Evidence for a pharmacokinetic interaction between itraconazole and tacrolimus in organ transplant patients. Br J Clin Pharmacol 1998;46:271–2.
57. Furlan V, Parquin F, Penaud JF, Cerrina J, Le Roy Ladurie F, Dartevelle P, Taburet AM. Interaction between tacrolimus and itraconazole in a heart-lung transplant recipient. Transplant Proc 1998;30:187–8.
58. Backman JT, Kivisto KT, Olkkola KT, Neuvonen PJ. The area under the plasma concentration-time curve for oral midazolam is 400-fold larger during treatment with itraconazole than with rifampicin. Eur J Clin Pharmacol 1998;54:53–8.
59. Jaruratanasirikul S, Sriwiriyajan S. Effect of rifampicin on the pharmacokinetics of itraconazole in normal volunteers and AIDS patients. Eur J Clin Pharmacol 1998;54:155–8.
60. Kawakami M, Suzuki K, Ishizuka T, Hidaka T, Matsuki Y, Nakamura H. Effect of grapefruit juice on pharmacokinetics of itraconazole in healthy subjects. Int J Clin Pharmacol Ther 1998;36:306–8.
61. Kanda Y, Kami M, Matsuyama T, Mitani K, Chiba S, Yazaki Y, Hirai H. Plasma concentration of itraconazole in patients receiving chemotherapy for hematological malignancies: the effect of famotidine on the absorption of itraconazole. Hematol Oncol 1998;16:33–7.
62. Jaruratanasirikul S, Sriwiriyajan S. Effect of omeprazole on the pharmacokinetics of itraconazole. Eur J Clin Pharmacol 1998;54:159–61.
63. Luurila H, Kivisto KT, Neuvonen PJ. Effect of itraconazole on the pharmacokinetics and pharmacodynamics of zolpidem. Eur J Clin Pharmacol 1998;54:163–6.
64. Raaska K, Neuvonen PJ. Serum concentrations of clozapine and *N*-desmethylclozapine are unaffected by the potent CYP3A4 inhibitor itraconazole. Eur J Clin Pharmacol 1998;54:167–70.
65. Palkama VJ, Neuvonen PJ, Olkkola KT. The CYP 3A4 inhibitor itraconazole has no effect on the pharmacokinetics of iv. fentanyl. Br J Anaesth 1998;81:598–600.
66. Varis T, Kaukonen KM, Kivisto KT, Neuvonen PJ. Plasma concentrations and effects of oral

methylprednisolone are considerably increased by itraconazole. Clin Pharmacol Ther 1998;64:363–8.
67. Gillies J, Hung KA, Fitzsimons E, Soutar R. Severe vincristine toxicity in combination with itraconazole. Clin Lab Haematol 1998;20:123–4.
68. Greenblatt DJ, Von Moltke LL, Harmatz JS, Mertzanis P, Graf JA, Durol ALB, Counihan M, Roth-Schechter B, Shader RI. Kinetic and dynamic interaction study of zolpidem with ketoconazole, itraconazole, and fluconazole. Clin Pharmacol Ther 1998;64:661–71.
69. Greenblatt DJ, Wright CE, Von Moltke LL, Harmatz JS, Ehrenberg BL, Harrel LM. Ketoconazole inhibition of triazolam and alprazolam clearance: differential kinetic and dynamic consequences. Clin Pharmacol Ther 1998;64:237–47.
70. Arlander E, Ekstrom G, Alm C, Carrillo JA, Bielenstein M, Bottiger Y, Bertilsson L, Gustafsson LL. Metabolism of ropivacaine in humans is mediated by CYP1A2 and to a minor extent by CYP3A4: an interaction study with fluvoxamine and ketoconazole as in vivo inhibitors. Clin Pharmacol Ther 1998;64:484–91.
71. Tiseo PJ, Perdomo CA, Friedhoff LT. Concurrent administration of donepezil HCl and ketoconazole: assessment of pharmacokinetic changes following single and multiple doses. Br J Clin Pharmacol 1998;46(Suppl 1):30–4.
72. Khoo SM, Porter JH, Edwards GA, Charman WN. Metabolism of halofantrine to its equipotent metabolite, desbutylhalofantrine, is decreased when orally administered with ketoconazole. J Pharm Sci 1998;87:1538–41.
73. De Backer M, De Vroey C, Lesaffre E, Scheys I, De Keyser P. Twelve weeks of continuous oral therapy for toenail onychomycosis caused by dermatophytes: a double-blind comparative trial of terbinafine 250 mg/day versus itraconazole 200 mg/day. J Am Acad Dermatol 1998;38:S57–63.
74. Gupta AK, Soori GS, Del Rosso JQ, Bartos PB, Shear NH. Severe neutropenia associated with oral terbinafine therapy. J Am Acad Dermatol 1998;38:765–7.
75. Ornstein DL, Ely P. Reversible agranulocytosis associated with oral terbinafine for onychomycosis. J Am Acad Dermatol 1998;39:1023–4.
76. Grunwald MH. Thrombocytopenia associated with oral terbinafine. Int J Dermatol 1998;37:634.
77. Fernandes NF, Geller SA, Fong TL. Terbinafine hepatotoxicity: case report and review of the literature. Am J Gastroenterol 1998;93:459–60.
78. Gupta AK, Del Rosso JQ, Lynde CW, Brown GH, Shear NH. Hepatitis associated with terbinafine therapy: three case reports and a review of the literature. Clin Exp Dermatol 1998;23:64–7.
79. Gupta AK, Lynde CW, Lauzon GJ, Mehlmauer MA, Braddock SW, Miller CA, Del Rosso JQ, Shear NH. Cutaneous adverse effects associated with terbinafine therapy: 10 case reports and a review of the literature. Br J Dermatol 1998;138:529–32.
80. Papa CA, Miller OF. Pustular psoriasiform eruption with leukocytosis associated with terbinafine. J Am Acad Dermatol 1998;39:115–17.
81. Condon CA, Downs AM, Archer CB. Terbinafine-induced acute generalized exanthematous pustulosis. Br J Dermatol 1998;138:709–10.
82. Wilson NJ, Evans S. Severe pustular psoriasis provoked by oral terbinafine. Br J Dermatol 1998;139:168.
83. Brooke R, Coulson IH, Al-Dawoud A. Terbinafine-induced subacute cutaneous lupus erythematosus. Br J Dermatol 1998;139:1132-3.
84. Murphy M, Barnes L. Terbinafine-induced lupus erythematosus. Br J Dermatol 1998;138:708–9.
85. Holmes S, Kemmett D. Exacerbation of systemic lupus erythematosus induced by terbinafine. Br J Dermatol 1998;139:1133.
86. Bong JL, Lucke TW, Evans CD. Persistent impairment of taste resulting from terbinafine. Br J Dermatol 1998;139:747–8.
87. Torrens JK, McWhinney PH. Parotid swelling and terbinafine. Br Med J 1998;316:440–1.
88. Gupta AK, Porges AJ. Hypersensitivity syndrome reaction to oral terbinafine. Australas J Dermatol 1998;39:171–2.
89. Humbert H, Denouel J, Cabiac MD, Lakhdar H, Sioufi A. Pharmacokinetics of terbinafine and five known metabolites in children, after oral administration. Biopharm Drug Disp 1998;19:417–23.
90. Jahangir M, Hussain I, Ul Hasan M, Haroon TS. A double-blind, randomized, comparative trial of itraconazole versus terbinafine for 2 weeks in tinea capitis. Br J Dermatol 1998;139:672–4.
91. Filho ST, Cuce LC, Foss NT, Marques SA, Santamaria JR. Efficacy, safety and tolerability of terbinafine for Tinea capitis in children: Brazilian multicentric study with daily oral tablets for 1, 2 and 4 weeks. J Eur Acad Dermatol Venereol 1998;11:141–6.
92. Trepanier EF, Nafziger AN, Amsden GW. Effect of terbinafine on theophylline pharmacokinetics in healthy volunteers. Antimicrob Agents Chemother 1998;42:695–7.
93. Gupta AK, Ross GS. Interaction between terbinafine and warfarin. Dermatology 1998;196:266–7.
94. Warwick JA, Corrall RJ. Serious interaction between warfarin and oral terbinafine. Br Med J 1998;316:440.
95. Gantmacher J, Mills-Bomford J, Williams T. Interaction between warfarin and oral terbinafine. Manufacturer does not agree that interaction was with terbinafine. Br Med J 1998;317:205.
96. Clarke MF, Boardman HS. Interaction between warfarin and oral terbinafine. Systematic review of interaction profile of warfarin is needed. Br Med J 1998;317:205–6.
97. Van der Kuy PH, Hooymans PM. Nortriptyline intoxication induced by terbinafine. Br Med J 1998;316:441.

Charles Woodrow, Isabela Ribeiro and Sanjeev Krishna

28 Antiprotozoal drugs

ANTIMALARIAL DRUGS

(SED-13, 799; SEDA-20, 257; SEDA-21, 293; SEDA-22, 302)

For a review of the current recommendations on the prevention and treatment of malaria see SEDA-20 (p. 257) and Newton and White (1[R]).

R ### *Antimalarial prophylaxis*

New antimalarial prophylactic regimens are urgently required, because of the spread of parasite resistance to established drugs, such as chloroquine, proguanil, and more recent additions such as mefloquine. Furthermore, factors other than efficacy may limit the use of prophylactic agents.

Quinine and artemisinin derivatives have relatively short half-lives and are reserved for treatment of established infection with P. falciparum.

Mefloquine causes severe neuropsychiatric symptoms in a significant minority of travellers.

Doxycycline requires daily dosing, may cause gastrointestinal adverse effects, vaginitis, and photosensitivity reactions and is contraindicated in children under 8 years of age and in pregnant women. Until recently it had not been extensively evaluated in Africa. Azithromycin, a semisynthetic macrolide derivative, has a longer half-life and fewer gastrointestinal adverse effects than erythromycin and has shown promise in phase II studies. In larger (phase III) studies in Kenya (in an area of intense P. falciparum malaria transmission), both doxycycline (100 mg od) and azithromycin (250 mg od) proved efficacious (93 and 83% respectively) in preventing parasitemia in semi-immune adults (2[C]). Both drugs were generally well tolerated, only one patient withdrawing because of a probable adverse effect (recurrent vaginitis in a doxycycline recipient). Azithromycin 1000 mg weekly was less efficacious than the daily regimen (64%). These results support the use of doxycycline as safe and effective prophylaxis for adults travelling to East Africa although studies in non-immune adults are required to confirm protective efficacy. Azithromycin is a potential prophylactic agent for groups who cannot take doxycycline and other antimalarial drugs.

Atovaquone acts synergistically with proguanil, and the combination of these two drugs (Malarone®) is highly efficacious in treatment of P. falciparum malaria in South-East Asia, Africa, and South America. Prophylaxis with either one or two tablets containing atovaquone 250 mg and proguanil hydrochloride 100 mg (one quarter or one half of the daily treatment dose), taken once daily for 10 weeks, prevented P. falciparum malaria in 100% of semi-immune adults in a highly endemic area of Kenya (3[C]). Children in Gabon taking daily Malarone at approximately one quarter of the treatment dose were similarly protected (4[C]). Gastrointestinal adverse effects including abdominal pain and vomiting, were relatively common in the initial parasite clearance phase of the pediatric study (when a full treatment course was given) and there was one case of repeated vomiting in the parasite clearance phase of the adult study. In both studies the regimens were well tolerated in the prophylaxis phase (no difference from placebo). This efficacy and tolerability profile may be applicable to malaria prevention outside Africa. The use of the combination is predicted to reduce the development of resistance to each drug. Furthermore, atovaquone eliminates parasites during the hepatic phase of infection (causal prophylaxis), potentially removing the requirement to continue prophylaxis for several weeks after return from a malarious area, a period when compliance with current regimens is likely to be poor.

Side Effects of Drugs, Annual 23
J.K. Aronson, ed.

ENDOPEROXIDES

Artemisia derivatives *(SED-13, 818; SEDA-20, 259; SEDA-21, 293; SEDA-22, 302)*

Artemisinin is an antimalarial constituent isolated from the traditional Chinese medicinal herb Qinghao (*Artemisia annua*). It is a sesquiterpene lactone with an endoperoxide bridge, structurally distinct from other classes of antimalarial agents. Several derivatives of the original compound have proved effective in the treatment of *P. falciparum* malaria and are currently available in a variety of formulations: artesunate (intravenous, rectal, oral), artelinate (oral), artemisinin (intravenous, rectal, oral), dihydroartemisinin (oral), artemether (intravenous, oral, rectal), and arteether (intravenous).

None of these medications has yet been registered for use in Europe or North America. In recent years there has been a substantial increase in our knowledge of their safety, efficacy, and pharmacokinetics. Higher cure rates are achieved when these compounds are combined with longer-acting antimalarial drugs, such as mefloquine. After years of continued use, the sequential use of artesunate and mefloquine remains an effective treatment in areas of multidrug resistance in South-East Asia and provides an impetus for the evaluation of other artesunate-containing combination regimens for the treatment of uncomplicated malaria, such as artemether + benflumetol (5[C]–9[C]). Reviews of clinical trials have reaffirmed the high tolerability of the artemisinins (10[R], 11[R]). Adverse effects have been chiefly limited to the GI tract. Most reported adverse events were described as mild and transient and none resulted in discontinuation of treatment. Although in animals several of the artemisinin derivatives have produced a characteristic neurological lesion, there is no good evidence of neurotoxicity in man. A recent study of mice suggested that intramuscular artemether is significantly more neurotoxic than intramuscular artesunate (12[C]).

Use in pregnancy Artemisinin derivatives (artesunate and artemether) for the treatment of multidrug resistant *Plasmodium falciparum* malaria have recently been evaluated in 83 Karen pregnant women in Thailand; 55 women were treated for recrudescent infection after quinine or mefloquine, 12 for uncomplicated hyperparasitemic episodes, and 16 had not declared their pregnancy when treated (13[C]). Artesunate and artemether were well tolerated and there was no drug-related adverse effect. Overall 73 pregnancies resulted in live births, three in abortions and two in still-births; five women were lost to follow-up before delivery. There was no congenital abnormality in any of the neonates, and the 46 children followed for more than 1 year all developed normally.

Interactions Recent pharmacokinetic studies have shown that artemisinin induces its own elimination and that of *omeprazole* through an increase in CYP2C19 activity and that of another enzyme, as yet to be identified (14[C]).

CHLOROQUINE AND CONGENERS *(SED-13, 801; SEDA-20, 260; SEDA-21, 294; SEDA-22, 303)*

Chloroquine

The efficacy of chloroquine as treatment for *Plasmodium falciparum* infection is now limited by parasite resistance in most parts of the world.

Cardiovascular Third-degree *atrioventricular conduction defects* have been reported in two patients with rheumatoid arthritis after prolonged administration of chloroquine (15[c], 16[c]).

Musculoskeletal Chloroquine-induced *neuromyopathy* is a complication of chloroquine treatment of autoimmune disorders or long-term use of chloroquine as a prophylactic antimalarial drug (17[c]).

Halofantrine *(SED-13, 820; SEDA-20, 260; SEDA-21, 295; SEDA-22, 304)*

Cardiovascular The *cardiotoxicity* of halofantrine has been previously well documented in patients in South-East Asia. African children receiving halofantrine (three doses of 8 mg/kg 6-hourly) for uncomplicated *P. falciparum* malaria had increases in both the PR interval and the QT_c interval; two children developed first-degree heart block and one child second-degree heart block out of 42 children in the study; the QT_c interval either increased by more than

125% of baseline value or by more than 0.44 seconds, an effect that persisted for at least 48 hours (18[C]).

Mefloquine *(SED-13, 808; SEDA-20, 261; SEDA-21, 296; SEDA-22, 304)*

Mefloquine remains useful in the treatment of uncomplicated malaria in areas of chloroquine resistance, but recommendations for mefloquine as prophylaxis in travellers are under constant review. In visitors to the Kruger National Park (South Africa), adverse effects were reported in 325 (25%) of 1300 subjects taking mefloquine; *gastrointestinal* and *neuropsychiatric* effects were dominant (19[C]). Four subjects required hospital attention for particularly severe *neuropsychiatric* reactions and 53 changed from mefloquine prophylaxis because of adverse effects. However in the same study chloroquine + proguanil prophylaxis led to reported adverse effects in 720 (29%) of 2488 subjects: one had a convulsion and 69 altered their prophylaxis because of adverse events or the dosing schedule. In this population mefloquine was as well tolerated as chloroquine + proguanil prophylaxis in general terms. This is in contrast to previous studies, in which the use of mefloquine led to higher rates of intolerance and severe adverse effects.

Gastrointestinal *Acute fatty liver* has recently been reported after malaria prophylaxis with mefloquine (20[c]).

A 46-year-old woman took five, weekly doses of mefloquine 250 mg before discontinuing treatment because of neuropsychiatric and gastrointestinal symptoms. Over the next month she had watery diarrhea, 11 kg weight loss, dependent edema, and abdominal fullness. On examination the liver was substantially enlarged; ultrasound imaging showed massive hepatomegaly with diffuse high-grade steatosis. Serological investigations for infective and autoimmune causes were negative. Her symptoms abated with fluid, electrolyte, and albumin replacement. A fine-needle liver biopsy showed features of diffuse macrovesical hepatic steatosis. Clinical and radiological changes subsided without sequelae.

Acute fatty liver in this case may have been an idiosyncratic adverse effect of mefloquine.

Skin and appendages Mefloquine has been previously associated with *erythema multiforme, Stevens–Johnson syndrome,* and *toxic epidermal necrolysis* (21[C]). A recent case report tentatively suggested that mefloquine may *exacerbate psoriasis* (as can other antimalarial drugs, such as quinidine, chloroquine, and proguanil) (22[c]).

Use in pregnancy A review of the use of mefloquine in pregnancy (23[C]) has not suggested that mefloquine has a worse effect in pregnancy than other antimalarials, such as chloroquine and pyrimethamine + sulfadoxine.

Overdosage Mefloquine has a relatively wide therapeutic margin, but can cause predictable and sometimes long-lasting toxicity in overdose. Two recent case reports have described how the antifungal drug terbinafine (Lamasil) was confused with Lariam, leading to accidental mefloquine overdosage and neuropsychiatric adverse effects, including ataxia, high-frequency hearing loss, depression, and paresthesia (24[c]).

Primaquine and congeners (8-aminoquinolines) *(SED-13, 810; SEDA-19, 264; SEDA-21, 296; SEDA-22, 305)*

Primaquine is an 8-aminoquinoline antimalarial used for many years to eradicate the hepatic stages of *P. vivax* and *P. ovale* and more recently as prophylaxis against *P. falciparum.* Primaquine can cause dose-dependent *hepatotoxicity,* as illustrated by a case of acute liver failure (with spontaneous recovery) caused by accidental overdosage (1260 mg on the second day of treatment for *Plasmodium vivax*) (24[c]).

Proguanil *(SED-13, 811, SEDA-22, 305)*

Proguanil (chloroguanide hydrochloride, Paludrine) has been used for many years as a prophylactic agent (in combination with chloroquine), and more recently in combination with atovaquone for therapy of uncomplicated *Plasmodium falciparum* infections (see section on atovaquone above). Proguanil has few, mostly mild, adverse effects (*gastrointestinal symptoms* and *mouth ulcers*) at therapeutic doses but can accumulate in patients with chronic renal insufficiency and cause *bone marrow toxicity.* Recently hepatitis with mild jaundice has been attributed to proguanil (25[c]).

Quinine *(SED-13, 814; SEDA-19, 265; SEDA-20, 261; SEDA-21, 297; SEDA-22, 306)*

Immunological and hypersensitivity reactions Quinine can cause a variety of *immune-mediated syndromes*, most commonly isolated *thrombocytopenia,* but rarely microangiopathic hemolytic anemia with thrombocytopenia and acute renal failure (*hemolytic-uremic syndrome,*). Two recent reports of immune-mediated syndromes following the use of quinine for leg cramps have helped to provide an immunopathological explanation for the diversity of such presentations (26[c], 27[c]). One patient presented with thrombocytopenic purpura, presumed to be idiopathic (which responded to corticosteroids and intravenous immunoglobulin) and subsequently presented again with hemolytic-uremic syndrome, and required intensive renal replacement and immunosuppressive therapy. Analysis of serum samples from the isolated thrombocytopenic stage of the presentation showed the presence of quinine-dependent antibodies specific for platelet surface glycoprotein GPIb/IX. Quinine-dependent antibody targets widened to include glycoprotein IIb/IIIa during the hemolytic-uremic phase of the illness, with additional binding to neutrophils and lymphocytes. In another case of acute systemic hypersensitivity to quinine, which mimicked septic shock, with little hemolysis or renal involvement, the patient presented twice with a virtually identical clinical picture: sudden fever, rigors, and back pain, followed by hypotension, metabolic acidosis, granulocytopenia, and disseminated intravascular coagulation. On each occasion clinical and laboratory indices recovered spontaneously within 36 hours. A retrospective analysis of the patient's serum showed the presence of neutrophil-specific, quinine-dependent antibodies. Glycoprotein epitopes involved in quinine-induced thrombocytopenia have been characterized (28[R]).

DRUGS USED FOR *PNEUMOCYSTIS CARINII* PNEUMONIA

The drugs used for the treatment and prophylaxis of *Pneumocystis carinii* pneumonia (PCP) have been reviewed (SEDA-20, 266; 29[R], 30[R]).

Atovaquone *(see also above) (SED-13, 828; SEDA-19, 266; SEDA-20, 264; SEDA-21, 298; SEDA-22, 307)*

Atovaquone is a hydroxynaphthaquinone with activity against a number of protozoa, such as *Pneumocystis carinii, P. falciparum,* and *Toxoplasma gondii.*

A study conducted by the AIDS Clinical Trials Group (ACTG) has shown that among patients who cannot tolerate treatment with co-trimoxazole, atovaquone and dapsone are similarly effective in preventing PCP. Among patients who did not originally take dapsone, atovaquone was better tolerated and it might be the preferred choice for prophylaxis of PCP in this setting (31[C]). Inexplicably the rate of PCP showed a greater fall in patients who discontinued the study drugs compared with those who continued to take them.

Co-trimoxazole (trimethoprim + sulfamethoxazole) *(see also Chapter 26) (SED-13, 826; SEDA-20, 264; SEDA 21, 299; SEDA-22, 307)*

Co-trimoxazole remains the drug of choice for the prophylaxis and treatment of a variety of opportunistic infections in HIV-infected patients (29[R], 32[R]). It is cheap and efficacious, and its use is limited only by the high incidence of adverse events in these patients.

Endocrine, metabolic Trimethoprim caused substantial *increases in fasting homocysteine concentrations,* up to concentrations associated with atherothrombotic complications (33[C]). The authors questioned the long-term administration of trimethoprim in patients with a high cardiovascular risk profile, cardiovascular disease, or a history of thrombosis, or in those who are being treated for hyperhomocysteinemia.

Urinary system The *nephrotoxicity* of anti-infective drugs and more specifically sulfonamides has recently been reviewed (34[R]). The main nephrotoxic effect of therapy with high-dose co-trimoxazole is *intratubular obstruction* caused by precipitation of the drug in the proximal renal tubule. The trimethoprim component of co-trimoxazole has also been implicated in an amiloride-like action on the distal tubule, leading to *hyperkalemia* and *metabolic acidosis.* A case of *hyperkalemic ascending paralysis,* mimicking Guillain–Barré syndrome, has been described after the administration of standard doses of co-trimoxazole to a patient with underlying type IV renal tubular acidosis (35[c]). High-dose intravenous co-trimoxazole caused significant *metabolic acidosis* in six of 15 HIV-infected patients treated for PCP (36[C]).

Immunological and hypersensitivity reactions This issue has been the subject of a number of recent papers and a review (37[R]). The acronyms DRESS (Drug Rash with Eosinophilia and Systemic Symptoms) and DIDMOHS (Drug-Induced Delayed Multi-Organ Hypersensitivity Syndrome) have been suggested to describe these reactions (38[r], 39[r]). A variety of mechanisms have been proposed for the skin reactions to co-trimoxazole and the increased incidence of these in patients with AIDS, in particular those with a high degree of immunosuppression. Glutathione and acetylator status appear to be involved in the pathogenesis of hypersensitivity (40[R]), while CD4 count may predict the likelihood of adverse reactions (41[C]). Desensitization protocols for non-life-threatening adverse reactions to co-trimoxazole have been increasingly advocated (42[C], 43[C]). Despite the number of articles published on this subject, there is still controversy on basic issues, such as whether reinstitution of full-dose therapy (rechallenge) or a dose escalation regimen ('desensitization') is preferable or desirable.

Rhabdomyolysis has not classically been considered part of the co-trimoxazole hypersensitivity syndrome. A recent review by scientists of the US Food and Drug Administration has described eight cases of rhabdomyolysis associated with co-trimoxazole in HIV-positive patients (44[C]). Six of these patients presented with other systemic symptoms consistent with a hypersensitivity syndrome. As this is a potentially fatal condition, rhabdomyolysis has since been added to the co-trimoxazole US labelling.

There has been a single report of *Stevens–Johnson syndrome, arthritis, and bilateral uveitis* complicating treatment with trimethoprim alone (45[c]). The case was clearly drug-induced, with a positive unintentional rechallenge. It brings to attention the fact that trimethoprim might be responsible for some of the serious adverse reactions described with the use of co-trimoxazole. This fact has been further underlined by a recent report of 13 cases of anaphylactic reactions after the use of trimethoprim alone for urinary infections (46[C]).

Interactions Two cases of a disulfiram-like reaction have been reported with the combined used of co-trimoxazole with *ethanol* (47[c]). It was hypothesized that co-trimoxazole might inhibit the elimination of acetaldehyde through an interaction with CYP2C9.

Dapsone *(SED-13, 826; SEDA-22, 309)*

A recent review has summarized the use of dapsone for the prevention and prevention of *P. Carinii* (48[R]). Dapsone is a synthetic sulfone with activity against *P. carinii* as monotherapy or when used in combination with trimethoprim or pyrimethamine. Dapsone has activity against other human pathogens, such as *Mycobacterium leprae* and *Plasmodium* species; other indications for its use include dermatitis herpetiformis. The combination with trimethoprim is recommended for the treatment of PCP in patients who cannot tolerate co-trimoxazole.

Respiratory There has been a second report of *eosinophilic pneumonia* associated with dapsone (49[c]).

A 60-year-old woman with chronic urticaria took dapsone (100 mg/day) after failure of the conventional treatment (antihistamines and corticosteroids). Two weeks later she developed wheezing, dyspnea, a productive cough, and fever. On examination she had pulmonary crackles. Laboratory tests showed a raised ESR (86 mm/hour), a leukocytosis (total white cell count 11.6×10^9/l) with a peripheral eosinophilia (9.4%), and a low hemoglobin (7.0 g/dl). Chest radiography showed bilateral infiltrates. Dapsone was withdrawn because of the anemia, and she was given ampicillin and erythromycin. As her symptoms rapidly abated and the lung infiltrates disappeared, a diagnosis of atypical pneumonia was made. Four months later, dapsone was again prescribed for worsening urticaria. A few hours later, she had a new episode of dyspnea, cough, and fever. Bronchoalveolar lavage fluid contained 136 800 cells/ml with 21% eosinophils. Dapsone was withdrawn and 8 months later she was well.

Hematological Dapsone-induced *methemoglobinemia* has been reviewed (50[R]), and in a recent case report the challenges of asymptomatic methemoglobinemia in a patient undergoing surgery have been discussed (51[c]).

DRUGS USED IN THE TREATMENT OF OTHER PROTOZOAL INFECTIONS

Metronidazole *(SED-13, 831; SEDA-21, 301; SEDA-22, 311)*

Metronidazole is an antimicrobial agent with broad activity, encompassing a number of bacterial and antiprotozoal infections, including amebiasis, giardiasis, *Trichomonas* infections, bacterial vaginosis, and anerobic infections. Metronidazole has been formulated as a vaginal gel (0.75%) for the treatment of bacterial vaginosis. A single daily 5-day regimen has been approved by the FDA and has been shown to be as effective as oral metronidazole (52[R]).

Nervous system Metronidazole can cause *peripheral neuropathy,* reportedly after chronic use and in high doses. A recent case of peripheral neuropathy was associated with intermittent use of metronidazole (2 g/day for 5 days every other month) (53[c]).

A 65-year-old white woman with small intestine bacterial overgrowth developed persistent numbness and tingling of her upper and lower extremities. She had been taking alternating courses of tetracycline and metronidazole for 5 days every other month for about 1 year. Other medications included amitriptyline, lisinopril, digoxin, omeprazole, and tamoxifen. Serum vitamin B_{12} and folate concentrations were within the reference ranges. She had reduced sensation in a stocking-glove distribution, reduced sensation to touch and pin-prick, intact reflexes, and no weakness. Neuropathy was attributed to metronidazole, which was withdrawn. After 4 months she reported improvement. On follow-up at 5 months, there was no evidence of peripheral neuropathy.

Skin and appendages A case of *fixed drug eruption* has been described after the administration of metronidazole (54[c]). A provocation test showed cross-reactivity with tinidazole but not secnidazole.

DRUGS USED FOR AMERICAN TRYPANOSOMIASIS

Chagas' disease, or American trypanosomiasis, is a zoonosis caused by the flagellate protozoan *Trypanosoma cruzi.* Acute Chagas' disease is a usually mild febrile illness that results from initial infection with the organism. After spontaneous resolution of the acute illness, most infected people remain for life in the indeterminate phase of chronic Chagas' disease, which is characterized by detectable parasitemia and antibodies to *T. cruzi* and an absence of symptoms. In a minority of chronically infected patients, the heart and gastrointestinal tract are affected, with significant associated morbidity and mortality.

Treatment options for *T. cruzi* infections remain suboptimal, owing to the toxicity and limited effectiveness of the available drugs. Nevertheless, new treatment regimens with lower doses and shorter durations of therapy have shown increased tolerability without apparent reduction of efficacy.

Nifurtimox is the only drug approved for use in the US, but is available exclusively on request from the Drug Service of the CDC. In acute Chagas' disease, it reduces both the duration of symptoms and parasitemia and mortality, but with limited efficacy in the eradication of parasites. Common adverse effects include *epigastric pain, nausea, vomiting, anorexia,* and *weight loss.* Neurological adverse events include *disorientation, insomnia, paresthesia, polyneuropathy,* and *convulsions.* Hematological adverse effects include *thrombocytopenia* and *granulocytopenia. Hypersensitivity cutaneous reactions* have also been reported (SED-13, 836-7).

Benznidazole, a nitroimidazole, has a similar efficacy and safety profile (SED-13, 833). This drug is widely used in Latin America, but is not available in the US. It also causes a disulfiram-like effect with ethanol.

There is growing consensus that patients with indeterminate phase infection, asymptomatic chronic cardiac Chagas' disease and children or young adults with positive serology should be treated (55[R]). In a recent double-blind, randomized, clinical trial benznidazole 5 mg/kg/day for 60 days was compared with placebo in children in the indeterminate phase of infection by *T. cruzi.* In general, treatment was well tolerated. The treated children had a significant reduction in mean titers of antibodies against *T. cruzi* measured by indirect hemaglutination, indirect immunofluorescence, and ELISA. On a 4-year follow-up, 62% of the benznidazole-treated children and no placebo-treated children were seronegative for *T. cruzi.* Xenodiagnosis after 48 months was positive in 4.7% of the benznidazole-treated children and in 51% of the placebo-treated children (56[C]).

Another potentially important development was the recently identified antitrypanosomal activity of other azole antimicrobial agents. The triazole itraconazole produced a parasitological cure rate of 53% in chronically infected patients compared with 44% in patients taking allopurinol, a result that may lead to more use of this family of drugs in *T. cruzi* infections (57[C]). Only four of 404 treatments were discontinued because of adverse effects that subsided after suspension of treatment.

Melarsoprol *(SED-13, 834)*

Melarsoprol is a trivalent arsenical with activity against East African and West African trypanosomiasis. It is the drug of choice in the case of *T. rhodesiense* infection with CNS involvement (stage II disease) and in stage I patients refractory or intolerant to suramin and pentamidine. Melarsoprol administered intravenously may cause a *reactive encephalopathy,* with a clinical picture consisting of high fever, headache, tremor, convulsions, and on occasion coma and death. The incidence of arsenic encephalopathy varies from 3 to 18% in various series (SED-12, 708; 58[R]). In a recent case-control study of physical growth, sexual maturity, and academic performance in 100 young subjects (aged 6–20 years) with and without a past history of sleeping sickness, melarsoprol-treated patients weighed less, were shorter, and had sexual maturity ratings significantly different from the corresponding controls (59[C]).

DRUGS USED IN VISCERAL LEISHMANIASIS

The current recommended treatment for visceral leishmaniasis consists of sodium stibogluconate in a dose of 20 mg/kg for 30 days. This achieves a cure in certain cases (60[C], 61[C]) and is reasonably safe, although transient pancreatitis, musculoskeletal pains, and loss of appetite have been reported. Primary unresponsiveness (cure not obtained by the first course of treatment) is being increasingly reported (62[C]) and is a particular problem in the Bihar region of North-East India, where a recent report documented primary unresponsiveness in 33% of cases (63[C]).

Cardiovascular *Myocarditis* with electrocardiographic changes has been well described, but the risk of *dysrhythmias* is usually small. Amphotericin B lipid complex (ABLC) 5–15 mg/kg total dose (given as five infusions) (64[C], 65[C]) has proved useful in the treatment of unresponsive cases; ultra-short courses of one or two infusions are being studied on economic grounds (66[C]) and show promise. Aminosidine (16 or 20 mg/kg/day for 21 days) has also proved significantly more efficacious than sodium stibogluconate in this area (67[C]).

As well as problems with drug resistance, there are increasing reports of severe cardiotoxicity, leading in some cases to death (68[C], 69[C]). This may largely be due to changes in physicochemical properties of the drug; one cluster of cases was associated with a high-osmolarity lot of sodium stibogluconate (68[C]). Furthermore, amphotericin may worsen stibogluconate-induced cardiotoxicity, so that a gap of at least 10 days between sodium stibogluconate and ABLC is recommended (69[C]).

REFERENCES

1. Newton P, White N. Malaria: new developments in treatment and prevention. Ann Rev Med 1999;50:179–92.
2. Andersen SL, Oloo AJ, Gordon DM, Ragama OB, Aleman GM, Berman JD, Tang DB, Dunne MW, Shanks GD. Successful double-blinded, randomized, placebo-controlled field trial of azithromycin and doxycycline as prophylaxis for malaria in Western Kenya. Clin Infect Dis 1998;26:146–50.
3. Shanks GD, Gordon DM, Klotz FW, Aleman GM, Oloo AJ, Sadie D, Scott TR. Efficacy and safety of atovaquone/proguanil as suppressive prophylaxis for *Plasmodium falciparum* malaria. Clin Infect Dis 1998;27:494–9.
4. Lell B, Luckner D, Ndjave M, Scott T, Kremsner PG. Randomised placebo-controlled study of atovaquone plus proguanil for malaria prophylaxis in children. Lancet 1998;351:709–13.
5. Von Seidlein L, Jaffar S, Pinder M, Haywood M, Snounou G, Gemperli B, Gathmann I, Royce C. Treatment of African children with uncomplicated falciparum malaria with a new antimalarial drug, CGP 56697. J Infect Dis 1997;176:1113–16.
6. Von Seidlein L, Bojang K, Jones P, Jaffar S, Pinder M, Obaro S, Doherty T, Haywood M, Snounou G, Gemperli B, Gathmann I, Royce C, McAdam K, Greenwood B. A randomized controlled trial of artemether/benflumetol, a new an-

timalarial and pyrimethamine/sulfadoxine in the treatment of uncomplicated falciparum malaria in African children. Am J Trop Med Hyg 1998; 58:638–44.

7. Hatz C, Abdulla S, Mull R, Schellenberg D, Gathmann I, Kibatala P, Beck H-P, Tanner M, Royce C. Efficacy and safety of CGP 56697 (artemether and benflumetol) compared with chloroquine to treat acute falciparum malaria in Tanzanian children aged 1–5 years. Trop Med Int Health 1998;3:498–504.
8. Van Vugt M, Brockman A, Gemperli B, Luxemberger C, Gathmann I, Royce C, Slight T, Looareesuwan S, White NJ, Nosten F. Randomized comparison of artemether–benflumetol and artesunate–mefloquine in treatment of multidrug-resistant falciparum malaria. Antimicrob Agents Chemother 1998;42:135–9.
9. Looareesuwan S, Wilairatana P, Chokejindachai W, Chalermrut K, Wernsdorfer W, Gemperli B, Gathmann I, Royce C. A randomized, double-blind, comparative trial of a new oral combination of artemether and benflumetol (CGP 56697) with mefloquine in the treatment of acute *Plasmodium falciparum* malaria in Thailand. Am J Trop Med Hyg 1999;60:238–43.
10. Price R, Van Vugt M, Phaipun L, Luxemburger C, Simpson J, McGready R, Ter Kuile F, Kham A, Chongsuphajaisiddhi T, White NJ, Nosten F. Adverse effects in patients with acute falciparum malaria treated with artemisinin derivatives. Am J Trop Med Hyg 1999;60:547–55.
11. Ribeiro IR, Olliaro P. Safety of artemisinin and its derivatives. A review of published and unpublished clinical trials. Med Trop 1998;58(Suppl 3):50–3.
12. Nontprasert A, Nosten-Bertrand M, Pukrittayakamee S, Vanijanonta S, Angus BJ, White NJ. Assessment of the neurotoxicity of parenteral artemisinin derivatives in mice. Am J Trop Med Hyg 1998;59:519–22.
13. McGready R, Cho T, Cho JJ, Simpson JA, Luxemburger C, Dubowitz L, Looareesuwan S, White NJ, Nosten F. Artemisinin derivatives in the treatment of falciparum malaria in pregnancy. Trans R Soc Trop Med Hyg 1998;92:430–3.
14. Svensson USH, Ashton M, Trinh NH, Bertilsson L, Dinh XH, Nguyen VH, Nguyen Thi Nieu, Nguyen Duy Sy, Lykkesfeldt J, Le Dinh Cong. Artemisinin induces omeprazole metabolism in human beings. Clin Pharmacol Ther 1998;64:160–7.
15. Veinot JP, Mai KT, Zarychanski R. Chloroquine related cardiac toxicity. J Rheumatol 1998; 25:1221–5.
16. Guedira N, Hajjaj-Hassouni N, Srairi JE, El Hassani S, Fellat R, Benomar M. Third-degree atrioventricular block in a patient under chloroquine therapy. Rev Rhum Eng Ed 1998;65:58–62.
17. Wasay M, Wolfe GI, Herrold JM, Burns DK, Barohn RJ. Chloroquine myopathy and neuropathy with elevated CSF protein. Neurology 1998; 51:1226–7.
18. Sowunmi A, Falade CO, Oduola AM, Ogundahunsi OA, Fehintola FA, Gbotosho GO, Larcier P, Salako LA. Cardiac effects of halofantrine in children suffering from acute uncomplicated falciparum malaria. Trans R Soc Trop Med Hyg 1998;92:446–8.
19. Durrheim DN, Gammon S, Waner S, Braack LE. Antimalarial prophylaxis—use and adverse events in visitors to the Kruger National Park. S Afr Med J 1999;89:170–5.
20. Grieco A, Vecchio FM, Natale L, Gasbarrini G. Acute fatty liver after malaria prophylaxis with mefloquine. Lancet 1999;353:295–6.
21. McBride SR, Lawrence CM, Pape SA, Reid CA. Fatal toxic epidermal necrolysis associated with mefloquine antimalarial prophylaxis. Lancet 1997;349:101.
22. Potasman I, Seligmann H. A unique case of mefloquine-induced psoriasis. J Travel Med 1998;5:156.
23. Phillips-Howard PA, Steffen R, Kerr L, Vanhauwere B, Schildknecht J, Fuchs E, Edwards R. Safety of mefloquine and other antimalarial agents in the first trimester of pregnancy. J Travel Med 1998;5:121–6.
24. Lobel HO, Coyne PE, Rosenthal PJ. Drug overdoses with antimalarial agents: prescribing and dispensing errors. J Am Med Assoc 1998;280: 1483.
25. Oostweegel LM, Beijnen JH, Mulder JW. Hepatitis during chloroguanide prophylaxis. Ann Pharmacother 1998;32:1023–5.
26. Glynne P, Salama A, Chaudhry A, Swirsky D, Lightstone L. Quinine-induced immune thrombocytopenic purpura followed by hemolytic uremic syndrome. Am J Kidney Dis 1999;33:133–7.
27. Schattner A. Quinine hypersensitivity simulating sepsis. Am J Med 1998;104:488–90.
28. Burgess JK, Lopez JA, Berndt MC, Dawes I, Chesterman CN, Chong BH. Quinine-dependent antibodies bind a restricted set of epitopes on the glycoprotein Ib-IX complex: characterization of the epitopes. Blood 1998;92:2366–73.
29. Fishman JA. Prevention of infection due to *Pneumocystis carinii*. Antimicrob Agents Chemother 1998;42:995–1004.
30. Fishman JA. Treatment of infection due to *Pneumocystis carinii*. Antimicrob Agents Chemother 1998;42:1309–14.
31. El-Sadr WM, Murphy RL, Yurik TM, Luskin-Hawk R, Cheung TW, Balfour HH Jr, Eng R, Hooton TM, Kerkering TM, Schutz M, Van Der Horst C, Hafner R. Atovaquone compared with dapsone for the prevention of *Pneumocystis carinii* pneumonia in patients with HIV infection who cannot tolerate trimethoprim, sulfonamides, or both. Community Program for Clinical Research on AIDS and the AIDS Clinical Trials Group. New Engl J Med 1998;339:1889–95.
32. Miller R. Clinical aspects of *Pneumocystis carinii* pneumonia in HIV-infected patients: 1997. Fems Immunol Med Microbiol 1998;22: 103–5.
33. Smulders YM, De Man AM, Stehouwer CD, Slaats EH. Trimethoprim and fasting plasma homocysteine. Lancet 1998;352:1827–8.

34. Schwarz A, Perez-Canto A. Nephrotoxicity of antiinfective drugs. Int J Clin Pharmacol Ther 1998;36:164–7.
35. McCarty M, Jagoda A, Fairweather P. Hyperkalemic ascending paralysis. Ann Emerg Med 1998;32:104–7.
36. Porras MC, Lecumberri JN, Castrillón JL. Trimethoprim/sulfamethoxazole and metabolic acidosis in HIV-infected patients. Ann Pharmacother 1998;32:185–9.
37. Moreno-Ancillo A, López-Serrano MC. Hypersensitivity reactions to drugs in HIV-infected patients. Allergic evaluation and desensitization. Clin Exp Allergy 1998;28(Suppl 4):57–60.
38. Bocquet H, Bagot M, Roujeau JC. Drug-induced pseudolymphoma and drug hypersensitivity syndrome (Drug Rash with Eosinophilia and Systemic Symptoms: DRESS). Semin Cutaneous Med Surg 1996;15:250–7.
39. Sontheimer RD, Houpt KR. DIDMOHS: a proposed consensus nomenclature for the drug-induced delayed multiorgan hypersensitivity syndrome. Arch Dermatol 1998;134:874–6.
40. Rose EW, McCloskey WW. Glutathione in hypersensitivity to trimethoprim/sulfamethoxazole in patients with HIV infection. Ann Pharmacother 1998;32:381–3.
41. Veenstra J, Veugelers PJ, Keet IPM, Van der Ven AJAM, Miedema F, Lange JMA, Coutinho RA. Rapid disease progression in human immunodeficiency virus type 1-infected individuals with adverse reactions to trimethoprim–sulfamethoxazole prophylaxis. Clin Infect Dis 1997;24:936–41.
42. Theodore CM, Holmes D, Rodgers M, McLean KA. Co-trimoxazole desensitization in HIV-seropositive patients. Int J STD AIDS 1998; 9:158–61.
43. Demoly P, Messaad D, Sahla H, Fabre J, Faucherre V, André P, Reynes J, Godard P, Bousquet J. Six-hour trimethoprim–sulfamethoxazole-graded challenge in HIV-infected patients. J Allergy Clin Immunol 1998;102:1033–6.
44. Singer SJ, Racoosin JA, Viraraghavan R. Rhabdomyolysis in human immunodeficiency virus-positive patients taking trimethoprim–sulfamethoxazole. Clin Infect Dis 1998;26:233–4.
45. Arola O, Peltonen R, Rossi T. Arthritis, uveitis, and Stevens–Johnson syndrome induced by trimethoprim. Lancet 1998;351:1102.
46. Bijl AM, Van der Klauw MM, Van Vliet AC, Stricker BH. Anaphylactic reactions associated with trimethoprim. Clin Exp Allergy 1998;28:510–2.
47. Heelon MW, White M. Disulfiram–cotrimoxazole reaction. Pharmacotherapy 1998;18:869–70.
48. Hughes WT. Use of dapsone in the prevention and treatment of *Pneumocystis carinii*pneumonia: a review. Clin Infect Dis 1998;27:191–204.
49. Jaffuel D, Lebel B, Hillaire-Buys D, Pene J, Godard P, Michel F-B, Blayac J-P, Bousquet J, Demoly P. Eosinophilic pneumonia induced by dapsone. Br Med J 1998;317:181.
50. Ward KE, McCarthy MW. Dapsone-induced methemoglobinemia. Ann Pharmacother 1998;32:549–53.
51. Chawla R, Kundra P, Bhattacharya A. Asymptomatic methaemoglobinaemia and its implications. Acta Anaesthesiol Scand 1998;42:736–8.
52. Wain AM. Metronidazole vaginal gel 0.75% (MetroGel–Vaginal): a brief review. Infect Dis Obstet Gynecol 1998;6:3–7.
53. Dreger LM, Gleason PP, Chowdhry TK, Gazzuolo DJ. Intermittent-dose metronidazole-induced peripheral neuropathy. Ann Pharmacother 1998;32:267–8.
54. Thami GP, Kanwar AJ. Fixed drug eruption due to metronidazole and tinidazole without cross-sensitivity to secnidazole. Dermatology 1998; 196:368.
55. Pays JF. Human American trypanosomiasis 90 years after its discovery by Carlos Chagas. II—Clinical aspects, physiopathology, diagnosis and treatment. Med Trop 1999;59:79–94.
56. Sosa Estani S, Segura EL, Ruiz AM, Velazquez E, Porcel BM, Yampotis C. Efficacy of chemotherapy with benznidazole in children in the indeterminate phase of Chagas' disease. Am J Trop Med Hyg 1998;59:526–9.
57. Apt W, Aguilera X, Arribada A, Pérez C, Miranda C, Sánchez G, Zulantay I, Cortes P, Rodriguez J, Juri D. Treatment of chronic Chagas' disease with itraconazole and allopurinol. Am J Trop Med Hyg 1998;59:133–8.
58. Pépin J, Milord F. The treatment of human African trypanosomiasis. Adv Parasitol 1994;33:1–47.
59. Aroke AH, Asonganyi T, Mbonda E. Influence of a past history of Gambian sleeping sickness on physical growth, sexual maturity and academic performance of children in Fontem, Cameroon. Ann Trop Med Parasitol 1998;92:829–35.
60. Karki P, Koirala S, Parija SC, Hansdak SG, Das ML. A thirty day course of sodium stibogluconate for treatment of Kala-azar in Nepal. Southeast Asian J Trop Med Public Health 1998;29:154–8.
61. Aronson NE, Wortmann GW, Johnson SC, Jackson JE, Gasser RA Jr, Magill AJ, Endy TP, Coyne PE, Grogl M, Benson PM, Beard JS, Tally JD, Gambel JM, Kreutzer RD, Oster CN. Safety and efficacy of intravenous sodium stibogluconate in the treatment of leishmaniasis: recent US military experience. Clin Infect Dis 1998;27: 1457–64.
62. Khalil EAG, El Hassan AM, Zijlstra EE, Hashim FA, Ibrahim ME, Ghalib HW, Ali MS. Treatment of visceral leishmaniasis with sodium stibogluconate in Sudan: management of those who do not respond. Ann Trop Med Parasitol 1998; 92:151–8.
63. Thakur CP, Sinha GP, Pandey AK, Kumar N, Kumar P, Hassan SM, Narain S, Roy RK. Do the diminishing efficacy and increasing toxicity of sodium stibogluconate in the treatment of visceral leishmaniasis in Bihar, India, justify its continued use as a first-line drug? An observational study of 80 cases. Ann Trop Med Parasitol 1998;92:561–9.

64. Sundar S, Murray HW. Cure of antimony-unresponsive Indian visceral leishmaniasis with amphotericin B lipid complex. J Infect Dis 1996; 173:762–5.
65. Sundar S, Agrawal NK, Sinha PR, Horwith GS, Murray HW. Short-course, low-dose amphotericin B lipid complex therapy for visceral leishmaniasis unresponsive to antimony. Ann Intern Med 1997;127:133–7.
66. Sundar S, Goyal AK, More DK, Singh MK, Murray HW. Treatment of antimony-unresponsive Indian visceral leishmaniasis with ultra-short courses of amphotericin-B-lipid complex. Ann Trop Med Parasitol 1998;92:755–64.
67. Jha TK, Olliaro P, Thakur CP, Kanyok TP, Singhania BL, Singh IJ, Singh NKP, Akhoury S, Jha S. Randomised controlled trial of aminosidine (paromomycin) v sodium stibogluconate for treating visceral leishmaniasis in North Bihar, India. Br Med J 1998;316:1200–5.
68. Sundar S, Sinha PR, Agrawal NK, Srivastava R, Rainey PM, Berman JD, Murray HW, Singh VP. A cluster of cases of severe cardiotoxicity among kala-azar patients treated with a high-osmolarity lot of sodium antimony gluconate. Am J Trop Med Hyg 1998;59:139–43.
69. Thakur CP. Sodium antimony gluconate, amphotericin, and myocardial damage. Lancet 1998; 351:1928–9.

P. Reiss and M.D. de Jong

29 Antiviral drugs

COMPOUNDS ACTIVE AGAINST DNA VIRUSES

Aciclovir *(SED-13, 872; SEDA-19, 273; SEDA-20, 269; SEDA-21, 306)*

Nervous system Neurotoxicity represents the only major adverse effect of aciclovir, and is strongly associated with high plasma aciclovir concentrations resulting from impaired renal function (1[R]).

Symptoms of neurotoxicity, which usually appear within the first 24–72 hours of administration, may include tremor, myoclonus, confusion, lethargy, agitation, hallucinations, dysarthria, asterixis, ataxia, hemiparesthesia, and seizures. While aciclovir-induced neurotoxicity is most prevalent with intravenous administration, it has also been reported after oral use in patients with terminal renal insufficiency on hemodialysis. A case of neurotoxicity possibly secondary to the topical use of aciclovir has also been described (2[CR]).

A 59-year-old woman on hemodialysis was treated with oral aciclovir 200 mg/24 hours for ophthalmic *Herpes zoster.* After a few days, an ophthalmic aciclovir cream was started (one application every 6 hours) because of ipsilateral *Herpes* keratitis. After 1 week of combined oral and topical treatment, she became confused, with dysarthria and audiovisual hallucinations. Aciclovir was withdrawn and hemodialysis was initiated. Complete resolution of symptoms was achieved after three hemodialysis sessions in 3 days. Aciclovir plasma concentrations before hemodialysis were high (45 μmol/l) and fell rapidly during hemodialysis.

There is no conclusive evidence for the contribution of the topically administered aciclovir to the high plasma concentrations and subsequent neurotoxicity in this case. However, the authors argued that the existence of high aciclovir plasma concentrations, in spite of careful adjustment of the oral dosage, pointed to significant topical absorption of the drug, especially since the absorption of aciclovir through the skin and mucous membranes may be unpredictable.

Hematological Neutropenia and thrombocytopenia occurred in an 8-year-old boy who was treated with aciclovir 200 mg bd for 5 months for 'chronic cold sores' (3[C]). After withdrawal of aciclovir, the absolute neutrophil and platelet counts normalized within days. There was no recurrence of oral herpes lesions during the ensuing month.

Cidofovir

Urinary system The main adverse effect associated with intravenous cidofovir is renal tubular damage, which can generally be prevented by assuring adequate hydration during and after drug administration and by co-administration of oral probenecid (SEDA-21, 306).

Special senses In a retrospective record review of 18 HIV-infected patients (30 eyes) who were being treated with intravenous cidofovir for complicated cytomegalovirus retinitis, eight patients developed anterior uveitis after a median of four (range 2–8) doses of cidofovir or a median of 55 (20–131) days after the start of therapy (4[C]). While they were receiving treatment with cidofovir, none of the patients showed any evidence of progression of CMV retinitis. Five of the eight had symptoms of photophobia and blurred vision at the onset of uveitis, and the other three were asymptomatic. There was no difference in the use of HIV-1 protease inhibitors between the patients who did or did not develop anterior uveitis. Baseline intraocular pressure measurements were available for 11/18 patients. With the introduction of cidofovir there was a fall in mean intraocular pressure, and a trend for this fall to be more pronounced in those who developed anterior

Side Effects of Drugs, Annual 23
J.K. Aronson, ed.

uveitis. Withdrawal of cidofovir was necessary in only one patient, after which all symptoms and signs disappeared and vision returned to baseline within 1 month. In two of the seven other patients, cidofovir had to be withdrawn because of nephrotoxicity. In the other five patients, cidofovir was continued and the uveitis was controlled with topical therapy, consisting of corticosteroids with or without a cycloplegic agent.

Famciclovir *(SEDA-19, 273; SEDA-20, 269; SEDA-21, 306)*

Famciclovir is an oral prodrug of penciclovir and is remarkably well tolerated. In a randomized placebo-controlled study of 455 patients oral famciclovir (125 or 250 mg tds or 250 mg bd) used to suppress recurrent genital *Herpes simplex* infections, the toxicity profile of famciclovir was comparable to placebo (5[cr]). The only serious adverse effects reported as being possibly related to famciclovir were raised bilirubin concentration and lipase activity in one patient after 10 months of treatment with famciclovir 125 mg tds. However, these laboratory abnormalities resolved on therapy after 7 days and did not recur during the rest of the study.

Ribavirin

The major toxic effect of ribavirin is hemolytic anemia, which is generally mild and reversible on withdrawal (SEDA-20, 271). The combination of interferon-α_{2b} with ribavirin has recently become the preferred treatment for patients with chronic hepatitis C virus infection. Two large randomized placebo-controlled comparisons of interferon-α_{2b} alone with the combination of interferon-α_{2b} with ribavirin have recently been published. In the initial treatment of chronic hepatitis C, 912 patients were randomly assigned to receive standard-dose interferon-α_{2b} alone or in combination with ribavirin (1000 or 1200 mg/day orally, depending on bodyweight) for 24 or 48 weeks (6[c]). As expected, dosage reduction for anemia was necessary in 8% of patients taking the combination therapy and in none of those treated with interferon alone. Dyspnea, pharyngitis, pruritus, rash, nausea, insommnia, and anorexia were adverse effects that were reported more often during combination therapy with ribavirin (6[c]). In patients whose chronic hepatitis had relapsed after therapy with interferon-α_{2b} alone, 345 patients were randomized to receive standard-dose interferon-α_{2b} alone or in combination with ribavirin (1000 or 1200 mg/day orally, depending on bodyweight) for 6 months (7[c]). Dosage reduction for anemia was required in 12/173 patients assigned to combination therapy and in none assigned to interferon alone. As was the case in the initial therapy study, dyspnea, nausea, and rash were significantly more common in patients treated with the combination of interferon and ribavirin (7[c]).

Valaciclovir *(SEDA-19, 275)*

Valaciclovir is the L-valyl ester of aciclovir. After oral administration, it is rapidly and extensively converted to aciclovir by first-pass metabolism, resulting in plasma aciclovir concentrations previously only attainable with intravenous administration. Like aciclovir, valaciclovir is generally well tolerated. In large placebo-controlled comparisons of the efficacy of valaciclovir and aciclovir in treating or suppressing recurrent genital *Herpes simplex* infections in immunocompetent people, dosages up to 2 g/day were well tolerated, with safety profiles comparable to aciclovir (8[c], 9[c]). In a comparison of high-dose valaciclovir (8 g/day) with two doses of aciclovir (0.8 and 3.2 g/day) for prophylaxis of cytomegalovirus disease in patients with advanced human immunodeficiency virus infection, intention-to-treat analysis showed a trend towards earlier mortality in those who received valaciclovir. In those who actually received valaciclovir, survival was significantly shorter. In view of the unexplained trend towards earlier mortality, as well as higher frequencies of renal toxicity (see below) and premature treatment discontinuation, the authors concluded that the dose of valaciclovir was too high and that better tolerated doses, which maintain a protective effect on cytomegalovirus disease, need to be identified (10[CR]).

Nervous system As evidenced by a reported case, high aciclovir concentrations attained with oral valaciclovir treatment in patients on hemodialysis may be neurotoxic (11[c]).

A 58-year-old man with chronic renal insufficiency, who was hemodialyzed twice a week, was treated with valaciclovir (1 g tds) for *Herpes zoster*. Two days later he became disoriented, dizzy, and dysarthric, and experienced hallucinations. The serum aciclovir concentration was 21 mg/l. Treatment was discontinued and he was treated with hemodialysis for 6 hours, resulting in marked clinical improvement. The next day his symptoms of dysarthria recurred, but immediately and completely resolved after a second hemodialysis.

Urinary system Aciclovir is excreted renally. High plasma concentrations of aciclovir can lead to precipitation in renal tubules, with resultant, generally reversible, impairment of renal function. Since oral valaciclovir can result in plasma aciclovir concentrations comparable to those attained with intravenous dosing, reversible impairment of renal function can also occur after prolonged use of high-dose valaciclovir. Indeed, in the above-mentioned study of high-dose valaciclovir for prevention of cytomegalovirus disease in HIV-infected persons, there was an association between treatment with valaciclovir and moderate nephrotoxicty (serum creatinine more than 1.5 time the upper limit of normal; estimated creatinine clearance under 50 ml/min) (10[CR]).

In the same study, high-dose valaciclovir was associated with an increased risk of a thrombotic microangiopathy-like syndrome, reported as thrombocytopenic purpura or hemolytic-uremic syndrome (10[CR]). This syndrome occurred in 14 out of 523 patients who received valaciclovir, and in only four out of 704 patients who received aciclovir after a median of 54 (range 8–84) weeks of treatment. The precise relation to valaciclovir remains unclear, since eight of 14 patients who were treated with valaciclovir had stopped treatment for at least 1 week before the onset of the syndrome. In addition, all patients with thrombotic microangiopathy-like syndromes had taken multiple concomitant medications, and most had other intercurrent illnesses, which could have explained the hematological and renal abnormalities. The authors concluded that additional data are required to understand the role of valaciclovir and other medications for thrombotic microangiopathy-like syndromes, which are recognized with increasing frequency in patients with advanced HIV disease.

COMPOUNDS ACTIVE AGAINST RNA VIRUSES

HIV PROTEASE INHIBITORS

Lipodystrophy and insulin resistance with HIV protease inhibitors

Several reports have confirmed that a syndrome of peripheral lipodystrophy, central adiposity, breast hypertrophy in women, hyperlipidemia, and insulin resistance is an adverse event associated with the use of potent combination antiretroviral therapy, particularly including HIV-1 protease inhibitors (12[C]–17[C]). Peripheral lipodystrophy in patients is characterized by fat wasting of the face, limbs, buttocks, and upper trunk, while central adiposity may cause an increase in belly size and an increase in the dorsocervical fat pad, creating the appearance of a 'buffalo hump' (18[C], 19[C]). The increase in belly size is often associated with symptoms of abdominal fullness, distension, and bloating. This is probably due to a change in body fat distribution, with selective accumulation of fat intra-abdominally (20[C]).

Indinavir

Respiratory system Shock and respiratory failure have been attributed to indinavir (21[C]).

A 36-year-old HIV-positive man had started to take zidovudine and zalcitabine 9 months earlier together with co-trimoxazole as primary prophylaxis against PCP, but switched to indinavir, stavudine, and lamivudine. Two hours after the first dose of indinavir he developed a high fever, generalized myalgia, and malaise and started to vomit. After the second dose he developed shock and cyanosis. A chest X-ray was compatible with adult respiratory distress syndrome. All cultures were negative for bacterial, viral, mycobacterial, and fungal pathogens. He recovered in 6 days and antiretroviral treatment without indinavir was reintroduced without recurrent problems.

The authors suggested that the severe shock and respiratory distress syndrome had been due to an idiosyncratic reaction to indinavir.

Urinary system The main clinically relevant adverse effect of the HIV-1 protease inhibitor indinavir is nephrolithiasis. Several reports have suggested that patients using indinavir may also develop a syndrome consisting of back or flank pain, accompanied by crystalluria, renal function abnormalities, and evidence of tubulointerstitial nephritis on renal biopsy, but without obvious renal calculus formation (22[C]–24[C]).

Skin and appendages In 337 patients who were given indinavir as part of combination antiretroviral therapy with nucleoside analogues, five patients (1.5%) developed severe alopecia a median of 50 days after starting indinavir. Three had diffuse shedding of hair involving the entire scalp, and two were initially aware of circumscribed circular areas of alopecia resulting in complete severe hair loss. Although indinavir was discontinued in all five cases, there was no regrowth a median of 30 days later (25[C]).

Nelfinavir

The main adverse event that has been consistently reported with nelfinavir is diarrhea and loose stools in 20–30% of patients. The frequency with which diarrhea is truly dose-limiting is not yet clear, but clinical experience suggests that in many cases treatment can be continued in conjunction with non-specific antidiarrheal medication (SEDA-22, 317; 26[c], 27[c]).

Nervous system Peripheral neuropathy has been reported with nelfinavir (28[C]).

A 40-year-old HIV-positive patient nelfinavir 750 mg tds to existing combination therapy with stavudine, lamivudine, and loviride. In the 4 years before he had taken various drugs, including zidovudine, zalcitabine, didanosine, stavudine, loviride, ritonavir, and saquinavir. Zalcitabine had been discontinued 3 years before because of pain and paresthesia in both feet after 4 weeks. Thereafter, he had persisting dysesthesia in the feet. One week after having started nelfinavir, this extended in both legs to the knees. He also had sharp pains in the Achilles tendons and bones and burning in the legs, which made walking impossible. He reduced the dosage to 1500 mg/day and felt an improvement within a few days; nelfinavir was then withdrawn, and his symptoms abated.

Although circumoral paresthesia has been a common adverse effect of ritonavir, peripheral neuropathy has not been previously reported with HIV-1 protease inhibitors. There has been another report of painful neuropathy in two patients who took ritonavir and indinavir respectively (29[c]).

Skin and appendages Three HIV-infected patients, who had all taken zidovudine, didanosine, and co-trimoxazole (for PCP prophylaxis) for over 12 months, developed generalized urticaria 8–10 days after starting nelfinavir 750 mg tds. Withdrawal of nelfinavir and treatment with antihistamines resulted in the disappearance of the lesions within 4–6 days. One patient restarted nelfinavir 250 mg tds without consulting his physician and had similar symptoms within 5 days. Desensitization by using a dose escalation protocol was attempted in all three patients after discontinuation of nelfinavir. This was successful in two cases; the third patient prematurely discontinued desensitization on his own request. During desensitization two of the patients had mild and transient pruritus and rash, reinforcing the diagnosis of a hypersensitivity skin reaction (30[C]).

Ritonavir

The adverse effects commonly observed with ritonavir in adults are reportedly similar in children (31[C]). Of 51 children aged 6 months to 18 years who took escalating doses of a liquid formulation of ritonavir (from 250 up to 400 mg/m^2 every 12 hours), seven withdrew because of gastrointestinal toxicity and four because of grade 3 hepatic transaminase rises. Both serum triglyceride and cholesterol concentrations increased significantly from baseline within 12 weeks of treatment.

Nervous system Myasthenia has been attributed to ritonavir (32[c]).

A 71-year-old man with an 8-year history of HIV infection developed slurred speech, difficulty in climbing stairs, bilateral ptosis, and lateral rectus weakness, 3 weeks after having started to take ritonavir (1200 mg/day). All his signs worsened with prolonged testing, and edrophonium produced improvement in ptosis and speech. Specific electromyographic testing confirmed myasthenia gravis. Computed tomography of the chest was normal. After withdrawal of ritonavir the signs and symptoms partly resolved by 3 months.

A definite causal link with ritonavir could not be established, but the authors speculated that ritonavir may have unmasked myasthenia gravis in this patient.

Urinary system In a retrospective analysis of 87 HIV-positive patients taking ritonavir in combination with two nucleoside analogues serum creatinine increased in 12 cases by 66 (5–242)% from 66 (range 46–102), with a median glomerular filtration rate (GFR) of 116 ml/min

(60–202). Ten of the 12 patients had other risk factors for nephrotoxicity, such as dehydration or use of nephrotoxic drugs (33[C]). It may be prudent to monitor renal function in patients receiving ritonavir, particularly in the presence of other risk factors for renal dysfunction.

Interactions An important consideration in the use of all HIV-1 protease inhibitors, but of ritonavir in particular, is their potential for drug interactions through their effects on cytochrome P450. The various interactions of ritonavir with other anti-HIV drugs have recently been reviewed (34[R]). Ritonavir can also produce clinically relevant interactions with recreational drugs (35[c]).

A 32-year-old HIV-positive man who added ritonavir 600 mg bd to his existing antiretroviral regimen of zidovudine and lamivudine became unwell within hours after having ingested two and a half tablets of Ecstasy, estimated to contain 180 mg of methylenedioxymethamfetamine (MDMA). He was hypertonic, sweating profusely, tachypneic, tachycardic, and cyanosed. Shortly after he had a tonic-clonic seizure and cardiorespiratory arrest. Attempts at resuscitation were unsuccessful. Blood concentrations obtained post-mortem showed an MDMA concentration of 4.56 mg/l, in the range of that reported in a patient with a life-threatening illness and symptoms similar to this patient after an overdose of 18 tablets of MDMA.

Ritonavir inhibits CYP2D6, which is the principal pathway by which MDMA is metabolized.

Saquinavir

Saquinavir, an HIV-1 protease inhibitor, is generally remarkably well tolerated. Diarrhea, usually of only moderate severity, occurring in 3–4% of patients, seems to be the most common single adverse effect (SEDA-22, 310). Several cases of patients with what may be unusual adverse effects have been reported over the last year.

A new soft gelatin capsule formulation of saquinavir with greater systemic availability than the hard gelatin capsule has become available. Of 442 patients who used the soft gelatin capsule 1200 mg tds, for 48 weeks, 8% withdrew because of adverse events, which were not necessarily related to saquinavir. No new adverse effects or laboratory abnormalities emerged compared with those previously observed with the hard gelatin capsule. The most frequent adverse effects were gastrointestinal, diarrhea being the most common (36[C]).

Psychiatric Saquinavir can occasionally be associated with acute paranoid psychotic reactions (37[C]).

A 41-year-old woman took zidovudine and didanosine for HIV-1 infection after an acute seroconversion illness. Zidovudine and didanosine had to be discontinued because of neutropenia and nausea, so she was given stavudine plus lamivudine without any adverse effects. Saquinavir (600 mg tds) was added 12 months later because of weight loss and a falling CD4 cell count. Within 24 hours saquinavir she developed agitated depression with paranoid ideation. After drug withdrawal her mental health returned to normal over 5 days. Over the next 6 weeks stavudine and lamivudine were reintroduced without any adverse effects and continued for a further 11 months. Saquinavir was then reintroduced at the previous dosage, and within 2 days she again became extremely mentally agitated with paranoid ideation. Saquinavir was withdrawn and she recovered within 7 days. She was later given indinavir without problems. Her mother had a history of major depressive illness.

Urinary system A renal stone has been attributed to saquinavir (38[c]).

A 42-year-old HIV-positive man with a prior history of *Pneumocystis carinii* pneumonia (PCP) who had been treated with zidovudine and dideoxycytidine started to take saquinavir 600 mg tds. His CD4 cell count rose from 28×10^6/l to 101×10^6/l and zidovudine and dideoxycytidine were replaced by stavudine and lamivudine, because of mild peripheral neuropathy. Saquinavir was continued unchanged. A few months later he developed left-sided loin pain and hematuria and a left renal calculus was seen on ultrasound. A month later the same signs and symptoms recurred and a few weeks later he passed a small black stone in the urine. Ultrasonic lithotrisy was performed, with a good result. Saquinavir was discontinued, after which he had no further renal problems.

This case suggests that saquinavir, like indinavir, may be associated with renal calculus formation in some individuals.

Skin and appendages Adverse skin reactions to saquinavir are exceptional, but erythema multiforme has recently been reported (39[c]).

A 32-year-old HIV-positive man who had been treated with didanosine and lamivudine, added saquinavir (600 mg tds) because of a rising plasma HIV-1 RNA viral load. Five days later he presented with a generalized maculopapular skin eruption, the lesions being centered on a bulla, and erosive lesions on the palate. Histological examination was compatible with erythema multiforme. Saquinavir was discontinued and all the mucocutaneous lesions healed within 15 days. Rechallenge was not attempted.

Interactions As with other HIV-1 protease inhibitors, saquinavir may be associated with drug interactions as a result of the effect of saquinavir on the hepatic cytochrome P450 oxidase system. Compared with other HIV protease inhibitors, saquinavir has less of an inhibitory effect on cytochrome P450 isoenzymes, but clinically relevant interactions can nevertheless occur. Drug interactions with saquinavir have recently been reviewed (40[R]).

In an HIV-1-positive kidney transplant recipient, saquinavir increased the trough concentration of ciclosporin 3-fold, resulting in fatigue, headache, and gastrointestinal discomfort. Ciclosporin, like saquinavir, is metabolized by CYP3A. Saquinavir plasma concentrations were likewise increased by ciclosporin. All the symptoms disappeared after downward adjustment of the doses of both ciclosporin and saquinavir (41[C]).

In 37 patients with HIV-associated non-Hodgkin's lymphoma who were treated with a 96-hour continuous intravenous infusion of cyclophosphamide, doxorubicin, and etoposide, severe (grade 3 or 4) mucositis occurred in eight of 12 patients who received concomitant saquinavir (600 mg tds) compared with three of 25 who did not receive saquinavir. Although the authors did not measure saquinavir plasma concentrations, they ssuggested that this finding may have been explained by inhibition of the metabolism of one or more of the cytotoxic drugs by saquinavir (42[c]).

HIV NUCLEOSIDE ANALOGUE REVERSE TRANSCRIPTASE INHIBITORS

Didanosine *(SEDA-18, 302; SEDA-19, 276; SEDA-20, 271; SEDA-21, 307)*

Special senses Extensive serial audiological studies in an HIV-infected child showed high-frequency hearing loss after 19 months of combined treatment with zidovudine and didanosine (dosages unknown), which were started at 24 months of age (43[CR]). Normal tympanograms indicated that this hearing loss was sensorineural. While no conclusive evidence was given for a causative role of either antiretroviral drug, the authors concluded that children taking antiretroviral therapy need to be monitored for possible ototoxicity.

Hearing loss attributed to didanosine has been reported in an HIV-infected adult (44[c]).

A 37-year-old HIV-infected man developed bilateral deafness while taking didanosine (400 mg/day), which had been started about 4 years before. He was also taking azithromycin, ciprofloxacin, and myambutol for about 1 month for a *Mycobacterium avium* infection. Otoscopic examination and tympanometry were normal. Audiometry showed a bilateral sensorineural hearing deficit of 40–60 dB. There were no other neurological abnormalities. An MRI scan of the brain was normal. Didanosine was withdrawn and replaced by alternative antiretroviral agents. All other medications were continued. His hearing improved progressively and returned to normal after 2 months.

In the absence of rechallenge, there was no conclusive evidence for a causative role of didanosine in the development of hearing loss in this case. However, the authors argued that the improvement on discontinuation of didanosine, which is known to cause neuritis, implicated the drug.

Lamivudine (3TC) *(SEDA-19, 276; SEDA-20, 271; SEDA-21, 308)*

Skin and appendages Paronychia has been reported in 12 HIV-infected patients who had taken lamivudine only for 3 months before the onset of symptoms (45[c]). Microbiological investigations for fungi or bacteria were negative. All were treated with topical antiseptics; surgical procedures were performed in four. Five patients healed without recurrence, while the paronychia recurred in six. There was no mention of withdrawal of lamivudine. The causative role of lamivudine in the development of paronychia in these patients remains obscure.

Stavudine (2′,3′-didehydro-3′-deoxy-thymidine, D4T) *(SEDA-20, 273)*

The most important adverse effects of stavudine are peripheral neuropathy and increases in hepatic transaminases, both of which usually resolve on withdrawal.

Sexual function Painful bilateral gynecomastia and hypersexuality, possibly related to the use of stavudine, have been reported (46[CR]).

A 25-year-old HIV-infected man reported hot flushes and headaches during the first days of treatment with stavudine (40 mg bd), followed by swelling and tenderness under both nipples. He also reported increased libido, premature ejaculation, and persistent erections. He denied illicit drug use. He had bilateral gynecomastia. Luteinizing hormone and testosterone concentrations were within the reference ranges, excluding primary causes of gynecomastia. One month after withdrawal of stavudine, the swelling and tenderness had abated and his sexual symptoms had resolved. The patient was not rechallenged with the drug.

The authors argued that although idiopathic gynecomastia could not be ruled out, the temporal relation between withdrawal of the drug and improvement in his symptoms suggested a causative role of stavudine.

Zidovudine *(SEDA-18, 303; SEDA-19, 278; SEDA-20, 273; SEDA-21, 310)*

Use in pregnancy As previously reported, zidovudine during pregnancy and delivery, followed by treatment of the infant for 6 weeks, shows promising efficacy in preventing materno-fetal transmission of HIV, and is associated with minimal short-term toxicity to both mother and child and no increased incidence of neonatal structural abnormalities (SEDA-19, 279). The only recognized toxic effect in infants is anemia within the first 6 weeks of life, which is not associated with premature delivery, duration of maternal treatment, degree of maternal immunosuppression, or maternal anemia. An 18-month follow-up of 342 children born to mothers who had taken zidovudine or placebo during pregnancy has recently been reported (47[CR]). There were no differences in growth parameters or immune function in uninfected children. In addition, no childhood neoplasias were reported in either group.

HIV NON-NUCLEOSIDE REVERSE TRANSCRIPTASE INHIBITORS

Nevirapine *(SEDA-19, 277; SEDA-21, 308)*

Liver The most frequent laboratory abnormality during nevirapine treatment is an increase in serum γ-glutamyl transferase activity, usually without changes in other measures of hepatic function. However, in a randomized, placebo-controlled comparison of zidovudine plus nevirapine, zidovudine plus didanosine, and the triple combination of zidovudine plus didanosine and nevirapine in 151 patients, there were abnormal liver function tests in increased frequency in the patients taking nevirapine (19 and 12 vs 6%) (48[cr]). Five of 98 patients taking nevirapine had to stop the drug permanently because of raised alanine aminotransferase activity, after which the laboratory abnormalities resolved completely.

Severe hepatitis has been attributed to nevirapine (49[cr]).

A 36-year-old woman with HIV and hepatitis C infection developed fever, right upper quadrant pain, headache, confusion, and a generalized skin rash. Her antiretroviral treatment included lamivudine (150 mg bd), stavudine (40 mg bd), and nevirapine (200 mg bd). The dose of nevirapine had been doubled 2 weeks before. Her laboratory results were as follows: white cell count 4.1×10^9/l with 18% eosinophils, aspartate aminotransferase 879 u/l, alanine aminotransferase 1424 u/l, lactate dehydrogenase 3268 u/l, activated prothrombin time 14 seconds, partial thromboplastin time 29 seconds. Abdominal ultrasound was normal. Her antiretroviral medications were stopped. She was given intravenous prednisolone (60 mg 6-hourly) and within 8 hours the signs of sepsis had abated and her liver function began to improve and resolved over the next few days. Several weeks later, she was rechallenged with lamivudine and zidovudine, without recurrence of liver toxicity or rash.

The authors argued that, although the syndrome could not be definitively attributed to nevirapine, several factors suggested that nevirapine was the most likely precipitant, including the fact that hepatic failure coincided with a systemic allergic response, which is commonly associated with nevirapine, especially after dose escalation. The rapid improvement with steroid therapy suggested that the hepatic failure was a manifestation of a systemic hypersensitivity reaction. However, since stavudine has also been associated with hepatitis, a causative role of stavudine cannot be excluded. The fact that lamivudine was given again without recurrence of hepatitis renders it an unlikely culprit.

Skin and appendages The principal adverse effect of nevirapine is skin rash, which occurs in about 20% of patients, and which progresses to

Stevens–Johnson syndrome in 0.5–1% of cases. An unusually high incidence of nevirapine-associated rash has been reported in Chinese HIV-infected patients (50[CR]). Of eight Chinese patients, five developed a rash within 4 weeks of treatment, resolving on withdrawal. Since the total number of patients in this report was small, it remains to be shown whether Chinese are indeed at increased risk of hypersensitivity reactions to nevirapine.

INFLUENZA VIRUS NEURAMINIDASE INHIBITORS

Zanamivir

Zanamivir is an inhibitor of influenza virus neuraminidase, an enzyme that is essential for viral replication in vitro. In vitro and in animals, it inhibits a range of strains of influenza A and B. It can be delivered directly to the site of viral replication by intranasal or oral inhalation. Phase II and III clinical studies have shown that zanamivir by inhalation, either orally or combined orally and intranasally, slightly shortened the duration and severity of influenza symptoms and in high-risk patients reduced the risk of complications (51[R], 52[cr]). Typical doses are 10 mg by oral inhalation and 6.4 mg by intranasal inhalation. Dosing frequency is 2–6 times/day. Zanamivir is well tolerated. In placebo-controlled studies, its toxicity profile was similar to placebo.

REFERENCES

1. Ernst ME, Franey RJ. Acyclovir- and ganciclovir-induced neurotoxicity. Ann Pharmacother 1998;32:111–13.
2. Gómez Campderá FJ, Verde E, Vozmediano MC, Valderrábano F. More about acyclovir neurotoxicity in patients on haemodialysis. Nephron 1998;78:228–9.
3. Grella M, Ofosu JR, Klein BL. Prolonged oral acyclovir administration associated with neutropenia and thrombocytopenia. Am J Emerg Med 1998;16:396–8.
4. Akler ME, Johnson DW, Burman WJ, Johnson SC. Anterior uveitis and hypotony after intravenous cidofovir for the treatment of cytomegalovirus retinitis. Ophthalmology 1998;105:651–7.
5. Diaz-Mitoma F, Sibbald G, Shafran SD, Boon R, Saltzman RL, and The Collaborative Famciclovir Genital Herpes Research Group. Oral famciclovir for the suppression of recurrent genital herpes. J Am Med Assoc 1998;280:887–92.
6. McHutchinson JG, Gordon SC, Schiff ER, Shiffman ML, Lee WM, Rustgi VK, Goodman ZD, Ling M-H, Cort S, Albrecht JK, for the International Hepatitis Interventional Therapy Group. Interferon alfa-2b alone or in combination with ribavirin as initial treatment for chronic hepatitis C. New Engl J Med 1998;339:1485–92.
7. Davis GL, Esteban-Mur R, Rustgi VK, Hoefs J, Gordon SC, Trepo C, Shiffman ML, Zeuzem S, Craxi A, Ling M-H, Albrecht J, for the International Hepatitis Interventional Therapy Group. Interferon alfa-2b alone or in combination with ribavirin for the treatment of relapse of chronic hepatitis C. New Engl J Med 1998;339:1493–9.
8. Reitano M, Tyring S, Lang W, Thoming C, Worm AM, Borelli S, Chambers LO, Robinson JM, Corey L, and the International Valaciclovir HSV Study Group. Valaciclovir for the suppression of recurrent genital herpes simplex virus infection: a large-scale dose range-finding study. J Infect Dis 1998;178:603–10.
9. Tyring SK, Douglas JM, Corey L, Spruance SL, Esmann J, and the Valaciclovir International Study Group. A randomized, placebo-controlled comparison of oral valacyclovir and acyclovir in immunocompetent patients with recurrent genital herpes infections. Arch Dermatol 1998;134:185–91.
10. Feinberg JE, Hurwitz S, Cooper D, Sattler FR, MacGregor RR, Powderly W, Holland GN, Griffiths PD, Pollard RB, Youle M, Gill J, Holland FJ, Power ME, Owens S, Coakley D, Fry J, Jacobson MA, and the AIDS Clinical Trials Group Protocol 204/Glaxo Wellcome 123-014 International CMV Prophylaxis Study Group. A randomized, double-blind trial of valacyclovir prophylaxis for cytomegalovirus disease in patients with advanced human immunodeficiency virus infection. J Infect Dis 1998;177:48–56.
11. Linssen-Schuurmans CD, Van Kan EJM, Feith GW, Uges DRA. Neurotoxicity caused by valacyclovir in a patient on hemodialysis. Ther Drug Monit 1998;20:385–6.
12. Roth VR, Kravcik S, Angel JB. Development of cervical fat pads following therapy with human immunodeficiency virus type 1 protease inhibitors. Clin Infect Dis 1998;27:65–7.
13. Striker R, Conlin D, Marx M, Wiviott L. Localized adipose tissue hypertrophy in patients re-

ceiving human immunodeficiency virus protease inhibitors. Clin Infect Dis 1998;27:218–20.
14. Viraben R, Aquilina C. Indinavir-associated lipodystrophy. AIDS 1998;12:F37–9.
15. Toma E, Therrien R. Gynecomastia during indinavir antiretroviral therapy in HIV infection. AIDS 1998;12:681–2.
16. Lui A, Karter D, Turett G. Another case of breast hypertrophy in a patient treated with indinavir. Clin Infect Dis 1998;26:1482.
17. Walli R, Herfort O, Michl GM, Demant T, Jäger H, Dieterle C, Bogner JR, Landgraf R, Goebel FD. Treatment with protease inhibitors associated with peripheral insulin resistance and impaired glucose tolerance in HIV-1-infected patients. AIDS 1998;12:F167–73.
18. Carr A, Samaras K, Burton S, Law M, Freund J, Chisholm DJ, Cooper DA. A syndrome of peripheral lipodystrophy, hyperlipidemia and insulin resistance in patients receiving HIV protease inhibitors. AIDS 1998;12:F51–8.
19. Lo JC, Mulligan K, Tai VW, Algren H, Schambelan M. 'Buffalo hump' in men with HIV infection. Lancet 1998;351:867–70.
20. Miller K, Jones E, Yanovski JA, Shankar R, Feuerstein I, Falloon J. Visceral abdominal-fat accumulation associated with use of indinavir. Lancet 1998;351:871–5.
21. Dieleman JP, In't Veld B, Borleffs JCC, Schreij G. Acute respiratory failure associated with the human immunodeficiency virus (HIV) protease inhibitor indinavir in an HIV-infected patient. Clin Infect Dis 1998;26:1012–13.
22. Kopp JB, Miller KD, Mican JA, Feuerstein IM, Vaughan E, Baker C. Crystalluria and urinary tract abnormalities associated with indinavir. Ann Intern Med 1997;127:119–25.
23. Tashima KT, Horowitz JD, Rosen S. Indinavir nephropathy. New Engl J Med 1997;336:138–40.
24. Chen SCA, Nankivell BJ, Dwyer DE. Indinavir-induced renal failure. AIDS 1998;12:440–1.
25. D'Arminio Monforte A, Testa L, Gianotto M, Gori A, Franzetti F, Sollima S, Bini T, Moroni M. Indinavir-related alopecia. AIDS 1998;12: 328.
26. Markowitz M, Conant M, Hurley A, Schluger R, Duran M, Peterkin J, Chapman S, Patick A, Hendricks A, Yuen GJ, Hoskins W, Clendeninn N, Ho DD. A preliminary evaluation of nelfinavir mesylate, an inhibitor of human immunodeficiency virus (HIV)-1 protease, to treat HIV infection. J Infect Dis 1998;177:1533–40.
27. Moyle GJ, Youle M, Higgs C, Monaghan J, Prince W, Chapman S, Clendeninn N, Nelson MR. Safety, pharmacokinetics, and antiretroviral activity of the potent, specific human immunodeficiency virus protease inhibitor nelfinavir: results of a phase I/II trial and extended follow-up in patients infected with human immunodeficiency virus. J Clin Pharmacol 1998;38:736–43.
28. Grunke M, Kraetsch HG, Löw P, Rascu A, Kalden JR, Harrer T. Nelfinavir associated with peripheral neuropathy in an HIV-infected patient. Infection 1998;26:252.
29. Colebunders R, De Droogh E, Pelgrom Y, Depraetere K, De Jonghe P. Painful hyperaesthesia caused by protease inhibitors? Infection 1998;26:250–1.
30. Demoly P, Messaad D, Trylesinski A, Faucherre V, Fabre J, Reynes J, Delmas, Dohin E, Godard P, Bousquet J. Nelfinavir-induced urticaria and successful desensitization. J Allergy Clin Immunol 1998;102:875–6.
31. Mueller BU, Nelson RP, Sleasman J, Zuckerman J, Heath-Chiozzi M, Steinberg SM, Balis FM, Brouwers P, Hsu A, Saulis R, Sei S, Wood LV, Zeichner S, Katz TK, Higham C, Aker D, Edgerly M, Jarosinski P, Serchuck L, Whitcup SM, Pizzuti D, Pizzo PA. Phase I/II study of the protease inhibitor ritonavir in children with human immunodeficiency virus infection. Pediatrics 1998;101:335–43.
32. Saadat K, Kaminski HJ. Ritonavir-associated myasthenia gravis. Muscle Nerve 1998;21:680–1.
33. Bochet MV, Jacquiaud C, Valantin MA, Katlama C, Deray G. Renal insufficiency induced by ritonavir in HIV-infected patients. Am J Med 1998;105:457.
34. Hsu A, Granneman GR, Bertz RJ. Ritonavir. Clinical pharmacokinetics and interactions with other anti-HIV agents. Clin Pharmacokinet 1998; 35:275–91.
35. Henry JA, Hill IR. Fatal interaction between ritonavir and MDMA. Lancet 1998;352:1751–2.
36. Gill MJ. On behalf of the NV15182 Study Team. Safety profile of soft gelatin formulation of saquinavir in combination with nucleosides in a broad patient population. AIDS 1998;12:1400–2.
37. Finlayson JA, Laing RBS. Acute paranoid reaction to saquinavir. Am J Health-Syst Pharm 1998;55:2016–17.
38. Green ST, McKendrick MW, Schmid ML, Mohsen AH, Prakasam SF. Renal calculi developing de novo in a patient taking saquinavir. Int J STD AIDS 1998;9:555.
39. Garat H, El Sayed F, Obadia M, Bazex J. Erythème polymorphe au saquinavir. Ann Dermatol Venereol 1998;125:42–3.
40. Vella S, Floridia M. Saquinavir. Clinical pharmacology and efficacy. Clin Pharmacokinet 1998;34:189–201.
41. Brinkman K, Huysmans F, Burger DM. Pharmacokinetic interaction between saquinavir and cyclosporine. Ann Intern Med 1998;129:914–15.
42. Sparano JA, Wiernik PH, Hu X, Sarta C, Henry DH, Ratech H. Saquinavir enhances the mucosal toxicity of infusional cyclophosphamide, doxorubicin, and etoposide in patients with HIV-associated non-Hodgkin's lymphoma. Med Oncol 1998;15:50–7.
43. Christensen LA, Morehouse CR, Powell TW, Alchediak T, Silio M. Antiviral therapy in a child with pediatric human immunodeficiency virus (HIV): case study of audiologic findings. J Am Acad Audiol 1998;9:292–8.
44. Colebunders R, Depraetere K. Deafness caused by didanosine. Eur J Clin Microbiol Infect Dis 1998;17:214–15.

45. Zerboni R, Angius AG, Cusini M, Tarantini G, Carminati G. Lamivudine-induced paronychia. Lancet 1998;351:1256.
46. Melbourne KM, Brown SL, Silverblatt FJ. Gynaecomastia with stavudine treatment in an HIV-positive patient. Ann Pharmacother 1998;32: 1108.
47. Sperling RS, Shapiro DE, McSherry GD, Britto P, Cunningham BE, Culnane M, Coombs RW, Scott G, Van Dyke RB, Shearer WT, Jimenez E, Diaz C, Harrison DD, Delfraissy JF, and the Pediatric AIDS Clinical Trial Group Protocol 076 Study Group. Safety of the maternal-infant zidovudine regimen utilized in the pediatric AIDS Clinical Trial Group 076 Study. AIDS 1998;12:1805–13.
48. Montaner JSG, Reiss P, Cooper D, Vella S, Harris M, Conway B, Wainberg MA, Smith D, Robinson P, Hall D, Myers M, Lange JMA, and the INCAS Study Group. A randomized, double-blind trial comparing combinations of nevirapine, didanosine, and zidovudine for HIV-infected patients. J Am Med Assoc 1998;279:930–7.
49. Leitze Z, Nadeem A, Choudhary A, Saul Z, Roberts I, Manthous CA. Nevirapine-induced hepatitis treated with corticosteroids. AIDS 1998; 12:1115–17.
50. Ho TTY, Wong KH, Chan KCW, Lee SS. High incidence of nevirapine-associated rash in HIV-infected Chinese. AIDS 1998;12:2082–3.
51. Waghorn SL, Goa KL. Zanamivir. Drugs 1998; 55:721–25.
52. The MIST (Management of Influenza in the Southern Hemisphere Trialists) Study Group. Randomised trial of efficacy and safety of inhaled zanamivir in treatment of influenza A and B virus infections. Lancet 1998;352:1877–81.

C.J. Ellis

30 Drugs used in tuberculosis and leprosy

DRUGS USED IN TUBERCULOSIS

Antituberculous drug-induced hepatotoxicity-increased risks with hepatitis C virus and HIV

Increasing age is known to predispose to *hepatotoxicity* from antituberculous drugs. Workers from Florida have reported a 5-fold increase in the likelihood of drug-induced hepatotoxicity in patients who are hepatitis C positive and a 4-fold increase in patients who are HIV-positive, compared with seronegative patients treated for tuberculosis (1^C). In all, 134 patients taking antituberculous drugs were monitored for drug-induced hepatotoxicity, defined as an increase in AST and/or ALT from normal to at least three times normal and/or an increase in bilirubin above normal. Of the 22 patients who developed drug-induced hepatotoxicity, only six developed drug-induced hepatotoxicity on reintroduction of treatment after an interval in which the abnormalities had resolved. Four of the six had liver biopsies, which showed active inflammation, attributed (at least in part) to hepatitis C. These were then treated with interferon-α, with improvement of liver chemistry. On improvement, antituberculous therapy was successfully reintroduced in the form of isoniazid and rifabutin, the latter being considered to be less hepatotoxic than rifampicin.

Isoniazid *(SED-13, 882; SEDA-20, 277)*

Lupus-like syndrome Expansion or new development of tuberculous lesions during ultimately successful therapy has been termed a 'paradoxical response'. It is most often reported in relation to intracranial tuberculomata, but is probably most common in tuberculous lymphadenopathy. It is also described in tuberculous pleurisy and in parenchymal lung disease. In most cases the problem eventually settles, but sometimes steroid therapy is used empirically. Two Japanese patients developed pleural effusions while taking antituberculous therapy and were believed to have isoniazid-induced lupus-like syndrome (2^c). This diagnosis was based on the presence of antinuclear antibody in the effusate and in one patient a positive lymphocyte stimulation test using isoniazid; in the other patient it was negative. Both had moderately strongly positive serum antinuclear antibodies (1 : 160). In the first patient the effusion disappeared 2 weeks after withdrawal of isoniazid; in the other treatment was continued but the effusion nevertheless resolved in 10 weeks. It would clearly be worth checking for evidence of lupus-like syndrome in patients with 'paradoxical responses' to antituberculous therapy and it remains to be seen how many cases would be explained by it.

Rifampicin *(SED-13, 892; SEDA-21, 313; SEDA-22, 322)*

Gastrointestinal A case of tablet-associated *esophagitis* has been reported in a 70-year-old white man on the fourth day of antibiotic therapy with vancomycin, gentamicin, and oral rifampicin for *Staphylococcus epidermidis* prosthetic valve endocarditis (3^c). The authors noted that age, bedridden state, gastro-esophageal reflux disease, simultaneous administration of several medications, and nasopharyngeal obstruction may have increased the risk of esophagitis. They found a second case of tablet-associated esophagitis caused by rifampicin in their review of the published literature.

Urinary system The most commonly reported association of rifampicin therapy with *acute renal insufficiency* occurs in the context of in-

Side Effects of Drugs, Annual 23
J.K. Aronson, ed.

termittent therapy or therapy that is resumed after an interval (re-treatment). The patient suddenly experiences a syndrome that typically comprises fever with chills, nausea, hemolytic anemia, thrombocytopenia with purpura, and acute renal insufficiency.

This course of events has been reported in a 71-year-old Belgian woman in whom rifampicin-dependent anti-I antibodies were detected (4[c]). The authors went on to review the literature, which yielded 48 cases of rifampicin-related acute renal insufficiency, of which 37 conformed to the pattern of illness in their patient. When biopsies were taken tubular lesions were detected, probably because the I antigen is expressed in tubular epithelium.

Less commonly reported causes of rifampicin-related acute renal insufficiency are *interstitial nephritis, light-chain proteinuria,* and rapidly progressive glomerulonephritis, one example of which has been reported from Japan (5[c]). A 64-year-old man who had received antituberculous therapy continuously for 5 weeks suddenly developed acute renal insufficiency and had crescentic glomerulonephritis. An antibody to rifampicin was detected in serum.

The largest series of patients with acute renal insufficiency secondary to rifampicin yet published comes from Romania (6[C]). All 60 patients developed acute renal insufficiency, with anuria in 57, immediately after the start of re-treatment with rifampicin. The immediacy is illustrated by the fact that the mean dose taken before the onset of first clinical symptoms was 600 mg, i.e. a single dose. The interval from the previous rifampicin treatment ranged from 21 days to 1 year. The authors remarked that the standard regimen for antituberculous treatment in Romania until 1995 included twice weekly rifampicin, a regimen that may be more likely to cause an immune-mediated process than continuous therapy. Over 120 000 cases of tuberculosis were treated in the area served by the reporting unit in the 9 years of the study, giving an incidence for post-rifampicin acute renal insufficiency of 0.05% of treated patients. The incidence in re-treated patients must be much higher, but unfortunately the figure was not given. Most patients reported flu-like symptoms, were anuric and anemic, and had a leukocytosis. Half had thrombocytopenia and a quarter had severe hemolysis. The prognosis was good—renal function recovered in 40% after 30 days and in 97% after 90 days.

Skin and appendages Rifampicin can cause a *fixed drug eruption* (7[c]).

Immunological and hypersensitivity reactions *Shock and cerebral infarction* have been reported in an HIV-positive patient after re-exposure to rifampicin (8[c]).

In 35 HIV-positive patients with previous *hypersensitivity reactions* to rifampicin, oral desensitization was safe and allowed the reintroduction of rifampicin in 60% of cases (9[C]).

Central venous catheters A prospective, randomized clinical trial in 12 high-risk adult patients has shown that the use of polyurethane, triple-lumen central venous catheters impregnated with minocycline and rifampicin (on both the luminal and external surfaces) is associated with a lower rate of infection than the use of catheters impregnated with chlorhexidine and silver sulfadiazine (on the external surface only) (10[C]). There were low rates of catheter-related bloodstream infection (0.3%) and catheter colonization (7.9%) with the use of catheters impregnated with minocycline and rifampicin. This favorable result may be explained either by differences in the coating of the catheters (internal and external surfaces versus external surface only), by microbiological advantages of minocycline and rifampicin over chlorhexidine and silver sulfadiazine, or even by an effect unrelated to the antibacterial activity. The additional costs of preventing an infection and a death would be about $3125 and $12 500 respectively (11).

Interactions Rifampicin may reduce plasma concentrations of *clozapine* and exacerbate psychotic symptoms (12[c]).

Interference with diagnostic tests Rifampicin metabolites in urine can cause a false positive test for *melanin* when assessed with the Von Jaksch Test (13).

A significantly *raised TSH concentration* during therapy with rifampicin has been reported in a man taking levothyroxine; TSH concentrations returned to baseline 9 days after withdrawal of rifampicin (14).

DRUGS USED IN LEPROSY

Dapsone *(SED-13, 894; SEDA-19, 284; SEDA-22, 321)*

Respiratory Two cases of *pulmonary eosinophilia* attributed to dapsone were reported in 1998. Four cases had previously been reported, in which the fixed combination of dapsone and pyrimethamine (a malaria prophylactic) had been implicated, but only one previous report had implicated dapsone alone.

The two patients, one a French woman treated for chronic urticaria (15[c]) the other an Indian man with lepromatous leprosy (16[c]), had a similar presentation, with fever, wheezing, and breathlessness. Both had peripheral eosinophilia and chest X-rays showed infiltrates. The woman's symptoms began 2 weeks after she started to take dapsone but recurred a few hours after a subsequent rechallenge. The man's symptoms arose a few hours after each daily dose. Symptoms in both cases resolved within a few days of stopping dapsone.

REFERENCES

1. Ungo JR, Jones D, Ashkin D, Hollender ES, Bernstein D, Albanese AP, Pitchenik AE. Antituberculous drug-induced hepatotoxicity. The role of hepatitis C virus and the human immunodeficiency virus. Am J Respir Crit Care Med 1998; 157:1871–6.
2. Hiraoka K, Nagata N, Kawajiri T, Suzuki, Kido M, Sakamoto N. Paradoxical pleural response to antituberculous chemotherapy and isoniazid-induced lupus. Respiration 1998;65:152–5.
3. Smith SJ, Lee AJ, Maddix DS, Chow AW. Pill-induced esophagitis caused by oral rifampin. Ann Pharmacother 1999;33:27–31.
4. De Vriese AS, Robbrecht DL, Vanholder RC, Ogelaers DP, Lameire NH. Rifampicin-associated acute renal failure: pathophysiologic, immunological and clinical features. Am J Kidney Dis 1998; 31:108–15.
5. Ogata H, Kubo M, Tamaki K, Hirakata H, Okuda S, Fujishima M. Crescentic glomerulonephritis due to rifampicin treatment. Nephron 1998;78:319–22.
6. Covic A, Goldsmith DJA, Segall L, Stoicescu C, Lungu S, Volovat C, Covic M. Rifampicin-induced acute renal failure: a series of 60 patients. Nephrol Dial Transplant 1998;13:924–9.
7. John SS. Fixed drug eruption due to rifampin. Lepr Rev 1998;69:397–9.
8. Martinez E, Collazos J, Mayo J. Shock and cerebral infarct after rifampicin re-exposure in a patient infected with human immunodeficiency virus. Clin Infect Dis 1998;27:1329–30.
9. Arrizabalaga J, Casas A, Camino X, Iribarren JA, Arrondo FR, Von Wichmann MA. Utilidad de la desensibilizacion a rifampicina en el tratamiento de enfermedades producidas por micobacterias en pacientes con SIDA. Med Clin 1998;111: 103–4.
10. Darouiche RO, Raad II, Heard SO, Thornby JI, Wenker OC, Gabrielli A, Berg J, Khardori N, Hanna H, Hachem R, Harris RL, Mayhall G. A comparison of two antimicrobial-impregnated central venous catheters. Catheter Study Group. New Engl J Med 1999;340:1–8.
11. Wenzel RP, Edmond MB. The evolving technology of venous access. New Engl J Med 1999; 340:48–50.
12. Joos AA, Frank UG, Kaschka WP. Pharmacokinetic interaction of clozapine and rifampicin in a forensic patient with an atypical mycobacterial infection. J Clin Psychopharmacol 1998;18: 83–5.
13. Altundag MK, Barista I. False-positive urine melanin pigment reaction caused by rifampin. Ann Pharmacother 1998;32:610.
14. Nolan SR, Self TH, Norwood JM. Interaction between rifampin and levothyroxine. South Med J 1999;92:529–31.
15. Jaffuel D, Lebel B, Hillaire-Buys D, Pene J. Eosinophilic pneumonia induced by dapsone. Br Med J 1998;317:181.
16. Arunthathi S, Raju S. Dapsone-induced pulmonary eosinophilia without cutaneous manifestations. Acta Leprol 1998;11:3–5.

A.G.C. Bauer

31 Antihelminthic drugs

Albendazole *(SED-13, 912; SEDA-20, 280; SEDA-21, 315; SEDA-22, 324)*

Albendazole is a benzimidazole derivative with a broad spectrum used in the treatment of gastrointestinal roundworms and strongyloidiasis, and in high doses in echinococcosis and neurocysticercosis. Its use has recently been reviewed (1[R]). The efficacy of albendazole in these conditions has again been confirmed, with few and usually minor adverse effects consisting of *gastrointestinal upsets, dizziness, rash*, and *alopecia*, which usually do not require drug withdrawal. About 15% of patients treated with albendazole in higher doses develop *raised serum transaminases*, necessitating closer follow-up and sometimes discontinuation of treatment after prolonged use. It has been emphasized that albendazole is *teratogenic* in animals and should not be used in pregnancy and lactation.

In another review albendazole was effective in neurocysticercosis in an optimal dosage of 15 mg/kg/day divided in two doses every 12 hours for 8 days (2[R]). Albendazole was generally well tolerated, although several patients had adverse reactions in the first days after the start of treatment, consisting of headache, vomiting, and exacerbation of neurological symptoms caused by an inflammatory reaction to antigens from degenerating cysts, necessitating the concomitant use of corticosteroids. In very large cysticerci, or cysticerci located in risky areas like the brainstem, these reactions may rarely be life-threatening.

In a further report on the use of albendazole 15 mg/kg/day in two divided doses for 14 days in the treatment of persistent neurocysticercosis (3[c]) adverse reactions were monitored in 43 patients with seizures and a solitary cysticercal cyst, who had not been treated before. In all patients CT scans confirmed the presence of a solitary cyst less then 2 cm in diameter. Antiepileptic treatment was continued. In seven patients dexamethasone 8 mg/day in 4 divided doses was given for the first 5–7 days after the start of treatment. Follow-up CT scans at 4–10 weeks after the start of treatment showed responses in 20 patients, with complete disappearance in seven patients and a reduction to 50% of the pre-treatment size in the other 13. There were adverse effects in 15 patients, with a maximum on the fifth day after the start of treatment. Six patients had severe *headaches*, 11 had *partial seizures*, and two had epileptic seizures and severe *postictal hemiparesis* that persisted for a week or more. Because of these serious adverse effects treatment was discontinued in seven patients and dexamethasone was added in those patients who were not already taking it, although its use proved questionable. Adverse effects were seen in three of seven patients who took prophylactic steroid therapy and in 12 of 36 patients who did not.

Albendazole has also been used in the treatment of human hookworm and trichuris infections. In a mass-treatment report from Western Australia (4[c]) 295 individuals in a remote rural area were treated with albendazole 400 mg/day for 5 days because of possible Giardia lamblia and hookworm infections. The 37% prevalence of Giardia fell to 12% between days 6 and 9, but rose again to 28% between days 18 and 30. The effect on hookworms (*Ankylostoma duodenale*) was more pronounced and more sustained with a reduction of the pretreatment prevalence of hookworm infections from 76% before treatment to 0% after 3–4 weeks. The tolerability of the drug was judged to be excellent by 89%, good by 1%, and moderately good by 1%, while 9% gave no response. Adverse effects were reported by five individuals and consisted of mild *abdominal pain* in two, mild or moderate *diarrhea* in two, moderate *fever* in one, and *weakness* in one.

In a randomized trial in Mexico (5[c]) 622 children with *Trichuris* were randomized to either albendazole 400 mg/day for 3 days, one dose of albendazole 400 mg, or one dose of py-

Side Effects of Drugs, Annual 23
J.K. Aronson, ed.

rantel 11 mg/kg. The aim was to study efficacy and the effects on growth. After three courses at 1 year the level of infection with *Trichuris* was reduced by 99% in the 3-day albendazole treatment group, by 87% in the single-dose albendazole treatment group, and by 67% in the pyrantel group. There were no significant differences in the increases in height, weight, or arm circumference, but contrary to expectations there was a *lower increase in the thickness of the triceps skin fold* in those given 3-day courses of albendazole. This was only found in the patients with lower pretreatment *Trichuris* stool egg counts. These findings suggest that although elimination of *Trichuris* may promote growth in children, albendazole in a dose of 1200 mg/kg every 4 months may have an independent negative effect on growth. In an accompanying commentary (6) it was concluded that the suggestion that relatively high doses of albendazole may affect growth deserves study, but that this possible effect must be weighed against the negative effect of prolonged helminthic infestation on children's health, growth, and cognitive function. However, it is unlikely that high-dose treatment will be standard in mass-treatment campaigns, and these results should not deter the use of single-dose albendazole in mass-treatment programs in high-risk populations.

Albendazole has also been used in the treatment and prophylaxis of microsporidiosis in patients with AIDS. In a small double-blind placebo-controlled trial from France (7[c]) the efficacy and safety of treatment with albendazole was studied in four patients treated with albendazole 400 mg bd for 3 weeks and in four patients treated with placebo. Microsporidia were cleared in all patients given albendazole but in none of those given placebo. Afterwards all eight patients were again randomized to receive either maintenance treatment with albendazole 400 mg bd or no treatment for the next 12 months; none of the three patients taking maintenance treatment had a recurrence, while three of the five who took no maintenance therapy developed a recurrence. During the double-blind part of the trial there were no serious adverse effects in the patients who took albendazole, although two complained of *headache*, one of *abdominal pain*, one had *raised transaminase activities*, and one had *thrombocytopenia*. However, half the patients were also taking anti-HIV triple therapy, which makes it difficult to assess these abnormalities. The authors concluded that the adverse effects were not serious and did not hinder maintenance therapy. The tentative conclusion derived from these findings is that albendazole may be useful in the treatment of microsporidiosis, which in patients with AIDS often leads to debilitating chronic diarrhea and is difficult to treat.

Hematological *Bone-marrow suppression*, usually transient and mainly affecting the white cell production, after treatment with albendazole has been noted in the past. Amegakaryocytic *thrombocytopenia* attributed to albendazole has recently been reported (8[c]).

A 25-year-old woman who had been taking albendazole 13 mg/kg/day for 5 months for hepatic and pulmonary echinococcosis developed fatigue, bleeding gums, and prolonged menstrual bleeding. She had ecchymoses and petechiae over her legs, a marked thrombocytopenia (10×10^9/l), a mild iron deficiency anemia, and a normal white blood cell count. There was no antiplatelet immunoglobulin. A bone-marrow aspiration showed absent megakaryocytes with normal granulocytes and mild erythroid hyperplasia. A cytogenetic study of the bone-marrow showed normal karyotype and immunophenotype. The albendazole was withdrawn and oral iron given. At follow-up 2 months later all laboratory abnormalities had resolved.

Ivermectin *(SED-13, 906; SEDA-20, 280; SEDA-21, 315; SEDA-22, 326)*

Ivermectin is a very effective microfilaricidal drug, used in the treatment of strongyloidiasis, all types of filariasis (except *Dipalonema perstans*), and also in scabies. It is generally considered to be safe, with only minor adverse effects, but more severe adverse effects can occur, through *allergic reactions* to dying worms, especially in loiasis. Recently the use of ivermectin and its adverse effects in patients infected with *Loa loa* have been reviewed (9[R]). It was concluded that ivermectin in a single dose of 150–300 μg/kg is effective in reducing microfilaria counts by over 90% with suppressed counts to 25% of pretreatment values after 1 year. An even more sustained effect can be reached by more frequent dosing. There is also some evidence that ivermectin in higher doses (400 μg/kg twice yearly) may have an effect on the adult *Loa loa*. Tolerance to ivermectin is generally excellent, but serious adverse effects, especially encephalopathy, can occur, principally in more heavily infected individuals. Ivermectin appears to promote the passage of *Loa loa* microfilaria into the cerebrospinal fluid, with a maximum after 3–5 days, followed by an intense allergic reaction to the dying microfilaria.

The Mectizan Expert Committee defined a definitive case of *Loa loa* encephalopathy related to ivermectin as having to satisfy two criteria:

- encephalopathy in which there is microscopic evidence of vasculopathy in the brain associated with *Loa loa* microfilaria;
- the onset of symptoms of disturbed CNS function within 5 days after treatment with ivermectin, progressing to coma without remission.

A probable case of *Loa loa* encephalopathy was defined as having to satisfy four criteria:

- coma in a previously healthy individual;
- the onset of CNS signs within 5 days of treatment with ivermectin progressing to coma;
- an initial microfilaremia of over 10 000/ml, or 1000/ml in a blood sample taken within 2 months of treatment;
- the presence of *Loa loa* microfilaria in the CSF.

Clinically common features of this condition are impaired consciousness appearing 3–4 days after treatment and lasting for 2–3 days.

There is no consensus on the proper management of ivermectin-associated *Loa loa* encephalopathy, and it is uncertain if co-administration of corticosteroids is of any use. In several patients with more severe reactions, *conjunctival hemorrhages* were seen. A systematic examination of the conjunctivae in 1682 patients complaining of any adverse reactions showed that these hemorrhages were closely correlated with the pretreatment microfilaria counts. This sign can be found 2 days after treatment and may thus single out patients prone to encephalopathy and needing closer follow-up. Although the incidence of such cases is very low (in the order of 1 in 10 000 treated patients), this serious adverse effect makes mass treatment of *Loa loa* infection problematic, and also mass treatment of onchocerciasis in areas in which *Loa loa* is endemic. To illustrate this point the same authors have presented three probable cases of *Loa loa encephalopathy* after ivermectin treatment for onchocerciasis (10^C). All three were young men treated with ivermectin 150 μg/kg in a mass-treatment campaign in onchocerciasis.

A 26-year-old, previously healthy, man developed CNS symptoms in the form of an inability to stand or eat and stiffness of the neck by the third day. On the fourth day he had difficulty swallowing and speaking. On the fifth day he couldn't speak and was incontinent of urine. He was given dexamethasone, diazepam, furosemide, and atropine. On the sixth day he became comatose. On the ninth day he developed a high fever, and was given penicillin and tube-feeding. His condition gradually worsened and he died on the 21st day. Serum microfilaria counts on day 13 after treatment were still high (3600/ml), and live *Loa loa* (10/ml) were found in the CSF.

A 32-year-old man with alcoholism had a very high pretreatment serum microfilaria count (50 000/ml). After starting ivermectin he took to his bed and wouldn't speak. On the third day he developed a fever, possibly attributed to malaria and treated with chloroquine. On the fourth day he was unable to stand, and alternately restless or somnolent; his CSF contained live *Loa loa* microfilaria. He became more incoherent and fidgety and had a marked grasp reflex. Later in the day he developed spastic hypertonia. On the fifth day he became incontinent and still wouldn't speak. Over the following days he gradually improved and 4 months later had no neurological abnormalities, although his relatives found that his behavior had changed and that he was much calmer then in the past. An electroencephalogram on day 15 showed periodic diffuse discharges of large amplitude during hyperventilation and on day 146 an asymmetric tracing with focal activity in the right parieto-occipital area, which worsened during hyperventilation. On day 233 the electroencephalogram was normal.

An 18-year-old previously healthy man was given ivermectin. On the second day he was unable to work and stayed at home. On the third day he was found unconscious in bed, incontinent of urine and feces. On the fourth day he did not move and had absent pain sensation. There was hypertonia in the arms with marked cogwheeling. On the fifth and sixth days there was a swinging horizontal movement of the eyeballs, but otherwise he appeared to improve. On the seventh day he could stay seated in bed with help and spoke several sentences. He could perform slow voluntary movements and his muscle strength and sensation returned to normal, although the cogwheel phenomenon still persisted. He gradually returned to normal over the following weeks. After 5 months the neurological examination was normal but he still complained of headaches and episodic amnesia. His pretreatment serum microfilaria counts were high (152 940/ml) and the CSF collected on the fourth day contained live *Loa loa* microfilaria. An electroencephalogram on the 19th day was slow with spontaneous, diffuse, paroxysmal, monomorphic theta activity, lasting 2–3 seconds. An electroencephalogram on the 105th day showed improvement, but focal abnormalities persisted in the left occipital region. On the 159th day all previously recorded abnormalities had disappeared.

Ivermectin and lymphatic filariasis In an open study from India (11[c]) 21 asymptomatic microfilaria carriers (with counts of 109–6934/ml of blood) were treated with a single oral dose of ivermectin 400 μg/kg and a single oral dose of diethylcarbamazine 6 mg/kg for infection with *Brugia Malayi*. Twelve hours after treatment microfilaria counts fell by 96–100% in all patients and 12 patients had become afilaremic. All had an adverse reaction, lasting up to 48 hours after treatment: fever in 20 patients, *myalgia* in 19, *headache* in 17, *lethargy* in 15, *chills* in 13, *sweating* in 11, *anorexia* in 11, *sore throat and pharyngeal congestion* in 10, *arthralgia* in six, *giddiness* in four, *nausea and vomiting* in three, *abdominal pain* in two, and *cough* in one. *Postural hypotension*, lasting 1 day, was noted in two individuals. Transient *dilated and painfully inflamed lymphatic channels*, which stood out in cords, were seen in two individuals. Most adverse effects were mild and self-limiting.

Ivermectin and scabies Another case of successful treatment of severe scabies with ivermectin has appeared (12[c]).

An 11-year-old girl developed severe crusted Norwegian scabies. Lindane lotion and topical keratolytics had no significant effect. She was given a single oral dose of ivermectin 6 mg/kg with dramatic effect. The pruritus subsided in 4 hours and the lesions started to clear 2 days later. A second dose of 6 mg was given after 3 weeks when no skin lesions were found anymore. The only adverse effect was some edema of the skin after the first dose, which did not occur after the second dose, suggesting that the reaction was more related to the intensity of the infection then to the effect of the drug itself.

Levamisole *(SED-13, 1135; SEDA-20, 348; SEDA-21, 317; SEDA-22, 328)*

Levamisole was originally developed as an antihelminthic drug, but is now mainly used as an immunomodulating drug in the adjuvant chemotherapy of Dukes B and C colonic cancer in combination with 5-fluorouracil, in the treatment of rheumatic diseases, and in the treatment of the nephrotic syndrome in children. Reports of the use of levamisole in the nephrotic syndrome have recently appeared.

In 11 children with nephrotic syndrome, of whom five were steroid-sensitive, six steroid-resistant, and all resistant to other immunosuppressive drugs, levamisole 2.5 mg/kg was given every 48 hours for up to 18 months (13[C]). Two patients were also given ciclosporin. All the patients in the steroid-sensitive group but none in the steroid-resistant group reacted favorably to levamisole, with disappearance of protein from the urine. There were serious adverse effects in two patients: one developed a transient *leukopenia* 2 months after the start of treatment and another developed a severe *exacerbation of pre-existing psoriasis*, although that may have been due to the withdrawal of cyclophosphamide.

Levamisole 2 mg/kg on alternate days was given to 25 steroid-dependent children with frequent relapses of idiopathic nephrotic syndrome (14[C]). The steroid was tapered, and continued for 3–14 months. During treatment with levamisole the relapse frequency was reduced by 40%. Two patients developed mild transient leukopenia, which disappeared 2 weeks after withdrawal. One had a slight rash that disappeared while treatment was continued and one complained of *epigastric pain*, which led to drug withdrawal.

Further reports on the use of levamisole combined with 5-fluorouracil in the adjuvant treatment of resected colon cancer have been published. In a prospective randomized trial (15[c]) 891 patients were randomized to receive either intensive fluorouracil and leucovorin combined with levamisole, or a standard regimen of fluorouracil plus levamisole. The patients were then again randomized to receive either 6 or 12 months of treatment. Standard fluorouracil plus levamisole was not as effective as fluorouracil, levamisole, and leucovorin, and treatment for 12 months was not superior to treatment for 6 months. Unfortunately, there was no treatment arm with fluorouracil and leucovorin only, which is now widely considered to be the treatment of choice. Serious grade 3–4 adverse effects were more frequent in the three-drug treatment groups, and consisted of *diarrhea* (13 vs 3 patients in the 6-month groups, 17 vs 7 in the 12-month groups) and *stomatitis* (10 vs 3 in the 6-month groups, 11 vs 6 in the 12-month groups). *Leukopenia* occurred more frequently in the standard treatment groups (10 vs 18, one of whom died, in the 6-month groups, and 13 patients, one of whom died, versus 14, one of whom died). There were four treatment-associated deaths.

In another study combined intravenous and intraperitoneal fluorouracil plus leucovorin was compared with standard treatment with fluorouracil and levamisole in 241 patients with resected stage 3 or high-risk stage 2 colon cancers (16[c]). In the combined treatment group there was an increased disease-free interval, an estimated 43% reduction in death rate, and a reduction in local tumor recurrence. Adverse effects were relatively uncommon and were generally judged to be mild to moderate; they were slightly more common in those treated with fluorouracil and levamisole, and consisted of nausea and vomiting (18 vs 14%), *diarrhea* (16 vs 10%), *mucositis* (17 vs 12%), *granulocytopenia* (29 vs 23%), and *thrombocytopenia* (5 vs 3%). Four cases of unspecified CNS toxicity were noted in those given fluorouracil plus levamisole. *Abdominal pain* during or shortly after intraperitoneal drug administration was noted in 19% of patients. Overall 53% of the patients given fluorouracil plus levamisole and 56% of those given fluorouracil plus leucovorin had mild to moderate adverse effects. Severe reactions, requiring a 20% dosage reduction of fluorouracil, were more common in the fluorouracil plus levamisole arm (13 vs 3%). There were no deaths. Unfortunately, in this study no patients were treated with fluorouracil and leucovorin intravenously only.

It is likely that most of these reported adverse effects, although perhaps enhanced by levamisole, except for the CNS toxicity noted in a few individuals, were caused by fluorouracil. This has been further emphasized by a dose-finding study to determine the maximum tolerated dose of levamisole in the treatment of colon cancer in 38 patients with advanced non-resectable colon cancer, treated with fluorouracil 450 mg/m^2 by rapid i.v. infusion for 5 days (17[c]). Levamisole was given orally three times daily for 5 days every 5 weeks until disease progression. The main dose-limiting toxic effects were *nausea and vomiting* and an unpleasant *metallic taste*. The dose used was about five times the total amount of levamisole given in the standard fluorouracil plus levamisole regimen. Levamisole enhances the gastrointestinal toxicity of fluorouracil, with *anorexia, nausea, vomiting*, and occasional *diarrhea*, but did not enhance the bone-marrow suppression associated with fluorouracil. Increasing the dose of levamisole to 150 mg/m^2 tds for 5 days resulted in significant CNS toxicity, with *confusion, vertigo*, and severe *vomiting*. None of the patients treated with this dosage were able to complete the course.

Psychiatric In the past, anxiety, sleep disturbances, and depression have all been associated with levamisole. Psychosis has also been reported (18[C]).

A 28-year-old man, without a psychiatric history, developed a paranoid psychosis. He had been taking levamisole twice a week in an unspecified dose for 2 years for a stage 4 melanoma and metastatic lymph nodes in the axilla. Physical examination, a CT scan, an electroencephalogram, and standard laboratory tests were all normal. He was treated with perphenazine, with partial success, but after tapering of the dose his symptoms reappeared. It was thought likely that the psychosis had been caused by levamisole, which was discontinued. Three weeks later he had recovered completely. Levamisole was not reintroduced.

Skin and appendages Levamisole-induced *cutaneous vasculitis* with histological features of leukocytoclastic vasculitis is consistent with a type III (immune complex-mediated) hypersensitivity reaction. In a recent series, five out of 160 children with nephrotic syndrome developed distinctive vascular purpura (19[C]). They had taken levamisole for a mean of 24 months when they developed purpuric erythematous macules, which evolved to ecchymotic and necrotic purpura. The lesions were mostly on the external ear. Biopsies obtained from the ear lesions in four patients showed vasculopathic reaction patterns, ranging from leukocytoclastic and thrombotic vasculitis to vascular occlusive disease without true vasculitis. There were anticardiolipin, antinuclear, and/or antineutrophil cytoplasmic antibodies in four patients. The lesions resolved within 2–3 weeks after levamisole withdrawal, whereas anticardiolipin and antineutrophil cytoplasmic antibodies disappeared after 2–14 months only. A direct effect of levamisole on the endothelial cells or levamisole-induced or unmasked latent immunological abnormalities were suspected.

Overdosage Acute overdosage of levamisole has been described (20[c]).

A 43-year-old man treated himself with a levamisole enema of 10 g (33 times the therapeutic dose) for a gastrointestinal worm infestation. Soon after he developed malaise, tachycardia, nausea, vertigo, and profuse diarrhea. He lost consciousness and developed generalized seizures and a respiratory arrest. He was intubated, ventilated, and treated with clonazepam. His condition improved after 4 hours. He remained somnolent for 6 hours, and was nauseated and vomited for 24 hours. There was hypokalemia after the diarrhea, raised CPK activity, and a leukocytosis. An electrocardiogram showed ST depression. By the fourth day all his symptoms had subsided.

The symptoms in this case were attributed to the cholinergic effect that levamisole has at this high dose.

Metrifonate *(see Chapter 1)*

Nitazoxanide

Nitazoxanide is a thiazolide derivative first described in 1975 and originally developed as a veterinary antihelminthic. Although rarely used in man, successful treatment of a large variety of helminthic and protozoal diseases has been described. Since it is also effective against *Fasciola hepatica* in vitro it has now been tried in the treatment of fasciola infections in man. In a village close to Alexandria in Egypt 137 patients were given nitazoxanide 500 mg bd for 6 days (21[c]). On the 30th day 113 patients (82%) were presumed cured, with stools free of fasciola eggs. Nitazoxanide was extremely well tolerated. Only three patients reported adverse effects: *abdominal pain* in two and *vomiting* in one. The symptoms were mild and disappeared without medication or discontinuation of treatment. Together with triclabendazole, nitazoxanide can be considered for the treatment of *Fasciola hepatica* infections in man.

Suramin *(SED-13, 915; SEDA-20, 213; SEDA-21, 318; SEDA-22, 330)*

Suramin is rarely used as a macrofilaricidal drug in the treatment of onchocerciasis, but is mainly used now in the treatment of hormone-refractory prostate cancer, in which it has shown some antitumor effect, although accompanied by extensive and sometimes severe adverse effects. Its neurological adverse effects have recently been reviewed in the context of a broad review of neuropathies associated with malignancy and chemotherapy (22[R]). Neurotoxicity is a dose-limiting adverse effect of suramin and there are two distinct types of neuropathy: a mild, length-dependent, *axonal polyneuropathy*, and a more serious subacute demyelinating, *Guillain–Barré-like polyneuropathy*. The reported incidence of neuropathy is 25–90% with a mean of about 50%. The more severe demyelinating neuropathies appear to be dose-related and occur when peak suramin plasma concentrations are maintained above 350 μg/ml. Milder neuropathies occurred in 50–70% of patients with plasma concentrations below 300 μg/ml, and severe motor neuropathy was rare in this category of patients. The milder axonal polyneuropathy is the most common neurological adverse effect of suramin and causes distal paresthesia, reduced pain and vibration sensation in the feet, weak toe extensors, and absent ankle jerks; this neuropathy is largely reversible. The more severe Guillain–Barré-like polyradiculoneuropathy occurs in 10–20% of patients after 1–5 months of treatment with a maximum at 2–9 weeks after the start of treatment. The first symptoms are distal limb and or facial paresthesia, followed by diffuse, symmetrical, proximal weakness and areflexia. About 25% of these patients eventually require ventilation. The CSF protein content may be raised. Electroencephalography shows slow motor conduction velocities and electromyography shows reduced recruitment in both proximal and distal muscles. In the more severe cases denervation emerges. Sural nerve biopsies have shown a reduced density of the large and small myelinated fibers, occasional axonal degeneration, and demyelination. Epineural and endoneural mononuclear inflammatory cell infiltrates are sometimes seen. After withdrawal of treatment symptoms may deteriorate further for several weeks with recovery, sometimes incomplete, after 1–2 months.

The precise mechanism of the toxicity of suramin is unknown, although both inhibition of the effects of nerve growth factors and a possible immune-mediated effect, consistent with the many immunomodulating effects, have been suggested. In a recent experimental study of dorsal root ganglion cell cultures suramin disrupted the transport and metabolism of glycolipids, with accumulation of the GM1 ganglioside and ceramide, leading to cell death (23).

Finally another two studies of the use of suramin in patients with hormone-refractory prostate cancer have appeared. In 24 patients with hormone-refractory prostate cancer given suramin twice weekly intravenously targeted to reach plasma concentrations of 50–100, 101–

150, 151–200, or 201–250 μg/ml plus doxorubicin, fatigue occurred in 18 and was dose-limiting in two (24[c]). Eight developed neurological symptoms, of whom three, all receiving the highest dose, developed grade III toxicity. There were five cases of *neuropathies*. Two patients had evidence of a demyelinating neuropathy, one of whom developed a Guillain–Barré-like syndrome and inflammatory myopathy. A further patient had a mixed axonal and demyelinating peripheral neuropathy. Two patients developed a motor neuropathy that exacerbated pre-existing neurological defects. Other frequent adverse events were *proteinuria, leukopenia*, and *alopecia*. However, the respective roles of suramin and doxorubicin in causing these adverse effects were uncertain.

In 81 patients intravenous suramin (peak plasma concentration 300 μg/ml trough concentration 175 μg/ml) combined with aminoglutethimide 250 mg qds in patients with progressive androgen-refractory prostate cancer after antiandrogen treatment had been discontinued, effectiveness was limited, whereas most adverse effects were attributed to suramin (25[C]). There were 38 episodes of grade 3 and 4 toxic effects in 29 patients. Severe *thrombocytopenia* occurred in four patients. There were four episodes of *atrial fibrillation*. One patient developed *uremia* which required dialysis. One patient developed grade 3 *neurosensory changes*, but none had neuromotor changes. There was one episode of grade 4 *rash*, which was probably attributable to aminoglutethimide, consisting of diffuse *erythematous exfoliating papules* over the chest, back, arms and face. All adverse effects were reversible.

Tiabendazole *(SED-13, 911; SEDA-22, 331)*

Tiabendazole is a benzimidazole derivative used in the treatment of strongyloidiasis. Several cases of severe *cholestasis*, even resulting in cirrhosis and liver transplantation, have previously been described, and two further cases have been reported (26[c]).

A 27-year-old patient from Surinam with β-thalassemia took tiabendazole 1250 mg bd for 2 days for strongyloidiasis. One week later she became icteric, with raised total and conjugated bilirubin, alkaline phosphatase, γ-glutamyltransferase, AsT, and AlT. Tests for antinuclear antibodies, parietal cells antibodies, smooth muscle antibodies, mitochondrial antibodies, hepatitis A, B, C, cytomegalovirus, Epstein–Barr virus, mumps, and measles were negative. Ultrasonography showed normal intrahepatic and extrahepatic bile ducts. Liver biopsy showed intrahepatic cholestasis and a slightly increased infiltrate in the portal areas. One week later she developed a generalized urticarial rash. She had mildly abnormal liver tests for the next 7 years, at which time a liver biopsy showed a slight lymphatic infiltrate in the portal fields, without signs of cirrhosis, chronic hepatitis, or primary biliary cirrhosis.

A 42-year-old woman, also from Surinam, with β-thalassemia and non-insulin dependant diabetes mellitus took tiabendazole 1250 mg bd for 2 days for strongyloidiasis. Five weeks later she developed general malaise, anorexia, weight loss, icterus, and a tender liver. She had raised total and direct bilirubin, γ-glutamyltransferase, and alkaline phosphatase, but only marginally raised transaminases. Tests for Hepatitis A, B, and C, cytomegalovirus, and schistosomiasis were negative. Tests for antinuclear antibodies and antibodies against liver cell membranes, smooth muscle, and mitochondria were negative, but there were parietal cell antibodies. Ultrasonography and ERCP showed normal intrahepatic and extrahepatic bile ducts. Liver biopsy showed severe centrally localized cholestasis. A year later all clinical and laboratory abnormalities had disappeared.

In view of these and previous cases of severe cholestasis after tiabendazole and the availability of less toxic equally effective drugs (albendazole or preferably ivermectin), tiabendazole must be considered obsolete in the treatment of strongyloidiasis.

Triclabendazole

Triclabendazole is a benzimidazole derivative used as a veterinary antihelminthic. Several reports have suggested that it may be of use in the treatment of *Fasciola hepatica* infection. In 20 patients with fascioliasis treated with two single doses of triclabendazole 10 mg/kg, the plasma concentrations of triclabendazole, its active metabolite triclabendazole-SO, and its sulfone metabolite were doubled by food (27[c]). There were no serious adverse effects, except for some *right-sided upper abdominal pain* in several patients, which could be relieved by oral spasmolytics. Triclabendazole should be administered with food.

REFERENCES

1. Venkatesan P. Albendazole. J Antimicrob Chemother 1998;41:145–7.
2. Sotelo J, Jung H. Pharmacokinetic optimisation of the treatment of neurocysticercosis. Clin

Pharmacokinet 1998;34:503–15.

3. Rajshekhar V. Incidence and significance of adverse effects of albendazole therapy in patients with a persistent solitary *Cysticercus* granuloma. Acta Neurol Scand 1998;98:121–3.
4. Reynoldson JA, Behnke JM, Gracey M, Horton RJ, Spargo RM, Hopkins RM, Constantine CC, Gilbert F, Stead C, Hobbs RP, Thompson RCA. Efficacy of albendazole against *Giardia* and hookworm in a remote aboriginal community in the north of Western Australia. Acta Trop 1998;71:27–44.
5. Forrester JE, Bailar III JC, Esrey SA, José MV, Castillejos BT, Ocampo G. Randomized trial of albendazole and pyrantel in symptomless trichuriasis in children. Lancet 1998;352:1103–8.
6. Winstantley P. Commentary: Albendazole for mass treatment of asymptomatic trichiuris infection. Lancet 1998;352:1080–1.
7. Molina JM, Chastang C, Goguel J, Michiels JF, Sarfati C, Desportes-Livage I, Horton J, Derouin F, Modaï J. Albendazole for treatment and prophylaxis of microsporidiosis due to *Encephalitozoon intestinalis* in patients with AIDS: a randomized double-blind controlled trial. J Infect Dis 1998;177:1373–7.
8. Yildiz BO, Haznedaroglu IC, Cöplü L. Albendazole-induced amegakaryocytic thrombocytopenic purpura. Ann Pharmacother 1998;32:842.
9. Boussinesq M, Gardon J. Challenges for the future: loiasis. Ann Trop Med Parasitol 1998;92:147–51.
10. Boussinesq M, GardonJ, Gardon-Wendel N, Kamgno J, Ngoumou P, Chippaux JP. Three probable cases of *Loa loa* encephalopathy following ivermectin treatment for onchocerciasis. Am J Trop Med Hyg 1998;58:461–9.
11. Shenoy RK, George LM, John A, Suma TK, Kumaraswami V. Treatment of microfilaraemia in asymptomatic brugian filariasis: the efficacy and safety of the combination of single doses of ivermectin and diethylcarbamazine. Ann Trop Med Parasitol 1998;92:579–85.
12. Jaramillo-Ayerbe F, Berrio-Muñoz J. Ivermectin for crusted Norwegian scabies induced by use of topical steroids. Arch Dermatol 1998;134:143–5.
13. Tenbrock K, Müller-Berghaus J, Fuchshuber A, Michalk D, Querfeld D. Levamisole treatment in steroid-sensitive and steroid-resistant nephrotic syndrome. Pediatr Nephrol 1998;12:459–62.
14. Kemper MJ, Amon O, Timmermann K, Altrogge H, Müller-Wiefel DE. Die Behandlung des häufig Rezidivierenden steroidsensiblen idiopathischen nephrotischen Syndroms im Kindersalter mit Levamisol. Dtsch Med Wochenschr 1998;123:239–43.
15. O'Connell MJ, Laurie JA, Kahn M, Fitzgibbons RJ, Ehrlichman C, Shepherd L, Moertel CG, Kocha WJ, Pazdur R, Wieand S, Rubin J, Vukov AM, Donohue JH, Krook JE, Figueredo A. Prospectively randomized trial of postoperative adjuvant chemotherapy in patients with high-risk colon cancer. J Clin Oncol 1998;16:295–300.
16. Scheithauer W, Kornek GV, Marczell A, Karner J, Salem G, Greiner R, Burger D, Stöger F, Ritschel J, Kovats E, Vischer HM, Schneeweiss B, Depisch D. Combined intravenous and intraperitoneal chemotherapy with fluorouracil + leucovorin vs fluorouracil + levamisole for adjuvant therapy of resected colon carcinoma Br J Cancer 1998;77:1349–54.
17. Reid JM, Kovach JS, O'Connell MJ, Bagniewski PG, Moertel CG. Clinical and pharmacokinetic studies of high-dose levamisole in combination with 5-fluorouracil in patients with advanced cancer Cancer Chemother Pharmacol 1998;41:477–84.
18. Jeffries JJ, Cammisuli S. Psychosis secondary to long-term levamisole therapy. Ann Pharmacother 1998;32:134–5.
19. Rongioletti F, Ghio L, Ginevri F, Bleidl D, Rinaldi S, Edefonti A, Gambini C, Rizzoni G, Rebora A. Purpura of the ears: a distinctive vasculopathy with circulating autoantibodies complicating long-term treatment with levamisole in children. Br J Dermatol 1999;140:948–51.
20. Joly C, Palisse M, Ribbe D, De Calmes O, Genevey P. Intoxication aiguë au lévamisole. Presse Med 1998;27:717.
21. Rossignoll JF, Abaza H, Friedman H. Successful treatment of human fascioliasis with nitazoxanide Trans R Soc Trop Med Hyg 1998;92:103–4.
22. Amato AA, Collins MP. Neuropathies associated with malignancy. Semin Neurol 1998;18:125–44.
23. Gill JS, Windebank AJ. Suramin induced ceramide accumulation leads to apoptotic cell death in dorsal root ganglion neurons. Cell Death Differ 1998;5:876–83.
24. Tu S-M, Pagliaro LC, Banks ME, Amato RJ, Millikan RE, Bugazia NA, Madden T, Newman RA, Logothetis CJ. Phase I study of suramin combined with doxorubicin in the treatment of androgen-independent prostate cancer. Clin Cancer Res 1998;4:1193–201.
25. Dawson N, Figg WD, Brawley OW, Bergan R, Cooper MR, Senderowicz A, Headlee D, Steinberg SM, Sutherland M, Patronas N, Sausville E, Linehan WM, Reed E, Sartor O. Phase II study of suramin plus aminogluthetimide in two cohorts of patients with androgen-independent prostate cancer; simultaneous antiandrogen withdrawal and prior antiandrogen withdrawal. Clin Cancer Res 1998;4:37–44.
26. Eland IA, Kerkhof SCMB, Overbosch D, Wismans PJ, Stricker BHCH. Cholestatische hepatitis toegeschreven aan her gebruik van tiabendazole. Ned Tijdschr Geneeskd 1998;142:1331–4.
27. Lecaillon JB, Godbillon J, Campestrini J, Naquira C, Miranda L, Pacheco R, Mull R, Poltera AA. Effect of food on the bioavailability of triclabendazole in patients with fascioliasis. Br J Clin Pharmacol 1998;45:601–4.

S. Dittmann

32 Vaccines

Editor's note: Abbreviations used in this chapter include:

- *ACIP: Advisory Committee on Immunization Practices;*
- *DT: diphtheria + tetanus toxoids (for pediatric use);*
- *DTaP: diphtheria + tetanus toxoids + acellular pertussis (for pediatric use);*
- *DTwP: diphtheria + tetanus toxoids (for pediatric use);*
- *Hib: Hemophilus influenzae type b;*
- *IPV: inactivated poliomyelitis vaccine;*
- *OspA: outer surface protein A [of Borrelia burgdorferi];*
- *PRP–D–Hib: conjugated Hib vaccine (a mutant polypeptide of diphtheria toxin covalently linked to Hib capsular polysaccharide);*
- *PRP-T-Hib: conjugated Hib vaccine (tetanus toxoid linked to Hib capsular polysaccharide);*
- *RRV-TV: tetravalent rhesus-based rotavirus vaccine, Rotashield;*
- *VAERS: Vaccine Adverse Events Reporting System;*
- *Vi: virulence antigen of Salmonella typhi;*
- *VSD: Vaccine Safety Datalink*

R Surveillance of adverse events after immunization

Currently, in many industrially highly developed countries that have markedly reduced the incidence of dangerous infectious diseases through immunization, there are controversial discussions about the benefit and risk of immunization. Vaccine adverse events, both those caused by vaccines (i.e. true adverse reactions) and those associated with immunization only by coincidence, become more visible than natural disease. Not surprisingly, vaccine safety concerns have become increasingly prominent in such successful immunization programs. Vaccines have been spuriously linked by various researchers to asthma, autism, diabetes, inflammatory bowel disease, multiple sclerosis, permanent brain damage, and sudden infant death syndrome. Modern communication is providing even more penetrating ways of communicating messages on the subject through the worldwide web. The result is a formidable challenge to immunization service providers. Neil Halsey, head of the Institute for Vaccine Safety at Johns Hopkins University, has summed up the features common to recent publications on vaccine adverse effects:

- *a causal link is usually claimed with a disease or condition of unknown or unclear cause;*
- *the association is claimed by one investigator or a group of investigators;*
- *the association is not confirmed by peers or by subsequent research;*
- *the claims are made with no apparent concern for potential harm from public loss of confidence and refusal to immunize;*
- *findings of subsequent studies that fail to confirm the original claim never get the publicity given to the 'original' finding, and so the public never gets a balanced view (1[R], 2[R]).*

A critical examination (3[R]) of a report (4[C]) of several children whose chronic bowel and behavioral abnormalities were linked to measles, mumps, and rubella (MMR) immunization can be used as an example to underline Halsey's comments. Without effective and credible systems for the detection of vaccine-associated adverse events through pharmacovigilance, for distinguishing causal reactions from coincidental reactions by pharmacoepidemiological or other studies, and for risk communication, vaccine safety concerns may confuse the media and the public.

Side Effects of Drugs, Annual 23
J.K. Aronson, ed.

A concerted effort is needed to improve communications at all levels regarding the real risks associated with vaccines and immunization and helping to reassure the public of the overwhelming safety record of vaccines. The medical community still holds pre-eminence as the advice giver to the public on matters of immunization and should play the key role in improved communication (1[R], 2[R]).

The US Vaccine Adverse Events Reporting System (VAERS) has already been described (SEDA-14, 919). The pros and cons of the system have again been discussed (5[R]). About 1000 reports per month are submitted by manufacturers (39%), state health coordinators (34%), health care professionals (25%), and parents (2%). Manufacturers' reports are primarily based on information received from health care providers or the parents of vaccinees. As a passive reporting system, VAERS is subject to numerous well-known deficiencies, such as under-reporting, incomplete and missing data, and recall bias. Resources are not adequate to allow follow-up for complete or accurate data in all cases. However, VAERS is useful to detect early warning signals and to generate hypotheses. For example, the information from a parent that her daughter had lost her hair after the second and third doses of hepatitis B vaccine, has initiated a study that found 59 similar cases, including three cases of positive rechallenge. As a result of this study, alopecia was added to the list of adverse reactions in the hepatitis B vaccine package insert. Individual case reports can also trigger a complete review of the VAERS database. For example, three reports of idiopathic thrombocytopenic purpura after measles-containing vaccine were received in a short period of time. The study of idiopathic thrombocytopenic purpura reported in the database found 54 other reports during the period 1990–95, including one case of positive rechallenge, which increased the likelihood that the association was causal.

Reports on adverse events after the administration of the two hepatitis B vaccines licensed in the US (Engerix-B and Recombivax HB) have been compared in two different surveillance systems: VAERS (mentioned above) and Vaccine Safety Datalink (VSD) (6[C]). VSD is a computerized record linkage system designed to permit more rigorous evaluation of causality of adverse events after immunization. Since 1989, VSD has actively maintained medical files on over 500 000 children, aged from birth to 6 years enrolled at four west coast health maintenance organizations. Immunization records, medical diagnoses, and diseases from clinic, hospitalization, and emergency room visits are coded. Whereas VAERS found that the reporting rate for events after brand 1 vaccine was at least three times higher than the reporting rate after brand 2 vaccine, VSD found no difference between rates of hospitalization or emergency room visits in recipients of the two vaccine brands. The authors concluded that the results of the VAERS database are subject to the inherent limitations of a passive surveillance system. The study underlines the importance of using other analytical studies, such as VSD, to evaluate preliminary results obtained by VAERS.

BACTERIAL VACCINES

Anthrax vaccine

Until recently, there has been little research into anthrax vaccines, other than that carried out for antibacteriological warfare purposes by the military. Currently, three human vaccines against *B. anthracis* (produced in Russia, the UK, and the US) are commercially available. The results of two field trials of two vaccines produced in Russia and the US have been analyzed (7[C]). The US killed vaccine was 93% effective in preventing cases of anthrax, and the Russian live attenuated vaccine afforded 75% protection when given by scarification and 84% when a jet-gun was used. The rates of local reactions (*erythema, induration*, and *edema*) and systemic reactions (*fever, malaise, arthralgia, rash, headache*) after the US vaccine were 5.75 and 0.4% respectively, compared with 0.54% local reactions and no systemic reactions after placebo. Adverse effects data on the Russian vaccine were not presented.

In the search for new vaccines against anthrax, manufacturers have aimed for better quality purified protective antigen vaccines with better adjuvants, vaccines made through recombinant gene technology, and mutant vaccines with altered protective antigens.

In a study by the Advisory Group of Medical Countermeasures of the UK Ministry of Defence only *mild discomfort at the injection site* was reported after the administration of a total of 55 000 doses of anthrax vaccine (8[C]).

Bacille Calmette–Guérin (BCG) vaccine *(SED-13, 920; SEDA-20, 287; SEDA-21, 326; SEDA-22, 336)*

A rare complication of intravesical BCG therapy, *a mycotic aneurysm*, has been reported (9[c]).

A 71-year-old man with bladder carcinoma in situ received six instillations of BCG at weekly intervals followed 3 months later by three booster instillations at weekly intervals. Four months later an inflammatory aortic aneurysm, which had ruptured into a pseudoaneurysm, was diagnosed and excised. *Mycobacterium bovis* was found. After treatment with isoniazid and rifampicin he recovered. There was no sign of tumor in the bladder at cystocopy 8 months after the last BCG instillation.

Arthritis and arthralgia are well-known adverse effects of intravesical BCG instillation as part of therapy of bladder cancer (SED-13, 925). The etiology and the different clinical pictures of BCG immunotherapy have been discussed (10[C]). Considering that mycobacteria are potent stimulators of the immune system and especially of T cells, it is not surprising to observe T cell mediated aseptic arthritis after BCG therapy. The authors suggested that the site of immune stimulation is critical, since intradermal injection produces a clinical presentation similar to reactive arthritis, and intravesical therapy causes a clinical picture identical to Reiter's syndrome.

In a large worldwide analysis of BCG adverse effects (1948–74) co-ordinated by the International Union Against Tuberculosis and Lung Disease (SED-12, 795) there have been 272 cases of lesions of bones and joints, including synovial lesions. However, case reports of arthritis after BCG vaccination in healthy individuals are rare. Now *polyarthritis* has been reported in a 33-year-old healthy woman 3 weeks after BCG vaccination (11[c]).

Haemophilus influenzae type b (Hib) vaccine *(SED-13, 927; SEDA-20, 288;SEDA-21, 329; SEDA-22, 337)*

Suspected association between type 1 diabetes mellitus and Hemophilus influenzae type b immunization The incidence of *diabetes mellitus* has been studied in Finnish children born between October 1983 and September 1985 compared with children born between October 1985 and 1987 (12[C]). Of the children born in the period 1985–87, 50% received Hib vaccine (diphtheria conjugated PRP-D-Hib vaccine) at 3, 4, and 6 months as a primary course and a booster dose at 14–18 months; the other 50% received one dose of the same vaccine at the age of 24 months. Taking into account the documented increase in diabetes in Finnish children, the small difference between the incidence rate of diabetes in children born during the period 1985–87 and immunized at 18 months and the incidence rate of children born in 1983–85 and not immunized against Hib disease was expected, with a slightly higher non-significant incidence in immunized children. In children over 4 years of age primed during the first year of life the incidence rate of diabetes was also slightly but non-significantly higher than in children immunized at 18 months of age. The authors concluded that early PRP-D-Hib immunization does not increase the risk of diabetes during the first 10 years of life.

This study has been criticized on the grounds that the authors did not present data comparing the incidence rates of children born in 1985–87 and primed during the first year of life with children born in 1983–85 and not immunized (13[C]). The critics presented significant differences in the incidence rate of diabetes between both groups of children and concluded that the immunization had increased the risk of diabetes. However, he did not mention that the relative risk of diabetes during the first 10 years of life in the immunized children born in 1985–87 was 1.19 compared to the non-immunized children born in 1983–85. We should also not forget to ask what is the biological plausibility of a causal relation between Hib vaccine and diabetes. And other epidemiological studies have presented data that could be used to show that Hib vaccine protects against diabetes. It should also be mentioned that the conjugated Hib vaccine (PRP-D-Hib) (12[C]–14[C]) has been almost completely replaced by different conjugated Hib vaccines.

We should also mention that the efficacy of Hib vaccines is very high. In countries in which universal Hib immunization has been implemented into the immunization schedule of children and where high coverage has been reported, the dangerous invasive disease causing many deaths and a high percentage of severe residual damage has been almost eliminated, e.g. in Scandinavia, Germany, the UK, and the US.

In 1997, US researchers suggested that immunization at 28 days after birth may cause type 1 diabetes mellitus in susceptible individuals. In May 1998, several institutions, including the National Institute of Allergy and Infectious Diseases, the Centers for Disease Control, the World Health Organization, and the UK's Department of Health, sponsored a workshop to assess the evidence of a possible link. Immunologists, diabetologists, epidemiologists, policymakers, and observers debated the available evidence and concluded that a causal link between immunization and type 1 diabetes is not supported. The results of the large randomized controlled trial of immunization against *Haemophilus influenzae* type b carried out in Finland in 1985–87 (mentioned above) were also reanalyzed and showed no association between the incidence of diabetes mellitus and the addition of another antigen to the schedule, irrespective of timing. Data reanalysis was made possible by prospective linking of individual information on exposure (in this case infant immunization or the administration of placebo) with the Finnish diabetes register (15[R]).

Lyme disease vaccine

Lyme disease is a tick-borne, spirochetal zoonosis characterized by a distinctive skin lesion, systemic symptoms, and neurological, rheumatological, and cardiac involvement, occurring in varying combinations over a period of months to years. *Borrelia burgdorferi* is the causative agent in North America, whereas in Europe three genomic groups of *B. burgdorferi* (named *B. burgdorferi* sensu stricto, *B. garinii*, and *B. afzelii*) have been identified. Endemic foci have been found in North America, Europe, the former USSR, Japan, and China. In many of these areas, Lyme disease is now the most common vector-borne disease. Because of this epidemiological problem and the severity of the disease, the development of a vaccine was initiated. High titers of antibody to outer surface protein A (OspA) of the spirochete prevented *B. burgdorferi* infection in mice and subsequently in immunized hamsters, dogs, and monkeys. Based on this experience, the development of a vaccine for human use (manufactured by SmithKline Beecham) was successful in the US. The Lyme disease vaccine (with adjuvant) is now licensed and commercially available in the US. Vaccines meeting the specific epidemiological situation in Europe are under development.

Table 1. *Percentage incidence of adverse effects within 7 days after injection (16[C])*

Adverse effect	Vaccine	Placebo
First injection		
Number of subjects	5156	5149
Any adverse effect	9.8	4.1
Musculoskeletal	6.4	1.3
Myalgia	5.5	0.6
General	1.8	0.9
Pain at injection site	0.3	0.04
Second injection		
Number of subjects	5050	5034
Any adverse effect	6.1	3.1
Musculoskeletal	3.3	1.1
Myalgia	2.5	0.4
General	1.7	0.8
Pain at injection site	0.8	0.1
Third injection		
Number of subjects	3745	3770
Any adverse effect	11.2	5.5
General	7.3	2.6
Tenderness	2.3	0.2
Pain at injection site	1.5	0.2
Unspecified pain	1.0	0.1
Reaction at injection site	0.8	0.2
Swelling	0.6	0.1
Pain in limb	0.5	0.02
Edema at injection site	0.5	0
Rigors	0.2	0
Skin or subcutaneous tissue	2.1	0.2
Erythematous rash	1.9	0.1

The results of two efficacy and safety trials using Lyme disease vaccine with or without adjuvant have been reported. In a double-blind trial, 10 305 subjects at least 18 years old, recruited at 14 sites in areas of the US where Lyme disease was endemic, were randomly assigned to receive either placebo (n = 5149) or OspA vaccine (n = 5156) (16[C]). The first two injections were given 1 month apart and 7515 subjects also received a booster dose at 12 months. The efficacy of the vaccine was 68% in the first year of the study in the entire population and 92% in the second year among the 3745 subjects who received a third injection. The vaccine was well tolerated. There was a higher incidence of mild, self-limiting, *local and systemic reactions* in the vaccine group, but only during the 7 days after vaccination (Table 1). There was no significant increase in the frequency of arthritis or neurological events in vaccine recipients. The authors concluded that OspA vaccine was safe and effective in the prevention of Lyme disease.

In another randomized double-blind trial in 10 936 subjects in areas of the US in which Lyme disease is endemic, either recombinant *B. burgdorferi* OspA with adjuvant or placebo was given initially and 1 and 12 months later (17[C]). In the first year, after two injections, 22 subjects given vaccine and 43 given placebo contracted definite Lyme disease; vaccine efficacy was 49% (95% CI = 15–69%). In the second year, after the third injection, 16 vaccine recipients and 66 placebo recipients contracted definite Lyme disease; vaccine efficacy was 76% (CI = 58–86%). The efficacy of the vaccine in preventing asymptomatic infection was 83% in the first year and 100% in the second year. Injection of the vaccine was associated with mild to moderate *local or systemic reactions* lasting a median of 3 days (Table 2).

Suspicions were expressed in the Mealey Publication's Drug and Medical Device Report that the Lyme disease vaccine LYMErix could cause an incurable form of *autoimmune arthritis*. It was hypothesized that blood concentrations of OspA after three doses of vaccine place vaccinees classified by genetic type HLA-DR4+ at risk of developing treatment-resistant Lyme arthritis. The pre-market trials for the vaccine have been assessed by an independent advisory committee, which found no link between Lyme disease immunization and autoimmune arthritis (18[R]). However, the committee stressed the need for long-term surveillance and further studies in those over 70 years and in children, and the effect of the vaccine in patients with chronic arthritis; the possible development of autoimmunity deserves particularly further study (19[R]). Since licensing of the vaccine, more than 1 million Americans have received it and no unusual adverse effects have been reported to the manufacturer (18[R]).

Meningococcal vaccine

(SED-13, 938; SEDA-20, 288; SEDA-21, 329; SEDA-22, 338)

Meningococcal vaccines have been comprehensively reviewed, distinguishing conventional polysaccharide vaccines, non-polysaccharide group B meningococcal vaccines, and conjugated meningococcal vaccines (20[R]).

Polysaccharide vaccines Polysaccharide vaccines are available in various combinations against meningococcal disease caused by group A, C, W_{135}, and Y meningococci. Meningococcal group B polysaccharide vaccine is poorly immunogenic in humans and therefore not available commercially. Studies mostly using a bivalent serogroup A + C vaccine carried out in about 15 countries including some millions of people have shown efficacy of 61–99%. Meningococcal group A vaccine is more immunogenic than group C vaccine in infants and small children. However, infants below 6 months of age produce a weak response, and meningococcal group C vaccine should not be used before the age of 2 years. With the quadrivalent vaccine used in Canada, *fever* was reported in less than 1%, *local reactions* in 6.3% and rash in 1.6% among those aged 11 years or older. Local reactions were also the most reported adverse effect in other reports.

Non-polysaccharide group B meningococcal vaccines Considering the poor immunogenicity of polysaccharide group B vaccines, different vaccines have been developed—a Norwegian outer membrane complex group B vaccine and a Cuban vaccine in which the group C polysaccharide is added to a mixture of high molecular weight B outer membrane proteins and proteoliposomes. Both vaccines have been used in clinical trials, mainly in Latin America, but more conclusive studies with these two products are awaited. Adverse reactions with the Cuban vaccine have been studied. Among 16 700 vaccinees, mostly older than 4 years, *local reactions* were observed in 62%, and *systemic reactions* in 4.3%.

Conjugated meningococcal vaccines Success with the protein–conjugate preparations of *Hemophilus influenzae* vaccines has facilitated research and development on conjugated meningococcal vaccines with preference for monovalent group C or bivalent group A/group C vaccines. Field trials in the UK and the Gambia have shown immunogenicity not only in adults but also in toddlers and even infants. Except for *local tenderness* in 30–75% of vaccinees, no conjugate vaccine evaluated to date has been associated with significant adverse effects (20[R]).

Table 2. *Percentages of subjects with symptoms with an overall incidence of at least 1% that were classified as related or possibly related to vaccination or unrelated to vaccination (17[C])*

Symptom	Vaccine	Placebo	P value
Related or possibly related to vaccination*			
Local at injection site			
Soreness	24.1	7.6	<0.001
Redness	1.8	0.5	<0.001
Swelling	0.9	0.2	<0.001
Systemic: early (<30 days)			
Total*	19.4	15.1	<0.001
Arthralgia	3.9	3.5	0.34
Headache	3.0	2.5	0.14
Myalgias	3.2	1.8	<0.001
Fatigue	2.3	2.0	0.37
Aching	2.0	1.4	0.01
Influenza-like illness	2.0	1.1	<0.001
Fever	2.0	0.8	<0.001
Chills	1.8	0.5	<0.001
Upper respiratory tract infection	1.0	1.1	0.69
Systemic: late (>30 days)			
Total*	4.1	3.4	0.06
Arthralgia	1.3	1.2	0.54
Unrelated to vaccination			
Early (<30 days)	27.1	27.9	0.37
Late (>30 days)	53.3	52.6	0.48

* Totals include all early or late related or possibly related systemic events, not just those with a frequency of at least 1%.

Pertussis vaccine (including diphtheria–tetanus–pertussis vaccine, DTP) *(SED-13, 940; SEDA-20, 289; SEDA-21, 329; SEDA-22, 338)*

Currently available whole-cell and acellular pertussis vaccines have been reviewed, with emphasis on the protectivity of the various virulence factors and antigens (21[R]). The authors summarized their review as follows: although *B. pertussis* has at least five proteins required for virulence and an additional two 'toxic' components, only serum neutralizing antibodies to pertussis toxin have been shown to confer immunity to pertussis.

Acellular pertussis vaccine Eight children developed *urticaria* within 30 minutes after administration of a diphtheria–tetanus–acellular pertussis (DTaP) vaccine that contained gelatin as a stabilizer (22[C]). None of the children had antigelatin IgE, and only two had detectable concentrations of antitoxoid IgE to diphtheria and pertussis toxoids. No methods to measure antithimerosal and antialum IgE were available. The authors recommended the development of such methods, which could improve research into the causality of adverse effects of this sort.

Whole-cell pertussis vaccine A follow-up study has been carried out in 105 children with collapse (a hypotonic–hyporesponsive episode or a shock-like syndrome) after their first immunization with DTwP–IPV vaccine (23[C]). Information about subsequent immunizations, health, and development in 101 of the children was supplied by child health care units. The parents of one child refused further immunization,

16 children completed their schedule with the combination diphtheria–tetanus–poliomyelitis vaccine (DT–IPV), and the other 84 children received further pertussis vaccine (DTP–IPV), totalling 236 doses; 74 children received the complete series of three additional doses. None of the children had recurrent collapse, and other adverse events were only minor. About half were given paracetamol prophylactically for the first subsequent dose; most of them did not take it for further doses. The authors suggested that it is unnecessary to withhold further doses of pertussis vaccine in a child with collapse after a previous dose. It has been suggested that the threat of natural pertussis in non-immunized children should be taken much more into account than the fear of developing a collapse reaction (24[R]). In another study (25[C]) in the US, one of the 14 children not completely immunized because of a hypotonic–hyporesponsive episode after a previous dose later developed natural pertussis, which lasted for 3 months and was transmitted to both her parents.

Acellular pertussis vaccine versus whole-cell pertussis vaccine In a randomized double-blind trial to determine the efficacy of vaccination against *Bordetella* infection, a multicomponent acellular pertussis has been compared with a whole-cell product and DT in 8532 infants aged 2–4 months, who received four doses of either DTwP or DTaP vaccine at 3, 4.5, 6, and 15–18 months of age, and 1739 controls, who received three doses of DT vaccine at 3, 4.5, 15–18 months of age (26[C]). All the vaccines were generally well tolerated. However, adverse reactions were significantly less common after DTaP compared with DTwP vaccine. *Persistent inconsolable crying* was four times more common in DTwP recipients than in DTaP recipients. High *fever*, 40.5°C or over, was three times more common in DTwP vaccinees than in DTaP vaccinees. Only one DTaP recipient had a *convulsion* in temporal relation to immunization.

Change in immunization policy The 2000 Childhood Immunization Schedule, proposed by the Advisory Committee of Immunization Practices (ACIP), the American Academy of Pediatrics, and the American Academy of Family Physicians, recommends exclusively acellular pertussis vaccines for routine use in the US (27).

Combination vaccines: DTaP or DTwP vaccine combined with other antigens such as *Haemophilus influenzae* type b [Hib] or inactivated poliovirus [IPV] or simultaneous administration of these vaccines *(SEDA-20, 290; SEDA-21, 330; SEDA-22, 342)*

Four-, five-, and even six-component combination vaccines based on DTaP or DTwP vaccine and including other antigens such as hepatitis B or Hib or IPV will play an important role in future immunization programs. Some such combination vaccines have already been licensed in some countries, others are expecting to be licensed soon or are under evaluation in clinical trials.

DTP and Hemophilus influenzae type B In a prospective randomized study 822 healthy infants were enrolled to receive three doses of either a candidate or a commercially available *Hemophilus influenzae* type b (Hib) vaccine concomitantly with diphtheria–tetanus–acellular pertussis (DTaP) vaccine (28[C]). They were randomly allocated to one of the following groups: (1) separate injection of DTaP and candidate Hib vaccine, (2) mixed injection of DTaP and candidate Hib vaccine, (3) separate injection of DTaP and commercial Hib vaccine. One year later the first 189 subjects received either separate or mixed injections of the same Hib and DTaP vaccines as booster doses. No serious adverse events occurred, and most local and systemic reactions were mild to moderate. Booster doses were more reactogenic than primary doses in all groups (Tables 3 and 4). The authors concluded that mixing DTaP and Hib vaccines for primary immunization did not result in increased reactogenicity.

In a similar study the safety and immunogenicity of a four-component DTaP–Hib vaccine (Lederle/Takeda) and the Lederle (HbOC) monocomponent Hib vaccine administered alone or together, have been studied in 126 children aged 12–15 months and 109 children aged 15–19 months. The only significant difference observed was in the rate of *local reactions*, which were more common in children who received the two separate injections: 23 vs 13%. There were no severe local reactions. *Fussiness, anorexia*, and/or *drowsiness* were reported by 0.2% of recipients of separ-

Table 3. *Numbers (percentages) of local symptoms occurring within 48 hours of immunization with separate injections of candidate or commercial Hib and DTaP vaccines or combined with mixed injections of candidate Hib and DTaP vaccines during the three-dose primary series and booster immunization (28[C])*

Vaccine group	Dose	No.	Redness		Swelling		Pain**
			Any	>20 mm	Any	>20 mm	Any
Candidate	Primary	702	83 (11.8)	0 (0.0)	37 (5.3)	4 (0.6)	23 (3.3)
Hib separate	Booster	40	13 (32.5)	5 (12.5)	6 (15.0)	2 (5.0)	4 (10.0)
Candidate	Primary	1429	231 (16.2)	2 (0.1)	96 (6.7)	2 (0.1)	69 (4.8)
Hib + DTaP mixed	Booster	138	48 (34.8)	16 (11.6)	36 (26.1)	6 (4.3)	20 (14.5)
Commercial	Primary	235	36 (15.3)	6 (2.6)	25 (10.6)	1 (0.4)	28 (11.9)
Hib separate	Booster	10	1 (10.0)	1 (10.0)	1 (10.0)	1 (10.0)	2 (20.0)
DTaP	Primary	937	141 (15.0)	1 (0.1)	81 (8.6)	3 (0.3)	47 (5.0)
Separate*	Booster	50	17 (34.0)	7 (14.0)	7 (14.0)	3 (6.0)	6 (12.0)

* Includes all subjects who received separate injections of candidate Hib or commercial Hib vaccine.
** There were no reports of severe pain, except for one case at the DTaP site when separately injected with commercial Hib.

Table 4. *General reactions (numbers and percentages) during the 48 hours after the separate injections of candidate Hib/commercial Hib and DTaP vaccines, and the combined injection of candidate Hib DTaP vaccine, after the three dose primary series and the booster dose (28[C])*

Vaccine groups	Dose	No.	Fever	Unusual crying	Vomiting	Diarrhea	Loss of appetite	Restlessness
Candidate Hib +	Primary	702	80 (11)	130 (19)	52 (7.4)	71 (10)	100 (14)	107 (15)
DtaP separate	Booster	40	12 (30)	4 (10)	2 (5.0)	4 (10)	7 (18)	9 (23)
Candidate Hib –	Primary	1429	101 (7.1)	220 (15)	115 (8.0)	140 (9.8)	160 (11)	214 (15.0)
DtaP mixed	Booster	138	34 (25)	12 (8.7)	2 (1.4)	14 (10)	17 (12)	21 (15)
Commercial Hib	Primary	235	38 (16)	57 (24)	18 (7.7)	32 (14)	25 (11)	34 (4.5)
and DTaP separate	Booster	10	3 (30)	1 (10)	1 (10)	2 (20)	1 (10)	1 (10)

ate vaccines and 43% of those who received the combination and by 43 and 40% of the younger and older children respectively (29[C]).

DTP–Hib–Polio vaccine The safety, immunogenicity, and lot consistency of five-component pertussis combination vaccine (DTaP–IPV–Hib [PRP-T]) in infants have been compared to those of whole cell pertussis combination vaccine (DTwP–IPV–Hib [PRP-T]), as have separate and combined injections of DTP–IPV and Hib. The combination vaccine DTaP–IPV–Hib was comparable or superior regarding safety and immunogenicity to the combination vaccine containing the whole cell pertussis component. There was no interaction between acellular pertussis and PRP-T, a feature that distinguishes this combination vaccine from some others, which depress anti-PRP responses. The combination vaccine DTaP–IPV–Hib produced significantly lower rates of local and systemic reactions than did the combination vaccine containing the whole-cell pertussis component. Local reactions, such as *redness, swelling*, and *tenderness* occurred two to three times more often after combination vaccine containing whole cell pertussis than after combination vaccines with acellular pertussis components. *Fever* was three times more common after whole cell combination vaccine. Fever over 40°C was rare in all vaccinees, because of the use of paracetamol prophylaxis. Systemic reactions, such *as fussiness, crying, reduced activity*, and *anorexia*, were about twice as frequent with whole cell vaccine as with acellular pertussis vaccine. Both local and systemic reactions persisted longer after whole cell vaccine than after acellular pertussis vaccine. There were no significant differences between reaction rates among infants given DTaP–IPV vaccine combined with Hib (PRP-T) vaccine in the same syringe compared with those given separate injections, except for local redness after the first dose (30[C]).

Pneumococcal vaccine *(SED-13, 942; SEDA-18, 332; SEDA-21, 330; SEDA-22, 344)*

Conjugated pneumococcal polysaccharide vaccines Pneumococcal polysaccharides are not immunogenic in infants, but polysaccharide-protein conjugates have improved immunogenicity. The immunogenicity of seven-valent pneumococcal-conjugate vaccine plus 23-valent pneumococcal vaccine in 11 children has been compared with the immunogenicity of 23-valent vaccine alone in 12 children up to 2 years of age with sickle cell disease (31[C]). IgG pneumococcal antibody concentrations were higher with combined administration, with no increase in adverse effects after immunization with 23-valent vaccine.

Suspected association between type 1 diabetes mellitus and pneumococcal vaccine When the FDA's Vaccines and Related Biological Products Advisory Committee has discussed whether it should recommend approval of a new conjugated pneumococcal vaccine intended for preventing meningitis and other infections in children, it heard testimony from Classen, an immunologist at Classen Immunotherapies, that the conjugated seven-valent pneumococcal vaccine was likely to cause a large epidemic of diabetes. The vaccine is similar in structure to conjugated vaccines used to prevent *Hemophilus influenzae* meningitis (see above under *Hemophilus influenzae* vaccine). The difference is that the seven-valent vaccine is composed of seven different vaccines, each to a separate strain of pneumococcus, so its toxicity may be seven times as great as the currently marketed *Hemophilus influenzae* vaccines (32[R]).

Sam Katz, a pediatrician of high repute, has commented on whether there is a causal relation between Hib and pneumococcal vaccines and diabetes: 'Classen has brought forth almost identical unsubstantiated hypotheses for each vaccine on which he has managed to insert his view at Congressional hearings, FDA meetings, etc. ... He persists in his distorted misinterpretation of the Finnish data, despite refutation of his statements by the Finnish investigators themselves. Classen's proposed first month of life schedule ignores the lack of or poor response of human (not murine) infants to the desired vaccines at that age' (Katz, personal communication).

Tetanus vaccine *(SED-13, 949)*

About 2 weeks after receiving a second dose of adsorbed tetanus toxoid a 50-year-old woman developed *generalized morphea*, a rare condition, in which multiple patches of skin sclerosis occur over much larger areas than in the localized variant. The cause of this condition is unknown, but an autoimmune mechanism triggered by endogenous and exogenous factors has been suggested. The patient denied taking any drugs. After prednisone therapy, a month later the lesions had dramatically improved (33[C]).

Typhoid fever vaccine *(SED-13, 950; SEDA-18, 332; SEDA-20, 290)*

The efficacy and safety of typhoid fever vaccine have been estimated in a meta-analysis in about 1.8 million vaccinees in efficacy trials and about 11 000 vaccinees in safety studies (34[R]). The 3-year cumulative efficacy for two doses of whole cell vaccines was 73 (65–80)%, 51 (35–63)% for three doses of Ty21 live attenuated vaccine, and 55 (30–71)% for one dose of Vi vaccine. After immunization, *fever* occurred in 16 (12–21)% of whole cell vaccine recipients, 2 (0.7–5.3)% of Ty21a vaccine recipients, and 1.1 (0.1–12.3)% of Vi vaccine recipients (Table 5).

VIRAL VACCINES

Hepatitis A vaccine *(SED-13, 928; SEDA-20, 290; SEDA-21, 330; SEDA-22, 344)*

In a paper dealing mainly with indications for the use of hepatitis vaccine, the data on the hepatitis A vaccines most widely used, HAVRIX (manufactured by SmithKline Biologicals) and VAQTA (manufactured by Merck), have been summarized (35[R]). The data are based on pre-licensure clinical trials and follow-up reports worldwide. No serious adverse effects have been attributed to hepatitis A vaccines. In children who received HAVRIX, soreness (15%) and induration (4%) at the injection site, feeding problems (8%), and headaches (4%) have been the most frequently observed adverse effects. In children who received VAQTA, the most common adverse effects were *pain* (19%), *tenderness* (17%), and *warmth* (9%) at the injection site. The reported frequencies are sim-

Table 5. *Local and systemic reactions after the administration of typhoid fever vaccines (34[R])*

Study	Age (years)	Type of study	Number vaccinated	Fever (%)	Swelling (%)	Vomiting (%)	Diarrhea (%)	Missed school or work (%)
Ty21a vaccine								
Gilman et al.	Adults	Clinic	155	1	NA	3	10	ND
Murphy et al.	0.5–2	Clinic	18	11	NA	17	11	ND
Rahman et al.	3–78	Clinic	157	2	NA	0	1	ND
Cryz et al.	2–6	Clinic	317	<1	NA	1	<1	ND
Cryz et al.	16–56	Clinic	30	2	NA	0	20	ND
Pooled estimate (95% CI)				2.0 (0.7–5.3)		2.1 (0.6–7.8)	5.1 (1.7–15)	
Vi vaccine								
Levin et al.	ND	Clinic	21	24	ND	NA	NA	ND
Tacket et al.	20–24	Clinic	19	0	ND	NA	NA	0
Klugman et al.	5–15	Field	253	<1	4	NA	NA	ND
Cumberland et al.	18–22	Clinic	388	<1	1	NA	NA	ND
Mirza et al.	5–15	Field	435	0	8	NA	NA	ND
Pooled estimate (95% CI)				1.1 (0.1–12)	3.7 (1.3–9.6)			
Whole-cell vaccine (heat inactivated)								
YTC	5–50	Field	214	9	5	NA	NA	11
Ashcroft et al.	5–15	Field	193	13	61	NA	NA	14
YTC	NA	Field	66	29	ND	NA	NA	17
Hejfez et al.	7–18	Field	2621	30	19	NA	NA	ND
Hejfez et al.	ND	Field	3463	26	21	NA	NA	ND
Hejfez et al.	7–20	Field	2157	13	13	NA	NA	ND
Dimache et al.	16–18	Field	94	27	ND	NA	NA	ND
Dimache et al.	21	Clinic	113	1	ND	NA	NA	ND
Dimache	20	Field	100	34	ND	NA	NA	2
Cumberland et al.	18–22	Clinic	390	2	20	NA	NA	ND
Pooled estimate (95% CI)					16 (21–21)	20 (13–30)		10 (6–16)

For references see (34[R]). YTC = Yugoslav Typhoid Commission. NA = not applicable. ND = not described in study.

ilar to the frequencies reported with hepatitis B vaccines.

Hepatitis B vaccine *(SED-13, 928; SEDA-19, 299; SEDA-21, 331; SEDA-22, 346)*

The reports of major adverse reactions that have been published since the introduction of the recombinant hepatitis B vaccine have been reviewed (36[R]). In the clinical trials with hepatitis B vaccine, the most frequent adverse effects were *soreness at the injection site*, sometimes accompanied by *erythema* (3–29%), *fatigue* (15%), *headache* (9%), and *temperature increase* higher than 37.7°C. The post-marketing surveillance literature (4.5 million doses) showed an overall rate of one adverse effect per 15 500 doses. Of these, *local reactions* were reported at a rate of 1 in 85 000 doses. Systemic reactions included *nausea, rash, headache, fever, malaise, fatigue, flu-like symptoms, diarrhea, urticaria, paresthesia*, and *somnolence*, all of which resolved, generally within 24–48 hours of vaccine administration. Reactions were less frequent with subsequent doses. Major adverse effects have been published as case reports: *anaphylaxis; urticaria, erythema nodosum, lichen planus; arthritis, Reiter's syndrome; pulmonary and cutaneous vasculitis; systemic lupus erythematosus; glomerulonephritis; Evan's syndrome, thrombocytopenic purpura; acute posterior multifocal placoid pigment epitheliopathy; Guillain–Barré syndrome, transverse myelitis, multiple sclerosis, acute cerebellar ataxia; chronic fatigue syndrome.* Table 6 summarizes the reports. Discussing the cause of the reported major adverse effects and a possible causal relation with vaccine administration, the authors considered that apart from *anaphylaxis* and *urticaria*, most of the reactions described were not allergic in nature and that the symptoms were those of immune-complex disease due to autoimmune mechanisms. Because of the extreme rarity of such serious adverse events, coincidence seems the simplest explanation, but an immune-complex mediated pathogenesis should not be excluded, given the close temporal relation between immunization and the onset of disease. Apart from immune-complex mechanisms, there may be reactions to other components of the vaccine, such as thimerosal, aluminium, or small quantities of yeast proteins.

Nervous system The current discussion on possible severe complications of hepatitis B immunization has been reviewed, with emphasis on *multiple sclerosis* (SEDA-22, 346; 37[R]). Some researchers and patient advocacy groups in France, the UK, and the US are particularly active in blaming the vaccine.

All available data that may throw light on the hypothesis that hepatitis B vaccine is causally linked to multiple sclerosis have been carefully reviewed (38[R]). The authors concluded that the most plausible explanation for the observed temporal association between immunization and multiple sclerosis is coincidence.

Skin and appendages Four cases of *urticaria* and one case of *angioedema* have been reported after hepatitis B immunization (39[c]). The results emphasize that urticaria can be due to sensitization to the hepatitis Bs antigen itself, hyperimmunization, or a non-allergic reaction.

Hematological A healthy 7-year-old girl developed *thrombocytopenic purpura* after hepatitis B immunization, three doses of vaccine every month followed by a booster (40[c]).

Subcutaneous nodules persisting for periods of 8 months to 2 years have been reported in four patients, in all of whom patch tests were positive with aluminum (41[c]).

Immunological and hypersensitivity reactions After hepatitis B immunization, three doses of vaccine every month followed by a booster, a healthy 24-year-old woman lost weight and developed migratory arthralgia. *Acute disseminated lupus erythematosus* was diagnosed. The authors discussed the possibility that immunization could have introduced an antigen that may have provoked an autoimmune reaction in genetically predisposed family members (40[c]).

Churg–Strauss *vasculitis* (allergic angiitis and granulomatosis) has been attributed to hepatitis B immunization (42[c]).

A 20-year-old woman developed chronic rhinitis 1 month after the last dose of hepatitis B, followed about 1 year later by severe asthma, nasal polyposis, petechial purpura in her fingernail beds and on her feet. A skin biopsy from the left leg showed infiltrates consistent with leukocytoclastic vasculitis.

The interval between immunization and the development of the vasculitis makes it very difficult to establish a causal relation.

Table 6. *Summary of important adverse reactions after recombinant hepatitis B vaccination (36[R])*

Reaction	Sex	Age (years)	No.	Time after vaccination	Duration of symptoms
Acute urticaria	F	24	1	30 minutes	30 minutes
Erythema nodosum	F	43	1	4 days	several weeks
Lichen planus	F	19	2	2 months	not reported
Lichen planus	M	50	2	1 month	3 months
Polyarthritis + erythema nodosum	M	31	1	1 day	6 weeks
Polyarthritis	F	41	1	2 weeks	7 months
Reiter's syndrome	M	29	2	4 weeks	4 months
Rheumatoid arthritis	F	49	1	24 hours	not reported
Pulmonary and cutaneous vasculitis	F	45	1	2 days	1 week
Systemic lupus erythematosus	F	43	1	2 weeks	not reported
Glomerulonephritis	M	21	3	6 weeks	a few days
Evans' syndrome	M	33	2	2 days	2 months
Thrombocytopenic purpura	F	15	3	4 weeks	4 months
Thrombocytopenic purpura	F	21	2	3 weeks	2 months at least
Acute posterior multifocal placoid pigment epitheliopathy	M	31	4	3 days	9 months (residual signs)
Acute posterior multifocal placoid pigment epitheliopathy	M	30	3	2 weeks	4 months (residual signs)
Central nervous system demyelination	F	26	3	6 weeks	3 weeks (residual signs)
Central nervous system demyelination	F	28	2	6 weeks	3 months (residual signs)
Acute transverse myelitis	M	40	1	2 weeks	6 weeks (residual signs)
Multiple sclerosis	F	43	1	7–10 days	4 weeks (residual signs)
Acute cerebellar ataxia	F	26	2	10 days	4 months
Median		31		14 days	8 weeks
Average		32		19 days	11 weeks

Third generation hepatitis B vaccines Between 5 and 15% of healthy immunocompetent individuals do not serocovert after receipt of the currently licensed hepatitis B vaccines containing only the major surface protein HbsAg without pre-S epitopes. In a study of a hepatitis B vaccine containing pre-S1, pre-S2, and antigenic components of both viral subtypes adw and ayw, all three antigenic components were produced in a continuous mammalian cell line, after transfection of the cells with recombinant hepatitis B surface antigen DNA (43[C]). The vaccine was manufactured as an aluminium hydroxide adjuvant formulation. The new vaccine (5, 10, 20, or 50 g). was given to 68 individuals with HBs antibody titers below 10 IU/l. Seroconversion rates in the four groups were 60, 76, 64, and 80%. There were local or systemic reactions in 15%. No dose-related incidence was seen.

Human immunodeficiency virus vaccine (including other immunization in HIV-infected persons) *(SED-13, 930; SEDA-20, 291; SEDA-21, 334; SEDA-22, 348)*

Immunization of HIV-infected persons In 1988, recognizing the severity of measles in immunodeficient individuals, the US Advisory Committee on Immunization Practices (ACIP) revised its measles immunization guidelines. It recommended that children with asymptomatic HIV infection should be immunized and that immunization should be considered for symptomatic HIV-infected children. Health authorities in many countries have made similar recommendations. Since then, many HIV-infected children have been safely immunized, and the ACIP recommendation has been expanded to all age groups of HIV-infected persons.

The first recognized serious complication of measles immunization, *measles giant-cell pneumonia*, has been described in a 21-year-old man with AIDS (44[c]).

A 21-year-old man developed AIDS followed by *Pneumocystis carinii* pneumonia. About a year after a booster immunization with measles–mumps–rubella (MMR) vaccine, he developed measles giant-cell pneumonia, confirmed by transbronchial and thoracoscopic lung biopsies. The entire genome of the isolated strain and that of the currently used vaccine strain Moraten were subsequently sequenced and were almost identical. However, taking into consideration the long interval between measles immunization and pneumonia, the causal relation was doubtful.

Meanwhile, the Committee on Infectious Diseases of the American Academy of Pediatrics and the Advisory Committee on Immunization Practices (ACIP) (45) have recommended that severely immunocompromised patients with HIV infection should not receive measles vaccine.

Response to immunization in HIV-infected persons The problems connected with pneumococcal disease and its prevention in HIV-infected individuals have been reviewed (46[R]). Pneumococcal disease occurs significantly more often in HIV-infected individuals, with pneumococcal pneumonia rates 5.5–17.5-fold greater than population-based estimates in the US, and the increasing rate of penicillin-resistant strains of *Streptococcus pneumoniae* highlight the need for improved prevention strategies. Studies of pneumococcal disease in HIV infection have repeatedly shown that over 85% of the isolates from bacteremic patients, in both the US and Africa, are of serotypes included in the 23-valent vaccine. However, the proportion of HIV-positive individuals who respond to 23-valent pneumococcal polysaccharide vaccine has been shown in some but not all studies to be slightly reduced compared with age-matched controls but comparable to other high-risk groups, such as elderly people, in whom clinical efficacy has been established. Some studies have suggested a trend towards a lower response rate as the CD4 cell count falls. The reason for concern about the safety of pneumococcal immunization in HIV-infected individuals is the reported association between immunization and increasing HIV virus load.

Much of this concern arises from extrapolation from published data on influenza immunization. However, there are some data on pneumococcal immunization alone. In 32 HIV-positive patients with a median CD4 cell count of 242×10^6/l, who received Pneumovax and tetanus toxoid there was no change in plasma HIV-1 RNA at 20–56 days after immunization (47[C]). In contrast there were marked increases in plasma viral RNA (1.6–586 times) reported in 12 asymptomatic HIV-positive individuals (mean CD4 cell count 374×10^6/l). More recently, a study of patients with more advanced disease found that HIV-1 RNA and DNA were unaffected by either conjugate or polysaccharide pneumococcal vaccine up to 309 days after immunization (48[C]). In summary, the authors of the review (46[R]) recommended that HIV-infected individuals be immunized with pneumococcal vaccine and that immunization should be carried out as early as possible in the course of HIV infection.

Influenza vaccine *(SED-13, 932; SEDA-21, 334; SEDA-22, 349)*

Skin and appendages Among at least 30 drugs believed to cause *bullous pemphigoid or cicatricial pemphigoid*, influenza vaccine is mentioned (three cases published) (49[R]).

Immunological and hypersensitivity reactions The question of whether egg allergy is a justified contraindication to influenza immunization has been studied in 80 individuals with egg allergy and 124 control subjects, who received influenza vaccine containing ovalbumin/ovomucoid 0.02, 0.1, or 1.2 g/ml (50[C]). The individuals with egg allergy received the vaccine in two doses 30 minutes apart; the first dose was one-tenth and the second dose nine-tenths of the recommended dose. The patients with egg allergy, even those with significant allergic reactions after egg ingestion, safely received influenza vaccine in this two-dose protocol with vaccine containing no more than 1.2 g/ml of egg protein.

Japanese encephalitis vaccine *(SED-13, 934; SEDA-20, 291; SEDA-21, 334; SEDA-22, 350)*

Japanese encephalitis vaccine has been reviewed (51[R]). Three types of Japanese encephalitis vaccine are currently produced: (1) mouse brain-derived inactivated vaccine, commercially available; (2) cell culture-derived inactivated vaccine; (3) cell culture-derived attenuated vaccine, produced and used exclusively in China. The mouse brain vaccine causes moderate transient local and systemic adverse effects.

Since 1989, *urticaria* and/or *angioedema* of the extremities, face, and oropharynx, and respiratory distress have been reported from Europe, North America, and Australia as a new pattern of adverse effects. Collapse due to hypotension has required hospitalization in several cases, and erythema multiforme and erythema nodosum have also occurred; the reported rates of such adverse effects varied markedly in different countries (respective ranges 0.7–12 per 10 000 and 50–104 per 10 000). The vaccine constituents responsible for the adverse effects have not yet been identified. The Chinese cell culture-derived inactivated vaccine is produced in primary hamster kidney cells; a highly purified Vero cell culture-derived inactivated vaccine is under clinical development in France. The Chinese live attenuated vaccine is also produced in primary hamster kidney cells. The efficacy of one dose is 80%, and the efficacy of two doses, given 1 year apart, is 97.5%. The vaccine reportedly causes very few adverse effects.

Measles vaccine, measles–mumps–rubella (MMR) vaccine (including measles–mumps and measles–rubella vaccines), and combination measles–mumps–rubella–varicella vaccine *(SED-13, 935, 937; SEDA-20, 291; SEDA-21, 335; SEDA-22, 351)*

A review of the data generated in the last 4 years has amply described the continued efforts of the scientific community to monitor and understand true measles vaccine-associated adverse events (52[R]). The rapidity and clarity of this same community's debunking of the spurious associations with Crohn's disease and autism (see below) suggests that those charged with vaccination programs have learned from past mistakes.

Neurological adverse effects of measles immunization R

Claims that cases of encephalopathy followed by permanent brain injury or death were due to measles immunization, submitted to the US National Vaccine Injury Compensation Program, have been reviewed (SED-13, 920; 53[C]). A total of 403 claims of encephalopathy and/or seizure disorders after measles, measles–rubella, measles–mumps–rubella, mumps, or rubella immunization were identified during the period 1970–93. The medical records of these cases were reviewed by physicians in the compensation program to determine, if possible, the cause of injury and the classification of the findings. The inclusion criteria established by the compensation program were met by 48 claims by patients with acute encephalopathy of undetermined cause 2–15 days after immunization with attenuated measles virus. The clustering and peak onset of encephalopathy occurred in 17 patients on days 8 and 9, and the encephalopathy was followed by permanent brain impairment or death. The patients ranged in age from 10 months to 49 months, with a median age of 15 months. There were no cases of encephalopathy of undetermined cause within 15 days after the administration of mumps or rubella vaccine. Table 7 shows the clinical findings and sequelae among the 48 cases. The authors concluded that manifestations of acute encephalopathy among these 48 children were similar to the clinical features of acute encephalopathy described after natural measles. Vaccine-associated measles encephalopathy may be a rare complication of measles immunization. From 1970 to 1993 in the US, about 75 million children received measles vaccine by age 4 years. The 48 cases of encephalopathy after measles immunization probably represented under-reporting to this passive compensation system. However, given the generous compensation offered in this program, it is reasonable to conclude that most serious cases temporally related to an immunization have been captured. The incidence of 48 cases of encephalopathy possibly caused by 75 million doses of vaccine can reasonably be described as low.

The 1994 report of the Institute of Medicine concluded that the evidence was inadequate to accept or reject a causal relation between MMR and encephalopathy, and it is known that the incidence of encephalitis after

Table 7. *Clinical effects of acute encephalopathy in 48 patients 2–15 days after the first dose of measles, measles–rubella, or measles–mumps–rubella vaccine, and sequelae, 1970–93 (53[C])*

Clinical onset	No.	Acute illness	No.	Neurological sequelae	No.
Ataxia	6				
Irritability	6	Ataxia	6	Ataxis (chronic)	4
Fever	5	Changd behavior	6	Mental retardation	3
Measles-like rash	3	Mental regression	4	Seizure disorder	1
		Hospitalization	3	Hearing loss	1
Behavior changes	8				
Lethargy	3	Mental regression	8	Mental retardation	6
Irritability	2	Coma	5	Spaastic paresis	5
Confusion	2	Hospitalization	6	Seizure disorder	1
Coma	1	Death	2	Choreoathetosis	1
Fever	6			Death (later)	1
Measles-like rash	1				
Seizures	34				
Fever	32	Hospitalization	33	Mental retardation	31
Status epilepticus	17	Mental regression	31	Seizure disorder	23
Generalized	14	Coma	29	Spastic paresis	10
Focal	3	Behavior changes	5	Death (later)	3
Measles-like rash	9	Death	2		

The clinical features of acute and chronic encephalopathy or death in these 48 patients were classified into three groups based on the initial findings of ataxia in six, behavior changes in eight, and seizures in 34. The onset of neurological findings varied in severity from ataxia or behavioral changes to prolonged seizures or coma. Fever preceded the onset of acute encephalopathy by several hours to several days in 43 of 48 children. A measles-like rash with a post-vaccination onset from day 6 to day 15 occurred in 13 children.

measles immunization of healthy children tends to be lower than the observed incidence of encephalitis of unknown cause. Two large studies have been negative. In a study analogous to the British Childhood Encephalopathy Study there were no increased risks of either encephalopathy or neurological sequelae after measles immunization (54[C]). A retrospective case-control study through the CDC Vaccine Safety Datalink assessing the risk for 300 000 doses of MMR and found not a single case of encephalitis/encephalopathy within 30 days of the administration of MMR (55[C]). In contrast, the review mentioned above (53[C]) reported an association between measles vaccine and encephalopathy. However, the conclusion of the report of the Institute of Medicine is still valid, namely that evidence is still inadequate to accept or reject a causal relation between measles vaccine and these diseases.

There are also no new findings to change the same conclusion of the report of the Institute of Medicine regarding transverse myelitis and Guillain–Barré syndrome.

In 1994, the US Institute of Medicine reviewed the world literature and published a comprehensive review of adverse events associated with childhood vaccines, including measles-containing vaccines (SEDA-18, 325). Since the Institute of Medicine report was published, a literature search for adverse events after measles immunization, limited to publications published in 1994–98 has unearthed a considerable amount of new data that strengthen the rare association of measles-containing vaccines with post-infectious encephalomyelitis (52[R]).

Recent studies on measles vaccine and subacute sclerosing panencephalitis have been discussed. Despite the compelling inverse relation between vaccine use and the incidence of subacute sclerosing panencephalitis, the authors referred to concerns raised at the first Public Conference on Vaccination in 1997 that measles vaccine may exacerbate existing subacute sclerosing panencephalitis and that a second dose of vaccine may be more likely to initiate it than the first.

Using RNA-templated sequencing, vaccine-strain measles virus has been implicated as the cause of death in three immunocompromised children with inclusion body encephalitis (52[R]). The authors referred to a case of measles vaccine virus-associated giant cell pneumonia in a patient with advanced HIV infection (see above).

R

Evidence against an association of measles/MMR immunization with Crohn's disease and autism

Inflammatory bowel disease (ulcerative colitis and Crohn's disease) is a general term for a group of chronic inflammatory disorders of unknown cause involving the gastrointestinal tract. Despite many attempts to confirm an infectious agent as the cause of disease, no bacterial, viral, or fungal agents have so far been isolated. There is strong evidence for a genetic predisposition.

Autism is characterized by absorption in self-centered subjective mental activities (such as day-dreams, fantasies, hallucinations), especially when accompanied by marked withdrawal from reality.

In 1993 and 1994, researchers in the UK and Sweden suggested that Crohn's disease might be a late result of measles infection at a critical time during early childhood (56[C], 57[C]). In a study of the outcome of maternal measles infection in 25 Swedish babies, three of four children exposed to measles in utero subsequently developed Crohn's disease (58[C]). Whereas wild measles virus was initially implicated, a controversial debate was initiated in 1995, when Thompson et al. suggested that attenuated measles vaccine virus might also cause inflammatory bowel disease, having found an increased risk of inflammatory bowel disease in about 3000 immunized individuals compared with about 11 000 non-immunized controls (59[C]). Furthermore, the Inflammatory Bowel Disease Study Group of the Royal Free Hospital, London (Wakefield and colleagues) suggested that measles virus is present in the bowel of patients with Crohn's disease (with evidence from transmission electron microscopy, immunohistochemistry, in situ hybridization, and immunogold electron microscopy) (56[C], 60[C], 61[C]).

Wakefield et al. then made two suggestions in a paper in the Lancet (4[C]): that autism is linked to a form of inflammatory bowel disease and that this new syndrome is associated with measles–mumps–rubella (MMR) immunization. Their hypothesis was that MMR vaccine causes non-specific gut injury, allowing the absorption of normally non-permeable peptides, which in turn cause serious developmental disorders. The authors stated that they had not proved an association between measles, mumps, and rubella vaccines and either autism or inflammatory bowel disease. However, there were enough references in the text to lead the reader to the assumption that there is sufficient evidence provided by the study, and by other scientific publications, that there is a link. This paper of Wakefield et al. resulted in a heated debate and a huge number of letters to the editor of the Lancet, in turn severely criticizing both the article and its implications for immunization programs, blaming the editor for publishing the article, and defending the obligation of clinical researchers to publish provocative findings. Considerable evidence, mainly microbiological and epidemiological, has been collected by others to suggest that the association with MMR does not exist.

The alleged association of measles vaccination with Crohn's disease and autism has also been criticized as being based on poor science and as having been largely refuted by a large volume of stronger work, three types of evidence against the hypothesis (biological, microbiological, and epidemiological) being considered in detail (52[R]).

Evidence against an association between MMR and Crohn's disease *Several groups have found no evidence of persistence of measles virus in the tissues of patients with Crohn's disease with a very sensitive test (polymerase chain reaction) (62[C]–65[C]). Furthermore, no viral genomic sequences of measles, mumps, and rubella viruses were found in intestinal specimens (62[C]). The results of Iizuka et al. (63[C], 64[C]) are particularly interesting—they used the same monoclonal antibody in their immunohistochemical studies that Wakefield et al. used. The antigen recognized could be a measles virus protein, but they considered it much more likely that the previous immunochemical observations were accounted for by antigen mimicry between measles virus and a host protein found in the intestinal tissue of* patients with Crohn's disease. Serological studies have also shown lower measles complement fixation titers in patients with Crohn's disease than in controls, not supporting an association of measles vaccine with Crohn's disease (66[C], 67[C]).

The major weaknesses of the epidemiological studies reported by the Inflammatory Bowel Disease Study Group have been discussed in a number of letters to the editor (68[R]) and editorials (3[CR]). On behalf of the World Health Organization Expanded Programme on Immunization, Lee et al. (68[R]) questioned the conclusion that there was a temporal association between immunization and the onset of symptoms, because the study of Wakefield et al. provided data on the interval between immunization and the onset of symptoms in only five of their 12 cases of so-called autism–bowel syndrome, and the age at which the vaccine was given was mentioned in only three. Furthermore, Lee et al. criticized the study on the grounds that no patient selection had been made by Wakefield et al., other than the 12 patients referred to them; there were no controls and no blinding of the investigators (68[R]). Payne and Mason (69[R]) made the same comment, that the cases reported by Wakefield et al. were highly selected and that the underlying population was unclear.

Several epidemiological studies have failed to confirm an association between measles/measles vaccine and Crohn's disease. For example:

- Copenhagen: in a study of 25 mothers with measles during pregnancy there were no cases of Crohn's disease in their children (70[C]);
- Finland: Peltola et al. (71[C]) reported on over a decade's effort to detect all severe adverse events associated with MMR vaccine distributed in Finland. There was no evidence to support the hypothesis that the vaccine could cause pervasive developmental disorders or inflammatory bowel disease. Comparing the incidence of Crohn's disease and the Finnish data for measles and measles immunization, Pebody et al. (72[C]) came to the same conclusion, namely that there is no association between Crohn's disease and measles vaccine.
- Japan: a nationwide survey of inflammatory bowel disease was carried out in 1979–93 in children under 16 years of age. From 1979 to 1992 the number of cases of inflammatory bowel disease was almost the same (ulcerative colitis rates 0.08–0.12 per 100 000, Crohn's disease 0.04–0.06 per 100 000). In 1992, the incidence of Crohn's disease rose to 0.10 and in 1993 to 0.12 per 100 000; the incidence rate of ulcerative colitis increased in 1993 to 0.18 per 100 000. Measles immunization (implemented in 1968) was 68% until 1993, and during the 1980s and early 1990s was relatively constant at about 70% (73[C]).
- UK: in close to 7 million children who received measles–rubella vaccine in a catch-up campaign there was no increase in the number of new cases or exacerbation of existing cases of Crohn's disease (74[R]).
- In an international case-control study of 499 patients with chronic inflammatory bowel disease and 998 control patients from nine countries, there was no difference in the risk of inflammatory bowel disease in association with either natural measles or measles immunization (75[C]).

Evidence against an association between MMR and autism Two studies have suggested a link between measles/MMR immunization and autism. Fudenberg (76[C]) reported that 15 of 40 patients with infantile autism developed symptoms within a week after MMR immunization. Wakefield et al. evaluated 12 children with chronic enterocolitis and regressive developmental disorders (4[C]). The onset of behavioral symptoms was associated with MMR immunization in eight cases, as reported by the parents. Both reports were non-comparative and anecdotal. By chance alone some cases of autism will occur shortly after immunization, and most children in developed countries receive their first measles or MMR vaccination in the second year of life, when autism typically manifests. The imprecision of the interval between immunization and the onset of behavioral symptoms in the study by Wakefield et al. makes these data suspect. Developmental delay is likely to be detected by a gradual awareness over a period of time, not on a particular day. Inaccuracies in the study of Fudenberg, for example referring to hepatitis B vaccine as a live vaccine, cast some doubts on the carefulness of the entire report. Epidemiological studies in various countries (UK, Sweden, Finland), comparing the introduction and use of vaccines and the *incidence of autism, have not supported a relation between measles/MMR vaccine and autism (68[C], 71[C], 72[C], 77[C]). Wing reviewed 16 studies in Europe, North America, and Japan and found no increase in autism with increasing use of measles or measles–mumps–rubella vaccines (78[C]). An analysis of two large European datasets produced similar results (79[C]). In early 1998, experts in various medical disciplines reviewed the work of the Inflammatory Disease Study Group of the Royal Free Hospital in detail and concluded that there is no evidence for a link between measles/MMR vaccine and either Crohn's disease or autism (80[R]).*

Publicity associated with the publication of the findings that measles immunization could be linked with Crohn's disease and autism *It has already been mentioned that the scientific and public response to the 1998 publication of Wakefield et al. (4[C]) was enormous and controversial. For example, Black et al. (81[R]) stated that the publicity generated by this paper was out of proportion to the strength of the evidence it contained; Beale (82[R]) suggested that the Lancet would bear a heavy responsibility for acting against the public health interest that the journal usually aims to promote; O'Brien et al. (83[R]) considered that the substantial amount of evidence that contradicts the findings of Wakefield et al. did not achieve the same prominence in the popular press.*

In replying to these letters, Wakefield (84) defended the clinician's duty to his patients and the researcher's obligation to test hypotheses. For his part, the editor of the Lancet pointed out that the paper had been presented with a commissioned commentary in the same issue; peer review had confirmed that the paper merited publication, with suitable revisions and editing, as an early report; finally, he considered that the press had presented the information in a balanced way (85).

The response to a newly published adverse event due to immunization must be rapid. If the reported association is correct, urgent re-evaluation of the immunization program is necessary. Otherwise, if the reported association is false, a credible counter-message is necessary to minimize the negative impact on the immunization program (52[R]). The rapidity of response to the 1998 publication of Wakefield et al., including the convening of an independent review panel in the UK, was very useful.

Skin and appendages New data support the already established causal relation between MMR vaccine and *thrombocytopenic purpura*, but not with the measles component itself (53[C]).

Gianotti–Crosti syndrome has been reported in a child immunized with MMR (86[c]).

Three days after MMR immunization a 15-month-old boy developed a rash, initially on the arms but later involving the legs. Six weeks later he had an extensive, symmetrical, non-follicular, papular eruption on his face, arms, and legs, with striking sparing of his trunk. This was labelled Gianotti–Crosti syndrome, a self-healing non-recurrent erythematous or skin-colored papular eruption with symmetrical distribution on the face, buttocks, and extremities in children.

A wide spectrum of infectious diseases has been associated with this syndrome, and preceding immunization against influenza, diphtheria, pertussis, and poliomyelitis has been reported.

Immunological and hypersensitivity reactions It has been suggested that hydrolyzed gelatin, rather than egg protein, is responsible for most episodes of *anaphylaxis* after measles immunization (52[R]). Egg allergy should no longer be a contraindication to measles immunization. However, a previous anaphylactic reaction to measles or MMR vaccine remains a contraindication.

Poliomyelitis vaccine *(SED-13, 943; SEDA-21, 336; SEDA-22, 352)*

Are polio researchers responsible for the AIDS epidemic? 'The River' by Edward Hooper picks up an old hypothesis

The hypothesis that oral polio vaccine played a key role in the current AIDS epidemic is more than 7 years old. This issue has been raised again by Edward Hooper, who has worked many years for the BBC and the UN in Africa and some years ago wrote a book called 'Slim', in which he described the AIDS epidemic in East Africa. His new book 'The River. A journey to the source of HIV and AIDS', published in 1999 (87), raised great public attention and has been discussed in BBC Press

Releases and in the New York Times. Leading experts in virology and AIDS research have published comments in Science and other scientific journals. 'The River' is a thoroughly researched, well-written book and deserves to be taken seriously. Hooper carefully collected data and events describing the first phases of HIV infection and AIDS, as well as the early development and implementation of polio vaccines. His book reflects some hundreds of interviews, including the leading researchers in the related fields, and he has documented more than 4000 references.

The hypothesis is based on the following facts and assumptions. In 1957 and 1958, Koprowski, from the Wistar Institute in Philadelphia, was administering oral polio vaccine in Africa (pre-licensure field trials in Burundi, Rwanda, and the North-east Congo) near Stanleyville (now Kisangani) in Congo. Not far from the base, chimpanzees for use in medical research were housed in Camp Lindi and might have carried a primate immunodeficiency virus (PIV). Chimpanzee kidneys for hepatitis research were shipped from Camp Lindi to the Virological Department of the Children Hospital in Philadelphia in 1958 and 1959. Hooper suggests that 'it could be that [kidneys from these chimpanzees] ended up at the Wistar', the laboratory in Philadelphia where polio vaccines were manufactured, where they contaminated vaccines with PIV. The poliovaccine that was supposed to be contaminated with PIV was then used in the Congo, transmitting the virus that evolved into HIV-1, the starting point of the worldwide HIV-1 epidemic. Over the next 20 years, infected humans progressed to AIDS, and the disease became visible in central Africa in the mid-to-late 1970s.

Does Hooper prove his hypothesis beyond a shadow of doubt? No, but he makes a powerful case for soberly and squarely addressing the issue.

There are strong arguments against the hypothesis. Poliovaccines were first propagated in kidney cultures of rhesus and cynomolgus macaques, and later in African green monkeys. Plotkin and Koprowski categorically stated in a letter to the editor of the New York Times (7 December 1999) that no chimpanzee tissues were used in the Wistar Institute for polivaccine production. They added that two independent analyses of the probable timing of the cross-over of HIV from chimpanzees into humans give dates earlier than 1957–59, the years in which the Wistar polio vaccine was used in the Congo (88). It should also be mentioned that the vaccine manufactured in Wistar at that time was not only used in Africa but also in Sweden, Poland, and the US. One vial of Wistar's oral polio vaccine stored in Stockholm has already tested negative. Garrett et al. in England experimentally examined the survival of human and simian immunodeficiency viruses in oral polio vaccine formulations; no live retrovirus came through the procedure. Recently, Wistar declared that they will release lab specimens from a polio vaccine project carried out at the end of the 1950s in Africa for examination in two independent laboratories, in order to dispel claims that Wistar scientists inadvertently caused the AIDS epidemic.

It should be mentioned that the majority of scientists believe that the AIDS epidemic began after the simian immunodeficiency virus was transmitted from chimpanzees to humans during the slaughter of chimpanzees as early as the 1930s (56, 89–91).

Finally, it is worth repeating the statement of the US Centers for Disease Control and Prevention, issued in 1992 but still valid (92): 'The suggestion that HIV, the AIDS virus, originated as a result of inadvertent inoculation of an HIV-like virus present in monkey kidney cell cultures used to prepare polio vaccine is one of a number of unsubstantiated hypotheses. The weight of scientific evidence does not support this idea and there is no more reason to believe this hypothesis than many others that have been considered and rejected on scientific grounds'.

Nevertheless, there are important lessons to be learned from Hooper's book. For many years, virologists and regulatory authorities have been worried that using permanent cell lines for vaccine virus propagation may somehow transfer cancer-causing properties and animal viruses. African green monkey kidneys are still used as the main cell substrate for oral polio vaccine. Millions of doses have been made from simian immunodeficiency virus (SIV)-positive monkeys before screening was introduced. Now there are well-tested non-oncogenic cell substrates, and it is time to reopen the debate on the use of primary cells versus cell lines for live attenuated virus vaccines. There is also a need to strengthen research on the sources of AIDS. However, the main focus of AIDS research should be prevention and treatment.

Change in immunization policy The US 2000 childhood immunization schedule, proposed by the Advisory Committee of Immunization Practices (ACIP), the American Academy of Pediatrics, and the American Academy of Family Physicians, recommends an all-IPV schedule for routine use in the US, aimed at the elimination of the rare vaccine-associated paralytic poliomyelitis (27).

Nervous system The available reports on a possible association between polio vaccine and *Guillain–Barré syndrome* have been reviewed (93[R]). The conclusion of a 1994 US Institute of Medicine committee that the evidence favored acceptance of a causal relation was mainly based on two reports from Finland (94[C], 95[C]). Kinnunen et al. (96[C]) have now extended their earlier study of Guillain–Barré syndrome and oral polio vaccine to include hospital reports from the whole of Finland for 1981–86, during which time an oral polio vaccine campaign was carried out to control an outbreak of poliomyelitis. Analyzing the monthly reports, they found out that the rise in the numbers of cases of Guillain–Barré syndrome had already started before the immunization campaign. Because there had also been an influenza epidemic during that time, the researchers acknowledged that the increase in the incidence of Guillain–Barré syndrome could also have been associated with influenza. Data from the Americas are also not supporting an association between oral polio immunization campaigns and Guillain–Barré syndrome (97[C]).

Rotavirus vaccine *(SEDA-20, 292; SEDA-21, 337)*

R *Intussusception due to Rotashield*

On 31 August 1998 a tetravalent rhesus-based rotavirus vaccine Rotashield (RRV-TV) was licensed in the US, and the Advisory Committee on Immunization Practices (ACIP), the American Academy of Pediatrics, and the American Academy of Family Physicians recommended its routine use in healthy infants. Rotashield was the first rotavirus vaccine ever licensed.

In pre-licensure studies of Rotashield, five cases of intussusception occurred among 10 054 vaccine recipients and one of 4633 controls, a difference that was not statistically significant. Three of the five cases in immunized children occurred within 6–7 days of receiving the vaccine. On the basis of these data, intussusception was included as a potential adverse reaction on the package insert, and the ACIP recommended post-licensure surveillance for this adverse event after immunization. Because of concerns about intussusception identified in pre-licensure trials, VAERS data were analyzed early in the post-licensure period (98).

From 1 September 1998 to 7 July 1999, 15 cases of intussusception in infants who had received rotavirus vaccine were reported to the Vaccine Adverse Event Reporting System (VAERS). Of the 15 infants, 13 developed intussusception after the first dose of the three-dose RRV-TV series, and 12 developed symptoms within 1 week of receiving any dose of RRV-TV. Thirteen concurrently received other vaccines. Eight infants required surgical reduction, and one required resection of 18 cm of distal ileum and proximal colon. Histopathological examination of the distal ileum showed lymphoid hyperplasia and ischemic necrosis. All the infants recovered. The dates of onset were from 21 November 1998 to 24 June 1999. The median age of the patients was 3 months (range 2–11 months). Ten were boys. The rate of hospitalization for intussusception among infants aged less than 12 months during 1991–97 (before RRV-TV licensure) was 51 per 100 000 infant-years in New York. The manufacturer had distributed about 1.8 million doses of RRV-TV as of 1 June 1999, and estimated that 1.5 million doses (83%) had been administered. Given this information, 14–16 cases of intussusception would have been expected by chance alone during the week following the receipt of any dose of RRV-TV. Fourteen of the 15 patients were immunized before 1 June, 1999, and of those 11 developed intussusception within 1 week of receiving RRV-TV. Based on these results, use of the vaccine was suspended (July 1999) pending the data review by the Advisory Committee on Immunization Practice (ACIP) (93[C]). Further studies detected more cases of intussusception (including two deaths) associated with the administration of Rotashield. Based on the results of an expedited review of the scientific data (indicating a strong association between Rotashield and intussusception) presented to the ACIP, it was recommended (22 October 1999) that Rotashield should no longer be used. The recommendation was made in co-operation with the FDA, NIH, and Public Health Service officials, along with the manufacturer, Wyeth–Lederle (99).

Varicella vaccine *(SED-13, 950; SEDA-20, 292; SEDA-21, 338; SEDA-22, 354)*

A 19-month-old girl was immunized against *Varicella* at 15 months of age and later developed *Herpes zoster* infection (100[c]). Viral cultures from various lesions isolated *Varicella zoster* virus. The OKA vaccine strain was revealed by polymerase chain reaction.

MISCELLANEOUS

Adjuvants—current status, problems, future prospect

Currently, the most common adjuvants for human use are still aluminium hydroxide and aluminium phosphate; calcium phosphate and oil emulsions have also some use in human vaccines. Much progress has been made on the development of alternative adjuvants, such as derivatives of muramyl dipeptide, monophosphoryl lipid A, liposomes, QS21, MF-59, and immunostimulating complexes (ISCOMS). Other areas of adjuvant research are the controlled release of vaccine antigens using biodegradable polymer microspheres (aiming to reduce the number of doses required for primary immunization) and reciprocal enhanced immunogenicity of protein–polysaccharide conjugates (useful for the development of combination vaccines). Two papers (101[R], 102[R]) have reviewed the current status, problems and future prospects in detail.

Vaccine-associated thrombocytopenic purpura Since 1994, the Pharmaceutical and Medical Safety Bureau has received 13 reports of acute *thrombocytopenic purpura* associated with immunization. These included eight cases after rubella vaccine, three after measles vaccine, and one after simultaneous administration of DTP and mumps vaccine (103[R]).

REFERENCES

1. Clements CJ, Evans G, Dittmann S, Reeler AV. Vaccine safety concerns everyone. Vaccine 1999; 17(Suppl 3):S90–4.
2. Jefferson T. Vaccination and its adverse effects: real or perceived. Br Med J 1998;317:159–60.
3. Chen RT, DeStefano F. Vaccine adverse events: causal or coincidental? Lancet 1998;351:611–12.
4. Wakefield AJ, Murch SH, Linnell AAJ, Casson DM, Malik M, Bewrelowitz M. Ileal–lymphoid–nodular hypoplasia, non-specific colitis and pervasive developmental disorder in children. Lancet 1998;351:637–41.
5. Varicchio F. The vaccine adverse event reporting system. J Toxicol Clin Toxicol 1998;36: 765–8.
6. Niu MT, Rhodes P, Salive M, Lively T, Davis DM, Black S, Shinefield H, Chen RT, Ellenberg SS, Braun M, Donlon J, Krueger C, Rastogi S, Varricchio F, Wise R, Haber P, Lloyd J, Terracciano G, Eltermann D, Gordon S, DeStefano F, Glasser J, Hadler S, Kimsey D Jr, Swint E, Fireman B, Hiatt R, Lewis N, Lieu T, and the VAERS and VSD Working Group. Comparative safety of two recombinant hepatitis B vaccines in children: data from the vaccine adverse event reporting system (VAERS) and vaccine safety datalink (VSD). J Clin Epidemiol 1998;51:503–10.
7. Demicheli V, Rivetti D, Deeks JJ, Jefferson T, Pratt M. The effectiveness and safety of vaccines against human anthrax: a systematic review. Vaccine 1998;9:880–4.
8. Blain P, Lightfoot N, Bannister B. Practicalities of warfare required service personnel to be vaccinated against anthrax. Br Med J 1998;317:1077–8.
9. Damm O, Briheim G, Hagstrom T, Jonsson B, Skau T. Ruptured mycotic aneurysm of the abdominal aorta: a serious complication of intravesical instillation BCG therapy. J Urol 1998;159: 984.
10. Buchs N, Chevrel G, Miossec P. BCG induced aseptic arthritis: an experimental model of reactive arthritis. J Rheumatol 1998;25:1662–5.
11. Kodali VRR, Clague RB. Arthritis after BCG vaccine in a healthy woman. J Intern Med 1998; 244:183–7.
12. Karvonen M, Cepaitis Z, Tuomilehto J. Association between type 1 diabetes and *Haemophilus influenzae* type b immunization: birth cohort study. Br Med J 1999;318:1169–72.
13. Classen JB, Classen DC. Association between type 1 diabetes and Hib vaccine: causal relation is likely. Br Med J 1999;319:1133.
14. Classen DC, Classen JB. The timing of pediatric immunization and the risk of insulin-dependent diabetes mellitus. Infect Dis Clin Pract 1997;6:449–54.
15. Jefferson T. Vaccination and its adverse effects: real or perceived. Br Med J. 1998;317:159–60.
16. Sigal LH, Zahradnik JM, Lavin P, Patella SJ, Bryant G, Haselby R, Hilton E, Kunkel M, Adler-Klein D, Doherty T, Evans J, Malawista SE, Molloy P, Seidner A, Sabetta J, Simon H, Klempner M,

Patella S, Mays J, Marks D. A vaccine consisting of recombinant *Borrelia burgdorferi* outer-surface protein A to prevent Lyme disease. New Engl J Med 1998;339:216–22.

17. Steere AC, Sikand VK, Meurice F, Parenti DL, Fikrig E, Schoen R, Nowakowski J, Schmid CH, Laukamp S, Buscarino C, Krause DS, Cohen S, Boyer J, Hanrahan K, Dalgin P, Dalgin J, Garrett A, Petelaba M, Feder H, Good S, Green J, Miller K, Spiegel M, Daniel G, Jacob R, Maderazo E, Maiorano M, Seidner A, Bruno L. Vaccination against Lyme disease with recombinant *Borrelia burgdorferi* outer-surface lipoprotein A with adjuvant New Engl J Med 1998;339:209–15.
18. SmithKline to vigorously defend itself against class action. Mealey Publications Report. Press Release Newswire Association Baltimore, 23 December 1999.
19. Marwick C. Guarded endorsement for Lyme virus vaccine. J Am Med Assoc 1998;279:1937–8.
20. Peltola H. Meningococcal vaccines. Drugs 1998;55:347–66.
21. Robbins JB, Schneerson R, Bryla DA, Trollfors B, Taranger J, Lagergard T. Immunity to pertussis: not all virulence factors are protective antigens. Adv Exp Med Biol 1998;452:207–18.
22. Sakaguchi M, Nakayama T, Inouye S. Cases of systemic immediate-type urticaria associated with acellular diphtheria–tetanus–pertussis vaccination. Vaccine 1998;16:1138–40.
23. Vermeer de Bondt PE, Labadie J, Rumke HC. Rate of recurrent collapse after vaccination with whole cell pertussis vaccine: Follow up study. Br Med J 1998;316:902–3.
24. Miller E. Collapse reactions after whole cell pertussis vaccination. Br Med J 1998;316:876.
25. Baraff LJ, Shields WD, Beckwith L, Strome G, Marcy SM, Cherry JD. Infants and children with convulsions and hypotonic–hyporesponsive episodes following diphtheria–tetanus–pertussis immunisation: follow-up evaluation. Pediatrics 1988; 81:789–94.
26. Stehr K, Cherry JD, Heininger U, Schmitt-Grohe S, Uberall M, Laussucq S, Eckhardt T, Meyer M, Engelhardt R, Christenson P, Muller W, Neugebauer A, Sailer K, Keller H, Kircher U, Netzel B, Sachsenhauser-Kratzer H, Thelen M, Buck KE, Nath G, Clapier E, Gelius P, Graf zu Castell B, Hess H-J, Maas-Doyle E, Mayer HPR, Renner K, Seltsam I, Seuwen G. A comparative efficacy trial in Germany in infants who received either the Lederle/Takeda acellular pertussis component DTP (DTaP) vaccine, the Lederle whole-cell component DTP vaccine, or DT vaccine. Pediatrics 1998;101:1–11.
27. Recommendations of the Advisory Committee on Immunization Practices (ACIP). The 2000 Immunization Schedule. Morb Mort Wkl Rep 2000; 49:25.
28. Schmitt HJ, Zepp F, Muschenborn S, Sumenicht G, Schuind A, Beutel K, Knuf M, Bock HL, Bogaerts H, Clemens R. Immunogenicity and reactogenicity of a *Haemophilus influenzae* type b tetanus conjugate vaccine when administered separately or mixed with concomitant diphtheria–tetanus–toxoid and acellular pertussis vaccine for primary and for booster immunizations. Eur J Pediatr 1998;157:208–14.
29. Rennels MB, Hohenboken MJ, Reisinger KS, Clements DA, Walter EB Jr, Blatter MM, Nonenmacher J, Hackell JG. Comparison of acellular pertussis–diphtheria–tetanus toxoids and *Haemophilus influenzae* type b vaccines administered separately vs. combined in younger vs. older toddlers. Pediatr Infect Dis J 1998;17:164–6.
30. Mills E, Gold R, Thipphawong J, Barreto L, Guasparini R, Meekison W, Cunning L, Russell M, Harrison D, Boyd M, Xie F. Safety and immunogenicity of a combined five-component pertussis–diphtheria–tetanus-inactivated poliomyelitis–*Haemophilus* b conjugate vaccine administered to infants at two, four and six months of age. Vaccine 1998;16:576–85.
31. Vernacchio L, Neufeld EJ, MacDonald K, Kurth S, Murakami S, Hohne C, King M, Molrine D. Combined schedule of 7-valent pneumococcal conjugate vaccine followed by 23-valent pneumococcal vaccine in children and young adults with sickle cell disease. J Pediatr 1998;133:275–8.
32. Classen JB. FDA told pneumococcal vaccine likely to cause epidemics of diabetes. Press release, Newswire Association, Baltimore, 9 November 1999.
33. Drago F, Rampini P, Lugani C, Rebora A. Generalized morphea after antitetanus vaccination. Clin Exp Dermatol 1998;23:142.
34. Engels EA, Falagas ME, Lau J, Bennish ML. Typhoid fever vaccines: a meta-analysis of studies on efficacy and toxicity. Br Med J 1998;316:110–16.
35. Rosenthal P. Hepatitis A vaccine: current indications. J Pediatr Gastroenterol Nutr 1998;27:111–13.
36. Grotto I, Mandel Y, Ephros M, Ashkenazi I, Shemer J. Major adverse reactions to yeast-derived hepatitis B vaccines—a review. Vaccine 1998; 16:329–34.
37. Marshall E. A shadow falls on hepatitis B vaccination effort. Science 1998;281:630–1.
38. Monteyne P, André FE. Is there a causal link between hepatitis B vaccination and multiple sclerosis? Vaccine 2000 (in press).
39. Barbaud A, Trechot P, Reichert-Penetrat S, Weber M, Schmutz JL. Allergic mechanisms and urticaria/angioedema after hepatitis B immunization. Br J Dermatol 1998;139:925–6.
40. Finielz P, Lam-Kam-Sang LF, Guiserix J. Systemic lupus erythematosus and thrombocytopenic purpura in two members of the same family following hepatitis B vaccine. Nephrol Dial Transplant 1998;13:2420–1.
41. Skowron F, Grezard P, Berard F, Balme B, Perrot H. Persistent nodules at sites of hepatitis B vaccination due to aluminium sensitization. Contact Dermatitis 1998;39:135–6.
42. Vanoli M, Gambini D, Scorza R. A case of Churg–Strauss vasculitis after hepatitis B vaccination. Ann Rheum Dis 1998;57:256–7.

43. Zuckerman JN. Hepatitis B third-generation vaccines: improved response and conventional vaccine non-response—third generation pre-S/S vaccines overcome non-response J Viral Hepatitis 1998;5(Suppl 2):13–15.
44. Angel J.B, Walpita P, Lerch RA, Sidhu MS, Masurekar M. DeLellis RA, Noble JT, Snydman DR, Udem SA. Vaccine-associated measles pneumonitis in an adult with AIDS. Ann Intern Med 1998;129:104–6.
45. Recommendations of the Advisory Committee on Immunization Practices (ACIP). Measles–mumps–rubella vaccine use and strategies for elimination of measles, rubella, and congenital rubella syndrome, and control of mumps. Morbid Mortal Wkly Rep 1998;47(No RR8):1–58.
46. Moore D, Nelson M, Henderson D. Pneumococcal vaccination and HIV infection. Int J STD AIDS 1998;9:1–7.
47. Katzenstein TL, Gerstoft J, Nielsen H. Assessments of plasma HIV RNA and CD4 cell counts after combined Pneumovax and Tetanus Toxoid vaccination: no detectable increase in HIV replication 6 weeks after immunization. Scand J Infect Dis 1996;28:239–41.
48. Kroon FP, Van Furth R, Bruisten SM. The effects of immunization on human immunodeficiency virus type 1 infection. New Engl J Med 1996;335:817–18.
49. Vassileva S. Drug-induced pemphigoid. Clin Dermatol 1998;16:379–87.
50. James JM, Zeiger RS, Lester MR, Fasano MB, Gern JE, Mansfield LE, Schwartz HJ, Sampson HA, Windom HH, Machtinger SB, Lensing S. Safe administration of influenza vaccine to patients with egg allergy. J Pediatr 1998;133:624–8.
51. Sabchareon A, Yoksan S. Japanese encephalitis. Ann Trop Paediatr 1998;18(Suppl):S67–71.
52. Duclos P, Ward BJ. Measles vaccines. A review of adverse events. Drug Saf 1998;19:435–54.
53. Weibel RE, Caserta V, Benor DE, Evans G. Acute encephalopathy followed by permanent brain injury or death associated with further attenuated measles vaccines: a review of claims submitted to the National Vaccine Injury Compensation Program. Pediatrics 1998;101:383–7.
54. Miller D, Wadsworth J, Diamond J. Measles vaccination and neurological events. Lancet 1997; 349:730–31.
55. Black S, Shinefield H, Ray P. Risk of hospitalization because of aseptic meningitis after measles–mumps–rubella vaccination in one- to two-year-old children: an analysis of the Vaccine Safety Datalink (VSD) Project. Pediatr Infect Dis J 1997;16:500–3.
56. Wakefield AJ, Pittilo RM, Sim R, Cosby SL, Stephenson JR, Dhillon AP, Pounder RE. Evidence of persistent measles virus infection in Crohn's disease. J Med Virol 1993;39:345–53.
57. Ekbom A, Wakefield AJ, Zack M, Adami HO. Perinatal measles infection and subsequent Crohn's disease. Lancet 1994;344:508–10.
58. Ekbom A, Daszak P, Kraaz W, Wakefield AJ. Crohn's disease after in utero measles virus exposure. Lancet 1996;348:515–17.
59. Thompson NP, Montgomery SM, Pounder RE, Wakefield AJ. Is measles vaccination a risk factor for inflammatory bowel disease? Lancet 1995; 345:1071–4.
60. Lewin J, Dhillon AP, Sim R, Mazure G, Pounder RE, Wakefield AJ. Persistent measles virus infection of the intestine: confirmation by immunogold electron microscopy. Gut 1995;36:564–9.
61. Daszak P, Purcell M, Lewin J, Dhillon AP, Pounder RE, Wakefield AJ. Detection and comparative analysis of persistent measles virus infection in Crohn's disease by immunogold electron microscopy. J Clin Pathol 1997;50:299–304.
62. Haga Y, Funakoshi O, Kuroe K, Kanazawa K, Nakajima H, Saito H, Murata Y, Munakata A, Yoshida Y. Absence of measles viral genomic sequences in intestinal tissues from Crohn's disease by nested polymerase chain reaction. Gut 1996; 38:211–15.
63. Iizuka M, Nakagomi O, Chiba M, Ueda S, Masamune O. Absence of measles virus in Crohn's disease. Lancet 1995;345:199.
64. Iizuka M, Masmune O. Measles vaccination and inflammatory bowel disease. Lancet 1997; 350:1775.
65. Afzal MA, Minor PD, Begley J, Bentey ML, Armitage E, Ghosh S, Ferguson A. Absence of measles virus genome in inflammatory bowel disease. Lancet 1998;351:646–7.
66. Fisher NC, Yee L, Nightingale P, McEwan R, Gibson JA. Measles virus serology in Crohn's disease. Gut 1997;41:66–9.
67. Touze I, Dubucquoi S, Cortot A, van Kruiningen HJ, Colombel J-F. IgM-specific measles-virus antibody in families with a high frequency of Crohn's disease. Lancet 1995;346:967.
68. Lee JW, Melgaard B, Clements CJ, Kane M, Mulholland EK, Olivé J-M. Autism, inflammatory bowel disease, and MMR vaccine. Lancet 1998; 351:905.
69. Payne C, Mason B. Autism, inflammatory bowel disease, and MMR vaccine. Lancet 1998; 351:907.
70. Nielsen LLW, Nielsen NM, Melbye M, Sodermann M, Jacobsen M, Aaby P. Exposure to measles in utero and Crohn's disease: a Danish register study. Br Med J 1998;316:196–7.
71. Peltola H, Patja A, Leinikki P, Valle M, Davidkin I, Paunio M. No evidence for measles, mumps, and rubella vaccine-associated inflammatory bowel disease or autism in a 14-year prospective study. Lancet 1998;351:1327–8.
72. Pebody RG, Paunio M, Ruutu P. Crohn's disease has not increased in Finland. Br Med J 1998; 316:1745.
73. Yamashito Y, Walker-Smith A, Shimizu T, Oguchi S, Ohtsuka Y. Measles vaccination and inflammatory bowel disease in Japanese children. J Pediatr Gastroenterol Nutr 1998;26:238.
74. Calman K. Measles, measles–mumps–rubella (MMR) vaccine, Crohn's disease and autism: Dear doctor letter from the Chief Medical Officer; March 1998, PL/CMO/98/2.

75. Gilat T, Hacohen D, Lilos, P, Langman MJS. Childhood factors in ulcerative colitis and Crohn's disease. Scand J Gastroenterol 1987;22:1009–24.
76. Fudenberg HH, Dialysable lymphocyte extract (DLyE) in infantile onset autism: a pilot study. Biotherapy 1996;9:143–7.
77. Gillberg C, Steffenburg S, Schaumann H. Is autism more common now than 10 years ago? Br J Psychiatry 1991;158:403–9.
78. Wing L. Autism spectrum disorders: no evidence for or against an increase in prevalence. Br Med J 1996;312:327–8.
79. Fombonne E. Inflammatory bowel disease and autism. Lancet 1998;351:955.
80. Department of Health, England and Wales. MMR vaccine is not linked to Crohn's disease or autism: conclusion of an expert scientific seminar. London: Press Release 98/109, 24 March, 1998.
81. Black D, Prempeh H, Baxter T. Autism, inflammatory bowel disease, and MMR vaccine. Lancet 1998;351:905–6.
82. Beale AJ. Autism, inflammatory bowel disease, and MMR vaccine. Lancet 1998;351:906.
83. O'Brien SJ, Jones IG, Christie P. Autism, inflammatory bowel disease, and MMR vaccine. Lancet 1998;351:906.
84. Wakefield AJ. Author's reply. Lancet 1998; 351:908.
85. Horton R. Editor's reply. Lancet 1998;351:908.
86. Velangi SS, Tidman MJ. Gianotti–Crosti syndrome after measles–mumps–rubella immunization. Br J Dermatol 1998;139:1122–3.
87. Hooper E. The River: a journey to the source of HIV and AIDS. Boston, New York, London: Little, Brown and Company, 1999.
88. Plotkin SA, Koprowski H. New York Times, 7 December 1999.
89. Moore JP. Up the river without a paddle. Lancet 1999;401:326–7.
90. Wain-Hobson S. Review of *The River*: a journey to the source of HIV and AIDS. Nature Med 1999;10:1117–18.
91. Weiss RA. Review of *The River*: a journey to the source of HIV and AIDS. Science, 1999; 286:1305–6.
92. US Department of Health and Human Services, Public Health Service, Centers for Disease Control. Origin of HIV. Press Release, 6 March 1992.
93. Salisbury DM. Association between oral poliovaccine and Guillain–Barré syndrome? Lancet 1998; 351:79–80.
94. Uhari M, Rantala H, Niemela M. Cluster of childhood Guillain–Barré syndrome after an oral poliovaccine campaign. Lancet 1989;2:440–1.
95. Kinnunen E, Farkkila M, Hovi T, Juntunen J, Weckstrom P. Incidence of Guillain–Barré syndrome during a nationwide oral poliovirus vaccine campaign. Neurology 1989;39:1034–6.
96. Kinnunen E, Junttila O, Haukka J, Hovi T. Nationwide oral poliovirus vaccination campaign and the incidence of Guillain–Barré syndrome. Am J Epidemiol 1998;147:69–73.
97. Olive JM, Castillo C, Castro RG, De Quadros CA. Epidemiologic study of Guillain–Barré syndrome in children <15 years of age in Latin America. J Infect Dis 1997;175(Suppl 1):160–4.
98. Anonymous. Intussusception among recipients of rotavirus vaccine—United States, 1998–1999. Morb Mortal Wkly Rep 1999;27:577–81.
99. Recommendations of the Advisory Committee on Immunization Practices (ACIP): US Rotavirus vaccine. CDC Media Relations, 22 October, 1999.
100. Liang MG, Heidelberg KA, Jacobson RM, McEvoy MT. *Herpes zoster* after varicella immunization J Am Acad Dermatol 1998;38:761–3.
101. Gupta RK, Siber GR. Adjuvants for human vaccines—current status, problems and future prospects. Vaccine 1995;13:1263–76.
102. Edelman R. Vaccine adjuvants. Rev Inf Dis 1980;2;370–83.
103. Anonymous. Vaccine-associated thrombocytopenic purpura. WHO Drug Inf 1998;12:240.

H.W. Eijkhout and W.G. van Aken

33 Blood, blood components, plasma, and plasma products

BLOOD PRODUCTS

Most patients do not react adversely to blood products. However, some have mild to severe effects immediately or delayed for 48 hours. Information on adverse reactions to blood products collected by the New Zealand Centre for Adverse Reactions Monitoring enables the identification of unusual or unpredictable adverse reactions; risk factors such as concomitant medications, underlying diseases, rate of administration; and batch problems (1[r]).

BLOOD SUBSTITUTES

The development of oxygen-carrying blood substitutes has progressed significantly in the last decade, and phase 1 and phase 2 clinical trials of both hemoglobin-based and perfluorocarbon-based oxygen carriers are nearing completion. As these products approach clinical use it is important for the laboratory medicine community to be aware of their effects on routine laboratory testing and the settings in which they might be used (2[r]).

However, perfluorocarbon blood substitutes are reported to have several adverse effects, the clinical significance of which is not currently fully understood. In healthy volunteers a transient *flu-like syndrome* has been described after Perfluorocarbon was administered as a contrast agent. Symptoms included back pain, malaise, flushing, and transient fever (3[R]). These symptoms are most likely cytokine-mediated, as the perfluorocarbon particles are cleared by cells of the reticuloendothelial system (4[c]).

One commonly observed adverse effect is transient *thrombocytopenia* 3–4 days after perfluorocarbon (3[R]). In several studies the fall in platelet count was 30–40%, and platelet counts returned to normal in 7–10 days. The use of radioactively labelled platelets showed increased platelet clearance, thought to be due to alteration of the platelet surface by the perfluorocarbon emulsion. Thus, current perfluorocarbon products are unlikely to be administered to thrombocytopenic patients.

Side Effects of Drugs, Annual 23
J.K. Aronson, ed.

BLOOD COMPONENTS

Aluminium in albumin solutions R

An Austrian manufacturer of human albumin 20% and 25% voluntarily recalled the products because the pharmacopoeial specification for aluminium (200 μg/l or less) for treatment of premature infants and dialysis patients cannot be guaranteed over the whole shelf life of 3 years when stored at temperatures above 8°C (5[R]).

The increase in aluminium content over the shelf-life period is due to the fact that the glass vial releases aluminium ions. This process is catalysed by the residual citrate content of albumin formulations and depends on the storage temperature as well as on the relation of the inner glass surface to the amount of liquid. For 10 ml bottles, stability of the aluminium content below 200 μg/l cannot be guaranteed for the shelf life, irrespective of storage conditions.

In 50 ml and 100 ml bottles stored at temperatures below 8°C, the increase in aluminium content is sufficiently slowed down, so that it does not rise beyond 200 μg/l within the 3-year shelf life. However, at storage temperatures exceeding 8°C, the aluminium content may increase beyond 200 μg/l. According to available stability studies, this threshold value is not surpassed before 12 months of storage at these higher temperatures.

A meta-analysis of virtually all existing randomized, controlled clinical studies of albumin or plasma protein fraction showed an excess mortality of about 6% for combined groups of patients with hypovolemia, burns, or hypoproteinemia who received albumin either instead of or in addition to crystalloid solutions. On the basis of their analysis, the authors concluded that albumin should not be given to critically ill patients outside of rigorously conducted randomized controlled trials (6[R]).

The FDA considers that the questions raised in these studies warrant serious consideration and that until the results of further studies are available physicians should exercise discretion in using albumin and plasma protein fraction. The importance of current treatment guidelines is stressed, although it is recognized that these guidelines may themselves require change.

Finally, the Paul Ehrlich Institut of Germany, has recalled certain batches of human albumin products (Human Albumin 20%, Human Albumin 20% Immuno, Human Albumin Immuno 20%, Human Albumin 25% Immuno), including batches that have exceeded 12 months of shelf life (7[r]). This action was taken after quality assurance tests had shown that the aluminium content of these batches had exceeded the maximum acceptable concentration of 200 μg/l. This could result in adverse effects, especially in neonates and dialysis patients, because of deposition in the brain and bones.

INTRAVENOUS IMMUNOGLOBULIN

Intravenous immunoglobulin is approved for the following indications: primary immune deficiencies, immune-mediated thrombocytopenia, Kawasaki disease, bone-marrow transplantation, chronic B cell lymphocytic leukemia, and pediatric HIV infection (8[c]). In addition, intravenous immunoglobulin is a promising immunomodulatory therapy for several neurological diseases, such as Guillain-Barré syndrome, chronic inflammatory demyelinating polyneuropathy, and multifocal motor neuropathy (9[R]). Intravenous immunoglobulin has also been used in the treatment of several other antibody-mediated diseases, such as dermatomyositis, autoimmune neutropenia, pemphigus vulgaris, and pemphigus foliaceus (10[c]–12[c]).

Mild adverse effects of intravenous immunoglobulin, such as *headache, chills, nausea, backache*, and *flushing*, occur at a rate of 5–10% (8[c], 13[R]). Most of these reactions are self-limiting and associated with over-rapid infusion (9[R]). In patients with adverse reactions to intravenous immunoglobulin there was a significant rise in plasma IL-6 and thromboxane B2 (14[C]).

Cardiovascular Intravenous immunoglobulin *expands the plasma volume and increases blood viscosity*, which may lead to volume overload in patients with cardiac insufficiency (9[R]). Increased blood viscosity has also been blamed for cerebral infarction and thromboembolic events (9[R], 15[R]).

Nervous system *Acute meningeal inflammation*, characterized by low-grade fever, headache, neck stiffness, nausea, vomiting, photophobia, and altered consciousness, has been described in 1–15% of patients receiving high dosages of intravenous immunoglobulin (16[c]). In addition, cerebrospinal fluid examination shows pleocytosis, with 10–90% polymorphonuclear cells and increased concentrations of several proteins (SEDA-22, 344; 17[c]). Recently, however, a 50-year-old man developed aseptic meningitis after a low dose of intravenous immunoglobulin (3.5 g) (16[c]). A few weeks after the first infusion, he received a second infusion and again developed symptoms of aseptic meningitis. The authors thought it unlikely that aseptic meningitis had been caused by a hypersensitivity reaction. They proposed that the mechanism of aseptic meningitis involved the entry of immunoglobulin molecules into the cerebrospinal fluid, causing an inflammatory reaction.

It has been reported that most patients with aseptic meningitis have a history of migraine (SEDA-22, 344; 15[R], 16[c]). To prevent aseptic meningitis, it has been advised that intravenous immunoglobulin should be infused at a slow rate and that diluted immunoglobulin solutions should be used (17[c]). Aseptic meningitis can be prevented by the administration of propranolol (9[R], 17[c]). In addition, prehydration and an antihistamine have been helpful in some patients (9[R], 17[c]).

Intravenous immunoglobulin causes severe *headache* in 56% of patients without a history of migraine (18[c]). The pathogenesis of this headache is unknown.

Hemiplegia has been observed on the third day of intravenous immunoglobulin therapy in a 58-year-old man treated for graft-versus-host disease after transfusion of non-leukocyte-depleted erythrocytes (19[c]). The hemiplegia resolved one day after discontinuation of intravenous immunoglobulin. A second case of hemiplegia has been described in a child treated with intravenous immunoglobulin for idiopathic thrombocytopenic purpura (20[c]). The authors of both reports suggested that the hemiplegia had been caused either by transient hyperviscosity or by vasospasm.

Endocrine, metabolic It has been advised that blood glucose should be monitored in patients with diabetes mellitus who receive glucose-containing intravenous immunoglobulin (9[R]).

Hematological Severe acute *hemolysis* due to high titers of blood donor-derived hemolysin has been reported (21[R], 22[C], 23[R]).

Although intravenous immunoglobulin is used to treat autoimmune neutropenia, it can also cause it (24[C]). The mechanism is not clear.

Liver Although transient *rises in liver enzymes* have been documented, they are not considered to be serious (22[C]).

Urinary system Since 1987 several cases of *acute renal insufficiency* have been described after the intravenous infusion of immunoglobulin (SEDA-22, 345; 24[C]).

The pathophysiology of acute renal insufficiency is probably related to hyperosmolar renal damage, due to sucrose present in 50 ml intravenous immunoglobulin formulations (15[R], 25[R], 26[R]). The histopathology of renal tissue shows osmotically-induced tubular injury, tubular vacuolization, and tubulointerstitial infiltrates (27[C]).

Studies in rats have suggested that after pinocytosis by renal tubular cells sucrose is incorporated into phagolysosomes. The intracellular accumulation of sucrose leads to vacuole formation and cellular swelling. On withdrawal of therapy renal insufficiency is self-limiting in most cases. However, sometimes hemodialysis is necessary (23[R], 27[C]). Risk factors for this adverse effect are pre-existing renal disease, age over 65 years, diabetes mellitus, hypertension, and a high infusion rate (SEDA-22, 345; 15[R], 26[R]). To minimize the risk of renal insufficiency it has been suggested that immunoglobulin should be diluted with hypotonic fluid, that the infusion rate should be reduced and the dosing intervals increased (27[C]).

Skin and appendages A few cases of *alopecia* in relation to intravenous immunoglobulin have been described (13[R], 28[c]). *Cutaneous vasculitis* has been reported in association with intravenous immunoglobulin (28[c]). Other reported skin reactions include *urticaria, maculopapular rashes, petechiae, eczema*, and *erythema multiforme* (28[c]).

Immunological and hypersensitivity reactions Selective IgA deficiency is a contraindication to intravenous immunoglobulin, because of the risk of *anaphylactic shock* in patients with IgA deficiency and anti-IgA antibodies (9[R], 21[R]).

Transmission of infection *Hepatitis C transmission* through certain immunoglobulin formulations for intravenous use has previously been described. However, since the introduction of additional viral inactivation steps, such as solvent detergent, intravenous immunoglobulin is not considered to pose an infectious risk (13[R]).

Neither hepatitis B nor HIV has been reported after the administration of intravenous immunoglobulin (13[R]). This is probably because of the high degree of viral inactivation of the cold ethanol fractionation and the screening of every donation for several viruses, such as HIV and hepatitis B and C (25[R]).

There has been some concern about possible transmission of *hepatitis G*. However, hepatitis G is an enveloped flavivirus with homology to hepatitis C and is probably also inactivated by the current procedures (25[R]).

Although transmission of *Creutzfeldt-Jakob disease* through blood components and plasma products has never been documented, the FDA has suggested that there is a theoretical possibility that blood products may carry the responsible agent (8[r]).

Use in pregnancy Intravenous immunoglobulin is indicated for idiopathic thrombocytopenic purpura in pregnancy. No fetal abnormalities have been reported (13[R]).

Interference with diagnostic routines *Pseudohyponatremia*, a laboratory artefact due to hyperproteinemia, has been observed during intravenous immunoglobulin treatment (29). As intravenous immunoglobulin increases the protein-containing non-aqueous phase of plasma, a relative decrease in plasma water volume can occur.

CLOTTING FACTORS

Recombinant activated factor VII is indicated for patients with inhibitors of clotting factors VIII and IX (30[r], 31[C]). It is also being used for patients with severe thrombocytopenia and bleeding (30[r]). In general this product is well tolerated, with an incidence of non-serious adverse events of 3.6% (30[r]). The most frequently reported adverse events are *hypertension, skin reactions, fever, headache, epistaxis, decreased plasma fibrinogen*, and *prolonged prothrombin time* (30[r], 31[C]).

Recombinant factor IX is used as substitution therapy in patients with hemophilia B. Mild adverse events include *discomfort at the infusion site, fever, dizziness, allergic rhinitis, and light-headedness* (32[R]).

Cardiovascular *Angina pectoris* and *tachycardia* have been reported after the use of recombinant factor VIIa (30[r]).

Two factor XI products, both containing antithrombin III and heparin, have been associated with evidence of coagulation activation and thrombotic events in patients with pre-existing vascular disease (33[R]). It has been recommended that doses of more than 30 units/kg and factor XI peak concentrations in severely deficient patients of more than 500–700 units/l should be avoided. In addition, the concurrent use of tranexamic acid or other antifibrinolytic drugs should be avoided.

Prothrombin complex is indicated for reversal of anticoagulation. Because of the potential adverse effects of this product, *including thromboembolism, myocardial infarction*, and *disseminated intravascular coagulopathy*, it is contraindicated in disseminated intravascular coagulopathy and hyperfibrinolysis. Relative contraindications for prothrombin complex concentrate are *liver disease, coronary heart disease, and factors that predispose to thrombosis* (34[R]).

Hematological Although the half-life of recombinant and plasma factor IX products are comparable, the in vivo recovery of recombinant factor IX is 28% lower than a highly purified plasma-derived product. To treat hemorrhage the dosage of recombinant factor IX needs to be 20% higher than plasma-derived products to increase the circulating factor IX activity to 1% per IU of recombinant factor IX given (32[R]).

Platelet membrane glycoprotein IIb/IIIa receptor inhibitor has been approved in various countries for the treatment of patients scheduled for percutaneous transluminal coronary angioplasty or coronary atherectomy to prevent ischemic complications (35[R]). Acute *thrombocytopenia*, at a rate of 0.5–3.2%, has been observed after glycoprotein IIb/IIIa receptor antagonist, probably induced by immune-mediated clearance of platelets (35[R]).

Urinary system During treatment with extremely high doses of factor IX concentrate, to induce immune tolerance, *nephrotic syndrome* has been described (36[c], 37[c]). Withdrawal or dosage reduction is of crucial importance for the resolution of nephrosis (36[c]). Renal biopsy in one of these patients showed peripheral capillary wall thickening and deposits throughout the basement membrane (37[c]). In addition, minimal interstitial fibrosis and tubular atrophy were present. There were no deposits of factor IX in the glomeruli, which the authors attributed to absence of free factor IX epitope in the tissue (37[c]).

Immunological and hypersensitivity reactions Inhibitor formation is one of the complications in patients who are treated for clotting factor deficiencies. Recombinant activated factor VII is indicated for patients with inhibitors. However *antibodies to factor VII* have been observed in a patient with factor VII deficiency, who received 40 times the recommended dose of recombinant activated factor VIIa (30[r]).

In 4% of patients with hemophilia B, factor IX inhibitor will develop. *Allergic and anaphylactic reactions* due to factor IX inhibitor have been described (SEDA-21, 343; 36[c]). Anaphylactic reactions occur particularly in patients with undetectable concentrations of factor IX, because of major disruptions in the factor IX gene (38[c]). In patients with factor IX inhibitor, IgG1 subclass antibodies have been found, which may activate complement, resulting in allergic reactions (SEDA-21, 343; 38[c]).

However, it has also been suggested that allergic reactions to factor IX products are IgE-mediated. In two patients with severe factor IX deficiency and high concentrations of factor IX inhibitors who developed anaphylaxis to factor IX, RAST and skin test reactions to factor IX were positive (38[c]). After desensitization, the circulating IgE antibodies to factor IX fell.

Inhibitor formation has been observed in only a few patients with factor XI deficiency. Like patients with hemophilia A and B, these patients may be treated with prothrombin complex concentrates or recombinant factor VIIa (33[R]).

Patients with hemophilia have various disturbances of immune function, resulting from infections with HIV and hepatitis, but also from chronic exposure to extraneous proteins in clotting factor concentrates (39[R]). Protein contaminants, such as immunoglobulins, fibrinogen, and fibronectin, can depress immune function. It has been postulated that high-purity concentrates in HIV-positive hemophiliacs are associated with better maintenance of CD4+ cells and other indicators of immune function compared with products of intermediate purity (39[R]).

Human antichimeric antibodies, specific to the murine epitope of Fab antibody fragments, have been observed in patients treated with glycoprotein IIb/IIIa receptor inhibitor. These antibodies are IgG antibodies and have so far not correlated with any adverse effects (35[R]).

Transmission of infection Hemophiliacs are at risk of *infection with HIV and hepatitis B and C* (39[R]). However, since viral inactivation methods, such as solvent detergent and heat pasteurization, have been implemented in the production process, the risks of HIV and hepatitis have virtually been eliminated. Nevertheless, many viral inactivation methods currently used do not completely eliminate certain (non-enveloped) viruses, e.g. parvovirus and hepatitis A (39[R], 40[R]). HIV appears to progress more rapidly in patients co-infected with hepatitis B and cytomegalovirus (39[R]). In addition, hepatitis C replicated more rapidly in patients infected with HIV (39[R]).

In a mortality study amongst hemophiliacs in the UK in 1977–91, AIDS was far the commonest cause of death, and liver disease ranked as the third commonest cause of death (40[R]).

It has recently been postulated that *transfusion-transmitted virus can be transmitted* through heat-treated blood products (41[c]). Transfusion-transmitted virus is a common DNA virus in healthy Japanese, and it lacks a lipid envelope, similar to parvovirus B19 (41[c], 42[c]). Transmission of transfusion-transmitted virus often occurs with blood transfusion and it can cause post-transfusion hepatitis with high postoperative peak AlT activity (42[c]). No patients with hepatitis due to transfusion transmitted virus have clinically apparent hepatitis (42[c]). The incidence of transfusion transmitted virus viremia in hemophiliacs was 43% of patients who received only virus-inactivated concentrates and 78% in those who received non-inactivated products before 1984 (41[c]).

APROTININIIN

Aprotinin, a naturally occurring serine protease inhibitor derived from bovine lung, which is indicated in cardiac surgery, reduces the risk of bleeding (43[C], 44[R]).

Hematological It has been postulated that aprotinin potentiates a *prothrombotic state* (44[R]). However, in randomized controlled studies no significant differences between aprotinin and placebo have been observed (44[R]).

Urinary system Aprotinin has a high affinity for renal tissue; 80–90% is stored in the proximal tubule cells after 4 hours and is excreted over 12–24 hours (44[R]). It has been hypothesized that aprotinin causes reversible overload of tubular reabsorption, resulting in *transient renal dysfunction* (44[R]). It has also been postulated that aprotinin has a direct toxic effect on the proximal tubule cells or alters intrarenal blood flow, through inhibition of renin and kallikrein activity (44[R]).

Immunological and hypersensitivity reactions *Allergic reactions* can occur on re-exposure. The incidence rates of aprotinin-related reactions are 2.7% in re-exposed adults (5/183) and 1.2% in children (3/354), with an overall incidence of 1.8% (8/437). The following advice has been given to reduce the risk and severity of these reactions: give a test dose of aprotinin; delay the first bolus injection until the surgeon starts the procedure; give an antihistamine before re-exposure; and avoid re-exposure within the first 6 months after the last exposure (43[C], 44[R]).

EPOETIN (ERYTHROPOIETIN)

The introduction of human recombinant epoetin has improved the treatment of anemia related to end-stage renal disease (45[C]). Epoetin is also very effective in children with chronic renal graft rejection and anemia (46[C]).

In patients with chemotherapy-induced anemia, epoetin increases hemoglobin concentration, reduces transfusion requirements, and improves quality of life (47[r], 48[c]). The response rate to epoetin in patients with multiple myeloma and anemia which is 55–85% (49[R]), will increase when GM-CSF or G-CSF is co-administered (50[R]). Epoetin is also approved for indications such as anemia induced by zidovudine in HIV-infected patients, the prevention of anemia in surgical patients, and anemia of prematurity (50[R], 51[R]). No acceleration of tumor growth by epoetin has been observed (52[R]).

The response to epoetin is abated in the presence of iron deficiency, infection, occult blood loss, hematological diseases, vitamin deficiencies, hemolysis, aluminium intoxication, and inflammation (53[R]).

After the first few doses of epoetin, *flu-like symptoms* occur transiently, with an incidence of 5.4–18% (53[R], 54[c]). It has been suggested that such symptoms can be avoided by dose escalation, starting with an ultra-low dose (54[c]). Other mild adverse effects, such as headache, conjunctival infection, nausea, vomiting, and diarrhea, have been documented (53[R]). Subcutaneous epoetin in patients undergoing hemodialysis can maintain the hematocrit at a desired target range using an average weekly dose lower than with intravenous administration (55[C]). Intravenous administration leads to higher initial epoetin concentrations compared with subcutaneous administration. However, after intravenous administration the half-life is only 4–5 hours, compared with 19–22 hours after subcutaneous administration (56[R]).

In the past subcutaneous epoetin-α resulted in more pain than epoetin-β, owing to citrate buffer in the product. Although the formulation of epoetin-α has been changed to a phosphate buffer, discomfort after epoetin-α administration is still greater than after epoetin-β (57[c], 58[C]).

Cardiovascular *Hypertension* is an important complication of epoetin during treatment of hemodialysis patients (59[C], 60[c]). In 25% of the patients with end-stage renal disease hypertension will develop, even accompanied by encephalopathy or seizures (59[C]). One of the possible mechanisms of epoetin-induced hypertension is an imbalance of local endothelial factors, such as endothelium-derived relaxation factor and endothelin (59[C]). When intravenous and subcutaneous epoetin were compared only intravenous epoetin was accompanied by hypertension (59[C], 60[c]). Plasma concentrations of proendothelin-1 and endothelin-1 increased after infusion of epoetin only in patients with hypertension. In addition, the molar ratio of endothelin-1 over proendothelin-1 was significantly higher in patients with hypertension than patients without (59[C]). The authors suggested that endothelin-converting enzyme may play a role in the pathogenesis of epoetin-induced hypertension (59[C]). Studies in rats have confirmed that epoetin stimulates endothelin release and synthesis of vascular tissue (61). There is a relation between the dose of epoetin and postdialysis blood pressure, but not predialysis blood pressure (60[c]). Risk factors for the development or worsening of hypertension are pre-existing hypertension, the presence of native kidney, a rapid increase in hematocrit, a low baseline hematocrit, high dosages of epoetin, and intravenous administration (60[c]).

There is an increased incidence of *peripheral vascular diseases* in diabetic patients who receive peritoneal dialysis and epoetin (45[C]). In these patients the time to a first vascular incident is shorter, the number of vascular events is increased, and more hospital days associated with vascular disease have been reported compared with patients receiving peritoneal dialysis without epoetin (45[C]). Significant risk factors for the development of peripheral vascular disease are epoetin therapy, epoetin dose, and smoking (45[C]). Peripheral vascular disease may be related to increased blood viscosity or other changes in blood rheology (45[C]).

Vascular access thrombosis has been reported in 14-26% of the patients treated with epoetin-α (53[R]). Most of the failures occurred in polytetrafluoroethylene grafts. There was no comparison with patients not treated with epoetin.

If epoetin is given preoperatively without autologous predonation, there is an increased risk of *hypertension*, an increased risk of *graft thrombosis* and *myocardial infarction* in cardiac surgery, and an increased risk of *venous thromboembolism* in orthopedic patients (44[R]).

Recently epoetin has been abused by athletes, increasing the risk of *hypertension* and *disseminated intravascular coagulopathy* (50[R]). In athletes epoetin causes increased blood viscosity, which will further increase during dehydration, leading to risks of myocardial infarction, cerebrovascular accident, or encephalopathy (50[R]). Epoetin induces accelerated fibrinolysis, and so epoetin doping can be detected by analysis of fibrin degradation products in urine (50[R]). In addition, hypochromic macrocytes are increased (50[R]).

Nervous system *Generalized tonic-clonic seizures* have been reported in 2–17% of dialysis patients treated with epoetin (62[C]). The mechanism is not known, but is most likely multifactorial, such as increased peripheral vascular resistance, reversal of hypoxic vasodilatation, and a direct pressor effect of epoetin mediated by enhanced production of serum endothelin-1 (62[c]).

Headache, probably due to intracranial hypertension, has been reported in 15% of patients with renal insufficiency treated with epoetin (52[R]).

Hematological In neonates *neutropenia* has been described after treatment with high doses of epoetin. Neutrophil counts increased in these neonates after discontinuation of epoetin therapy (63[c]).

Epoetin can cause significant *leukopenia*, especially affecting lymphocytes (64[C]). The fall in lymphocyte count in patients with renal insufficiency is less significant. Pretreatment with imidazole-2-hydroxybenzoate, which inhibits the synthesis of prostaglandins, causes a less marked and delayed reduction of lymphocytes (64[C]).

Endocrine, metabolic In two patients with uremic non-insulin-dependent diabetes, *glucose control deteriorated* after the introduction of epoetin, requiring insulin therapy (65[c]).

Skin and appendages *Generalized skin rash* and *local swelling at the injection site* have been reported after subcutaneous epoetin (48[c]).

Sexual function In a 25-year-old man with chronic renal insufficiency, treated with epoetin, recurrent *veno-occlusive priapism* has been reported. The episodes resolved after the epoetin dosage was reduced (66[c]). The exact mechanism is not known. In the past several cases of priapism have been reported, and it has been hypothesized that androgen therapy probably contributes (66[c]).

Immunological and hypersensitivity reactions *Anti-epoetin antibodies* have never been found in patients treated with epoetin (67[C]).

THROMBOPOIETIN

Thrombopoietin increases the number of megakaryocyte colonies in bone-marrow and also induces maturation of megakaryocytes (68[R]). Recombinant thrombopoietin, which is not yet licensed, is indicated for correction of thrombocytopenia, induced by chemotherapy or radiotherapy (68[R]). It has been tested in subcutaneous doses up to 5 μg/kg/day, resulting in increased numbers of platelets at 7 days, with a peak count at 17 days (68[R]).

So far *thrombotic complications* (deep venous thrombosis, pulmonary embolism, and superficial vein thrombosis) have been described in five patients receiving thrombopoietin (69[R]). In none was thrombosis related to the platelet count, since none had more than 1000 × 10^9/l platelets. It could not be determined if the thrombosis was due to thrombopoietin or if an underlying malignancy predisposed these patients to thrombosis (69[R]).

In in vitro studies thrombopoietin stimulates leukemic cell growth, but in clinical studies restimulation of leukemia has not been observed (69[R]).

REFERENCES

1. Anonymous. Blood products (manufactured)—reporting adverse reactions. WHO Pharm Newslett 1998;5/6:6–7.

2. Scott MG, Kucik DF, Goodnough LT, Monk TG. Blood substitutes: evolution and future applications. Clin Chem 1997;43:1724–31.

3. Spence RK. Perfluorocarbons in the twenty-first century: clinical applications as transfusion alternatives. Artif Cells Blood Substitutes Immobilization Biotechnol 1995;23:367–80.
4. Flaim SF, Hazard DR, Hogan J, Peters RM. Characterization and mechanism of side-effects of Oxygent HT in swine. Biomater Artif Cells Immobilization Biotechnol 1991;19:383–5.
5. Anonymous. Albumin (human) batches withdrawn: increase in aluminium levels. WHO Newsletter 1998;9/10:1.
6. Anonymous. Albumin and plasma protein fraction-safety concerns. WHO Newsletter 1998; 9/10:6.
7. Anonymous. Albumin (human) batches withdrawn: increase in aluminium levels. WHO Newsletter 1999;1/2:1.
8. Milgrom H. Shortage of intravenous immunoglobulin. Ann Allergy Asthma Immunol 1998;81:97–100.
9. Stangel M, Hartung HP, Marx P, Gold R. Intravenous immunoglobulin treatment of neurological autoimmune diseases. J Neurol Sci 1998;153:203–14.
10. Hern S, Harman K, Bhogal BS, Black MM. A severe persistent case of pemphigoid gestationis treated with intravenous immunoglobulins and cyclosporin. Clin Exp Dermatol 1998;23:185–8.
11. Enk AH, Knop J. Adjuvante Therapie von Pemphigus vulgaris und Pemphigus foliaceus mit intravenösen Immunoglobulinen. Hautartz 1998; 49:774–6.
12. Colonna L, Cianchini G, Frezzolini A, De Pita O, Di Lella G, Puddu P. Intravenous immunoglobulins for pemphigus vulgaris: adjuvant or first choice therapy. Br J Dermatol 1998;138:1102–3.
13. Silver RM. Management of idiopathic thrombocytopenic purpura in pregnancy. Clin Obstet Gynecol 1998;41:436–48.
14. Bagdasarian A, Tonetta S, Harel W, Mamidi R, Uemura Y. IVIG adverse reactions: potential role of cytokines and vasoactive substances. Vox Sang 1998;74:74–82.
15. Machkhas H, Harati Y. Side effects of immunosuppressant therapies used in neurology. Neurol Clin 1998;16:171–88.
16. Attout H, Mallet H, Desmurs H, Berthier S, Gil H, De Waziéres B, Dupond JL. Méningite aseptique au course d'un traitement par immunoglobulines intraveineuses a très faibles doses. Rev Med Interne 1998;19:140–1.
17. Jolles S, Hill H. Management of aseptic meningitis secondary to intravenous immunoglobulin. Br Med J 1998;316:936.
18. Finkel AG, Howard JF, Douglas Mann J. Successful treatment of headache related to intravenous immunoglobulin with antimigraine medications. Headache 1998;38:317–21.
19. Hazouard E, Sauvagnac X, Corcia Ph, Legras A, Dequin PF, Ginies G. Accident vasculaire transitoire possiblement lié aux immunoglobulines intraveneineuses. Presse Med 1998;27:161.
20. Tsiouris J, Tsiouris N. Hemiplegia as a complication of childhood immune thrombocytopenic purpura with intravenously administered immunoglobulin. J Pediatr 1998;133:717.
21. Choudhry VP, Mahapatra M, Kashyap R. Immunoglobulin therapy in immunohematological disorders. Indian J Pediatr 1998;65:681–90.
22. Stangel M, Müller M, Marx P. Adverse events during treatment with high-dose intravenous immunoglobulins for neurological disorders. Eur Neurol 1998;40:173–4.
23. Wills AJ, Unsworth DJ. A practical approach to the use of intravenous immunoglobulin in neurological disease. Eur Neurol 1998;39:3–8.
24. Lee YC, Woodfield DG, Douglas R. Clinical usage of intravenous immunoglobulins in Auckland. NZ Med J 1998;111:48–50.
25. Jolles S, Hughes J, Whittaker S. Dermatological uses of high-dose intravenous immunoglobulin. Arch Dermatol 1998;134:80–6.
26. Stahl M, Schifferi JA. The renal risks of high-dose intravenous immunoglobulin treatment. Nephrol Dial Transplant 1998;13:2182–5.
27. Ahsan N. Intravenous immunoglobulin induced-nephropathy: a complication of IVIG therapy. J Nephrol 1998;11:157–61.
28. Howse M, Bindoff L, Carmichael A. Facial vasculitic rash associated with intravenous immunoglobulin. Br Med J 1998;317:1291.
29. Lawn N, Wijdicks EFM, Burritt MF. Intravenous immune globulin and pseudohyponatremia. New Engl J Med 1998;339:632.
30. Roberts HR. Clinical experience with activated factor VII: focus on safety aspects. Blood Coagul Fibrinolyses 1998;9(Suppl 1):S115–18.
31. Key NS, Aledort LM, Beardsley D, Cooper HA, Davignon G, Ewenstein BM, Gilchrist GS, Gill JC, Glader B, Hoots WK, Kisker CT, Lusher JM, Rosenfield CG, Shapiro AD, Smith H, Taft E. Home treatment of mild to moderate bleeding episodes using recombinant factor VIIa (Novoseven) in haemophiliacs with inhibitors. Thromb Haemost 1998;80:912–18.
32. White G, Shapiro A, Ragni M, Garzone P, Goodfellow J, Tubridy K, Courter S. Clinical evaluation of recombinant factor IX. Semin Hematol 1998;35(Suppl 2):33–8.
33. Bolton-Maggs PHB. The management of factor XI deficiency. Haemophilia 1998;4:683–8.
34. Butler AC, Tait RC. Management of oral anticoagulant-induced intracranial haemorrhage. Blood Rev 1998;12:35–44.
35. Ferguson JJ, Kereiakes DJ, Adgey AAJ, Fox KAA, Hillegass WB, Pfisterer M, Vassanelli C. Safe use of platelet GP IIb/IIIa inhibitors. Am Heart J 1998;135:S77–89.
36. Tengborn L, Hansson S, Fasth A, Lübeck P-O, Berg A, Ljung R. Anaphylactoid reactions and nephrotic syndrome – a considerable risk during factor IX treatment in patients with haemophilia B and inhibitors: a report in the outcome in two brothers. Haemophilia 1998;4:854–9.
37. Dharnidharka VR, Takemoto C, Ewenstein BM, Rosen S, Harris HW. Membranous glomerulonephritis and nephrosis post factor IX infusion in hemophilia B. Pediatr Nephrol 1998;12:654–7.

38. Dioun AF, Ewenstein BM, Geha RS, Schneider LC. IgE-mediated allergy and desensitization to factor IX in hemophilia B. J Allergy Clin Immunol 1998;102:113–17.
39. Hoots K, Canty D. Clotting factor concentrates and immune function in haemophilic patients. Haemophilia 1998;4:704–13.
40. Giangrande PLF. Hepatitis in haemophilia. Br J Haematol 1998;103:1–9.
41. Sumazaki R, Yamada-Osaki M, Kajiwara Y, Shirahata A, Matsui A. Transfusion transmitted virus. Lancet 1998;352:1308–9.
42. Fujiwara T, Iwata A, Iizuka H, Tanaka T, Okamoto H. Transfusion transmitted virus. Lancet 1998;352:1310.
43. Dietrich W. Incidence of hypersensitivity reactions. Ann Thorac Surg 1998;65(Suppl 6):S60–4.
44. Faught C, Wells P, Fergusson D, Laupacis A. Adverse effects of methods for minimizing perioperative allogeneic transfusion: a critical review of the literature. Transfus Med Rev 1998;12:206–25.
45. Wakeen M, Zimmerman SW. Association between human recombinant EPO and peripheral vascular disease in diabetic patients receiving peritoneal dialysis. Am J Kidney Dis 1998;32:488–93.
46. Aufricht C, Marik JL, Ettenger RB. Subcutaneous recombinant human erythropoietin in chronic renal allograft dysfunction. Pediatr Nephrol 1998;12:10–13.
47. Barosi G, Marchetti M, Liberato NL. Cost-effectiveness of recombinant human erythropoietin in the prevention of chemotherapy-induced anaemia. Br J Cancer 1998;78:781–7.
48. Csáki C, Ferencz T, Schuler D, Borsi JD. Recombinant human erythropoietin in the prevention of chemotherapy-induced anaemia in children with malignant solid tumors. Eur J Cancer 1998;34:364–7.
49. Dalton WS. Anemia in multiple myeloma and its management. Cancer Control 1998;5:S46–50.
50. Veys N. Use and abuse of erythropoietin. Tijdschr Geneeskd 1998;54:1315–22.
51. Cazzola M. How and when to use erythropoietin. Curr Opin Hematol 1998;5:103–8.
52. Beguin Y. A risk-benefit assessment of epoetin in the management of anaemia associated with cancer. Drug Saf 1998;19:269–82.
53. MacKinnon GE, Singla D. Epoetin alfa in chronic renal failure. P&T 1998;23:437–46.
54. Ohira N, Takasugi K, Takasugi N, Yorioka N, Ito T, Kushihata S, Takemasa A. Dose escalation induces tolerance to side-effects of erythropoietin in a patient with dialysis anaemia: case report. J Int Med Res 1998;26:102–5.
55. Kaufman JS, Reda DJ, Fye CL, Goldfarb DS, Henderson WG, Kleinman JG, Vaamonde CA. Subcutaneous compared with intravenous epoetin in patients receiving hemodialysis. New Engl J Med 1998;39:578–83.
56. Goodnough LT. Guidelines for the treatment of preoperative anaemia with epoetin. Biodrugs 1998;10:183–91.
57. Cumming MN, Sharkey IM, Sharp J, Plant ND, Coulthard MG. Subcutaneous erythropoietin alpha (Eprex) is more painful than erythropoietin beta (Recormon). Nephrol Dial Transplant 1998;13:817.
58. Veys N, Dhondt A, Lameire N. Pain at the injection site of subcutaneously administered erythropoietin: phosphate-buffered epoetin alpha compared to citrate-buffered epoetin alpha and epoetin beta. Clin Nephrol 1998;49:41–4.
59. Kang D-K, Yoon K-I, Han D-S. Acute effects of recombinant human erythropoietin on plasma levels of proendothelin-1 and endothelin-1 in haemodialysis patients. Nephrol Dial Transplant 1998;13:2877–83.
60. Ifudu O, Dawood M, Homel, P. Erythropoietin-induced elevation in blood pressure is immediate and dose dependent. Nephron 1998;79:486–7.
61. Tuskahara H, Hori C, Tsuchida S, Hiraoka, Fujisawa K, Mayumi M. Role of endothelin in erythropoietin-induced hypertension in rats. Nephron 1998;79:499–500.
62. Beccari M. Erythropoietin-induced epilepsy in hemodialysis patients? Nephron 1998;78:354.
63. Latini GM Rosati E. Transient neutropenia may be a risk of treating neonates with high doses of recombinant erythropoietin. Eur J Pediatr 1998;157:443–4.
64. Buemi M, Allegra A, Corica F, Cavallaro G, Aloisi C, Pettinato G, Frisina N. Rapid and transient lymphocytopenia after i.v. administration of high doses of human recombinant erythropoietin. Hematol Pathol Mol Hematol 1998;11:13–17.
65. Rigalleau V, Blanchetier V, Aparicio M, Baillet L, Sneed J, Dabadie H, Gin H. Erythropoietin can deteriorate glucose control in uraemic non-insulin-dependent diabetic patients. Diabetes Metab 1998;24:62–5.
66. Brown JA, Nehra A. Erythropoietin-induced recurrent veno-occlusive priapism associated with end-stage renal disease. Urology 1998;52: 328–30.
67. Ten Bokkel Huinink WW, De Swart CAM, Van Toorn DW, Morack G, Breed WPM, Hillen HFP, Van Der Hoeven JJM, Reed NS, Fairlamb DJ, Chan SYT, Godfey KA, Kristensen GB, Van Tinteren H, Ehmer B. Controlled multicentre study the influence of subcutaneous recombinant human erythropoietin on anaemia and transfusion dependency in patients with ovarian carcinoma treated with platinum-based chemotherapy. Med Oncol 1998;15:174–82.
68. Ramsey G. Hematopoietic growth factors and transfusion medicine. Transfus Med Rev 1998;12:195–205.
69. Archimbaud E, Thomas X. Thrombopoietic factors potentially useful in the treatment of acute leukemia. Leuk Res 1998;22:1155–64.

P.I. Folb

34 Intravenous infusions: solutions and emulsions

PLASMA SUBSTITUTES

Gelofusine

Gelofusine is a colloidal plasma volume expander used in the treatment of hypotension. It is prepared from bovine collagen. Severe *anaphylactoid reactions* after gelofusine occur with an incidence that has been reported at between 0.066 and 0.345% of cases. They are more common in those with known drug allergy and in men. The mechanism may be triggering of non-immune complement C3 activation by colloid particles in the gelatine formulation or by combination with components in the patient's blood (1[C]).

Hypotension has been described in a patient who received 500 ml of gelofusine during surgery for infrarenal abdominal aneurysm (2[c]). Within 5 minutes there was a significant fall in blood pressure, in the absence of surgical bleeding and ischemic changes on the electrocardiogram. There was no change in oxygenation. A further 500 ml of gelofusine was rapidly infused, with an additional fall in blood pressure to 50/30. Subsequently, after recovery, a small test dose (100 ml) of gelofusine reproduced the transient hypotension.

Hydroxyethyl starch *(SED-13, 992; SEDA-20, 311; SEDA-21, 351; SEDA-22, 371)*

Urinary system The potential effects of hydroxyethyl starch on renal function are controversial. Although hydroxyethyl starch appears to protect against ischemic damage in kidney transplants when added to kidney transplant perfusion solutions, it rarely causes *renal insufficiency*. Two healthy, full-term primigravidae with uneventful pregnancies and without a previous history of renal disease developed acute transient non-oliguric renal insufficiency after caesarean section under epidural anesthesia. During the procedure hydroxyethyl starch 6% (molecular weight 70 000 Da, molar substitution 0.5) was administered, 500 ml to one patient and 1000 ml to the other, for volume substitution after moderate blood loss (less than 800 ml). Acute non-oliguric renal insufficiency occurred on day 3 in the first patient and on day 2 in the second after caesarean section. Renal function recovered spontaneously. Hydroxyethyl starch is a known cause of histological renal lesions resembling osmotic nephrosis. These lesions involve the proximal and distal tubules. Severe changes in proximal tubules have been described in dogs after complete blood exchange with hydroxyethyl starch. It is believed that smaller molecules (molecular weight less than 50 000 Da) are excreted unchanged by glomerular filtration, leading to a large amount of osmotically active small molecules in the ultrafiltrate. As a result of reduced glomerular filtration in these patients, a highly viscous ultrafiltrate, complicated by tubular stasis and osmotic nephrosis of tubular cells, may have been caused by re-absorption of hydroxyethyl starch, resulting in acute renal insufficiency. In the two cases described in this report, and in the absence of either significant hypotension or oliguria, acute renal insufficiency due to purely pre-renal (hypovolemic) causes was improbable (3[c]).

Skin and appendages A 68-year-old woman developed marked and persistent *periocular swelling* after infusion of hydroxyethyl starch for sudden hearing loss. In the affected periocular skin and in normal skin lysosomal storage of hydroxyethyl starch could be detected with a specific antibody in histiocytes, endothelial cells, basal keratinocytes, and small nerves. In the periocular skin, there was more depo-

---

Side Effects of Drugs, Annual 23
J.K. Aronson, ed.

sition of hydroxyethyl starch, in addition to distinct xanthomatous changes and features of lymphoedema. In addition, there was a 50% reduction in the pH-dependent activity of the lysosomal α-glucosidase in cultured fibroblasts. This finding is consistent with a heterozygous glycogenosis type II (Pompe's disease) and it is potentially of pathogenetic relevance for the intralysosomal accumulation of hydroxyethyl starch. It is possible that α-glucosidase has a role in the elimination of tissue-stored hydroxyethyl starch. Patients with reduced α-glucosidase activity may be at risk of unusual adverse effects after extraordinary and prolonged tissue storage of hydroxyethyl starch, especially if it is infused in large quantities. There may be unusual lysosomal accumulation of hydroxyethyl starch in endothelial cells and macrophages in this situation, which may in turn account for the higher risk of pruritus and other unusual adverse effects (4[c]).

In a prospective, randomized, controlled, epidemiological comparison of the safety and tolerance of 6% hydroxyethyl starch (200/0.5) solution with Ringer's lactate solution, hydroxyethyl starch was associated with no more serious complications with the former than the latter. There was a greater than 10% incidence of *pruritus* in both groups (5[C]).

Immunological and hypersensitivity reactions The cause of adverse *immunological reactions* to hydroxyethyl starch, which are uncommon, is not clear. Of 1004 patients at least 14 days after starch administration, using a highly sensitive enzyme-linked immunoadsorbent assay technique, one had a low titer (1 : 10) of hydroxyethyl starch-reactive antibodies of the immunoglobulin M (IgM) class. Despite repeated infusions, no clinical reaction could be detected in this patient. The authors concluded that hydroxyethyl starch-reactive antibodies are extremely rare and that they do not necessarily cause anaphylaxis. This low antigenicity of hydroxyethyl starch might explain its excellent tolerance, compared with other plasma expanders (6[c]).

The reason for the tolerability of hydroxyethyl starch may be the raw material: hydroxyethyl starch is synthesized from amylopectin, a waxy starch derived from maize, by attaching hydroxyethyl groups to the starch molecule. Amylopectin is very similar to glycogen. Whereas glycogen occurs in the cells of warm-blooded organisms, amylopectin is the lower-branched analogue in cells of plant origin. The human immune system is replete with this molecular structure. This may explain why the hydroxyethyl starch-induced antibody is directed against the hydroxyethyl group and not against the starch molecule itself.

TOTAL PARENTERAL NUTRITION *(SED-13, 994; SEDA-20, 310; SEDA-21, 353; SEDA-22, 373)*

The benefits and safety of total parenteral nutrition have been considerably improved in recent years by innovative strategies, such as supplementation with medium-chain triglycerides, glutamine, or branch-chain amino acids. Increasing efforts have been made to avoid adverse effects associated with total parenteral nutrition, such as *hyperglycemia, central venous catheter infection,* and *hepatic dysfunction.* Major developments in the future are likely to be achieved with the identification of nutrients, hormones, or other active compounds that can positively influence outcome beyond the safe provision of 40 essential nutrients in proper amounts, which is what principally has been achieved to date (7[R]).

Endocrine, metabolic *Insulin secretion and sensitivity* Some children receiving total parenteral nutrition have abnormal glucose tolerance. When this was studied in 12 patients, aged 5.7–19 years, receiving cyclic nocturnal total parenteral nutrition, patients with normal glucose tolerance had an insulin response to intravenous glucose tolerance testing similar to that of normal persons of the same age (8[C]). Two patients with abnormal glucose tolerance had a reduced capacity to release insulin, whereas insulin sensitivity was unchanged in one of them. Patients with a limited capacity to release insulin, either constitutional or acquired, may not be able to produce enough insulin in these conditions and they may develop glucose intolerance during total parenteral nutrition. Insulin sensitivity was not a key factor in the alteration of glucose tolerance in this study.

Fatty acids Patients undergoing home parenteral nutrition for severe malabsorption or reduced oral intake may exhaust their stores of essential fatty acids, causing clinical effects, mainly dermatitis. In a comparative study of fatty acid profiles in 37 healthy control subjects and 56 patients receiving home parenteral nutrition, reduced small bowel length was associated with aggravated biochemical signs of essential fatty acid deficiency (9[C]). This applied to total *n*-6 fatty acids and not to *n*-3 fatty acids. There were skin problems in 25 of the 56 patients receiving home parenteral nutrition. Patients receiving home parenteral nutrition had biochemical signs of essential fatty acid deficiency. Parenteral fluids did not increase the concentration of essential fatty acids to values comparable with those of control subjects. However, 500 ml of 20% Intralipid once a week was sufficient to prevent an increase in the Holman index (an indicator that reflects optimum proportions of polyunsaturated fatty acids).

Mineral and fluid balance Since chronic renal insufficiency is frequently complicated by *rises in serum potassium, phosphate, and magnesium,* parenteral nutrition solutions used to treat malnourished patients with chronic renal insufficiency are usually prepared with little supplementation of these cations. Four patients with chronic renal insufficiency developed significant hypophosphatemia 3–5 days after starting parenteral nutrition. Other electrolyte abnormalities included *hypomagnesaemia* (1 patient) and *hypokalemia* (3 patients) (10[c]). It would appear that *hypophosphatemia* might be considered the most significant of the electrolyte risks in this clinical setting, and the electrolytes of such patients should be monitored closely when nutritional support is begun.

Increased excretion of calcium in the urine, *hypercalciuria,* often occurs in patients receiving total parenteral nutrition. The pathogenesis of this particular form of hypercalciuria is not readily explicable on the basis of endocrine or metabolic effects. After persistent hypercalciuria, osteopenia can develop, causing ‘metabolic bone disease’, pathological fractures, and immobilization. Hypercalciuria can also lead to nephrolithiasis and nephrocalcinosis, factors that can impair renal function. Intravenous chlorothiazide has been successfully used for its hypocalciuric effect, with remarkable effect over a period of 6 months in a 13-year-old child who had received total parenteral nutrition for 6 years. Calcium excretion and tubular reabsorption of phosphate returned to normal (11[c]). What is not clear from this study is whether the drug actually has a positive long-term beneficial effect on metabolic bone disease.

Increasing the inorganic phosphorus content of total parenteral nutrition formulas decreases hypercalciuria due to total parenteral nutrition in experimental animals and man. Urinary calcium excretion is significantly lower when patients receive higher inorganic phosphorus formulae, without changing the load of ultrafilterable calcium or filtered calcium, but significantly reducing fractional calcium excretion. There were no differences in serum concentrations of ionized calcium, parathyroid hormone, 25-hydroxycholecalciferol, 1,25-dihydroxycholecalciferol, or urinary cAMP between different treatments with inorganic phosphorus formulae. Thus, increasing the inorganic phosphorus content of the total parenteral nutrition formula reduces urinary calcium content by increasing renal tubular calcium resorption. This effect is not due to alterations in the parathormone-1,25-dihydroxycholecalciferol axis, but more likely reflects a direct action of inorganic phosphorus on the renal tubules (12[c]).

Micronutrient deficiency *Selenium deficiency* caused by total parenteral nutrition has resulted in heart failure (13[c]).

A 38-year-old man with Crohn’s disease had been receiving total parenteral nutrition for 16 years, from the age of 22 years. After 6 years of parenteral nutrition he developed heart failure and ventricular extra beats associated with selenium deficiency. A serum concentration of 62 μg/l was measured (reference range 80–230 μg/l). Selenium supplements improved his condition but did not normalize left ventricular function. He was given selenium supplements and was free from heart failure for 11 years, but the echocardiographic findings gradually deteriorated and he died of congestive heart failure at the age of 38 years. At autopsy, his heart showed linear fibrosis in the interventricular septum, confined to the right side. The subendocardial region and the right ventricular free wall were relatively spared.

The authors proposed that the cardiac changes in this case were characteristic of the cardiomyopathy related to selenium deficiency. Once fully developed, left ventricular dysfunction may be irreversible, even after the use of selenium supplements.

Selenium deficiency has also been reported to have caused a myopathy (14[c]).

A 35-year-old man developed selenium deficiency after repeated administration of total parenteral nutrition for 13 years. The deficiency syndrome manifested as muscle weakness but not pain in both arms and legs, especially the thighs. There was a dominant proximal muscle weakness and reduced deep tendon reflexes. There was a progressive rise in serum CK activity, mainly of the MM type. Serum aldolase and lactate dehydrogenase were significantly raised. Peripheral muscle electromyography showed a myogenic pattern of short duration and amplitude. Muscle biopsy showed myopathic changes, with mild variation in size, regeneration of muscle fibers and muscle cell necrosis. There was no infiltration of inflammatory cells. The serum concentration of selenium was very low (1 μg/l compared with the reference range of 97–160 μg/l). After treatment for 3 months with selenium infusions the muscle weakness began to resolve and the CK activity improved. The muscle weakness did not disappear completely and serum selenium concentrations did not return to normal for more than 4 months after treatment. Eventually, after about 5 months, there was virtually complete resolution of the muscle weakness and serum CPK abnormality

Selenium is a constituent of glutathione peroxidase, an enzyme that catalyses the oxidation of reduced glutathione by hydrogen peroxide and other hydroperoxides to form oxidized glutathione and water. In addition, glutathione peroxidase reduces phospholipid hydroperoxide in cell membranes. Selenium deficiency, as well as glutathione depletion, reduces resistance against oxidative stress, resulting in lipid peroxidation. Selenium via glutathione peroxidase may be one of the key mediators in response to oxidative stress. Cardiomyopathy and hyperglycemia are additional possible complications of selenium deficiency, but they were not noted in this case.

Choline deficiency developed in a 41-year-old woman with advanced cervical cancer who underwent prolonged total parenteral nutrition, manifesting with rising liver function test abnormalities (15[c]). She became jaundiced and complained of nausea and vomiting. There was steady improvement with oral choline supplementation, 3 g/day, and with an oral glutamine supplement 15 g/day. There was a 45% improvement in serum choline concentration over baseline.

Amino acids In septicemic patients with multi-organ dysfunction syndrome serum carnitine concentrations are in the reference range, and they remain unchanged over treatment for 10 days with parenteral nutrition without carnitine supplementation. This has been established in a study of 28 adult septicemic patients, whose mean APACHE II on admission was 17. Of these patients, ten had septicemia with multi-organ dysfunction syndrome and 18 had uncomplicated septicemia. There were no differences in patients given long-chain triglycerides (16) and a 1 : 1 mixture of long-chain and medium-chain triglycerides (12 patients). It does not appear from these findings that carnitine deficiency plays a significant role in the pathogenesis of multi-organ dysfunction syndrome complicating septicemia, whether or not parenteral nutrition is given in the acute phase of the illness (16[C]).

Hematological To test the hypothesis that infection facilitates activation of coagulation during parenteral nutrition, healthy subjects were injected intravenously with endotoxin (2 ng/kg) after they had received either standard parenteral nutrition for 1 week (n = 7) or normal enteral feeding (n = 8) (17[c]). Compared with enteral feeding, parenteral nutrition was associated with selectively enhanced activation of the coagulation system (plasma concentrations of thrombin-antithrombin III complexes) during endotoxemia. Activation of the fibrinolytic system (plasminogen activator activity, tissue-type plasminogen activator, plasminogen activator inhibitor type 1) proceeded similarly in both groups. Bacterial infection, a common complication in patients receiving parenteral nutrition, may aggravate the occurrence of another common complication (venous thrombosis) by synergistic stimulation of the coagulation system. Lipids were not included in the parenteral nutrition in this study, and it is possible that the shift towards thrombogenesis may be even more pronounced in patients receiving parenteral nutrition containing lipids.

Liver, biliary tract Intestinal transplantation is combined with liver transplantation in 46% of cases, because of terminal liver failure (18[cr]). Of 78 patients who had received parenteral nutrition for more than 2 years and/or had short bowel syndrome and could not be weaned from parenteral nutrition (12 patients), 58 developed chronic *cholestasis* and 37 developed one or more severe liver complications (*serum bilirubin concentration 60 μmol/l, factor V (proaccelerin) 50%, portal hypertension, encephalopathy, ascites, bleeding from the gastrointestinal tract,* or *histological findings consisting of extensive fibrosis and cirrhosis*) after 6 (3–132) months and 17 (2–155) months respectively. Liver disease was responsible for deaths in 6.5% of the patients (22% of deaths).

The high incidence of cholestatic liver disease associated with long-term parenteral nutrition in infants who have undergone major gut resection is linked to high plasma concentrations of phytosterols, compounds that resemble cholesterol but have an alkylated side-chain (19[R]). The phytosterols that accumulate in patients receiving parenteral nutrition are derived from the soya oil and/or soya lecithin that is used to make the intravenous lipid emulsion. There is a strong association between phytosterolemia and cholestatic liver disease, which suggests a possible causative association. Experiments in neonatal piglets have suggested that phytosterols, given without any of the other components of parenteral nutrition, can reduce bile flow. The authors suggested that increasing the content of phytosterols in cell membranes may interfere with the function of important transport proteins involved in the secretion of bile. If a 20% lipid emulsion is infused at a rate of more than 50 ml/kg/week into a premature neonate who has had a major gut resection, and if this rate of infusion is continued for 2 months, the plasma phytosterol concentration is likely to rise to a value close to 25% of the total plasma sterols. The mechanism of the liver injury and effect on bile flow caused by total parenteral nutrition is likely to be more complex than a simple sterol-induced change in membrane fluidity. Intravenous lipid emulsions that do not contain phytosterols may be safer.

In a retrospective study conducted to determine the incidence of cholestasis and liver failure in 42 patients with intestinal resection in the neonatal period who subsequently became dependent on parenteral nutrition support, the effect of various associated clinical factors on the incidence and severity of cholestasis was determined (20[C]). Cholestasis developed in 28 while they were receiving parenteral nutrition. In 21 patients, the raised direct bilirubin concentration returned to normal while they continued to receive parenteral nutrition. Seven patients progressed to liver failure. Patients without cholestasis had been dependent on parenteral nutrition for longer than patients with cholestasis. It was clear from this study that cholestasis in neonates with intestinal resection is not simply a function of the duration of exposure to intravenous nutrition. The results instead suggested that infection early in life, when the developing liver may be uniquely sensitive to cholestatic injury and additionally stressed by intravenous nutrition, may play an important role.

Immunological and hypersensitivity reactions *Hypersensitivity reactions* have been reported infrequently in children receiving parenteral nutrition. The length of exposure before the reaction, the severity of the response, and the component responsible are variable. An anaphylactic reaction occurred in a 4-year-old boy when parenteral nutrition was resumed after a 5-day interruption (21[c]). The diagnosis of the underlying condition was presumed small bowel obstruction, with a previous history of surgery and radiotherapy for Wilms' tumor. The authors considered the reaction to have been an IgE-mediated allergic response, although the causative agent was not identified with certainty. They raised the question of whether a history of cancer or anticancer therapy may modulate immune function, placing children at greater risk of hypersensitivity reactions.

Immune function has been studied in ten surgical infants (aged under 6 months) requiring parenteral nutrition in two consecutive phases: (a) after 31 days with no enteral feeding (total parenteral nutrition); and (b) after 4.7 days from the addition to parenteral nutrition of small volumes of enteral feeding. Host bactericidal activity against coagulase-negative staphylococci, measured by an in vitro whole blood model, was lowest in the patients who received total parenteral nutrition, and it increased significantly after the addition of small enteral feeds, approaching the levels measured in controls. Production of tumor necrosis factor-α (TNF-α) was low during total parenteral nutrition and rose significantly after the addition of small enteral feeds in patients on parenteral nutrition. The increase in killing of coagulase-negative staphylococci after the addition of small enteral feeds correlated significantly with the duration of enteral feeding. The mechanism causing impaired immune function during total parenteral nutrition is not known, and it is probably multifactorial. Neither is it understood how small additional enteral feeds affect host bactericidal activity (22[C]).

Infections Evidence that lipids are associated with an increase risk of clinically documented infections is sparse. In a prospective comparison in 512 patients with hematological malignancies who were undergoing bone-marrow transplantation, the incidences of bacteremia and fungemia during the first month after the transplant were studied. The patients were randomly assigned to receive 6–8% (low dose) or 25–30% (standard dose) of total energy as a 20% lipid emulsion. An adaptive randomization scheme, stratified for various treatments and transplant type, ensured that confounding treatment variables did not differ between the groups. Of 482 evaluable patients, 55 in the standard-dose group developed bacteremia or fungemia compared with 54 in the low-dose group. There was no association between the incidence of bacteremia or fungemia and intravenous lipid. Similar results were obtained when the results were analysed according to intention-to-treat, when bacterial or fungal infections at all sites were included, and when the observation period was extended to 60 days. These results suggest that moderate amounts of intravenous lipid rich in linoleic acid are not associated with an increased incidence of bacterial or fungal infections in patients undergoing bone-marrow transplantation and receiving total parenteral nutrition (23[C]).

In infants of very low birth weight, *fungal colonization* and the association between fungal colonization and systemic fungal diseases was significantly linked to prolonged administration of antibiotics, parenteral nutrition, and Intralipid emulsion (24[C]). Of 116 infants with birth weights under 1500 g, fungal colonization was detected in 25, of whom 17 developed colonization by 2 weeks of life. *Candida albicans* (61%) and *Candida parapsilosis* (29%) were the two most common organisms. The rectum (76%) was the most frequent site of colonization. Cultures were taken from the oropharynx, rectum, skin (groin and axilla), urine, and endotracheal aspirates in the first 24 h after birth and weekly thereafter. There was an association between colonization and subsequent fungemia in one infant, representing 4% of colonized infants. It was also noted that although fungal colonization represents a risk factor for invasive candidiasis in infants of very low birth weight, candidiasis in this population is not invariably associated with prior colonization. Factors other than fungal colonization can also contribute to the occurrence of invasive candidiasis.

In a study of the independent risk factors for nosocomial coagulase-negative staphylococcal bacteremia among neonates of very low birth weight, after adjusting for the severity of the underlying illness, there was a significant association between coagulase-negative staphylococcal bacteremia and exposure during hospitalization to intravenous lipids (25[C]). The study was conducted in 590 consecutively admitted neonates with birth weights under 1500 g, in two neonatal intensive care units, with a case-control study of 74 cases of coagulase-negative staphylococcal bacteremia and 74 pairs of matched controls. The independent risk factors for bacteremia were intravenous lipids (odds ratio 9.4), mechanical ventilation (odds ratio 2.0), and short peripheral venous catheters (odds ratio 2.6). It would appear that exposure to intravenous lipids at any time during hospitalization remains and has possibly become an increasingly important risk factor for coagulase-negative staphylococcal bacteremia. In neonates of very low birth weight 85% of these bacteremias are now attributable to lipid therapy. In contrast, the relative importance of intravenous catheters as independent risk factors has declined. Mechanical ventilation in the week before bacteremia has emerged as a risk factor for bacteremia.

Local complications *Catheter-related complications* A preterm infant developed total parenteral nutrition ascites after infusion through a low umbilical vein catheter. In a follow-up study of eight patients, all of whom developed hypotension and ascites, each had an umbilical vein catheter overlying the liver on plain film. Catheters had been in place for a mean of 8.9 days before extravasation. Ultrasound in four patients showed hepatic parenchymal damage around the umbilical vein catheter tip. Total parenteral nutrition given through abnormally placed umbilical vein catheters is not without risk, and correct placing of the catheter is paramount (26[c]).

Extravasation Two cases of extravasation of parenteral nutrition in adult patients have been reported (27[cr]). In both cases there was an intense inflammatory reaction after the incident as a result of tissue injury. Each was successfully managed with multiple subcutaneous applications of chondroitin sulfatase, an enzyme that is very similar to the mucopolysaccharide hyaluronidase that depolymerizes chondroitin sulfate. There were no sequelae to the extravasation. The exact mechanism of tissue toxicity by extravasated parenteral nutrition is not understood, but it seems to be related to osmolarity, pH, and ions. The osmolarity of parenteral nutrition is an important factor that contributes to the toxicity of extravasation. Special care should be taken when peripheral parenteral nutrition solutions of high osmolarity (1000–1700 mOsm/l) are used. The authors recommended that 600–900 mOsm/l should not be exceeded. Fat emulsions are harmless to the tissues if extravasated. The area affected may become blistered, with darkening of the skin, or ischemic, depending on whether the skin thickness is partially or fully damaged. In children, extravasation can have devastating consequences, such as deep necrosis, amputation, severe sequelae in the affected limb, or other complications, such as subdural collection of fat emulsion, liporrhachis, and acute abdomen after intra-abdominal extravasation. Children are at special risk, because very young infants and children are unable to communicate the pain that results from the pressure of extravasated fluid. Other individuals in this situation are comatose patients, those under general anesthesia, and patients who are being resuscitated. Other risk factors that predispose to extravasation are related to venepuncture technique, state of the patient, and medication delivery.

Risk factors In a prospective study of the effects of parenteral medium- chain and long-chain triglycerides on lymphocyte subpopulations and function in severely malnourished patients with acquired immunodeficiency syndrome (AIDS), long-chain triglycerides were compared with a balanced emulsion of long-chain and medium-chain triglycerides (28[C]). Administration was over 6 days. With 2 g/kg/day of lipids, long-chain triglycerides cause significant abnormalities in lymphocyte function, expressed as a reduction in phytohemagglutinin A response. Such abnormalities were not observed with long-chain plus medium-chain triglycerides, which reduced IgM and increased the C3 fraction.

Interactions Patients treated with *interleukin*-2 (IL-2) develop profound anorexia, malaise, loss of energy, mucositis, nausea, and vomiting, which may contribute to poor nutrition. In 21 patients who took a normal diet (controls) and 16 who received total parenteral nutrition during IL-2 treatment, total parenteral nutrition improved serum calcium and potassium concentrations, particularly during spontaneous diuresis after completion of IL-2 treatment (29[C]). Unexpectedly, total parenteral nutrition reduced the frequency and severity of cholestatic jaundice caused by IL-2, the pathophysiological basis of which is unknown. A brief period of total parenteral nutrition during IL-2 treatment was well tolerated and it corrected the calorie and protein malnutrition. Total parenteral nutrition also improved control of serum electrolytes, particularly calcium, potassium, and magnesium concentrations, although there was more marked hypophosphatemia during IL-2 treatment. The reason for this change is not clear.

Warfarin resistance Warfarin resistance has been described in a patient with short bowel syndrome receiving intravenous lipid (30[c]). Up to 20 mg of warfarin was given daily without increase in the INR. Although intravenous lipid has been reported anecdotally to account for warfarin resistance, this report suggests that the more likely explanation was the reduced surface area for drug absorption secondary to total surgical removal of the patient's duodenum and gastrojejunostomy. However, several other reports have refuted a correlation between warfarin resistance and short bowel syndrome. Conversely, warfarin resistance has occurred secondary to intravenous lipid administration in a patient with only 12 cm of small bowel; the patient had been given oral warfarin while he received daily Intralipid fat emulsion to prevent fatty acid deficiency (31[c]).

CATHETERS

Cardiovascular *Superior vena cava thrombosis* has been described after frequent central venous catheterization and total parenteral nutrition (32[c]). The possible etiological factors included the catheter material, catheter-related sepsis, endothelial trauma, osmotic injury, and hypercoagulability. Although thrombosis of the great veins of the thorax is rare, it is life-threatening, characterized clinically by swelling of the head, upper limbs, and torso, and on chest X-ray by mediastinal widening. Confirmation of thrombosis is best achieved by contrast venography or contrast-enhanced CT scan. In this patient there was eventual partial recovery.

Respiratory The clinical differentiation of *chylothorax* from *leakage of parenteral nutrition into the pleural space* can be difficult.

However, in one case the diagnosis of leakage of parenteral nutrition fluid was made by additional tests of electrolytes, showing very high potassium (11.3 mmol/l) and glucose (128 mmol/l) concentrations, ruling out chylothorax (33[c]).

Infections The incidence and type of complications related to central venous catheters in 71 patients with AIDS have been studied and compared with two control groups of patients without AIDS (65 immunocompromised patients and 14 immunocompetent patients receiving home total parenteral nutrition) (34[C]). Three groups of patients requiring permanent venous access for administration of virustatics and/or total parenteral nutrition were investigated retrospectively. The Port-A-Cath system of implantation was used in all cases. Catheter-related mortality was low in all groups (0–1%). Infectious complications could not be related to the degree of immunosuppression (CD4+ lymphocyte counts or white blood cell count). The incidence of both infectious and non-infectious complications was significantly higher in the immunocompetent subjects than in the others, probably because of the type of medium used and/or differences in handling of the catheter. The overall conclusion was that central venous catheters are safe and well tolerated by patients with AIDS and that they present no greater risk than they do to other categories of patients, regardless of levels of immune competence. This conclusion would need to be regarded with some caution, given the retrospective nature of the study and the imbalance in the number of subjects studied in each category. However, it would appear that totally implantable central venous catheters are safe and well tolerated by patients with AIDS, no differently to other immunocompromised patients and immunocompetent patients.

REFERENCES

1. Laxenaire MC, Charpentier C, Feldman L. Reactions anaphylactoídes aux substituts colloidaux du plasma: incidence, facteurs de risque, mecanismes. Enquete prospective multicentrique Francaise. Groupe Francais d'Etude de la Tolerance des Substituts Plasmatiques. Ann Fr Anesth Réanim 1994;13:301–10.
2. Walker SR, MacSweeney ST. Plasma expanders used to treat or prevent hypotension can themselves cause hypotension. Postgrad Med J 1998;74: 492–4.
3. Dickenmann MJ, Filipovic M, Schneider MC, Brunner FP. Hydroxyethylstarch-associated transient acute renal failure after epidural anaesthesia for labour analgesia and caesarean section. Nephrol Dial Transplant 1998;13:2706.
4. Kiehl P, Metze D, Kresse H, Reimann, Kraft D, Kapp A. Decreased activity of acid alpha-glucosidase in a patient with persistent periocular swelling after infusions of hydroxyethyl starch. Br J Dermatol 1998;138:672–7.
5. Bothner U, Georgieff M, Vogt NH. Assessment of the safety and tolerance of 6% hydroxyethyl starch (200/0.5) solution: a randomized, controlled epidemiology study. Anesth Analg 1998;86: 850–5.
6. Dieterich H-J, Kraft D, Sirtl C, Laubenthal H, Schimetta W, Polz W, Gerlach E, Peter K. Hydroxyethyl starch antibodies in humans: incidence and clinical relevance. Anesth Analg 1998;86: 1123–6.
7. McCowen KC, Chan S, Bistrian BR. Total parenteral nutrition. Curr Opin Gastroenterol 1998; 14:157–63.
8. Lienhardt A, Rakotoambinina B, Colomb V, Souissi S, Sadoun E, Goulet O, Robert J-J, Ricour C. Insulin secretion and sensitivity in children on cyclic total parenteral nutrition. J Parenter Enter Nutr 1998;22:382–6.
9. Jeppesen PB, Hoy C-E, Mortensen PB. Essential fatty acid deficiency in patients receiving home parenteral nutrition. Am J Clin Nutr 1998;68:126–33.
10. Duerksen DR, Papineau N. Electrolyte abnormalities in patients with chronic renal failure receiving parenteral nutrition. J Parenter Enter Nutr 1998;22:102–4.
11. Muller D, Eggert P, Krawinkel M. Hypercalciuria and nephrocalcinosis in a patient receiving long-term parenteral nutrition: the effect of intravenous chlorothiazide. J Pediatr Gastroenterol Nutr 1998;27:106–10.
12. Berkelhammer C, Wood RJ, Sitrin MD. Inorganic phosphorus reduces hypercalciuria during total parenteral nutrition by enhancing renal tubular calcium absorption. J Parenter Enter Nutr 1998;22:142–6.
13. Inoko M, Konishi T, Matsusue S, Kobashi Y. Midmural fibrosis of left ventricle due to selenium deficiency. Circulation 1998;98:2638–9.
14. Tsuda K, Yokoyama Y, Morita M, Nakazawa Y, Onishi S. Selenium and chromium deficiency during long-term home total parenteral nutrition in chronic idiopathic intestinal pseudoobstruction. Nutrition 1998;14:291–5.
15. Hager L. Choline deficiency and TPN associated liver dysfunction: a case report. Nutrition 1998;14:60–2.

16. Montero JG, Leyba CO, Jiminez FJJ, Villar JM, VegaMDF, Garmendia JLG. L-carnitine levels in critical septicemic patients with parenteral nutrition. Nutr Hosp 1998;13:77–80.
17. Van Der Poll T, Levi M, Braxton CC, Coyle SM, Roth M, Ten Cate JW, Lowry SF. Parenteral nutrition facilitates activation of coagulation but not of fibrinolysis during human endotoxaemia. J Infect Dis 1998;177:793–5.
18. Cavicchi M, Crenn P, Beau P, Degott C, Boutron MC, Messing B. Severe liver complications associated with long-term parenteral nutrition are dependent on lipid parenteral input. Transpl Proc 1998;30:2547.
19. Clayton PT, Whitfield P, Iyer K. The role of phytosterols in the pathogenesis of liver complications of pediatric parenteral nutrition. Nutrition 1998;14:158–64.
20. Sondheimer JM, Asturias E, Cadnapaphornchai M. Infection and cholestasis in neonates with intestinal resection and long-term parenteral nutrition. J Pediatr Gastroenterol Nutr 1998;27:131–7.
21. Market AD, Lew DB, Schropp KP, Hak EB. Parenteral nutrition-associated anaphylaxis in a 4-year-old child. J Pediatr Gastroenterol Nutr 1998;26:229–31.
22. Okada Y, Klein N, Van Saene HKF, Pierro A. Small volumes of enteral feedings normalise immune function in infants receiving parenteral nutrition. J Pediatr Surg 1998;33:16–19.
23. Lenssen P, Bruemmer BA, Bowden RA, Gooley T, Aker SN, Mattson D. Intravenous lipid dose and incidence of bacteremia and fungemia in patients undergoing bone marrow transplantation. Am J Clin Nutr 1998;67:927–33.
24. Huang Y-C, Chung-Chen LI, Tzou-Yien Lin, Rey-In Lien, Yi-Hong C, Jue-Lan W, Chuen Hsueh. Association of fungal colonization and invasive disease in very low birth weight infants. Pediatr Infect Dis J 1998;17:819–22.
25. Avila-Figueroa C, Goldmann DA, Richardson DK, Gray JE, Ferrari A, Freeman J. Intravenous lipid emulsions are the major determinant of coagulase-negative staphylococcal bacteremia in very low birth weight newborns. Pediatr Infect Dis J 1998;17:10–17.
26. Coley BD, Seguin J, Cordero L, Hogan MJ, Rosenberg E, Reber K. Neonatal total parenteral nutrition ascites from liver erosion by umbilical vein catheters. Pediatr Radiol 1998;28:923–7.
27. Gil M-A, Mateu J. Treatment of extravasation from parenteral nutrition solution. Ann Pharmacother 1998;32:51–5.
28. Gelas P, Cotte L, Poitevin- F, Pichard C, Leverve X, Barnoud D, Leclercq P, Touraine-Moulin F, Trepo C, Bouletreau P. Effect of parenteral medium- and long-chain triglycerides on lymphocytes subpopulations and functions in patients with acquired immunodeficiency syndrome: a prospective study. J Parenter Enter Nutr 1998;22:67–71.
29. Samlowski WE, Wiebke G, McMurry M, Mori M, Ward JH. Effects of total parenteral nutrition (TPN) during high-dose interleukin-2 treatment for metastatic cancer. J Immunother 1998;21:65–74.
30. Brophy DF, Ford SL, Crouch MA. Warfarin resistance in a patient with short bowel syndrome. Pharmacotherapy 1998;18:646–9.
31. Lutomski DM, Palascak JE, Bower RH. Warfarin resistance associated with intravenous lipid administration. J Parenter Enter Nutr 1987;11: 316–18.
32. Muckart DJJ, Neijenhuis PA, Madiba TE. Superior vena caval thrombosis complicating central venous catheterisation and total parenteral nutrition. S Afr J Surg 1998;36:48–51.
33. Wolthuis A, Landewe RBM, Theunissen PHMH, Westerhuis LWJJM. Chylothorax or leakage of total parenteral nutrition? Eur Resp J 1998;12:1233–5.
34. Consten ECJ, Van Lanschot JJB, Movig FM, Rijsman L, Oosting J, Danner SA. Safety and complications of central venous catheters in AIDS patients. Clin Microbiol Infect 1998;4:508–13.

K. Peerlinck and J. Vermylen

35 Drugs affecting blood coagulation, fibrinolysis, and hemostasis

COUMARIN CONGENERS

(SED-13, 1033; SEDA-20, 313; SEDA-21, 358; SEDA-22, 386)

Interactions In a prospective case-control study, designed to determine causes of INRs greater than 6.0 in an out-patient anticoagulant unit, there was a clear dose-dependent association between the use of *paracetamol (acetaminophen)* and having an INR greater than 6.0 (1[C]). The authors studied 93 patients with INRs over 6.0 (cases) and 196 patients with INRs of 1.7–3.3 (controls) during warfarin therapy. The likelihood of an INR greater than 6.0 increased from an odds ratio of 3.5 for doses of 2275–4549 mg per week, to 6.9 for doses 4550–9099 mg per week, to a 10-fold increase at a dose of over 9100 mg per week.

Potentiation of the effect of warfarin by *danshen* (the root of *Salvia miltiorrhiza*), a widely used traditional Chinese herbal medicine, particularly for cardiovascular complaints, has been described in a 62-year-old man with a mechanical mitral valve prosthesis (2[c]).

HEPARINS *(SED-13, 1028; SEDA-20, 313; SEDA-21, 358; SEDA-22, 386)*

Hematological An FDA Health Advisory warning was issued in December 1997 after a total of 30 cases of *spinal hematoma* had been reported in patients undergoing spinal or epidural anesthesia while receiving low molecular weight heparin perioperatively. In the European literature the risk of spinal hematoma in patients receiving low molecular weight heparin was not considered clinically significant. In Europe low molecular weight heparin is given once a day and with a smaller total daily dose; this enables the placement (and removal) of needles and catheters during periods of reduced low molecular weight heparin activity. Identification of further risk factors is difficult, owing to the rarity of spinal hematoma. However, several possible risk factors have been suggested: about 75% of the patients were elderly women, in 22 patients an epidural catheter was used, and in 17 patients the first dose of low molecular weight heparin was administered while the catheter was indwelling; 12 patients received antiplatelet drugs and/or warfarin in addition to low molecular weight heparin (3[R]). The authors formulated recommendations for minimizing the risk of spinal hematoma, including using the smallest effective dose of low molecular weight heparin perioperatively, delaying heparin therapy as long as possible postoperatively, and removing catheters when anticoagulant activity is low. Furthermore, they warned against the combination of low molecular weight heparin with antiplatelet drugs or oral anticoagulants.

DRUGS THAT ALTER PLATELET FUNCTION

Abciximab *(SED-13, 1039; SEDA-21, 359;SEDA-22, 387)*

Another case of profound *thrombocytopenia* after abciximab has been reported, but with a delayed onset (6 days after abciximab therapy), whereas the previously reported cases occurred within 24 hours (4[c]). The authors speculated that preceding treatment with

Side Effects of Drugs, Annual 23
J.K. Aronson, ed.

methylprednisolone may have delayed the onset of thrombocytopenia.

Clopidogrel *(SED-13, 1039; SEDA-20, 314; SEDA-21, 359; SEDA-22, 387)*

In a review of the antiplatelet effects of clopidogrel, adverse effects were also reviewed (5[R]). Major *bleeding* seems to be rare with clopidogrel and it does not cause bone-marrow toxicity. Other adverse effects of clopidogrel include *pruritus* and *urticaria.*

Ticlopidine *(SED-13, 1039; SEDA-20, 314; SEDA-21, 359; SEDA-22, 387)*

Respiratory A case of *bronchiolitis obliterans organizing pneumonia* associated with ticlopidine has been reported (6[c]).

A 76-year-old non-smoking woman with giant-cell arteritis who had a normal chest radiograph was taking prednisone 45 mg/day and ticlopidine 250 mg bd for persistence of cloudy vision. After 1 month of ticlopidine therapy, she developed increasing dyspnea and a pruritic rash. Chest radiography showed diffuse interstitial infiltrates, predominantly affecting the peripheries of both lungs. Transbronchial biopsy showed widening of the alveolar fields with a mixed inflammatory infiltrate. Ticlopidine was withdrawn; prednisone was continued in the same dosage. Her symptoms completely resolved within 3 months and her chest radiograph normalized within 5 months.

Hematological In a review of the antiplatelet effects of ticlopidine, adverse effects were also reviewed (5[R]). Major *bleeding* seems to be rare with ticlopidine. Ticlopidine can be associated with *neutropenia,* and severe neutropenia occurs in about 1% of treated patients. Neutropenia typically occurs in the first few months after the start of therapy, but is seen infrequently in the first 2–3 weeks.

Another serious and often fatal side effect of ticlopidine is *thrombotic thrombocytopenic purpura,* 60 cases of which have been reviewed (7[R]). Ticlopidine had been prescribed for less than 1 month in 80% of the patients, and platelet counts were normal within 2 weeks of the onset of thrombotic thrombocytopenic purpura in most patients. Mortality rates were higher among patients who were not treated with plasmapheresis than among those who underwent plasmapheresis (50% compared with 24%). The authors concluded that the onset of ticlopidine-associated thrombotic thrombocytopenic purpura is difficult to predict, despite close monitoring of platelet counts.

THROMBOLYTIC AGENTS

(SED-13, 1035; SEDA-20, 314; SEDA-21, 359; SEDA-22, 387)

Secondary *intraventricular hemorrhage* has been described in two patients who received intraventricular tissue-type plasminogen activator to hasten the lysis of intraventricular hemorrhage (8[c]).

ANTIFIBRINOLYTIC DRUGS

(SED-13, 1060; SEDA-20, 314)

Repeated *anaphylactic reactions* to aprotinin in fibrin sealant have been described (9[c]). Fibrin tissue adhesives are efficient in many surgical and endoscopic procedures. They contain fractions of pooled human plasma and human thrombin and small amounts of aprotinin for the prevention of early fibrinolysis in vivo. In the described case repeated instillation of fibrin sealant resulted in repeated anaphylactic reactions, and aprotinin-specific antibodies could be detected.

REFERENCES

1. Hylek MH, Heiman H, Skates SJ, Sheehan MA, Singer DE. Acetaminophen and other risk factors for excessive warfarin anticoagulation. J Am Med Assoc 1998;279:657–62.
2. Izzat MB, Yim APC, El-Zufari MH. A taste of Chinese medicine! Ann Thorac Surg 1998;66:941–2.
3. Horlocker TT, Wedel DJ. Spinal and epidural blockade and perioperative low molecular weight heparin: smooth sailing on the Titanic. Anesth Analg 1998;86:1153–6.
4. Schwartz S, Schwab S, Steiner H-H, Hacke W. Secondary hemorrhage after intraventricular fibrinolysis: a cautionary note: a report of two cases. Neurosurgery 1998;42:659–63.
5. Sharis PJ, Cannon CP, Localzo J. The antiplatelet effects of ticlopidine and clopidogrel. Ann Intern Med 1998;129:394–405.
6. Alonso-Martinez JL, Elejalde-Guerna JI, Larrinaga-Linero D. Bronchiolitis obliterans-organizing pneumonia caused by ticlopidine. Ann Intern Med 1998;129:71–2.

7. Bennett CL, Weinberg PD, Rozenberg-Ben-Dror K, Yarnold PR, Kwaan HC, Green D. Thrombotic thrombocytopenic purpura associated with ticlopidine. A review of 60 cases. Ann Intern Med 1998;128:541–4.
8. Jenkins LA, Lau S, Crawford M, Keung Y-K. Delayed profound thrombocytopenia after c7E3 Fab (abciximab) therapy. Circulation 1998;97:1214–15.
9. Scheule AM, Beierlein W, Lorenz H, Ziemer G. Repeated anaphylactic reactions to aprotinin in fibrin sealant. Gastrcintest Endosc 1998;48:83–5.

H.J. de Silva

36 Gastrointestinal drugs

ANTACIDS *(SED-13, 1066; SEDA-20, 316)*

There is an unsubstantiated belief that calcium-containing antacids cause a *rebound increase in gastric acid secretion* that is more intense than with other antacids. This was thought to be due to absorption of calcium, the resultant hypercalcemia leading to increased acid secretion. This has been investigated in two trials. One (1^C) was an open, randomized, cross-over study in 12 healthy volunteers who were given calcium carbonate and magnesium carbonate (Rennie) and hydrotalcite (Talcid). The other (2^C) was a double-blind, cross-over trial in 12 healthy volunteers who were given placebo, Maalox liquid, and Rennie liquid. All the antacids used had similar efficacy and there was no evidence of acid rebound with the calcium-containing antacid.

Severe *hypermagnesemia* has been attributed to magnesium hydroxide (3^c).

A 42-year-old Hispanic woman with normal renal function took magnesium hydroxide (as milk of magnesia) 30 ml each night with Maalox 30 ml tds for about 5 days for abdominal pain and constipation. She developed confusion, vomiting, hypothermia, hypotension, and abdominal distention. Additional medications included lithium carbonate, chlorpromazine, benzatropine, and docusate sodium. Her serum magnesium concentration was 4.5 mmol/l (reference range 0.7–1.0). This was treated with intravenous calcium gluconate and fluids. At surgery for abdominal distention she was found to have adhesions from a previous oophorectomy. On the second postoperative day she developed a cardiac dysrhythmia and died in asystole.

ANTIEMETICS

Cisapride *(SED-13, 1067; SEDA-20, 316; SEDA-21, 361; SEDA-22 389)*

Gastrointestinal The effect of cisapride in a dose of 10 mg bd on gastroduodenal reflux and gall bladder motility has been assessed in 77 patients with gallstones in a double-blind, placebo-controlled trial (4^C). Cisapride increased gall bladder motility but did not have any effect on gastroduodenal reflux. *Diarrhea, abdominal cramps,* and *increased bladder frequency* were its common adverse effects.

A multicenter trial in 353 patients assessed the efficacy and tolerance of sodium alginate (four 10 ml sachets a day) compared with cisapride (5 mg qds) in the symptomatic treatment of uncomplicated gastro-esophageal reflux without severe esophagitis (5^C). Sodium alginate, which costs less than cisapride, was more effective in relieving symptoms. Adverse effects were rare and not serious. Constipation was the most common adverse effect of alginate while *diarrhea* was the commonest adverse effect of cisapride.

Risk factors *Children* The clinical use of cisapride and its risk:benefit ratio in children has been reviewed (6^R). Overall it is well tolerated. The most common adverse effects are diarrhea, abdominal cramps, borborygmi, and colic. Serious adverse events are rare and include isolated cases of extrapyramidal reactions, seizures in epileptic patients, cholestasis, QT segment prolongation and ventricular dysrhythmias, anorexia, and enuresis. Interactions of cisapride with other drugs are similar to those reported in adults. Co-administration with drugs that inhibit CYP3A4, such as imidazoles, macrolide antibiotics, the antidepressant nefazodone, and protease inhibitors such as ritonavir, is contraindicated. Furthermore, co-administration of anticholinergic drugs may compromise the beneficial effects of cisapride.

Side Effects of Drugs, Annual 23
J.K. Aronson, ed.

Elderly patients The pharmacokinetic properties of cisapride have been studied in eight elderly patients (mean age 85 years) (7[C]). There were no adverse effects, apart from a slightly increased stool frequency. There were no changes in the corrected QT interval. However, plasma cisapride concentrations became higher than expected. Thus, in extremely elderly patients cisapride should be administered once or twice a day rather than three times.

Interactions A possible interaction of cisapride 20 mg/day with *diltiazem* has been reported for the first time in a 45-year-old woman (8[c]) who developed near syncope and had QT interval prolongation. The QT interval returned to normal after withdrawal of cisapride. Rechallenge was not attempted. Diltiazem inhibits CYP3A4, and should therefore probably be avoided in combination with cisapride.

Domperidone *(SED-13, 1069; SEDA-22, 389)*

The mechanism of action and clinical use of domperidone and its specific use in diabetic gastroparesis have been reviewed (9[r], 10[R]). Domperidone is generally well tolerated and has a low incidence of adverse effects. Adverse effects after oral administration include *headache, dry mouth, diarrhea, itching, muscle cramps,* and *anxiety. Galactorrhea, breast tenderness,* and *pseudopregnancy* can occur in women because of a dopamine-induced increase in serum prolactin concentration. Intravenous domperidone is no longer recommended, as it has been associated with an *increased risk of cardiovascular events,* including cardiac arrest.

Interactions No clinically significant drug interactions have been reported with domperidone. However, concomitant administration of *anticholinergic drugs* may antagonize its beneficial effects. Furthermore, because domperidone is metabolized mainly by CYP3A4, interactions between azole antifungals and domperidone can occur. Since *cimetidine and antacids* can interfere with the systemic availability of domperidone (SEDA-22, 389) they should not be given together with domperidone.

5-HT3 receptor antagonists
(SED-13, 1070; SEDA-20, 316; SEDA-22, 390)

5-HT3 receptor antagonists are used as antiemetics in patients receiving highly emetogenic chemotherapy. In 59 patients who were given intravenous granisetron 1 mg 30 minutes before treatment on days of chemotherapy, the most common adverse effects were *headache, somnolence,* and *weakness* (11[c]). In a large double-blind study comparison of single-dose oral granisetron versus intravenous ondansetron in the prevention of nausea and vomiting induced by chemotherapy in 1085 patients, the drugs were equally effective and gave rise to a similar frequency of adverse effects, commonly *headache, weakness,* and *constipation* (12[C]). *Dizziness* and *blurred vision* were reported by significantly more of the patients who received ondansetron. Granisetron and ondansetron were also effective in controlling nausea and vomiting related to emetogenic chemotherapy in a cross-over study in 40 oriental patients (13[c]). Adverse effects were similar to those reported in Western studies, *constipation* and *headache* being the commonest. In another placebo-controlled study of the efficacy and safety of granisetron (3 mg), droperidol (1.25 mg), and metoclopramide (10 mg) intravenously for the prevention of nausea and vomiting in 120 parturients undergoing cesarean section under spinal anesthesia, granisetron was the most effective antiemetic (14[C]). The adverse events profiles of all three drugs were similar to that of placebo. In a cross-over study in 90 patients receiving cisplastin-based chemotherapy, prednisolone 50 mg significantly improved the antiemetic effects of granisetron (3 mg intravenously) compared with placebo (15[C]).

ULCER HEALING DRUGS
(SED-13, 1071; SEDA-20, 317; SEDA-21, 362; SEDA-22, 390)

Previous studies have suggested an increased risk of nosocomial pneumonia associated with histamine receptor antagonists in critically ill patients. The mechanism is unclear. To investigate this further, two randomized studies have been performed. One compared ranitidine (0.25 mg/kg/h intravenously) with sucralfate (1 g every 6 h via nasogastric tube) for prophylaxis against stress-induced gastritis in 96 severely injured patients (16[C]). Ranitidine was associated with a 1.5 times increased risk of developing any infection compared with sucralfate. Furthermore, of the 49 patients who received ranitidine, 14 developed 26 separate episodes of pneumonia, while of the 47 patients who received sucralfate, ten developed 14 episodes of pneumonia. The other study, placebo-controlled, compared intravenous ranitidine (50 mg tds) and pirenzepine (10 mg tds) in 158 patients who were being mechanically ventilated; the pneumonia rates were similar in the three groups (17[C]).

In another study of stress ulcer prophylaxis, 53 critically ill patients were randomized to receive sucralfate 1 g 6-hourly, cimetidine 300 mg 8-hourly, or cimetidine 900 mg/day by continuous intravenous infusion (18[C]). Although bacterial colonization was increasingly likely in patients with a persistent alkaline gastric environment, gastric luminal pH and the degree of bacterial colonization of the stomach were similar in the three groups.

Several treatments are available for promoting the healing of gastric and duodenal ulcers associated with the use of non-steroidal anti-inflammatory drugs (NSAIDs). They include histamine receptor antagonists, proton pump inhibitors, and prostaglandin analogues. Two large randomized, double-blind, multicenter trials in a total of 1456 patients have compared the efficacy of ranitidine 150 mg bd with omeprazole 20 or 40 mg/day (ASTRONAUT study) (19[C]) and omeprazole 20 or 40 mg/day with misoprostol 200 μg qds (OMNIUM study) (20[C]) in the treatment of NSAID-induced ulcers. The proportions of the patients with treatment success at 8 weeks were 77% with both doses of omeprazole, 63% with ranitidine, and 71% with misoprostol. The most frequent adverse effects were *diarrhea* in 11% and *abdominal pain* in 8% of patients taking misoprostol. Both these adverse effects were 2–4 times more frequent with misoprostol than with omeprazole. Withdrawal from the study owing to adverse effects was also more frequent in the misoprostol arm of the OMNIUM study.

HISTAMINE H_2-RECEPTOR ANTAGONISTS *(SED-13, 1071; SEDA-20, 317; SEDA-21, 362; SEDA-22, 391)*

Musculoskeletal In 33 patients taking cimetidine, ranitidine, or famotidine for more than 2 years there was little effect on the degree of bone mineral density (21[C]).

Interactions A meta-analysis of 24 studies has been performed to determine the effects, if any, of histamine H_2 receptor antagonists on blood *alcohol* (22[C]). Cimetidine and ranitidine, but not famotidine or nizatidine, cause small increases in blood alcohol concentrations. The mechanism is unclear, but one possibility is inhibition of gastric alcohol dehydrogenase. However, relative to accepted legal definitions of intoxication the effect of any histamine receptor antagonist on blood alcohol concentrations is unlikely to be clinically significant.

Cimetidine

A second case of cimetidine-induced *climacteric symptoms* has been reported (23[c]).

A 31-year-old white man on maintenance hemodialysis had frequent episodes of hot flushes, sweating, palpitation, and dizziness, which started after about 1 month of treatment with cimetidine 400 mg/day. When the drug was temporarily discontinued and later when it was totally withdrawn, he noted marked improvement in 2–5 days.

Famotidine

Histamine receptor antagonists can cause a variety of reactions involving the central nervous system. These are rare with famotidine. Five elderly patients (61–85 years old) developed acute central nervous system reactions consisting of *confusion, agitation, hallucinations,* and *disorientation* 24 h to a few days after starting to take famotidine in a dosage of 40 mg/day (24[C]). These features resolved completely 24–48 hours after withdrawal. Rechallenge was not attempted.

Ranitidine

Cholestatic liver damage due to ranitidine has been reported (25[c]).

A 29-year-old man developed cholestasis (confirmed histologically) while taking ranitidine 150 mg bd for about two weeks. The drug was withdrawn and the patient was treated with corticosteroids and ursodeoxycholic acid. Three months later he had recovered completely. Rechallenge was not attempted.

PROTON PUMP INHIBITORS

(SED-13, 1075; SEDA-20, 318; SEDA-21, 363; SEDA-22, 391)

The use of proton pump inhibitors in acid-related disorders has been extensively reviewed (26[R]–28[R]). The adverse effects profile during short-term administration (under 12 weeks) is similar to that reported with short-term use of histamine receptor antagonists. The type and frequency of adverse effects reported with lansoprazole, omeprazole, pantoprazole, and rabeprazole appear to be comparable. The most common adverse effects include *headache, diarrhea, nausea, abdominal pain, constipation, dizziness,* and *skin rash.*

Tumor-inducing effects of proton pump inhibitors

The adverse effects of long-term proton pump inhibitors are generally similar to those observed during short-term treatment. However, of concern is the potential for enterochromaffin-like cell hyperplasia, gastric carcinoid tumors and gastric cancers, colorectal polyps and adenocarcinoma, atrophic gastritis, and intestinal metaplasia in patients with Helicobacter pylori infection, and bacterial overgrowth.

Therapeutic doses of proton pump inhibitors usually produce somewhat higher serum gastrin concentrations than histamine receptor antagonists. However, except for small intestinal bacterial overgrowth, there is no convincing evidence yet to implicate proton pump inhibitors in the development of malignant or premalignant lesions in the human gastrointestinal tract. Nevertheless, although omeprazole has been used for more than 14 years and lansoprazole for more than 10 years, longer term data are required to completely rule out the possibility of increased risk of gastric tumor formation.

An increasing number of gastric polyps (and now carcinoid tumors) is being reported in patients taking proton pump inhibitors. Although these may be coincidental and may only account for a minority of sporadic cases (29[c]), it is too early to disregard the possibility that they are treatment induced (30[c]). Long-term prospective controlled trials including investigation of the effects of stopping and restarting proton pump inhibitors on the evolution of gastric polyps will have to be done before a firm causal relation can be established.

An uncontrolled retrospective study of patients who had taken proton pump inhibitors for an average of 33 months found gastric polyps in 17 of 231 patients who underwent two or more endoscopies for complicated gastro-esophageal reflux disease (31[C]). The polyps were generally small (under 1 cm), sessile, and multiple, and were present in the proximal or mid gastric body. Of the 15 polyps removed endoscopically, nine were fundic gland type, four were hyperplastic, and two were inflammatory. None had any dysplasia or carcinoma.

Gastric carcinoid tumor, detected during long-term anti-ulcer therapy with a histamine receptor antagonist and proton pump inhibitors, has been reported for the first time (32[c]).

A 31 year old Japanese man with recurrent duodenal ulcer was treated with famotidine, omeprazole, and lansoprazole at different times over 3 years. Gastroscopy showed a small carcinoid tumor in the upper cardia after 35 months. The lesion became larger while the patient was taking lansoprazole.

Interactions Proton pump inhibitors can interact with other drugs by increasing gastric pH, inhibiting hepatic cytochrome P450, or inducing specific isoforms of this enzyme system. However, drug interactions involving these isoenzymes and omeprazole or lansoprazole are uncommon and generally appear to be clinically unimportant. Omeprazole can interact with *diazepam, phenytoin,* and possibly *warfarin.* Lansoprazole has been reported to increase *theophylline* clearance by 10%, but does not appear to inhibit the metabolism of a number of drugs metabolized by cytochrome P450. Pantoprazole seems to have a lower drug interaction potential than either omeprazole or lansoprazole.

Omeprazole *(SED-13, 1075; SEDA-22, 392)*

The effects of omeprazole 40 mg/day on the pharmacokinetics of *itraconazole* 200 mg have been studied in 11 healthy volunteers (33[C]). Omeprazole reduced the absorption of itraconazole. As the absorption of itraconazole is pH dependent (it requires a pH of under 3.0 for complete dissolution and absorption) the likely explanation for this interaction is the effect of omeprazole on gastric pH.

OTHER ULCER-HEALING AGENTS

Liquorice *(SED-13, 1077)*

Liquorice-induced pseudohyperaldosteronism can cause *hypokalemic myopathy* (34[c]).

A 65-year-old man, diabetic and alcoholic, developed pseudohyperaldosteronism with hypokalemia, myopathy, and a reversible dilated cardiomyopathy associated with a small dose of liquorice-containing stomachics (liquorice extract in total granules of 3 g/day) over a few years for gastritis and a total of 800 mg of glycyrrhizin intravenously over 2 months for worsening liver dysfunction.

Helicobacter pylori eradication regimens *(SEDA-20, 320; SEDA-21, 362; SEDA-22, 392*

The antimicrobial treatment of *Helicobacter pylori* has been reviewed (35[r]). Generally two antimicrobials with bismuth or ranitidine or a proton pump inhibitor such as omeprazole are required to achieve a cure rate of over 90% and avoid the resistance that occurs when clarithromycin or metronidazole is the single antimicrobial used. Compliance is one of the most important factors associated with cure rates, and this will depend on the adverse effects of individual drugs used and the length of treatment. Bismuth plus metronidazole is effective, but causes more adverse effects than omeprazole plus amoxicillin plus either clarithromycin or metronidazole. Clarithromycin raises the blood concentrations of *carbamazepine* and *digoxin*. In developing countries resistance to metronidazole can reach 95%. To ensure high cure rates treatment may be required for 10 days, although 7-day regimens are also known to be successful.

EMETICS *(SED-13, 1078)*

A case of Munchausen's syndrome by proxy involving syrup of ipecacuanha has been reported in an 18-month-old child who was brought by his mother with persistent vomiting for 4 weeks with generalized myopathy and pneumonia (36[c]). Its over-the-counter availability, low cost, and effective emetic properties give this drug a high appeal for such abuse.

Gastrointestinal decontamination in acute toxic ingestion has been reviewed (37[R]).

- Although ipecac generally seems to have a good safety profile, it may be associated with protracted vomiting. Other reported adverse effects include *drowsiness, agitation, abdominal cramps, diarrhea, aspiration pneumonia, cerebral hemorrhage, pneumoperitoneum,* and *pneumomediastinum.*
- Gastric lavage may be useful in some patients who have taken life-threatening doses of highly toxic substances. However, toxin absorption may be enhanced by gastric lavage. Reported adverse effects mainly include *laryngospasm, hypoxemia, aspiration pneumonia, bradycardia, electrocardiographic ST segment elevation,* and rarely *mechanical injury to the gastrointestinal tract.*
- Activated charcoal has gained popularity as a first choice for gut decontamination, based on its efficacy and relative lack of adverse effects. Poor patient acceptance is a disadvantage, and frequent vomiting can become a problem.
- Saline laxatives (magnesium citrate, magnesium sulfate, sodium sulfate, and disodium phosphate) or saccharide laxatives (sorbitol, mannitol, lactulose) are also used in poisoned patients. Common adverse effects are *abdominal cramps, excessive diarrhea,* and *abdominal distention. Dehydration* and *electrolyte imbalance* in children, and *hypermagnesemia* and *magnesium toxicity* (with magnesium-based cathartics) have also been reported.
- Whole bowel irrigation to wash the entire gastrointestinal tract rapidly and mechanically is similar to the methods used by gastroenterologists to prepare patients for colonic investigation or bowel surgery. It is safe, even in children, pregnant women, and patients with cardiac or respiratory failure. Polyethyleneglycol-isotonic electrolyte solution is the commonly used substance. Complications are usually minor and include *nausea, vomiting, abdominal distention and cramps, and anal irritation.*

LAXATIVES *(SED-13, 1080; SEDA-21, 361; SEDA-22, 393)*

Anatomical changes in the colon have been reported in patients taking chronic stimulant laxatives, defined as laxative ingestion more than three times a week for a year or more (38[C]). Loss of haustra, which suggests neuronal injury, or damage to colonic longitudinal musculature was seen in eight of 29 patients who used a variety of diphenylmethane and anthraquinolone laxatives and none of the 26 patients who were not using these drugs. In 18 consecutive patients who were chronic users of stimulant laxatives, there was loss of haustra in 15 who took bisacodyl, phenolphthalein, senna, or casanthranol.

The efficacy, speed of action, and acceptability of ispaghula husk, lactulose, and other laxatives in the treatment of simple constipation in 394 patients have been studied by 65 general practitioners (39[C]). Ispaghula was used by 224 and other laxatives by 170. After 4 weeks of treatment ispaghula husk was assessed by the GPs to be superior to other laxatives. In the assessment by patients, ispaghula users had a higher proportion of normal stools and less soiling than patients using other laxatives. *Abdominal pain and gripes* and *diarrhea* were less common with ispaghula. *Distention, flatulence, indigestion,* and *nausea* were equally frequent in the two groups.

Colonic ulceration has been attributed to the use of hydrogen peroxide in an enema (40[c]).

A 13-year-old girl was given 10% hydrogen peroxide as an enema for constipation. She developed severe rectal bleeding, and colonoscopy showed mucosal ulceration up to the splenic flexure. Histology confirmed ulceration due to traumatic burns. She improved gradually on conservative treatment, and 2 months later a repeat colonoscopy was normal.

Dantron

In Canada, after a review of the benefits and risks associated with the use of dantron-containing stimulant laxatives, it has been concluded that dantron is a genotoxic animal carcinogen and that the risks of using it outweigh the therapeutic benefits (41[r]). Dantron is a synthetic anthraquinone and although there is no direct evidence that it has caused cancer in humans, it may have carcinogenic potential. The manufacturers have voluntarily withdrawn their products.

Phenolphthalein

Various reports have appeared in relation to withdrawal of laxatives. Two are concerned with products containing phenolphthalein.

The Federal Institute for Drugs and Medical Devices in Germany has recommended that marketing authorizations for these products be renounced, in view of the latest findings regarding its potential toxic effects (42[r]).

Further to the actions taken in the US and France to withdraw laxative products containing phenolphthalein, because of concerns about its potential *genotoxicity* and *carcinogenicity,* the following measures have been taken (43[r]).

Canada After reviewing the benefits and risks associated with the use of phenolphthalein-containing laxatives, Health Canada has concluded that there is a risk that phenolphthalein may cause cancer in humans; therefore authority to sell and distribute these products will be revoked.

European Union At a Pharmacovigilance Working Party meeting in September 1997, it was indicated that national competent authorities were either considering immediate suspension of phenolphthalein or were discussing with the relevant marketing authorization holders voluntary withdrawal down to the wholesale level. If voluntary action was not agreed by marketing authorization holders, the national competent authorities concerned would consider suspension of the products.

Japan Manufacturers have voluntarily withdrawn products containing phenolphthalein.

Phosphates

Sodium phosphates are considered to be dangerous (44[R]). The FDA has limited the container size for oral solutions of sodium phosphates (dibasic sodium phosphate/monobasic sodium phosphate) to not more than 90 ml in over-the-counter laxatives. The FDA has taken this action because of reports of deaths associated with overdosage of sodium phosphate oral solution when the product was packaged in a larger container and a larger than intended dose was taken inadvertently. The agency has also required warning and direction statements to inform consumers that exceeding the recommended dose of oral and rectal sodium phosphates products in a 24-hour period can be harmful.

Two studies have compared different bowel preparations for colonic investigations. In one, 68 patients were randomly assigned to receive either sulfate-free polyethylene glycol electrolyte lavage or sodium picosulfate plus magnesium sulfate, the day before colonoscopy (45[C]). Bowel cleansing was significantly better with picosulfate plus magnesium. Adverse effects were more common with polyethylene glycol electrolyte lavage, especially *nausea, vomiting,* and *palpitation,* and four patients did not complete treatment owing to adverse effects. In the other trial (46[C]), 194 patients were randomized to receive either picolax or fleet phosphate soda before barium enema. There was no difference in the quality of bowel preparation, but picosulfate was easier to take and better tasting and it provoked less nausea and vomiting.

Senna

The safety and efficacy of senna has been reviewed (47[R]). Its rhein-anthrone-induced laxative effects occur through two distinct mechanisms – an increase in intestinal fluid transport, which causes accumulation of fluid intraluminally, and an increase in intestinal motility. Senna can cause mild abdominal complaints, such as *cramps* or *pain.* Other adverse effects are *discoloration of the urine* and *hemorrhoidal congestion.* Prolonged use and overdose can result in *diarrhea,* extreme *loss of electrolytes, especially potassium, damage to the surface epithelium,* and *impairment of bowel function by damage to autonomic nerves.* Abuse of senna has also been associated with *melanosis coli,* but resolution occurs 8–11 moths after withdrawal. The development of tolerance and genotoxicity do not seem to be problems associated with senna, especially when used periodically in therapeutic doses.

AMINOSALICYLATES *(SED-13, 1082; SEDA-20, 320; SEDA-21, 364; SEDA-22, 393)*

In a randomized double-blind study of 99 patients with ulcerative colitis, balsalazide 3 g/day and mesalazine 1.2 g/day effectively maintained remission (48[C]). Adverse events were equally common in the two groups, and the common ones reported were *headache, abdominal pain and diarrhea, respiratory infections, body pains,* and *flu-like symptoms.*

In a 12-week trial in 168 patients with mild to moderate ulcerative colitis, olsalazine 3 g/day was as effective as mesalazine 3 g/day in inducing remission (49[C]). There were more adverse effects in patients taking olsalazine (41 of 88) than mesalazine (29 of 80). The majority of adverse effects related to bowel disturbances—*diarrhea, vomiting, discomfort, heartburn, flatulence,* and *nausea.* Diarrhea was more common in patients taking olsalazine. One patient taking mesalazine developed a *lupus-like syndrome.*

In a double-blind multicenter study in 182 patients with active Crohn's disease affecting the ileum and/or ascending colon, a modified-release formulation of budesonide (9 mg/day) was more effective in inducing remission than mesalazine 2 g bd (50[C]). Adverse events were similar in the two groups. Mild *abnormalities of adrenal function tests* were slightly more common with budesonide, but the clinical significance of these was unclear.

The dose response relation of oral mesalazine in inflammatory bowel disease has been briefly reviewed (51[r]). Higher doses (3 g/day) are more effective in inducing and maintaining remission than lower doses (1.5 g/day). None of the known adverse effects of mesalazine is clearly dose related.

Cardiovascular *Pericarditis* has been reported in a 16-year-old boy with inflammatory bowel disease taking mesalazine (52[c]). It resolved on withdrawal, but recurred after starting sulfasalazine 500 mg tds.

Severe symptomatic *bradycardia* has been reported in a 29-year-old woman with ulcerative colitis who was taking mesalazine (53[c]). Bradycardia resolved on withdrawal. Six weeks later mesalazine was restarted for a relapse of her colitis, and symptomatic bradycardia recurred. Again this resolved on withdrawal.

Respiratory *Pleural effusion with pulmonary infiltration* has been reported in a 72-year-old woman with ulcerative colitis taking mesalazine 800 mg tds (54[c]). The lung pathology resolved after drug withdrawal.

Hematological A possible association between mesalazine and *pancytopenia* has been reported in a 23-year-old man with Crohn's disease (55[c]). The pancytopenia resolved after withdrawal.

Gastrointestinal Severe *diarrhea,* which was associated with changes in fecal eicosanoid content, that mimicked the effects expected with the use of non-steroidal anti inflammatory drugs, has been reported in a 57-year-old man with non-granulomatous enterocolitis who took mesalazine 4 g/day (56[c]). The diarrhea resolved dramatically on withdrawal.

Urinary system There have been several reports of *tubulo-interstitial nephritis* in patients with inflammatory bowel disease, possibly due to mesalazine (57[c]–60[c]). In addition, there has been a report of a possible association between mesalazine and *nephrotic syndrome due to minimal change nephropathy,* which resolved after withdrawal (61[c]).

Interactions An interaction of mesalazine with *warfarin* has been reported (62[c]).

A 55-year-old woman was taking warfarin 5 mg/day for deep venous thrombosis when she was also given mesalazine 800 mg tds for a solitary cecal ulcer. Four weeks later she developed worsening of her venous thrombosis. Her serum warfarin concentrations were undetectable and the INR was 0.9. Mesalazine was discontinued; her INR rose to 1.8 on the following day and was 2.1 five days later.

CHOLELITHOLYTIC AGENTS—BILE ACIDS *(SED-13, 1085; SEDA-22, 395)*

The results of contact dissolution of gall stones using infusions of methyl tert-butyl ether via percutaneous transhepatic gallbladder puncture have been assessed in 803 patients (63[C]). Stones were dissolved in 724 of 761 patients in whom gall bladder puncture was successful. The 30 day mortality was 0.4%. Common complications were *biliary leak, fever, leukocytosis, abdominal pain,* and *mild increases in transaminases.* Toxic effects due to ether were not reported.

PANCREATIC ENZYME SUPPLEMENTS *(SED-13, 1086; SEDA-20, 322; SEDA-21, 366; SEDA-22, 395)*

The effect of high-dose pancreatic enzymes on pancreatic function has been assessed in a double-blind study in 12 healthy volunteers, six of whom were given 18 capsules of Panzytrat (20 000 units of lipase, 18 000 units of amylase and 1000 units of protease per capsule) daily for 4 weeks (64[C]). There were no morphological or functional changes in the pancreas in those treated. None of the subjects had severe adverse effects. Two had transient *mild nausea, epigastric pain,* and *heartburn.* There were no abnormalities in liver function tests.

A case of *fibrotic injury of the entire colon* has been reported in an 8-year-old boy with cystic fibrosis who took pancreatic enzymes 12000 IU/kg at each meal (65[c]). He had earlier been taking 5000 IU/kg. The first colonic symptoms occurred 1 year after the increase in dose.

SCLEROSANT INJECTIONS
(SED-13, 1086)

Ethanol injection

There have been three studies of the effects of percutaneous ethanol injections in the treatment of hepatocellular carcinoma, either alone (66[R], 67[C]) or in combination with transcatheter arterial embolization (68[C]). The procedure was effective and safe and improved long-term survival. Adverse effects were generally mild and of short duration, and commonly *included abdominal pain, fever, intoxication (especially among non-drinkers), transient rises in serum transaminases,* and *chemical thrombosis of the tributary branch of the portal vein.*

Hepatic infarction has been reported in two patients with hepatocellular carcinoma after percutaneous ethanol injection of the tumors (69[c]). Both patients had previously been treated with transcatheter arterial infusion using a suspension of styrene maleic acid neocarzinostatin, perhaps through a combination of arterial damage due to the neocarzinostatin and vasculitis caused by flow of the injected ethanol into a portal vein branch.

REFERENCES

1. Simoneau G. Absence of rebound effect with calcium carbonate. Eur J Drug Metab Pharmacokinet 1996;24:351–7.
2. Hurlimann S, Michel K, Inauen W, Halter F. Effect of Rennie liquid versus Maalox liquid on intragastric pH in a double blind, randomized, placebo controlled, triple crossover study in healthy volunteers. Am J Gastroenterol 1996;91:1173–80.
3. MacLaughlin SA, McKinney PE. Antacid induced hypermagnesemia in a patient with normal renal function and bowel obstruction. Ann Pharmacother 1998;32:312–15.
4. Baxter PS, Maddern GJ. Effect of cisapride on gastroduodenal reflux and gall bladder motility in patients with gallstones. Dig Surg 1998;15:35–41.
5. Poynard T, Vernisse B, Agostini H, for a multicenter group. Randomized multicenter comparison of sodium alginate and cisapride in the symptomatic treatment of uncomplicated gastroesophageal reflux. Aliment Pharmacol Ther 1998;12:159–65.
6. Vandenplas Y. Clinical use of cisapride and its risk benefit in pediatric patients. Eur J Gastroenterol Hepatol 1998;10:871–81.
7. Yamamoto T, Takano K, Sanaka M, Kuyama Y, Yamanaka M, Koike Y, Mineshita S. Pharmacokinetic characteristics of cisapride in elderly patients. Int J Clin Pharmacol Ther 1998;36:432–4.
8. Thomas AR, Chan L-N, Bauman JL, Olopade CO. Prolongation of QT interval related to cisapride-diltiazem interaction. Pharmacotherapy 1998;18:381–5.
9. Barone JA. Domperidone: mechanism of action and clinical use. Hosp Pharm 1998;33:191–7.
10. Prakash A, Wagstaff AJ. Domperidone: a review of its use in diabetic gastropathy. Drugs 1998; 56:429–45.
11. Trovato JA, Stull DM, Finley RS. Outcomes of antiemetic therapy after the administration of high dose antineoplastic agents. Am J Health Sys Pharm 1998;55:1269–74.
12. Perez EA, Hesketh P, Sandbach J, Reeves J, Chawla S, Markman M, Hainsworth J, Bushnell W, Friedman C. Comparison of single-dose oral granisetron versus intravenous ondansetron in the prevention of nausea and vomiting induced by moderately emetogenic chemotherapy: A multicentre, double-blind, randomized parallel study. J Clin Oncol 1998;16:754–60.
13. Poon RTP, Chow LWC. Comparison of antiemetic efficacy of granisetron and ondansetron in oriental patients: a randomized crossover study. Br J Cancer 1998;77:1683–5.
14. Fujii Y, Tanaka H, Toyooka H. Prevention of nausea and vomiting with granisetron, droperidol and metoclopramide during and after spinal anesthesia for cesarean section: a randomized, double blind, placebo controlled trial. Acta Anaesthesiol Scand 1998;42:921–5.
15. Handberg J, Wessel V, Larsen L, Herrstedt J, Hansen HH. Randomized, double blind comparison of granisetron plus prednisolone as antiemetic prophylaxis during multi-day cisplastin based chemotherapy. Supportive Care Cancer 1998; 6:63–7.
16. O'Keefe GE, Gentilello LM, Maier RV. Incidence of infectious complications associated with the use of histamine 2 receptor antagonists in critically ill trauma patients. Ann Surg 1998;227:120–5.
17. Hanisch EW, Encke A, Naujoks F, Windolf J. A randomized, double blind trial for stress ulcer prophylaxis shows no evidence of increased pneumonia. Am J Surg 1998;176:453–7.
18. Ortiz JE, Sottile FD, Sigel P, Nasraway SA. Gastric colonization as a consequence of stress ulcer prophylaxis: a prospective, randomized trial. Pharmacotherapy 1998;18:486–91.
19. Yeomans ND, Tullasay Z, Juhasz L, Racz I, Howard JM, Van Rensburg CJ, Swannell AJ, Hawkey CJ. A comparison of omeprazole with ranitidine for ulcers associated with non steroidal anti inflammatory drugs. New Engl J Med 1998;338:719–26.
20. Hawkey CJ, Karrasch JA, Szczepanski L, Walker DG, Barkun A, Swannell AJ, Yeomans ND. Omeprazole compared with misoprostol for ulcers associated with nonsteroidal antiinflammatory drugs. New Engl J Med 1998;338:727–34.
21. Adachi Y, Matsumata T, Iso Y, Yoh R, Kitano S. Bone mineral density in patients taking H2 receptor antagonists. Calcif Tissue Int 1998;62:283–5.
22. Weinberg DS, Burnham D, Berlin JA. Effect of histamine 2 receptor antagonists on blood alcohol levels: a meta-analysis. J Gen Intern Med 1998;13:594–9.
23. Bastani B, Galli D, Gellens ME. Cimetidine induced climacteric symptoms in a young man maintained on chronic hemodialysis. Am J Nephrol 1998;18:538–40.
24. Odeh M, Oliven A. Central nervous system reactions associated with famotidine: report of five cases. J Clin Gastroenterol 1998;27:253–4.
25. Ramrakhiani S, Brunt EM, Bacon BR. Possible cholestatic injury from ranitidine with a review of the literature. Am J Gastroenterol 1998;93:822–6.
26. Berardi RR, Welage LS. Proton pump inhibitors in acid related diseases. Am J Health Syst Pharm 1998;55:2289–98.
27. Garnett W. Considerations for long term use of proton pump inhibitors. Am J Heath Syst Pharm 1998;55:2268–79.
28. Israel D, Hassall E. Omeprazole and other proton pump inhibitors: pharmacology, efficacy, and safety, with special reference to use in children. J Pediatr Gastroenterol Nutr 1998;27:568–79.
29. Declich P, Farrara A, Galati F, Caruso S, Baldacci MP, Ambrosiani L. Do fundic gland polyps develop under long term omeprazole therapy? Am J Gastroenterol 1998;93:1393.
30. Naegels S, Urbain D. Omeprazole and fundic gland polyps. Am J Gastroenterol 1998;93:855.
31. Choudhry U, Boyce HW, Coppola D. Proton pump inhibitor associated gastric polyps. A retrospective analysis of their frequency, and endo-

scopic, histologic, and ultrastructural characteristics. Am J Clin Pathol 1998;110:615–21.
32. Haga Y, Nakatsura T, Shibata Y, Sameshima H, Nakamura Y, Tanimura M, Ogawa M. Human gastric carcinoid detected during long term anti ulcer therapy of H2 receptor antagonist and proton pump inhibitor. Dig Dis Sci 1998;43:253–7.
33. Jaruratanasirikul S, Sriwiriyajan S. Effect of omeprazole on the pharmacokinetics of itraconazole. Eur J Clin Pharmacol 1998;54:159–61.
34. Hasegawa J, Suyama Y, Kinugawa T, Morisawa T, Kishimoto Y. Echocardiographic findings of the heart resembling dilated cardiomyopathy during hypokalemic myopathy due to licorice induced pseudoaldosteronism. Cardiovasc Drugs Ther 1998;12:599–600.
35. Goodwin CS. Antimicrobial treatment of *Helicobacter pylori* infection. Clin Infect Dis 1998;25:1023–6.
36. Cooper C, Kilham H, Ryan M. Ipecac – a substance of abuse. Med J Aust 1998;168:94–5.
37. Lheureux P, Askenasi R, Paciorkowski F. Gastrointestinal decontamination in acute toxic ingestions. Acta Gastro-enterol Belg 1998;61:461–7.
38. Joo JS, Ehrenpreis ED, Gonzalez L, Kaye M, Breno S, Wexner SD, Zaitman D, Secrest K. Alterations in colonic anatomy induced by chronic stimulant laxatives. The cathartic colon revisited. J Clin Gastroenterol 1998;26:283–6.
39. Dettmar PW, Sykes J. A multicenter, general practice comparison of ispaghula husk with lactulose and other laxatives in the treatment of simple constipation. Curr Med Res Opin 1998;14:227–33.
40. Bollen P, Goossens A, Hauser B, Vandenplas Y. Colonic ulcerations caused by an enema containing hydrogen peroxide. J Pediatr Gastroenterol Nutr 1998;26:232–3.
41. Anonymous. Laxatives containing dantron-voluntary withdrawal. WHO Pharm Newslett 1998; 112:4.
42. Anonymous. Laxatives containing phenolphthalein-recommendation to revoke marketing authorization. WHO Pharm Newslett 1997;112:3.
43. Anonymous. Laxatives containing phenolphthalein-voluntary withdrawal. WHO Pharm Newslett 1998;112:4–5.
44. Anonymous. Laxatives containing sodium phosphates-package size limitations and warnings. WHO Pharm Newslett 1998;112:2.
45. Regev A, Fraser G, Delpre G, Leiser A, Neeman A, Maoz E, Anikin V, Niv Y. Comparison of two bowel preparations for colonoscopy: sodium picosulphate with magnesium citrate versus sulphate free polyethylene glycol lavage solution. Am J Gastroenterol 1998;93:1478–82.
46. Macleod AJM, Duncan KA, Pearson RH, Bleakney RR. A comparison of fleet phospho soda with picolax in the preparation of the colon for double contrast barium enema. Clin Radiol 1998;53:612–14.
47. Mascolo N, Capasso R, Capasso F. Senna. A safe and effective drug. Phytother Res 1998; 12(Suppl 1):S143–5.
48. Green JRB, Gibson JA, Kerr GD, Swarbrick ET, Lobo AJ, Holdsworth CD, et al. Maintenance of remission of ulcerative colitis: a comparison between balsalazide 3 g daily and mesalazine 1.2 g daily over 12 months. Aliment Pharmacol Ther 1998;12:1207–16.
49. Kruis W, Brandes JW, Schreiber S, Theuer D, Krakamp B, Schutz E, Otto P, Lorenz-Mayer H, Ewe K, Judmaier G. Olsalazine versus mesalazine in the treatment of mild to moderate ulcerative colitis. Aliment Pharmacol Ther 1998;12:707–15.
50. Thomsen OO, Cortot A, Jewell D, Wright JP, Winter T, Veloso FT, Vatn M, Persson T, Pettersson E. A comparison of budesonide and mesalazine for active Crohn's disease. New Engl J Med 1998; 339:370–4.
51. Mulder CJJ, Van den Hazel SJ. Drug therapy: dose response relationship of oral mesalazine in inflammatory bowel disease. Mediators Inflamm 1998;7:135–6.
52. Sentongo TAS, Piccoli DA. Recurrent pericarditis due to mesalamine hypersensitivity: a pediatric case report and review of the literature. J Pediatr Gastroenterol Nutr 1998;27:344–7.
53. Asirvatham S, Sebastian C, Thadani U. Severe symptomatic sinus bradycardia associated with mesalamine use. Am J Gastroenterol 1998;93:470–1.
54. Sesin PG, Mucciardi N, Almeida S, Levanda M. Mesalamine associated pleural effusion with pulmonary infiltration. Am J Health Syst Pharm 1998;55:2304–5.
55. Kotanagi H, Ito M, Koyama K, Chiba M. Pancytopenia associated with 5-amino salicylic acid use in a patient with Crohn's disease. J Gastroenterol 1998;33:571–4.
56. Fine KD, Sarles HE, Cryer B. Diarrhea associated with mesalamine in a patient with chronic nongranulomatous enterocolitis. New Engl J Med 1998;338:923–5.
57. Calvino J, Romero R, Pintos E, Losada E, Novoa D, Guimil D, Mardaras J, Sanchez-Guisande D. Mesalazine associated tubulo-interstitial nephritis in inflammatory bowel disease. Clin Nephrol 1998;49:265–7.
58. Popoola J, Muller F, Pollock L, O'Donnell P, Carmichael P, Stevens P. Late onset interstitial nephritis associated with mesalazine treatment. Br Med J 1998;317:795–7.
59. Brouillard M, Gheerbrant J-D, Gheysens Y, Fleury D, Devred M, Hazzan M, Colombel J-F. Interstitielle chronique et mesalazine: 3 nouveaux cas? Gastroenterol Clin Biol 1998;22:724–6.
60. Howard G, Lynn KL. Renal dysfunction and the treatment of inflammatory bowel disease (IBD): a case for monitoring. Aust NZ J Med 1998:28:346.
61. Skhiri H, Knebelmann B, Martin-Lefevre L, Grunfeld JP. Nephrotic syndrome associated with inflammatory bowel disease treated by mesalazine. Nephron 1998;79:236.
62. Marinella M. Mesalamine and warfarin therapy resulting in decreased warfarin effect. Ann Pharmacother 1998;32:841–2.

63. Hellstern A, Leuschner U, Benjaminov A, Ackermann H, Heine T, Festi D, et al. Dissolution of gallbladder stones with methyl tert-butyl ether and stone recurrence. A European survey. Dig Dis Sci 1998;43:911–20.
64. Friess H, Kleeff J, Malfertheiner P, Muller MW, Homuth K, Buchler MW. Influence of high dose pancreatic enzyme treatment on function in healthy volunteers. Int J Pancreatol 1998;23:115–23.
65. Moss RL, Musemeche CA, Feddersen RM. Progressive pan colonic fibrosis secondary to oral administration of pancreatic enzymes. Pediatr Surg Int 1998;13:168–70.
66. Livraghi T. Percutaneous ethanol injection in the treatment of hepatocellular carcinoma in cirrhosis. Minimally Invasive Ther Allied Technol 1998;7:553–8.
67. Livraghi T, Benedini V, Lazzaroni S, Meloni F, Torzilli G, Vettori C. Long term results of single session percutaneous ethanol injection in patients with large hepatocellular carcinoma. Cancer 1998;83:48–57.
68. Tanaka K, Nakamura S, Numata K, Kondo M, Morita K, Kitamura T, Saito S, Kiba T, Okazaki H, Sekihara H. The long term efficacy of combined transcatheter arterial embolization and percutaneous ethanol injection in the treatment of patients with large hepatocellular carcinoma and cirrhosis. Cancer 1998;82:78–85.
69. Seki T, Wakabayashi M, Nakagawa T, Imamura M, Tamai T, Nishamura A, Yamashiki N, Okamura A, Inoue K. Hepatic infarction following percutaneous ethanol injection therapy for hepatocellular carcinoma. Eur J Gastroenterol Hepatol 1998;10:915–18.

Thierry Vial and Jacques Descotes

37 Drugs acting on the immune system

INTERFERONS *(SED-13, 1090; SEDA-20, 326; SEDA-21, 369; SEDA-22, 399)*

Interferon-α

Although the adverse effects profiles of the currently available formulations of interferon-α are very similar, patients who have adverse effects with one formulation can be successfully retreated with another type of interferon-α. This has been shown in 22 patients in whom lymphoblastoid interferon-α was discontinued because of severe adverse effects *(leukopenia, thrombocytopenia, thyroid disorders*, or *psychiatric disturbances)* and were successfully retreated with similar dosages of leukocyte interferon-α (1^C). Only one of these patients had severe leukopenia again.

The FDA has expanded the indications for a drug/biological combination product to include patients with chronic hepatitis C who have not been treated with interferon-α. This product, Rebetron® Combination Therapy (Schering), contains recombinant interferon-α_{2b} for injection (Intron A®) and ribavirin (Rebetol®) in capsules, and was previously only approved for patients who had relapsed after treatment with interferon alone (2^r). Serious adverse effects have occurred with this treatment and patients should be closely monitored by their physicians. Rebetol® can cause significant adverse reproductive effects, including *fetal death* or *structural malformations*, in several animal species. Women must therefore not become pregnant during therapy and for 6 months after completing therapy. All women of childbearing potential and their partners should practise effective means of birth control, and any pregnancies should be reported to the manufacturer's pregnancy register immediately.

Side Effects of Drugs, Annual 23
J.K. Aronson, ed.

Rebetol® causes anemia, which can be serious, especially in patients with underlying cardiovascular disease. Intron A® has been associated with *psychiatric disorders*, including depression and suicidal behavior (suicidal thoughts, suicide attempts, and completed suicides). Depression, suicidal ideation, and suicides occurred in patients treated with Rebetron®.

Most patients who take Intron A® complain of *flu-like symptoms*, fevers, chills, and body aches. These symptoms are often relieved by non-prescription medicines, such as paracetamol (acetaminophen) or ibuprofen.

Cardiovascular Patients with a pre-existing cardiac disease are more likely to develop cardiovascular toxicity while receiving interferon-α, but these complications are rare and are usually not clinically relevant in patients without a history of cardiac disease. Among 89 patients treated for chronic hepatitis C, a 12-lead electrocardiogram performed monthly during a 12-month treatment period and a 6-month follow-up showed only minimal and non-specific abnormalities in five patients (two had *right bundle branch block*, one *left anterior hemiblock*, and two *unifocal ventricular extra beats*) (3^C). None of these disorders required treatment withdrawal, and complete non-invasive cardiovascular assessment was normal. Overall, the role of interferon-α was uncertain and the 5.6% incidence of electrocardiographic abnormalities was suggested to be similar to that expected in the general population. Nevertheless, severe cardiac dysrhythmias are still possible in isolated cases, as illustrated by the development of third-degree atrioventricular block, reversible on withdrawal, in a 57-year-old man with lower limb arteritis but no other cardiovascular disorder (4^c).

Although most patients with mild-to-moderate clinical manifestations of hepatitis C virus-associated mixed cryoglobulinemia improved during treatment with interferon-α, acute worsening of ischemic lesions has been reported in three patients who had prominent cryoglobulinemia-related ischemic manifestations (5[c]). All three had acute progression of pre-existing peripheral ischemia or leg ulcers within the first month of treatment, and transmetatarsal or right toe amputations were required in two. The lesions healed after interferon-α withdrawal. It was therefore suggested that the anti-angiogenic activity of interferon-α may also impair revascularization and healing of ischemic lesions in patients with initially severe ischemic manifestations.

Respiratory The respiratory adverse effects of interferon-α include *interstitial pneumonitis*, which is rare. Now acute exacerbation of asthma has been reported in two men aged 27 and 57 years with a previous history of mild asthma (6[c]). They developed progressive aggravation of asthma within 8–10 weeks of treatment for chronic hepatitis C, and finally required emergency treatment with systemic corticosteroids and inhaled β_2 agonists. Severe asthma recurred 2–3 weeks after interferon-α rechallenge in both patients. Although these cases are anecdotal, they strongly suggest that interferon-α should be regarded as a possible cause of asthma exacerbation in predisposed patients.

Nervous system Although the anti-angiogenic effects of interferon-α have been successfully used to treat severe hemangiomas in infants, the possibility of *spastic diplegia* is a matter of recent concern (SEDA-22, 404). These findings have recently been re-emphasized by an additional report of persistent, severe, spastic diplegia after 1 year of treatment in a 5-month-old boy (7[c]). Because the immature central nervous system of infants may be more susceptible to interferon-α toxicity, it has been stressed that this treatment should be reserved for infants with life-threatening hemangiomas (8[r]). That interferon-α can play a role in the occurrence of this acute neurological complication has been further substantiated by the finding of abnormally high interferon serum concentrations in 45% of neonates with spontaneous cerebral palsy compared with control children (9[C]).

Interferon-α can cause *seizures*. They are usually generalized tonic-clonic seizures, but reversible photosensitive seizures have also been reported (10[c]).

A 62-year-old man without a personal or family history of epilepsy received interferon-α (3 MU three times a week) for 2 years for multiple myeloma. He had frequent episodes of myoclonic jerks in the face, especially when the sun was shining while driving his car. He also had one generalized seizure. Electroencephalography showed a paroxysmal response to intermittent photic stimulation and magnetic resonance imaging was normal. The seizures disappeared and his electroencephalogram normalized after interferon-α withdrawal.

In this case the possible role of interferon-α was suspected only late during treatment, indicating that patients should be regularly questioned about neurological symptoms, because more severe complications might have occurred.

Akathisia occurred in two patients shortly after they had started to take interferon-α; one improved after the frequency of injections was reduced (11[cr]). Unfortunately, this report did not provide sufficient convincing evidence for a causal relation; the development of akathisia may have been coincidental.

Psychiatric Experience of the neuropsychiatric effects of interferon-α has been increasing in recent years, but several questions regarding the identification of vulnerable patients, the mechanisms, the medical management, and the long-term outcome are still not clearly answered. In 10 patients with melanoma and no previous psychiatric disorders, depression scores measured on the Montgomery-Asberg Depression Rating Scale were significantly increased after 4 weeks of high-dose interferon-α (12[c]). Patients whose scores were higher before treatment developed the worst symptoms of depression during treatment. While this has to be confirmed by larger studies, this positive correlation provides striking evidence that baseline and regular assessment of mood and cognitive functions are necessary to detect disorders as early as possible. Whereas psychiatric adverse effects usually disappeared after withdrawal, interferon-α was suggested as a possible cause of persistent *manic-depressive illness* for more than 4 years in a 40-year-old man (13[c]). Although the manic episodes may have been coincidental, the negative history and the age of onset are in keeping with a possible role of interferon-α treatment.

The management of the psychiatric complications of interferon-α has not been carefully investigated, but multiple approaches are theoretically possible. Various pharmacological and non-pharmacological interventions have recently been discussed (14[R]), and prompt intervention should be carefully considered in every patient who develops significant neuropsychiatric adverse effects while receiving interferon-α. Depending on the clinical manifestations, proposed treatment options include antidepressant, psychostimulant, or antipsychotic drugs, but formal studies are awaited. Opioid antagonists have also been regarded as a possible alternative for cognitive impairment.

Endocrine, metabolic *Thyroid* Thyroid disorders relatively often complicate treatment with interferon-α, and detailed clinical and biological features have been described in recent case reports (15[c]–17[c]). Two of these reports also mentioned associated adverse effects that developed concomitantly, namely myelosuppression and severe proximal myopathy (Hoffmann's syndrome).

In 175 patients treated for hepatitis B or C virus infection, women with chronic hepatitis C and patients with previously high titers of antithyroid autoantibodies were more prone to developing thyroid disorders (18[C]). After 6 months of treatment, 12% of patients with chronic hepatitis C had thyroid disorders compared with 3% of patients with chronic hepatitis B. This study also suggested a possible relation between low free triiodothyronine serum concentrations before treatment and the subsequent occurrence of thyroid dysfunction. After a follow-up of 6 months after the end of interferon-α treatment, 60% of affected patients with chronic hepatitis C still had persistent thyroid dysfunction; all had been positive for thyroid peroxidase antibodies before treatment. Long-term surveillance is therefore needed in these patients.

The immunological predisposition to thyroid disorders has been studied in 17 of 439 Japanese patients who had symptomatic autoimmune thyroid disorders during interferon-α treatment (19[C]). There was a significantly higher incidence of human leukocyte antigen (HLA)-A2 haplotype compared with the general Japanese population (88% versus 41%), suggesting that HLA-A2 is a possible additional risk factor for the development of interferon-α induced autoimmune thyroid disease.

Among other potential predisposing factors, treatment with iodine for 2 months in 21 patients with chronic hepatitis C receiving interferon-α did not increase the likelihood of thyroid abnormalities compared with eight patients who received iodine alone, but abnormal thyroid tests were more frequent compared with 27 patients who received interferon-α alone (20[C]). This suggests that excess iodine had no synergistic effects on the occurrence of thyroid dysfunction induced by interferon-α.

Parathyroid Exacerbation of secondary hyperparathyroidism occurred in a 20-year-old renal transplant patient who also developed psoriasis during interferon-α treatment (21[c]). Both disorders resolved after withdrawal.

Dyslipidemia Very severe but asymptomatic and reversible hypertriglyceridemia (more than ten times higher than the top of the reference range) has been repeatedly reported in association with interferon-α, particularly in patients with previously high serum triglyceride concentrations (22[c], 23[c]). In a prospective study of lipid changes in 36 patients with chronic hepatitis C treated with interferon-α for 6 months the most prominent findings included an increase in triglycerides, VLDL cholesterol, and apolipoprotein B, and a fall in HLD cholesterol and apolipoprotein A1 (24[C]). Three patients also developed chylomicronemia, and two of those had severe hypertriglyceridemia. All three patients had triglycerides over 2 g/l before treatment, suggesting that patients with abnormal triglyceride serum concentrations at baseline are more likely to develop marked hypertriglyceridemia.

Hematological The well-known hematological toxicity of interferon-α is often investigated. Increasing evidence suggests that serum thrombopoietin concentrations in patients who have had *thrombocytopenia* during interferon-α treatment for chronic viral hepatitis C either do not increase (in patients with compensated cirrhosis) or increase only moderately and less than expected (in non-cirrhotic patients) (25[C]). The authors proposed that interferon-α impairs liver production of thrombopoietin, raising the possibility of testing thrombopoietin administration in patients with severe thrombocytopenia before or during treatment with interferon-α (26[r]).

In a retrospective study of 158 patients with chronic viral hepatitis treated for 6–12 months, lymphoblastoid interferon-α produced the largest fall in leukocyte and platelet counts (−38% and −32% versus baseline values), recombinant interferon-α was associated with intermediate toxicity (−32% and −26%), and leukocyte interferon-α produced the smallest reduction (−27% and −22%) (27[C]). The lowest mean values were observed after an average of 4–5 months. However, the clinical relevance of these differences is probably minimal, because the overall reduction in leukocyte and platelet numbers was small, and no patients developed clinical symptoms of cytopenia.

Thrombotic thrombocytopenic purpura is a possible complication of interferon-α in patients with chronic myelogenous leukemia, and may develop even after a successful prolonged (2–3 years) treatment (28[c]). Complete recovery is expected after prompt medical management with plasma exchange and corticosteroids.

Liver Even moderate but continuing alcohol consumption needs to be taken seriously in patients receiving interferon-α, and *exacerbation of previous acute alcohol hepatitis* has been reported in two patients with chronic hepatitis C, despite reduced alcohol consumption (29[c]). Liver transaminases subsequently normalized after withdrawal of interferon-α in both patients.

Positive serological markers of autoimmune hepatitis before treatment in patients with concomitant chronic hepatitis C are sometimes associated with further exacerbation of an underlying autoimmune liver disease during interferon-α treatment. Of three patients with raised antimitochondrial antibodies (over 1:160), only the two patients with M2 (with or without M4 or M8) subtypes had biochemical exacerbation of cholestasis and an unfavorable response to interferon-α (30[c]). Although very few patients were investigated, determination of antibodies against submitochondrial particles may help to identify patients who are likely to have no benefit and even exacerbation of liver disease with interferon-α.

Urinary system Acute renal complications are repeatedly described in cancer patients receiving interferon-α who have received prior chemotherapy. In two patients with chronic myelogenous leukemia, acute renal insufficiency and massive proteinuria developed after 3–4 weeks of interferon-α treatment (31[cR]). Both improved after hemodialysis, but proteinuria persisted. Renal biopsies showed *focal segmental glomerulosclerosis.* A review of 15 other available reports of renal insufficiency and proteinuria in patients with chronic myeloid leukemia or other malignancies confirmed that the histological spectrum of renal lesions associated with interferon-α is varied, and includes membranous glomerulonephritis, minimal change glomerulonephritis, acute interstitial nephritis, hemolytic-uremic syndrome, and thrombotic microangiopathy. Renal complications were reversible in nine patients; three patients had persistent proteinuria and four persistent renal dysfunction, of whom three required chronic hemodialysis. Two-thirds of the patients developed renal complications within 1 month of interferon-α treatment, and one-third had received a relatively low dosage of interferon-α (9–15 MU/week).

Skin and appendages *Cutaneous sarcoidosis* has previously been reported (SED-13, 1097). In another case, a 60-year-old woman receiving interferon-α developed cutaneous sarcoid foreign body granulomas at the sites of a previous childhood skin injury (32[c]). This suggests that interferon-α may facilitate the development of cutaneous sarcoid granuloma from particulate foreign matter.

Hypertrichosis of the eyelashes (trichomegaly) has rarely been noted, but it developed in two of 36 patients with chronic viral hepatitis who were examined for ocular complications during treatment with high-dose interferon-α (18–30 MU/week) (33[c]). These two patients had received the highest dose of interferon-α.

Meyerson's phenomenon, multiple focal and transient eczematous eruptions around melanocytic nevi, has been reported in a 24-year-old man when the dosage of interferon-α for Behçet's disease was doubled (34[c]).

Special senses Retinal complications of interferon-α in patients with chronic viral hepatitis are well described, and this has been reviewed (35[R]). *Retinopathy* consisting of cotton-wool spots and/or superficial retinal hemorrhages has been reported with a variable incidence (18–86%), and the available data suggest that the increased incidence can be influenced by a high initial dose of interferon-

α. Whereas diabetes mellitus and systemic hypertension have been identified as possible risk factors, the incidence of retinopathy was not significantly increased in 19 patients with chronic renal insufficiency, compared with 17 patients without chronic renal insufficiency (33[C]). However, it was felt that renal insufficiency may be associated with the most severe cases, i.e. those requiring dosage reductions. Although retinopathy due to interferon-α is usually asymptomatic and spontaneously reversible and does not require withdrawal, uncommon ocular complications have been reported (35[R]), as exemplified in a further case report (36[c]).

A 60-year-old smoker was treated with interferon-α (100 MU/week for 2 months and 9 MU/week for 15 weeks) for cutaneous melanoma. Ocular examination was normal before treatment, but he developed acute loss of peripheral vision in his left eye after 23 weeks. Examination was consistent with anterior ischemic optic neuropathy and there was optic disc edema, a pupillary defect, and circular visual field constriction in the left eye. There was renal artery constriction in both eyes. Despite treatment with aspirin, high-dose dexamethasone, heparin, and finally withdrawal of interferon-α, loss of visual function progressed and affected both eyes. Ciclosporin was started, but he was considered to have irreversible loss of visual function.

This report shows that interferon-α can be a potent precipitator of extremely severe ocular disorders and also argues for careful ocular surveillance in patients receiving adjuvant interferon-α for high-risk resected melanoma.

The pathogenesis of retinopathy associated with interferon-α is unclear. In 45 patients with chronic hepatitis C (25 treated with interferon) there was an association between retinal hemorrhages caused by interferon-α (six patients) and a concomitant significant increase in plasma-activated complement (C5a), compared with baseline C5a serum concentrations (37). However, the significance and contribution of raised C5a concentrations in the pathogenesis of ocular complications needs to be clarified.

Sudden hearing loss has previously been reported (SEDA-21, 372). In another report of promptly reversible hearing loss on interferon-α withdrawal, the presence of anti-endothelial cell antibodies was suggested to play a role in the development of autoimmune microvascular damage (38[c]).

Immunological and hypersensitivity reactions The significance of pretreatment autoantibodies as a risk factor for autoimmune clinical disorders during treatment with interferon-α is strongly debated. A study in 83 patients with chronic hepatitis C identified one or more pre-existing autoantibodies (mostly low-titer antinuclear antibodies) in 35 patients (group I), of whom seven had clinical evidence of immune-mediated disorders, whereas five of 48 patients without pre-existing autoantibodies (group II) had similar disorders (39[C]). After 12–48 weeks of interferon-α treatment in 44 patients, six of 20 patients from group I developed new *immune-mediated disorders* (thyroid disorders in three, arthropathy in two, and psoriasis in one), but none of the 24 patients in group II. Patients positive for autoantibodies before interferon-α may therefore be much more likely to develop autoimmune diseases, particularly thyroid disorders, during interferon-α treatment. The possible role of interferon-α in the development of *rheumatoid arthritis* or *systemic lupus erythematosus* has again been described in isolated cases (40[c], 41[c]).

Risk factors *Interferon-α and transplantation* Possible deleterious effects of interferon-α on renal graft function are repeatedly reported (42[c]).

A 43-year-old man with stable renal graft function, taking ciclosporin, methylprednisolone, and azathioprine, developed chronic myelogenous leukemia and received interferon-α (3 MU/day). Seven weeks later, he became tired and had increased proteinuria and a raised serum creatinine concentration (574 μmol/l). Interferon-α was withdrawn and he received high-dose methylprednisolone for suspected acute graft rejection. This was unsuccessful and a first renal biopsy showed widespread interstitial edema that could not be correctly interpreted. Hemodialysis was restarted, and he finally developed a catheter infection and died from sepsis. Histology of the explanted renal graft showed severe predominantly acute vascular rejection.

The rapid occurrence of renal dysfunction after interferon-α in this case suggested a causal relation.

In a retrospective study of 153 patients who underwent bone-marrow transplantation for chronic myelogenous leukemia, pretransplant interferon-α treatment for more than 12 months was associated with a significant increase in transplant-related mortality during the first 2 years when compared with patients who received pretransplant interferon-α for less than 12 months (28 of 46 patients versus nine of 38) (43[C]). This adverse outcome was also more frequent in patients who discontinued treatment less than 3 months before transplantation.

Interferon-α in hemodialysis High daily dosage or serum concentrations of interferon-α may be associated with more frequent and more severe adverse effects during the treatment of chronic hepatitis C in hemodialysis patients. In one study, three of ten hemodialysis patients had severe neurological adverse effects (generalized seizures or posterior leukoencephalopathy) (44[C]). In another study, three of six patients receiving daily injections had to discontinue treatment because of depression, loss of consciousness and persistent high-grade fever, while no serious adverse effects was reported in three other patients who received interferon-α three times a week (45[C]). In both studies there were significant changes in interferon-α pharmacokinetics (higher Cmax, AUC, and half-life) in hemodialysis patients compared with patients with normal renal function, consistent with altered clearance of interferon-α.

Interactions Severe synergistic hemotoxicity sometimes results from combining interferon-α with *cytotoxic drugs*, such as busulfan and cyclophosphamide. This was again demonstrated in a patient who developed refractory bone-marrow aplasia after combined interferon-α and low-dose cytosine arabinoside maintenance for chronic myelogenous leukemia (46[c]). Complete recovery was achieved after allogeneic bone-marrow transplantation.

The combination of interferon-α with *ribavirin* is one of the most promising treatments for chronic hepatitis C. Although no synergistic effects have yet been identified in large controlled trials, two patients developed rapid and particularly severe anemia within 4 and 6 weeks of combined treatment (47[c]). One patient required erythrocyte transfusions, and both recovered after withdrawal. The combination of pure red cell aplasia due to interferon-α and hemolytic anemia due to ribavirin was suggested to account for this possible interaction.

Interferon-β

Nervous system The possible deleterious effects of interferon-β_{1b} on increased *spasticity* have been examined in 19 patients with primary progressive multiple sclerosis, 19 untreated matched patients, and ten patients treated with interferon-β_{1b} for relapsing-remitting multiple sclerosis (48[C]). Patients with primary progressive multiple sclerosis had frequent (68%) and clinically relevant increased spasticity (seven required oral baclofen), usually after about 2 months of treatment, whereas only two (11%) of the untreated patients and none of the patients with relapsing-remitting multiple sclerosis had similar disabling spasticity. Seven patients had to discontinue treatment after 6 months because of spasticity, and symptoms improved over several months after withdrawal. The authors suggested that this possible adverse effect should be taken into account in clinical trials because it could mask the positive clinical effects of interferon-β_{1b}.

Psychiatric The possible link between interferon-β and *depression* is debated (SEDA-20, 332; SEDA-22, 404). The emotional state of 90 patients with relapsing-remitting multiple sclerosis has been carefully assessed with a battery of psychological tests at baseline and after 1 and 2 years of interferon-β_{1b} treatment (49[C]). In contrast to what was expected, and despite the lack of controls, there was significant improvement in emotional state, as shown by significant reductions in scores of anxiety and depression over time. In addition, there was no effect of low-dose oral steroids in a subgroup of 46 patients.

Endocrine, metabolic Our knowledge of the possible effects of interferon-β on autoimmune disorders is growing with more extensive use of this cytokine. *Thyroid disorders* before and during the first 9 months of interferon-β_{1b} treatment have been systematically investigated in eight patients with relapsing remitting multiple sclerosis (50[C]). Before treatment, one patient had positive thyroperoxidase antibodies and one was taking thyroxine for multinodular goiter. After 3 months three other patients developed sustained positive titers of thyroperoxidase antibodies, of whom one developed hypothyroidism after 9 months. These results are in accordance with a previous similar study and isolated case reports (SEDA-21, 374; SEDA-22, 405), and suggest that interferon-β, like interferon-α, can cause thyroid autoimmunity.

Urinary system *Hemolytic-uremic syndrome* associated with interferon-β has been recently described (SEDA-22, 405). Two women aged 24 and 44 years whose primary diagnosis was relapsing multiple sclerosis also developed a thrombotic thrombocytopenic purpura-like syndrome within 2–4 weeks after starting interferon-β_{1a} (51[c]). Thrombocytopenia and renal function normalized in the first patient, whereas the second patient had thrombotic angiopathy on renal biopsy and required dialysis while awaiting renal transplantation. As interferon-α has also been suggested to produce hemolytic-uremic syndrome with thrombotic thrombocytopenic purpura, it is tempting to speculate that either interferons or other cytokines may play a role in this syndrome.

Skin and appendages *Granulomatous dermatitis* with disseminated pruritic papules and histological features resembling those of sarcoid granulomas has been described in a 57-year-old man who received interferon-β_{1b} (52[c]). The first lesions were observed after 2 months of treatment, persisted for 2 years, and slowly improved after interferon-β withdrawal and treatment with hydroxychloroquine PUVA.

Immunological and hypersensitivity reactions The clinical relevance of neutralizing antibodies to recombinant interferon-β is uncertain. The systemic availability of interferon-β_{1b}, measured by a myxovirus protein A assay, was completely inhibited in patients with neutralizing antibodies (53[C]). The presence of increased titers of serum-binding antibodies increased the likelihood of neutralizing antibodies. Unfortunately, the study provided no information on the clinical outcome in these patients. From a recent in vitro study of nine patients who developed neutralizing antibodies against the available formulations of recombinant interferon-β (three on interferon-β_{1a} and six on interferon-β_{1b}), it appears that these antibodies systematically cross-react in both binding and biological assays (54[C]). Although the sample size was small and lacked clinical confirmation, these results suggest that clinical benefit will not be obtained by switching to an alternative formulation when the absence of response or relapse during treatment is due to neutralizing antibodies.

Another study has shown that antibodies can spontaneously disappear in patients receiving long-tem treatment. Of 24 of 51 patients who initially developed neutralizing antibodies, generally during the first year of treatment, only five still had antibodies after a mean treatment duration of 102 months (55[C]). The mean time to antibody disappearance was 20 months. This confirms that treatment decisions should be based on clinical grounds rather than on the isolated identification of neutralizing antibodies.

An *anaphylactoid* reaction to interferon-β_{1b} has been reported only once before (SEDA-20, 332). In a further report, a 21-year-old woman had a severe anaphylactic-like reaction with laryngospasm and undetectable blood pressure within 10 minutes after interferon-β_{1a} injection (56[c]). It is still uncertain that anaphylaxis was definitely attributable to interferon, because rechallenge and skin tests were not performed in this patient, who had tolerated the treatment for the 6 previous months. Owing to the complex effects of interferon-β on the immune system and the paucity of reports of allergic reaction to steroids, another isolated case history has suggested that interferon-β_{1b} might have favored the development of an anaphylactoid reaction to previously well-tolerated injections of methylprednisolone (57[c]).

Tumor-inducing effects It has been suspected that interferon-β can accelerate *hepatocellular carcinoma* (58[c]).

A 62-year-old man with severe chronic hepatitis and positive serum anti-HCV, HBs, and HBc antibodies underwent unsuccessful treatment with interferon-α for 3 months and then received interferon-β for 6 months with a partial response. During treatment his α-fetoprotein (normal before treatment) progressively increased to seven-fold the upper limit of the reference range. There was also a slight increase in IL-6 serum concentration. A hepatocellular carcinoma was diagnosed 9 months later.

Liver carcinoma is an unexpected consequence of interferon-β in patients with chronic hepatitis C. However, the authors cited other published Japanese reports of hepatocellular carcinoma during or after interferon treatment. It is worth noting that interferon-β, but not interferon-α, significantly increased serum IL-6 concentrations in patients with chronic hepatitis C (59[C]), and that IL-6 has been suggested to promote the growth of hepatocellular carcinoma.

Interferon-γ

Although interferon-γ treatment is currently limited to patients with chronic granulomatous disease, it has recently been investigated in systemic sclerosis. The majority of 27 patients randomized to receive interferon-γ for 12 months complained of symptoms consistent with *influenza-like syndrome*, namely headache (85%), fever (81%), and arthralgia and myalgia (70%) (60[C]). There were adverse events (one or more per patient) leading to treatment discontinuation in four, including arthralgia, cardiac pain, atrioventricular block, reversible loss of hearing, and impotence; however, a causal relation with interferon-γ was not documented.

INTERLEUKINS *(SED-13, 1101; SEDA-20, 338; SEDA-21, 375; SEDA-22, 406)*

Interleukin-2 (IL-2)

The use of low-dose IL-2 as an adjunct to continuous antiretroviral therapy in HIV-infected patients with CD4 cell counts of 200–500 × 10^6/l is the major recent therapeutic advance for this immunoenhancing agent. In two recent randomized controlled studies (44 patients given subcutaneous IL-2, 58 given a modified-release polyethylene glycol-modified formulation, 27 given continuous intravenous IL-2, and 50 controls), IL-2 was well tolerated and a minority of patients required drug withdrawal because of adverse events (61[C], 62[C]). The overall adverse effects profile of both routes of administration was very similar, but was substantially less severe than previously described with high-dose IL-2. It consisted mostly of *fatigue, nasal/sinus congestion, fever above 38°C, headache, gastrointestinal disorders, stomatitis, somnolence*, and *mood change*. Increased bilirubin and alanine aminotransferase activities were more frequent than in the control group. None of the patients developed the capillary leak syndrome or significant hypertension, but *cardiomyopathy, attempted suicide, ulcerative colitis*, and *exacerbation of hepatitis B* were identified in one patient each among 85 patients treated with IL-2 (61[C]). *Erythema* and *injection site reactions* were observed in 66–69% of patients who received subcutaneous IL-2, and skin biopsies showed a perivascular infiltrate with lymphocytes and some eosinophils.

Liver, biliary *Gall-bladder changes* have been previously reported in patients given IL-2 and should be promptly recognized to avoid unnecessary intervention in symptomatic patients (SED-13, 1105). A further systematic ultrasonography examination performed in 25 HIV-infected patients treated with low-dose IL-2 (6-18 MU per day) confirmed that most patients had gall-bladder wall thickening (80%), abnormal echo texture (64%), and intramural fluid (52%) or pericholecystic fluid (20%) (63[C]). The frequency or severity of ultrasonographic abnormalities correlated with a higher dose of IL-2, as did complaints of right upper quadrant pain (24%). Although these findings mimicked those observed with acute cholecystitis, clinical symptoms and ultrasonographic abnormalities rapidly reversed after IL-2 withdrawal or between two cycles.

Interleukin-3 (IL-3)

The potential hemopoietic benefits of post-chemotherapy IL-3 are limited. In a phase III trial in 185 ovarian cancer patients treated with *carboplatin and cyclophosphamide*, premature discontinuation was significantly more frequent in patients randomized to received recombinant IL-3 (5 μg/kg from day 3 to day 12) than in the placebo group (64[C]). The most frequent adverse effects were allergic reactions (50% versus 23%), which required IL-3 discontinuation in 21 patients compared with one in the placebo group, and headache (46% versus 19%). In this setting, IL-3 stimulated hemopoiesis, but did not reduce platelet transfusions or increase adherence to the chemotherapeutic regimen. Similar toxic effects related to IL-3 occurred in a comparison of G-CSF alone, GM-CSF alone, and sequential IL3 and GM-CSF in 48 patients with cancer (16 in each group) receiving high-dose cyclophosphamide (65[C]). In particular, fever above 38.5°C, skin rash, and headaches were more frequent during IL-3 administration. As a result, 90% of patients receiving IL-3 required pharmacological treatment for adverse effects.

COLONY-STIMULATING FACTORS *(SED-13, 1111; SEDA-20, 342; SEDA-21, 377; SEDA-22, 407)*

Granulocyte colony-stimulating factor (G-CSF; filgrastim, lenograstim) and granulocyte-macrophage colony-stimulating factor (GM-CSF; molgramostim, sargramostim)

The potentially new clinical applications of GM-CSF have been lengthily reviewed (66[R]). Whereas it has been repeatedly stated that GM-CSF produced more frequent adverse effects than G-CSF, there were no significant differences in the adverse effects profiles and severity in 181 patients with cancers randomized to receive sargramostim or filgrastim for chemotherapy-induced myelosuppression (67[C]).

Use in healthy donors G-CSF and GM-CSF are both used in the short term in healthy volunteers to mobilize peripheral blood progenitor cells or granulocytes before allogeneic transplantation. However, this procedure has not been yet compared with bone-marrow donation and is not free from adverse effects. The effects and the safety of a 5-day regimen of G-CSF (nine patients) or GM-CSF (eight patients) have been compared (68[C]). Most patients complained of flu-like symptoms in both groups (six and seven respectively), but rash at the injection site was observed only in four patients treated GM-CSF. In the G-CSF group, there was a fall in platelet count (below 150×10^9/l) in five patients, raised serum lactic dehydrogenase activity, and raised uric acid concentrations; three patients required transient treatment with allopurinol. Treatment with G-CSF in 26 healthy donors for 5–7 days produced *transient changes in endothelial cell and clotting activation markers* (69[C]). Although these abnormalities may indicate a risk of thrombotic complications, their clinical relevance to healthy donors is unknown.

Several further case reports have stressed the possible occurrence of severe and unexpected adverse effects. Another case of spontaneous *splenic rupture* with histological evidence of massive extramedullary myelopoiesis after splenectomy has been reported in a 33-year-old healthy donor who received G-CSF for 6 days (70[c]). In a healthy woman, G-CSF was suggested to have transiently reactivated an alloantibody to an erythrocyte antigen (anti-Jk[a] antibody) (71[c]). This antibody was apparently passively transferred to the transplant recipient, who developed a high-titer of anti-Jka antibody during the first month after transplantation. This report raised the possibility that transplant recipients may develop hemolytic reactions to G-CSF subsequent to erythrocyte transfusion.

Use in children Guidelines for the appropriate use of hemopoietic growth factors in children have been proposed by a panel of European experts, who carefully summarized the potential indications and recommendations, and concluded that adult guidelines are applicable to children in most cases (72[R]). The authors considered that growth factors should be used in children for only a limited number of circumstances (prophylaxis or treatment in low-risk patients treated with chemotherapy, routine use in aplastic anemia, mobilization of peripheral blood progenitor cells in healthy pediatric donors).

In a recent large randomized placebo-controlled trial in 264 very low-birth weight neonates, treatment with GM-CSF for 28 days was not associated with specific toxic effects, but the incidence of nosocomial infections was not reduced (73[C]).

Use in drug-induced agranulocytosis Drug-induced agranulocytosis is a severe condition with a mortality rate of 6–10% despite the use of recently introduced potent antibiotics. Hemopoietic growth factors are therefore expected to reduce the duration of neutropenia and mortality. Two recent reviews have examined the available data, which mostly consisted of isolated case reports or small series of patients (74[R], 75[R]). Overall, the authors reached contrasting opinions, suggesting that hemopoietic growth factors might or might not be of interest in patients with severe drug-induced agranulocytosis. Adverse effects were noted in 13 of 118 case reports (74[R]). Although most of them were benign, *pulmonary toxicity* or *acute respiratory distress syndrome* have been noted in a few patients.

Use in HIV-infected patients The safety and activity of subcutaneous GM-CSF (300 μg/day for one week and 150 μg twice weekly for 11 weeks) has been compared with no treatment in 244 leukopenic HIV-infected patients (76[C]). Adverse effects were reported in most of the patients treated with GM-CSF and consisted of *flu-like symptoms* (98%), *bone pain* (42%), and *injection site reactions* (85%). There was a two-fold increase in serum transaminase and alkaline phosphatase activities in 5.7% of patients. There was a moderate, but not significant, increase in HIV p24 antigen concentration.

Respiratory A further report described acute febrile *interstitial pneumonitis* within less than 48 hours after the second to fourth cycles of chemotherapy (doxorubicin, cyclophosphamide, bleomycin, methotrexate, and methylprednisolone) in five patients with non-Hodgkin's lymphoma who were receiving prophylactic G-CSF (three patients) or GM-CSF (two patients) (77[c]). Lymphocytic alveolitis was confirmed in four of these patients and all three patients tested had an increased number of CD8+ T cells. Even though all the patients received high dose methylprednisolone, two died as a result of diffuse and extensive interstitial pulmonary fibrosis on post-mortem lung examination. Although both G-CSF and GM-CSF can cause acute pneumonitis in patients being treated for cancer, it is still unknown to what extent hemopoietic growth factors are involved in this complication. Another case suggested that G-CSF alone can cause severe pulmonary toxicity (78[c]).

A 72-year-old man with a normal chest X-ray was unnecessarily treated with G-CSF (5 μg/kg/day) for very moderate cytopenia. Five days later, he complained of dyspnea and fatigue, but without fever. His chest X-ray showed diffuse bilateral alveolar opacities and he had low oxygen saturations. Blood cultures were negative, and infectious pneumonitis (*Mycobacterium tuberculosis, Pneumocystis carinii, Herpes simplex*, and *cytomegalovirus*) was ruled out. Despite corticosteroid and antibiotic treatment, he required mechanical ventilation and died 12 days after the onset of symptoms.

Gastrointestinal (see also Use in healthy donors) There has been another case of life-threatening *splenic rupture* in a 22-year-old woman with acute myeloid leukemia (79[c]). The rupture was diagnosed in the presence of abdominal pain and signs of hypovolemic shock, 10 days after she started G-CSF treatment to support peripheral blood stem cell transplantation. Histology after splenectomy showed only small clusters of myeloblasts and no specific cause for the rupture. In particular, she was still pancytopenic at the time of splenic rupture.

Musculoskeletal There are still uncertainties about the role of G-CSF in the development of *bone changes* during long-term G-CSF maintenance therapy. There was bone mineral loss with features of osteopenia/osteoporosis in 15 of 30 patients treated with G-CSF for a mean of 5.8 years for severe chronic neutropenia (80[C]). However, six of nine patients investigated before G-CSF treatment had evidence of osteopenia/osteoporosis. Bone mineral loss is therefore frequent in children with congenital neutropenia, but it is not currently possible to rule out acceleration of bone mineral loss in patients taking maintenance G-CSF.

Immunological and hypersensitivity reactions Both G-CSF and GM-CSF can cause *anaphylactoid reactions*, and this has again been illustrated in two patients. One had acute bronchospasm after subcutaneous GM-CSF injection around a lower limb ulcer (81[c]). The other developed dyspnea, hypotension, and a pruritic erythematous skin rash within minutes of G-CSF injection, and later tolerated GM-CSF uneventfully (82[c]).

Tumor-inducing effects Although not yet proven, concerns have arisen over the prolonged use of G-CSF in children with aplastic anemia and the possible increased or accelerated risk of *myelodysplasia* (SED-14, 1117). This problem has been analysed in a retrospective study of 72 adults with aplastic anemia, of whom 18 received G-CSF and 23 ciclosporin (83[C]). Of the five who developed myelodysplastic syndrome, four had received G-CSF/ciclosporin. All four had monosomy 7, and the hematological disease was diagnosed within 16–31 months after the diagnosis of aplastic anemia and 12–20 months after the start of G-CSF treatment. Two died from acute leukemia. The incidence of myelodysplastic syndrome in this subgroup of patients was therefore 8.3% after 2 years and 39% after 3 years, whereas no case was observed over a 20-year period in patients not receiving this combined treatment. Univariate analysis showed that G-CSF plus ciclosporin and G-CSF treatment for more than 1 year were the most significant risk factors for the short-term development of monosomy 7 myelodysplastic syndrome. Myelodysplastic syndrome with monosomy 7 was also associated with G-CSF treatment in another patient, with a reduction in the number of monosomy 7 positive cells after G-CSF withdrawal and another increase after readministration (84[c]).

Stem cell factor *(SEDA-22, 406)*

Stem cell factor produces direct mast cell stimulation with subsequent *allergic-type reactions*. Despite careful premedication with diphenhydramine, ranitidine, inhaled salbutamol, and pseudoephedrine, such reactions were still observed in 3% of patients (85[C]).

MONOCLONAL ANTIBODIES

(SED-13, 1131; SEDA-20, 353; SEDA-21, 379; SEDA-22, 409)

Monoclonal antibodies in transplantation Daclizumab, a humanized anti-IL2 receptor monoclonal antibody, is being investigated for initial immunosuppression in transplant patients. Results of a phase III trial in 275 patients who received ciclosporin, corticosteroids, and daclizumab or placebo, evidenced no specific adverse effects associated with daclizumab (186[C]). In particular, the cytokine-release syndrome did not occur, and there was no difference in the incidence of fungal or cytomegalovirus infections between the two groups.

Monoclonal antibodies in cancer Rituximab, a chimeric monoclonal antibody directed against the CD20 antigen of normal and malignant B lymphocytes has been approved for the treatment of refractory or relapsing follicular lymphoma. A wide range of adverse events has been reported in most patients (87[R]). A transient *flu-like syndrome* is very common (50–90%), particularly after the first infusion of rituximab, and is often associated with various hypersensitivity-like symptoms (5–20%). In the most severe cases, patients had life-threatening *cytokine release syndrome* with dyspnea, bronchospasm, hypoxia, hypotension, urticaria, and angio-edema. Deaths have been reported in eight of 12 000–14 000 patients after drug launch. In recent case reports, rituximab was suggested as a possible cause in the development of aggressive peripheral T-cell lymphoma in two patients 15 and 18 months after receiving rituximab for low-grade B-cell non-Hodgkin's lymphoma (88[c], 89[c]).

Edrocolomab (17-1A antibody), a mouse monoclonal antibody, is used as an adjuvant treatment in patients with colorectal cancer. *Hypersensitivity and anaphylactic reactions* have been noted, and *urticaria* prolonged over a 4-month period was reported in one patient (90[c]).

An additional study in 50 patients with advanced, low-grade non-Hodgkin's lymphoma has confirmed that CAMPATH-1H, a humanized monoclonal antibody directed against the CD52 antigen of normal lymphocytes and B cell or T-cell lymphomas, produced marked *lymphopenia* and *neutropenia*, which were the probable cause of frequent severe infections (91[C]). Seven patients developed opportunistic infections and nine had bacterial septicemia; three patients died from infectious complications. Severe resistant *autoimmune thrombocytopenia* has also been noted in one patient, but the evidence that CAMPATH-1H was involved was limited (92[c]).

IMMUNOSUPPRESSIVE DRUGS

Azathioprine and 6-mercaptopurine

(SED-13, 1120; SEDA-20, 346; SEDA-21, 381; SEDA-22, 409)

There have been additional reports to suggest that measures of thiopurine methyltransferase (TPMT) activity can predict the occurrence of severe adverse effects in patients taking azathioprine. In one study, 14 of 33 patients with rheumatoid arthritis had severe adverse effects (mostly gastrointestinal toxicity, flu-like reactions or fever, pancytopenia, and hepatotoxicity) within 1–8 weeks after azathioprine was started (93[C]). Adverse effects subsided after withdrawal in all patients, but all eight patients who were rechallenged developed the same adverse effect. A baseline reduction in TPMT activity was significantly associated with the occurrence of these toxic effects in seven of eight patients, with a relative risk of 3.1 (95% CI = 1.6–6.2) compared with patients with high TPMT activity (seven of 25 patients). Another prospective evaluation in 67 patients with rheumatic disorders showed that TPMT genotype analysis is useful in identifying patients at risk of azathioprine toxicity (94[C]). Treatment duration was significantly longer in patients with the wild-type TPMP alleles than in those with mutant alleles, and that was due to the early occurrence of *leukopenia* in the latter.

Hematological Double therapy with ciclosporin and prednisone has been compared with triple therapy with ciclosporin, prednisone, and azathioprine in a randomized trial in 250 renal transplant patients (95[C]). Patients in the triple therapy group had less frequent severe episodes of acute rejection and more frequent episodes of *leukopenia* than the double therapy group (28% vs 4%). There were no other differences in the adverse effects profiles, in particular the incidence of infectious complications.

Liver Azathioprine *hepatotoxicity* is well known, and one previous study suggested an increased risk in renal transplant patients infected by hepatitis B or C (SEDA-20, 341). In 79 renal transplant patients with chronic viral hepatitis, azathioprine maintenance (34 patients) was associated with a poorer outcome of the liver disease than in 45 patients who discontinued azathioprine (96[C]). Cirrhosis was more frequent in the first group (six versus one), and more patients died with a functioning graft (14 vs two), mostly because of liver dysfunction (five patients) or infection (six patients). These results suggest that azathioprine further accelerates the course of the liver disease in these patients.

Azathioprine-induced *veno-occlusive disease of the liver* is a life-threatening complication, particularly in renal transplant patients. Another case report described the successful use of a transjugular intrahepatic portosystemic shunt over 26 months in a 33-year-old man who developed veno-occlusive disease, with progressive worsening 15 months after renal transplantation (97[c]).

Immunological and hypersensitivity reactions The distinction between relapse of the treated disease, systemic sepsis, and acute azathioprine hypersensitivity may be difficult, as has again been demonstrated in three patients with vasculitic disorders (98[c]).

Infections The frequency, course, and severity of *shingles* have been retrospectively evaluated in a sample of 550 patients treated with 6-mercaptopurine for inflammatory bowel disease (99[C]). Twelve patients aged 14–73 years developed shingles after an average of 921 days, an incidence that was about two-fold higher than in the general population. Only three patients were still taking corticosteroids at the time of onset of the shingles, and leukopenia was not associated with the occurrence of shingles. In nine patients, the course of shingles was 7–71 days, and was uncomplicated. Two patients had more severe symptoms and suffered from post-herpetic neuralgia. The last patient, a 14-year-old boy, had a brief episode of *Herpes zoster* during initial treatment and had *Herpes zoster* encephalitis at the age of 23 years, 16 months after 6-mercaptopurine had been restarted. From this report, it appears that 6-mercaptopurine can be restarted after brief discontinuation in patients who are expected to benefit from it.

Interactions Owing to the increased risk of hematological toxicity from the combination of azathioprine with *allopurinol*, it is usually recommended that the dosage of azathioprine be reduced by two-thirds. Because of the possible risks of decreased immunosuppression, cyclic urate oxidase may be safely given, as has been shown in six hyperuricemic transplant patients treated with azathioprine (100[C]).

Ciclosporin *(SED-13, 1123; SEDA-20, 348; SEDA-21, 382; SEDA-411)*

A previous meta-analysis whose aim was to compare the safety of Neoral® (the microemulsion formulation) and Sandimmune® (the standard formulation) suggested that Neoral® offered significant advantages over Sandimmune® (SEDA-22, 411). As the data were subject to many potential biases, the same authors reanalysed their results, taking into account only randomized prospective studies (101[C]). The incidence of adverse effects was higher with Sandimmune® in open-label studies (840 patients) and higher with Neoral® in blinded studies (3006 patients). In accordance with other investigators, these authors concluded that de novo immunosuppression with Neoral® is beneficial without significant differences in the incidence of adverse effects, whereas conversion from Sandimmune® to Neoral® in previously stable patients is associated with significantly more adverse effects with Neoral®.

Cardiovascular The incidence, clinical features, consequences, and management of ciclosporin-induced *hypertension* have been reviewed (102[R]). The prevalence was 29–54% in non-transplant patients and 65–100% in heart and liver transplant patients also taking corticosteroids. Disturbed circadian rhythm with a loss of nocturnal blood pressure fall was the main characteristic, and patients therefore had higher risks of left ventricular hypertrophy, cerebrovascular damage, microalbuminuria, and other target organ damage.

Respiratory *Hypersensitivity pneumonitis* has been reported for the first time (103[c]).

A 35-year-old woman taking glibenclamide and mesalazine for Crohn's colitis was given ciclosporin for severe disease exacerbation. Within 6 weeks, she developed arthralgia and moderate thrombocytopenia, and ciclosporin was discontinued. Acute fever (41°C) and dyspnea were noted several days later, and a chest X-ray showed diffuse bilateral infiltrates. Bronchoalveolar lavage showed neutrophil preponderance and plasma cells, and a lung biopsy strongly suggested an acute hypersensitivity pneumonitis. All her symptoms subsided after a short course of prednisolone and oxygen.

Both the absence of an infectious cause and the rapid improvement without withdrawal of other drugs, suggested that ciclosporin was the likely cause.

Nervous system From the results of a retrospective study of 227 liver transplant patients who received Neoral® as the primary immunosuppressive agent, it has been suggested that this formulation may reduce the risk of severe neurotoxicity (104[C]). Mild-to-moderate symptoms, i.e. *headache* (24 patients), *mild hand tremor* (13 patients), and *paresthesia* (five patients), were the most frequent, whereas *generalized seizures* were reported in only two patients.

A retrospective study identified a significantly higher incidence of central nervous system symptoms in patients with Behçet's disease (105[C]). There were *headache, fever, paralysis, ataxia, dysarthria*, or *disturbed consciousness* in 12 of 47 ciclosporin-treated patients compared with nine of 270 patients not treated or taking other drugs. CT and/or MRI scans were abnormal in all 12 patients. As the clinical findings were very similar to the neurological effects of Behçet's disease, it was suggested that ciclosporin can promote the development of neurological complications in this population.

Ciclosporin neurotoxicity is particularly frequent in liver and bone-marrow transplant patients, and patients usually recover after temporary dosage reduction or withdrawal. However, a fatal outcome has been reported (106[c]).

A 54-year-old man was given ciclosporin and methotrexate after allogeneic bone-marrow transplantation. He noted blurred vision during several days and became confused 11 weeks after transplantation. Generalized tonic-clonic seizures occurred the day after and he was given phenytoin and empirical antibiotics. His neurological condition deteriorated during the next 5 days, despite ciclosporin withdrawal, and he died from respiratory failure. Postmortem examination showed white matter edema and astrocyte injury without demyelination.

Most studies have focused on the central nervous system adverse effects of ciclosporin, and there have been few reports of *peripheral neuropathy*. In two patients, ciclosporin was suggested as a possible cause of an entrapment neuropathy, and surgery was required in both patients (107[c]). However, the report did not provide sufficient evidence to assess the causal relation fully. Another patient developed a symmetric polyneuropathy with flaccid paraplegia while her ciclosporin serum concentrations were about twice normal (108[c]). Electromyography showed features of axonal degeneration in the peripheral nerves and neurological symptoms improved on ciclosporin dosage reduction. Peripheral optic neuropathy, with visual loss, nystagmus, and ophthalmoplegia, has also been reported (109[c]). Finally, bilateral optic disc edema is sometimes associated with ciclosporin given for bone-marrow transplantation, but unilateral papilledema with otherwise asymptomatic raised intracranial pressure can occur (110[c]).

Migraine associated with ciclosporin is sometimes resistant to classical treatment and the consequences can be even more severe. Three young adult renal transplant patients, including two with a previous history of moderate migraine, had severe attacks of unilateral throbbing migraine associated with vomiting during ciclosporin treatment (111[c]). In two patients, vomiting was severe enough to reduce compliance with the immunosuppressive regimen, and both patients subsequently lost their grafts. The same sequence of events was again observed after retransplantation. Replacement with tacrolimus may be beneficial in such cases.

Mineral and fluid balance *Hypomagnesemia* is infrequently noted during ciclosporin treatment, and no specific complications have been so far reported. In a 43-year-old renal transplant patient, hypomagnesemia was associated with muscle weakness and a near four-fold increase in serum creatine kinase activity (112[c]). Both disorders resolved after magnesium supplementation, and ciclosporin was continued.

Urinary system The potential long-term consequences of ciclosporin *nephrotoxicity* constitute a major disadvantage in non-transplant patients. Renal function was assessed 7 years after the end of a 1-year ciclosporin treatment period in 36 young patients from a randomized placebo-controlled trial of ciclosporin in diabetes mellitus, 19 taking ciclosporin and 17 taking placebo (113[C]). Blood pressure did not differ between the groups. Compared with baseline values, urinary albumin excretion rate was significantly higher and estimated glomerular filtration rate significantly lower with ciclosporin. The results in the placebo group showed no change or increases. In addition, there was progression to micro- or macroalbuminuria in four ciclosporin-treated patients, and two of five patients who underwent renal biopsy had arteriolar hyalinosis. It is as yet not known whether these changes will translate to an increased risk of nephropathy, but they suggest that ciclosporin might enhance it.

Hemolytic-uremic syndrome is a rare complication of ciclosporin that usually appears between the second and fourth weeks after transplant, with associated fever, thrombocytopenia, erythrocyte fragmentation, neurotoxicity, and renal impairment. Uncommon clinical features have been reported. In two women hemolytic-uremic syndrome was apparently revealed by an episode of severe acute depression (114[c]). In another patient, the authors discussed the possibility that a single injection of ciclosporin might have induced the development of fibrin thrombi seen in the perioperative graft biopsy (115[c]). Later on, she was confirmed to have clinical and biological features of hemolytic-uremic syndrome, which reversed after ciclosporin withdrawal.

Skin and appendages In two patients, ciclosporin-associated soft tissue proliferation with an abnormal hyperplastic reaction has been suggested to account for the development of *hyperplastic pseudofolliculitis barbae* (116[c]) and *eruptive angiomatosis* (117[c]), not previously reported with ciclosporin. There has also been a rare report of acute *generalized pustular psoriasis* 1 week after ciclosporin withdrawal in a 32-year-old woman who had taken ciclosporin for 12 weeks for chronic plaque psoriasis (118[c]). This is in keeping with a similar phenomenon sometimes observed after corticosteroid withdrawal.

A white-headed man noted progressive *darkening of the hair* while taking ciclosporin (119[c]).

Immunological and hypersensitivity It has been suggested that *anaphylactoid reactions* to intravenous ciclosporin were probably due to improper mixing of the formulation, which may result in an unexpectedly large bolus of Cremophor EL (120).

Tumor-inducing effects It is generally considered that malignancies in patients taking immunosuppressive drugs are a direct consequence of immunosuppression rather than due to a specific drug. In a recent in vitro and in vivo experiment, ciclosporin promoted tumor growth by a direct cellular effect (121). This was suggested to be due to increased synthesis of transforming growth factor-β (TGF-β) as anti-TGF-β antibodies blocked the increased spread of cancer cells. The clinical relevance of these data awaits further careful clinical confirmation. At the moment, continuing analysis of clinical experience has not provided clear evidence for a ciclosporin-specific effect and has instead supported an immunosuppressive effect (122[C]).

Interactions Only interactions that have not previously been reported or interactions that add significant information will be discussed here.

A reciprocal interaction between ciclosporin and *saquinavir* has been reported in an HIV-positive kidney transplant patient (123[c]). Whereas ciclosporin concentrations were previously acceptable, there was a three-fold increase in ciclosporin trough concentrations after 3 days of saquinavir (3600 mg/day). In addition the saquinavir AUC was four times higher than that usually observed in patients taking similar dosages.

The interaction of ciclosporin with *troglitazone* has been confirmed in four heart transplant patients with a 30–60% fall in ciclosporin concentrations within days of taking troglitazone 200 mg/day (124[c]).

The interaction of ciclosporin with *acetazolamide* was previously supported by a single case report only. In three further patients, the addition of acetazolamide produced a near seven-fold increase in ciclosporin blood concentrations within 3 days (125[c]).

High-dose chemotherapy with *cyclophosphamide, vincristine, prednisolone, and intrathecal methotrexate* given for post-transplant lymphoproliferative disease was suggested to have favored the occurrence of acute ciclosporin neurotoxicity (headache, fever, seizures, and visual agnosia) in a 9-year-old cardiac transplant patient (126[c]). Ciclosporin serum concentrations were normal and a further similar episode occurred on ciclosporin readministration.

Cyclophosphamide *(SED-13, 1122; SEDA-20, 347; SEDA-21, 386; SEDA-22, 410)*

The relative benefits and risks of continuous oral or pulse intravenous use of cyclophosphamide are still debated. Whereas pulsed cyclophosphamide has been repeatedly presented as being less toxic, its effects have been questioned. An additional study in 47 patients has shown that intravenous pulsed cyclophosphamide was as effective as daily oral cyclophosphamide, but caused fewer adverse effects (127[C]). The patients were randomized to receive monthly intravenous pulses of cyclophosphamide (0.75 g/m^2, 22 patients) or daily oral cyclophosphamide (2 mg/kg/day, 25 patients) for at least 1 year. Both groups received corticosteroids. Whereas efficacy end-points did not show significant differences between the two groups, leukopenia (18% versus 60%) and severe infections (14% with no deaths versus 40% with three deaths) were significantly less frequent with intravenous pulsed cyclophosphamide. As a result, the probability of freedom from adverse effects (no deaths, severe infections, leukopenia, or thrombocytopenia) over a 12-month period was only about 25% in the oral daily group, compared with 70% in the intravenous pulse group. In addition, and based on the findings of a significantly lower serum follicle-stimulating hormone concentration at 3 and 6 months and a 57% reduction in the total dose in the intravenous pulse group, the intravenous pulse regimen was expected to produce fewer adverse gonadal effects and a reduced risk of malignancies.

Urinary system Cyclophosphamide was thought to have favored the development of emphysematous *cystitis* in a 73-year-old man (128[c]).

Infections Severe opportunistic infections are regarded as a major consequence of cyclophosphamide treatment, and a wide spectrum of organisms is involved.

A 72-year-old man with autoimmune thrombocytopenia had taken prednisone (30 mg/day) for 1 year, when he was found to have systemic lupus erythematosus (129[c]). Prednisone was continued and he started to take chloroquine (250 mg/day) and monthly cyclophosphamide (0.75 g/m^2). Three weeks after the first bolus of cyclophosphamide, he complained of fever and dyspnea, and chest X-rays showed bilateral pulmonary infiltrates. Despite prompt medical management, he died 5 days after admission with cytomegalovirus-induced interstitial pneumonia.

In addition to cyclophosphamide, this patient had several risk factors of developing fatal infection, namely age (older than 50 years), low leukocyte nadir (2900 $\times$ 10^6/l) after treatment with cyclophosphamide and prednisone.

Tumor-inducing effects Cyclophosphamide can cause *myelodysplastic syndromes*, particularly after prolonged treatment. The type of myelodysplastic syndromes and cytogenetic abnormalities that developed after treatment with alkylating agents for rheumatic diseases have been described in eight patients (mean age 57 years), of whom seven had received oral cyclophosphamide and one chlorambucil (130[C]). The mean cumulative dose of cyclophosphamide was 118 g for a mean cumulative duration of 4.4 years, and the myelodysplastic syndrome was diagnosed 0–4 years (mean 2.4 years) after the end of treatment. Concomitant immunosuppressive drugs were given in four of seven cyclophosphamide-treated patients. Cytogenetic abnormalities of chromosome 5 and/or 7, which are characteristic of treatment-related myelodysplastic syndromes, were found in all patients. Only two patients were still alive at the time of the report, and the outcome was remarkably poor in patients with chromosome 5 deletion. This study suggested that a high cumulative dose of cyclophosphamide is a risk factor for hematological malignancies, and that patients require long-term surveillance.

Methotrexate *(SEDA-21, 387; SEDA-22, 416; see also Chapter 45)*

A reduced incidence of several adverse effects of low-dose methotrexate may be achieved by using folic or folinic acid. In a meta-analysis of 307 patients with rheumatoid arthritis from seven randomized clinical trials, of whom 147 received folate supplementation, hematological adverse effects did not appear to be significantly reduced in the folate group (131[C]). However, there was a 79% reduction in mucosal and gastrointestinal adverse effects in patients taking folic acid and a non-significant trend toward a reduction (42%) in patients taking folinic acid. Disease activity was not modified by low doses of folate. Finally, the authors noted that folinic acid is more expensive.

Respiratory *Pulmonary endoalveolar hemorrhage* has not been previously described as a feature of methotrexate pneumonitis. It has been reported as a possible complication in a 57-year-old woman who voluntarily increased her dosage of methotrexate from 7.5 mg once a week to 7.5 mg/day for 15 days (132[c]).

Nervous system Neurological disorders are often under-recognized in patients taking low-dose methotrexate. Nevertheless, occasional cases of neurotoxicity are sometimes noted, as illustrated by the following report of acute *dysarthria* (133[c]).

A 71-year-old man was given oral methotrexate (15 mg/week) for cutaneous T-cell lymphoma. Within 3 weeks he developed progressive dysarthria and incoordination, and neurological examination showed mild buccofacial dyskinesia. Complete examination was otherwise normal, and he fully recovered 6–8 weeks after methotrexate withdrawal.

This case is reminiscent of other previously reported neurological abnormalities with low-dose methotrexate.

Skin and appendages *Yellow nail pigmentation* without paronychia has been noted in a patient treated for psoriasis (134[c]).

Tumor-inducing effects Some of the mechanisms and risk factors of methotrexate-associated *non-Hodgkin's lymphoma* in patients with rheumatoid arthritis have been reviewed, including an analysis of the characteristic features of 25 detailed published cases (135[R]). Although the epidemiological evidence is limited, several reports of spontaneous remission of lymphomas after methotrexate withdrawal strongly support a cause-and-effect relation.

Mycophenolate mofetil

(SED-13, 1130; SEDA-20, 351; SEDA-21, 389; SEDA-22, 418)

Mycophenolate is being used increasingly in primary immunosuppressive regimens for organ transplantation and can be useful in patients who have had complications from other immunosuppressive drugs. In 16 renal transplant patients with suspected ciclosporin nephrotoxicity, the addition of mycophenolate allowed safe reduction in the dosage of ciclosporin, with subsequent improvement in renal function and arterial blood pressure over 6 months (136[C]). It might allow the rapid withdrawal of corticosteroids in patients taking ciclosporin or tacrolimus, and therefore reduce the incidence of corticosteroid-induced post-transplant diabetes, hypercholesterolemia, and hypertension (137[C]). There have been several reports of patients with ciclosporin-associated thrombotic microangiopathy/hemolytic uremic syndrome in whom mycophenolate was successfully substituted (138[c], 139[c]). However, frequent and sometimes severe gastrointestinal adverse effects often required dosage reduction. The possible, but as yet unproven, negative consequences of increased immunosuppression (i.e. infections and neoplasms) produced by the addition of mycophenolate requires careful attention.

Gastrointestinal Gastrointestinal adverse effects, particularly *diarrhea*, are undoubtedly the most frequent and dose-limiting toxic effects of mycophenolate. Pooled data from the tricontinental and the US studies in kidney transplant patients showed incidences of diarrhea of 31% and 36% in patients taking 2 and 3 g/day respectively (140[R]). In a retrospective study, 29% of 109 mycophenolate-treated patients had diarrhea that required hospitalization, and 12% developed upper intestinal symptoms (i.e. *gastritis, esophagitis*) (141[C]). Frequent dosage reduction was necessary and only 28% of patients were still taking full doses after 1 year.

Gastrointestinal toxicity was confirmed to be the most frequent adverse effect (53%) in 120 pancreas transplant patients who received a triple immunosuppressive regimen consisting of mycophenolate, tacrolimus, and prednisone (142[C]). As a result, conversion from mycophenolate to azathioprine at 1 year was mostly due to gastrointestinal toxicity, and that was significantly more frequent in recipients of pancreas transplantation alone (49%) compared with recipients of pancreas transplantation after previous kidney transplantation (26%) or recipients of simultaneous pancreas and kidney transplants (14%). In another study in 120 kidney transplant patients randomized to receive tacrolimus and prednisone with or without mycophenolate there was a high rate of mycophenolate withdrawal (43%) during the first 6 months, again mostly because of gastrointestinal toxicity (143[C]). In both of these studies, the withdrawal rate was higher than in the pivotal trials in kidney transplant patients (4–10% after 6 months) (140[r]). As both studies used the combination of tacrolimus with mycophenolate rather than mycophenolate plus ciclosporin, a synergistic effect on the gastrointestinal tract or more probably higher serum concentrations of mycophenolic acid due to an interaction with tacrolimus might be suspected (SEDA-21, 390; SEDA-22, 421). The latter is in accordance with dose-related gastrointestinal toxicity.

The mechanism of gastrointestinal toxicity is not well understood.

A 42-year-old woman with a renal transplant taking triple immunosuppression (azathioprine, ciclosporin, and corticosteroids) was converted after 7 years from azathioprine plus ciclosporin to mycophenolate (2 g/day) because of ciclosporin nephrotoxicity (144[c]). Within 2 months she had developed severe and persistent watery diarrhea (5–10 stools per day) and lost 7 kg over 2 months. Investigations ruled out an infectious cause and there were features of duodenal villous atrophy on histological examination. Diarrhea disappeared after mycophenolate withdrawal and two subsequent duodenal biopsies showed improvement 2 months later and further complete recovery 6 months later.

This report suggests that loss of normal villous structure is one of the possible mechanisms of mycophenolate-induced severe diarrhea.

Infections The role of mycophenolate in the occurrence of opportunistic infections is debated. In a retrospective comparison of 358 simultaneous pancreas plus kidney transplant patients who received a ciclosporin-based immunosuppressive regimen, the rate of opportunistic infections was similar in patients treated with mycophenolate ($n = 109$) and azathioprine ($n = 249$) (141[C]). However, very few patients taking mycophenolate were available for long-term comparison. In contrast, another retrospective comparison of 135 renal transplant patients (69 prophylactic treatment and 66 rescue therapy) showed that the combination of mycophenolate, tacrolimus, and prednisone (49 patients) produced fewer rejection episodes, but a significantly higher incidence of infectious episodes than the combination of mycophenolate, ciclosporin, and prednisone (145[C]). In a randomized trial of 120 renal transplant patients, there was a significantly higher rate of asymptomatic or symptomatic cytomegalovirus infection in patients who took mycophenolate, tacrolimus, and prednisone than in patients who took tacrolimus plus prednisone (20 versus 5%) (143[C]). Overall, both of these studies suggest that mycophenolate plus tacrolimus has a more potent immunosuppressive effect, with an increased risk of infections (and theoretically lymphoproliferative disorders), as the counterpart of a possible greater effect on acute rejection prophylaxis.

Tumor-inducing effects There has been one report of recurrence of *Kaposi's sarcoma* 4 months after starting mycophenolate in a 58-year-old renal transplant patient who 7 years before had had similar lesions that reversed on withdrawal of ciclosporin (146[c]).

Sirolimus (rapamycin)

(SEDA-21, 390)

Sirolimus is primarily used for the prevention of allograft rejection, and its potential negative effects mostly consist of dose-related *hyperlipidemia* and a moderate *myelosuppressive effect.* In a 1-year follow-up of 40 renal transplant patients treated with various dosages of sirolimus (0.5–7 mg/m^2/day) in addition to a ciclosporin-based regimen, there were significant *increases in serum cholesterol and trigly-*

cerides, and significant *falls in white blood cell and platelet counts*, compared with historical controls (147[C]). These effects correlated with sirolimus trough concentrations but not dosages. One patient had to discontinue sirolimus because of hyperlipidemia refractory to treatment. Two case reports have recently suggested that sirolimus can produce features of the capillary leak syndrome in patients with psoriasis (148[c]).

A 53-year-old woman with severe psoriasis for 3 years, who had previously taken ciclosporin, sulfasalazine, and topical corticosteroids, was given sirolimus (8 mg/m^2/day), and 3 days later had fever, leg edema, dyspnea, weight gain, anemia, and hypotension. Chest X-ray showed pulmonary congestion and cardiomegaly. Empirical antibiotics were unsuccessful, and all symptoms progressively disappeared after sirolimus withdrawal.

A 58-year-old man took sirolimus (8 mg/m^2/day) for severe psoriasis with arthritis. He also took ibuprofen, co-trimoxazole, and paracetamol. Within 1 month he developed nocturnal fever, dizziness, orthostatic hypotension, leg edema, and anemia. All his symptoms subsided after sirolimus withdrawal, furosemide treatment, and erythrocyte transfusion.

No other causes were found, and the authors noted that of 34 psoriatic patients given sirolimus, three had *leg edema* and a *reduced hematocrit*. Based on limited in vitro findings, they suggested that sirolimus might enhance apoptosis of activated lymphocytes and thereby cytokine release.

Tacrolimus *(SED-13, 1130; SEDA-20, 351; SEDA-21, 390; SEDA-22, 419)*

Long-term follow-up (mean of 93 months) of tacrolimus-based immunosuppression has been reported in 121 adult patients with liver transplants (149[C]). *Infections* were the most common causes of deaths (17 patients out of 42), and half of them occurred during the first year after transplantation. *Cardiovascular events* (seven patients) or de novo malignancies (three patients) were also important causes of death. *End-stage renal disease* related to tacrolimus nephrotoxicity was noted in two patients who required renal transplantation. At 7 years, other important adverse effects included *hyperkalemia* (30%) or *hypertension* (31%) requiring treatment, and *insulin-dependent diabetes mellitus* (13%). Seven patients developed de novo *malignancies* and six had post-transplant *lymphoproliferative disorders*. The risks of tacrolimus in renal transplantation have been discussed (150[R]).

Cardiovascular Several reports have previously focused on the possible occurrence of *cardiomyopathy* in tacrolimus-treated transplant patients, particularly children. In two further liver transplant children aged 2.5 and 14 years who died from multiorgan system failure due to sepsis and end-stage liver failure, pathological examination showed prominent concentric left ventricular hypertrophy (151[c]). Although tacrolimus was regarded as a possible cause of asymptomatic hypertrophic cardiomyopathy in these patients, a direct causal relation was difficult to establish. The cause is probably multifactorial, and potential confounding factors (e.g. hypertension, corticosteroids) are numerous in this population. In a retrospective review of 89 pediatric heart transplant patients who had survived for at least 6 months, repeated echocardiography showed signs of cardiac hypertrophy, particularly early after transplantation and in very young infants (152[C]). However, there was no evidence of progressive hypertrophy on follow-up examinations, and no significant differences in the degree of cardiac hypertrophy between patients aged over 1 year at the time of transplantation who received ciclosporin (26 patients) or tacrolimus (41 patients).

In a retrospective study, the prevalence of *hypertension* 2 years after adult liver transplantation was significantly lower in patients treated with tacrolimus (64% of 28 patients) than in patients treated with ciclosporin (82% of 131 patients) (153[C]). In addition, hypertension occurred later with tacrolimus. A similar benefit of tacrolimus over ciclosporin was found in a randomized comparative trial in 85 heart transplant patients, and 41% of 39 tacrolimus-treated patients developed new-onset hypertension requiring treatment, compared with 71% of 46 ciclosporin-treated patients (154[C]).

Nervous system Tacrolimus-induced acute *neurotoxicity* is very similar to that caused by ciclosporin. This has again been shown in six patients (including five children) who developed signs of *encephalopathy* with generalized or focal seizures, reduced visual acuity or cortical blindness, altered mental status, and white matter lesions on MRI scan, particularly in the parieto-occipital regions (155[c], 156[c], 157[C]). Three patients had tacrolimus blood concentrations above the target range before the neurological adverse event. Although there was complete resolution after tacrolimus withdrawal or reduction in dosage in four patients, two children still had persistent brain imaging abnormalities and recurrent episodes of seizures.

Endocrine, metabolic In a pooled analysis of four randomized trials of tacrolimus versus ciclosporin after renal transplantation, the prevalence of post-transplant *diabetes mellitus* at 1 year (two studies, 532 patients) was five times higher with tacrolimus than with ciclosporin (odds ratio: 5.0; 95% CI = 2.0–12.4) (158[C]). In the opinion of the US FDA, post-transplant diabetes mellitus was a significant hazard in tacrolimus-treated patients, even though about half of the patients were no longer taking insulin at 2 years after transplantation (159). The exact mechanisms of tacrolimus-induced diabetes are unknown. In one renal transplant patient with genetic susceptibility, tacrolimus was associated with insulin-dependent diabetes mellitus and the simultaneous occurrence of anti-glutamic acid decarboxylase antibody (160[c]). Within 2 months after conversion from tacrolimus to ciclosporin, the antibody was no longer detected and the patient's insulin requirements fell dramatically. Tacrolimus-induced direct beta cell toxicity, with subsequent development of β-cell autoimmunity, was therefore suggested as a possible mechanism in patients with genetic susceptibility for type I diabetes.

In contrast to its effects on glucose metabolism, tacrolimus offers potential advantages over ciclosporin for lipid disorders (146[C]).

Gastrointestinal The first case of tacrolimus-associated *Clostridium difficile diarrhea* has been reported (161[c]).

A 29-year-old man was given mycophenolate and tacrolimus for an episode of renal transplant rejection that occurred 6.5 years after transplantation. Four weeks after tacrolimus was begun, he had diarrhea, nausea, and malaise. There was *C. difficile* toxin in the stools, and his symptoms abated with metronidazole. About 1 month later, he developed diarrhea, fever, and severe dehydration. *C. difficile* toxin was again detected in the stools, and his symptoms completely resolved with oral vancomycin and withdrawal of tacrolimus.

Similar cases have been reported to the manufacturers. A possible relation between the macrolide molecular structure of tacrolimus and the development of *C. difficile* colitis remains to be established.

Urinary system The nephrotoxic adverse effects of tacrolimus and ciclosporin are clinically indistinguishable. The pathological features of renal biopsies at 2 years of treatment in patients enrolled in a large multicenter comparison of tacrolimus and ciclosporin in renal transplantation have been reported (162[C]). Of 412 patients initially randomized, renal biopsies were available from 79 treated with tacrolimus and 65 treated with ciclosporin. There were features of tacrolimus or ciclosporin nephrotoxicity (hyaline arteriolar change, tubular vacuolization) in 19 and 11 patients respectively. There were no differences in the rates of biopsy-proven acute rejection (8.9% versus 9.2%) or chronic allograft nephropathy (62% and 72%). In addition, the histological features of chronic allograft nephropathy were very similar. An older age of the donor, acute rejection, cytomegalovirus infection, and ciclosporin- and tacrolimus-associated nephrotoxicity during the first year of transplantation were the most significant factors associated with the occurrence of chronic nephropathy.

As with ciclosporin, tacrolimus used as the primary immunosuppressive drug has sometimes been associated with de novo *thrombotic microangiopathy/hemolytic-uremic syndrome*. Its role has been clearly confirmed in a 52-year-old heart transplant patient in whom hemolytic-uremic syndrome recurred 6 days after tacrolimus readministration (163[c]). From a report of two additional cases and a review of 19 other reported cases, the incidence of tacrolimus-associated thrombotic microangiopathy has been suggested to be 1.0–4.7%; 15 cases were reported in renal transplant patients (164[cR]). The mean time to diagnosis was 9 months (4 days to 31 months), and the tacrolimus trough concentrations were usually within the target range. Most patients had the clinical features of hemolytic-uremic syndrome. Final outcomes were known in 18 patients: 10 had tacrolimus dosage reduction only (six recovered, three had an acute cellular rejection, one lost his renal graft); one stopped taking tacrolimus and recovered; seven had tacrolimus dosage reduction or discontinuation and underwent plasmapheresis, fresh-frozen plasma exchange, high-dose steroids, or anticoagulation (three died of sepsis and multiorgan failure, one lost her renal graft, and three recovered). Furthermore, and in contrast to previous reports (SEDA-19, 353), a change from ciclosporin to tacrolimus in patients with ciclosporin-associated hemolyticuremic syndrome is not always successful. This has been again shown in two renal transplant patients who developed resistant late acute rejection while taking ciclosporin (165[c]). After a switch to tacrolimus, they had clinical and histological features of hemolytic-uremic syndrome, with biopsy-proven thrombotic microangiopathy within 2 and 12 days after conversion. Both finally required explantation of their renal allografts.

Skin and appendages A brief case report has suggested that tacrolimus may cause *gingival hyperplasia* (166[c]).

Second-generation effects Although reassuring results have been obtained (SEDA-21, 392), experience with tacrolimus in pregnant women is still limited. One report has described congestive heart failure with *dilated cardiomyopathy* in twin boys born to a woman with a renal transplant who took tacrolimus throughout her pregnancy (167[c]). One twin died from irreversible cardiac failure, and autopsy findings showed thrombogenic cardiomyopathy and degeneration of cardiac muscle. The other twin was more actively treated and had only mild tricuspid insufficiency on follow-up. This report is in keeping with the possible and debated role of tacrolimus in the development of cardiomyopathy in children (see Cardiovascular).

Overdosage A further report has confirmed that even large accidental overdosage of tacrolimus does not result in marked acute toxicity (168[c]). The inadvertent administration of 25 times the intended dose in a 22-month-old infant produced minimal consequences, with only a five-fold reversible increase in serum amylase activity.

Interactions Further reports have confirmed that drugs that inhibit ciclosporin metabolism have similar effects on the metabolism of tacrolimus; this includes nefazodone (169[c]).

A 16-year-old boy had a five-fold increase in tacrolimus blood concentrations and a two-fold increase in creatinine concentrations within 4 weeks of nefazodone treatment. Complete normalization occurred after replacement with paroxetine and a transient reduction in tacrolimus dosage.

Mibefradil, another potent inhibitor of CYP3A, which is no longer in use, increased tacrolimus blood concentrations dramatically (170[c]).

It has been confirmed that *metronidazole* can produce a two-fold increase in blood concentrations of ciclosporin and tacrolimus, with a subsequent increase in serum creatinine in both cases (171[c]).

IMMUNOENHANCING DRUGS

(SEDA-20, 348; SEDA-22, 421)

Levamisole

See Chapter 31.

OK-432 (Picibanil)

Hyponatremia related to a *syndrome of inappropriate secretion of antidiuretic hormone* (SIADH) has been attributed to picibanil (172[c]).

A 59-year-old woman with a previous history of squamous cell carcinoma of the esophagus developed a metastatic lung tumour 4 years later. A right lower lobectomy was performed, and intrapleural picibanil instillation was performed on postoperative days 4, 5, and 9 for pulmonary fistula with prolonged air leakage. On day 13 she had fatigue, nausea, and drowsiness. Her serum sodium was 106 mmol/l and there was a 2.5-fold increase in serum antidiuretic hormone concentration. Complete recovery was noted after fluid restriction and sodium supplementation.

The author thought that SIADH had resulted from severe pleurisy secondary to intrapleural administration of picibanil rather than to direct stimulation of antidiuretic hormone release.

REFERENCES

1. Cacopardo B, Benanti F, Brancati G, Romano F, Nunnari A. Leucocyte interferon-α retreatment for chronic hepatitis C patients previously intolerant to other interferons. J Viral Hepatitis 1998;5:333–9.
2. Anonymous. Interferon-α-2b and ribavirin combination therapy-indications extended: previously untreated hepatitis C patients. WHO Newsletter 1999;1/2;9.
3. Colivicchi F, Magnanimi S, Sebastiani F, Silvestri R, Magnanimi R. Incidence of electrocardiographic abnormalities during treatment with human leukocyte interferon-alfa in patients with chronic hepatitis C but without preexisting cardiovascular disease. Curr Ther Res Clin Exp 1998;59:692–6.
4. Parrens E, Chevalier JM, Rougier M, Douard H, Labbé L, Quiniou G, Broustet A, Broustet J-P. Apparition d'un bloc auriculo-ventriculaire du troisième degré sous interféron α: à propos d'un cas. Arch Mal Coeur Vaiss 1999;92:53–6.
5. Cid MC, Hernandez-Rodriguez J, Robert J, Del Rio A, Casademont J, Coll-Vinent B, Grau JM, Kleinman HK, Urbano-Marquez A, Cardellach F. Interferon-α may exacerbate cryoglobulinemia related ischemic manifestations. Arthritis Rheum 1999;42:1051–5.
6. Bini EJ, Weinshel EH. Severe exacerbation of asthma: a new side effect of interferon-α in patients with asthma and chronic hepatitis C. Mayo Clin Proc 1999;74:367–70.
7. Wörle H, Maass E, Köhler B, Treuner J. Interferon alpha-2a therapy in haemangiomas of infancy : spastic diplegia as a severe complication. Eur J Pediatr 1999;158:344.
8. Enjolras O. Neurotoxicity of interferon-α in children treated for hemangiomas. J Am Acad Dermatol 1998;39:1037-8.
9. Grether JK, Nelson KB, Dambrosia JM, Phillips TM. Interferons and cerebral palsy. J Pediatr 1999;134:324–32.
10. Brouwers PJ, Bosker RJI, Schaafsma M, Wilts G, Neef C. Photosensitive seizures associated with interferon alfa-2a. Ann Pharmacother 1999;33:113–14.
11. Horikawa N, Yamazaki T, Sagawa M, Nagata T. A case of akathisia during interferon-α therapy for chronic hepatitis type C. Gen Hosp Psychiatry 1999;21:134–40.
12. Capuron L, Ravaud A. Prediction of the depressive effects of interferon alfa therapy by the patient's initial affective state. New Engl J Med 1999;340:1370.
13. Monji A, Yoshida I, Tashiro KI, Hayashi Y, Tashiro N. A case of persistent manic depressive illness induced by interferon-alfa in the treatment of chronic hepatitis C. Psychosomatics 1998;39:562–4.
14. Valentine AD. Managing the neuropsychiatric adverse effects of interferon treatment. BioDrugs 1999;11:229–37.
15. Fortis A, Christopoulos C, Chrysadakou E, Anevlavis E. De Quervain's thyroiditis associated with interferon-α-2b therapy for non-Hodgkin's lymphoma. Clin Drug Invest 1998;16:473–5.
16. Ghilardi G, Gonvers JJ, So A. Hypothyroid myopathy as a complication of interferon alpha therapy for chronic hepatitis C virus infection. Br J Rheumatol 1998;37:1349–51.
17. Schmitt K, Hompesch BC, Oeland K, Von Straehr WG, Thürmann PA. Autoimmune thyroiditis and myelosuppression following treatment with interferon-α for hepatitis C. Int J Clin Pharmacol Ther 1999;37:165–7.
18. Fernandez-Soto L, Gonzalez A, Escobar-Jimenez F, Vazquez R, Ocete E, Olea N, Salmeron J. Increased risk of autoimmune thyroid disease in hepatitis C vs hepatitis B before, during, and after discontinuing interferon therapy. Arch Intern Med 1998;158:1445–8.
19. Kakizaki S, Takagi H, Murakami M, Takayama H, Mori M. HLA antigens in patients with interferon-α-induced autoimmune thyroid disorders in chronic hepatitis C. J Hepatol 1999;30:794–800.
20. Minelli R, Braverman LE, Valli MA, Schianchi C, Pedrazzoni M, Fiaccadori F, Salvi M, Magotti MG, Roti E. Recombinant interferon α (rIFN-α) does not potentiate the effect of iodine excess on the development of thyroid abnormalities in patients with HCV chronic active hepatitis. Clin Endocrinol 1999;50:95–100.
21. Calvino J, Romero R, Suarez-Penaranda JM, Arcocha V, Lens XM, Mardaras J, Novoa D, Sanchez-Guisande D. Secondary hyperparathyroidism exacerbation: a rare side-effect of interferon-alpha? Clin Nephrol 1999;51:248–51.
22. Elisaf M, Tsianos EV. Severe hypertriglyceridaemia in a non-diabetic patient after α-interferon. Eur J Gastroenterol Hepatol 1999;11:463.
23. Junghans V, RĄnger TM. Hypertriglyceridaemia following adjuvant interferon-α treatment in two patients with malignant melanoma. Br J Dermatol 1999;140:168–92.
24. Fernandez-Miranda C, Castellano G, Guijarro C, Fernandez I, Schöebel N, Larumbe S, Gomez-Izquierdo T, Del Palacio A. Lipoprotein changes in patients with chronic hepatitis C treated with interferon-α. Am J Gastroenterol 1998;93:1901–4.
25. Peck-Radosavljevic M, Wichlas M, Pidlich J, Sims P, Meng G, Zacherl J, Garg S, Datz C, Gangl A, Ferenci P. Blunted thrombopoietin response to interferon alfa-induced thrombocytopenia during treatment for hepatitis C. Hepatology 1998;28:1424–9.
26. Martin TG, Shuman MA. Interferon-induced thrombocytopenia: is it time for thrombopoietin? Hepatology 1998;28:1430–2.
27. Toccaceli F, Rosati S, Scuderi M, Iacomi F, Picconi R, Laghi V. Leukocyte and platelet lowering by some interferon types during viral hepatitis treatment. Hepato-Gastroenterology 1998;45:1748–52.
28. Rachmani R, Avigdor A, Youkla M, Raanani P, Zilber M, Ravid M, Ben Bassat I. Thrombotic

thrombocytopenic purpura complicating chronic myelogenous leukemia treated with interferon-α. A report of two successfully treated patients. Acta Haematol 1998;100:204–6.
29. Zylberberg H, Fontaine H, Thépot V, Nalpas B, Bréchot C, Pol S. Triggering of acute alcohol hepatitis by α-interferon therapy. J Hepatol 1999;30:722–5.
30. Garrido Palma G, Sanchez Cuenca JM, Olaso V, Pina R, Urquijo JJ, Lopez Viedma B, Bustamante M, Berenguer M, Berenguer J. Response to treatment with interferon-alfa in patients with chronic hepatitis C and high titers of -M2, -M4 and -M8 antimitochondrial antibodies. Rev Esp Enferm Dig 1999;91:175–81.
31. Shah M, Jenis EH, Mookerjee BK, Schriber JR, Baer MR, Herzig GP, Wetzler M. Interferon-α-associated focal segmental glomerulosclerosis with massive proteinuria in patients with chronic myeloid leukemia following high dose chemotherapy. Cancer 1998;83:1938–46.
32. Eberlein-König B, Hein R, Abeck D, Engst R, Ring J. Cutaneous sarcoid foreign body granulomas developing in sites of previous skin injury after systemic interferon-alpha treatment for chronic hepatitis C. Br J Dermatol 1999;140:370–2.
33. Kadayifcilar S, Boyacioglu S, Kart H, Gursoy M, Aydin P. Ocular complications with high-dose interferon alpha in chronic active hepatitis. Eye 1999;13:241–6.
34. Krischer J, Pechère M, Salomon D, Harms M, Chavaz P, Saurat JH. Interferon alfa-2b-induced Meyerson's nevi in a patient with dysplastic nevus syndrome. J Am Acad Dermatol 1999;40:105–6.
35. Hayasaka S, Nagaki Y, Matsumoto M, Sato S. Interferon associated retinopathy. Br J Ophthalmol 1998;82:323–5.
36. Lohmann CP, Kroher G, Bogenrieder T, Spiegel D, Preuner J. Severe loss of vision during adjuvant interferon alfa-2b treatment for malignant melanoma. Lancet 1999;353:1326.
37. Sugano S, Suzuki T, Watanabe M, Ohe K, Ishii K, Okajima T. Retinal complications and plasma C5a levels during interferon alpha therapy for chronic hepatitis C. Am J Gastroenterol 1998;93:2441–4.
38. Cadoni G, Marinelli L, de Santis A, Romito A, Manna R, Ottaviani F. Sudden hearing loss in a patient hepatitis C virus (HCV) positive on therapy with alpha-interferon: a possible autoimmune-microvascular pathogenesis. J Laryngol Otol 1998;112:962–3.
39. Bell TM, Bansal AS, Shorthouse C, Sandford N, Powell EE. Low-titre auto-antibodies predict autoimmune disease during interferon-α treatment of chronic hepatitis C. J Gastroenterol Hepatol 1999;14:419–22.
40. Boonen A, Stockbrügger RW, Van der Linden S. Pericarditis after therapy with interferon-α for chronic hepatitis C. Clin Rheumatol 1999; 18:177–9.
41. Johnson DM, Hayat SQ, Burton GV. Rheumatoid arthritis complicating adjuvant interferon-α therapy for malignant melanoma. J Rheumatol 1999;26:1009–10.
42. Bren A, Kandus A, Ferluga D. Rapidly progressive renal graft failure associated with interferon-α treatment in a patient with chronic myelogenous leukemia. Clin Nephrol 1998;50:266–7.
43. Beelen DW, Elmaagacli AH, Schaefer UW. The adverse influence of pretransplant interferon-α (IFN-α) on transplant outcome after marrow transplantation for chronic phase chronic myelogenous leukemia increases with the duration of IFN-α exposure. Blood 1999;93:1779–80.
44. Rostaing L, Chatelut E, Payen JL, Izopet J, Thalamas C, Ton-That H, Pascal JP, Durand D, Canal P. Pharmacokinetics of αIFN-2b in chronic hepatitis C virus patients undergoing chronic hemodialysis or with normal renal function: clinical implications. J Am Soc Nephrol 1998;9:2344–8.
45. Uchihara M, Izumi N, Sakai Y, Yauchi T, Miyake S, Sakai T, Akiba T, Maumo F, Sato C. Interferon therapy for chronic hepatitis C in hemodialysis patients: increased serum levels of interferon. Nephron 1998;80:51–6.
46. Fiegl M, Chott A, Seewann HL, Lechner K, Gisslinger H. Persisting bone marrow aplasia following interferon-alpha combined with Ara-C for chronic myelogenous leukemia. Leuk Lymphoma 1999;34:191–5.
47. Tappero G, Ballaré M, Farina M, Negro F. Severe anemia following combined α-interferon/ribavarin therapy of chronic hepatitis C. J Hepatol 1998;29:1033–4.
48. Bramanti P, Sessa E, Rifici C, D'Aleo C, Floridia D, Di Bella P, Lublin F. Enhanced spasticity in primary progressive MS patients treated with interferon beta-1b. Neurology 1998;51:1720–3.
49. Borras C, Rio J, Porcel J, Barrios M, Tintoré M, Montalban X. Emotional state of patients with relapsing-remitting MS treated with interferon beta-1b. Neurology 1999;52:1636–9.
50. Rotondi M, Oliviero A, Profice P, Mone CM, Biondi B, Del Buono A, Mazziotti G, Sinisi AM, Bellastella A, Carella C. Occurrence of thyroid autoimmunity and dysfunction throughout a nine-month follow-up in patients undergoing interferon-β therapy for multiple sclerosis. J Endocrinol Invest 1998;21:748–52.
51. Herrera WG, Balizet LB, Harberts SW, Brown ST. Occurrence of a TTP-like syndrome in two women receiving beta interferon therapy for relapsing multiple sclerosis. Neurology 1999;52:135.
52. Mehta CL, Tyler RJ, Cripps DJ. Granulomatous dermatitis with focal sarcoidal features associated with recombinant interferon β-1b injections. J Am Acad Dermatol 1998;39:1024–8.
53. Deisenhammer F, Reindl M, Harvey J, Gasse T, Dilitz E, Berger T. Bioavailability of interferon beta 1b in MS patients with and without neutralizing antibodies. Neurology 1999;52:1239–43.
54. Khan OA, Dhib-Jalbut SS. Neutralizing antibodies to interferon β-1a and interferon β-

1b in MS patients are cross-reactive. Neurology 1998;51:1698–702.
55. Rice GPA, Paszner B, Oger J, Lesaux J, Paty D, Ebers G. The evolution of neutralizing antibodies in multiple sclerosis patients treated with interferon β-1b. Neurology 1999;52:1277–9.
56. Corona T, Leon C, Ostrosky-Zeichner L. Severe anaphylaxis with recombinant interferon beta. Neurology 1999;52:425.
57. Clear D. Anaphylactoid reaction to methyl prednisolone developing after starting treatment with interferon β-1b. J Neurol Neurosurg Psychiatry 1999;66:690.
58. Malaguarnera M, Restuccia S, Di Fazio I, Di Marco R, Pistone G, Trovato BA. Rapid evolution of chronic viral hepatitis into hepatocellular carcinoma after beta-interferon treatment. Panminerva Med 1999;41:59–61.
59. Furusyo N, Hayashi J, Ohmiya M, Sawayama Y, Kawakami Y, Ariyama I, Kinukawa N, Kashiwagi S. Differences between interferon-α and -β treatment for patients with chronic hepatitis C virus infection. Dig Dis Sci 1999;44:608–17.
60. Grassegger A, Schuler G, Hessenberger G, Walder-Hantich B, Jabrowski J, Macheiner W, Salmhofer W, Zahel B, Pinter G, Herold M, Klein G, Fritsch PO. Interferon-gamma in the treatment of systemic sclerosis : a randomized controlled multicentre trial. Br J Dermatol 1998;139:639–48.
61. Carr A, Emery S, Lloyd A, Hoy J, Garsia R, French M, Stewart G, Fyfe G, Cooper DA. Outpatient continuous intravenous interleukin-2 or subcutaneous, polyethylene glycol-modified interleukin-2 in human immunodeficiency virus-infected patients: a randomized, controlled, multicenter study. J Infect Dis 1998;178:992–9.
62. Hengge UR, Goos M, Esser S, Exner V, Dötterer H, Wiehler H, Borchard C, MĄller K, Beckmann A, Eppner MT, Berger AM, Fiedler M. Randomized, controlled phase II trial of subcutaneous interleukin-2 in combination with highly active antiretroviral therapy (HAART) in HIV patients. AIDS 1998;12:F225–34.
63. Premkumar A, Walworth CM, Vogel S, Daryanani KD, Venzon DJ, Kovacs JA, Feuerstein IM. Prospective sonographic evaluation of interleukin-2-induced changes in the gallbladder. Radiology 1998;206:393–6.
64. Hofstra LS, Kristensen GB, Willemse PHB, Vindevoghel A, Meden H, Lahousen M, Oberling F, Sorbe B, Crump M, Sklenar I, Sluiter WJ, Kiese B, Trope CG, De Vries EGE. Randomized trial of recombinant human interleukin-3 versus placebo in prevention of bone marrow depression during first-line chemotherapy for ovarian carcinoma. J Clin Oncol 1998;16:3335–44.
65. Ballestrero A, Ferrando F, Garuti A, Basta P, Gonella R, Stura P, Mela GS, Sessarego M, Gobbi M, Patrone F. Comparative effects of three cytokine regimens after high-dose cyclophosphamide: granulocyte colony-stimulating factor, granulocyte-macrophage colony-stimulating factor (GM-CSF), and sequential interleukin-3 and GM-CSF. J Clin Oncol 1999;17:1296–303.
66. Armitage JO. Emerging applications of recombinant human granulocyte-macrophage colony-stimulating factor. Blood 1998;92:4491–508.
67. Beveridge RA, Miller JA, Kales AN, Binder RA, Robert NJ, Harvey JH, Windsor K, Gore I, Cantrell J, et al. A comparison of efficacy of sargramostim (yeast-derived RhuGM-CSF) and filgrastim (bacteria-derived RhuG-CSF) in the therapeutic setting of chemotherapy-induced myelosuppression. Cancer Invest 1998;16:366–73.
68. Fischmeister G, Kurz M, Haas OA, Micksche M, Buchinger P, Printz D, Ressmann G, Stroebel T, Peters C, Fritsch G, Gadner H. G-CSF versus GM-CSF for stimulation of peripheral blood progenitor cells (PBPC) and leukocytes in healthy volunteers: comparison of efficacy and tolerability. Ann Hematol 1999;78:117–23.
69. Falanga A, Marchetti M, Evangelista V, Manarini S, Oldani E, Giovanelli S, Galbusera M, Cerletti C, Barbui T. Neutrophil activation and hemostatic changes in healthy donors receiving granulocyte colony-stimulating factor. Blood 1999;93:2506–14.
70. Falzetti F, Aversa F, Minelli O, Tabilio A. Spontaneous rupture of spleen during peripheral blood stem-cell mobilisation in a healthy donor. Lancet 1999;353:555.
71. Norol F, Bonin P, Charpentier F, Bierling P, Beaujean F, Cartron JP, Bories D, Kuentz M. Apparent reactivation of a red cell alloantibody in a healthy individual after G-CSF administration. Br J Haematol 1998;103:256–8.
72. Schaison G, Eden OB, Henze G, Kamps WA, Locatelli F, Ninane J, Ortega J, Riikonen P, Wagner HP. Recommendations on the use of colony-stimulating factors in children: conclusions of a European panel. Eur J Pediatr 1998;157:955–66.
73. Cairo MS, Agosti J, Ellis R, Laver JJ, Puppala B, deLemos R, Givner L, Nesin M, Wheeler JG, Seth T, Van De Ven C, Fanaroff A. A randomized, double-blind, placebo-controlled trial of prophylactic recombinant human granulocyte-macrophage colony-stimulating factor to reduce nosocomial infections in very low birth weight neonates. J Pediatr 1999;134:64–70.
74. Beauchesne MF, Shalansky SJ. Nonchemotherapy drug-induced agranulocytosis: a review of 118 patients treated with colony-stimulating factors. Pharmacotherapy 1999;19:299–305.
75. Vial T, Gallant C, Choquet-Kastylevsky G, Descotes J. Treatment of drug-induced agranulocytosis with haematopoietic growth factors. A review of the clinical experience. BioDrugs 1999;11:185–200.
76. Barbaro G, Di Lorenzo G, Grisorio B, Soldini M, Barbarini G. Effect of recombinant human granulocyte-macrophage colony-stimulating factor on HIV-related leukopenia: a randomized, controlled clinical study. AIDS 1997;11:1453–61.
77. Couderc LJ, Stelianides S, Frachon I, Stern M, Epardeau B, Baumelou E, Caubarrere I, Hermine O. Pulmonary toxicity of chemotherapy and G/GM-CSF: a report of five cases. Respir Med 1999;93:65–8.

78. Ruiz-Argüelles G, Arizpe-Bravo D, Sanchez-Sosa S, Rojas-Ortega S, Moreno-Ford V, Ruiz-Argüelles A. Fatal G-CSF-induced pulmonary toxicity. Am J Hematol 1999;60:82–3.
79. Kasper C, Jones L, Fujita Y, Morgenstern GR, Scarffe JH, Chang J. Splenic rupture in a patient with acute myeloid leukemia undergoing peripheral blood stem cell transplantation. Ann Hematol 1999;78:91–2.
80. Yakisan E, Schirg E, Zeidler C, Bishop NJ, Reiter A, Hirt A, Riehm H, Welte K. High incidence of significant bone loss in patients with severe congenital neutropenia (Kostmann's syndrome). J Pediatr 1997;131:592–7.
81. Dupre D, Schoenlaub P, Cologner M, Plantin P. Réaction anaphylactique après injection locale de GM-CSF au cours d'un ulcère veineux de jambe. Ann Dermatol Vénéréol 1999;126:160–1.
82. Keung YK, Suwanvecho S, Cobos E. Anaphylactoid reaction to granulocyte colony-stimulating factor used in mobilization of peripheral blood stem cell. Bone Marrow Transplant 1999;23:200–1.
83. Kaito K, Kobayashi M, Katayama T, Masuoka H, Shimada T, Nishiwaki K, Sekita T, Otsubo H, Ogasawara Y, Hosoya T. Long-term administration of G-CSF for aplastic anaemia is closely related to the early evolution of monosomy 7 MDS in adults. Br J Haematol 1998;103:297–303.
84. Nishimura M, Yamada T, Andoh T, Tao T, Emoto M, Ohji T, Matsuda K, Kameda N, Satoh Y, Matsutani A, Azuno Y, Oka Y. Granulocyte colony-stimulating factor (G-CSF) dependent hematopoiesis with monosomy 7 in a patient with severe aplastic anemia after ATG/CsA/G-CSF combined therapy. Int J Hematol 1998;68:203–11.
85. Shpall EJ, Wheeler CA, Turner SA, Yanovich S, Brown RA, Pecora AL, Shea TC, Mangan KF, Williams SF, LeMaistre CF, Long GD, Jones R, Davis MW, Murphy-Filkins R, Parker WRL, Glaspy JA. A randomized phase 3 study of peripheral blood progenitor cell mobilization with stem cell factor and filgrastim in high-risk breast cancer patients. Blood 1999;8:2491–501.
86. Charpentier B, Thervet E. Placebo-controlled study of a humanized anti-TAC monoclonal antibody in dual therapy for prevention of acute rejection after renal transplantation. Transplant Proc 1998;30:1331–2.
87. Onrust SV, Lamb HM, Barman Balfour JA. Rituximab. Drugs 1999;58:79–88.
88. Micallef INM, Kirk A, Norton A, Foran JM, Rohatiner AZS. Peripheral T-cell lymphoma following rituximab therapy for B-cell lymphoma. Blood 1999;93:2427–8.
89. Tetreault S, Abler SL, Robbins B, Saven A. Peripheral T-cell lymphoma after anti-CD20 antibody therapy. J Clin Oncol 1998;16:1635–6.
90. Sizmann N, Korting HC. Prolonged urticaria with 17-1A antibody. Br Med J 1998;317:1631.
91. Lundin J, Osterborg A, Brittinger G, Crowther D, Dombret H, Engert A, Epenetos A, Gisselbrecht C, Huhn D, Jaeger U, Thomas J, Marcus R, Nissen N, Poynton C, Rankin E, Stahel R, Uppenkamp M, Willemze R, Mellstedt H. CAMPATH-1H monoclonal antibody in therapy for previously treated low-grade non-Hodgkin's lymphomas: a phase II multicenter study. J Clin Oncol 1998;16:3257–63.
92. Otton SH, Turner DL, Frewin R, Davies SV, Johnson SA. Autoimmune thrombocytopenia after treatment with CAMPATH-1H in a patient with chronic lymphocytic leukaemia. Br J Haematol 1999;106:252–62.
93. Stolk JN, Boerbooms AMT, De Abreu RA, De Koning DGM, Van Beusekom HJ, Muller WH, Van De Putte LBA. Reduced thiopurine methyltransferase activity and development of side effects of azathioprine treatment in patients with rheumatoid arthritis. Arthritis Rheum 1998;41:1858–66.
94. Black AJ, McLeod HL, Capell HA, Powrie RH, Matowe LK, Pritchard SC, Collie-Duguid ESR, Reid DM. Thiopurine methyltransferase genotype predicts therapy-limiting severe toxicity from azathioprine. Ann Intern Med 1998;129:716–18.
95. Amenabar JJ, Gomez-Ullate P, Garcia-Lopez FJ, Aurrecoechea B, Garcia-Erauzkin G, Lampreabe I. A randomized trial comparing cyclosporine and steroids with cyclosporine, azathioprine, and steroids in cadaveric renal transplantation. Transplantation 1998;65:653–61.
96. David-Neto E, Da Fonseca JA, De Paula FJ, Nahas WC, Sabbaga E, Ianhez LE. Is azathioprine harmful to chronic viral hepatitis in renal transplantation? A long-term study on azathioprine withdrawal. Transplant Proc 1999;31:1149–50.
97. Azoulay D, Castaing D, Lemoine A, Samuel D, Majno P, Reynes M, Charpentier B, Bismuth H. Successful treatment of severe azathioprine-induced hepatic veno-occlusive disease in a kidney-transplanted patient with transjugular intrahepatic portosystemic shunt. Clin Nephrol 1998;50:118–22.
98. Stratton JD, Farrington K. Relapse of vasculitis, sepsis, or azathioprine allergy? Nephrol Dial Transplant 1998;13:2927–8.
99. Korelitz BI, Fuller SR, Warman JI, Goldberg MD. Shingles during the course of treatment with 6-mercaptopurine for inflammatory bowel disease. Am J Gastroenterol 1999;94:424–6.
100. Ippoliti G, Negri M, Campana C, Vigano M. Urate oxidase in hyperuricemic heart transplant recipients treated with azathioprine. Transplantation 1997;63:1370–1.
101. Shah MB, Martin JE, Schroeder TJ, First MR. Validity of open labelled versus blinded trials: a meta-analysis comparing Neoral and Sandimmune. Transplant Proc 1999;31:217–19.
102. Taler SJ, Textor SC, Canzanello VJ, Schwartz L. Cyclosporin-induced hypertension. Incidence, pathogenesis and management. Drug Saf 1999;20:437–49.
103. Roelofs PM, Klinkhamer PJ, Gooszen HC. Hypersensitivity pneumonitis probably caused by cyclosporine. A case report. Resp Med 1998;92: 1368–70.
104. Wijdicks EFM, Dahlke LJ, Wiesner RH. Oral cyclosporine decreases severity of neuro-

toxicity in liver transplant recipients. Neurology 1999;52:1708–10.

105. Kotake S, Higashi K, Yoshikawa K, Sasamoto Y, Okamoto T, Matsuda H. Central nervous system symptoms in patients with Behçet disease receiving cyclosporine therapy. Ophthalmology 1999;105: 586–9.

106. Gopal AK, Thorning DR, Back AL. Fatal outcome due to cyclosporine neurotoxicity with associated pathological findings. Bone Marrow Transplant 1999;23:191–3.

107. Kaito K, Kobayashi M, Otsubo H, Ogasawara Y, Sekita T, Shimada T, Hosoya T. Cyclosporine and entrapment neuropathy. Report of two cases. Acta Haematol 1998;100:159.

108. Terrovitis IV, Nanas SN, Rombos AK, Tolis G, Nanas JN. Reversible symmetric polyneuropathy with paraplegia after heart transplantation. Transplantation 1998;65:1394–413.

109. Porges Y, Blumen S, Fireman Z, Sternberg A, Zamir D. Cyclosporine-induced optic neuropathy, ophthalmoplegia, and nystagmus in a patient with Crohn disease. Am J Ophthalmol 1998;126:607–9.

110. Saito J, Kami M, Taniguchi F, Kanda Y, Takeda N, Mitani K, Hirai H, Araie M, Fujino Y. Unilateral papilledema after bone marrow transplantation. Bone Marrow Transplant 1999;23:963–5.

111. Maghrabi K, Bohlega S. Cyclosporine-induced migraine with severe vomiting causing loss of renal graft. Clin Neurol Neurosurg 1998;100:224–7.

112. Cavdar C, Sifil A, Sanli E, Gülay H, Camsari T. Hypomagnesemia and mild rhabdomyolysis in living related donor renal transplant recipient treated with cyclosporine A. Scand J Urol Nephrol 1998;32:415–17.

113. Parving HH, Tarnow L, Nielsen FS, Rossing P, Mandrup-Poulsen T, Osterby R, Nerup J. Cyclosporine nephrotoxicity in type 1 diabetic patients. A 7-year follow-up study. Diabetes Care 1999;22:478–83.

114. Van der Molen L, Van Son WJ, Tegzess AM, Stegeman CA. Severe vital depression as the presenting feature of cyclosporin-A-associated thrombotic microangiopathy. Nephrol Dial Transplant 1999;14:998–1000.

115. Kohli HS, Sud K, Jha V, Gupta KL, Minz M, Joshi K, Sakhuja V. Cyclosporin-induced haemolytic-uraemic syndrome presenting as primary graft dysfunction. Nephrol Dial Transplant 1998;13:2940–2.

116. Lear J, Bourke JF, Burns DA. Hyperplastic pseudofolliculitis barbae associated with cyclosporin. Br J Dermatol 1997;136:132–48.

117. De Felipe I, Redondo P. Eruptive angiomas after treatment with cyclosporine in a patient with psoriasis. Arch Dermatol 1998;134:1487–8.

118. Mahendran R, Grech C. Generalized pustular psoriasis following a short course of cyclosporin (Neoral). Br J Dermatol 1998;139:934.

119. Rebora A, Delmonte S, Parodi A. Cyclosporin A-induced hair darkening. Int J Dermatol 1999;38:229–30.

120. Liau-Chu M, Theis JGW, Koren G. Mechanism of anaphylactoid reactions: improper preparation of high-dose intravenous cyclosporine leads to bolus infusion of Cremophor EL and cyclosporine. Ann Pharmacother 1997;31:1287–91.

121. Hojo M, Morimoto T, Maluccio M, Asano T, Morimoto K, Lagman M, Shimbo T, Suthanthiran M. Cyclosporine induces cancer progression by a cell-autonomous mechanism. Nature 1999;397:530–4.

122. Jensen P, Hansen S, Moller B, Leivestad T, Pfeffer P, Geiran O, Fauchald P, Simonsen S. Skin cancer in kidney and heart transplant recipients and different long-term immunosuppressive therapy regimens. J Am Acad Dermatol 1999;40:177–86.

123. Brinkman K, Huysmans F, Burger DM. Pharmacokinetic interaction between saquinavir and cyclosporine. Ann Intern Med 1998;129:914–15.

124. Park MH, Pelegrin D, Haug IMT, Young JB. Troglitazone, a new antidiabetic agent, decreases cyclosporine level. J Heart Lung Transplant 1998;17:1139–40.

125. Tabbara KF, Al-Faisal Z, Al-Rashed W. Interaction between acetazolamide and cyclosporine. Arch Ophthalmol 1998;116:832–3.

126. Tweddle DA, Windebank KP, Hewson QC, Yule SM. Cyclosporin neurotoxicity after chemotherapy. Br Med J 1999;318:1113.

127. Haubitz M, Schellong S, Göbel U, Schurek HJ, Schaumann D, Koch KM, Brunkhorst R. Intravenous pulse administration of cyclophosphamide versus daily oral treatment in patients with antineutrophil cytoplasmic antibody-associated vasculitis and renal involvement. Arthritis Rheum 1998;41:1835–44.

128. Abuzarad H, Gadallah MF, Rabb H, Vermess M, Ramirez G. Emphysematous cystitis: possible side-effect of cyclophosphamide therapy. Clin Nephrol 1998;50:394–6.

129. Garcia-Porrua C, Gonzalez-Gay MA, Pérez De Llano LA, Alvarez-Ferreira JA. Fatal interstitial pneumonia due to cytomegalovirus following cyclophosphamide treatment in a patient with systemic lupus erythematosus. Scand J Rheumatol 1998;27:465–6.

130. McCarthy CJ, Sheldon S, Ross CW, McCune WJ. Cytogenetic abnormalities and therapy-related myelodysplastic syndromes in rheumatic disease. Arthritis Rheum 1998;41:1493–6.

131. Ortiz Z, Shea B, Suarez Almazor ME, Moher D, Wells GA, Tugwell P. The efficacy of folic acid and folinic acid in reducing methotrexate gastrointestinal toxicity in rheumatoid arthritis. A metaanalysis of randomized controlled trials. J Rheumatol 1998;25:36–43.

132. Kokelj F, Plozzer C, Muzzi A, Ciani F. Endoalveolar haemorrhage due to methotrexate overdosage in a patient treated for psoriatic arthritis. J Dermatol Treat 1999;10:67–9.

133. Aplin CG, Russell-Jones R. Acute dysarthria induced by low dose methotrexate therapy in a patient with erythrodermic cutaneous T-cell lymphoma: an unusual manifestation of neurotoxicity. Clin Exp Dermatol 1999;24:23–4.

134. Malka N, Reichert S, Trechot P, Barbaud A, Schmutz JL. Yellow nail pigmentation due to methotrexate. Dermatology 1998;197:276.
135. Georgescu L, Paget SA. Lymphoma in patients with rheumatoid arthritis. What is the evidence of a link with methotrexate? Drug Saf 1999;20:475-87.
136. Hueso M, Bover J, Seron D, Gil-Vernet S, Sabate I, Fulladosa X, Ramos R, Coll O, Alsina J, Grinyo JM. Low-dose cyclosporine and mycophenolate mofetil in renal allograft recipients with suboptimal renal function. Transplantation 1998;66:1727–31.
137. Stegall MD, Wachs ME, Everson G, Steinberg T, Bilir B, Shrestha R, Karrer F, Kam I. Prednisone withdrawal 14 days after liver transplantation with mycophenolate. Transplantation 1997;64:1755–60.
138. Lecornu-Heuze L, Ducloux D, Rebibou JM, Martin L, Billerey C, Chalopin JM. Mycophenolate mofetil in cyclosporin-associated thrombotic microangiopathy. Nephrol Dial Transplant 1998;13:3212–13.
139. McGregor DO, Robson RA, Lynn KL. Haemolytic-uraemic syndrome in a renal transplant recipient treated by conversion to mycophenolate mofetil. Nephron 1998;80:365–6.
140. Simmons WD, Rayhill SC, Sollinger HW. Preliminary risk-benefit assessment of mycophenolate mofetil in transplant rejection. Drug Saf 1997;17:75–92.
141. Odorico JS, Pirsch JD, Knechtle SJ, D'Alessandro AM, Sollinger HW. A study comparing mycophenolate mofetil to azathioprine in simultaneous pancreas-kidney transplantation. Transplantation 1998;66:1751–9.
142. Gruessner RWG, Sutherland DER, Drangsteivt MB, Wrenshall L, Humar A, Gruessner AC. Mycophenolate mofetil in pancreas transplantation. Transplantation 1998;66:318–23.
143. Shapiro R, Jordan ML, Scantlebury VP, Vivas C, Gritsch HA, Casavilla FA, McCauley J, Johnston JR, Randhawa P, Irish W, Hakal TR, Fung JJ, Starzl TE. A prospective, randomized trial to compare tacrolimus and prednisone with and without mycophenolate mofetil in patients undergoing renal transplantation: first report. J Urol 1998;160:1982–6.
144. Ducloux D, Ottignon Y, Semhoun-Ducloux S, Labbé S, Saint-Hillier Y, Miguet JP, Carayon P, Chalopin JM. Mycophenolate mofetil-induced villous atrophy. Transplantation 1998;66:1115–16.
145. Daoud AJ, Schroeder TJ, Shah M, Hariharan S, Peddi VR, Weiskittel P, First MR. A comparison of the safety and efficacy of mycophenolate mofetil, prednisone and cyclosporine and mycophenolate mofetil, and prednisone and tacrolimus. Transplant Proc 1998;30:4079–81.
146. Gomez E, Aguado S, Rodriguez M, Alvarez-Grande J. Kaposi's sarcoma after renal transplantation—disappearance after reduction of immunosuppression and reappearance 7 years after start of mycophenolate mofetil treatment. Nephrol Dial Transplant 1998;13:3279–80.
147. Kahan BD, Podbielski J, Napoli KL, Katz SM, Meier-Kriesche HU, Van Buren CT. Immunosuppressive effects and safety of a sirolimus/cyclosporine combination regimen for renal transplantation. Transplantation 1998;66:1040–6.
148. Kaplan MJ, Ellis CN, Bata-Csorgo Z, Kaplan RS, Endres JL, Fox DA. Systemic toxicity following administration of sirolimus (formerly rapamycin) for psoriasis. Association of capillary leak syndrome with apoptosis of lesional lymphocytes. Arch Dermatol 1999;135:553–7.
149. Jain AB, Kashyap R, Rakela J, Starzl TE, Fung JJ. Primary adult liver transplantation under tacrolimus: more than 90 months actual follow-up survival and adverse events. Liver Transplant Surg 1999;5:144–50.
150. Kliem V, Brunkhorst R. Tacrolimus in kidney transplantation. A clinical review. Nephron 1998;79:8–20.
151. Chang RKR, Alzona M, Alejos J, Jue K, McDiarmid SV. Marked left ventricular hypertrophy in children on tacrolimus (FK506) after orthotopic liver transplantation. Am J Cardiol 1998;81:1277–80.
152. Scott JS, Boyle GJ, Daubeney PE, Miller SA, Law Y, Pigula F, Griffith BP, Webber SA. Tacrolimus: a cause of hypertrophic cardiomyopathy in pediatric heart transplant recipients? Transplant Proc 1999;31:82–3.
153. Canzanello VJ, Textor SC, Taler SJ, Schwartz LL, Porayko MK, Wiesner RH, Krom RAF. Late hypertension after liver transplantation: a comparison of cyclosporine and tacrolimus (FK506). Liver Transplant Surg 1998;4:328–34.
154. Taylor DO, Barr ML, Radovancevic B, Renlund DG, Mentzer RM, Smart FW, Tolman DE, Frazier OH, Young JB, Van Veldhuisen P. A randomized, multicenter comparison of tacrolimus and cyclosporine immunosuppressive regimens in cardiac transplantation: decreased hyperlipidemia and hypertension with tacrolimus. J Heart Lung Transplant 1999;18:336–45.
155. Steg RE, Kessinger A, Wszolek ZK. Cortical blindness and seizures in a patient receiving FK506 after bone marrow transplantation. Bone Marrow Transplant 1999;23:959–62.
156. Tomura N, Kurosawa R, Kato K, Takahashi S, Watarai J, Takeda O, Watanabe A, Takada G. Transient neurotoxicity associated with FK506: MR findings. J Comput Assisted Tomogr 1998;22:505–7.
157. Torocsik HV, Curless RG, Post J, Tzakis AG, Pearse L. FK506-induced leukoencephalopathy in children with organ transplants. Neurology 1999;52:1497–500.
158. Knoll GA, Bell RC. Tacrolimus versus cyclosporin for immunosuppression in renal transplantation: meta-analysis of randomised trials. Br Med J 1999;318:1104–7.
159. Cavaillé-Coll MW, Elashoff MR. Commentary on a comparison of tacrolimus and cyclosporine for immunosuppression after cadaveric renal transplatation. Transplantation 1998;65:142–5.
160. Yoshioka K, Sato T, Okada N, Ishii T, Imanishi M, Tanaka S, Kim T, Sugimoto T, Fujii S. Post-transplant diabetes with anti-glutamic acid de-

carboxylase antibody during tacrolimus therapy. Diabetes Res Clin Pract 1998;42:85–9.

161. Sharma AK, Holder FE. *Clostridium difficile* diarrhea after use of tacrolimus following renal transplantation. Clin Infect Dis 1998;27:1540–1.

162. Solez K, Vincenti F, Filo RS. Histopathologic findings from 2-year protocol biopsies from a U.S. multicenter kidney transplant trial comparing tacrolimus versus cyclosporine. A report of the FK506 kidney transplant study group. Transplantation 1998;66:1736–40.

163. Walder B, Ricou B, Suter PM. Tacrolimus (FK 506)-induced hemolytic uremic syndrome after heart transplantation. J Heart Lung Transplant 1998;17:1004–6.

164. Trimarchi HM, Truong LD, Brennan S, Gonzalez JM, Suki WN. FK506-associated thrombotic microangiopathy. Transplantation 1999; 67:539–44.

165. Schmidt RH, Lenz T, Gröne HJ, Geiger H, Scheuermann EH. Haemolytic-uraemic syndrome after tacrolimus rescue therapy for cortisone-resistant rejection. Nephrol Dial Transplant 1999; 14:979–83.

166. Basile C, Marangi AL, Montanaro A, Giordano R, De Padova F, Ligorio VA, Santese D, Di Marco L, Semeraro A, Vernaglione L. Tacrolimus and gingival hyperplasia. Nephrol Dial Transplant 1998;13:2980–1.

167. Vyas S, Kumar A, Piecuch S, Hidalgo G, Singh A, Anderson V, Markell MS, Baqi N. Outcome of twin pregnancy in a renal transplant recipient treated with tacrolimus. Transplantation 1999;67:490–2.

168. Odoul F, Talbotec C, Boussa N, Le Guellec C, Furet Y, Maurage C, Breteau M. Massive ingestion of tacrolimus in a young liver transplant patient. Transplant Proc 1998;30:4327–9.

169. Campo JV, Smith C, Perel JM. Tacrolimus toxic reaction associated with the use of nefazodone: paroxetine as an alternative agent. Arch Gen Psychiatry 1998;55:1050–2.

170. Krähenbühl S, Menafoglio A, Giostra E, Gallino A. Serious interaction between mibefradil and tacrolimus. Transplantation 1998;66:1113–15.

171. Herzig K, Johnson DW. Marked elevation of blood cyclosporin and tacrolimus levels due to concurrent metronidazole therapy. Nephrol Dial Transplant 1999;14:521–3.

172. Hanagiri T, Muranaka H, Hashimoto M, Nagashima A. A syndrome of inappropriate secretion of antidiuretic hormone associated with pleuritis caused by OK-432. Respiration 1998;65:310–12.

H.D. Reuter

38 Vitamins

VITAMIN A (RETINOL)

(SED-13, 1167; SEDA-18, 380; SEDA-21, 433)

A few case reports have suggested an association between the use of high doses of vitamin A (retinol and retinyl esters) during pregnancy and *birth defects* (1[r]). These malformations are similar to those produced by the vitamin A derivative isotretionin (13-*cis*-retinoic acid [Accutane]). The minimum human teratogenic daily dose is estimated to be 25 000–50 000 IU, and a recent report (2[c]) has suggested that it may be as little as 10 000 IU. The National Research Council's Committee on Dietary Allowance advocates a recommended daily allowance (RDA) of 800 retinol equivalents/day for non-pregnant women of childbearing age and pregnant women. The RDA is equivalent to 2700 IU of vitamin A obtained from a supplement as retinol or 4800 μg of β-carotene. The committee of the American College of Obstetricians and Gynecologists recommends supplementation with 5000 IU/day as the maximum intake before and during pregnancy. This is well below the probable minimum human teratogenic dose. Prenatal multivitamin formulations in common use contain 5000 IU or less vitamin A, but vitamin tablets containing 25 000 IU or more of vitamin A are available as over-the-counter formulations. Pregnant women or those planning to become pregnant should be cautioned about the potential teratogenicity of high doses of vitamin A supplements.

The benefits and safety of maternal and infant vitamin A supplementation administered with each of the three diphtheria-tetanus-pertussis (DPT) and poliomyelitis immunizations and with a fourth dose of measles immunization have been assessed in a randomized double-blind, placebo-controlled study in 9424 mother-infant pairs from Ghana, India, and Peru (3[C]). Vitamin A 200 000 IU was given to 4716 mothers and 25 000 IU to their infants with each of the first three doses of DPT/poliomyelitis immunization at 6, 10, and 14 weeks. Placebo was given to 4708 mothers and their infants. At 9 months, with measles immunisation infants in the vitamin A group were given a further dose of 25 000 IU and those in the placebo group received 100 000 IU. At 6 months there was a small reduction in vitamin A deficiency in the vitamin A group compared with controls; this effect was no longer apparent at 9 months. There were no significant differences in mortality throughout the study.

Adverse effects were a *bulging fontanelle* (in under 1% of the infants) and vomiting. Among the infants without a bulging fontanelle before the start of the study, more of the vitamin A recipients than placebo recipients had a bulging fontanelle within 48 h of the dose at 6, 10, and 14 weeks. After the fourth dose at 9 months, a bulging fontanelle was more common among the controls than among the infants given vitamin A. However, after each dose under 1% of the infants in either group had a bulging fontanelle. Of the 62 infants in the vitamin A group who had a bulging fontanelle reported at 24 h after a dose, the bulging had resolved within 48 hours in 445 (73%). Among the controls, in whom almost of all the instances of bulging were reported with the 100 000 IU dose, 25 of 42 had resolution of bulging within 48 hours. Under 3% of mothers in each group reported a bulging fontanelle after each dose. *Vomiting* occured only within 48 h after administration of the fourth dose in 167 (4.9%) infants in the vitamin A group versus 236 (6.5%) in the control group. There were no significant differences in convulsions or raised temperature at any dose.

All-*trans* retinoic acid (ATRA)

All-*trans* retinoic acid 70, 110, 150, 190, or 230 mg/m^2/day has been given to 26 patients with advanced potentially hormone-responsive breast cancer taking tamoxifen 20 mg/day (4[C]).

Side Effects of Drugs, Annual 23
J.K. Aronson, ed.

At all doses *headaches, nausea, skin changes,* and *bone pain* occured. The headaches were most severe during the first week of treatment, peaking at the end of the first week. They were sometimes associated with nausea and occasionally with vomiting, although there was no other evidence of raised cerebrospinal fluid pressure. Headaches and nausea tended to subside during the weeks when all-*trans* retionic acid was not given and recurred during the weeks of all-*trans* retionic acid reintroduction, although their severity tended to wane with subsequent cycles of treatment. Similarly, skin reactions, such as erythema and desquamation, were dose related and were most severe during the initial cycles of treatment. Bone pain occurred intermittently. There was life-threatening hypercalcemia in one patient, but it was felt to be due to disease progression. The dose of 230 mg/m^2/day produced unacceptable headache and skin toxicity, but doses of up to 190 mg/ m^2/day were tolerable.

The incidence, clinical features, and outcome of *all-trans retionic acid syndrome* have been analysed in 413 cases of newly diagnosed acute promyelocytic leukemia (5[C]). Patients under 65 years old with a white blood cell count below 5 × 10^9/l were initially randomized to all-*trans* retionic acid followed by chemotherapy or to all-*trans* retionic acid with chemotherapy started on day 3. In patients with white cell counts over 5 × 10^9/l chemotherapy was rapidly added if the white cell count was greater than 6, 10, and 15 × 10^9/l by days 5, 10, and 15 of all-*trans* retionic acid treatment. The retionic acid syndrome occured during induction treatment in 64 of 413 patients (15%). Clinical signs developed after a median of 7 (range 0–35) days. In two cases they were present before the start of treatment; in 11 they occured on recovery from the phase of aplasia due to the addition of chemotherapy. Respiratory distress (98% of patients), fever (81%), pulmonary infiltrates (81%), weight gain (50%), pleural effusion (47%), renal failure (39%), pericardial effusion (19%), cardiac failure (17%), and hypertension (12%) were the main clinical signs. Mechanical ventilation was required in 13 patients and dialysis in two. A total of 55 patients (86%) who experienced the all-*trans* retionic acid syndrome achieved complete remission, compared with 94% of patients who had no all-*trans* retionic acid syndrome, and nine died of the syndrome. None of the patients with complete remission who received all-*trans* retionic acid for maintenance had recurrence of the syndrome. The syndrome was associated with a lower event-free survival and survival at 2 years.

A case of all-*trans* retionic acid syndrome has been reported in a patient who developed diffuse alveolar hemmorhage while being treated with all-*trans* retionic acid for acute promyeloic leukemia (6[c]).

An 18-year-old woman developed promyelocytic leukemia and was given all-*trans* retionic acid and dexamethasone. At 15 days she developed significant hemoptysis and respiratory failure, requiring mechanical ventilation. Her temperature was 39.1°C and she had disseminated intravascular coagulation. A lung biopsy showed diffuse interstitial neutrophilic infiltration, interstitial fibrinoid necrosis, and diffuse alveolar hemorrhage; pulmonary capillaritis was diagnosed. She was given intravenous methylprednisolone 1 g /day for 3 days followed by a tapering dose of oral prednisolone. She subsequently completed a full 45-day course of all-*trans* retionic acid.

VITAMINS OF THE B GROUP

(SED-13, 1171; SEDA-18, 381; SEDA-19, 369; SEDA-20; 364)

Thiamine (vitamin B$_1$)

Recent investigations have shown that thiamine is directly involved in ribose synthesis in pancreatic adenocarcinoma cells through transketolase catalysed non-oxidative pentose phosphate reactions. In addition, the chemically modified co-factor oxythiamine inhibited tumor cell proliferation in vitro and in vivo by 40% and 91% in two distinct tumor models (7[C]). According to a review of thiamine supplementation in cancer patients this raises serious suspicions that routine thiamine administration may not be warranted and could possibly be harmful (8[R]). Thiamine deficiency in cancer patients is most often observed during or shortly after chemotherapy. Clinical and experimental data have shown increased thiamine utilization by human tumors and its interference with experimental chemotherapy. Current thiamine adminsitration protocols oversupply thiamine by 200–20 000% of the RDA, because it is considered harmless and needed by cancer patients. However, since the thiamine-dependent transketolase pathway is the main reaction which supplies ribose phosphate for nucleic acids in tumors, excessive thiamine supplementation may be responsible for failed therapeutic attempts to terminate cancer cell proliferation. The authors therefore recommended that cancer management should include regular evaluation of thiamine status of the patient, especially during chemotherapy, and that dosages of thiamine should not exceed 1.2 mg/day unless necessary. Future studies should clarify if oxythiamine as an inhibitor of transketolase is really safe and if it is especially effective against cancer.

Pyridoxine (vitamin B_6)

(SED-13, 1173; SEDA-21, 407)

℞ *Debate on vitamin B_6 continues*

Under the headline 'Still time for rational debate about vitamin B_6' the controversial debate on the safety of vitamin B_6 has been revived (9[r]). Vitamin B_6 is marketed for stress in general, for depression associated with premenstrual syndrome and oral contraceptives, and for carpal tunnel syndrome, although it is doubtful that it has more than a placebo effect. It is legitimately prescribed in general deficiency states in doses starting at 150 mg/day. Adverse events include sensory neuropathy at oral doses about 2–3 g/day or more.

The editorial refers to the attempts of the UK Government's Committee on Toxicity to find the safe level of daily consumption of vitamin B_6. In July 1997 the committee recommended that the sale of vitamin B_6 in, for instance, health-food shops should be restricted to doses of 10 mg/day. Doses between 10 and 50 mg should be restricted to sale at pharmacies; and doses of 50 mg and above would be available only on prescription. Contrary to these UK recommendations the Committee of the US National Academy of Science concluded that there were no convincing reports of adverse events at doses of up to 200 mg/day. Paying attention to the fact that recommendations tend to be more cautious than might seem necessary from the available evidence, the US experts halved the 200 mg/day dose to define their limit as 100 mg/day.

The author of the editorial found fault with the fact that the US experts have based their recommendations on the slimmest of evidence. The main human study was a self-recall series of 172 patients presenting to a private practice in London (10[C]). In a letter to the editor Beckett (11[r]) pointed out that daily doses of 200 mg or less have been taken by millions of people world wide for several decades without evident toxicity and that testimonials from clinicians expert in the use of vitamin B_6 have attested to its safety in these doses (12[R]). Referring to the editorial, the author of the study in question stated that their study referred to 172 women with raised blood concentrations of pyridoxine that reverted to normal within 4 days of stopping vitamin B_6, and was not a 'self-recall series'. In a recent follow-up of these women who had raised blood concentrations (compared with controls from the same practice who had had a blood test in 1985–6 and whose record showed that they were not taking vitamin B_6 or multivitamins at that time or since, 16 of 50 respondents had subsequently had autoimmune disease, compared with one of the 38 controls. The autoimmune diseases included thyroid disease (n = 5), rheumatoid arthritis (n = 3), diabetes (n = 2), Sjögren's syndrome (n = 2), primary biliary cirrhosis (n = 1), polymyalgia rheumatica (n = 1), and polyarteritis nodosum (n = 1). In the controls there was one case of diabetes.

In another letter to the editor (13[r]) it was mentioned that the suspicion of partiality about the Committee on Toxicity becomes more plausible when one considers the issue of homocysteine. This intermediate metabolite may well turn out to be of greater importance as a risk factor than cholesterol and blood pressure. Raised homocysteine concentrations appear to be accessible to treatment with vitamin B_6 (100 mg/day) together with vitamin B_{12} and folic acid (14[C]). Furthermore, the statement that there is no good evidence for the efficacy of vitamin B_6 in any disease, apart from depression, was criticized, because this ignores important studies in autism, pregnancy outcome, asthma, and sickle-cell anaemia (13[r]).

Nervous system In an article on current perspectives of pyridoxine-dependent seizures the risks of pyridoxine have been reviewed (15[R]). *Sensory neuropathy* has been described in certain individuals taking high daily doses of pyridoxine on a long-term basis. Although this condition is generally reversible, a chronic painful neuropathy has developed in some patients. Besides individual patient susceptibility, the risk of pyridoxine neurotoxic effects is related to both the daily dose and the duration of administration. Peripheral neuropathy did not develop in individuals taking 500 mg/day for up to 2 years, whereas it did develop almost universally in patients who took more than 1000 mg/day for variable periods (16[R]). In an adult, a daily dose of 500 mg/day is about 7.1 mg/kg/day. Therefore a child with pyridoxine-dependency taking 5 mg/kg/day may not be at risk of neuropathy. Only one patient with pyridoxine-dependent seizures in whom a sensory neuropathy developed has been described (17[c]). It is recommended that patients with this disorder who will require life-long pharmacological doses of pyridoxine should be assessed for signs of a sensory peripheral neuropathy.

Nicotinic acid (niacin), nicotinamide

Treatment of dyslipidemia with nicotinic acid can be accompanied by adverse effects that include *gastrointestinal irritation, flushing* and *itching of the skin, raised transaminases, hyperglycemia,* and *hyperuricemia.*

In two trials of accelerated radiotherapy with carbogen and nicotinamide in patients with cancer the adverse effects of nicotinamide have been documented (18[C], 19[C]). In the first 62 patients with stage III–IV laryngeal carcinoma were treated with accelerated radiotherapy (total radiation 64 Gy) combined with carbogen breathing in 11 patients and with both carbogen and nicotinamide (Arcon) in 51 patients. Adverse effects attributed to nicotinamide in the 51 patients were *nausea* in 35 patients, *vomiting* in 20, *flushing, dizziness, epigastric pain, and headache* in two patients each, *and gastrointestinal bleeding, sweating, fatigue, and emotional disturbances* in one patient each.

In the second trial nicotinamide (Nicobion) 6 g was given in tablet form to 15 patients with advanced head and neck and non-small cell lung carcinomas 90 min before radiotherapy. Toxicity (*nausea and vomiting*) did not correlate with any of the pharmacokinetic parameters, such as t_{max}, C_{max}, $t_{1/2}$, or AUC. Gastrointestinal toxicity reached grade 1 (nausea not requiring antiemetics) in four patients, grade 2 (nausea and/or vomiting requiring antiemetics) in four patients, and grade 3 (nausea and/or vomiting requiring nasogastric intubation or parenteral support) in two patients.

Modified-release niacin The efficacy and tolerability of a modified-release formulation of niacin (Niaspan) has been investigated in a double-blind, placebo-controlled study in 128 patients (20[C]). There was no statistical difference between nicacin and placebo in relation to adverse events such as headche, abdominal pain, diarrhea, dyspepsia, nausea, vomiting, pharyngitis, and rhinitis. *Pruritus* was reported in 10 patients taking niacin (11%) and *rash* in 9 patients (10%); there were no similar effects in those taking placebo.

In another study the efficacy and tolerability of Niaspan has been evaluated in 122 patients (21[C]). Niaspan had only a 5% discontinuation rate for *flushing*, and most of the episodes were mild and well-tolerated. Liver enzymes (AST, AlT, alkaline phosphatase) in patients taking nicacin 1 or 2 g/day did not differ significantly from those taking placebo.

In a study of the efficacy and tolerability of Niaspan in 517 patients the most commonly reported adverse events were *headache* in 92 patients (13%), *pain* in any part of the body except the abdomen in 46 (6%), abdominal pain in 54 (8%), *diarrhea* in 97 (13%), *dyspepsia* in 46 (6%), *nausea* in 72 (10%), *vomiting* in 38 (5%), *rhinitis* in 30 (4%), *pruritus* in 56 (8%), and *rash* in 51 (7%) (22[C]).

In a study of the efficacy and tolerability of Niaspan in 269 adults and 230 additional adults for whom short-term safety data were available, 4.8% of the patients withdrew because of *flushing* (13 of 269) (23[C]). During the first 4 weeks about half had flushing. The mean intensity was about 4.0 on a visual analog scale (representing 'none' to 'intolerable'). Patients were encouraged to use aspirin prophylactically to minimize flushing. Other niacin-related adverse effects leading to withdrawal included *nausea* (3.3%) sometimes with *vomiting, other gastrointestinal symptoms* (1.5%), and *pruritus* (2.6%). Once case each of *gout, acanthosis nigricans, headache, palpitation, raised glucose concentrations,* and *shoulder pain* led to patient withdrawal. Certain adverse events thought to be associated with niacin were uncommon in the study group. There was one case of *peptic ulcer, amblyopia* occurred in three patients, and *leg aches and myalgias* in one patient taking Niaspan with simvastatin, with a normal creatine kinase activity.

Liver Three cases of *hepatic dysfunction* in patients taking crystalline nictonic acid 1.5–3.0 g/day have been reported (24[c]). The cases were all associated with reduced ratio of esterified cholesterol to free cholesterol in LDL, a reduction in lecithin cholesteryl acyl transferase activity (LCAT) and other evidence of liver dysfunction, including prolonged prothrombin time. Transaminases were in the reference ranges. On reduction of the dosage or withdrawal of nicotinic acid all abnormalities resolved within 4 weeks. Others have pointed out that some observations suggest that lipid-lowering with niacin always is part of a generalized hepatotoxic effect (25[C]).

Special senses Ocular adverse effects of niacin include *sicca syndrome, blurred vision,* and *eyelid edema.* A few cases of advanced *'cystoid' macular edema,* reported in two reports in the 1970s and 1980s, took months to resolve after niacin had been withdrawn (SEDA-20, 191). Four new cases have now been added in patients who took niacin 2–4.5 g/day (26[c], 27[c]). The first symptoms of blurred vision appeared 1–18 months after the start of therapy. Discontinuation of niacin resulted in improvement of visual acuity and resolution of the cystoid macular edema within 1–2 months. A particular feature that distinguishes this form of maculopthy is the absence of leakage on fluorescein angiography. Retinal edema, when it occurs, will abate on withdrawal of niacin (28[R]).

Three cases of *impaired vision* occurred after the administration of high-dose niacin (29[c]).

A 51-year old man increased his dose of niacin from 1 to 4.5 g/day. Within four weeks, he noted blurred vision in both eyes. Niacin was discontinued and his vision improved within a month.

A 53-year old man increased his dose of niacin from 1 to 3 g/day over a year. After he had been taking 3 g/day for 6 months, he noticed a gradual darkening of vision. His symptoms improved within 3 days of withdrawal.

A 51-year old man took niacin 2 g bd. After 18 months he noted visual symptoms, which resolved within two months of withdrawal.

Skin and appendages Two patients complained of *dental and gingival pain,* not previously reported adverse effects of niacin (30[c]). The pain abated on withdrawal and in one case recurred on rechallenge.

Vitamin B_{12} (hydroxocobalamin, cyanocobalamin) Severe *hypersensitivity* to one of the cobalamins has been reported in two patients who took the other cobalamin together with anti-allergy prophylaxis without further allergic reactions (31[c]).

A 42-year-old woman who had received monthly intramuscular cyanocobalamin for 4 years developed Quincke's edema. She was given hydroxocobalamin instead, each injection being preceded by 4 mg of dexamethasone. After 13 years of this treatment she had not had any allergic reactions.

A 35-year-old woman who had received monthly intramuscular hydroxocobalamin for 6 years developed anaphylactic shock immediately after a dose. Later she was given cyanocobalamin with terfenadine 120 mg/day for 2 days before each injection. After 3 years she had not had any allergic reactions.

Skin prick and intradermal tests, with increasing concentrations of hydroxocobalamin and cyanocobalamin, and histamine release tests on blood basophils with hydroxocobalamin and cyanocobalamin were negative in both patients.

Folic acid

One aspect of folate mebatolism concerns the recycling of the putatively atherogenic amino acid, homocysteine (32[R]). For reasons that are not clear, homocysteine accumulates in the blood of dialysis patients, and this accumulation is inversely related to folate status. Because of the association of folate with a risk factor for atherosclerosis—it is the major cause of morbidity and mortality in dialysis patients—folate supplementation has been widely recommended as a strategy to reduce homocysteine concentrations.

Nervous system *Worsening of seizure frequency and severity* has been reported in relation to folic acid (33[c]).

A 26-year-old woman with a family history of spinal amyotrophy and multiple sclerosis sought prepregnancy counselling and was given folic acid 0.8 mg/day to prevent neural tube defects. At 2 years of age, 6 months after a chickenpox infection, she had had recurrent fits and language regression, successfuly treated with ethosuximide. At 12 years of age she developed seizures nearly every month, characterized by sensations of fear, loss of contact, fixed eyes, motor automatism, and post-ictal aphasia. This had responded to carbamazepine. After starting to take folic acid she had a generalized tonic-clonic seizure for the first time and a significant increase in seizure frequency.

Because of the temporal relation between the seizure worsening and the administration of folic acid, a role of folic acid in provoking seizures was supposed. The first report of an epileptic patient with megaloblastic anemia in whom folate therapy resulted in an exacerbation of seizures was published in 1960. Although several subsequent controlled studies have failed to show any adverse effect on seizure frequency linked to folic acid supplementation, case reports and uncontrolled studies have documented worsening seizure frequency in some patients given folic acid. The case reported here shows that this adverse effect can occur with a dose as low as 800 μg/day.

VITAMIN C (ASCORBIC ACID)

(SED-13, 1175; SEDA-21, 407; SEDA-22, 438)

Urinary system As long-term or high-dosage consumption of vitamin C is suggested to play a role in calcium oxalate kidney stone formation, a study was undertaken to determine the biochemical and physicochemical risks of high doses of vitamin C (34[C]). A man with no history of nephrolithiasis took ascorbic acid 2 g qds while following his normal diet. The study was planned to last 9 days. However, he developed significant hematuria on the eigth day. *Urinary oxalate and ascorbic acid concentrations were increased.* The intestinal absorption of vitamin C falls from almost 100% at normal doses to 20% at a dose of 5 g/day (35[C]), and the high concentrations of ascorbic acid in this study suggest that, irrespective of the quantity converted to oxalate, at least 35% of the ingested ascorbic acid has been absorbed. The relative supersaturation of oxalate and the Tiselius risk index both increased. Increases in the calcium oxalate relative supersaturation (36[r]) and Tiselius index (37[C]) are powerful physicochemical indicators of increases in the crystal-forming potential of the urine. In this case the increases in both measures were impressively substantiated by scanning electron microscopy, which showed large crystals and crystal aggregates in the urine. The authors suggested that the passage of these crystals caused irritation and epithelial injury manifesting as hematuria.

Tubulointerstitial nephropathy has been associated with prolonged massive doses of vitamin C 3 g/day (38[c]).

VITAMIN D (CALCIFEROL) AND ANALOGS *(SED-13, 1177; SEDA-20, 366; SEDA-21, 438)*

Calcitriol (1,25-dihydroxycholecalciferol)

Calcium combined with vitamin D_3 in one tablet (Orocal) has been compared with calcium administered in a sachet (Ostram) plus vitamin D_3 as a separate tablet (Devaron) in 119 elderly women (39[C]). Three patients taking the combined formulation withdraw because of adverse effects (all *gastrointestinal disturbances*), but none of those taking the separate tablets. Of those taking the combined tablet (n = 59) 43 and 39 patients had adverse effects at 6 and 12 months respectively, compared with 46 and 41 of the 60 patients taking separate tablets. For the most part, patients complained of *arthralgia* and *gastrointestinal complaints.* None of the patients had symptomatic calcium nephrolithiasis.

VITAMIN K (PHYTOMENADIONE)

(SED-13, 1182; SEDA-21, 409; SEDA-22, 439)

In a worldwide post-marketing surveillance program a conventional vitamin K_1 formulation (Konakion), which contains Cremophor EL (polyethoxylated castor oil), has been compared with a new mixed micellar formulation (Konakion MM) (40[C]). During 1974–95 an estimated 635 million adults and 728 million children were given Konakion or Konakion MM. Of the 404 adverse events reported in 286 subjects (see Table 1) 387 (98%) were associated with Konakion, which had 95% of sales. Konakion MM accounted for 4% (n = 17) of the reported adverse effects and 5% of sales. Of the 17 adverse events 13 reported with Konakion MM were minor *injection site reactions.* Overall, 120 of the adverse events were serious, of which 117 (98%) were associated with Konakion. There were 85 probable *anaphylactoid reactions* (of which six were fatal) with conventional Konakion, compared with one non-fatal anaphylactoid reaction with Konakion MM. During the last 12 months of post-marketing surveillance, there were 14 serious adverse events reported in an estimated 21 million individals treated with Konakion, but none in the 13 million who received Konakion

Table 1. *The distribution of 404 adverse events associated with vitamin K_1 in 286 patients, by system; the figures in parantheses refer to serious adverse events*

System	Konakion (Cremophor EL)	Konakion (mixed micelles)	Total	% of total (n = 404)
General disorders	83 (37)	2 (1)	85 (38)	21.0
Cardiovascular	31 (10)	1 (0)	32 (10)	7.9
Cardiovascular: heart rate and rhythm disorders	18 (11)		18 (11)	4.5
Cardiovascular: vascular (extracardiac)	8 (3)		8 (3)	2.0
Cardiovascular: myocardial, endocardial, pericardial and valve disorders	1 (1)		1 (1)	0.2
Respiratory	31 (15)	1 (1)	32 (16)	7.9
Nervous system: central nervous and peripheral nervous systems	10 (4)		10 (4)	2.5
Nervous system: autonomic nervous system	3 (0)		3 (0)	0.7
Endocrine, metabolic, nutritional	1 (0)		1 (0)	0.2
Hematological: platelet, bleeding, and clotting disorders	5 (2)		5 (2)	1.2
Hematological: erythrocyte disorders	3 (1)		3 (1)	0.7
Hematological: white cell and reticuloendothelial system disorders	2 (2)		2 (2)	0.5
Liver, biliary	14 (3)		14 (3)	3.4
Gastrointestinal	14 (2)		14 (2)	3.4
Urinary system	3 (3)		3 (3)	0.7
Skin and appendages	90 (9)	5 (0)	95 (9)	23.5
Special senses: hearing and vestibular disorders	2 (0)		2 (0)	0.5
Musculoskeletal	2 (1)		2 (1)	0.5
Neonates and infants	13 (7)		13 (7)	3.2
Application site disorders	53 (6)	8 (1)	61 (7)	15.1
Totals	387 (117)	17 (3)	404 (120)	100%

MM. These results suggest that formulations of vitamin K_1 that are solubilized with Cremophor EL have a higher profile of adverse events, including anaphylactoid reactions, than the newer mixed micellar formulation Konakion MM.

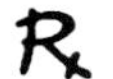

Vitamin K and cancer

The relation between neonatal vitamin K administration and childhood cancer has been investigated in three case-control studies.

In the first retrospective study 685 children who developed cancer before their 15th birthday were compared with 3442 controls matched for date and hospital of birth (41[C]). There was no association between the administration of vitamin K and the development of all childhood cancers (unadjusted odds ratios 0.89; 95% CI = 0.69–1.15) or for all acute lymphoblastic leukemia (1.20; 0.75–1.92), but there was a raised odds ratio for acute lymphoblastic leukemia 1–6 years after birth (1.79; 1.02–3.15).

However, no such association was seen in a separate cohort-based study not dependent on case-note retrieval, in which the rates of acute lymphoblastic leukemia in children born in hospital units in which all babies received vitamin K were compared with those born in units in which less than a third received prophylaxis. It was concluded that on the basis of currently published evidence neonatal intramuscular vitamin K administration does not increase the risk of early childhood leukemia.

In a second study children aged 0–14 years with leukemia (n = 150), lymphomas (n = 46), central nervous system tumors (n = 79), a range of other solid tumours (n = 142), and a subset of acute lymphoblastic leukemia (n = 129) were compared with 777 children matched for age and sex (42[C]). Odds ratios showed no significant positive association for leukemias (1.30; 0.83–2.03), acute lympho-

blastic leukemia (1.21; 0.74–1.97), lymphomas (1.06; 0.46–2.42), central nervous system tumors (0.74; 0.40–1.34), and other solid tumors (0.59; 0.37–0.96). There was no association with acute lymphoblastic leukemia in children aged 1–6 years. The authors concluded that they had not confirmed the observation of an increased risk of childhood leukemia and cancer associated with intramuscular vitamin K.

In a third study 597 cases and matched controls were compared. The association between cancer generally and intramuscular vitamin K was of borderline significance (odds ratio 1.44); the association was strongest for acute lymphoblastic leukemia (1.73) (43[C]). However, there was also an effect of abnormal delivery. The authors suggested from the lack of consistency between the various studies so far published, including their own, and the low relative risks found in most of them, that the risk, if any, attributable to the use of vitamin K cannot be large, but that the possibility that there is some risk cannot be excluded. They recommended that prophylaxis using the commonly used intramuscular dose of 1 mg should be restricted to babies at particularly high risk of vitamin K deficiency; alternatively, a lower dose might be given to a larger proportion of those at risk.

Analysis of ecological studies of the relation between hospital policies on neonatal vitamin K administration and subsequent occurrences of childhood cancer has been carried out using data from selected large maternity units in Scotland, England, and Wales (44[C]). The study covered 94 hospitals, with a total of 2.3 million births during periods when intramuscular vitamin K was routinely used and 1.4 million births when a selective policy was in operation. An increased risk was occasionally associated with vitamin K (highest odds ratio 1.25 for acute lymphoblastic leukemia in one hospital), but the overall results were not significant, and there was no evidence to support the previouly suggested doubling of the risk of childhood cancer.

On the basis of all these results it is unlikely that there is a greatly increased risk of childhood cancer attributable to intramuscular vitamin K given to newborns, if indeed there is any risk at all.

REFERENCES

1. American College of Obstetricians and Gynecologists. vitamin A supplementation during pregnancy. Intern J Gynecol Obstet 1998;61:205–6.
2. Rothman KJ, Moore LL, Singer MR, Nguyen US, Mannino S, Milunsky A. Teratogenicity of high vitamin A intake. New Engl J Med 1995;333:1369–73.
3. Arthur P, Bahl P, Bhan MK, Kirkwood BR, Martines J, Moulton LH, Panny ME, Ram M, Ram M, Underwood B. Randomised trial to assess benefits and safety of vitamin A supplementation linked to immunisation in early infancy. Lancet 1998;352:1257–63.
4. Budd GT, Adamson PC, Gupta M, Homayoun P, Sandstrom SK, Murphy RF, McLain D, Tuason L, Peereboom D, Bukowski RM, Ganapathi R. Phase I/II trial of all-trans retionic acid and tamoxifen in patients with advanced breast cancer. Clin Canc Res 1998;4:635–42.
5. De Botton S, Dombret H, Sanz M, San Miguel J, Caillot D, Zittoun R, Gardembas M, Stamatoulas A, Condé E, Guerci A, Gardin C, Geiser K, Cony Makhoul D, Reman O, De La Serna J, Lefrere F, Chomienne C, Chastang C, Degos L, Fenaux P, and the European APL Group. Incidence, clinical features, and outcome of all-trans retionic acid syndrome in 413 cases of newly diagnosed acute promyelocytic leukemia. Blood 1998;92:2712–18.
6. Nicolls MR, Terada LS, Tuder RM, Prindiville SA, Schwarz MI. Diffuse alveolar hemorrhage with underlying pulmonary capillaritis in the retionic acid syndrome. Am J Respir Crit Care Med 1998;158:1302–5.
7. Boros LG, Brandes JL, Lee W-NP, Cascante M, Puigjaner J, Revesz E, Bray TM, Schirmer WJ, Melvin WC. Thiamine supplementation to cancer patients: a double edged sword. Anticancer Res 1998;18:595–602.
8. Boros LG, Puijaner P, Cascante M, Lee WP, Brandes JL, Bassilian S, Yusuf FI, Williams RD, Muscarella P, Melvin WS, Schirmer WJ. Oxythiamine and dehydroepiandrosterone inhibit the nonoxidative synthesis of ribose and tumor cell proliferation. Cancer Res 1997;57:4242–9.
9. Anonymous. Still time for rational debate about vitamin B_6. Lancet 1998;351:1523.
10. Dalton K, Dalton MJT. Characteristics of pyridoxine overdose neuropathy syndrome. Acta Neurol Scand 1997;76:8–11.
11. Beckett A. Debate continues on vitamin B_6. Lancet 1998;352:62.
12. IPCS International Programme on Chemical Safety in cooperation with the joint FAO/WHO Expert Committee on Food Additives (JECFA). Environmental Health Criteria 70. Geneva: WHO, 1987.
13. Downing D. Debate continues on vitamin B6. Lancet 1998;352:63.
14. Selhub J, Jaques PF, Wilson PWF, Sha JR, Stabler SP, Allen RH. Vitamin status and intake as primary determinants of homocysteinemia in

an elderly population. J Am Med Assoc 1993; 270:2693–8.
15. Gospe SM Jr. Current perspectives on pyridoxine-dependent seizures. J Pediatr 1998; 132:919–23.
16. Bendich A, Cohen M. vitamin B_6 safety issues. Ann NY Acad Sci 1990;585:321–30.
17. McLachlan RS, Brown WF. Pyridoxine-dependent epilepsy with iatrogenic neuropathy. Can J Neurol Sci 1995;22:50–1.
18. Kaanders JHAM, Pop LAM, Marres HAM, Liefers J, Van Den Hoogen FJA, Van Daal WAJ, Van Der Kogel AJ. Accelerated radiotherapy with carbogen and nicotinamide (ARCON) for laryngeal cancer. Radiother Oncol 1998;48:115–22.
19. Bernier J, Stratford MRL, Denekamp J, Dennis MF, Bieri S, Hagen F., Kocagöncü O, Bolla M, Rojas A. Pharmacokinetics of nicotinamide in cancer patients treated with accelerated radiotherapy: the experience of the co-operative group of radiotherapy of the European Organization for Research and Treatment of Cancer. Radiother Oncol 1998;48:123–33.
20. Goldberg AC. Clinical trial experience with extended-release niacin (Niaspan): dose-escalation study. Am J Cardiol 1998;82:35U–38U.
21. Morgan JM, Capuzzi DM, Guyton JR. A new extended-release niacin (Niaspan): efficacy, tolerability, and safety in hypercholesterolemic patients. Am J Cardiol 1998;82:29U–34U.
22. Capuzzi DM, Guyton JR, Morgan JM, Goldberg AC, Kreisberg RA, Brusco OA, Brody J. Efficacy and safety of an extended-release nicacin (Niaspan): a long-term study. Am J Cardiol 1998;82:74U–81U.
23. Guyton JR, Goldberg AC, Kreisberg RA, Sprecher DL, Superko HR, O'Connor CM. Effectiveness of once-nightly dosing of extended-release niacin alone and in combination for hypercholesterolemia. Am J Cardiol 1998;82:737–43.
24. Tatò F, Vega GL, Grundy SM. Effects of crystalline nicotinic acid-induced hepatic dysfunction on serum low-density lipoprotein cholesterol and lecithin cholesteryl acyl transferase. Am J Cardiol 1998;81:805–7.
25. Tato F, Vega GL, Grundy SM. Effects of crystalline nicotinic acid-induced hepatic dysfunction on serum low-density lipoprotein cholesterol and lecithin cholesteryl acyl transferase. Am J Cardiol 1998;81:805–7.
26. Callanan D, Blodi BA, Martin DF. J Macular edema with nicotinic acid (niacin). J Am Med Assoc 1998;279:1702.
27. Devaney DM. Maculopathy induced by nicotinic acid. Clin Eye Vis Care 1998;10:67–71.
28. Carlson LA. The broad spectrum hypolipidaemic drug nicotinic acid. J Drug Dev Suppl 1990;3:223–6.
29. Anonymous. Nicotinic acid–visual loss. WHO Newsletter 1998;11/12:6.
30. Leighton RF, Gordon NF, Small GS, Davis WJ, Ward ES Jr. Dental and gingival pain as side effects of niacin therapy. Chest 1998;114:1472–4.
31. Guillevin L. Reintroduction of vitamin B_{12} in 2 patients with prior B_{12}-induced anaphylaxis. Br J Haematol 1998;60:269–70.
32. Westhuyzen J. Folate supplementation in the dialysis patient—fragmentary evidence and tentative recommendations. Nephrol Dial Transplant 1998;13:2748–50.
33. Guidolin L, Vignoli A, Canger R. Worsening in seizure frequency and severity in relation to folic acid administration. Eur J Neurol 1998;5: 301–3.
34. Auer BL, Auer D, Rodgers AL: Relative hyperoxaluria, crystalluria and haematuria after megadose ingestion of vitamin C. Eur J Clin Invest 1998;28:695–700.
35. Marcus R, Coulston AM. The vitamins. In: Goodman Gilman A, Rall TN, Nies AS, Taylor P, editors. The Pharmacological Basis of Therapeutics, 8th edition. New York: Pergamon Press, 1990:1530–52.
36. Werness PG, Brown CM, Smith LH, Finlayson B. EQUIL 2: a basic computer program for the calculation of urinary saturation. J Urol 1985;134:1242–4.
37. Tiselius HG. An improved method for the routine biochemical evaluation of patients with recurrent calcium oxalate stone disease. Clin Chim Acta 1982;122:409–18.
38. Nakamoto Y, Motohashi S, Kasahara H, Numazawa K. Irreversible tubulointerstitial nephropathy associated with prolonged massive intake of vitamin C. Nephrol Dial Transplant 1998;13:754–6.
39. Deroisy R, Collette J, Chevallier T, Breuil V, Reginster JY. Effects of two 1-year calcium and vitamin D_3 treatments on bone remodeling markers and femoral bone density in elderly women. Curr Ther Res Clin Exp 1998;59:850–62.
40. Pereira SP, Williams R. Adverse events associated with vitamin K_1: Results of a worldwide postmarketing surveillance programme. Pharmacoepidemiol Drug Saf 1998;7:173–82.
41. Parker L, Cole M, Craft AW, Hey EN. Neonatal vitamin K administration and childhood cancer in the north of England: retrospective case-control study. Br Med J 1998;316:189–93.
42. McKinney PA, Juszczak E, Findlay E, Smith K. Case-control study of childhood leukemia and cancer in Scotland: findings for neonatal intramuscular vitamin K. Br Med J 1998;316:173–7.
43. Passmore SJ, Draper G, Brownbill P, Kroll M. Case-control studies of relation between childhood cancer and neonatal vitamin K administration. Br Med J 1998;316:178–84.
44. Passmore SJ, Draper G, Brownbill P, Kroll M. Ecological studies of relation between hospital policies on neonatal vitamin K administration and subsequent occurence of childhood cancer. Br Med J 1998;316:184–9.

J. Costa and M. Farré

39 Corticotrophins, corticosteroids, and prostaglandins

SYSTEMIC GLUCOCORTICO-STEROIDS *(SED-13, 1193; SEDA-20, 368; SEDA-21,412; SEDA-22, 443)*

In this section adverse effects arising from the oral or intravenous administration of corticosteroids are covered. Other routes of administration are dealt with in the next section, apart from inhalation and nasal administration, which are dealt with in Chapter 16.

Cardiovascular Patients with seropositive rheumatoid arthritis taking long-term systemic corticosteroids are at risk of accelerated *cardiac rupture* in the setting of transmural acute myocardial infarction treated with thrombolytic drugs (1^c). Two women and one man, aged 53–74 years, died after they received thrombolytic therapy for acute myocardial infarction. All three had a long history of seropositive rheumatoid arthritis treated with prednisone 5–20 mg/day for many years.

Fatal *myocardial infarction* occurred after intravenous methylprednisolone for an episode of ulcerative colitis (2^c).

A day after a dose of intravenous methylprednisolone 60 mg a 79-year-old woman developed acute thoracic pain and collapsed. An electrocardiogram showed signs of a myocardial infarction and her cardiac enzyme activities were raised. She died within several hours. Autopsy showed a anterior transmural myocardial infarction and mild atheromatous lesions in the coronary arteries.

This report highlights the risk of cardiovascular adverse effects with short courses of corticosteroid therapy in elderly patients with inflammatory bowel disease, even with rather low-dosage regimens.

Serious cardiac dysrhythmias and sudden death have been reported with pulsed methylprednisolone. Now oral methylprednisolone has been implicated as a possible cause of *sinus bradycardia* (3^c).

A 14-year-old boy received an intravenous dose of methylprednisolone 30 mg/kg for progressive glomerulonephritis. After 5 hours his heart rate had fallen to 50 beats/min and an electrocardiogram showed sinus bradycardia. His heart rate then fell to 40 beats/min and a temporary transvenous pacemaker was inserted and methylprednisolone discontinued. His heart rate increased to 80 beats/min over 3 days. After a further 3 days, he was treated with oral methylprednisolone 60 mg/m^2/day and his heart rate fell to 40 beats/min in 5 days. Oral methylprednisolone was stopped on day 8 of treatment and his heart rate normalized.

Dilated cardiomyopathy caused by occult pheochromocytoma has been described infrequently. A 34-year-old woman had *acute congestive heart failure* 12 hours after administration of dexamethasone 16 mg for an atypical migraine (4^c). The authors postulated that the acute episode had been induced by the dexamethasone, which increased the production of adrenaline causing β_2-adrenoceptor stimulation, peripheral vasodilatation, and congestive heart failure. In an addendum they reported another similar case.

Respiratory A 59-year-old man had intractable *hiccups* during treatment with dexamethasone for multiple myeloma (5^c). The authors commented that hiccups are an uncommon adverse effect of high-dose corticosteroid administration. Low-dose metoclopramide is effective and may allow a patient to continue beneficial therapy without the discomfort

Side Effects of Drugs, Annual 23
J.K. Aronson, ed.

and exhaustion that can accompany intractable hiccups.

Nervous system *Epidural thoracic lipomatosis* has been associated with long-term steroid treatment (6[c]).

A 78-year-old man was given methylprednisolone (60 mg/day reducing to 8 mg/day) for temporal arteritis. After 4 months he developed numbness and paresis of the legs and hyperalgesia at dermatomes T3 and T4. After 10 months he had marked disturbance of proprioception combined with spinal ataxia and an increasing loss of motor bladder control. There was an intraspinal epidural lipoma in the dorsal part of the spine from T1–10. The fat was removed surgically and within 4 weeks his gait disturbance and proprioception improved, the sensory deficit abated, and the bladder disorder disappeared completely.

Psychiatric Pulsed intravenous methylprednisolone (2.5 g over 5 days, 5 g over 7 days, or 10 g over 5 days) caused *impaired memory* in patients with relapsing-remitting multiple sclerosis, but this effect is reversible, according to results of an Italian study (7[C]). Compared with ten control patients, there was marked selective impairment of explicit memory in 14 patients with relapsing-remitting multiple sclerosis treated with pulsed intravenous methylprednisolone. However, this memory impairment completely resolved 60 days after methylprednisolone treatment. According to the authors, this is the first report that corticosteroid-induced memory impairment is fully reversible.

Intravenous methylprednisolone was associated with a spectrum of adverse reactions, most frequently *behavioral disorders,* in 213 children with rheumatic disease, according to the results of a US study (8[C]). However, intravenous methylprednisolone was generally well tolerated. The children received their first dose of intravenous methylprednisolone 30 mg/kg over at least 60 minutes, and if the first dose was well tolerated they were given further infusions at home under the supervision of a nurse. There was at least one adverse reaction in 46 children (22%), of whom 18 had an adverse reaction within the first three doses. The most commonly reported adverse reactions were behavioral disorders (21 children), including mood changes, hyperactivity, hallucinations, disorientation, and sleep disorders. Other adverse reactions are listed in Table 1. Several children had serious acute reactions, which were readily controlled. Most of them were able to continue methylprednisolone therapy with premedication or were given an alternative corticosteroid. The researchers emphasized the need to monitor treatment closely and to have appropriate drugs readily available to treat adverse reactions.

Table 1. *Adverse reactions in 213 children given intravenous methylprednisolone*

Adverse effect	Number of patients
Behavioral changes	21
Abdominal disorders	11
Pruritus	9
Hives	5
Hypertension	5
Bone pain	3
Dizziness	3
Fatigue	2
Fracture	2
Hypotension	2
Lethargy	2
Tachycardia	2
Anaphylactoid reaction	1
'Grey appearance'	1

Endocrine, metabolic *Empty sella syndrome* occurred in a boy who developed hypopituitarism after long-term pulse therapy with prednisone for nephrotic syndrome (9[c]).

A 16-year-old Japanese boy's growth and development was normal until the age of 2 years. He then developed nephrotic syndrome and was treated with pulsed corticosteroid therapy nine times over the next 14 years. After the age of 3 years, his rate of growth had fallen. At 16 years, when he was taking prednisone 60 mg/m^2/day he was given prednisone on alternate days and the dose was gradually tapered. The secretion of pituitary hormones, except antidiuretic hormone, was impaired and an MRI scan of his brain showed an empty sella and atrophy of the pituitary gland.

When markedly impaired growth is noted in patients treated with corticosteroids long-term or in pulses, it is necessary to assess pituitary function and the anatomy of the pituitary gland. Children who receive steroid pulse therapy may develop an empty sella more frequently than is usually recognized.

Liver Three children developed *hepatomegaly* and raised liver enzymes after receiving high-dose dexamethasone therapy (0.66–1.09 mg/kg/day) (10[c]).

Gastrointestinal A 47-year-old woman developed a *gastrocolic fistula* during treatment with aspirin (dosage and duration of therapy not stated) and prednisone for chronic rheumatoid arthritis (11[c]). The author commented that recent reports have shown that 50–75% of gastrocolic fistulas are related to benign gastric ulcers secondary to the use of NSAIDs. The use of aspirin and prednisone, as in this patient, increases the risk of complication of the peptic ulcer disease two-fold to four-fold.

Perforation of the sigmoid colon has been described in 61-year-old Caucasian man with rheumatoid arthritis treated with pulses of methylprednisolone 1000 mg and colonic diverticular disease (12[c]). The authors suggested that methylprednisolone pulses should be used carefully in patients over 50 years of age and/or people with demonstrated or suspected diverticular disease.

Musculoskeletal *Osteoporosis* is a well-recognised adverse effect of corticosteroid therapy. The effect of intermittent cyclical therapy with etidronate has been investigated in the prevention of bone loss in 117 patients taking high-dose corticosteroid therapy (a mean daily dose of at least 7.5 mg for 90 days followed by at least 2.5 mg/day for at least 12 months) (13[C]). The patients were randomized to oral etidronate 400 mg/day or placebo for 14 days, followed by 76 days of oral calcium carbonate (500 mg elemental calcium), cycled over 12 months. The mean lumbar spine bone density changed 0.30% and −2.79% in the etidronate and placebo groups respectively. The mean difference between the groups after 1 year (3.0%) was significant. The changes in the femoral neck and great trochanter were not different between the groups. There was a reduction in pyridinium cross-links, significant from baseline at both 6 and 12 months, in the etidronate group. Osteocalcin increased in the placebo group, and the differences between the groups at 6 and 12 months were −25% and −35% respectively. There was no significant difference between the groups in the number of adverse events, including gastrointestinal disorders.

In a placebo-controlled study of the effects of 104 weeks of intermittent cyclical etidronate therapy in 49 patients, the same dose and cycles were used as in the previous study, but calcium (97 mg/day) was given with vitamin D (400 IU) (14[C]). Intermittent cyclical etidronate therapy with vitamin D supplementation significantly increased lumbar spine bone mineral density by 4.5 in patients with osteoporosis resulting from long-term treatment with corticosteroids.

Femoral head necrosis in kidney transplant recipients who receive postoperative immunosuppression with prednisone can be prevented, at least to some extent, by minimizing the dosage of prednisone whenever feasible (15[C]). Of 750 patients (445 men and 305 women) who had undergone kidney transplantation in 1968–95, 374 had received an average of 12.5 g of prednisone during the first year after surgery (high-dose prednisone group) and 276 had received an average of 6.5 g during this time (low-dose prednisone group) plus ciclosporin. Femoral head necrosis occurred in 42/374 patients (11%) in the high-dose prednisone group, an average of 26 months after transplantation. In contrast, femoral head necrosis occurred in only 19/376 patients (5.1%) in the low-dose group an average of 21 months after transplantation. The difference between the high-dose and low-dose groups was highly significant.

Immunological and hypersensitivity reactions An *anaphylactoid reaction* (angioedema, generalized urticaria, worsening bronchospasm, and marked hypotension) occurred in a 68-year-old woman after treatment with intravenous methylprednisolone for asthma. She had developed urticaria with the agent 1 year earlier, but the reaction had been thought to be related to the solvent in the formulation (16[c]).

A girl with asthma had *anaphylaxis* with loss of consciousness after a single dose of prednisone (17[c]).

Forty minutes after a first dose of prednisone 25 mg, a 17-year-old girl with a history of aspirin intolerance had generalised flushing, hives, hypogastric pain, and abdominal cramps, followed by vomiting and diarrhea. She lost consciousness and developed arterial hypotension. She responded to intravenous diphenhydramine and hydrocortisone. Intradermal skin tests were positive for prednisone and negative for methylprednisolone and hydrocortisone. An oral challenge test with prednisone led to flushing, nausea, dizziness, tachycardia, and hypotension and responded to intravenous diphenhydramine and hydrocortisone. Challenge tests with intravenous methylprednisolone and hydrocortisone were negative.

Infections and infestations Fatal *aspergillosis* with a thyroid gland abscess occurred in a 74-year-old man after treatment with prednisolone for polymyalgia rheumatica (18[c]). The authors commented that in patients at risk of fungal infections, local findings in the thyroid region may arouse suspicion of aspergillosis.

The cumulative and mean daily dosages of corticosteroids in patients treated for systemic lupus erythematosus, inflammatory myopathy, overlap syndrome, or mixed connective tissue disease were the most important risk factors for the development of tuberculosis, according to a study conducted in Korea (19[c]). Records were analysed from 269 patients who had been hospitalized during a 5-year period. In 21 patients active tuberculosis developed after a mean duration of 27 months from diagnosis of their rheumatic disease, an incidence rate of 20 cases per 1000 patient-years. The mean cumulative and daily dosages of prednisolone during the follow-up period were 31 594 mg and 25 mg respectively in patients who developed tuberculosis, compared with 17 043 mg and 18 mg in patients who did not. Corticosteroid pulse therapy was a risk factor for the development of tuberculosis.

A 43-year-old woman developed *cavitary lung tuberculosis* after she received methotrexate and corticosteroid pulse therapy for rheumatoid arthritis (20[c]). The authors commented that the onset of the lung infection appeared to be closely related to methotrexate and corticosteroid pulse therapy, because of the interval between drug administration and the onset of tuberculosis, and the lack of other risk factors for opportunistic infections.

Tumor-inducing effects Patients (mean age 39 years, $n = 1862$) who underwent 1924 renal transplantations from March 1995 to May 1997 were followed for 3–150 months. They received one of the following regimens: prednisolone and azathioprine (group 1; $n = 100$); prednisolone, azathioprine, and ciclosporin (group 2; $n = 1464$); and the same therapy as group 2 plus either muromonab-CD3 or antithymocyte globulin as induction or antirejection therapy (group 3; $n = 298$). The mean time to appearance of neoplasia after renal transplantation was 48 months. Malignancies developed earlier in group 3 patients (mean time to appearance 31 months) than in group 2 (39 months) and in group 1 (90 months). Seven of the patients who developed malignancies had also received pulse methylprednisolone for acute rejection. The authors concluded that the treatment of acute rejection with pulsed methylprednisolone and the use of muromonab-CD3 and antithymocyte globulin may lead to an increased incidence of malignancies after renal transplantation. They recommended that strategies be implemented for the early detection of malignancy (21[C]).

Genetic effects First trimester in utero exposure to a corticosteroid is associated with a small risk of major *neonatal malformations,* according to the results of a Canadian meta-analysis (22[C]). Six cohort studies and one case-control study were analysed, and the results showed that women who had taken long-term corticosteroid therapy during pregnancy were more likely to have a baby with a major malformation than women who had not; odds ratio 2.46 (95% CI = 1.41–4.29).

A *hydatidiform mole* during pregnancy may have been due to the corticosteroids used in an immunosuppressive regimen (23[c]).

A 33-year-old woman was receiving immunosuppressive therapy after renal transplantation: ciclosporin (dosage adjusted to achieve blood concentrations of 120–160 ng/ml), azathioprine 1 mg/kg (frequency of administration not stated), and methylprednisolone 40 mg/day from day 1 after transplantation, tapered weekly by 4–8 mg/day. Because of rejection symptoms at weeks 1, 4, and 7, she received three cycles of intravenous methylprednisolone 250 mg/day, each cycle lasting 5–7 days; she also received a bolus dose of methylprednisolone 500 mg on day 0. Pregnancy was diagnosed on day 12 after transplantation (9 weeks after conception). At week 6 after transplantation she had a missed abortion. Curettage was performed and a partial hydatidiform mole was detected. She was discharged at week 10 and immunosuppressive therapy was tapered.

Interactions *Itraconazole* 200 mg/day markedly increased plasma methylprednisolone concentrations and reduced morning plasma cortisol concentrations by over 80% in ten healthy volunteers (24[C]). The maximum concentration, AUC and half-life of methylprednisolone were increased 1.9, 3.9 and 2.4 times respectively. The authors recommended that care be taken when methylprednisolone is prescribed in combination with itraconazole or other potent inhibitors of CYP3A4.

Steroid-induced catatonic psychosis has been reported, with unexpected arousal after the administration of *etomidate* (25[c]).

A 27-year-old woman with myasthenia gravis taking prednisolone 100 mg/day became unresponsive and had respiratory difficulties. She was given etomidate 20 mg intravenously to facilitate endotracheal intubation. One minute later she became alert and oriented, with normal muscle strength, and became very emotional. Eight hours later she again became catatonic and had a similar response to etomidate 10 mg. Steroid-induced catatonia was diagnosed, her steroid dosage was reduced, and she left hospital uneventfully 4 days later.

The effect of etomidate on catatonia, similar to that of amobarbital, is thought to be due to enhanced GABA receptor function in patients with an overactive reticular system.

SPECIAL ROUTES OF ADMINISTRATION OF CORTICOSTEROIDS *(SED-13, 1204; SEDA-20, 378; SEDA-21, 419; SEDA-22, 451)*

Women should be warned about the possibility of *menstrual disorders* after local triamcinolone injections (26[C]). Premenopausal women received their first injection of triamcinolone intra-articularly ($n = 46$), injected into soft tissue ($n = 24$), or epidurally ($n = 7$). The patients were specifically asked to report flushing or menstrual irregularities during a mean follow-up period of 6 weeks. Of the 77 women in the study, 39 reported menstrual disorders. The onset of menstruation was later than expected in ten women and earlier in 16 women. There was reduced loss of blood and/or a shorter duration of menstruation in four women and increased loss of blood and/or a longer duration of menstruation in 18. Also, 22 women had flushing. Menstrual disorders occurred significantly less often in women who were taking oral contraceptives.

Epidural and intrathecal administration Bilateral posterior *subcapsular cataracts* have been reported after treatment with epidural methylprednisolone for low back pain secondary to degenerative joint disease and disk protrusion (27[c]).

A 42-year-old man had received 15 epidural injections of methylprednisolone 80 mg over 10 year. About 6 weeks after his last injection, he developed progressively worsening 'cloudy' vision. He had bilateral posterior subcapsular cataracts and subsequently underwent bilateral cataract removal.

The authors commented that it is possible that multiple epidural steroid injections had contributed to cataract formation. The patient also had several other risk factors for cataracts (cigarette smoking, alcohol consumption, exposure to ultraviolet radiation, low socioeconomic class, and low intake of antioxidant vitamins). However, the role of these other risk factors is speculative.

Post-lumbar puncture syndrome with abducent nerve palsy followed the use of intrathecal prednisolone for the treatment of low back pain and sciatica (28[c]).

A 38-year-old woman received intrathecal prednisolone 3 ml (strength not stated) and a day later developed a postural headache, nausea, and dizziness. She was treated with intravenous fluids and analgesics. Eight days later she suddenly developed a complete palsy of the right abducent nerve. An MRI brain scan with contrast showed contrast meningeal enhancement typical of post-lumbar puncture syndrome. She was treated with oral glucocorticoids and blood patching was performed. Her headache began to resolve a week later. Four months later she had almost completely recovered function of her abducent nerve and a repeat MRI scan was normal.

Inhalation The use of corticosteroids by inhalation and nasal administration is covered in Chapter 16.

Intra-articular administration An *erythema multiform-like eruption* has been reported after intra-articular triamcinolone, with cross-sensitivity to budesonide (29[c]).

A 70-year-old man had received 3 intra-articular injections of triamcinolone (dose not stated) into the same knee over 3 months without any allergic reaction. However, 12–24 hours after the last injection he developed pruritus and erythema at the injection site. This eruption was treated with topical budesonide, but within the next few hours, acute eczema developed. The lesions spread to his legs and abdomen, and were erythematous, edematous, and erythema multiform-like. He was treated with boric acid solution dressings, emollients, and oral antihistamines. His lesions gradually resolved and did not recur during 8 months of follow-up. A month after the lesions had resolved, he underwent patch testing, which was positive for triamcinolone 1% and budesonide 1% pet, but negative for other corticosteroids.

Rectal administration *Cushing's syndrome* occurred in a 65-year-old woman with ulcerative colitis who received a daily beta-methasone enema (30[c]). The authors reported the pharmacokinetics of beta-methasone after rectal dosing, with plasma concentrations of beta-methasone high enough to cause Cushing's syndrome. Suppression of the hypothalamus-pituitary-adrenal axis disappeared after the dosage schedule was changed from daily to three times a week. These findings suggest that a considerable amount of beta-methasone is absorbed after rectal dosing.

A 48-year-old woman developed *avascular necrosis* 9 months after she had completed a 3-month course of hydrocortisone 100 mg retention enemas once or twice daily for ulcerative proctitis (31[c]). An MRI scan showed multiple bony infarcts in her distal femora, proximal tibiae, and posterior proximal right fibular head, extending from the diaphysis to the epiphysis, consistent with avascular necrosis.

Topical administration The percutaneous absorption of high-potency topical steroids has been documented, but *hypothalamic-pituitary-adrenal axis suppression* leading to clinically significant adrenal insufficiency or Cushing's syndrome is infrequent. Two patients developed adrenal suppression after the unregulated use of betamethasone dipropionate 0.05% ointment (about 80 g/week) or clobetasol 0.05% ointment (up to 100 g/week), obtained without prescription to treat psoriasis (32[c]).

A 58-year-old woman, who had been involved in the manufacturing of corticosteroid creams and ointments for over 10 years, developed occupational *contact sensitisation* to topical corticosteroids (33[c]). Patch tests were positive to hydrocortisone, hydrocortisone butyrate, and tixocortol pivalate. Intradermal tests were positive to hydrocortisone succinate, methylprednisolone, and prednisolone. An oral challenge with betamethasone 0.75 mg, 2.5 mg, and 8 mg on three consecutive days resulted in no adverse reactions. She was therefore advised to use betamethasone if required and to avoid handling corticosteroid creams and ointments.

Acute anaphylaxis occurred in an 18-year-old man after the third course of intradermal injections of triamcinolone suspension ('Kenalog' 10 mg per treatment) for alopecia areata (34[c]). Subsequent rechallenge with intradermal triamcinolone 1 ml resulted in the same anaphylactic reaction as before and his serum IgE concentration was increased.

Although immediate hypersensitivity reactions to paramethasone acetate, causing widespread eruptions, have been described in at least four cases, a *delayed allergic reaction* has not previously been described (35[c]).

A woman had received intralesional paramethasone and other topical corticosteroids several times for her alopecia between the ages of 7 and 18 years. When she was 30 she was again treated with intralesional paramethasone for a relapse of alopecia. She developed pruritus after the first intralesional injection and erythema, edema, and vesicles 6–8 hours later. A biopsy showed spongiform lymphocytic folliculitis with spongiosis and exocytosis in the sweat gland ducts and in the pilosebaceous unit. She was treated with triamcinolone cream and her skin lesions resolved. Patch tests were positive for paramethasone, with cross-reactivity to tixocortol pivalate, hydrocortisone, and hydrocortisone butyrate.

Chronic lichenified eczema has been attributed to prolonged use of topical methylprednisolone aceponate and budesonide (strength and duration of therapy not stated) in a 26-year-old woman (36[c]). Patch tests were positive for methylprednisolone aceponate and budesonide cream, but negative for all other topical corticosteroids.

MINERALOCORTICOIDS

(SED-13, 1206; SEDA-21, 420)

Congestive heart failure occurred in a 47-year-old woman after she had taken fludrocortisone 100 μg/day for 2 weeks for Addison's disease (37[c]). Ten months later fludrocortisone 25 μg/day was restarted, and the dosage was increased to 100 μg/day over 2 months. At follow-up after 4 months, she was well, without fluid retention or electrolyte abnormalities.

PROSTAGLANDINS *(SED-13, 1316; SEDA-18, 422; SEDA-21, 420; SEDA-22, 452)*

Alprostadil (Prostaglandin E_1)

Neonates with hypoplastic left heart syndrome awaiting heart transplantation are given continuous prostaglandin E_1 perfusion for a prolonged period of time, which can result in various adverse effects. Of 15 neonates with hypoplastic left heart syndrome (nine boys and six girls; median weight 3123 g) included in a cardiac transplant program between January 1993 and August 1996, who received continuous endovenous perfusion of prostaglandin E_1 from the time of diagnosis of the cardiomyopathy, 13 received transplants and six died in the operating room (38[C]). All had short-term adverse effects from the continuous perfusion of prostaglandin E_1, including slight *fever* and *irritability*. However, none had apneic pauses. *Cortical hyperostosis* occurred in 13 and *antral hyperplasia* in 12, but in all transplanted cases regression of the antral hyperplasia was seen after 6 months and regression of the cortical hyperostosis was seen after 12 months.

Urinary system Intracavernosal alprostadil (prostaglandin E_1) is effective and well tolerated in the treatment of erectile dysfunction, according to the results of a 6-month study (funded by Pharmacia & Upjohn) in 848 men (mean age 52 years) with at least a 4-month history of erectile dysfunction (39[C]). This is provided that the individual dose is established by titration and patients receive training in injection techniques and periodic supervision during treatment. An initial dose was established for each patient and the patients then administered the alprostadil themselves at home. Of 727 evaluable patients, 682 (94%) had at least one erectile response after the injection of alprostadil, and 88% of injections lead to a satisfactory sexual response. The most commonly reported adverse event was *penile pain,* reported by 44% of patients, but only after 8% of injections. In just over half of the patients who had penile pain, the condition was reported as mild. *Prolonged erection, penile fibrosis,* and *priapism* occurred in 8, 4, and 0.9% of patients respectively. Treatment was withdrawn because of medical events in 4% of patients and drug-related events accounted for treatment withdrawal in 2% of patients.

The impact of treatment with transurethral alprostadil for erectile dysfunction on the quality of life of 249 men and their partners has been evaluated (40[C]). The men who had organic erectile dysfunction of more than 3 months' duration, self-administered transurethral alprostadil in an open-label, dose-escalating, outpatient study. Patients with a sufficient response ($n = 159$) were randomly assigned double-blind to either active medication or placebo for 3 months at home. Drug-related *urogenital pain* was reported by 12% of patients during outpatient dosing. However, this pain was usually mild, and only five patients (2%) during outpatient dosing discontinued treatment. One patient reported minor urethral bleeding/spotting. The transurethral administration of alprostadil was associated with minimal or no discomfort in 83–88% of patients. In the out-patient study, *dizziness* occurred in one patient and *hypotension* in one patient. During home treatment drug-related *urogenital pain* was reported by 11 patients (14%), minor *urethral bleeding/spotting* by one (1.3%), and *dizziness* by two (2.6%). One patient reported *prolonged erections* on two occasions during home treatment, each lasting less than 5 hours.

The incidence of *priapism* after intracorporeal administration of alprostadil is 1%. The first case report of priapism after medicated urethral system for erection (MUSE) has been published (41[c]).

A 57-year-old man with erectile impotence, who had previously been treated with intracorporeal injections of papaverine and alprostadil, resulting in recurrent episodes of priapism necessitating aspiration, decided to try intraurethral alprostadil (MUSE). The dose needed to achieve a full erection in the clinic was titrated to 1 μg, but after 5 months this was found to be inadequate unless supplemented by a hot bath before MUSE administration. The patient stated that with MUSE alone the erection lasted for 5–10 minutes but on the two previous occasions when he had had a hot bath for 20 minutes and then used MUSE, the erection had lasted 3–4 hours. However, on the third occasion, priapism lasted 20 hours and necessitated corporeal aspiration for detumescence.

Skin and appendages Penile shaft *lichen sclerosus* has been reported in a 63-year-old man in association with alprostadil intracavernous injection for erectile dysfunction (42[c]). The authors suggested that the lichen sclerosus had been caused by (1) an isomorphic response to the trauma of repeated needle injection; (2) a local cutaneous response to alprostadil-induced collagen synthesis or alprostadil-induced fibroblast production of IL-6, with secondary paracrine/autocrine-induced collagen synthesis by improper skin exposure due to direct injection into the skin or by retrograde flow of alprostadil through the needle puncture tract; or (3) a random occurrence of separate events.

Iloprost

A multicenter, randomized, parallel-group comparison of two different doses of oral iloprost and placebo has been conducted, to identify the optimal dose of oral iloprost on the basis of efficacy and tolerability in patients with

Raynaud's phenomenon secondary to systemic sclerosis (43[C]). A total of 103 patients were given total daily doses of iloprost of 100 μg (n = 33), or 200 μg (n = 35), or placebo (n = 35) for 6 weeks. The mean percentage reductions in the frequency, total daily duration, and severity of Raynaud's attacks were greater in the iloprost groups at the end of treatment and at the end of follow-up. Adverse effects were reported by 80% of patients taking placebo, 85% taking oral iloprost 100 μg/day, and 97% taking oral iloprost 100 μg/day. There were significant differences in the frequency of five types of adverse events. *Headache, flushing, nausea,* and *trismus* were all more common with increasing iloprost dose, while flu-like illnesses were most commonly reported in the placebo group. Treatment was prematurely discontinued in 9, 30, and 51% respectively, and discontinuation was precipitated by adverse events 6, 27, and 51%.

The use of iloprost has been proposed in patients with systemic sclerosis, a disease that is often characterized by pulmonary hypertension and Raynaud's phenomenon. Three patients with systemic sclerosis who were treated with iloprost developed *acute thrombotic events* (44[cr]). In one case, intestinal infarction occurred 1 day after infusion of iloprost. In another patient the left kidney was not perfused 22 days after the last infusion of iloprost because of thrombosis of the left renal artery. The last patient, 9 months after the start of treatment with iloprost, and 5 days after the last infusion, had an anterolateral myocardial infarction. The authors commented that their observations did not allow them to conclude that there is a direct relation between infusion of iloprost and thrombotic events. However, they said that this possibility should be considered, and they suggested that risk factors for thromboembolism should be carefully evaluated in each patient with systemic sclerosis who is receiving iloprost.

Latanoprost

Cardiovascular Two patients in their seventies developed *hypertension* during treatment with topical latanoprost (dosage not stated) for open-angle glaucoma; both were also taking tocopherol (vitamin E) supplements. Neither had a previous history of hypertension (45[c]). The authors commented that it is likely that systemic absorption of topically applied latanoprost could cause hypertension. Self-medication with vitamin E has been reported to aggravate or precipitate hypertension.

Skin and appendages *Increased pigmentation of the eyelashes* has been reported in a patient treated with latanoprost (46[c]).

Heavy sweating occurred in a 6-year-old boy with aniridia and glaucoma during treatment with latanoprost eye-drops (47[c]). Other combinations of antiglaucoma eye-drops had been ineffective in reducing the intraocular pressure. He was given latanoprost (dose not stated) eye-drops at night in combination with a beta-blocker during the day. However, at night he had very heavy sweating. His pyjamas had to be changed regularly about 1–2 hours after he went to sleep. When latanoprost was discontinued, the heavy sweating resolved. When it was restarted, the heavy sweating recurred. The author commented that systemic absorption occurred for the most part through the mucous membranes of the nose and throat, since the sweating was less severe when the boy's lachrymal points were compressed for 10 minutes after the administration of latanoprost.

Special senses *Cystoid macular edema* developed in two patients treated with topical latanoprost for glaucoma (48[c]). Latanoprost was withdrawn, and the cystoid macular edema was treated with topical corticosteroids and ketorolac, with improvement in visual acuity. The macular edema resolved in both cases. Cystoid macular edema may be related to a prostaglandin-like action. Cystoid macular edema has been reported in four other patients shortly after they started to use latanoprost (49[c]). Other reports of the same complication of latanoprost have appeared (50[c]–52[c]).

In four patients with complicated open-angle glaucoma in whom *anterior uveitis* appeared to be associated with latanoprost, the uveitis was unilateral and occurred only in the eye receiving latanoprost in three patients. In one patient, latanoprost was used in both eyes, and the uveitis was bilateral (53[c]). Four of five eyes had a history of prior inflammation and/or prior incisional surgery. All patients were rechallenged. The uveitis improved after withdrawal and recurred after rechallenge in all eyes. The authors concluded that topical prostaglandin analogs may be relatively contraindicated in patients with a history of uveitis or prior ocular surgery. There may also be a risk in eyes that have not had previous uveitis or incisional surgery.

The incidence of *iris pigmentation* differs between eyes with differently colored irises: green-brown, yellow-brown, and blue-brown eyes, in that order, have the highest incidence, whereas eyes with uniformly blue, grey, or green irises are much less affected even after 2 years of treatment. About 60% of eyes with an initial green-brown iris will have increased pigmentation within 1 year. The corresponding figure for initially blue-brown eyes is about 20%. All patients who have developed increased pigmentation of the iris have been withdrawn from studies, and during follow-up for up to almost 3 years the change in iris pigmentation has been stable without signs of reversibility or further increase. Nevi and freckles have not changed color or size. Apart from the change in color the iris looks normal and pigmentation dispersion has not been observed. No cell proliferation is involved and the change in color is due to melanogenesis. It has been concluded that the change in iris pigmentation is unlikely to cause any long-term consequence besides the cosmetic one. The possibility of late loss of pigment and induction of a pigmentary glaucoma also seems unlikely; melanocytes in the iris are continent and do not release melanin (54[R]).

The time of onset of the *changes in iris pigmentation* can be as early as 3 months. The earliest reported change in iris color occurred in a 78-year-old woman, whose iris color changed from blue-green to brown-green within 4 weeks (55[c]).

Misoprostol

Misoprostol, an analog of prostaglandin E_1 licensed for use in the management of gastroduodenal ulceration, is uterotonic and provides an effective alternative to gemeprost, the most widely used prostaglandin pessaries after mifepristone. Extra-amniotic prostaglandin $F_{2\alpha}$ and intracervical misoprostol have been compared for termination of pregnancy in 40 women at 16–24 weeks of gestation (56[C]). All women given $PGF_{2\alpha}$ aborted within 28 hours, and 16 within 20 hours; termination of pregnancy was complete in 13 cases. With misoprostol all the women aborted within 20 hours, 18 within 13 hours; termination of pregnancy was complete in 17 cases. The mean time to induction of abortion was 16 hours for extra-amniotic $PGF_{2\alpha}$ and 10 hours for intracervical misoprostol (significantly quicker). The incidence of prostaglandin-associated *pyrexia, vomiting,* and *diarrhea* was significantly higher with $PGF_{2\alpha}$. Abdominal pain was similar in the two groups.

Recent data from Brazil, where misoprostol has been used orally and vaginally as an abortifacient, have suggested a relation between the use of misoprostol by women in an unsuccessful attempt to terminate pregnancy and *Möbius' syndrome* (congenital facial paralysis) in their infants (57[C]). The frequency of misoprostol use during the first trimester by mothers of infants in whom Möbius' syndrome was diagnosed and mothers of infants with neural-tube defects have been compared. There were 96 infants with Möbius' syndrome and 96 with neural-tube defects. The mean age at the time of the diagnosis of Möbius' syndrome was 16 (range 0.5–78) months and the diagnosis of neural-tube defects was made within 1 week of birth in most cases. Of the mothers of the infants with Möbius' syndrome, 47 had used misoprostol in the first trimester of pregnancy, compared with 3 of the mothers of the infants with neural-tube defects (odds ratio 30; 95% CI = 12–76). Of the mothers of the infants with Möbius' syndrome 20 had taken misoprostol only orally (odds ratio, 39; CI = 9.5–159), 20 had taken misoprostol both orally and vaginally, three had taken it vaginally, and four did not report how they had taken it. The authors concluded that attempted abortion with misoprostol is associated with an increased risk of Möbius' syndrome in infants.

The common phenotypical effects of exposure of the fetus to misoprostol in utero have been defined in 42 infants who were exposed to misoprostol during the first 3 months of gestation, and then born with congenital abnormalities (58[C]). *Equinovarus with cranial nerve defects* occurred in 17 infants. Ten children had equinovarus as part of more extensive *arthrogryposis.* The most distinctive phenotypes were arthrogryposis confined to the legs (five cases) and terminal transverse limb defects (nine cases), with or without Möbius' syndrome. The most common dose of misoprostol was 800 μg (range 200–16000). Deformities attributed to vascular disruption were found in these children. The authors suggested that the uterine contractions induced by misoprostol cause vascular disruption in the fetus, including brain-stem ischemia. Information on the effects of taking misoprostol during pregnancy should be made more widely available, to dissuade women from misusing the drug. Additional information on the risk associated with continuing a pregnancy to term after a failure of mifepristone and prostaglandin has been provided (59[C]).

Oral misoprostol 400 μg has been compared with placebo in the routine management of the third stage of labor. In this study *shivering* was a specific adverse effect of oral misoprostol in the puerperium (19% vs 5%, relative risk 3.69; 95% CI = 2.05–6.64) (60[C]).

Use in pregnancy *Uterine rupture* has been described after the use of transvaginal misoprostol for induction of labor in a 26-year-old patient with a previous low transverse cesarean delivery (61[c]). Other reports include two cases of disruption of prior uterine incisions after misoprostol (62[c]) and two cases of uterus rupture, after inappropriate use (63[c]). In one case the dose 200 μg was too high. In the other case oxytocin was started 5 hours after the second misoprostol tablet, while the usual recommendation is to wait at least 12 hours. One patient had also had a previous dilatation and curettage for spontaneous abortion, which is a predisposing factor for uterine rupture in labor.

Sulprostone

Sulprostone is a synthetic prostaglandin analog of dinoprostone (PGE_2) used for inducing uterine contraction. In large series, it has had good tolerability with a very low complication rate. The most severe complication is *myocardial infarction* secondary to coronary spasm, with a frequency of 1 in 20 000, usually in smokers and women over 35 years of age with cardiovascular disease. Myocardial infarction has been reported in a woman aged 35 years with normal coronary arteries and good left ventricular function (64[c]). Several experimental studies have provided support for the hypothesis that coronary spasms play a major role in the pathophysiology of myocardial infarction during the administration of sulprostone. However, the possibility of myocardial infarction is not mentioned in the product information.

A 38-year-old woman developed complete *heart block, ventricular fibrillation,* and subsequent *asystole* about 7 minutes after intravenous sulprostone 30 μg over 5 minutes, after she had previously been given a total dose of intramyometrial sulprostone 500 μg at seven different points for postpartum hemorrhage after cesarean section (65[c]). The time course suggested that the most likely cause of the arrest was the intravenous sulprostone. Contributory causes may have been hemorrhagic shock, electrolyte abnormalities, and hypothermia (from massive blood transfusion).

Cardiac arrest occurred in a 39-year-old woman 3.5 hours after the administration of sulprostone 250 μg directly into the uterine wall for post-partum hemorrhage after manual removal of the placenta (66[c]). She had specific contraindications to sulprostone, as formulated by the French authorities: age over 35 years, heavy cigarette smoking, and cardiovascular risk factors. In the Netherlands sulprostone is registered for intravenous administration only. The authors strongly advised against administration directly into the uterine wall.

PROSTACYCLIN ANALOGS

(SEDA-22, 454)

Epoprostenol

Epoprostenol has become the preferred long-term treatment for patients with primary pulmonary hypertension who continue to have symptoms in spite conventional therapy. However, *tolerance,* which always occurs, has made dosing uncertain. The effectiveness of epoprostenol given according to an aggressive dosing strategy for longer than 1 year has been investigated in these patients (67[c]). The dose of epoprostenol was increased by 2.4 ng/kg/min each month to the maximum tolerated dose. Adverse effects were common and included *diarrhea, jaw pain, headaches,* and *flushing* in all patients.

Pulmonary veno-occlusive disease is a rare form of pulmonary hypertension associated with fibrotic occlusion of the smaller pulmonary veins. Although vasodilator therapy is effective in many patients with primary pulmonary hypertension, the role of vasodilators in veno-occlusive disease is unclear, because of concerns about precipitating pulmonary edema. There have been reports of successful therapy with oral vasodilators or intravenous prostacyclin. In contrast, there has been a description of a patient who developed *acute pulmonary edema* and respiratory failure 15 minutes after the start of a low-dose prostacyclin infusion 2 ng/kg/min, leading to death an hour later (68[c]).

This case has several important implications for the management of patients with pulmonary hypertension. Although previous reports suggested that prostacyclin may be safe in patients with pulmonary veno-occlusive disease, the experience reported here suggests that even in very low doses prostacyclin can produce acute decompensation. Thus, consideration must be given to the diagnosis of pulmonary veno-occlusive disease in all patients with suspected primary pulmonary hypertension.

Two further cases of *pulmonary edema* have been reported during continuous intravenous epoprostenol in patients with severe pulmonary hypertension and pulmonary capillary hemangiomatosis, a rare condition characterized by proliferation of thin-walled microvessels in the alveolar walls (69[c]). This report suggests that epoprostenol should not be used in such patients.

REFERENCES

1. Kotha P, McGreevy MJ, Kotha A, Look M, Weisman MH. Early deaths with thrombolytic therapy for acute myocardial infarction in corticosteroid-dependent rheumatoid arthritis. Clin Cardiol 1998;21:853–6.
2. Baty V, Blain H, Saadi L, Jeandel C, Canton PH. Fatal myocardial infarction in an elderly woman with severe ulcerative colitis: what is the role of steroids? Am J Gastroenterol 1998;93:2000–1.
3. Küçükosmanoglu O, Karabay A, Ozbarlas N, Noyan A, Anarat A. Marked bradycardia due to pulsed and oral methylprednisolone therapy in a patient with rapidly progressive glomerulonephritis. Nephron 1998;80:484.
4. Kothari SN, Kisken WA. Dexamethasone-induced congestive heart failure in a patient with dilated cardiomyopathy caused by occult pheochromocytoma. Surgery 1998;123:102–5.
5. Cersosimo RJ, Brophy MT. Hiccups with high dose dexamethasone administration: a case report. Cancer 1998;82:412–14.
6. Pinsker MO, Kinzel D, Lumenta CB. Epidural thoracic lipomatosis induced by long-term steroid treatment case illustration. Acta Neurochir 1998;140:991–2.
7. Oliveri RL, Sibilia G, Valentino P, Russo C, Romeo N, Quattrone A. Pulsed methylprednisolone induces a reversible impairment of memory in patients with relapsing-remitting multiple sclerosis. Acta Neurol Scand 1998;97:366–9.
8. Klein Gitelman MS, Pachman LM. Intravenous corticosteroids: adverse reactions are more variable than expected in children. J Rheumatol 1998;25:1995–2002.
9. Kamoda T, Nakahara C, Matsui A. A case of empty sella after steroid pulse therapy for nephrotic syndrome. J Rheumatol 1998;25:822–3.
10. Verrips A, Rottevell JJ, Lippens R. Dexamethasone-induced hepatomegaly in three children. Pediatr Neurol 1998;19:388–91.
11. Suazo Barahona J, Gallegos J, Carmona Sánchez R, Martínez R, Robles Díaz G. Nonsteroidal anti-inflammatory drugs and gastrocolic fistula. J Clin Gastroenterol 1998;26:343–5.
12. Candelas G, Jover JA, Fernández B, Rodríguez Olaverri JC, Calatayud J. Perforation of the sigmoid colon in a rheumatoid arthritis patient treated with methylprednisolone pulses. Scand J Rheumatol 1998;27:152–3.
13. Roux C, Oriente P, Laan R, Hughes RA, Ittner J, Goemaere S, Di Munno O, Pouilles JM, Horlait S, Cortet B. Randomized trial of effect of cyclical etidronate in the prevention of corticosteroid-induced bone loss. J Clin Endocrinol Metab 1998;83:1128–33.
14. Pitt P, Li F, Todd P, Webber D, Pack S, Moniz C. A double blind placebo controlled study to determine the effects of intermittent cyclical etidronate on bone mineral density in patients on long term oral corticosteroid treatment. Thorax 1998;53:351–6.
15. Lausten GS, Lemser T, Jensen PK, Egfjord M. Necrosis of the femoral head after kidney transplantation. Clin Transplant 1998;12:572–4.
16. Vanpee D, Gillet J-B. Allergic reaction to intravenous methylprednisolone in a woman with asthma. Ann Emerg Med 1998;32:754.
17. Polosa R, Prosperini G, Pintaldi L, Rey JP, Colombrita R. Anaphylaxis after prednisone. Allergy 1998;53:330–1.
18. Vogeser M, Haas A, Ruckdeschel G, Von Scheidt W. Steroid-induced invasive aspergillosis with thyroid gland abscess and positive blood cultures. Eur J Clin Microbiol Infect Dis 1998;17:215–16.
19. Kim HA, Yoo CD, Baek HJ, Lee EB, Ahn C, Han JS, Kim S, Lee JS, Choe KW, Song YW. Mycobacterium tuberculosis infection in a corticosteroid-treated rheumatic disease patient population. Clin Exp Rheumatol 1998;16:9–13.
20. Di Girolamo C, Pappone N, Melillo E, Rengo C, Giuliano F, Melillo G. Cavity lung tuberculosis in a rheumatoid arthritis patient treated with low-dose methotrexate and steroid pulse therapy. Br J Rheumatol 1998;37:1136–7.
21. Thiagarajan CM, Divakar D, Thomas SJ. Malignancies in renal transplant recipients. Transpl Proc 1998;30:3154–5.

22. Beique LC, Friesen, MH, Park LY, Díaz-Citrin O, Koren G, Einarson TR. Major malformations associated with corticosteroid exposure during the first trimester: a meta-analysis. Can J Hosp Pharm 1998;51:83.
23. Markert UR, Klemm A, Flossmann E, Werner W, Sperschneider H, Fünfstück R. Renal transplantation in early pregnancy with acute graft rejection and development of a hydatidiform mole. Clin Nephrol 1998;49:391–2.
24. Varis T, Kaukonen KM, Kivistö KT, Neuvonen PJ. Plasma concentrations and effects of oral methylprednisolone are considerably increased by itraconazole. Clin Pharmacol Ther 1998;64:363–8.
25. Ilbeigi MS, Davidson ML, Yarmush JM. An unexpected arousal effect of etomidate in a patient on high-dose steroids. Anesthesiology 1998;89:1587–9.
26. Mens JMA, Nico De Wolf A, Berkhout BJ. Disturbance of the menstrual pattern after local injection with triamcinolone acetonide. Ann Rheum Dis 1998;57:700.
27. Chen YCJ, Gajraj NM, Clavo A, Joshi GP. Posterior subcapsular cataract formation associated with multiple lumbar epidural corticosteroid injections. Anesth Analg 1998;86:1054–5.
28. Dumont D, Hariz H, Meynieu P, Salama J, Dreyfus P, Boissier M-C. Abducens palsy after an intrathecal glucocorticoid injection: evidence for a role of intracranial hypotension. Rev Rhum Engl Ed 1998;65:352–4.
29. Valsecchi R, Reseghetti A, Leghissa P, Cologni L, Cortinovis R. Erythema-multiforme-like lesions from triamcinolone acetonide. Contact Dermatitis 1998;38:362–3.
30. Tsuruoka S, Sugimoto K, Fujimura A. Drug-induced Cushing syndrome in a patient with ulcerative colitis after betamethasone enema: evaluation of plasma drug concentration. Ther Drug Monit 1998;20:387–9.
31. Braverman DL, Lachmann EA, Nagler W. Avascular necrosis of bilateral knees secondary to corticosteroid enemas. Arch Phys Med Rehabil 1998;79:449–52.
32. Gilbertson EO, Spellman MC, Piacquadio DJ, Mulford MI. Super potent topical corticosteroid use associated with adrenal suppression: clinical considerations. J Am Acad Dermatol 1998;38:318–21.
33. Lauerma AI. Occupational contact sensitization to corticosteroids. Contact Dermatitis 1998; 39:328–9.
34. Downs AMR, Lear JT, Kennedy CTC. Anaphylaxis to intradermal triamcinolone acetonide. Arch Dermatol 1998;134:1163–4.
35. Miranda Romero A, Bajo del Pozo C, Sánchez Sambucety P, Martínez Fernández M; García Muñoz M. Delayed local allergic reaction to intralesional paramethasone acetate. Contact Dermatitis 1998;39:31–2.
36. Corazza M, Virgili A. Allergic contact dermatitis from 6-alpha-methylprednisolone aceponate and budesonide. Contact Dermatitis 1998; 38:356–7.
37. Bhattacharyya A, Tymms DJ. Heart failure with fludrocortisone in Addison's disease. J R Soc Med 1998;91:433–4.
38. Caballero S, Torre I, Arias B, Blanco D, Zabala JI, Sánchez Luna M. Efectos secundarios de la prostaglandina E_1 en el manejo del síndrome de corazón izquierdo hipoplastico en espera de trasplante cardiaco. An Esp Pediatr 1998;48:505–9.
39. Alvarez E, Andrianne R, Arvis G, Boezaart F, Buvat J, Czyzyk A, et al. The long-term safety of alprostadil (prostaglandin-E_1) in patients with erectile dysfunction. Br J Urol 1998;82:538–43.
40. Williams G, Abbou C-C, Amar ET, Desvaux P, Flam TA, Lycklama à Nijeholt GAB, et al. The effect of transurethral alprostadil on the quality of life of men with erectile dysfunction, and their partners. MUSE Study Group. Br J Urol 1998;82:847–54.
41. Bettocchi C, Ashford L, Pryor JP, Ralph DJ. Priapism after transurethral alprostadil. Br J Urol 1998;81:926.
42. English JC 3rd; King DH; Foley JP. Penile shaft hypopigmentation: lichen sclerosus occurring after the initiation of alprostadil intracavernous injections for erectile dysfunction. J Am Acad Dermatol 1998;39:801–3.
43. Black CM, Halkier-Sørensen L, Belch JJF, Ullman S, Madhok R, Smit AJ, Banga J-D, Watson HR. Oral iloprost in Raynaud's phenomenon secondary to systemic sclerosis: a multicentre, placebo-controlled, dose-comparison study. Br J Rheumatol 1998;37:952–60.
44. Tedeschi A, Meroni PL, Del Papa N, Salmaso C, Boschetti C, Miadonna A. Thrombotic events in patients with systemic sclerosis treated with iloprost. Arthritis Rheum 1998;41:559–60.
45. Peak AS, Sutton BM. Systemic adverse effects associated with topically applied latanoprost. Ann Pharmacother 1998;32:504–5.
46. Reynolds A, Murray PI, Colloby PS. Darkening of eyelashes in a patient treated with latanoprost. Eye 1998;12:741–3.
47. Schmidtborn F. Systemic side effects of latanoprost therapy in a child with aniridia and glaucoma. Ophthalmologe 1998;95:633–4.
48. Callanan D, Fellman RL, Savage JA. Latanoprost-associated cystoid macular edema. Am J Ophthalmol 1998;126:134–5.
49. Ayyala RS, Cruz DA, Margo CE, Harman LE, Pautler SE, Misch DM, Mines JA, Richards DW. Cystoid macular edema associated with latanoprost in aphakic and pseudophakic eyes. Am J Ophthalmol 1998;126:602–4.
50. Avakian A, Renier SA, Butler PJ. Adverse effects of latanoprost on patients with medically resistant glaucoma. Arch Ophthalmol 1998;116:679–80.
51. Gaddie IB, Bennett DW. Cystoid macular edema associated with the use of latanoprost. J Am Optom Assoc 1998;69:122–8.
52. Heier JS, Steinert RF, Frederick AR Jr. Cystoid macular edema associated with latanoprost use. Arch Ophthalmol 1998;116:680–2.

53. Fechtner RD, Khouri AS, Zimmerman TJ, Bullock J, Feldman R, Kulkarni P, Michael AJ, Realini T, Warwar R. Anterior uveitis associated with latanoprost. Am J Ophthalmol 1998;126:37–41.
54. Alm A. Prostaglandin derivates as ocular hypotensive agents. Prog Retinal Eye Res 1998; 17:291–312.
55. Pappas RM, Pusin S, Higginbotham EJ. Evidence of early change in iris color with latanoprost use. Arch Ophthalmol 1998;116:1115–16.
56. Ghorab MN, El Helw BA. Second-trimester termination of pregnancy by extra-amniotic prostaglandin $F_{2\alpha}$ or endocervical misoprostol. A comparative study. Acta Obstet Gynecol Scand 1998;77:429–32.
57. Pastuszak AL, Schüler L, Speck Martins CE, Coelho K-EFA, Cordello SM, Vargas F, Brunoni D, Schwarz IVD, Larrandaburu M, Safattle H, Meloni VFA, Koren G. Use of misoprostol during pregnancy and Möbius' syndrome in infants. New Engl J Med 1998;338:1881–5.
58. Gonzalez CH, Marques-Dias MJ, Kim CA, Sugayama SMM, Da Paz JA, Huson SM, Holmes LB. Congenital abnormalities in Brazilian children associated with misoprostol misuse in first trimester of pregnancy. Lancet 1998;351:1624–7.
59. Sitruk-Ware R, Davey A, Sakiz E. Fetal malformation and failed medical termination of pregnancy. Lancet 1998;352:323.
60. Hofmeyr GJ, Nikodem VC, De Jager M, Gelbart BR. A randomised placebo controlled trial of oral misoprostol in the third stage of labour. Br J Obstet Gynaecol 1998;105:971–5.
61. Sciscione AC, Nguyen L, Manley JS, Shlossman PA, Colmorgen GH. Uterine rupture during preinduction cervical ripening with misoprostol in a patient with a previous Caesarean delivery. Aust NZ J Obstet Gynaecol 1998;38:96–7.
62. Wing DA, Lovett K, Paul RH. Disruption of prior uterine incision following misoprostol for labor induction in women with previous cesarean delivery. Obstet Gynecol 1998;91:828–30.
63. Fletcher H, McCaw-Binns A. Rupture of the uterus with misoprostol (prostaglandin E_1) used for induction of labour. J Obstet Gynaecol 1998;18:184–5.
64. Feenstra J, Borst F, Huige MC, Oei SG, Stricker BH. Acuut myocardinfarct na toediening van sulproston. Ned Tijdschr Geneeskd 1998;142:192–5.
65. Chen FG, Koh KF, Chong YS. Cardiac arrest associated with sulprostone use during caesarean section. Anaesth Intensive Care 1998;26:298–301.
66. Beerendonk CC, Massuger LF, Lucassen AM, Lerou JG, Van Den Berg PP. Circulatiestilstand na gebruik van sulproston bij fluxus post partum. Ned Tijdschr Geneeskd 1998;142:195–7.
67. McLaughlin VV, Genthner DE, Panella MM, Rich S. Reduction in pulmonary vascular resistance with long-term epoprostenol (prostacyclin) therapy in primary pulmonary hypertension. New Engl J Med 1998;338:273–7.
68. Palmer SM, Robinson LJ, Wang A, Gossage JR, Bashore T, Tapson VF. Massive pulmonary edema and death after prostacyclin infusion in a patient with pulmonary veno-occlusive disease. Chest 1998;113:237–40.
69. Humbert M, Maitre S, Capron F, Rain B, Musset D, Simonneau G. Pulmonary edema complicating continuous intravenous prostacyclin in pulmonary capillary hemangiomatosis. Am J Respir Crit Care Med 1998;157:1681–5.

A. Buitenhuis and C.J. van Boxtel

40 Sex hormones and related compounds, including hormonal contraceptives

FEMALE SEX HORMONES

Estrogens and progestogens

(SED-13, 1255; SEDA-21, 426, SEDA-22, 458)

The estradiol-containing vaginal ring delivery system offers efficacy, safety, and tolerability with improved comfort and acceptability. The most frequent adverse events were *vaginitis, breast tenderness, abdominal pain, pruritus,* and *vaginal discomfort* (1^R). However, the incidence of these adverse events was similar to those of other estrogen vaginal delivery systems.

Potential adverse effects of estrogen/androgen therapy, which are usually reversible on early withdrawal of treatment include mild *hirsutism, acne,* and *voice changes.* Under 5% of women experience acne or facial hirsutism with the esterified estrogen/methyl testosterone combination. In the Estratest Working Group study, the incidence of hirsutism in the women who took esterified estrogens plus a low dose of methyltestosterone was not significantly different from the incidence of hirsutism in the women who took conjugated estrogens 0.625 mg/day. Women had significantly less *nausea* with estrogen/androgen treatment than with conjugated estrogen therapy. *Cancers, cardiovascular disease, thromboembolism,* and *liver disease* are rare among users of the combination of esterified estrogens and methyltestosterone (Estratest®). The only adverse events exceeding 4% of total reports were *alopecia, acne, weight gain,* and *hirsutism* (2^C).

Compounds with tissue-selective estrogenic effects, known as SERMs (selective estrogen receptor modulators), are currently being evaluated. One of these is raloxifene, whose pharmacological profile appears favorable: the only adverse effect so far directly attributable to raloxifene is *hot flushes* (3^r).

Endocrine, metabolic Hyperlipidemic postmenopausal women taking combined sequential estrogen and progestogen replacement therapy have large *fluctuations in lipid and lipoprotein concentrations.* These fluctuations depend on the hormonal phase, i.e. estrogen alone or combined with progestogen. Progestogens blunt or even overwhelm the estrogenic effects on lipoproteins (4^{cr}).

The impact of a new formulation of low-dose micronized medroxyprogesterone plus 17-β-estradiol on lipid profiles in menopausal women has been studied for 12 months. Total cholesterol concentrations fell 8.4%, low density lipoprotein cholesterol fell 18%, and high density lipoprotein cholesterol increased 6.9%; total triglycerides increased 12%. The most frequently reported adverse events were *menorrhagia, breast tenderness, cervical polyps or cysts, bloating, fatigue or lethargy, influenza or a flu-like syndrome, back pain, headaches, irritability,* and *depression* (5^C).

Skin and appendages *Melasma* (the macular hyperpigmentation associated with increased estrogen states) occurred in a 54-year-old woman who developed it in atypical sites after starting to take HRT; on withdrawal it began to fade (6^c). This adverse effect has not been described before.

The reported incidence of adverse skin reactions to transdermal estradiol varies from 2% to over 25%, depending on the transdermal system, climatic conditions, and individual sensitivity. In a recent study of 78 women 29 repor-

Side Effects of Drugs, Annual 23
J.K. Aronson, ed.

ted one or more adverse events and eight discontinued prematurely (7[c]). The main reasons for premature withdrawal included *problems of adhesion, skin reactions, or undesirable systemic effects, such as headache, breast tenderness, weight gain, leg cramps,* and unacceptable *withdrawal bleeding.*

Genital system Continuous administration of an estrogen and a progestogen is effective in achieving amenorrhea with prolonged use (75% at 6 months). An adverse effect of such a regimen is a high incidence of unpredictable *break-through bleeding,* particularly during the initial months of treatment (8[cr]).

Of 206 postmenopausal women who took the oral combination of estradiol valerate plus norethisterone (9[C]) eight discontinued because of bleeding during year one; during years two and three there were no discontinuations because of bleeding. By the end of year three 133 patients had completed the study. There were serious adverse effects in 24, but there was no definite relation to therapy. The numbers of adverse events reported each year by the patients who completed the study are shown in Table 1. The authors concluded that this combination was effective in the majority of patients and was well tolerated.

Table 1. *The numbers of adverse events each year in patients taking estradiol valerate plus norethisterone*

	Year 1 $n = 164$	Year 2 $n = 144$	Year 3 $n = 133$
Bleeding/spotting	91	60	24
Breast tenderness	63	4	3
Weight gain	10	5	2
Fractures	7	1	1
Joint/bone pain	6	3	6
Palpitation	5	3	–
Hypertension	4	4	3
Menopausal symptoms	4	1	5
Phlebitis	3	–	–
Breathlessness	3	0	1
Abdominal pain	2	2	–
Breast lumps	2	4	2
Ovarian cysts	1	1	4
Abnormal smear	–	2	–
Other adverse affects	105	53	34
Total	306	143	85

Mammary tension and *mastodynia* are adverse effects related to the action of estrogens (10[cr]). In postmenopausal women estrogen plus progestogen replacement therapy may be associated with an increase in mammographic density and with the onset or worsening of mastodynia. Tibolone, a steroid with estrogenic, progestogenic, and some androgenic activity, does not seem to affect breasts of normal structure and may be considered a first-rate replacement therapy in women whose breasts are rather dense or who have benign mastopathy (10[cr]).

Tumor-inducing effects The most important and controversial potential adverse effect of hormone therapy is an *increased risk of breast cancer,* the most common cancer in women. Four meta-analyses showed no increased risk of breast cancer in women who had ever taken estrogen, compared with non-users. A majority of studies suggest an increased risk of breast cancer among women who take estrogen for 5–10 years or longer. The summary relative risk estimate based on the findings of these studies is 1.32 (95% C1 = 1.16–1.51) for women who reported long-term use compared to never users. An increased risk of breast cancer may not persist after estrogen therapy is discontinued, suggesting that estrogen acts as a promoter rather than a cause of breast cancer (11[R]). In one publication from the Nurse's Health Study (12[C]), the estimated risk of breast cancer associated with estrogen alone was 1.36 compared with 1.50 for estrogen plus progestogen therapy. A more recent analysis from the same cohort found that women who took unopposed estrogen had a 5% per year increased risk of breast cancer compared with 9% per year in women taking estrogen plus progestogen. The most promising marker is the increase in breast density that occurs in 15–50% of women who take replacement estrogen (11[R]).

Adverse effects in men Estrogen therapy in men with prostate cancer may be superior to castration in terms of efficacy, but orally administered estrogens are associated with adverse effects: *gynecomastia, loss of sexual function,* and unacceptable *cardio-vascular toxicity* (13[r]). Low-dose estrogens in combination with antiandrogens or antithrombotic agents may be better tolerated.

Progestogens *(SED-13, 1262; SEDA-21, 431; SEDA-22, 462)*

The effectiveness, adverse events, and acceptability of the FDA-approved variant of levonorgestrel capsule implants in the US over 5 years and the determinants of these outcomes have been studied (14[C]). There were three pregnancies, yielding a 5-year cumulative rate of 1.3 per 100 users, an average annual rate of three per 1000 women. *Ectopic pregnancy* occurred at a rate of 0.6 per 1000 woman-years. There were no pregnancies in women who weighed less than 79 kg. Medical conditions that most often led to removal of the implant were *prolonged or irregular menstrual bleeding,* followed by *headache, weight gain,* and *mood changes.* Weight gain averaged 1 kg/year.

In 140 women using the Norplant-2® contraceptive subdermal implant system there were no accidental pregnancies over 3 years (15[C]). Adverse effects that caused withdrawal from the study were *acne, headache, and pain at the implant site.* The termination rate for these medical reasons in year 3 of the study was 4.6%. The other main reason for termination was *prolonged menstrual flow*; the 3-year cumulative termination rate for menstrual irregularities was 3.8%.

Two regimens for emergency contraception started within 72 h of unprotected coitus have been studied: (a) the progestagen levonorgestrel in two separate doses each of 0.75 mg; (b) the Yuzpe regimen of combined oral contraceptives—ethinylestradiol 100 μg plus levonorgestrel 0.5 mg repeated 12 hours later (16[C]). The relative risk of pregnancy for levonorgestrel compared with the Yuzpe regimen was 0.36 (95% C1 = 0.18–0.70). Nausea and vomiting were significantly less frequent with the levonorgestrel regimen. Adverse effects of both regimens were *nausea, vomiting, dizziness, fatigue, headache, breast tenderness,* and *low abdominal pain.* However, all of these adverse effects were less frequent with levonorgestrel.

Cardiovascular The incidence of *hepatic veno-occlusive disease* in 249 consecutive women treated with norethisterone who underwent allogenic hemopoietic stem cell transplantation was 27% compared with 3% in women without this treatment (17[C]). One-year survival rates were 17% and 73% in patients with (n = 24) or without veno-occlusive disease (n = 225) respectively. Because of this adverse effect, norethisterone should not be used in patients undergoing bone-marrow transplantation. Heparin prophylaxis does not affect the risk of death from veno-occlusive disease.

Oral contraceptives *(SED-13, 1211; SEDA-21, 433; SEDA-22, 462)*

Venous thromboembolism and oral contraceptives: second-generation and third-generation formulations compared

It has been confirmed that the incidence and mortality rates of thrombotic diseases among young women are low (18[C]). In women aged 15–29 years who used oral contraceptives containing third-generation progestogens, venous thromboembolism was twice as common as arterial complications. In women aged 30–44 years of age the number of arterial complications exceeded the number of venous complications by about 50%. However, in women under 30 years, deaths from arterial complications were 3.5 times more common than deaths from venous complications and in women aged 30–44 years 8.5 times more common. Women over 30 years of age who take oral contraceptives containing third-generation progestogens may have a lower risk of thrombotic morbidity, disability, and mortality than users of second-generation progestogens. However, a weighted analysis such as this does not result in any consistent recommendation of a particular progestogen type.

In a recent study the incidence of venous thromboembolic disease in about 540 000 women born between 1941 and 1981 and taking oral contraceptives was 4.1–4.2 cases/10 000 woman-years (19[Cr]).

Users of oral contraceptives with second-generation progestogens have 30% greater increased risk of thrombotic diseases, a 260% greater increased risk of thrombotic deaths, and a 220% greater increased risk of post-thrombotic disability than users of oral contraceptives with third-generation progestogens (18[R]).

Hemostatic variables have been reviewed in women taking oral contraceptives containing desogestrel and gestodene in comparison with oral contraceptives containing levonorgestrel

(20[R]). The database of 17 comparative studies was homogeneous. There were no differential effects for coagulation and fibrinolysis parameters, except for factor VII, which was consistently increased by 20% among users of third-generation oral contraceptives than among users of second-generation oral contraceptives. Factor VII is not a risk marker for venous thrombotic disease.

We believe that women with risk factors for venous thromboembolism should not be treated with a third-generation progestogen but that a third-generation drug is the first choice for all other women. However, currently proof of this hypothesis is lacking.

The efficacy and adverse effects of oral cyproterone acetate 2 mg in combination with ethinylestradiol 35 μg in facial acne tarda have been studied in 890 women aged 15–50 years, of whom 96 withdrew prematurely from the study (21[C]). Of these 96 women only 30 withdrew because of adverse events: *menstrual problems* (11), *headache* (10), *increased body weight* (3), and *thrombophlebitis* (1). Five women withdrew because of poor efficacy. In all, 260 patients had adverse events during treatment. The incidence fell as the study progressed. Of those events that first occurred during treatment, the most frequently cited were *breast tension* (12%), *headache* (8.9%), *nausea* (5.8%), *nervousness* (4.0%), and *dizziness* (2.6%). There were no serious adverse events. There were no clinically significant changes in body weight or blood pressure.

Interactions The effect of the protease inhibitor *ritonavir* 600 mg every 12 hours (i.e. only slightly lower than the therapeutic dose intended for the treatment of AIDS/ARC) on the single-dose and steady-state pharmacokinetics of ethinylestradiol has been studied in 23 healthy women. Ritonavir reduced ethinylestradiol concentrations (C_{max} and AUC) by 30–40% (22[C]).

The effect of *fluconazole* 150 mg on circulating ethinylestradiol concentrations has been studied on day 6 of one of two cycles in women taking oral contraceptives (23[C]). The serum concentrations of ethinylestradiol (C_{max} and AUC) were significantly increased by fluconazole; the t_{max} was not affected. These findings suggest that there is a potential for a clinically significant interaction between fluconazole and ethinylestradiol in oral contraceptives, by inhibition of estrogen metabolism.

Post-coital contraceptives

The US FDA has approved a marketing application for the Preven® Emergency Contraceptive Kit (Gynetics) containing tablets for postcoital emergency contraception, packaged with a urinary pregnancy test. The application is based on a regimen that consists of two tablets containing ethinylestradiol and levonorgestrel to be taken within 72 hours of unprotected intercourse and two tablets to be taken 12 hours later. This regimen is about 75% effective in preventing pregnancy. The most common adverse effects are *nausea, vomiting, menstrual irregularities, breast tenderness, headache, abdominal pain and cramps,* and *dizziness* (24[r]). Although emergency contraception is not as effective as proper use of a regular contraceptive method, it substantially reduces the chances of pregnancy when used within 72 hours after unprotected sexual intercourse.

ANTIESTROGENS *(SED-13, 1260; SEDA-21, 426)*

Tamoxifen

The use of tamoxifen to prevent breast cancer has been reviewed (25[r]). For this indication the long-term toxicity of tamoxifen is very important. The available data after 5, 10, and 15 years of follow up have confirmed the increase in the incidence of *endometrial cancer* and of *thromboembolic complications* and provide some suggestion of *ocular toxicity,* but these effects are not common and should be more than balanced by the reduced risk of coronary heart disease and osteoporosis (25[r]).

Tamoxifen also has beneficial side effects: it protects the myocardium, reduces the incidence of ischemic heart disease, reduces the loss of bone mineral density, and has beneficial effects on lipids (26[r]).

Genital system A *leiomyoma of the breast* occurred in a 50-year-old woman taking tamoxifen. This leiomyoma appeared as a discrete mass and had a microscopic pattern akin to leiomyomas at other sites (27[c]). Tamoxifen has been shown to cause a sudden rapid increase in the growth rate of uterine leiomyomas (28[cr]).

Tumor-inducing effects The effects of norethisterone on endometrial abnormalities have been studied in 463 post-menopausal women taking tamoxifen or placebo (29[C]). As in other studies, the results showed that any increased risk of *endometrial cancer* caused by tamoxifen is low and that transvaginal ultrasound screening is probably not justified for asymptomatic women taking tamoxifen. The authors found that 26% of women taking tamoxifen have *endometrial thickening* of 8 mm or more. It is possible to identify cysts in 7% of these women, polyps in 3%, and both cysts and polyps in 8%. These changes are characteristic of tamoxifen and unlike those seen with estrogen replacement therapy.

GONADOTROPHINS AND OVULATION-INDUCING DRUGS

(SED-13, 1259; SEDA-20, 388; SEDA-22, 465)

The efficacy of recombinant human luteinizing hormone (rhLH) for supporting follicular development induced by recombinant human follicle-stimulating hormone (rhFSH) has been investigated in hypogonadotropic hypogonadal women (30[C]). A total of 42 adverse events were reported in 14 of the 53 cycles in this study. Of these, 32 adverse events occurred in 11 of the 42 cycles treated with rhLH, and ten occurred in three of the 11 cycles not treated with rhLH. The most frequent adverse events were *pelvic and abdominal pain, headache, breast pain, nausea, ovarian enlargement,* and *somnolence.* These adverse events are similar to those reported during therapy with FSH alone (30[C]).

The short- and long-term effects of ovulation induction have also been reported (31[R]). In the short term clomiphene and gonadotrophins cause *ovarian hyperstimulation syndrome* (ovarian enlargement, bloating, and nausea) and *multiple pregnancies;* gonadotrophins also cause *ectopic pregnancy.* In the long term clomiphene may cause an *increased risk of ovarian cancer.*

Clomiphene citrate

The antiestrogenic adverse effects of clomiphene citrate are *hot flushes* (10%), *mood swings, depression, headaches* (1%), *pelvic pain* (5.5%), *nausea* (2%), *breast tenderness* (2–5%), *dryness and loss of hair* (0.3%), *visual symptoms, halos and streaks around lights (particularly at night), blurring,* and *scotoma* (1.5%) (31[R]).

The European Metrodin HP Study Group has assessed the efficacy and safety of a highly purified urinary FSH in combination with human chorionic gonadotrophin (hCG) in inducing spermatogenesis in 28 men with primary complete isolated hypogonadotrophic hypogonadism, of whom 25 achieved spermatogenesis (33[c]). Mean testicular volume increased by about 7 ml during treatment. Adverse events considered to be related to hCG were acne (n = 3), weight gain (n = 2), and *gynecomastia* (n = 1). Acne can be attributed to increased testosterone. Gynecomastia is an adverse effect of hCG treatment (32[C]) and may be caused by raised serum estradiol concentrations.

MALE SEX HORMONES

Androgenic and anabolic steroids and related compounds

(SED-13, 1265; SEDA-21, 434; SEDA-22, 463)

Androgen therapy should be considered for postmenopausal women who complain of poor libido, poor energy, or a feeling of malaise (34[R]). Because of its *adverse effects on serum lipids* (see below), it should be given in association with estrogens.

Male hormone replacement therapy, a topic of growing interest, has been reviewed (35[R]). Hypogonadism can be accompanied by hot flushes, similar to those seen in postmenopausal women, and gynecomastia. The potential risks of testosterone replacement in adult men are *precipitation or worsening of sleep apnea, hastened onset of clinical significant prostate disease, benign prostatic hyperplasia, prostatic carcinoma, gynecomastia, fluid retention, polycythemia, exacerbation of hypertension, edema,* and *increased risk of cardio-vascular disease.*

The adverse effects of long-term testosterone therapy in HIV-positive men are *irritability, weight gain, fatigue, hair loss, reduced volume of ejaculate, testicular atrophy, truncal acne, breast tenderness,* and *increased aggression* (36[c]).

The effects and adverse effects of testosterone replacement with a non-genital transdermal system, Androderm, have been studied in 41 HIV-positive men with low testosterone concentrations (37[C]). Nine men taking placebo and 11 taking testosterone reported adverse events. Five men taking testosterone had *reactions at the site of administration;* other adverse events in this group included problems related to resistance mechanisms (2), gastrointestinal system (2), and skin and appendages (1); there was one severe adverse event (a suicidal amitriptyline overdose). There were skin reactions at the site of application of the placebo or testosterone patch in 19% of participants. One man had *blisters* on one occasion, related to rupture of the patch. The mean red cell counts increased with testosterone and fell with placebo. Hemoglobin concentrations increased with testosterone, but fell with placebo.

Supraphysiological androgen hormone concentrations may cause *acne, hirsutism,* and *deepening of the voice.*

Endocrine, metabolic Androgens alone have *unfavorable effects on lipids* and are *atherogenic* (34[R]). However, the simultaneous administration of estrogens appears to have a protective effect on the lipid profile. Androgen implants combined with estrogens cause a fall in total cholesterol and of LDL cholesterol, without significant effects on HDL cholesterol or triglycerides. There is a similar reduction in total cholesterol in postmenopausal women treated with estrogen plus methyltestosterone, with a reduction in HDL_2 cholesterol and triglycerides but no change in LDL cholesterol. Testosterone replacement therapy should therefore be given to women only if they are concurrently using estrogen replacement therapy.

Potential adverse effects of oxandrolone are *acceleration of puberty and skeletal maturation* (38[c]).

A 9 year-old boy with early puberty took oxandrolone for 22 months because of constitutional delay of growth. His height velocity increased above the 97th percentile and his bone age developed twice as fast as his chronological age. The oxandrolone was withdrawn, but his growth velocity did not decrease and his bone age continued to accelerate.

The authors hypothesized that oxandrolone could have induced early puberty. They concluded that in young children oxandrolone should be used with caution for short periods only.

Hematological A 26-year-old woman developed severe *aplastic anemia,* complicated by superior sagittal sinus thrombosis, while taking fluoxymesterone 30 mg/day (39[c]). Anabolic steroids have been reported to be thrombogenic (40[r], 41[C], 42[c]).

Tumor-inducing effects Danazol inhibits pituitary gonadotropin with weak androgenic effects, and is currently used in the treatment of endometriosis, fibrocystic disease of the breast, idiopathic thrombocytopenic purpura, and hereditary angioedema. Its hepatotoxic effects include reversible rises in serum aminotransferases and cholestasis hepatitis; a few cases of *hepatocellular tumors* have been reported.

A 34-year-old woman who had taken danazol 400 mg/day for 13 years for hereditary angio-edema developed a mass in the right hypochondrium. Her alcohol intake was under 20 g/day. She had a large heterogeneous hepatic tumor, a well-differentiated hepatocellullar carcinoma in a non-cirrhotic liver.

The hypothesis that hepatocellular carcinoma had been caused by danazol was accepted in the absence of other causes (43[c]). This is the third report of hepatocellular carcinoma associated with long-term danazol.

ANTIANDROGENS *(SED-13, 1267; SEDA-20, 387; SEDA-22, 464)*

The effects of antiandrogens in 34 patients with benign prostatic hypertrophy have been studied (44[C]). The adverse effects of allylestrenol (50 mg/day for 16 weeks) were *reduced libido* (8.1%), *rash* (2.7%), *a rise in lactate dehydrogenase* (8.1%) and a *rise in triglycerides* (2.9%). After 16 weeks the medication was withheld and the patients were monitored for a further 16 weeks.

The efficacy of non-steroidal anti-androgen monotherapy (bicalutamide, flutamide, or nilutamide) has been evaluated in the treatment of advanced prostate cancer (45[R]). Because of a high incidence of drug-related adverse effects, nilutamide monotherapy is limited and it is not recommended by the manufacturer. Adverse effects of these anti-androgens are listed in Table 2.

The efficacy and tolerability of two antiandrogens, bicalutamide and flutamide, each combined with monthly depot injections of leuprolide or goserelin have been assessed in 813 patients with stage D2 prostatic cancer

Table 2. *Adverse effects of bicalutamide, flutamide, and nilutamide in patients with prostatic cancer (56[R])*

Adverse effect	Bicalutamide	Flutamide	Nilutamide
Hot flushes	15%	15%	30–50%
Breast tenderness, gynaecomastia	70%	40–50%	50%
Nausea	3%	3%	3%
Diarrhea	<5%	5–30%	6%
Hepatotoxicity	0.5%	4–6%	8%
	one case nearly fatal	3/10 000 fatal or serious	1 case fatal
Dyspnea	NR	NR	2–4%
Visual problems	NR	NR	20–65%
Alcohol intolerance	NR	Anecdotal	20%
Impotence	20%	20%	50%
Treatment withdrawal	<5%	10–20%	NR

NR, not reported.

Table 3. *Adverse effects of bicalutamide and flutamide, each combined with leuprorelide or goserelin in patients with prostatic cancer (57[C])*

Adverse event	I	II	III	IV
Hot flashes	55	55	52	52
Pain	35	30	36	32
back pain	30	25	23	26
pelvic pain	24	17	20	17
abdominal pain	9	10	13	12
bone pain	9	9	10	12
Constipation	22	19	21	16
Weakness	14	25	26	20
Dyspnea	14	5	12	9
Nausea	13	12	15	14
Peripheral edema	13	11	14	11
Nocturia	12	14	12	13
Hematuria	11	7	12	6
Diarrhea	10	30	13	24
Dizziness	9	14	11	6
Anemia	8	12	10	10
Abnormal liver function tests	8	9	7	12
Flu-like illness	7	11	7	6

I, Bicalutamide + leuprolide (n = 135).
II, Flutamide + leuprolide (n = 138).
III, Bicalutamide + goserelin (n = 266).
IV, Flutamide + goserelin (n = 269).

(46[C]). Flutamide plus leuprolide had a significantly poorer outcome than the other three therapies. *Diarrhea* was more common among patients treated with flutamide, and *hematuria* was more common among patients treated with bicalutamide. The adverse events recorded in this study are listed in Table 3.

Bicalutamide

Bicalutamide appears to be a logical first-choice antiandrogen (47[R]). It has demonstrated efficacy and a favorable adverse effect profile compared with the known safety profiles of other antiandrogens (48[C]).

The effects and adverse effects of a high dose of bicalutamide 150 mg/day have been studied in 31 patients with progressive androgen-independent prostate cancer (49[R]). Bicalutamide was modestly effective, particularly in patients previously treated with long-term flutamide. The most frequent adverse effect was mild *exacerbation of hot flushes* (40%), *gynecomastia* (5%), *breast tenderness* (5%), *nausea* (10%), *fatigue* (10%), and *pruritus* (5%). One patient had fever, chills, and rigors during the first month of therapy and another with a history of severe chronic obstructive pulmonary disease had respiratory compromise within 30 days of stopping the drug. In neither case was a clear cause of these symptoms detected.

Other adverse effects mentioned in another review (50[R]) were *breast pain, diarrhea, vomiting, hematuria, weakness, skin rash, and transient rises in liver enzyme activities.*

Bicalutamide has statistically significant benefits over castration with respect to sexual interest and physical capacity (51[C]).

Interactions Bicalutamide is highly bound to plasma proteins and can displace *warfarin and other coumarin anticoagulants* from binding sites in vitro (50).

Table 4. *Adverse effects of flutamide in 1387 patients with prostatic cancer (47[C]); number of patients (%)*

	Flutamide	Placebo
Hot flushes	69 (10.3)	65 (9.7)
Anemia	57 (8.5)	36 (5.4)
Diarrhea	42 (6.3)	18 (2.7)
Hepatic dysfunction	16 (2.4)	13 (1.9)
Nausea	15 (2.2)	17 (2.5)
Vomiting	12 (1.8)	13 (1.9)

Flutamide

The effects of flutamide have been studied in 1387 patients with metastatic prostate cancer after bilateral orchidectomy (52[C]). The incidence of toxic effects was minimal. The only notable differences in adverse effects between flutamide and placebo were the greater rates of *diarrhea* and *anemia* with flutamide. A total of 43 patients (33 taking flutamide and ten taking placebo) were withdrawn from the study because of drug toxicity. The numbers of patients with adverse effects are shown in Table 4.

Skin and appendages *Pseudoporphyria* has been attributed to flutamide (53[c]).

A 68-year-old man presented with a 9-week history of skin fragility and blisters on the back of the hands. He had prostatic carcinoma treated with flutamide. A diagnosis of pseudoporphyria associated with androgen therapy was considered. Flutamide was replaced by bicalutamide, resulting in a permanent healing of the lesions.

Pseudoporphyria is characterized by blisters, increased skin fragility, and erosions in sun-exposed areas. It has been associated with some drugs, particularly amiodarone, dapsone, diflunisal, furosemide, ketoprofen, nalidixic acid, naproxen, pyridoxine, and tetracycline hydrochloride.

DRUGS USED IN BENIGN PROSTATIC HYPERPLASIA

The long-term implications of medical therapy on benign prostatic hyperplasia have been reviewed (54[R]). Efficacy over placebo in 1-year studies can be achieved by the α-blockers and 5-α-reductase inhibitors. Both groups of drugs have demonstrated long-term safety. The duration of therapy for benign prostatic hyperplasia should be considered life-long. Therefore safety must be a primary concern. The results of three recent long-term, randomized, placebo-controlled studies are available and suggest that finasteride may prevent further progression of benign prostatic hyperplasia (55[C]–57[C]). Prostate volume fell by 20% with finasteride, compared with an increase of 8–11% with placebo (54[R]).

Table 5. *Adverse effects of finasteride with or without dibenyline in benign prostatic hyperplasia (60[C])*

Adverse effect	Finasteride	Dibenyline	Combination
Light-headedness	1.9%	25%	19%
Nasal stuffiness	–	9.9%	11%
Impotence	9.3%	17%	17%

Finasteride

The long-term efficacy and safety of finasteride (58[C]) have been studied in 102 patients with benign prostatic hyperplasia. Overall finasteride has a good safety profile with few adverse effects. However, adverse experiences due to sexual dysfunction continued throughout the study. The low continuous dropout rate due to sexual disturbances (erectile dysfunction) might have reflected a natural process in this aged population and was not necessarily drug related.

Finasteride is poorly effective in patients with small prostate glands (59[R]). In patients with glands larger than 40 ml it produces significant improvement. Early intervention with finasteride can reduce the number of surgical procedures. 5-α-dihydrotestosterone potentiates erectile capacity. Because finasteride inhibits the production of 5-α-dihydrotestosterone, adverse effects, such as *impotence* (3–4%), *gynecomastia* (0.4%), and *decreased ejaculatory volume,* can occur.

The therapeutic and adverse effects of dibenyline, finasteride, and a combination of the two in 190 patients with symptomatic benign prostatic hyperplasia have been evaluated (60[C]). Adverse effects were more common with dibenyline than with finasteride alone or in combination with dibenyline. The dropout rate was higher with dibenyline (16%) than finasteride alone (7.5%) or in combination (4.6%). The reported adverse effects are listed in Table 5.

cardio-vascular The long-term effects and adverse effects of finasteride have been studied in a multicenter study of 3270 men (61^{C}). There was a background history of cardio-vascular disease in 40% of the patients at baseline, and *myocardial infarction* was reported in 1.5% of those taking finasteride and 0.5% of those taking placebo.

Sexual function In the long-term study of finasteride cited above (61^{C}) the numbers of serious adverse events and withdrawals because of adverse events were significantly higher with placebo. Drug-related adverse effects in 1% or more of patients were *reduced libido, ejaculation disorders,* and *impotence.* A total of 273 patients, 165 (10%) taking finasteride and 108 (7%) taking placebo, reported a sexual adverse event, including *change in libido, ejaculation disorders, impotence,* or *orgasmic dysfunction* during the treatment period.

The benefit of combining an α-blocker with a 5-α-reductase inhibitor has been assessed (62^{C}). Modified-release alfuzosin was more effective than finasteride with no additional benefit in combining both drugs. The adverse effects of α-blockade were *postural hypotension, hypotension, headache, dizziness,* and *malaise;* the adverse effects of finasteride were *ejaculatory disorders* and *impotence.*

REFERENCES

1. Bachman G. Estradiol-releasing vaginal ring delivery system for urogenital atrophy. J Reprod Med Obstet Gynecol 1998;43:991–8.
2. Barrett-Connor E. Efficacy and safety on estrogen/androgen therapy: menopausal symptoms, bone and cardio-vascular parameters. J Reprod Med Obstet Gynecol 1998;43;746–52.
3. Compston JE. Selective oestrogen receptor modulators: potential therapeutic applications. Clin Endocrinol 1998;48;389–91.
4. Weintraub MS, Grosskopf I, Charach G, Eckstein N, Ringel Y, Maharshak N, Rotmensch HH, Rubinstein A. Fluctuations of lipid and lipoprotein levels in hyperlipidemic post menopausal women receiving hormone replacement therapy. Arch Intern Med 1998;158:1803–6.
5. Harrison RF, Magill P, Kilminster SG. Impact of a new formulation of low-dose micronised medroxyprogesterone and 17-beta estradiol, on lipid profiles in menopausal women. Clin Drug Invest 1998;16:93–9.
6. Johnston GA, Sviland L, Mc Lellan DJ. Melasma of the arms associated with hormone replacement therapy. Br J Dermatol 1998;139:932.
7. Bhathena RK, Anklesaria BS, Ganatra AM. Skin reactions with transdermal estradiol therapy in a tropical environment. Int J Gynecol Obstet 1998;60:177–9.
8. Cameron ST, Critchley HOD. Continuous oestrogen and interrupted progestogen in HRT bleed-free regimens. Contemp Rev Obstet Gynecol 1998; 10:151–5.
9. Perry W, Wiseman RA, Cullen NM. Combined oral estradiol valerate-norethisterone treatment over three years in postmenopausal women. Gynecol Endocrinol 1998;12:109–22.
10. Colacurci N, Mele D, De Franciscus P, Costa V, Fortunato N, De Seta L. Effects of tibolone on the breast. Eur J Obstet Gynecol Reprod Biol 1998;80:235–8.
11. Barrett-Connor E, Grady D. Hormone replacement therapy, heart disease and other considerations. Ann Rev Public Health 1998;19:55–72.
12. Colditz GA, Hankinson SE, Hunter DJ, Willet WC, Manson JE, Stampfer MJ, Hennekens C. The use of estrogens and progestins and the risk of breast cancer in postmenopausal women. New Engl J Med 1995;332:1589–93.
13. Iversen P. Orchidectomy and estrogen therapy revisited. Eur Urol 1998;34(Suppl 3):7–11.
14. Sivin I, Mishell DR, Darney P. Levenorgestrel capsule implants in the United States: a 5-year study. Obstet Gynecol 1998;92:337–44.
15. Chompootaweep S, Kochagarn E, Tang-Usana J, Theppitaksak B. Experience of Thai women in Bangkok with Norplant-2-implants. Contraception 1998;58:221–5.
16. Grimes D, Von Hertzen H, Piaggio G, Van Look PFA. Randomised controlled trial of levonorgestrel versus the Yuzpe regimen of combined oral contraceptives for emergency contraception Lancet 1998;352:428–33.
17. Hägglund H, Remberger M, Klaesson S, Lonnqvist B, Lungman P, Ringden O. Norethisterone treatment, a major risk-factor for veno-occlusive disease in the liver after allogenic bone marrow transplantation. Blood 1998;92:4568–72.
18. Lidegaard O. Thrombotic diseases in young women and the influence of oral contraceptives. Am J Obstet Gynecol 1998;179;S62–7.
19. Farmer RDT, Lawrenson RA. Oral contraceptives and venous thromboembolic disease: the findings from database studies in the United Kingdom and Germany. Am J Obstet Gynecol 1998;179:S78–86.
20. Winkler UH. Effects on hemostatic variables of desogestrel- and gestodene-containing oral contraceptives in comparison with levonorgestrel containing oral contraceptives: a review. Am J Obstet Gynecol 1998;179:S51–61.
21. Gollnick H, Albring M, Brill K. The efficacy of oral cyproterone acetate in combination with ethinylestradiol in acne tarda of the facial type. J Dermatol Treat 1998;9:71–9.
22. Ouellet D, Hsu A, Qian J, Locke CS, Eason CJ, Cavanaugh JH, Leonard JM, Granneman GR. Ef-

fect of ritonavir on the pharmacokinetics of ethinyl estradiol in healthy female volunteers. Br J Clin Pharmacol 1998;46:111–16.
23. Sinofsky FE, Pasquale SA. The effect of fluconazole on circulating ethinyl estradiol levels in women taking oral contraceptives Am J Obstet Gynecol 1998;178:300–4.
24. Anonymous. Oral contraceptives—approved for emergency use. WHO Newslett 1998;9/10:12.
25. Bruzzi P. Tamoxifen for the prevention of breast cancer. Important questions remain unanswered and existing trials should continue. Br Med J 1998;316:1181–2.
26. Baum M. Tamoxifen—the treatment of choice. Why look for alternatives? Br J Cancer 1998;78 Suppl 4:1–4.
27. Son EJ, Oh KK, Kim EK, Son HJ, Jung WH, Lee HD. Leiomyoma of the breast in a 50-year old woman. Am J Roentgenol 1998;171:1684–6.
28. Leo L, Lanza A, Re A, Tessarolo M, Bellino R, Lauricella A, Wierdis T. Leiomyoma in patients receiving tamoxifen. Clin Exp Obstet Gynecol 1994;21:94–8.
29. Powles TJ, Bourne T, Athanasiou S, Chang J, Grubock K, Ashley S, Oakes L, Tidy A, Davey J, Viggers J, Humphries S, Collins W. The effects of norethisterone on endometrial abnormalities identified by transvaginal ultrasound screening of healthy post-menopausal women on tamoxifen or placebo. Br J Cancer 1998;78:272–5.
30. Loumaye E, Piazzi A, Warne D, Kalubi M, Cox P, Lancaster S, Rotere S, Sauvage M, Ursicino G, Baird D, et al. Recombinant human luteinizing hormone (LH) to support recombinant follicle-stimulating hormone (FSH)-induced follicular development and FSH-deficient anovulatory women: a dose finding study. J Clin Endocrinol Metab 1998;83:1507–14.
31. Vollenhoven BJ, Healy DL. Short and long-term effects of ovulation induction. Endocrinol Metab Clin North Am 1998;27:903–14.
32. European Metrodin HP Study Group, Geneva Switzerland. Efficacy and safety of highly purified urinary follicle-stimulating hormone with human chorionic gonadotropin for treating men with isolated hypogonadotropic hypogonadism. Fertil Steril 1998;70:256–62.
33. Kirk JMW, Savage MO, Grant DB, Bouloux P-MG, Besser GM. Gonadal function and response to human chorionic and menopausal gonadotrophic therapy in male patients with idiopathic hypogonadotrophic hypogonadism. Clin Endocrinol 1994;41:57–63.
34. Vermeulen A. Plasma androgens in women. J Reprod Med Obstet Gynecol 1998;43:725–33.
35. Tenover JL. Male hormone replacement therapy including ‘Andropause’. Endocrinol Metab Clin North Am 1998;27:969–87.
36. Maguen S, Wagner GJ, Rabkin JG. Long-term testosterone therapy in HIV-positive men: side effects and maintenance of clinical benefit. AIDS 1998;12:327–8.
37. Bhasin S, Storer TW, Asbel-Sethin N, Kilbourne A, Hays R, Sinha-Hikim I, Shen R, Arver S, Beall G. Effects of testosterone replacement with a nongenital transdermal system, Androderm, in human immunodeficiency virus-infected men with low testosterone levels. J Clin Endocrinol Metab 1998;83:3155–62.
38. Doeker B, Muller-Michaels J, Andler W. Induction of early puberty in a boy after treatment with oxandrolone? Horm Res 1998;50:46–8.
39. Kaito K, Kobayashi M, Otsubo H, Ogasawara Y, Sekita T, Shimada T, Hosoya T. Superior sagittal sinus thrombosis in a patient with aplastic anemia treated with anabolic steroids. Int J Hematol 1998;68:227–9.
40. Ferenchick GS. Are androgenic steroids thrombogenic? New Engl J Med 1990;322:476.
41. Lowe GDO, Thomson JE. Mesterolone: thrombosis during treatment, and a study of its prothrombotic effects. Br J Clin Pharmacol 1979;7:107.
42. Toyama M, Watanabe S, Kobayashi T, Iida K, Koseki S, Yamaguchi I, Sugishita T. Two cases of acute myocardial infarction associated with aplastic anemia during treatment with anabolic steroids. Jpn Heart J 1994;35:369–73.
43. Crampon D, Barnoud R, Durand M, et al. Danazol therapy: an unusual aetiology of hepatocellular carcinoma. J Hepatol 1998;29:1035–6.
44. Noguchi K, Harada M, Masuda M, Takeda M, Kinoshita Y, Fukushima S, Miyai K, Fukuoka H, Hosaka M. Clinical significance of interruption of therapy with allylestrenol in patients with benign prostatic hypertrophy. Int J Urol 1998;5:466–70.
45. Boccon-Gibod L. Are non-steroidal anti-androgens appropriate as monotherapy in advanced prostate cancer? Eur Urol 1998;33:159–64.
46. Sarosdy MF, Schellhammer PF, Sharifi R, Block NL, Soloway MS, Venner PM, Patterson AL, Vogelzang NJ, Chodak GW, Klein EA, Schellenger JJ, Kovenbag GJCM. Comparison of goserelin and leuprolide in combined androgen blockade therapy. Urology 1998;52:82–8.
47. Kolvenbag GJCM, Blackledge GRP, Gotting-Smith K. Bicalutamide (Casodex) in the treatment of prostate cancer: history of clinical development. Prostate 1998;34:61–72.
48. Tyrrel CJ, Denis L, Newling D. Casodex™ 10-200 mg daily used as monotherapy for the treatment of patients with advanced prostate cancer. Eur Urol 1998;33:39–53.
49. Joyce R, Fenton MA, Rode P, Constantine M, Gaynes L, Kolvenbag G, DeWolf W, Balk S, Taplin ME, Bubley GJ. High dose bicalutamide for androgen independent prostate cancer: effect of prior hormonal therapy. J Urol 1998;159:149–53.
50. Goa KL, Spencer CM. Bicalutamide in advanced prostate cancer: a review. Drugs Aging 1998;12;401–22.
51. Iversen P, Tyrrell CJ, Kaisary AV, Anderson JB, Baert L, Tammela T, Chamberlain M, Carroll K, Gotting-Smith K, Blackledge GRP. Casodex (bicalutamide) 150 mg monotherapy compared with castration in patients with previously untreated nonmetastatic prostate cancer: results from two multicenter randomized trials at a median follow-up of 4 years. Urology 1998;51:389–96.

52. Eisenberger MA, Blumenstein BA, Crawford D, Miller G, McLeod DG, Loehrer PJ, Wilding G, Sears K, Culkin DJ, Thompson IM, Bueschen AJ, Lowe BA. Bilateral orchiectomy with or without flutamide for metastatic prostate cancer. New Engl J Med 1998;339;1036–42.
53. Borroni G, Brazelli V, Baldini F. Flutamide-induced pseudoporphyria. Br J Dermatol 1998;138: 711–12.
54. Nickel JC. Long-term implications of medical therapy on benign prostatic hyperplasia end points. Urology 1998;51 Suppl A: 50–7.
55. Nickel JC, Fradet Y, Boake C, Pommerville PJ, Perreault J-P, Afridi SK, Elhilali MM, Barr RE, Beland GA, Bertrand PE, et al. Efficacy and safety of finasteride therapy for benign prostatic hyperplasia; results of a 2-year randomized controlled trial (the PROSPECT study). Can Med Assoc J 1996;155:1251–9.
56. Andersen JT, Ekman P, Wolf H, Beisland HO, Johansson JE, Kontturi M, Lehtonen T, Tveter K, Bodker A, Vedel O, et al. Can finasteride reverse the progress of benign prostatic hyperplasia? A two year placebo-controlled study. Urology 1995;46:631–7.
57. Marberger JM, Marshall VR, Navarrete RV, et al. Continuous improvement with finasteride in symptomatic benign prostatic hyperplasia. J Urol 1997;157(Suppl 4):133A.
58. Ekman P. Maximum efficacy of finasteride is obtained within 6 months and maintained over 6 years. Eur Urol 1998;33:312–17.
59. Ekman P. A risk-benefit assessment of treatment with finasteride in benign prostatic hyperplasia. Drug Saf 1998;18:161–70.
60. Kuo HC. Comparative study for therapeutic effect of dibenyline, finasteride and combination drugs for symptomatic benign prostatic hyperplasia. Urol Int 1998;60:85–91.
61. Margerger MJ. Long-term effects of finasteride in patients with benign prostatic hyperplasia;a double-blind, placebo-controlled multicenter study. Urology 1998;51:677–86.
62. De Bruyne FMJ, Jardin A, Colloi D, Resel L, Witjes WPJ, Delauche-Cavallier MC, McCarthy C, Geffriaud-Ricouard C. Sustained release alfuzosin, finasteride and the combination of both in the treatment of benign prostatic hyperplasia. Eur Urol 1998;34:169–75.

J.A. Franklyn

41 Thyroid hormones and antithyroid drugs

THYROID HORMONES

(SED-13, 1275; SEDA-20, 393; SEDA-21, 437; SEDA-22, 469)

The routine use of sensitive assays for serum thyrotrophin (TSH) has led to the recognition that many patients taking standard doses of thyroxine (T_4) are biochemically 'overtreated'. Most attention continues to be focused on the potential detrimental effect of such mild thyroid hormone excess on the bones and heart. There have been further cross-sectional studies examining the effect of thyroxine on bone mineral density. In one study bone mineral density was compared in 50 women taking T_4 either for primary thyroid failure or for hypothyroidism secondary to radioiodine treatment for hyperthyroidism. These two groups did not differ in terms of bone density at the hip or spine and did not differ from the reference population. In addition, there was no correlation between bone density and circulating thyroid hormone concentrations or duration of T_4 replacement (1[C]). These findings are reassuring for those taking and prescribing T_4, although large studies of fracture risk in such patients are required, in view of previous evidence of an adverse effect of T_4 on bone mineral density, especially in post-menopausal women (2[C]).

Whether T_4 therapy has an adverse effect on the cardiovascular system, and in particular on the risk of dysrhythmias, continues to be debated. Evidence from the Framingham population that suppression of serum TSH is a risk factor for *atrial fibrillation* has heightened concern that subclinical hyperthyroidism secondary to T_4 therapy has a similar adverse effect (3[C]). Five women taking T_4 who reported frequent bouts of *palpitation* were investigated while taking T_4 and again after T_4 withdrawal (4[C]). There was a clear *increase in mean 24-h heart rate* during T_4 treatment, as well as an *increase in atrial extra beats and the number of episodes of re-entrant AV nodal tachycardia.* Four of these patients had evidence of abnormal conduction pathways even when they were not taking T_4 therapy, as evidenced by a short PR interval, but exacerbation of atrial dysrhythmias in these predisposed subjects is consistent with the view that thyroid hormones increase atrial excitability and may increase the risk of cardiac morbidity, especially if given in doses sufficient to suppress serum TSH.

While biochemical evidence of mild thyroid hormone excess is common in subjects taking T_4, it is uncommon to induce symptoms, signs, or biochemical changes of overt thyroid hormone excess by taking thyroid hormones. A report has described self-induced thyrotoxicosis associated with a marked rise in circulating free T_4 and free tri-iodothyronine concentrations in a pregnant woman with an eating disorder who was abusing both T_4 treatment and furosemide (5[c]). This case reminds us that if the cause for thyrotoxicosis remains obscure, T_4 abuse should be explored and considered.

ANTITHYROID DRUGS

(SED-13, 1279; SEDA-20, 394; SEDA-21, 437; SEDA-22, 469)

Hematological The most feared complication of thionamide drugs is *bone-marrow suppression.* Agranulocytosis is the most common presentation of this idiosyncratic complication. Two further reports of agranulocytosis have appeared (6[c]). One unusually occurred after a second exposure to the drug, in this case propylthiouracil. Aplastic anemia is very rare and has been said to occur as an adverse effect of thionamide therapy with about one-tenth of the

Side Effects of Drugs, Annual 23
J.K. Aronson, ed.

frequency of agranulocytosis. A report has described the development of aplastic anemia in a 58-year-old woman taking methimazole for the third time; she responded well to drug withdrawal and treatment with human granulocyte colony stimulating factor (7[c]).

Immunological and hypersensitivity reactions *Vasculitis* is another important adverse effect that is often poorly recognized as being drug related, leading to a delay in diagnosis. Several recent reports have described propylthiouracil-induced ANCA-associated small vessel vasculitis (8[c], 9[c]), crescentic glomerulonephritis (10[c]), and Wegener's granulomatosis (11[c]). More common, however, may be a condition termed 'antithyroid arthritis syndrome', which is a transient migratory polyarthritis occurring within 2 months of starting thionamides and resolving within 4 weeks of stopping therapy (12[cR]).

Interactions Since thionamides block the organification of iodine and incorporation of iodine into iodotyrosines, administration of thionamides inhibits the uptake of iodine-131 used therapeutically in hyperthyroidism. For this reason, thionamides are generally withdrawn for a period of up to a week before radioiodine therapy is planned and re-introduction is similarly delayed until several days after radioiodine therapy. A recent retrospective study (13[C]) has compared the effect of treatment with either methimazole or propylthiouracil before radioiodine, the thionamide being withdrawn 5–55 days before radioiodine administration. The findings confirmed the view that propylthiouracil, although not methimazole, significantly reduced the cure rate after radioiodine compared with that found in subjects not pretreated with propylthiouracil, and that discontinuation for 4 months was required for the cure rates to be similar. These findings highlight the relative *'radio-resistance'* induced by thionamide therapy, determining that prolonged drug withdrawal or an increased dose of radioiodine may be required to produce an acceptable cure rate.

IODINE AND THE IODIDES

(SED-13, 1281; SEDA-21, 438; SEDA-22, 470)

It has been estimated that in 1994 some 1.5 billion people in 118 countries were at risk of iodine deficiency, this being regarded as the world's most significant cause of preventable brain damage and mental retardation. Fortification of all salt for animal and human consumption has been chosen as the preferred method for the prevention of iodine deficiency disorders, and this approach is proving effective in reducing the incidence of such disorders. However, iodine supplementation is not without risks, which have been discussed (14[R]) and which include *allergic reactions* and iodine-induced *hyperthyroidism.* It has been clearly shown that the benefits of iodine deficiency outweigh the risks on a population basis, but it is nevertheless evident that introduction of iodine supplementation is associated with clinical problems in individual subjects.

A summary of the occurrence and epidemiology of iodine-induced hyperthyroidism has been published (15[R]), based on the authors' experience in Tasmania, Zaire, Zimbabwe, and Brazil. Another review has more specifically examined the cardiac features of iodine-induced hyperthyroidism and has emphasized the importance of awareness, monitoring, and treatment of such hyperthyroidism in areas in which iodine supplementation has been recently introduced (16[R]).

The complexity of the interaction between iodine intake and *autoimmune thyroid disease* has been highlighted by reports of evidence that iodide (compared with thyroxine) induces thyroid autoimmunity in patients with endemic (iodine deficient) goiter (17[R]), while in those with pre-existing thyroid autoimmunity, evidenced by the presence of antithyroid (thyroid peroxidase) antibodies, administration of iodine in an area of mild iodine deficiency led to subclinical or overt hypothyroidism (18[R]).

More importantly, in a study from Italy the use of iodine-containing disinfectants was responsible for transient neonatal hypothyroidism in more than 50% of cases identified (another common cause being transfer of maternal antibodies) (19[C]). These findings led the authors to conclude that pregnant women should be advised of the adverse effects of using iodine-containing products and that their use should be generally discouraged.

REFERENCES

1. Hanna FWF, Pettit RJ, Ammari F, Evans WD, Sandeman D, Lazarus JH. Effect of replacement doses of thyroxine on bone mineral density. Clin Endocrinol 1998;48:229–34.
2. Uzzan B, Campos J, Cucherat M, Nony P, Boissel JP, Perret GY. Effects on bone mass of long-term treatment with thyroid hormones:a meta-analysis. J Clin Endocrinol Metab 1996;81:4278–89.
3. Sawin CT, Geller A, Wolf PA, Belanger AJ, Baker E, Bacharach P, Wilson PWF, Benjamin EJ, A'Agostino RB. Low serum thyrotropin concentration as a risk factor for atrial fibrillation in older persons. New Engl J Med 1994;331:1249–52.
4. Biondi B, Fazio S, Coltorti F, Palmieri EA, Carella C, Lombardi G, Sacca L. Clinical case seminar. Reentrant atrioventricular nodal tachycardia induced by levothyroxine. J Clin Endocrinol Metab 1998;83:2643–5.
5. Wark H, Wallace EM, Wigg S, Tippett C. Thyroxine abuse: an unusual case of thyrotoxicosis in pregnancy. Aust NZ J Obstet Gynaecol 1998;38:221–3.
6. Roeloffzen WWH, Verhaegh JJ, Van Poelgeest AE, Gansevoort RT. Fever or a sore throat after start of antithyroidal drugs? A medical emergency. Neth J Med 1998;53:113–17.
7. Mezquita P, Luna V, Muñoz-Torres M, Torres-Vela E, Lopez-Rodriguez F, Callejas JL, Escobar-Jimenez F. Methimazole-induced aplastic anaemia in third exposure: successful treatment with recombinant human granulocyte colony-stimulating factor. Thyroid 1998;8/9:791–4.
8. Harper L, Cockwell P, Savage COS. Case of propylthiouracil-induced ANCA associated small vessel vasculitis. Nephrol Dial Transplant 1998;13:455–8.
9. Miller RM, Savige J, Nassis L, Cominos BI. Antineutrophil cytoplasmic antibody (ANCA)-positive cutaneous leucocytoclastic vasculitis associated with antithyroid therapy in Graves' disease. Australas J Dermatol 1998;39:96–9.
10. Fujieda M, Nagata M, Akioka Y, Hattori M, Kawaguchi H, Ito K. Antineutrophil cytoplasmic antibody-positive crescentic glomerulonephritis associated with propylthiouracil therapy. Acta Paediatr Jap Overs Ed 1998;40:286–9.
11. Pillinger M, Staud R. Wegener's granulomatosis in a patient receiving propylthiouracil for Graves' disease. Sem Arthritis Rheum 1998; 28:124–9.
12. Bajaj S, Bell MJ, Shumak S, Briones-Urbina R. Antithyroid arthritis syndrome. J Rheumatol 1998;25:1235–9.
13. Imseis RE, Van Middlesworth L, Massie JD, Bush AJ, Van Middlesworth NR. Pretreatment with propylthiouracil but not methimazole reduces the therapeutic efficacy of iodine-131 in hyperthyroidism. J Clin Endocrinol Metab 1998;83:685–7.
14. Delange F. Risks and benefits of iodine supplementation. Lancet 1998;351:923–4.
15. Stanbury JB, Ermans AE, Bourdoux P, Todd C, Oken E, Tonglet R, Vidor G, Braverman LE, Medeiros-Neto G. Iodine-induced hyperthyroidism: occurrence and epidemiology. Thyroid 1998;8:83–100.
16. Dunn JT, Semigran MJ, Delange F. The prevention and management of iodine-induced hyperthyroidism and its cardiac features. Thyroid 1998;8:101–6.
17. Kahaly GJ, Dienes HP, Beyer J, Hommel G. Iodine induces thyroid autoimmunity in patients with endemic goitre: a randomised, double-blind, placebo-controlled trial. Eur J Endocrinol 1998;139:290–7.
18. Reinhardt W, Luster M, Rudorff KH, Heckmann C, Petrasch S, Lederbogen S, Haase R, Saller B, Reiners C, Reinwein D, Mann K. Effect of small doses of iodine on thyroid function in patients with Hashimoto's thyroiditis residing in an area of mild iodine deficiency. Eur J Endocrinol 1998;139: 23–8.
19. Weber G, Vigone MC, Rapa A, Bona G, Chiumello G. Neonatal transient hypothyroidism: aetiological study. Arch Dis Child Fetal Neonat Ed 1998;79:F70–2.

H.M.J. Krans

42 Insulin, glucagon, and hypoglycemic drugs

INSULIN *(SED-13, 1290; SEDA-20, 396; SEDA-21, 440; SEDA-22, 472)*

Endocrine, metabolic *Hypoglycemia* is the most frequent adverse effect of insulin therapy. To avoid hypoglycemia the methods of insulin administration and the types of insulin used need further improvement (1).

Impaired hypoglycemic awareness was associated with an increased rate of severe hypoglycemia in 130 children and adolescents (aged 3–17 years) (2^R). One-third of the severe episodes developed without warning symptoms. Impaired awareness, young age, and recent attacks of hypoglycemia were independent risk factors.

In a teaching hospital in Edinburgh, 56 admissions of 51 patients for hypoglycemia were registered during 12 months; 41 patients had diabetes mellitus and 33 were using insulin (3^R). There was a high incidence of neurological effects. Psychiatric illness or alcoholism was common. Four patients died but only one as a direct consequence of hypoglycemia. A further six patients died within 15 months, not related to hypoglycemia.

The concentrations of the counter-regulatory hormones adrenaline and glucagon were higher before treatment of coma in insulin-treated persons admitted to hospital for hypoglycemia than in the fasting state. However, concentrations of adrenaline, glucagon, cortisol, and growth hormone are lower during a hypoglycemic episode in a diabetic than when these hormones are measured during induced hypoglycemia in non-diabetics (4^r). There was an inverse correlation between glucose and adrenaline in hypoglycemia, but no direct relation to blood glucose values for the other hormones. The addition of intramuscular glucagon during intravenous glucose therapy did not result in different glucose concentrations at any time (4^r). In type 2 diabetes counter-regulatory hormones are reduced compared with controls, but the patients release the hormones at higher blood glucose concentrations than type 1 diabetics, and the glucagon response is not blunted (5^r, 6^r).

Low responses of counter-regulatory hormones on induced hypoglycemia in a 27-year-old woman with poorly controlled diabetes (HbA_{1c} 11%), with frequent hypoglycemic instances of which she was not aware, improved dramatically after 3 months of good regulation (7^c); only growth hormone showed no reaction.

Hypoglycemia inceased beta-adrenoceptor sensitivity in normal subjects but reduced it in type 1 diabetes (8^C).

In 20 insulin-treated diabetic patients with episodes of severe hypoglycemia in 1982–4 re-evaluated in 1992–4 emergency visits were reduced from 1.05/year to 0.42/year between 1984 and 1994 (9^R). There were no cases of fatal hypoglycemia. There was no association with HbA_{1c}. Multiple daily insulin doses reduced the frequency of hypoglycemia to one-third. In 1984 unawareness was a predisposing factor and most of the patients had deficient counter-regulation (adrenaline). Most patients had a long history of insulin injections (mean 29 years). In 1994 six patients were partly and eight patients totally retested and compared with ten matched control patients with type 1 diabetes. Hypoglycemia was induced by insulin and the patients with frequent hypoglycemia reached values under 3.0 mmol much faster and in six patients the test had to be stopped before the normal duration of 3 hours for hypoglycemia; this never happened in the control patients. Counter-regulation was deficient in both 1984 and 1994, indicating that reduced counter-regulation can be permanent and does not only depend on specific circumstances.

Side Effects of Drugs, Annual 23
J.K. Aronson, ed.

Avoidance of hypoglycemia during 3 months can improve hypoglycemic unawareness for a period over 3 years (10[C]). In contrast, supervised induction of brief hypoglycemia twice weekly reduced the clinical awareness of hypoglycemia by 33% and reduced the important adrenaline response, so reducing the behavioral and physiological defenses against hypoglycemia (11[C]).

No effects of repeated hypoglycemia on cognitive function could be found in patients included in the Diabetes Control and Complications Trial, a large American study that included more than 1400 patients, which showed that normalization of blood glucose prevents or delays the development of secondary (microvascular) complications in type 1 diabetes (12[R]).

Immunological and hypersensitivity reactions It has been suggested that increased concentrations of corticotropin releasing hormone, which has an immunomodulatory effect and causes vasodilatation and mast cell degranulation, could play a role in urticaria that develops during hypoglycemic periods in type 1 diabetes (see SEDA-13; 381). Adrenal hyperandrogenemia is found in many diseases with hypersensitivity (13[r]).

A *biphasic hypersensitivity reaction* to human insulin (or another component of the injection fluid) was described in a 45-year-old woman who had used insulin for 4 years. Within 20 minutes after the injection a swelling developed and in a later phase papular lesions with lichenoid features and post-inflammatory hyperpigmentation emerged (14[c]). Histopathologically, there was neutrophilic infiltration with erythrocyte extravasation and eosinophilic amorphous material on two occasions only surrounded by neutrophilic infiltrate. Saline injection did not elicit an effect. IgE anti-insulin antibodies were not found. There was no Arthus reaction (type IV allergy).

Continuous intraperitoneal infusion of insulin causes *increased insulin immunogenicity,* but it is not known if this is accompanied by an increased frequency of autoimmune diseases. Antibodies against insulin, thyroglobulin, thyroperoxidase, gastric parietal cells, smooth muscle, mitochondria, liver and kidney micosomes, endomysium, and gliadin, and anti-nuclear antibodies were determined before and yearly after transfer to continuous intraperitoneal infusion of insulin in 28 patients; 19 remained negative for all investigated antibodies and in the other nine the anti-insulin titer increased but other anti-body titers remained constant or fluctuated (15[r]). They concluded that during continuous intraperitoneal infusion of insulin in type 1 diabetes the frequency of other autoimmune diseases like hyperthyroidism was not increased. However, this conclusion was criticized, as the small numbers did not allow a positive or negative conclusion (16).

Interactions *β-blockers* can block the symptoms of hypoglycemia, as illustrated in a recent report (17[c]).

A 68-year-old woman with diabetes and hypertension using 42 units of NPH insulin and 4 times 20 mg of propranolol died with a blood glucose concentration below 1.4 mmol/l without any symptoms of hypoglycemia.

An older report of hypoglycemia induced by topical timolol eye drops (18[c]) was mentioned in this paper.

Maprotiline, a tetracyclic antidepressant, repeatedly induced hypoglycemia in a 39-year-old woman with type 1 diabetes even when the insulin dose was reduced from 20 U/day to 4–10 U/day. Maprotiline seems to prolong the half-life of insulin. A glucagon stimulation test showed a maximum C-peptide concentration of only 0.22 nmol/l (19[c]).

Olanzapine has been reported to have precipitated diabetes (20[c]).

The antipsychotic drug induced diabetic ketoacidosis in a 31-year-old man with a treatment-refractory psychiatric disorder without prior diabetes. He got olanzapine 10 mg/day. After 3 months he developed hyperglycemia and an acidosis (pH 7.11). After metabolic compensation he needed at least 64 U of insulin, but 15 days after stopping olanzapine his insulin requirements fell and after 15 days later insulin was withdrawn.

Severe insulin resistance with ketoacidosis (pH 6.9) has also been reported with clozapine (21[C]). After withdrawal insulin requirements fell. Reinstitution of clozapine induced an identical increase in insulin need.

NEW SYNTHETIC INSULINS

Lispro insulin

Lispro insulin acts more rapidly than human insulin, but its half-life and blood glucose lowering activity are shorter. It is not necessary to delay a meal until sufficient insulin is absorbed. It can be given immediately before or during the meal and can be used when rapid action is important, as in out-patient treatment of ketonuria (22[r]) or in continuous subcutaneous insulin infusion (23[R]). In an open randomized crossover study, 113 patients with at least 6 months of continuous subcutaneous insulin infusion before the study were treated with regular insulin or lispro (23[R]). Postprandial blood glucose was lower and HbA_{1c} fell more with lispro. There were no differences hypoglycemic episodes, catheter obstruction, or adverse effects. Satisfaction with treatment was better with lispro.

There were no differences between human NPH or human ultralente insulin when the long-acting insulin was added once or twice daily to lispro (24[r]). When either lispro or regular insulin was given during the evening meal in a randomized double-blind study in insulin-using adolescents, lispro reduced the number of hypoglycemic episodes at night but redistribution of evening carbohydrate might be necessary to reduce postprandial hypoglycemia (25).

Premeal hyperglycemia is common. The short action of lispro can then be extended by the addition of NPH insulin. In a 3-month study in which besides the once daily injection of NPH insulin at each meal, lispro or lispro + NPH insulin was injected, the postprandial blood glucose concentration was lower, but the post-absorptive glucose concentration was higher in the lispro only group; there was no difference in HbA_{1c}. The addition of NPH insulin (30% at breakfast, 40% at lunch, and 10% at dinner) improved post-absorptive glucose and HbA_{1c} (26[C]), although the additions increased the number of injections substantially. Insulin Mix 25 (25% lispro and 75% neutral protamine lispro) reduced the glucose response to a standardized breakfast meal better than premixed 30% regular/70% NPH when 22 patients with type 2 diabetes were studied three times in a double-blind fashion (27[Cr]). Protamine-lispro mixed with lispro insulin has the same action profile of lispro, with the continuing action of the long-acting component (28[C]). The same mixture given three or four times daily provides acceptable control (29[r]), but gives no possibility of adjusting the short-acting insulin regularly. NPH-lispro must be mixed with lispro immediately before the meal in the syringe (30). The mixture is not stable for a longer period as a partial exchange of the rapid-acting analog and the protamine-bound human insulin takes place. Instant mixing is no solution when pens are used.

Insulin lispro may be successful in patients with subcutaneous insulin resistance, as demonstrated in a 61-year-old woman (31[c]).

Rapid improvement of regulation by lispro during pregnancy causes *proliferative diabetic retinopathy* more often. In 14 patients treated with lispro to improve control before or at the beginning of pregnancy, six of the ten patients with normal optic fundi remained negative. However, three patients developed bilateral progressive retinopathy with marked vision impairment, in two cases with vitreous hemorrhage; one patient with a negative examination 6 months before pregnancy, but with minimal lesions 18 months earlier, developed progressive retinopathy with vitreous hemorrhages in spite of multiple coagulations (32[r]). The authors advised care when starting lispro in patients with a history of retinal lesions and to look for those at risk by performing fluorescein angiography, which distinguishes incipient changes better.

Insulin aspart

Insulin aspart is a new rapid-acting synthetic insulin in which proline is exchanged for aspartate. There was an intraindividual variation in metabolic effect of 10–20% in healthy people (33[r]). In a double-blind cross-over design using insulin aspart or soluble human insulin before meals and NPH insulin before bedtime, 90 of 104 patients with type 1 diabetes completed the trial (34[r]). Insulin aspart improved postprandial control by reducing hyperglycemic and hypoglycemic variations, but night-time control was inferior. There were 547 hypoglycemic episodes in the aspart period compared with 615 in the regular insulin period (no significant difference). However, there were only 20 major hypoglycemic events in 16 patients using aspart versus 44 events in 24 patients using human insulin. One patient was withdrawn with fatigue and anorexia during aspart. Convulsions during hypoglycemia occurred once in each group.

In a double-blind cross-over study with aspart and human insulin in type 1 diabetes, human insulin was given 30 minutes before a meal with placebo immediately before the meal, or placebo was given 30 min before the meal with aspart insulin or human insulin immediately before the meal (35[r]). On average insulin aspart was absorbed twice as fast as human insulin. Postprandial glucose control improved on aspart. There were no episodes of serious hypoglycemia.

A new development is the binding of two 9-fluorenylmethoxy-carbonyl moieties to two amino acids in the structure of aspart insulin, phenylalanine and lysine (36[r]). This compound has no biological activity but gradually releases its groups and keeps diabetic animals in a good metabolic state over 2–3 days. Experiments in humans have not yet been reported.

MODES OF ADMINISTRATION OF INSULIN

In 48 children and adolescents pen devices were more accurate than syringes when under 5 U of insulin had to be injected; for higher doses pens and syringes were comparable (37[Cr]).

Implantable insulin infusion pumps have been reviewed (38[R]). In 31 centers 914 pumps were implanted, representing 2121 patient-years. Some commonly reported pump complications were:

- *hematoma* or *seroma,* usually resolved by needle aspiration;
- *pump migration,* the frequency lessening with experience; surgical intervention is necessary;
- rare *pump pocket infections;* the causes were difficult to determine, but in two patients coagulase-negative staphylococci were found, suggesting contamination with skin flora during refill;
- progressive *thinning of the skin* 1–30 months after implantation in 2 per 100 patient-years; pain and skin erosion often followed; the cause is unclear; only a correlation with physical activity could be found.

Pump failures were rare (2 per 100 patient-years). Almost all recent pumps are programmable. Catheter malfunction was the most frequent event (obstruction, total occlusion, and peritoneal adhesions—13, 10, and 3.1 events per 100 patient-years respectively). Flushing sometimes prevented occlusion. Better tip design had a big effect. Adhesion formation decreased with daily injections of heparin. Ketoacidosis frequency was comparable to that reported with continuous subcutaneous insulin infusion and was usually related to catheter obstruction. It diminished in the review period. Severe hypoglycemic episodes were lower than during intensive subcutaneous therapy.

INSULIN-LIKE GROWTH FACTOR (IGF) *(SEDA-21, 397)*

The structures of the IGF molecule and the IGF I receptor are comparable to insulin and the insulin receptor. Insulin and IGF I can bind to both receptors but insulin can only transfer 1% of the IGF message on the IGF receptor and IGF I only 1% of the insulin message on the insulin receptor. IGF I was given as co-therapy with insulin in 223 patients for 12 weeks twice daily (39[Cr]). The doses of IGF I were 40/40, 80/40, or 80/60 g/kg, Patients who received co-therapy were able to reduce their daily insulin doses. The number of episodes of hypogycemia was the same, but glucose regulation was tighter during IGF I co-therapy. The fall in HbA_{1c} was higher with co-therapy (−1.2%) than with intensive therapy only (−0.7%). The dosage regimen of 40/40 g/kg, was well tolerated. Higher doses had no greater effect but were associated with edema, jaw pain, headache, palpitation, tachycardia, syncope, or early worsening of retinopathy.

ORAL HYPOGLYCEMIC DRUGS

SULFONYLUREAS *(SED-13, 1297; SEDA-20, 398; SEDA-21, 443; SEDA-22, 475)*

Cardiovascular Transient myocardial ischemia, as seen in myocardial infarction, augments postischemic myocardial function and prevents dysrhythmias. K_{ATP} channels play a role in this so-called ischemic precondition. In 48 atrial trabeculae, obtained during catheterization, the recovery of the developed muscle force in patients treated with a sulfonylurea was only half of what was found in non-diabetics or diabetics treated with insulin. This suggests that inhibition of K_{ATP} channels by oral sulfonylureas may contribute to *increased cardiovascular mortality* (40[r]). The question of whether the findings obtained mainly with glibenclamide can be generalized to all sulfonylureas has been discussed, since sulfonylureas differ greatly in their ability to interfere with vascular or cardiac K_{ATP} channels (41[r]). Both glimiperide and glibenclamide (42[r]) improved glycemia in 29 patients in a randomized, double-blind, placebo-controlled, cross-over study of a number of risk factors for ischemic heart disease (plasminogen activator inhibitor activity, plasminogen activator inhibitor antigen, LDL-cholesterol, C-peptide, proinsulin, des-31,32 proinsulin, etc), but K_{ATP} channels were not investigated.

Endocrine, metabolic Factitious *hypoglycemia* was found in a 20-year-old woman, who even had a exploratory laparotomy with pancreatic biopsy, which showed a histological picture compatible with hyperplasia (43[C]). Glipizide was detected in the blood at a concentration of 0.72 (usual target range 0.1–0.49) μg/ml.

There have been recent reviews of oral antihyperglycemic drugs and perioperative consequences (44[R]) and the currently available oral antihyperglycemic drugs (45[R]). Gliclazide is now available in more formulations with different kinetics in vivo and in vitro. When comparing identical doses of Diamicron™ and Diabrezide™ in an open coss-over study of two times 6 months Diabrezide had a larger acute and mid-term hypoglycemic effect than Diamicon (46[r]).

The previous conclusion (6[Cr]) (SEDA-22, 475) that fasting is well tolerated and that old age is no contraindication to sulfonylurea therapy has not been accepted by others (47[r], 48[r]), as the previous study included only a small number of relatively healthy patients with type 2 diabetes.

Severe hypoglycemia induced by long-acting and short-acting sulfonylureas in Basel (200 000 inhabitants) has been analysed in a retrospective study in 28 patients (median age 73 years) (49[R]); 11 men and 5 women were treated (2.24 per 1000 person-years) with long-acting sulfonylureas (15 glibenclamide, one chlorpropamide) and two men and ten women (0.75 per 1000 person-years) with short-acting sulfonylureas (ten glibornuride, two gliclazide). Metformin was only involved when combined with a sulfonylurea. There were no deaths. Reduced food intake (9 patients), increased activity (2), impaired renal function (2), alcohol (2), too many tablets (3), and no obvious factor (10) were the causes. ACE inhibitors (5 patients), beta-blockers (5), trimethoprim (1), and acenocoumarol (1) were co-medications that may have contributed to hypoglycemia.

Liver *Cholestasis* has been attributed to glibenclamide (50[C]) gliclazide (51[c]).

A 64-year-old man who had taken glibenclamide 10 mg/day for 4 years developed cholestasis. There was no extrahepatic obstruction on ERCP and serological tests for hepatitis A, B, and C, Helicobacter pylori, and antimitochondrial or antinuclear antibodies were all negative. Liver biopsy showed portal and periportal inflammation, edema, and prominent centrilobular hepatocanalicular cholestasis. When glibenclamide was withdrawn and insulin given, the laboratory values normalized within 8 weeks. Rechallenge was considered unethical.

Use in pregnancy *Hypoglycemia* has been reported in a neonate whose mother had taken tolbutamide (52[c]).

A woman with pre-existing hypertension took labetalol 600 mg/day and tolbutamide for gestational diabetes and had long-standing hypoglycemia. She had started to take tolbutamide 500 mg/day in week 23 and increased the dosage to 1500 mg/day in week 29. Her HbA_{1c} concentration was 5.0–5.8%. She felt no intrauterine movements during week 34, and emergency cesarean section was performed. The baby had diabetic fetopathy (details not specified) and a blood glucose concentration of 0.8 mmol/l. Despite the administration of 20% glucose 10 ml as a bolus and then 8 ml/h, the blood glucose remained below 1 mmol/l, and 10 hours after birth octreotide, a somatostatin analog, was given. Intravenous glucose was discontinued after 3 days and octreotide on day 9. There were no signs of encephalopathy. C-peptide, proinsulin, and insulin in the child were inappropriately high. Serum tolbutamide in the child was 141 μmol/l at 3 hours and the half-life was 46 hours.

The half-life of tolbutamide in this case was much longer than the reported half-life in adults of 7 hours, but the normal half-life in neonates is not known. The activity of CYP2C9, which metabolizes tolbutamide, may be reduced in the first two days of life.

BIGUANIDES *(SED-13, 1301; SEDA-20, 398; SEDA-21, 445; SEDA-22, 475)*

Metformin

The blood glucose lowering effect of metformin was comparable to that of sulfonylureas, according to a meta-analysis, but body weight increases with sulfonylurea therapy and decreases with metformin, leading to a mean weight change difference of 2.9 kg (53[R]).

An extensive review of metformin has recently been published (54[R]).

Metformin and lactic acidosis

The most life-threatening complication of metformin treatment, lactic acidosis, is rare (3 per 100 000 patient-years) and is most often seen when contraindications to metformin (impaired kidney or liver function, alcoholism, circulatory problems, old age) are neglected or not detected (54[R]).

Experience with metformin in a large American health organization in 9875 patients has been presented (55[C]). There was one probable case of lactic acidosis in an 82-year-old woman who developed renal impairment during treatment with metformin 500 mg/day.

In 11 797 patients (22 296 person-years) in Saskatchewan who took metformin in 1980–95 there were 9 cases of lactic acidosis per 100 000 patient-years (56[C]), much lower than the estimated rate of 40–64 cases for phenformin.

The lower frequency of lactic acidosis during treatment with metformin compared with other biguanides may be caused by its short non-polar hydrophobic side chains substituted with two CH_3 groups. This has a lower affinity for hydrophobic structures, such as phospholipid in mitochondrial and cellular membranes, than the longer monosubstituted side-chains of the other biguanides (54[R]).

In reaction to a previously reported case of lactic acidosis at a therapeutic metformin concentration (SEDA-22, 476), in which a mitochondrial defect (increased susceptibility to metformin) was supposed, it has been observed that diabetes itself may dispose to hyperlactatemia (57[r]). Others (58[r]) have taken issue with the opinion (SEDA-22, 476) that the association of lactic acidosis and metformin may be coincidental, as lactic acidosis can also emerge during critical illnesses (type A lactic acidosis, caused by circulatory insufficiency). However, patients with type B lactic acidosis, with high biguanide concentrations, will also develop circulatory insufficiency after some hours.

Lactic acidosis occurred in a man with only mild renal impairment having an operation for a sigmoid volvulus (59[c]).

A 65-year-old man with a creatinine clearance of 67 ml/min taking metformin 850 mg bd developed lactic acidosis (lactate 25 mmol/l, pH 7.13, bicarbonate 5 mmol/l). Despite the relatively small dosage of metformin he had unexplained very high metformin concentrations (61 mg/ml).

A possible explanation for the high metformin concentration in this case was that an unknown substance related to intestinal inclusion inhibited its tubular excretion.

Phenformin-induced lactic acidosis has again been reported (60[c]).

A 67-year-old man who had taken phenformin and glibenclamide for 2 years became lethargic and confused. His pH was 6,91, serum lactate 25 mmol/l and later 30 mmol/l, and his blood glucose very low (0.5 mmol/l), possibly because of vomiting, anorexia, and glibenclamide. Hemodialysis was advised but not performed, since he recovered spontaneously.

The results of hemodialysis in biguanide-induced lactic acidosis are variable. Metformin and buformin are dialysable, but phenformin is poorly eliminated. Successful continuous veno-venous hemofiltration has been reported (61[c]).

A 68-year-old woman with type 2 diabetes and hypertension took phenformin 90 mg/day and glibenclamide 6 mg/day. She developed a urinary tract infection and oliguria followed by respiratory distress and mental confusion without neurological defects. Her pH was 6.84, serum lactate 28 mmol/l, creatinine 186 μmol/l, glucose 10.4 mmol/l, and there were no ketone bodies. She received assisted ventilation, bicarbonate, dopamine + dobutamine, glucose + insulin, and antibiotics. Her serum lactate increased to 44 mmol/l and continuous venovenous hemofiltration was started. After 5 days her lactate concentration was in the reference range (0.5–2.2 mmol/l). The serum phenformin concentration was almost 600 ng/ml (10 times the therapeutic value).

Drug interactions can precipitate metformin-induced lactic acidosis, as has been reported after the addition of indomethacin (62[C]).

A 57-year-old woman, who had taken metformin 500 mg bd for 15 years, took indomethacin 50 mg qds for 2 months. She developed oliguria and acidosis (pH 6.82, serum lactate 21 mmol/l, creatinine 480 μmol/l). After stopping metformin and indomethacin she improved and left hospital with stable impaired kidney function.

The authors reported that two other cases of metformin-associated lactic acidosis with concurrent NSAID therapy have been reported to the Committee on Safety of Medicines in the UK. Indomethacin can impair kidney function and may have done so in this case. Phenformin can cause tubular damage and oliguria in animals (63) and so it is conceivable that metformin-induced renal damage may also have contributed.

The official warning in Canada to withdraw metformin 48 hours before the administration of contrast media for radiological investigation, since co-administration can cause acute renal insufficiency, has been discussed (64). The following protocol has been suggested:

- *take a blood sample for creatinine baseline estimation before giving a contrast medium;*
- *withdraw metformin 48 hours before the investigation;*
- *if the urine output is normal for 48 hours after the radiological procedure the patient can resume metformin;*
- *when it is discovered after a procedure that the preinvestigation creatinine was raised (since the procedure may be carried out before the creatinine is known), the patient's physician should be contacted and the creatinine must be measured again within 48 hours.*

Since January 1998 the package insert approved by the FDA states: 'Glucophage (metformin) should be discontinued at the time of or prior to the procedure and withheld for 48 hours subsequent to the procedure and reinstituted only after renal function has been reevaluated and found to be normal' (65).

Hematological *Megaloblastic anemia* is rare with metformin, but vitamin B_{12} can be reduced and pre-existing deficiency may be exacerbated (54[R]).

Liver A 52-year-old woman took glipizide and enalapril and then, because of persistent hyperglycemia, metformin 1000 mg/day (66[c]). Her liver enzymes were normal, and after 2 weeks the dosage of metformin was increased to 2000 mg/day. Two weeks later she became icteric and her bilirubin and liver enzymes were increased. Serological studies were negative. All drugs were withdrawn. A liver biopsy was consistent with toxic hepatitis. She had normal liver enzymes after a month. This may be the first reported case of metformin-induced *hepatitis,* although a case was published in Turkish in 1991. Hepatitis after sulfonylureas is known, and this patient had taken glipizide for several years. The combination of glipizide and metformin may have been to blame. However, it is difficult to decide specifically after reading the next report (67[c]).

A 75-year-old man taking insulin about 40 units/day was given metformin 500 mg bd. He also used enteric-coated aspirin, diltiazem XR, ibuprofen, and lovastatin. Two months later his liver enzymes were increased, but he felt well. Hepatitis antibodies were negative. After withdrawal of metformin his liver enzymes became normal. He agreed to restart metformin. His liver enzymes remained normal, but he finally preferred insulin monotherapy.

It is not clear what caused the hepatitis in this case, although it seems that metformin was not to blame.

Gastrointestinal The well-known gastrointestinal adverse effects of metformin (*diarrhea, flatulence, abdominal bloating, anorexia, nausea, vomiting, and metallic taste*), which occur in up to 29% of patients, can be reduced by giving metformin during or immediately after meals starting with a low dose and increasing it gradually (54[R]).

ALPHA-GLUCOSIDASE INHIBITORS *(SED-13, 1302; SEDA-20, 399; SEDA-21, 446; SEDA-22, 477)*

Acarbose

In a 2-year study of the tolerability and safety of acarbose in 2035 patients the incidence of adverse effects was 7.5% and of withdrawals 2.5% (68[r]). Of 1907 patients, 444 (23%) reported one or more adverse events. In 143 patients the physician considered the relation between the adverse event (all gastrointestinal) and acarbose probable or possible. There were 77 deaths, but none was considered to be related to acarbose; 52 stopped taking acarbose because of an adverse event, and 45 were considered to be related to acarbose. Laboratory analyses were all within the reference ranges. HbA_{1c} fell by 1.92%.

The effect of adding acarbose or placebo to insulin (69[C]) or metformin (70[C]) has been investigated in patients with type 2 diabetes. The results were comparable with the results of the UK Prospective Diabetes Study (71[r]). In this study 1946 patients were randomized to acarbose (maximum 100 mg tds) or placebo. After 3 years, 39% were still using acarbose compared with 58% using placebo. The main reasons for stopping were *flatulence* (30% vs 12%) or *diarrhea* (16% vs 8%). After 3 years the HbA_{1c} was 0.5% lower (median 8.1 vs 8.6). Acarbose was equally effective when added to diet, sulfonylurea, metformin, or insulin.

When acarbose or placebo was given to patients with type 1 diabetes treated with insulin, acarbose reduced postprandial blood glucose but there was no difference in HbA_{1c}; only gastrointestinal adverse effects were present (72[C]).

The addition of metformin to acarbose in 49 patients produced a synergistic effect (73[C]).

Endocrine, metabolic Extreme *weight loss* has been attributed to acarbose (74[c]).

A 47-year-old woman weighing 59 kg took acarbose 50 mg tds. Her blood glucose improved but she lost about 1 kg/month. She had a sore tongue without oral ulcers and no evidence of malabsorption. Later she developed general weakness and iron deficient anemia but no other evidence of malabsorption. After she had lost 7 kg in 5 months acarbose was withdrawn. Her complaints disappeared, her weight normalized, and she had no signs of iron deficiency anemia, even without iron therapy.

Extreme weight loss due to acarbose is rare. In this case the mechanism was unclear.

Liver In addition to a previous report (SEDA-22, 477) three established (75[c]) and one probable (76[c]) case of liver toxicity by acarbose have been described in women aged 52–57. All had signs of liver impairment within 2–8 months after starting acarbose and the changes subsidized within a month after withdrawal. The first patient was given acarbose again; her liver enzymes increased after 3 days and normalized within 10 days after withdrawal. The second and third patients had liver biopsies, which confirmed hepatic changes. Two other cases have been reported (77[c]).

A 45-year-old man took acarbose 50 mg tds for a year and developed an AsT of 62 U/l and an AlT of 127 U/l, with negative serology; 3 months later the AlT was 153 U/l. After withdrawal of acarbose his liver enzymes normalized.

A 54-year-old woman had fatigue and dark urine after taking acarbose 50 mg tds for 5 months. Her AsT was 2436 U/l, AlT 2556U/l, gamma-GT 601 U/l, and alkaline phosphatase 174 U/l; serology was negative and she had a normal liver and gall-bladder on ultrasound. Her liver enzymes normalized 5 months after withdrawal.

Another patient taking acarbose also had a serum AlT three times the upper limit of the reference range, but she had positive serology for hepatitis A (70[c]).

Gastrointestinal Long-term acarbose had a good effect on late dumping syndrome in six patients with type 2 diabetes; one patient complained of increased *flatulence* (78[c]).

Miglitol

The effects of miglitol 25 or 50 mg tds have been compared with placebo and various doses of glibenclamide in 411 patients aged over 60 years (mean 68 years) with mild type 2 diabetes insufficiently controlled by diet for 56 weeks (79[r]). HbA_{1c} fell after one year by 0.92% (glibenclamide), 0.49% (miglitol 25 mg) and 0.40% (miglitol 50 mg). Gastrointestinal events were most common in patients taking miglitol. Most (88%) of the hypoglycemic events were minor and occurred in the patients taking glibenclamide. Mean body weight increased continuously and significantly in those taking glibenclamide. In the other groups weight fell by more than 1 kg. The rate of withdrawal was the same in all groups; withdrawal was mostly occasioned by cardiovascular effects in those taking glibenclamide and by *hyperglycemia, flatulence,* or *diarrhea* in those taking miglitol.

THIAZOLIDINEDIONES

(SED-13, 1302; SEDA-20, 399; SEDA-21, 446; SEDA-22, 478)

The thiazolidinediones have recently been reviewed (80[R]). Troglitazone is available in the US and Japan, rosiglitazone in the US, and pioglitazone in Japan; darglitazone is still in a developmental phase, and ciglitazone and englitazone have been discontinued owing to adverse effects on the liver. These drugs reduce insulin resistance, stimulate glucose uptake in muscle, and reduce glucose outflow from the liver. They can be given as single drugs or in combination with other antihyperglycemic therapy. They seem to promote fat accumulation in subcutaneous tissue (81[C]) rather than in the abdominal region, which plays such a bad role in the insulin resistance syndrome. They may ameliorate albuminuria in incipient diabetic nephropathy (82[C]).

Troglitazone

Troglitazone 100 or 200 mg/day or placebo was given for 16 weeks to 259 patients already taking sulfonylurea therapy (83[C]). HbA_{1c} was 0.4% and 0.7% lower and blood glucose concentrations fell. The most common event was hypoglycemia, but this did not occur more often when troglitazone was added. Liver enzymes increased to the same extent in the three groups and never rose above normal. No patients withdrew because of drug related effects.

Nervous system *Ataxia* has been attributed to troglitazone in two patients aged about 80 years (a man and a woman) (84[c]). The ataxia developed during treatment and disappeared in one case 2–3 days after withdrawal and in the other within 2 weeks. In one the ataxia was accompanied by a dementia-like syndrome, which completely disappeared within 8 weeks. One of the patients was rechallenged and developed ataxia again.

Gastrointestinal Troglitazone can cause *fulminant hepatitis* (85[c]).

A 58-year-old man developed severe hepatitis after taking troglitazone 400 mg/day and glibenclamide 5 mg/day. Glibenclamide was stopped after 6 weeks as his HbA_{1c} was 7.0%. About 2 weeks later he developed malaise and 1 week later jaundice. His bilirubin, AsT, and AlT were greatly raised and there was ascites. He had taken about 34 g of troglitazone. Drug induced lymphocyte stimulation test was strongly positive for troglitazone and not for other drugs. Troglitazone was withdrawn and 3 days later the plasma concentration was below the limit of detection. Notwithstanding intensive therapy he died after 5 weeks. At autopsy the liver showed yellow atrophy and massive hepatocellular coagulation necrosis with moderate neutrophil, monocyte, and eosinophil infiltration.

The positive lymphocyte stimulation test, the eosinophils, and the low blood concentrations 3 days after withdrawal suggest that hypersensitivity to troglitazone was the underlying cause. The authors reported that another patient with hepatitis after troglitazone had had a subacute course after withdrawal of the drug.

Hepatotoxicity has delayed the registration of troglitazone in Europe. In the US patient with diabetes who used troglitazone in a study, developed hepatic failure necessitating liver transplantation and died. Troglitazone was withdrawn from a major National Institutes of Health evaluation of various regimens for preventing type 2 diabetes. In Japan the government recommended in December 1997 that liver function tests should be assessed every month in patients taking troglitazone.

Less severe liver damage can be caused by troglitazone (86[C]).

A 62-year-old woman with normal liver function tests took troglitazone 400 mg/day in combination with gliclazide 80 mg/day and pravastatin. After 9 months her AsT and AlT were slightly above normal, but the HbA_{1c} was 7.0% and treatment was continued. Her liver enzymes were measured monthly and after 19 months rose abruptly. Troglitazone was withdrawn immediately and she received insulin. Her liver enzymes improved rapidly. A biopsy showed hepatic necrosis round the central vein and a mild inflammatory infiltrate and fibrosis in the portal area compatible with protracted acute hepatitis. A lymphocyte stimulation test and a skin test were negative for troglitazone.

MISCELLANEOUS DRUGS

Repaglinide *(SEDA-22, 479)*

Repaglinide is a non-sulfonylurea drug that stimulates insulin secretion but binds to binding sites other than the sulfonylurea binding sites and has a short half-life after absorption. Patients with type 2 diabetes with unsatisfactory control after taking metformin for 6 months, were randomized to metformin alone, repaglinide alone, or metformin + repaglinide (each 27 patients) (87[C]). Combined therapy reduced HbA_{1c} after 3 months by 1.4% and fasting glucose by 2.2 mmol/l. Repaglinide alone or in combination increased insulin concentrations. The most common adverse effects were *hypoglycemia, diarrhea,* and *headache.* Gastrointestinal adverse effects were common in those taking metformin alone and *body weight increased* in both groups taking repaglinide.

In 424 patients in a European multicenter randomized double-blind study for 1 year two-thirds of the patients used repaglinide (0.5–4 mg tds) and the others glibenclamide (1.75–10.5 mg/day) (88). HbA_{1c} first fell but later increased. The same trends were seen in fasting blood glucose. There were no differences in hypoglycemia. A comparable American study of 576 patients (89^C) showed essentially the same result.

The effect of a missed meal during repaglinide and glibenclamide therapy has been compared in 83 randomized patients (90^C). During two meals there were six separate hypoglycemic events in those taking glibenclamide. Blood glucose fell from 4.3 mmol/l to 3.4 mmol/l in those taking glibenclamide when lunch was omitted. There were no changes in blood glucose in those taking repaglinide.

REFERENCES

1. Amiel SA. Hypoglycaemia avoidance-technology and knowledge. Lancet 1998;352:502–3.
2. Barkai L, Vámosi I, Lukcás K. Prospective assessment of severe hypoglycaemia in diabetic children and adolescents with impaired and normal awareness of hypoglycaemia. Diabetologia 1998;41:898–903.
3. Hart SP, Frier BM. Causes, management and morbidity of acute hypoglycaemia in adults requiring hospital admission. Q J Med 1998;51:505–10.
4. Hvidberg A, Christensen NJ, Hilsted J. Counterregulatory homones in insulin-treated diabetic patients admitted to an accident and emergency department with hypoglycaemia. Diabetic Med 1998;15:199–204.
5. Levy CJ, Kinsley BT, Bajaj M, Simonson DC. Effect of glycemic control on glucose counterregulation during hypoglycemia in NIDDM. Diabetes Care 1998;21:1330–9.
6. Burge MR, Schmitz-Fiorentino K, Fischette C, Qualis CR, Schade DS. A prospective trial of risk factors for sulfonylurea-induced hypoglycemia in type 2 diabetes mellitus. J Am Med Assoc 1998;279:137–43.
7. Kaneto H, Ikeda M, Kishimoto M, Iiada M, Hoshi A, Watarai T, Kubota M, Kajimoto Y, Yamasaki Y, Hori M. Dramatic recovery of counterregulatory hormone response to hypoglycaemia after intensive insulin therapy in poorly controlled type 1 diabetes mellitus. Diabetologia 1998; 41:982–3.
8. Fritsche A, Stumvoll M, Grüb M, Sieslack S, Renn W, Schmülling R-M, Häring H-U, Gerich JE. Effect of hypoglycemia on beta-adrenergic sensitivity in normal and type 1 diabetic subjects. Diabetes Care 1998;21:1505–10.
9. Oskarson P, Adamson U, Clausen Sjöbom N. Lins P-E. Long-term follow-up of insulin-dependent diabetes mellitus with recurrent episodes of severe hypoglycemia. Diabetes Res Clin Pract 1999;44:165–74.
10. Dagogo-Jack S, Fanelli CG, Cryer PE. Durable reversal of hypoglycemia unawareness in type 1 diabetes. Diabetes Care 1999;22:866–7.
11. Ovalle F, Fanelli CG, Paramore DS, Hershey T, Craft S, Cryer PE. Brief twice-weekly episodes of hypoglycemia reduce detection of clinical hypoglycemia in type 1 diabetes mellitus. Diabetes 1998;47:1472–9.
12. Austin EJ, Deary IJ. Effects of repeated hypoglycemia on cognitive function (in the DCCT). Diabetes Care 1999;22:1273–7.
13. Sacerdote AS. Hypoglycemic urticaria revisited. Diabetes Care 1999;22:861.
14. Al-Sheik OA. Unusual local cutaneous reactions to insulin injections: a case report. Saudi Med J 1998;19:199–201.
15. Lassmann-Vague V, SanMarco M, LeJeune P-J, Alessis C, Vague P, Belicar P. Autoimmunity and intraperitoneal insulin treatment by programmable pumps. Diabetes Care 1998;21:2041–3.
16. Charles MA. Autoimmunity and intraperitoneal insulin. Diabetes Care 1998;21:2043–4.
17. Cooper JW. Fatal asymptomatic hypoglycemia in an elderly insulin-dependent diabetic patient taking an oral beta-blocking medication. Diabetes Care 1998;21:2197–8.
18. Silverstone BZ, Marcus T. Hypoglycemia due to ophthalmic timolol in a diabetic. Harefuah 1990; 118:693–4.
19. Isotani H, Kameoka K. Hypoglycemia associated with maprotiline in a patient with type 1 diabetes. Diabetes Care 1999;22:862–3.
20. Gatta B, Rigalleau V, Gin H. Diabetic ketoacidosis with olanzapine treatment. Diabetes Care 1999;22:1002–3.
21. Colli A, Cocciolo M, Francobandiera G, Rogantin F, Cattalini N. Diabetic acidosis associated with clozapine treatment. Diabetes Care 1999;22:176–7.
22. Travaglini MT, Garg SK, Chase HP. Use of insulin lispro in the outpatient management of ketonuria. Arch Pediatr Adolesc Med 1998;152:672–5.
23. Renner R, Peutzner A, Trautmann M, Harzer O, Sauter K, Landgraf R. Use of insulin lispro in continuous subcutaneous insulin infusion treatment. Diabetes Care 1999;22:784–8.
24. Zinman B, Ross S, Campos RV, Strack T, the Canadian Lispro Study Group. Effectiveness of human ultralente versus NPH insulin in providing basal insulin replacement for an insulin lispro multiple daily injection regimen. Diabetes Care 1999;22:603–8.
25. Mohn A, Matyka KA, Harris DA, Ross KM, Edge JA, Dunger DB. Lispro or regular insulin for multiple injection therapy in adolescence. Diabetes Care 1999;22:27–32.

26. Ciofetta M, Lalli C, Del Sindaco P, Torlone E, Pampanelli S, Mauro L, Chiara DL, Brunetti P, Bolli GB. Contribution of postprandial versus interprandial blood glucose to HbA_{1c} in type 1 diabetes on physiologic intensive therapy with lispro insulin at mealtime. Diabetes Care 1999;22:795–800.
27. Koivisto VA, Tuominen JA, Ebeling P. Lispro Mix25 insulin as premeal therapy in type 2 diabetic patients. Diabetes Care 1999;22:459–62.
28. Rave K, Heinemann L, Puhl L, Gudat U, Woodworth JR, Weyer C, Heise T. Premixed formulations of insulin lispro. Diabetes Care 1999;22:865–6.
29. Lalli C, Ciofetta M, Del Sindaco P, Torlone E, Pampanelli S, Compagnucci P, Cartechini MG, Bartocci L, Brunetti P, Bolli GB. Long-term intensive treatment of type 1 diabetes with the short-acting insulin analog lispro in variable combination with NPH insulin at mealtime. Diabetes Care 1999;22:468–77.
30. Joseph SE, Korzon-Burakowska A, Woodworth JR, Evans M, Hopkins D, Janes JM, Amiel SA. The action profile of lispro is not blunted by mixing in the syringe with NPH insulin. Diabetes Care 1998;21:2098–102.
31. Darmon P, Curtillet C, Boullu S, Laugier A, Dutour A, Oliver C. Insulin analog lispro decreases insulin resistance and improves glycemic control in an obese patient with insulin-requiring type 2 diabetes. Diabetes Care 1998;21:1575.
32. Kitzmiller JL, Main E, Ward B, Theiss T, Peterson DL. Insulin lispro and the development of proliferative diabetic retinopathy during pregnancy. Diabetes Care 1999;22:874–6.
33. Heinemann L, Weyer C, Rauhaus M, Heinrichs S, Heise T. Variability of the metabolic effect of soluble insulin and the rapid-acting insulin analog insulin aspart. Diabetes Care 1998;21:1910–14.
34. Home PD, Lindholm A, Hylleberg B, Round P, UK Insulin Aspart Group. Improved glycemic control with insulin aspart. Diabetes Care 1998;21:1904–9.
35. Lindholm A, McEwen J, Riis AP. Improved postprandial glycemic control with insulin aspart. Diabetes Care 1999;22:801–5.
36. Gershonov E, Shechter Y, Fridkin M. New concept for long-acting insulin. Diabetes 1999;48: 1437–42.
37. Lteif AN, Schwenk WF. Accuracy of pen injectors versus insulin syringes in children with type 1 diabetes. Diabetes Care 1999;22:137–40.
38. Pinget M, Jeandidier N. Long term safety and efficacy of intraperitoneal insulin infusion by means of implantable pumps. Horm Metab Res 1998;30:475–86.
39. Thrailkill KM, Quattrin T, Baker L, Kuntze JE, Compton PG, Martha PM Jr. Cotherapy with recombinant human insulin-like growth factor I and insulin improves glycemic control in type 1 diabetes. Diabetes Care 1999;22:585–92.
40. Cleveland JC Jr, Meldrum DR, Cain BS, Banerjee A, Harken AH. Oral sulfonylurea hypoglycemic agents prevent ischemic preconditioning in human myocardium. Circulation 1997;96:29–32.
41. Wascher TC. Sulfonylureas and cardiovascular mortality in diabetes:a class effect? Circulation 1998;97:1427–8.
42. Britton ME, Denver AE, Mohamed-Ali V, Yudkin JS. Effects of glimepiride vs glibenclamide on ischaemic heart disease risk factors and glycaemic control in patients with type 2 diabetes mellitus. Clin Drug Invest 1998;16:303–17.
43. Gorgojo GG, Cancér E, Andreu M, Camblor M, Lajo T, Álvarez V, Moreno B. Hipoglucemia factitia induca por glipizida en una paciente con síndrome de Münchhausen. Endocrinologia 1998;45:38–42.
44. DeWitt DE, Evans TC. Perioperative management of oral antihyperglycemic agents: special consideration for metformin. Semin Anesth 1998;17:267–72.
45. Anonymous. New oral antihyperglycaemic agents expand armamentarium in the battle against type 2 diabetes mellitus. Drugs Ther Perspect 1998;12:6–9.
46. Galeone F, Fiore G, Mannucci E. Medium-term hypoglycaemic effects of two different oral formulations of gliclazide. Diabetic Med 1999;16:618–19.
47. Shorr RI. Hypoglycemia from glipizide and glyburide. J Am Med Assoc 1998;279:1441–3.
48. Gambassi G, Carbonin P, Bernabei R. Hypoglycemia from glipizide and glyburide. J Am Med Assoc 1998;279:1441–3.
49. Stahl M, Berger W. Higher incidence of severe hypoglycaemia leading to hospital admission in type 2 diabetic patients treated with long-acting versus short-acting sulphonylureas. Diabet Med 1999;16:586–90.
50. Tholakanahalli VN, Potti A, Heyworth MF. Glibenclamide-induced cholestasis. West J Med 1998;168:274–7.
51. Dourakis SP, Tzemanakis E, Sinani C, Kafari G, Hadziyannis S. Gliclazide induced acute hepatitis. Arch Hell Med 1998;15:87–9.
52. Christesen HBT, Melander A. Prolonged elimination of tolbutamide in a premature newborn with hyperinsulinaemic hypoglycaemia. Eur J Endocrinol 1998;138:698–701.
53. Johansen K. Efficacy of metformin in the treatment of NIDDM. Meta-analysis. Diabetes 1999; 48:33–7.
54.. Cusi K, DeFronzo RA. Metformin: a review of its metabolic effects. Diabetes Rev 1998;6:89–131.
55. Selby JV, Ettinger B, Swain BE, Brown JB. First 20 months' experience with use of metformin for type 2 diabetes in a large health maintenance organization. Diabetes Care 1999;22:38–44.
56. Stang M, Wysowski DK, Butler-Jones D. Incidence of lactic acidosis in metformin users. Diabetes Care 1999;22:925–7.
57. Chan NN, Darko D, O'Shea D. Lactic acidosis with therapeutic metformin blood level in a low-risk diabetic patient. Diabetes Care 1999;22:178.
58. Cohen RD, Woods HF. Metformin and lactic acidosis. Diabetes Care 1999;22:1010–11.

59. Lalau JD, Race J-M, Brinquin L. Lactic acidosis in metformin therapy. Diabetes Care 1998; 21:1366–7.
60. Kwong SC, Brubacher J. Phenformin and lactic acidosis: a case report and review. J Emerg Med 1998;16:881–6.
61. Mariano F, Benzi L, Cecchetti P, Rosatello A, Merante D, Goia F, Capra L, Lanza G, Curto V, Cavalli PL. Efficacy of continuous haemofiltration (CVVH) in the treatment of severe phenformin-induced lactic acidosis. Nephrol Dial Transplant 1998;13:1012–15.
62. Chann NN, Fauvel NJ, Feher MD. Non-steroidal anti-inflammatory drugs and metformin. A cause for concern? Lancet 1998;352:201.
63. Schwarzbeck A. Non-steroidal anti-inflammatory drugs and metformin. Lancet 1998;352: 818.
64. Rasuli P, Hammond DI. Metformin and contrast media: where is the conflict? Can Assoc Radiol J 1998;49:161–6.
65. Hammond DI, Rasuli P. Metformin and contrast media. Clin Radiol 1998;53:933–4.
66. Babich MM, Pike I, Shiffman ML. Metformin induced acute hepatitis. Am J Med 1998;104:490–2.
67. Swislocki ALM, Noth R. Pseudohepatotoxity of metformin. Diabetes Care 1998;21:677–8.
68. Mertes G. Efficacy and safety of acarbose in the treatment of type 2 diabetes: data from a 2-year surveillance study. Diabetes Res Clin Pract 1998;40:63–70.
69. Kelley DE, Bidot P, Freedman Z, Haag B, Podlecki D, Rendell M, Schimel D, Weiss S, Taylor T, Krol A, Magner J. Efficacy and safety of acarbose in insulin-treated patients with type 2 diabetes. Diabetes Care 1998;21:2056–61.
70. Rosenstock J, Brown A, Fischer J, Jain A, Littlejohn T, Nadeau D, Sussman A, Taylor T, Krol A, Magner J. Efficacy and safety of acarbose in metformin-treated patients with type 2 diabetes. Diabetes Care 1998;21:2050–5.
71. Holman RR, Cull CA, Turner RC. A randomized double-blind trial of acarbose in type 2 diabetes shows improved glycemic control over 3 years (UKPDS 44). Diabetes Care 1999;22:960–4.
72. Riccardi G, Giacco R, Parillo M, Turco S, Rivellese AA, Ventura MA, Contadini S, Marra G, Monteduro M, Santeusanio F, Brunetti P, Librenti MC, Pontiroli AE, Vedani P, Pozza G, Bergamini L, Bianchi C. Efficacy and safety of acarbose in the treatment of type 1 diabetes mellitus: a placebo-controlled, double-blind, multicentre study. Diabetic Med 1999;16:228–32.
73. Hanefeld M, Bär K. Efficacy and safety of combined treatment of type 2 diabetes with acarbose and metformin. Diabetes Stoffwechsel 1998;7:186–90.
74. Yoo W-H, Park T-S, Baek H-S. Marked weight loss in a type 2 diabetic patient treated with acarbose. Diabetes Care 1999;22:45–6.
75. Fujimoto Y, Ohhira M, Miyokawa N, Kitamori S, Kohgo Y. Acarbose-induced hepatic injury. Lancet 1998;351:340.
76. Diaz-Gutierrez FL, Ladero JM, Diaz-Rubio M. Acarbose-induced acute hepatitis. Am J Gastroenterol 1998;93:481.
77. Andrade RJ, Lucena M, Vega JL, Torres M, Salmeron FJ, Bellot V, Garcia-Escaño MD, Moreno P. Acarbose-associated hepatotoxicity. Diabetes Care 1998;21:2029–30.
78. Hasegawa T, Yoneda M, Nakamura K, Ohnishi K, Harada H, Kyouda T, Yoshida Y, Makino I. Long-term effect of alpha-glucosidase inhibitor on late dumping syndrome. J Gastroenterol Hepatol 1998;13:1201–6.
79. Johnston PS, Lebovitz HE, Coniff RF, Simonson DC, Raskin P, Munera CL. Advantages of alpha-glucosidase inhibition as monotherapy in elderly type 2 diabetic patients. J Clin Endocinol Metab 1998;83:1512–22.
80. Day C. Thiazolidinediones: a new class of antidiabetic drugs. Diabetic Med 1999;16:179–92.
81. Mori Y, Murakawa Y, Okada K, Horikoshi H, Yokoyama J, Tajima N, Ikeda Y. Effect of troglitazone on body fat distribution in type 2 diabetic patients. Diabetes Care 1999;22:908–12.
82. Imano E, Kanda T, Nakatani Y, Nishida T, Arai K, Motomura M, Kajimoto Y, Yamasaki Y, Hori M. Effect of troglitazone on microalbuminuria in patients with incipient diabetic nephropathy. Diabetes Care 1998;21:2135–9.
83. Buysschaert M, Bobbioni E, Starkie M, Frith L, Troglitazone Study Group. Troglitazone in combination with sulphonylurea improves glycaemic control in type 2 diabetic patients inadequately controlled by sulphonylurea therapy alone. Diabet Med 1999;16:147–53.
84. Maher TD, Mirza SA. Ataxia and reversible dementia-like syndrome associated with troglitazone. Diabetes 1999;48 (Suppl 1):A85.
85. Shibuya A, Watanabe M, Fujita Y, Saigenji K, Kuwao S, Takahashi H, Takeuchi H. An autopsy case of troglitazone-induced fulminant hepatitis. Diabetes Care 1998;21:2140–3.
86. Iwase M, Yamaguchi M, Yoshinari M, Okamura C, Hirahashi T, Tsuji H, Fujishima M. A Japanese case of liver dysfunction after 19 months of troglitazone treatment, Diabetes Care 1999;22:1382–4.
87. Moses R, Slobodniuk R, Boyages S, Colagiuri S, Kidson W, Carter J, Donnelly T, Moffitt P, Hopkins H. Effect of repaglinide addition to metformin monotherapy on glycemic control in patients with type 2 diabetes. Diabetes Care 1999;22:119–24.
88. Wolffenbuttel BHR, Landgraf R. A 1-year multicenter randomized double-blind comparison of repaglinide and glyburide for the treatment of type 2 diabetes. Diabetes Care 1999;22:463–7.
89. Marbury T, Huang W-C, Strange P, Lebovitz H. Repaglinide versus glyburide: a one-year comparison trial. Diabetes Res Clin Pract 1999;43:155–66.
90. Damsbo P, Clauson P, Marbury TC, Windfeld K. A double-blind randomized comparison of meal-related glycemic control by repaglinide and glyburide in well-controlled type 2 diabetic patients. Diabetes Care 1999;22:789–94.

P. Coates

43 Miscellaneous hormones

Calcitonin *(SED-13, 1307; SEDA-20, 402; SEDA-21, 451; SEDA-22, 483)*

Calcitonin is well established in the treatment of disorders of high bone turnover, such as Paget's disease and postmenopausal osteoporosis. *Tachyphylaxis* develops if it is used continuously at high doses for more than a few months. Intranasal calcitonin has a systemic availability of only 3% of the subcutaneous form but is associated with fewer adverse effects. The role of calcitonin in treating acute pain due to osteoporotic crush fractures has been reviewed, but the mechanism of its analgesic effect is not known (1^R). Adverse effects are common but are usually mild and dose related. These include gastrointestinal effects (*nausea, cramps, and vomiting*), *dizziness and flushing,* and local reactions either at the injection site (*rash, pruritus*) or in the nose (*rhinitis, dryness, sneezing, and rarely epistaxis*).

Interactions Plasma *lithium* concentrations were significantly reduced in four women within 3 days of starting calcitonin, and there was increased renal clearance of lithium in two of these patients (2^c).

Follicle-stimulating hormone (FSH)

The first gonadotropins available for clinical use were extracted from the urine of postmenopausal women. Human menopausal gonadotropin (hMG) is in limited supply and contains other proteins, which may be allergenic, as well as luteinizing hormone. Purified FSH preparations (urofollitropin and highly purified urofollitropin) are also extracted from human urine. Recombinant FSH from a Chinese hamster ovarian cell line (follitropin alpha) has recently become available and is likely to replace other gonadotropins because of its purity and ease of patient self-administration. FSH treatment for infertility has been reviewed in detail (3^R, 4^R). *Multiple pregnancy* occurs in 20% of patients, 80% being twin pregnancies. There is no documented increase in congenital abnormalities in children conceived after ovulation induction with FSH.

Endocrine, metabolic *Ovarian hyperstimulation syndrome* is characterized by massive ovarian enlargement and a fluid shift from the intravascular space to the peritoneal, pleural, and pericardial cavities. Rates of up to 20% for all grades and 1–2% for severe ovarian hyperstimulation syndrome have been documented and do not differ between FSH preparations. Women with polycystic ovarian syndrome are at a higher risk of developing this complication (3^R). In rare cases women have died of pulmonary embolism, disseminated intravascular coagulation, or adult respiratory distress syndrome (4^R). If the patient is pregnant, ovarian hyperstimulation syndrome is more severe and prolonged (4^R). Generally, it resolves within 7 days if the patient is not pregnant or in 10-20 days if she is. The underlying cause of this adverse effect is not known.

Gonadotropin-releasing hormone (gonadorelin, GnRH) and analogs

Gonadorelin has different effects according to its duration of use. If given continuously, it first stimulates gonadotropin release, but later inhibits it by down-regulation of hypophyseal receptors. The therapeutic indications for gonadorelin and its analogs have been summarized before (SED-13, 1311). Long-acting and depot formulations have the same adverse effects profile as shorter-acting analogs.

Cardiovascular Gonadorelin has *an inhibitory effect on nitric oxide-mediated arterial relaxation,* which disappears within 3 months after stopping treatment. This effect was abolished with 'add-back' hormone replacement in

Side Effects of Drugs, Annual 23
J.K. Aronson, ed.

a prospective randomized study of 50 women treated for 6 months (5[C]).

Psychiatric *Depressed mood and emotional lability* have been reported in up to 75% of patients receiving gonadorelin analogs, and there have been occasional reports of more severe mood disturbance (6[CR]). Successful treatments of this symptom include 'add-back' estrogen (6[CR]) and sertraline (7[C]).

Endocrine, metabolic Virtually all women who receive long-term gonadorelin have *hypoestrogenic symptoms,* which include *hot flushes, vaginal dryness, reduced libido,* and *mood changes.* 'Add-back' estrogen replacement reduces the frequency and severity of these symptoms without apparently compromising the effectiveness of gonadorelin in women with endometriosis (7[C], 8[C]). Similarly, almost all men on this treatment experience reduced libido and impotence.

A woman with type 2 diabetes had *worse glycemic control* while receiving buserelin (9[c]). Her blood glucose returned to its previous concentration after withdrawal. This is only the second such report in a diabetic patient.

Ovarian hyperstimulation syndrome (ovarian enlargement, abdominal pain and tenderness, and ascites) has been reported in a woman with polycystic ovarian syndrome, 3 weeks after an intramuscular injection of leuprorelin acetate for endometriosis (10[c]). She was later given further courses of the drug without this complication. This is the second report of this syndrome in a patient who did not receive concomitant gonadotropin treatment.

Tumor modifying effects *Tumor flare* occurred more commonly in women treated with goserelin than after oophorectomy in a randomized multicenter trial of 136 patients; however there was no difference in survival (11[C]).

Human growth hormone (hGH, somatotropin)

Recombinant human growth hormone is well established in the treatment of childhood growth hormone deficiency, Turner's syndrome, and chronic renal insufficiency. Experimental indications include idiopathic short stature in children, adult growth hormone deficiency, osteoporosis, and catabolic states associated with acute and chronic illnesses. Adverse effects differ in adults and children. In adults, adverse effects are commoner in men, in heavier patients, and in adult-onset growth hormone deficiency, but efficacy is no greater. This is because of the higher dose of growth hormone when calculated according to body weight, and also to lower growth hormone sensitivity in women (10[R], 11[C]). Adverse effects are more frequent with rapid dosage escalation and are reversible after dosage reduction. To minimize adverse effects, it is recommended that treatment be started at a low dose i.e. 0.4–0.8 units/day, and titrated according to the age-specific concentration of insulin-like growth factor-1 (12[R], 13[C], 14[R]).

Cardiovascular *Hypertension* and *edema* (including generalized or peripheral edema and carpal tunnel syndrome) are commoner in adults and in adult onset growth hormone deficiency. Edema is three times more frequent with a dose of 0.025 mg/kg/day than 0.0125 mg/kg/day (12[R]). In a randomized controlled study of 33 obese women, three of nine who received growth hormone and two of seven who received growth hormone plus insulin-like growth factor-1 withdrew from the study, because of intolerable edema, compared to none in the placebo group. Most patients receiving growth hormone required diuretic treatment for edema in this study, in which dose was calculated according to body weight (15[C]). In a randomized placebo-controlled trial of growth hormone replacement in 166 hormone-deficient adults, 48% of the treated group and 30% of the placebo group reported mild to moderate edema, which resolved in 70% of subjects despite continued treatment (16[C]).

Nervous system *Carpal tunnel syndrome* is probably dose-related, as it is commoner in adults than in children.

Headache, vomiting or visual disturbances early in treatment may indicate *idiopathic intracranial hypertension* (pseudotumor cerebri) and require further investigation, as loss of visual acuity and visual fields have been reported in untreated patients; 30 cases have been reported worldwide (17[C]). Chronic renal insufficiency, Turner's syndrome, obesity, and biochemical growth hormone deficiency are all associated with an increased risk. Most cases occur within the first 8 weeks of treatment, and withdrawal or dose reduction of recombinant growth hormone gives complete resolution. Fundoscopy is recommended before starting treatment and regularly during the first few months, although the absence of papilledema does not exclude the diagnosis. Up to 48% of children with intracranial hypertension due to growth hormone also develop a sixth nerve palsy (17[C]).

Endocrine, metabolic *Hyperinsulinemia* is common in patients treated with growth hormone, but its long-term effect has not yet been determined. In a 5-year study, 67 children treated with growth hormone all showed a sustained increase in fasting and oral glucose-stimulated insulin concentrations. This was most significant in children on dialysis and with renal transplants (18[C]). In another study, insulin secretion in response to intravenous glucose was increased in 14 children with renal insufficiency, but returned to baseline after 12 months. However, increased insulin concentrations persisted in nine girls with Turner's syndrome (19[C]). Concomitant glucocorticoid and growth hormone treatment in children with juvenile arthritis caused a small but significant rise in blood glucose and glycosylated hemoglobin, which returned to pretreatment concentrations after growth hormone was withdrawn (20[C]). Hyperglycemia not requiring specific treatment has been reported more frequently in adult patients (16[C]) and in patients receiving high-dose growth hormone to treat wasting associated with burns or HIV infection (21[C], 22[C]). A single case report documented diabetes 2 months after growth hormone was begun in a 14-year-old girl, with restoration of normoglycemia after it was withdrawn (23[c]). Post-marketing reports have previously shown 3-fold incidence of type 2 diabetes in patients treated with growth hormone; this is thought to represent earlier onset rather than an increase in de novo cases (24[R]).

Skin and appendages A 12-year-old boy developed *lipohypertrophy* at the site of growth hormone injection (25[c]). Site rotation gave partial resolution and is recommended to prevent this complication.

Special senses *Retinopathy* has been reported in two nondiabetic patients treated with growth hormone (26[C]). The first, an obese 31-year-old man, developed non-proliferative retinopathy and macular edema with reduced visual acuity after 14 months' therapy, which improved after growth hormone was stopped. The second, an 11-year-old girl with Turner's syndrome, developed unilateral neovascularization after 22 months.

Musculoskeletal *Arthralgia* in small and large joints and *myalgia* in proximal muscle groups are common, especially with high doses of growth hormone or if dosage escalation is rapid (12[R], 13[C], 15[C], 22[C]).

There are conflicting reports on a possible *increased fracture risk* in children with osteogenesis imperfecta treated with growth hormone, many of whom have a qualitative collagen defect (27[C], 28[c]).

Immunological and hypersensitivity reactions In a 15-year-old boy with previously quiescent lupus nephritis, laboratory markers of disease activity rose during growth hormone treatment and returned to baseline concentrations within 3 months after withdrawal (29[c]).

Growth hormone and the risk of malignancy

The incidence of malignancy is increased in acromegaly, in which growth hormone is present in excess. Patients treated with growth hormone have therefore been carefully monitored. The first report of leukemia in Japanese children treated with growth hormone (30[C]) prompted a world wide survey. There have now been reports of 44 new cases of leukemia in growth hormone recipients, of which only 20 were acute lymphoblastic leukemia. This is much less than the expected 80–85% of new childhood leukemia (31[R]). A recent review of Japanese patients found that of the 15 patients who had developed hematological malignancy since 1975, six had other risk factors for leukemia, such as Fanconi's syndrome or prior chemotherapy or radiotherapy. The incidence of leukemia in this study was 3 per 100 000, similar to that in the general population of the same age (32[C]). The National Cooperative Growth Study (NCGS: a post marketing database that includes 19 846 patient-years since the time of growth hormone exposure) similarly reported no increase in the incidence of new leukemia when patients with other risk factors were excluded from the analysis (33[R]).

The recurrence rate of intracranial tumors has been addressed in a number of large observational studies. Reports from the NCGS database (which includes 1262 children with brain tumors) and from England have shown no increase in intracranial tumor recurrence in patients treated with growth hormone (34[C], 35[C]). For patients with craniopharyngioma, postoperative irradiation reduced the recurrence rate, but growth hormone therapy did not increase the risk (36[C]).

In the NCGS study extracranial non-leukemia malignancy rates were similarly not increased in patients treated with growth hormone compared with those who were not (37[C]).

Conclusions *There is no evidence that growth hormone treatment increases the risk of new or recurrent malignancy at any site. Despite this, certain precautions are still recommended for children who have previously been treated for cancer. The diagnosis of growth hormone deficiency should be clearly established (31[R]) and it is recommended that treatment be delayed for at least a year after tumor therapy is completed (24[R]).*

Growth hormone-release inhibiting hormone (somatostatin) and analogs

Somatostatin acts as a neurotransmitter, in the regulation of growth hormone and thyrotropin release, as a regulator of gastrointestinal and pancreatic function, and as an immune modulator. Its effects are mediated through at least five different receptors, which are present in varying concentrations in different organs. The synthetic analogs of somatostatin have different receptor affinities, and thus different clinical and adverse effect profiles to the native hormone, as well as having longer half-lives.

Cardiovascular *Sinus bradycardia* (less than 50 beats per minute) is reported in up to 25% of acromegalic patients taking octreotide, and conduction abnormalities are also commonly reported in these patients. This adverse effect is reported only rarely in other recipients of somatostatin or octreotide, probably reflecting the high rate of cardiac abnormalities due to acromegaly (38[cR]).

Biliary *Biliary sludge and gallstones* are frequent adverse effects of both octreotide (39[C]) and its longer acting analogs (40[C]). Ursodiol appeared to reverse gallbladder abnormalities in seven of ten patients given both medications and monitored with serial ultrasound. Data from this study also showed earlier development of sludge in recipients of higher doses of octreotide (40[C]).

Interactions *Morphine* analgesia appeared to be significantly reduced during somatostatin infusions in three patients with cancer. Opioid antagonist properties have previously been reported for somatostatin and its analogs (41[cr]).

In a controlled study of octreotide and *midodrine* (an alpha-adrenoceptor agonist) in patients with orthostatic hypotension, the pressor effect of the two drugs was synergistic (42[C]).

Vasopressin and analogs

Vasopressin has both antidiuretic and vasoconstrictor properties. The use of the native hormone and of triglycyl-lysine vasopressin (terlipressin) to treat acute variceal bleeding has been reviewed (43[R], 44[R]).

Desmopressin (*N*-deamino-8-*D*-arginine vasopressin, DDAVP) is an analog that has little vasoconstrictor effect but has potent antidiuretic action and hemostatic properties. Its use in bleeding disorders has been reviewed (45[R]).

Cardiovascular *Thromboembolic complications* have been rarely reported in recipients of DDAVP. Most events occurred in elderly men with other risk factors. One child developed cerebral ischemia after *Varicella* infection and DDAVP for enuresis (45[R]).

Cardiac adverse effects dictate the need for withdrawal in 20–30% of patients treated with vasopressin for variceal bleeding (44[R]). These *include increased systemic vascular resistance with bradycardia, reduced cardiac blood flow, myocardial ischemia, heart failure, and dysrhythmias.*

Hematological Mild to moderate *thrombocytopenia* has been reported in uremic patients treated with DDAVP. In the first case report of more severe thrombocytopenia, a 50-year-old uremic woman's platelet count fell from 149 $\times$ 10^9/l to 45 $\times$ 10^9/l after an abdominal hysterectomy with prophylactic DDAVP, and she developed a fatal subdural hemorrhage (46[cr]). DDAVP also stimulates fibrinolysis, and this may have contributed to the outcome in this patient (44[R]).

Mineral, fluid balance *Hyponatremia* and generalized convulsions have been reported in DDAVP recipients. The risk is increased in infants and patients receiving hypotonic intravenous fluids, and such patients need to be carefully monitored. Mild hyponatremia, which did not cause symptoms, was found in five of 399 children in an open multicenter trial (47^C).

REFERENCES

1. Maksymowych WP. Managing acute osteoporotic vertebral fractures with calcitonin. Can Fam Phys 1998;44:2160–6.
2. Passiu G, Bocchetta A, Martinelli V, Garau P, Del Zompo M, Mathieu A. Calcitonin decreases lithium plasma levels in man. Preliminary report. Int J Clin Pharm Res 1998;18:179–81.
3. Goa KL, Wagstaff AJ. Follitropin alpha in infertility. Biodrugs 1998;9:235–60.
4. Vollenhoven BJ, Healy DL. Short- and long-term effects of ovulation induction. Endocrinol Metab Clin North Am 1998;27:903–14.
5. Yim SF, Lau TK, Sahota DS, Chung TKH, Chang AMZ, Haines CJ. Prospective randomized study of the effect of 'add-back' hormone replacement on vascular function during treatment with gonadotropin-releasing hormone agonists. Circulation 1998;98:1631–5.
6. Warnock JK, Bundren JC, Morris DW. Depressive symptoms associated with gonadotropin-releasing hormone agonists. Depression Anxiety 1998;7:171–7.
7. Moghissi KS, Schlaff WD, Olive DL, Skinner MA, Yin H. Goserelin acetate (Zoladex) with or without hormone replacement therapy for the treatment of endometriosis. Fertil Steril 1998;69:1056–62.
8. Freundl G, Godtke K, Gnoth Ch, Godehardt E, Kienle E. Steroidal 'add-back' therapy in patients treated with GnRH agonists. Gynecol Obstet Invest 1998;45 Suppl 1:22–30.
9. Imai A, Takagi A, Horibe S, Fuseya T, Takagi H, Tamaya T. A gonadotropin-releasing hormone analogue impairs glucose tolerance in a diabetic patient. Eur J Obstet Gynecol Reprod Biol 1998;76:121–2.
10. Jirecek S, Nagele F, Huber JC, Wenzl R. Ovarian hyperstimulation syndrome caused by GnRH-analogue treatment without gonadotropin therapy in a patient with polycystic ovarian syndrome. Acta Obstet Gynecol Scand 1998;77:940–1.
11. Taylor CW, Green S, Dalton WS, Martino S, Rector D, Ingle JN, Robert NJ, Budd GT, Paradelo JC, Natale RB, Bearden JD, Mailliard JA, Osborne CK. Multicenter randomized clinical trial of goserelin versus surgical ovariectomy in premenopausal patients with receptor-positive metastatic breast cancer: an intergroup study. J Clin Oncol 1998;16:994–9.
12. Blethen S. Dosing, monitoring, and safety of growth hormone-replacement therapy in adults with growth hormone deficiency. Endocrinologist 1998;8:36S–40S.
13. Drake WM, Coyte D, Camacho-Hubner C, Jivanji NM, Kaltsas G, Wood DF, Trainer PJ, Grossman AB, Besser GM, Monson JP. Optimizing growth hormone replacement therapy by dose titration in hypopituitary adults. J Clin Endocrinol Metab 1998;83:3913–19.
14. Meling TR. Growth hormone deficiency in adults: the role of replacement therapy. Biodrugs 1998;9:351–62.
15. Thompson JL, Butterfield GE, Gylfadottir UK, Yesavage J, Marcus R, Hintz RL, Pearman A, Hoffman AR. Effects of human growth hormone, insulin-like growth factor 1, and diet and exercise on body composition of obese postmenopausal women. J Clin Endocrinol Metab 1998;83:1477–84.
16. Cuneo RC, Judd S, Wallace JD, Perry-Keene D, Burger H, Lim- Tio S, Strauss B, Stockigt J, Topliss D, Alford F, Hew L, Bode H, Conway A, Handelsman D, Dunn S, Boyages S, Cheung NW, Hurley D. The Australian multicenter trial of growth hormone (GH) treatment in GH-deficient adults. J Clin Endocrinol Metab 1998;83:107–16.
17. Crock PA, McKenzie JD, Nicoll AM, Howard NJ, Cutfield W, Shield LK, Byrne G. Benign intracranial hypertension and recombinant growth hormone therapy in Australia and New Zealand. Acta Paediatr Int J Paediatr 1998;87:381–6.
18. Haffner D, Nissel R, Wuhl E, Schaeffer F, Bettendorf M, Tonshoff B, Mehls O. Metabolic effects of long-term growth hormone treatment in prepubertal children with chronic renal failure and after kidney transplantation. Pediatr Res 1998;43:209–15.
19. Filler G, Amendt P, Kohnert K-D, Devaux S, Ehrich JHH. Glucose tolerance and insulin secretion in children before and during recombinant growth hormone treatment. Horm Res 1998;50:32–7.
20. Touati G, Prieur AM, Ruiz JC, Noel M, Czernichow P. Beneficial effects of one-year growth hormone administration to children with juvenile chronic arthritis on chronic steroid therapy. I. Effects on growth velocity and body composition. J Clin Endocrinol Metab 1998;83:403–9.
21. Singh KP, Prasad R, Chari PS, Dash RJ. Effect of growth hormone therapy in burn patients on conservative treatment. Burns 1998;24:733–8.
22. Nguyen B-Y, Clerici M, Venzon DJ, Bauza S, Murphy WJ, Longo DL, Baseler M, Gesundheit N, Broder S, Shearer G, Yarchoan R. Pilot study of the immunologic effects of recombinant human growth hormone and recombinant insulin-like growth factor in HIV-infected patients. AIDS 1998;12:895–904.

23. Filler G, Franke D, Amendt P, Ehrich JHH. Reversible diabetes mellitus during growth hormone therapy in chronic renal failure. Pediatr Nephrol 1998;12:405–7.
24. Frisch H. Pharmacovigilance: the use of KIGS (Pharmacia and Upjohn international growth database) to monitor the safety of growth hormone treatment in children. Endocrinol Metabol 1997;4 Suppl B:83–6.
25. Ruvalcaba RHA, Kletter GB. Abdominal lipohypertrophy caused by injections of growth hormone: a case report. Pediatrics 1998;102:408–10.
26. Koller EA, Green L, Gertner JM, Bost M, Malozowski SN. Retinal changes mimicking diabetic retinopathy in two nondiabetic, growth hormone-treated patients. J Clin Endocrinol Metab 1998;83:2380–3.
27. Antoniazzi F, Bertoldo F, Mottes M, Valli M, Sirpresi S, Zamboni G, Valentini R, Tato L. Growth hormone treatment in osteogenesis imperfecta with quantitative defect of type I collagen synthesis. J Pediatr 1996;129:432–9.
28. Kodama H, Kubota K, Abe T. Osteogenesis imperfecta: are fractures and growth hormone treatment linked? J Pediatr 1998;132:559.
29. Yap H-K, Loke K-Y, Murugasu B, Lee B-W. Subclinical activation of lupus nephritis by recombinant human growth hormone. Pediatr Nephrol 1998;12:133–5.
30. Anonymous. Leukemia in patients treated with growth hormone. Lancet 1988;1:1159–60.
31. Moshang T Jr. Use of growth hormone in children surviving cancer. Med Pediatr Oncol 1998;31:170–2.
32. Nishi Y, Tanaka T, Takano K, Fujieda K, Igarashi Y, Hanew K, Hirano T, Yokoya S, Tacibana K, Saito T, Watanabe S. Recent status in the occurrence of leukemia in growth hormone-treated patients in Japan. J Clin Endocrinol Metab 1999;84:1961–5.
33. Allen DB, Rundle AC, Graves DA, Blethen SL. Risk of leukemia in children treated with human growth hormone: review and reanalysis. J Pediatr 1997;131:S32–6.
34. Moshang T Jr, Rundle AC, Graves DA, Nickas J, Johanson A, Meadows A. Brain tumor recurrence in children treated with growth hormone: the National Cooperative Growth Study experience. J Pediatr 1996;128 (Suppl):S4–7.
35. Ogilvy-Stuart AL, Ryder WDJ, Gattamaneni HR, Clayton PE, Shalet SM. Growth hormone and tumour recurrence. Br Med J 1992;304:1601–5.
36. Price DA, Wilton P, Jonsson P, Albertsson-Wikland K, Chatelain P, Cutfield W, Ranke MB. Efficacy and safety of growth hormone treatment in children with prior craniopharyngioma: an analysis of the Pharmacia and Upjohn international growth database (KIGS) from 1988 to 1996. Horm Res 1998;49:91–7.
37. Tuffli GA, Johanson A, Rundle AC, Allen DB. Lack of increased risk of extracranial, nonleukemic neoplasms in recipients of recombinant deoxyribonucleic acid growth hormone. J Clin Endocrinol Metab 1995;80:1416–22.
38. Herrington AM, George KW, Moulds CC. Octreotide-induced bradycardia. Pharmacotherapy 1998;18:413–16.
39. Davies PH, Stewart SE, Lancranjan I, Sheppard MC, Stewart PM. Long-term therapy with long-acting octreotide (Sandostatin-LAR) for the management of acromegaly. Clin Endocrinol 1998; 48:311–16.
40. Avila NA, Shawker TH, Roach P, Bradford MH, Skarulis MC, Eastman R. Sonography of gallbladder abnormalities in acromegaly patients following octreotide and ursodiol therapy: incidence and time course. J Clin Ultrasound 1998;26:289–94.
41. Ripamonti C, De Conno F, Boffi R, Ascani L, Bianchi M. Can somatostatin be administered in association with morphine in advanced cancer patients with pain? Ann Oncol 1998;9:921–3.
42. Hoeldtke RD, Horvath GG, Bryner KD, Hobbs GR. Treatment of orthostatic hypertension with midodrine and octreotide. J Clin Endocrinol Metab 1998;83:339–43.
43. Avgerinos A. Approach to the management of bleeding esophageal varices: role of somatostatin. Digestion 1998;59 Suppl 1:1–22.
44. Burroughs AK, Planas R, Svoboda P. Optimizing emergency care of upper gastrointestinal bleeding in cirrhotic patients. Scand J Gastroenterol Suppl 1998;33:14–24.
45. Sutor AH. Desmopressin (DDAVP) in bleeding disorders of childhood. Semin Thromb Hemost 1998;24:555–66.
46. Sun HL, Chien CC. Thrombocytopenia and subdural hemorrhage after desmopressin administration. Anesthesiology 1998;88:1115–17.
47. Hjalmas K, Hanson E, Hellstrom A-L, Kruse S, Sillen U. Long- term treatment with desmopressin in children with primary monosymptomatic nocturnal enuresis: an open multicenter study. Br J Urol 1998;82:704–9.

I. Aursnes

44 Drugs affecting lipid metabolism

FIBRATES *(SED-13, 1324; SEDA-21, 458; SEDA-22, 490)*

Liver *Hepatitis* has been observed with etofibrate (1[c]), and one case of liver failure probably due to beclobrate has been reported (SED-13, 1324). Liver biopsies have shown a lymphoplasmocytic infiltrate in all of five cases with chronic hepatitis associated with fibrates (2[C]).

Skin and appendages *Photosensitivity* due to fenofibrate (3[c]) has been confirmed with systemic photochallenge (4[c]). *Chronic radiodermatitis* after cardiac catheterization has been observed in a 62-year-old woman taking ciprofibrate. A second catheterization performed when she had stopped taking it did not provoke new lesions (5[c]).

Musculoskeletal Reduced renal function in the elderly appears to be a risk factor for *myopathy.* A 73-year-old woman taking long-acting bezafibrate had an increase in serum creatinine and again when she was rechallenged by self-medication (6[c]).

Sexual function Gemfibrozil has been suspected to cause *reduced libido* in two cases (7[c], 8[c]) and four cases with loss of libido and impotence involving gemfibrozil have previously been reported (SED-13, 1325). Recently there has been another report of impotence (9[C]).

Interactions Several interactions between *warfarin* and hypolipidemic drugs have been described (SEDA-21, 459). This now also includes clinically important potentiation of warfarin by bezafibrate (10[c]) and gemfibrozil (11[c]). In the latter report the hypoprothombinemia was profound and the authors speculated that this interaction may often be overlooked. Two other patients developed significant intensification of the anticoagulant effect of warfarin while taking fenofibrate, and the authors supported the idea that coagulation factors in the blood are lowered 5–10 days after the start of therapy (12[c]).

HMG COENZYME-A REDUCTASE INHIBITORS *(SED-13, 1327; SEDA-22, 490)*

Nervous system *Peripheral neuropathy* occurs with statins, and perhaps with all cholesterol-lowering drugs, and may be related to reduced production of ubiquinone, as suggested by a recent review (13[CR]). Moreover, it appears that once a statin produces a neuropathy, rechallenge with any other statin is likely to cause a recurrence. This is reported to occur 1–3 weeks after rechallenge, whereas the resolution takes 4–6 weeks after withdrawal (13[CR]).

Endocrine, metabolic *Vascular collapse* may be related to low production of cortico-ster oids (14[C]). In a study of 521 patients taking simvastatin 40–80 mg/day, serum cortisol concentrations were on average reduced by 3–7% (15[C]). In the men there was a 10% fall in serum testosterone. However, there were no reports of *sexual dysfunction.*

After short-term treatment with pravastatin, a 77-year-old woman transiently developed symptoms diagnosed as *porphyria cutanea tarda* (16[c]).

Skin and appendages Adverse effects of statins on the skin are rarely seen. Potentially life-threatening *toxic epidermal necrolysis* oc-

Side Effects of Drugs, Annual 23
J.K. Aronson, ed.

curred in a 73-year-old moderately obese woman with type 2 diabetes and hypertension after she had taken 40 mg of atorvastatin (17[c]).

Musculoskeletal The number of patients with *rhabdomyolysis,* according to post-marketing reporting from the first million individuals taking lovastatin, was 24, of whom 17 had taken other medications that are known to increase this risk (18[R]). Rhabdomyolysis due to a short course of erythromycin in a 73-year-old man who had taken lovastatin for 7 years was accompanied by signs of multiple organ toxicity so severe as to mimic sepsis (19[c]). There is some evidence that patients with other illnesses may be at greater risk of myopathy than would be anticipated from the experience in controlled trials (20[C]).

Immunological and hypersensitivity reactions There were 25 serious hypersensitivity reactions (such as *arthralgia* and *thrombocytopenia*) among the first million patients taking lovastatin, at least some of which were considered to be due to the drug (21[R]). Severe *thrombocytopenia* occurred in a 75-year-old woman taking simvastatin 5 mg/day and was resistant to therapy until she developed a pneumonia. Recovery from the thrombocytopenia coincided with an increased interleukin concentration in the blood (22[C]). There was a close temporal association with *thrombotic thrombocytopenic purpura* in a 43-year-old man after his second dose of simvastatin (23[c]). *Thrombocytopenia* likewise occurred in a 46-year-old man coinciding with atorvastatin treatment (24[c]). The same patient had tolerated simvastatin, which led the authors to speculate whether there was idiosyncrasy directed specifically at atorvastatin.

Lupus-like symptoms have been reported in patients taking statins and a 67-year-old woman had a fatal reaction which started 1 week after she took fluvastatin 20 mg/day. When the drug was withdrawn 10 weeks later she had arthralgia, pains in the muscles, an erythematous maculopapular rash, and breathlessness due to a widespread alveolitis (25[c]). Simvastatin-induced *lupus erythematosus* was suspected in a 79-year-old white man after 3 months of treatment (26[C]). He had signs of pleuropericarditis that resolved within 2 weeks of withdrawal.

Interactions With the exception of fluvastatin and pravastatin, the statins are metabolized by CYP3A4. Other drugs metabolized by this enzyme can greatly enhance the concentration of the statin in the body and thereby precipitate rhabdomyolysis. With *itraconazole* there is a different susceptibility to interaction with statins through CYP3A4, in that simvastatin is more affected than pravastatin (27[C]). In another study the blood concentration of fluvastatin was not significantly increased, whereas that of lovastatin was (28[C]). Concomitant use of simvastatin with itraconazole should be avoided, and the same holds true according to another report for atorvastatin (29[C]). Similarly, *diltiazem* interacts with lovastatin but not with pravastatin (30[C]). These potential interactions have not been studied systematically for all statins.

INDIVIDUAL HMG COENZYME-A REDUCTASE INHIBITORS

Atorvastatin *(SEDA-20, 409; SEDA-21, 460; SEDA-22, 491)*

Pooled data from 21 completed and 23 continuing trials representing 3000 patient-years have shown that *constipation, flatulence, dyspepsia, abdominal pain, headache,* and *myalgia* occur in 1–3% of patients. Under 2% of atorvastatin-treated patients discontinued treatment secondary to an adverse effect (31[R]). Serious events in this review amounted to one patient with *pancreatitis* and one with *cholestatic jaundice* (31[R]).

Interactions Atorvastatin, although a substrate for CYP3A4, does not affect blood terfenadine concentrations to a clinically significant extent (32[C]).

Cerivastatin *(SEDA-22, 491)*

A summary of the phase IIb/III studies on this drug has shown a similarity to other statins concerning *hepatic and renal toxicity.* At dosages of 0.3–0.4 mg/day after 8 weeks in 349 patients there were no rises in creatine phosphokinase activity above 10 times the upper limit of the reference range, and asymptomatic increases (to over three times the upper limit of the reference range) occurred more often with placebo (2.8%) than with cerivastatin (1.4% with 0.4 mg; none with 0.3 mg) (33[R]).

Lovastatin *(SED-13, 1329)*

Lovastatin in combination with gemfibrozil caused a *rise in creatine kinase* activity to 234 000 U/l, with complete remission after both drugs had been discontinued (34[c]).

Pravastatin *(SED-13, 1329; SEDA-21, 460)*

Although myopathy is rarely seen with pravastatin in clinical trials, it does occur and *rhabdomyolysis* was suspected in a 67-year-old obese man having an acute myocardial infarction (35[C]).

Simvastatin *(SED-13, 1329; SEDA-22, 492)*

Respiratory Hypersensitivity reactions can occur with statins (SED-13,1328), and an otherwise unexplained case of *interstitial lung disease and pleural effusion* developed during treatment with simvastatin for six months (36[c]).

Skin and appendages A 66-year-old man had persistent photosensitivity after using simvastatin intermittently (37[c]). The clinical, histopathological, and photobiological features met the criteria for *chronic actinic dermatitis.*

Interactions Simvastatin should be avoided in patients taking other drugs with effects on CYP3A4 (28[C]) and in patients using *grapefruit juice* (38[C]). Severe rhabdomyolysis occurred in a 52-year-old woman taking a combination of gemfibrozil and simvastatin (39[c]). Raised serum lactic dehydrogenase activity often follows the rise in creatine kinase. In a patient with steroid-resistant nephrotic syndrome, an increase in lactic dehydrogenase activity indicated tissue injury in the absence of an increase in creatine kinase (40[c]).

REFERENCES

1. Macedo G, Ribeiro T. Etofibrate induced acute hepatitis mimicking biliary tract disease. Arq Med 1996;10:185–6.
2. Ganne-Carrie N, De Leusse A, Guetter C, Castera L, Levecq H, Bertrand H-J, Plumet Y, Trinchet J-C, Beaugrand M. Auto-immune hepatitis associated with fibrate treatment. Gastroenterol Clin Biol 1998;22:525–9.
3. Leroy D, Dompmartin A, Lorier E, Leport Y, Audebert C. Photosensitivity induced by fenofibrate. Photodermatol Photoimmunol Photomed 1990;7:136–8.
4. Leenutaphong V, Manuskiatti W. Fenofibrate-induced photosensitivity. J Am Acad Dermatol 1996;35:775–7.
5. Gironet NJANV, Machet M-C, Machet L, Lorette G, Vaillant L. Chronic radiodermatitis after cardiac catheterization induced by ciprofibrate (Lipanor)? Ann Dermatol Venereol 1998;125:598–600.
6. Terrovitou CT, Milionis HJ, Elisaf MS. Acute rhabdomyolysis after bezafibrate re-exposure. Nephron 1998;78:336–7.
7. Bain SC, Lemon M, Jones AF. Gemfibrozil-induced impotence. Lancet 1990;336:1389.
8. Pizarro S, Bargay J, D'Agosto P. Gemfibrozil-induced impotence. Lancet 1990;336:1135.
9. Pedrajas JNA, Pardal JLP. Gemfibrozil-induced impotence. An Med Interna 1998;15:175–6.
10. Beringer TR. Warfarin potentiation with bezafibrate. Postgrad Med J 1997;73:657–8.
11. Rindone JP, Keng H-C. Gemfibrozil-warfarin drug interaction resulting in profound hypoprothrombinemia. Chest 1998;114:641–2.
12. Ascah KJ, Rock GA, Wells PS. Interaction between fenofibrate and warfarin. Ann Pharmacother 1998;32:765–8.
13. Ziajka PE, Wehmeier T. Peripheral neuropathy and lipid-lowering therapy. South Med J 1998;91:667–8.
14. French J, White H. Transient symptomatic hypotension in patients on simvastatin. Lancet 1989;2:807–8.
15. Stein EA, Davidson MH, Dobs AS, Schrott H, Dujovne CA, Bays H, Weiss SR, Melino MR, Stapanavage ME, Mitchel YB. Efficacy and safety of simvastatin 80 mg/day in hypercholesterolemic patients. Am J Cardiol 1998;82:311–16.
16. Schindl A, Trautinger F, Pernerstorfer-Schon H, Konnaris C, Honigsmann H. Porphyria cutanea tarda induced by the use of pravastatin. Arch Dermatol 1998;134:1305–6.
17. Pfeiffer CM, Kazenoff S, Rothberg HD. Toxic epidermal necrolysis from atorvastatin. J Am Med Assoc 1998;279:1613–14.
18. Mantell G, Burke MT, Staggers J. Extended clinical safety profile of lovastatin. Am J Cardiol 1990;66:11–15.
19. Wong PWK, Dillard TA, Kroenke K. Multiple organ toxicity from addition of erythromycin to long-term lovastatin therapy. South Med J 1998;91:202–5.
20. Duell PB, Connor WE, Illingworth DR. Rhabdomyolysis after taking atorvastatin with gemfibrozil. Am J Cardiol 1998;81:368–9.
21. Tobert JA, Shear CL, Chremos AN, Mantell GE. Clinical experience with lovastatin. Am J Cardiol 1990;65:23–6.

22. Yamada T, Shinohara K, Katsuki K. Severe thrombocytopenia caused by simvastatin in which thrombocyte recovery was initiated after severe bacterial infection. Clin Drug Invest 1998;16:172–4.
23. McCarthy LJ, Porcu P, Fausel CA, Sweeney CJ, Danielson CFM. Thrombotic thrombocytopenic purpura and simvastatin. Lancet 1998;352:1284–5.
24. Gonzalez-Ponte ML, Gonzalez-Ruiz M, Duvos E, Gutierrez-Iniguez MA, Olalla JI, Conde E. Atorvastatin-induced severe thrombocytopenia. Lancet 1998;352:1284.
25. Sridhar MK, Abdulla A. Fatal lupus-like syndrome and ARDS induced by fluvastatin. Lancet 1998;352:114.
26. Khosla R, Butman AN, Hammer DF. Simvastatin-induced lupus erythematosus. South Med J 1998;91:873–4.
27. Neuvonen PJ, Kantola T, Kivisto KT. Simvastatin but not pravastatin is very susceptible to interaction with the CYP3A4 inhibitor itraconazole. Clin Pharmacol Ther 1998;63:332–41.
28. Kivisto KT, Kantola T, Neuvonen PJ. Different effects of itraconazole on the pharmacokinetics of fluvastatin and lovastatin. Br J Clin Pharmacol 1998;46:49–53.
29. Kantola T, Kivisto KT, Neuvonen PJ. Effect of itraconazole on the pharmacokinetics of atorvastatin. Clin Pharmacol Ther 1998;64:58–65.
30. Azie NE, Brater DC, Becker PA, Jones DR, Hall SD. The interaction of diltiazem with lovastatin and pravastatin. Clin Pharmacol Ther 1998;64:369–77.
31. Yee HS, Fong NT. Atorvastatin in the treatment of primary hypercholesterolemia and mixed dyslipidemias. Ann Pharmacother 1998;32:1030–43.
32. Stern RH, Smithers JA, Olson SC. Atorvastatin does not produce a clinically significant effect on the pharmacokinetics of terfenadine. J Clin Pharmacol 1998;38:753–7.
33. Davignon J, Hanefeld M, Nakaya N, Hunninghake DB, Insull W Jr, Ose L. Clinical efficacy and safety of cerivastatin: Summary of pivotal phase IIb/III studies. Am J Cardiol 1998;82:32J–39J.
34. Deltoro MG, Rocati G, Cavanilles CR, Cervellera AG-C, Catala JC, Belda JEB, De Lelis FP, Rodena JVP, Gonzalez EO, Ballester AH. Rhabdomyolysis and renal failure due to lovastatin-gemfibrozil. A case report. Endocrinologia 1998; 45:35–7.
35. Offman EM, Sabawi N, Melendez LJ. Suspected pravastatin-induced rhabdomyolysis in a patient experiencing a myocardial infarction. Can. J Hosp Pharm 1998;51:233–5.
36. De Groot RE, Willems LN, Dijkman JH. Interstitial lung disease with pleural effusion caused by simvastatin. J Intern Med 1996;239:361–3.
37. Granados MTRDE, La Torre C, Cruces MJ, Pineiro G. Chronic actinic dermatitis due to simvastatin. Contact Dermatitis 1998;38:294–5.
38. Lilja JJ, Kivisto KT, Neuvonen PJ. Grapefruit juice-simvastatin interaction: effect on serum concentrations of simvastatin, simvastatin acid, and HMG-CoA reductase inhibitors. Clin Pharmacol Ther 1998;64:477–83.
39. Tal A, Rajeshawari M, Isley W. Rhabdomyolysis associated with simvastatin-gemfibrozil therapy. South Med J 1997;90:546–7.
40. Ogawa D, Maruyama K, Miyatake N, Kashihara N, Makino H. Concomitant use of simvastatin and cyclosporin A increases LDH in nephrotic syndrome. Nephron 1998;80:351–2.

Andrew Stanley

45 Cytostatic drugs

Author's note: *The wide range of cytostatic drugs, the multitude of their toxic effects, and the fact that they are generally used in combinations of several agents all make it impossible to provide as detailed an overview of adverse reactions in this field as the Annual gives in others. This year most of this chapter is devoted to a special review of the adverse effects of fluorouracil.*

R ## *Fluorouracil*

Fluorouracil is a fluorinated pyrimidine, which is converted intracellularly to the active form, fluorodeoxyuridine monophosphate, which inhibits thymidylate synthetase and hence reduces the production of thymidylic acid, the deoxyribonucleotide of thymine (5-methyluracil), a DNA pyrimidine base, blocking DNA synthesis. Fluorouracil is specific to the S phase of the cell cycle. It is used to treat carcinoma of the breast, ovary, and skin, and adenocarcinoma of the gastrointestinal tract, and it can be given intravenously or topically.

Cardiovascular *The cardiotoxicity of fluorouracil was first identified in 1975 (1[C]). Of 140 patients treated with intravenous 5-fluorouracil, four developed ischaemic chest pain within 18 hours of either the second or third dose. In three of these patients the pain recurred after subsequent doses. Predose electrocardiograms in two cases were normal. None of the four patients had a history of ischaemic heart disease, although all had received left ventricular irradiation (2[c]). A survey of 1083 patients in 1982 reported cardiotoxicity in 1.1% of all patients and in 4.6% of patients with prior evidence of heart disease (3[C]). The association is more striking in those patients who receive a continuous infusion of fluorouracil and in patients who receive concomitant cisplatin (4[c], 5[c]). For example, myocardial ischemia and infarction occur in about 10% of patients who receive fluorouracil by infusion and sudden death has occurred (6[R]).*

More frequent use of fluorouracil by continuous infusion, increased awareness of the problems, and more sophisticated monitoring have increased the reported incidence. By 1990 there were more than 67 clinical cases described (7[C]) and an incidence ranging up to 68% of silent ischemic electrocardiographic changes was identified in patients monitored by continuous 24-hour ambulatory electrocardiography during fluorouracil infusion (8[C]). The clinical features include the following:

- *Precordial pain (both non-specific and anginal) (7[c]).*
- *Electrocardiographic ST-T wave changes (non-specific and ischemic) (7[c], 8[c]).*
- *Acute myocardial infarction (rare) (9[c], 10[c]).*
- *Atrial dysrhythmias (including atrial fibrillation) and less often, ventricular extra beat (including refractory ventricular tachycardia and fibrillation) (8[c]–10[c]).*
- *Ventricular dysfunction (usually global, less frequently segmental).*
- *Cardiac failure, pulmonary edema, and cardiogenic shock (with and without ischemic symptoms) (10[c]–13[c]).*
- *Sudden death (10[c]).*

These events occur in patients who have no known underlying coronary vessel disease and the pathogenesis seems to be coronary artery spasm. Anginal symptoms are often a precursor, and can be relieved by discontinuing the fluorouracil. In most cases, the dysrhythmia was treatable and the ischemic-like symptoms and electrocardiographic changes disappeared (if the infusion was discontinued) or responded

Side Effects of Drugs, Annual 23
J.K. Aronson, ed.

to nitrates, allowing the infusion to continue. The abnormalities of segmental and global ventricular function reverted to normal within days to weeks of withdrawal. Some patients needed intravenous inotropic and vasodilator support during the initial period (11[c]–14[c]). In most patients with chest pains, with or without electrocardiographic changes, the creatinine kinase MB fraction remained normal (7[c], 10[c], 12[c]).

Five cases of paroxysmal atrial fibrillation and sinus bradycardia attributed to fluorouracil have been reported (15[c]). These are probably the least well documented cardiac complications associated with fluorouracil and this work is therefore of particular importance.

Acute pulmonary edema leading to lethal cardiogenic shock has been reported with fluorouracil. This is believed to be the first reported case and it occurred despite the fact that the patient had received eight infusions of leucovorin 100 mg/m^2 at weekly intervals (16[c]). Most often the patient developed cardiotoxicity during the second or later course of treatment, but some had problems during the first course (7[c]). Those who developed cardiac toxicity and recovered usually had symptoms again when re-challenged with another infusion (7[c], 10[c]).

The mechanism of fluorouracil cardiotoxicity is still uncertain. The ischemic-like pains and electrocardiographic findings, lack of changes in creatine kinase (MB fraction) and frequent responses to nitrates and at times to calcium antagonists in the setting of anatomically normal coronary angiography, plus reversible contractility defects, suggest coronary vasospasm as a mechanism of fluorouracil cardiotoxicity. However, the global dysfunction possibly due to stunned myocardium and the lack of universal response to coronary vasodilators leaves some questions about this hypothesis. Some investigators have postulated myocarditis or myocardiopathy (17–19). In 43 patients it did not interfere with the electrical properties of myocardial fibers (20[C]).

With regard to risk factors for cardiotoxicity with fluorouracil, there was no influence of age or sex on incidence (7[c]). Symptoms have been reported in a 38-year-old man (13[c]) and in several women in their 40s (7[c], 11[c]) with no prior cardiac history. Cardiac findings have occurred when fluorouracil was given by infusion or bolus as a single agent or with cisplatin and other drugs (7[c], 21[c]). Although some felt that cardiac irradiation and pre-existing heart disease were risk factors (3[C], 8[c]), others did not (7[c], 22[c]). Several investigators documented normal coronary arteries in patients with severe symptoms (10[c], 11[c]). Findings on autopsy and endomyocardial biopsy have shown diffuse, interstitial edema, intracytoplasmic vacuolization of myocytes, and no inflammatory infiltrate (23[c]). Acute myocardial infarction has been demonstrated pathologically in some, but not all, patients with clinical infarction (7[c]).

Some investigators have reported success in preventing cardiotoxicity with calcium antagonists, such as nifedipine and diltiazem (24[c]), while others had less success (12[c], 25[c]). Two patients with proven fluorouracil cardiotoxicity did not have cardiotoxicity when treated with the specific thymidylate synthase inhibitor raltitrexed 3 mg/m^2 every 3 weeks (26[c]). The authors commented that fluorouracil cardiotoxicity is therefore not mediated via thymidylate synthase.

Careful observation for cardiac symptoms and dysrhythmias is warranted during fluorouracil infusion, especially in patients who were symptomatic during prior courses.

Vascular *Fluorouracil has been associated with a number of vascular effects, particularly thromboembolic or circulatory in nature (27[c]). Although Raynaud's phenomenon has been reported after cisplatin-based chemotherapy, the first case of digital ischemia and Raynaud's phenomenon has been reported with fluorouracil given in a De Gramond type schedule (28[c]).*

Respiratory Fibrosing alveolitis *Pulmonary toxicity in the form of fibrosing alveolitis has been reported in a 55-year-old man with gastric adenocarcinoma, treated with fluorouracil (29[c]). The patient received fluorouracil 1 g intravenously each week for 9 weeks and mitomycin 10 mg intravenously every 3 weeks. After 12 treatments the patient developed severe dyspnea. Although mitomycin C was most likely the agent responsible for pulmonary toxicity in this patient, combined use with fluorouracil as a contributing factor cannot be ruled out. Necropsy confirmed that the patient had interstitial fibrosis (30[c]).*

Nervous system *Fluorouracil has been known to cause neurotoxicity since the earliest clinical trials (31[c]). The incidence of neurotoxicity is 5–15% and occurs with all schedules of ad-*

ministration in common use (32[R], 33[R]). The toxicity is acute in onset and a cumulative dose-dependency has not been observed.

Acute cerebellar dysfunction, with gait ataxia, nystagmus, dysmetria, and dysarthria, is the most common form of neurotoxicity (31[c], 32[R]). Confusion and cerebral cognitive defects have also been reported (32[R], 34[c]). A rare problem is optic neuropathy and impaired vision (35[c]).

The acute cerebellar syndrome is considered to be associated with peak concentrations of fluorouracil (31[c], 36[R]). Continuous 5-day infusions appear not to cause neurological toxicity, even when the total dose is higher, although high-dose infusions can cause encephalopathy, with symptoms varying from lethargy to coma (37[R]).

A single case of cerebral demyelination has been reported in a patient receiving fluorouracil and levamisole (38[c]).

Two patients showing some of the classic fluorouracil neurological complications have been reported. One had a cerebellar syndrome in association with global motor weakness and bulbar palsy and the other a bilateral third cranial nerve palsy (39[c]).

The first two cases of peripheral neuropathy possibly caused by fluorouracil have been reported (40[c]).

Five patients developed ischemic stroke within 2–5 days of finishing a 4-day course of fluorouracil plus low-dose cisplatin by continuous infusion (41[c]). Whilst cisplatin has been implicated as having produced central ischemic events, most commonly in combination with vindesine and bleomycin, there has only been one other report involving fluorouracil. Although the casual link was not conclusive, the circumstantial evidence was strong. The cause of neurotoxicity is not well understood. Acute neurological symptoms, including somnolence, cerebellar ataxia, and upper motor neuron signs, are primarily seen in patients receiving intracarotid infusions for head and neck tumors and also in patients receiving fluorouracil monotherapy in high doses. This syndrome has been reproduced in animals by a neurotoxic metabolite of fluorouracil, fluorocitrate, which has been believed to cause neurotoxicity (42, 43). However, several patients have developed severe toxic symptoms due to deficiency of dihydropyrimidine dehydrogenase the enzyme that is mainly responsible for metabolizing fluorouracil (44[C]). This toxicity appears to be due to the parent compound and not metabolites. Patients with complete or partial deficiency of the enzyme are particularly subject to fluorouracil neurotoxicity.

The neurotoxicity is usually reversible by withdrawing fluorouracil. Since there is no cumulative effect, therapy can be resumed later if desired, usually with either a lower dose or a less frequent dosing schedule to prevent recurrence.

Endocrine, metabolic *Patients with poorly controlled diabetes are at risk of greater or more severe fluorouracil toxicity, causing hyperglycemia, which has been fatal. This toxic effect seems to be independent of previous diabetic control and/or schedules of the fluorouracil (45[C]).*

There have been attempts to unravel the mechanism of fluorouracil-induced hyperammonemia, lactic acidosis, and encephalopathy, a rare toxic effect associated with high dose therapy. The various authors seem not to be able to reach a single causative mechanism, although Krebs cycle metabolism is almost certainly involved (46[c]–48[c]).

Hematological *The hematological toxicity of fluorouracil is dose-dependent and schedule-dependent (49[R]). Leukocytes and platelets are affected, although the latter less so. Myelosuppression begins 4–7 days after the first dose, with recovery usually 14 days after the last dose (50[R]). With continued treatment anemia can develop in 3–4 months (51[C]). Severe bone-marrow depression causing death has been reported (52[C]).*

Leukopenia *Leukopenia is the most common blood dyscrasia secondary to fluorouracil and usually occurs after every course. The lowest white cell counts are usually seen between the 9th and the 14th day after the first course of treatment, but can be delayed for up to 20 days (53[C], 54[C]). Leukopenia usually resolves after drug withdrawal. This rapid onset leukopenia is often followed by megaloblastic anemia (55[C]). Agranulocytosis has been reported during fluorouracil therapy (54[c]).*

Thrombocytopenia *Thrombocytopenia has occurred during fluorouracil therapy but is much less frequent than leukopenia (44[c]). The following summarizes the dose-dependency of the hematological effects of fluorouracil (56[C], 57[C]):*

- *with a daily bolus of 12 mg/kg for 5 days, leukopenia (under 4 × 10^9/l) occurred in all of 70 patients; 31% had marked leukopenia (under 2 × 10^9/l);*
- *with a continuous infusion of 30 mg/kg/day for 5 days, the leukopenia was mild and occurred in only 12% of patients;*
- *a protracted continuous infusion of 300 mg/m²/day caused one case of moderate leukopenia and four cases of mild/moderate thrombocytopenia;*
- *with a daily bolus of 500 mg/m² for 5 days there was in a 38% incidence of leukopenia (with 20% below 2 × 10^9/l and an 8% incidence of thrombocytopenia (1% severe)).*

Liver Hepatic fibrosis *It has been suggested that handling cytostatic agents may insidiously cause hepatic damage and possibly irreversible fibrosis. Three case reports of hepatic injury in nurses after years of handling cytotoxic drugs (bleomycin, vincristine, cyclophosphamide, doxorubicin, dacarbazine, fluorouracil, and methotrexate) have been described (58[c]). All had neurological symptoms associated with raised serum alanine aminotransferase and alkaline phosphatase activities. Liver biopsy showed portal hepatitis, with piecemeal necrosis in one and hepatic fibrosis and fat accumulation in the others.*

Hepatic necrosis *Diffuse hepatic necrosis has been described in a 29-year-old man receiving 500 mg/day for 4 days (route of administration unspecified) for adenocarcinoma (59[c]). The patient developed nausea, vomiting, diarrhea, and massive and diffuse hepatic necrosis. The drug was withdrawn and the patient died 2 days later (6 days after starting medication). However, the role of fluorouracil in inducing hepatic disease in this patient is unclear.*

Ascites *In a retrospective analysis of a study of N-phosphonoacetyl-L-aspartate (250 mg/m²) followed by weekly boluses of fluorouracil (600–800 mg/m²) in 44 patients with metastatic colorectal cancer, five of 17 patients with complete or partial responses to therapy developed transient ascites (with or without associated hypoalbuminemia) compared with one of 27 without such a response (60[C]). Other significant findings in some of the responders included raised bilirubin concentrations and transaminase activities from metastasis. The authors cautioned that the adverse effects observed do not necessarily represent disease progression.*

Biliary Biliary sclerosis causing cholestatic jaundice *Cholestatic jaundice associated with biliary sclerosis is a serious complication of intra-hepatic infusion and is believed to result from perfusion of the blood supply to the gall bladder and upper bile duct with high local concentrations of the drug. Continuous intrahepatic infusion of fluorouracil is a useful alternative to intravenous therapy in patients with hepatic metastases. The response rate reported for the treatment of colon cancer patients with hepatic metastases approaches 50%. Because at least 50% of fluorouracil is cleared in the first pass through the liver, systemic toxicity with this form of therapy is mild, consisting primarily of oral mucositis and gastrointestinal symptoms, such as nausea, vomiting, diarrhea, and less often myelosuppression. The median time to onset of biliary sclerosis is three treatment cycles, and although fluorouracil may be re-instituted at a lower dose after normalization of serum hepatic enzyme activities, most patients become progressively less tolerant.*

Gastrointestinal *Any site along the gastrointestinal tract can be affected, resulting in symptoms such as nausea and vomiting, stomatitis, dysphagia, retrosternal burning, abdominal pain, diarrhea, and proctitis.*

The spectrum of toxic effects associated with fluorouracil varies considerably according to the dose, dosage schedule, and route of administration. Stomatitis and diarrhea are frequent adverse effects, particularly in patients who received a 5-day regimen. An alternative regimen using continuous intravenous infusion of fluorouracil at doses of 30 mg/kg/day for 5 days gives equivalent therapeutic results but a different pattern of toxicity (61[C]). Gastrointestinal symptoms, such as stomatitis and diarrhea, are the principal dose-limiting toxic effects, but myelosuppression is less intense. When fluorouracil is given in combination with leucovorin in patients with metastatic colon cancer, there is enhanced gastrointestinal toxicity, irrespective of the fluorouracil schedule.

Stomatitis is common and can be severe and life-threatening (54[C]). Stomatitis may be preceded by a dry mouth and erythema of the mucosa followed by a white patchy membrane.

In severe cases this is followed by ulceration and necrosis. Breakdown of the mucosa is very painful and can act as a focus for infection (50[R]). Xerostomia at the start of therapy and a baseline neutrophil count of under 4 × 10^9/l are significantly associated with dose-limiting oral mucositis later in chemotherapy, according to the results of a logistic regression analysis of 63 patients (62[C]). Mouth-cooling with oral ice chips for 30 minutes starting immediately before fluorouracil substantially reduced the severity of mucositis.

Nausea and vomiting is frequent but generally mild (54[C]).

Gastric ulceration has been reported in patients receiving fluorouracil by intrahepatic infusion via percutaneous catheterization in doses of 20–30 mg/kg for 4 days followed by 15 mg/kg over 17 days. Symptoms were observed from 4–20 days after starting therapy (63[C]). Gastrointestinal bleeding in three patients and death in one patient were also reported following intra-arterial fluorouracil (64[C]).

Diarrhea is common, particularly in patients who receive a 5-day regimen. The diarrhea my be watery or bloody and life-threatening in severe cases. Repeated episodes of watery diarrhea (more than 3 movements per day) for several days should alert the oncologist to the potential dangers of dehydration and sepsis, which represent potentially fatal adverse effects. Life-threatening diarrhea with hematemesis, high intestinal obstruction, melena, septicemia, and shock have been reported after total doses of 4–4.5 g of fluorouracil (65[c]). Similarly, diarrhea followed by neutropenia and life-threatening or fatal sepsis occurred in two of 55 patients with advanced colorectal carcinoma in a pilot study of continuous infusion of fluorouracil (750 mg/m²/day for 5 days) plus subcutaneous recombinant interferon alfa 2a (6–18 million units/day) (66[C]). Severe diarrhea and mucosal ulceration of the colon with necrosis has also been reported (67[c]).

A 53-year-old man had a side-to-side ileo-descending colostomy for disseminated carcinoma. Fluorouracil was given in doses of 15 mg/kg for 4 days, then 7.5 mg/kg intravenously on days 6 and 8. He developed severe diarrhea and severe ulceration of the by-passed portion of the colon, resulting in necrosis, and death occurred as the result of bronchopneumonia. Autopsy showed ulcers from the ileocecal valve to the ileo-colostomy site. The mucosa of the stomach, small intestine, and colon distal to the colostomy were not involved.

In two cases the diarrhea and colitis associated with fluorouracil therapy were caused by toxigenic Clostridium difficile. Both patients responded to oral vancomycin (68[c]). Colitis has been reported as a rare complication of fluorouracil treatment. Two cases have been reported after intra-arterial chemotherapy (69[c]). A further case has been reported, described by the authors as neutropenic enterocolitis, presenting as abdominal pain, diarrhea, and neutropenia (70[c]). Proven pseudomembranous colitis followed 36 weekly doses of fluorouracil (700 mg) and folinic acid (150 mg); the authors believed that this was only the second reported case (71[c]).

Skin and appendages *Two types of skin rashes occur with fluorouracil. The more common form involves erythema of exposed skin areas. With continued fluorouracil therapy the skin becomes hyperpigmented, thin, and atrophic (52[C]). Patients treated with fluorouracil also have an increased susceptibility to sunburn (72[C]). Less commonly (about 1.5%), a severe seborrheic pruritic dermatitis occurs (52[C]). These rashes are usually reversible on withdrawal of fluorouracil.*

Asymptomatic hyperpigmentation *Serpentine supravenous hyperpigmentation is a peculiar dermatological effect seen with continuous infusions of fluorouracil (52[C]). Hyperpigmentation occurs only in the tissues overlying the veins proximal to the infusion site in the limb used. The veins are not sclerosed and usually remain patent (73[C]). This has also been reported in a 56-year-old black man after intravenous fluorouracil 750 mg/m²/week over 24 weeks for stage D prostatic carcinoma (74[c]). The patient developed nasal mucosal friability, diffuse pigmentation of the face and hands, and markedly increased pigmentation of the skin immediately overlying the veins that had been used for multiple fluorouracil infusions. Many irregular dark streaks were noted, extending from the hand to the shoulder. These streaks were 1–1.5 cm wide and serpiginous in their course.*

Linear serpentine erythematous eruption overlying the superficial veins on both arms after infusion of fluorouracil has been reported (75[c]). There was residual macular pigmentation, which persisted for 3 months after withdrawal of the fluorouracil.

Contact dermatitis *Topical fluorouracil has been associated with allergic contact dermatitis in patients with actinic keratosis and basal cell epitheliomas (76[c]). Topical fluorouracil ointment (5%) was reported to exacerbate dermatitis when it was mistakenly given instead of fluocinonide ointment (77[c]).*

Hair changes *Partial reversible alopecia is common after systemic fluorouracil therapy (54[C]).*

Nail changes *Diffuse blue superficial pigmentation, onycholysis, dystrophy, pain and thickening of the nail bed, transverse striations, half and half nail changes, paronychial inflammation, hyperpigmentation, and nail loss have all been reported with fluorouracil therapy (78[c]–80[c]). It has further been reported that the blue pigment may be scraped off (78[c]).*

Telangiectasia *Telangiectasia and herpes labialis have been reported in four patients receiving topical 1% fluorouracil in propylene glycol applied three times a day for 7–28 days. Two patients developed herpes labialis 7–10 days after the start of therapy and two developed persistent telangiectasia at the application site (81[c]).*

Potentiation of tumor response and cutaneous toxicity by ionizing radiation *Fluorouracil not only augments the therapeutic effect of ionizing radiation on tumors but also increases its mucocutaneous toxicity. The likelihood of severe toxicity within the radiation field is increased significantly and relates to the area irradiated (e.g. oral stomatitis, esophagitis, enteritis, and skin desquamation). The onset of these effects is within 7 days of the start of radiation.*

Hand-foot syndrome or palmar-plantar erythrodysesthesia *Fluorouracil, alone or in combination regimens, via continuous or intermittent infusions or bolus doses, has been associated with a rare syndrome of unknown cause, characterized by varying degrees of painful, erythematous, swollen palms of the hand and soles of the feet (82). Tingling, tenderness, and desquamation can also occur. Pain can be so severe as to inhibit walking and hand grasping (82[c]). The onset of the reaction has ranged from 3 days to 10 months (82[c], 83[c]). Severity appeared to be dose-related in one case (84[c]). The condition gradually subsides over 5–7 days when the drug is withdrawn (84[c]). However, it may recur on rechallenge (83[c]). Pyridoxine 100–150 mg/day has been used to manage this syndrome, allowing continued treatment in a small number of patients (85[c], 86[c]).*

Bullous pemphigoid *A case of bullous pemphigoid was reported in an 84-year-old man after topical therapy with fluorouracil 1% solution daily over several days for actinic keratosis. All treated lesions became bullous, with the development of a few bullae on untreated areas of normal skin. Bullous lesions were pruritic and sore and some contained hemorrhagic fluid. There was a leukocytosis (11.7×10^9/l). The blister fluid contained predominantly eosinophils, and immunofluorescent studies of the serum and blister fluid showed anti-basement membrane antibody titers of 1 : 640 and 1 : 160 respectively. Fluorouracil was discontinued and the patient was treated with steroids and saline compresses, with abatement of symptoms (87[c]).*

Special senses Excessive lacrimation and conjunctivitis *Excessive lacrimation and other ocular disturbances have been reported secondary to intravenous fluorouracil (88[c]–90[c]). In a review of this subject, blurred vision, excessive lacrimation, excessive nasal discharge, and conjunctivitis were the most commonly reported ocular effects of fluorouracil (91[R]). Patients may find that their symptoms, eye irritation and excessive tear production, are aggravated by cold weather. The onset of symptoms varies from 15 minutes to 14 months after the start of treatment (88[c]). Symptoms usually resolve 2–3 weeks after withdrawal of therapy, with or without the use of topical antibiotic-steroid combinations (88[c], 91[R]).*

Tear duct fibrosis (dacryostenosis) and eversion of lower eyelid (ectropion) *More severe toxic effects including tear duct fibrosis and eversion of the lower eye lid have been reported (88[c]). Tear duct fibrosis develops in one of six patients with excessive lacrimation from fluorouracil (92[c]). The eversion of the lower eye lid is reversible with conservative management (93[c]), whilst the tear duct fibrosis may not be (94[c]). Persistent lacrimation has been described in six patients receiving intraven-*

ous fluorouracil weekly for 6–10 months (94[c]). Lacrimation persisted in five patients after the withdrawal of fluorouracil suggesting an irreversible dacryostenosis. Lacrimal duct stenosis has also been reported (95[c]). Bilateral cicatricial ectropion was also reported in a patient after topical administration of fluorouracil for the treatment of multiple facial actinic keratoses (96[c]). If ectropion and tear duct stenosis progress, surgical correction may be required.

Three women developed lacrimal outflow obstruction while receiving fluorouracil, cyclophosphamide, and methotrexate for breast cancer (97[c]). The authors reported on the severity of the adverse effect. They commented on both the high incidence of excessive tearing in patients given fluorouracil, a probable pre-condition, and the rarity of permanent damage (12 patients reported world wide), but counselled on the need for vigilance and early referral to an ophthalmologist. Others have suggested that the prevalence of tearing and canalicular fibrosis in patients receiving fluorouracil is related to total dose and duration of treatment, and that the risks become significant at 20–60 weeks of therapy and a total fluorouracil dose of 20–50 g (98[C]).

Ankyloblepharon *Ankyloblepharon (adherence of the eyelids resulting in narrowing of palpebral apertures) was reported in a 59-year-old man during fluorouracil therapy for metastatic adenocarcinoma of the stomach (99[c]). It appeared that bilateral conjunctival ulcers, secondary to fluorouracil and ulcerative blepharitis, resulted in ankyloblepharon. Withdrawal of chemotherapy resulted in improvement and re-initiation of therapy resulted in recurrence of ocular lesions.*

Sexual function *Vaginitis (shedding of the vaginal epithelium) may be nearly as common as mucositis in women receiving systemic fluorouracil-based chemotherapy regimens (100[C]).*

Chromosomal damage *An increased incidence in the number of chromosomally aberrant lymphocytes was observed in nurses handling cytostatic agents (cyclophosphamide, doxorubicin, vincristine, fluorouracil, and methotrexate) (101[C]).*

Immunological and hypersensitivity reactions Anaphylaxis *An anaphylactic reaction with shock after a tenth dose of fluorouracil 900 mg intravenously was reported in a 60-year-old man with colorectal adenocarcinoma (102[c]). Two minutes after his tenth dose of fluorouracil he became cyanotic and collapsed, with a rapid thready pulse of 120. His blood pressure was 30/0 mmHg. Adrenaline 1 : 1000, 1 ml, was given, with immediate and prompt signs of recovery. Within 25 minutes, his blood pressure, pulse, and skin color had returned to normal.*

Miscellaneous *Fluorouracil increases the activity and toxicity of ionizing radiation (50[R]).*

Risk factors ***Age and sex as independent predictors of fluorouracil toxicity*** *Cancer is most common in older people, but little information is available with regard to the impact of age on the toxicity of chemotherapy. A study has been undertaken to determine if age is an independent risk factor for fluorouracil toxicity (103[C]). Toxicity data from a prospective, randomized, multi-institution trial of fluorouracil-based treatment for advanced colorectal carcinoma were analysed. Toxicity for each organ system was graded. The results showed that advanced age was significantly associated with the occurrence of any severe toxicity (58 vs 36%), leukopenia (24 vs 10%), diarrhea (24 vs 14%), vomiting (15 vs 5%), severe toxicity in more than two organ systems (10 vs 3%), and treatment mortality (9 vs 2%). Age and sex were independent predictors of severe toxicity. Advanced age does not contraindicate the use of this type of chemotherapy, but monitoring for multiple organ toxicity and vigorous supportive care of those with toxicity are required.*

Dosing decisions in older patients are difficult and must integrate assessments of organ function, co-morbidity, overall physical status and goals of treatment, in an effort to ensure the best possible outcome for these patients.

Dihydropyrimidine dehydrogenase deficiency *During the past 30 years, extensive research on the mechanism of fluorouracil has shown that anabolism of fluorouracil to pyrimidine nucleotide analogs is required for its cytotoxic effects. More recent studies have emphasized the importance of pyrimidine catabolism in the regulation of fluorouracil availability and its subsequent anabolism. Dihydropyrimidine dehydrogenase is the initial enzyme of pyrimidine catabolism accounting* *for degradation of greater than 80% of a dose of fluorouracil. The importance of catabolism and particularly dihydropyrimidine dehydrogenase in fluorouracil chemotherapy has previously been demonstrated in studies with competitive inhibitors of dihydropyrimidine dehydrogenase and in patients with suspected or proven dihydropyrimidine dehydrogenase deficiency. Before 1991, only two cases of dihydropyrimidine dehydrogenase deficiency associated with fluorouracil toxicity in adults were reported, and in both cases it was the fluorouracil toxicity that focused attention on pyrimidine catabolism. In 1991 a third case of dihydropyrimidine dehydrogenase deficiency was reported (104[c]), suggesting that it may be more frequent than initially thought. There was complete deficiency of dihydropyrimidine dehydrogenase in the affected patient, with evidence of partial deficiency in the patient's parents, daughter, brother, and the brother's children. This pattern of dihydropyrimidine dehydrogenase activity was consistent with the previous two reports, suggesting an autosomal recessive pattern of inheritance.*

A 35-year-old woman with breast carcinoma treated with doses of fluorouracil that were not unusually high. Chemotherapy with cyclophosphamide, fluorouracil, and methotrexate started 3 weeks after surgery. Following day 8 of the protocol, the patient had severe gastrointestinal adverse effects (nausea, prolonged vomiting, diarrhea, stomatitis), hematological toxicity (neutropenia), and fever. She also had mild neurological toxicity causing unsteadiness and difficulty in spelling simple words, which persisted for about 2 weeks.

The neurotoxicity of fluorouracil seems to be more prolonged and severe in patients with dihydropyrimidine dehydrogenase deficiency (105[c]).

Only a few cases of dihydropyrimidine dehydrogenase deficiency have been identified: however, all cases exhibited remarkable toxicity. Enhanced toxicity occurring at normal doses is what usually sets these patients apart. The authors suggested that monitoring dihydropyrimidine dehydrogenase activity may be appropriate in the management of those who have severe toxicity from fluorouracil (104[c]).

Additional studies are needed to characterize this genetic defect, in order to answer the following question. What is the frequency of this gene defect in the general population? Does dihydropyrimidine dehydrogenase deficiency correlate with the occurrence of severe fluorouracil toxicity? Do individuals with partial dihydropyrimidine dehydrogenase deficiency (i.e. heterozygotes) have altered metabolism of fluorouracil? Is monitoring dihydropyrimidine dehydrogenase activity helpful in the management of patients experiencing severe toxicity to fluorouracil chemotherapy?

Circadian variation in toxicity *If the rhythm in fluorouracil toxicity is linked to the asleep-awake circadian cycle across species, the least toxic time in man would correspond to 0400 h. This hypothesis has been tested using a single-reservoir programmable-in-time external ambulatory pump (Chronopump, Autosyringe, Hooksett, USA) in 35 patients with metastatic colorectal cancer (106[C]). Fluorouracil was infused for 5 days via an implanted venous access port, with peak drug delivery at 0400 hours and no infusion from 1800 to 2200 hours. Each course was repeated after a drug-free interval of 16 days. Intrapatient dose escalation was planned from 4 to 9 g/m^2/course (800 to 1800 mg/m^2/day $\times$ 5 days) if toxicity was less than grade 2 according to the World Health Organization (WHO). There was grade 2 or greater toxicity in under 5% of the courses, indicating adequate control of toxicity via dose escalation, and their incidence was dose dependent. The median maximal tolerated dose was 7.5 mg/m^2/course in 30 patients assessed for this end point.*

Cellular glutathione concentrations and fluorouracil toxicity *Little is known about whether components of the diet can modulate the efficacy of fluorouracil in patients with colon carcinoma. Glutathione, an important antioxidant and anticarcinogen, is present in many foods in varying amounts.*

The effect of cellular glutathione concentration on the growth of human colon adenocarcinoma cells HT-29 and on the cytotoxic activity of fluorouracil in these cells has been studied (107). Glutathione and buthionine sulfoximine were used respectively to enhance or reduce the glutathione concentration in these cells. A 34% increase in cellular glutathione concentration had no effect on the growth of HT-29 cells, nor on the cytotoxic activity of fluorouracil. A 50% reduction in the cellular glutathione concentration enhanced fluorouracil cytotoxicity by 20–31%, depending on the fluorouracil concentration.

Use in pregnancy *Fluorouracil is contraindicated throughout pregnancy. The literature on pregnancy and cytotoxic drugs is necessarily limited, but it appears in general that risk of teratogenesis diminishes with the advancement of pregnancy. Therefore most cytotoxic drugs are absolutely contraindicated in the first trimester, and when fluorouracil has been used in the first trimester it has been reported to cause multiple congenital abnormalities (108[c]).*

Fluorouracil is teratogenic in a number of species, but the mechanisms of its developmental toxicity are not fully understood. Administration of fluorouracil to pregnant rats on day 14 of gestation results in dose-dependent growth retardation and numerous malformations in near-term fetuses, including hind limb defects and cleft palate. After treatment, a number of rapid biochemical and cellular alterations are detectable in embryonic hind limbs and in craniofacial and other tissues, including inhibition of thymidylate synthetase and altered cell cycle progression. In order to assess the importance of these early events in fluorouracil-induced dysmorphogenesis, embryonic midfacial tissues and hind limbs were dissected 3 or 6 hours after administration of fluorouracil to the dam and placed in explant culture. After 5 days in culture, craniofacial explants were evaluated morphologically for palatal closure, and growth was assessed by measuring total protein and DNA contents. Hind-limb explants were stained for cartilage using alcian blue to evaluate development of digits. Craniofacial explants cultured at either 3 or 6 hours after exposure showed dose-dependent growth retardation and defects of palatal fusion at the end of the culture period. Deficits in protein and DNA content were similar to those in craniofacial tissues that continued to develop in utero after treatment, although morphological defects in cultured explants did not correlate well with the incidence of cleft palate in vivo. Dose-dependent deficits in metatarsal and phalanx development were observed in hind-limb explants dissected either 3 or 6 hours after maternal treatment (109).

Overdosage *Cases of deliberate overdosage are unknown, but excessive duration or dosage of therapy will produce life-threatening toxicity because of the hematological effects and other symptoms and signs that are qualitatively similar to the adverse effects. There is no specific antidote to fluorouracil toxicity; treatment consists of supportive care.*

Interactions *The pharmacokinetics of fluorouracil have been studied with escalating doses as a 72-hour intravenous infusion alone or in combination with a fixed dose of dipyridamole, a nucleoside transport inhibitor and an enhancer of fluorouracil cytotoxicity (110[C]). Stomatitis was dose-limiting at a fluorouracil dose of 2300 mg/m^2/day. For courses given with fluorouracil alone, the pharmacokinetics were linear for doses of 185–2300 mg/m^2/day; however, above this dose total body clearance fell significantly. Dipyridamole increased the total body clearance of fluorouracil, resulting in significantly lower mean steady-state fluorouracil plasma concentrations over the dose range studied. The clinical observation that dipyridamole did not appear to modulate fluorouracil-induced mucositis or leukopenia may be explained by lower fluorouracil drug exposure. The basis for this pharmacokinetic interaction is not understood but serves to underscore the importance of incorporating pharmacokinetic analysis in clinical trials involving new drug combinations.*

Dose-dependency of fluorouracil toxicity *The dose-limiting toxicity of fluorouracil varies with the dose and mode of administration.*

- *With five consecutive daily bolus injections of 450–600 mg/m^2, the dose-limiting toxicities are myelosuppression, mucositis, and diarrhea.*
- *With weekly injections of 450–600 mg/m^2, myelosuppression is dose-limiting.*
- *With continuous five-day infusion of 1000 mg/m^2/day, mucositis and diarrhea are dose-limiting.*
- *With protracted continuous infusion of 200–400 mg/m^2/day, mucositis and palmar-plantar erythrodysesthesia syndrome are the most common dose-limiting adverse effects (50[R]).*
- *Some very high-dose short-exposure studies have been reported, including 14 g over 24 hours (111) and 2.6 g/m^2 weekly (112[C]); in the latter study neurotoxicity was dose-limiting.*

Routes of administration ***Intra-arterial*** *Intravenous administration of fluorouracil 1 g has been compared with hepatic arterial infusion (113[C]). When fluorouracil was administered over 2 hours, systemic drug exposure was 0.7 times lower and clearance 1.5 times higher with* *hepatic arterial infusion. When the duration of infusion was extended to 24 hours, systemic drug exposure was 0.4 times lower and the clearance was 2- to 3-fold higher with hepatic arterial infusion. For the 24-hour infusion, co-treatment with angiotensin II (given temporarily to increase tumor blood flow) and albumin microspheres, given to increase drug uptake by liver via the hepatic artery produced an additional two-fold reduction in systemic fluorouracil exposure. Further evaluation is planned to determine if this will improve the therapeutic index of regionally administered fluorouracil.*

Intraperitoneal *Intraperitoneal administration of fluorouracil has been reported to produce a desirable regional advantage (114[C]). The results of a phase I trial of intraperitoneal fluorouracil in escalating concentrations for 4 hour, along with a fixed dose of cisplatin 90 mg/m^2 every 28 days, has been used (115[C]). There was dose-limiting neutropenia at a fluorouracil concentration of 20 mmol/l, although individual patients tolerated concentrations as high as 30 mmol/l. Other toxic effects included mild-to-moderate nausea and vomiting; diarrhea occurred less often. Peak plasma concentrations occurred 1 hour after instillation and there was a significant linear relation between the intraperitoneal fluorouracil dose and the peak plasma fluorouracil concentration. At every dose, the mean peak intraperitoneal fluorouracil concentration exceeded that in the plasma by two to three log units.*

Relation of toxicity to pharmacokinetics *Fluorouracil pharmacokinetics have been determined in 19 patients receiving fluorouracil by protracted venous infusion at doses of 190–600 mg/m^2/day (116[C]). The steady-state fluorouracil plasma concentration and AUC were significantly lower in the nine patients who experienced WHO grade 2 toxicity or less compared with the nine patients who experienced greater than grade 2 toxicity. In contrast, there was no difference in fluorouracil plasma concentrations between the ten responders and the nine patients who had no evidence of a clinical response. These investigations confirm previous observations that correlations can be drawn between fluorouracil pharmacokinetics and clinical toxicity (117[C]). Furthermore, the data suggest that pharmacokinetic monitoring might permit identification of patients at increased risk of toxicity.*

Interactions Allopurinol *Concurrent administration of allopurinol with fluorouracil inhibits the intracellular formation of fluorouridine monophosphate from fluorouracil in normal tissues. In tumor cells that activate fluorouracil by alternative pathways, antitumor responses are still seen (50[R]). Allopurinol increased the half-life of high-dose fluorouracil when it was given by intravenous bolus but not when it was given by 5-day continuous infusion (50[R]).*

Allopurinol ameliorates fluorouracil-induced granulocytopenia and possibly lessens the severity of mucositis (118[C]). Allopurinol mouthwash (450 mg total in methylcellulose) given immediately and 1, 2, and 3 hours after fluorouracil reduced the incidence and severity of mucositis in six patients (119[C]) and in another study of 42 patients there was significant reduction of oral toxicity and prolonged pain relief (120[C]). In a randomized double-blind, placebo-controlled trial in 44 patients allopurinol mouthwashes resolved stomatitis in nine of 22 treated patients, and diminished its intensity in ten (121[C]). However, in another randomized, double-blind, cross-over study of allopurinol mouthwash in 77 patients did not ameliorate fluorouracil-induced mucositis (122[C]). Nor did allopurinol reduce the toxicity of intravenously administered fluorouracil (123[C]).

Cimetidine *Pre-treatment for 4 weeks with cimetidine 1 g/day increased the oral systemic availability of fluorouracil by 74%; the AUC was increased by 27% and total body clearance was reduced by 28% (124[C]).*

Interferons *Initial studies have suggested that interferons may have synergistic activity with fluorouracil (125[C], 126[C]). Interferon-α_{2b} has also been associated with an 80% increase in fluorouracil AUC (127[C]).*

Leucovorin *When combined with fluorouracil, leucovorin enhances the binding of the fluorouracil metabolite fluorouridine monophosphate to thymidylate synthetase. DNA-directed toxicity is increased, whilst RNA-directed toxicity is not affected (127[C]).*

A qualitative alteration in toxicity is reported with increased gastrointestinal toxicity (50[R]).

Methotrexate *There is sequence-dependent synergy between fluorouracil and methotrexate. Pre-treatment with methotrexate enhances the formation of fluorouridine monophosphate and hence fluorouridine triphosphate and RNA-directed toxicity. In studies in which methotrexate has been given 1 h before fluorouracil, response rates did not differ significantly. However, when it was given 4 hours or more before, there were significantly better response rates (129[C]).*

Metronidazole *Pre-treatment with metronidazole increased the toxicity of fluorouracil given by daily bolus dose (130[C]). The clinical significance of this is yet to be determined.*

Pyridoxine *The dose and duration of protracted infusional fluorouracil is limited by mucositis, diarrhea, and/or palmar-plantar erythrodysesthesia. Typically, palmar-plantar dysesthesia begins several weeks to months after starting treatment. Although the dysesthesia abates within several weeks of discontinuing the infusion, it rapidly recurs when the infusion is resumed. Five patients who developed palmar-plantar dysesthesia during infusion of fluorouracil were treated with oral pyridoxine, 50 or 150 mg/day, once it reached moderate severity (131[C]). The severity of the skin toxicity improved, with resolution of pain in four of the five patients, despite continued administration of fluorouracil. The ability of pyridoxine to modulate fluorouracil-induced cutaneous toxicity is currently undergoing evaluation in the randomized trial (132[C]).*

ANNUAL REVIEW

Table 1 lists some review articles that have recently contributed to our overall understanding of cytostatic induced drug toxicity, its occurrence, predictability, significance, and management.

Table 1. *Some recent review articles on cytostatic induced drug toxicity*

Specific or comparative toxic effects of single or multiple cytostatic drugs

Amenorrhea induced by adjuvant chemotherapy in early breast cancer patients: prognostic role and clinical implications (133[R])

Cardiotoxicity of the antiproliferative compound fluorouracil (134[R])

New developments in cancer treatment with the novel thymidylate synthase inhibitor raltitrexed ('Tomudex') (135[R])

Doxorubicin vs epirubicin: report of a second-line randomized phase II/III study in advanced breast cancer (136[R])

Toxicity of fluorouracil in patients with advanced colorectal cancer: effect of administration schedule and prognostic factors (137[R])

Toxicity that is modified by the treatment schedule

The pharmacokinetics and metabolism of ifosfamide during bolus and infusion administration: a randomized cross-over study (138[R])

A phase I study of docetaxel and ifosfamide in patients with advanced solid tumors (139[R])

Bolus injection (2–4 min) versus short-term infusion (10–20 min) of fluorouracil in patients with advanced colorectal cancer: a prospective randomized trial (140[R])

The efficacy of intravenous continuous infusion of fluorouracil compared with bolus administration in advanced colorectal cancer (141[R])

Predictability of general chemotherapy toxic effects

Hematological and non-hematological toxicity after fluorouracil and leucovorin in patients with advanced colorectal cancer: significant association with sex, increasing age, and cycle number (142[R])

CARDIOVASCULAR

Anthracyclines It has been suggested that monitoring B type natriuretic peptide concentrations after anthracycline administration can reflect cardiac tolerance, and through serial monitoring allow a picture of the degree of *left ventricular dysfunction* to be established (143[C]).

RESPIRATORY

Bleomycin Bleomycin has long been known to be a primary cause of *pulmonary toxicity*. A fatal pulmonary toxicity rate of 2.8% (n = 194) has been described. The authors further noted that the incidence of fatal pulmonary toxicity increased with each decade of life above 30 and that the lower the glomerular filtration rate at the time of administration the greater the death rate. They concluded that the death rate may exceed 10% in those over 40 years of age (144[C]).

NERVOUS SYSTEM

Methotrexate Treatment with chemotherapy of children with acute lymphoblastic leukemia (irrespective of drugs involved in their specific regimen) and intrathecal methotrexate before 5 years of age has structural and functional effects on the developing neocerebellar-frontal subsystem (145[C]). There was a significantly higher risk of *late cognitive impairment* (concentration and memory) in patients (n = 39) treated with adjuvant cyclophosphamide, fluorouracil, and methotrexate than in age/disease/surgery/radiation matched controls (146[C]).

LIVER

Methotrexate Dexamethasone increased the *hepatotoxicity* of methotrexate in 57 children with brain tumors (147[C]). The hepatotoxicity was not related to differences in serum concentrations and was independent of bone-marrow toxicity or mucositis

URINARY SYSTEM

Carboplatin Ultra-high-dose carboplatin can be safely administered as long as clinicians individualize and adjust the therapy to renal function using ^{51}Cr-EDTA glomerular filtration rate; there was only one death attributed to carboplatin in 31 patients who died of *acute renal insufficiency* (148[C]).

Cisplatin The nephrotoxicity of cisplatin is well documented in both adults and children. However, there have been few longitudinal studies. In 35 children who had received cisplatin for a maximum of 2 years *nephrotoxicity* was not related to total dose but was less severe in children who received cisplatin in doses under 40 mg/m^2/day (149[C]). During follow-up for 2 years there was partial but significant recovery in renal function.

Raltitrexed Whilst raltitrexed dose not cause *renal toxicity,* its pharmacokinetics and hence its toxic effects, particularly on the bone-marrow and gut, are directly related to creatinine clearance (150[C]). It is recommended that the dose be reduced and dosage interval increased in patients with mild to moderate renal impairment.

SKIN AND APPENDAGES

Hydroxyurea The incidence of skin lesions in patients taking hydroxyurea varies from 10 to 35%. They usually occur after several years of maintenance therapy. However, a patient has been described who developed lichen planus-like dermatitis on hands after just 15 days of treatment (151[c]). The degeneration of these skin lesions into full-blown ulcers has been described in 14 patients who developed extremely painful leg ulcers most commonly on the malleoli. The patients had been taking hydroxyurea for an average of 6 years and nine had multiple ulcers (152[C]).

SPECIAL SENSES

Carboplatin Audiological testing has been recommended for patients receiving high-dose carboplatin therapy, following *hearing problems* in a series of ten patients with ovarian cancer (153[C]).

Cisplatin In 86 patients treated with cisplatin-based chemotherapy for testicular cancer cumulative exposure (over 400 mg/m^2) and a previous history of noise exposure were significant risk factors for irreversible *ototoxicity* (154[C]). In addition, high doses of vincristine (greater than 6 mg/m^2) significantly increased the risk of reversible ototoxicity.

MUSCULOSKELETAL

Paclitaxel The severity of *myalgia and arthralgia* correlated significantly with the total cumulative dose of paclitaxel 210 mg/m^2/cycle by 3-hour infusion in 247 patients with a median cumulative dose of 630 mg/m^2 (155[C]).

MISCELLANEOUS

Cisplatin Fatal acute *tumor lysis syndrome* has been reported in a 74-year-old woman who received cisplatin (50 mg/m^2 on day 1) and fluorouracil (1000 mg/m^2 by continuous infusion for 5 days) for vulvar carcinoma (156[c]). Whilst this is a well known complication of chemotherapy, particularly with hematological tumors, it is extremely rare as a complication of neoadjuvant chemotherapy for gynecological tumors.

Mesna *(SED-13, 431)*

Mesna has been used for over a decade in the prevention of hemorrhagic cystitis induced by ifosfamide and cyclophosphamide. It has also been used as an aerosol mucolytic. In a randomized, cross-over study 25 volunteers received single doses of intravenous mesna and four different formulations of oral mesna (68). One subject withdrew from the study because of *ocular inflammation* followed by *loss of appetite, nausea, and vomiting.* Another developed a rash during the period in which three of his four oral doses were given. Two further subjects developed *loose stools* after one of the oral doses. Another reported *dizziness* after an oral dose. One reported *pain at the site of the intravenous infusion.* The adverse effects were all considered to be mild or moderate and resolved spontaneously without treatment.

Interactions *Platinum agents* are now combined with ifosfamide in the treatment of cancer. The possibility that mesna may interfere with the anticancer effects of platinum agents has been investigated using cultured malignant glioma cells (69). Mesna protected tumor cell lines from the cytotoxic effect of the platinum agents. This in vitro study emphasizes the importance of specifying in detail the infusion schedules of mesna and platinum agents.

REFERENCES

1. Dent RG, McColl I. 5-Fluorouracil and angina. Lancet 1975;1:347–8.
2. Pottage A, Holt S, Ludgate S, Langlands AO. Fluorouracil cardiotoxicity. Br Med J 1978;1:547.
3. Labianca R, Beretta C, Clerici M, Fraschini P, Luporini G. Cardiotoxicity of 5-fluorouracil: a study on 1083 patients. Tumori 1982;68:505–10.
4. De Forni M, Malet-Martino MC, Jaillais P, Shubinski RE, Bachaud JM, Lemaire L, Canal P, Chevreau C, Carrie D, Soulie P, Roche H, Boudjema B, Mihura J, Martino R, Bernadet P, Bugat R. Cardiotoxicity of high-dose continuous infusion fluorouracil: a prospective clinical study. J Clin Oncol 1992;10:1795–1801.
5. Ensley J, Kish J, Tapazoglou E, et al. 5-FU infusions associated with an ischaemic cardiotoxicity syndrome. Proc Am Soc Clin Oncol 1986;5:142.
6. Gradishar WJ, Vokes EE. 5-Fluorouracil cardiotoxicity: a critical review. Ann Oncol 1990;1:409–14.
7. Lomeo AM, Avolio C, Iacobellis G, Manzione L. 5-Fluorouracil cardiotoxicity. Eur J Gynaecol Onol 1990;11:237–41.
8. Rezkalla S, Kloner RA, Ensley J, Al Sarraf M, Revels S, Olivenstein A, Bhasin S, Kerpel-Fronious S, Turi ZG. Continous ambulatory ECG monitoring during 5-fluorouracil therapy: a prospective study. J Clin Oncol 1989;7:509–14.
9. Collins C, Weiden PL. Cardiotoxicity of 5-fluorouracil. Cancer Treat Rep 1987;71:733–6.
10. Freeman NJ, Costanza ME. 5-Fluorouracil-associated cardiotoxicity. Cancer 1988;61:36–45.
11. McKendall GR, Anamur M, Most AS, Shurman A. Toxic cardiogenic shock associated with infusion of 5-fluorouracil. Am Heart J 1989;118:184–6.
12. Patel B, Kloner RA, Ensley J, Al Sarraf M, Kish J, Wynne J. 5-Fluorouracil cardiotoxicity: left ventricular dysfunction and effect of coronary vasodilators. Am J Med Sci 1987;294:238–43.
13. Misset B, Escudier B, Leclercq B, Rivara D, Rougier P, Nitenberg G. Acute mycocardiotoxicity during 5-fluorouracil therapy. Intensive Care Med 1990;16:210–11.
14. Coronel B, Madonna O, Mercatello A, Caillette A, Moskovtchenko JF. Myocardiotoxicity of 5-fluorouracil. Intensive Car Med 1988;14:429–30.
15. Aziz SA, Tramboo NA, Mohi-ud-Din K, Iqbal K, Jalal S, Ahmed M. Supraventricular arrhythmia: a complication of 5-fluorouracil therapy. Clin Oncol R Coll Radiol 1998;10:377–8.
16. Wang WS, Hsieh RK, Chiou TJ, Liu JH, Fan FS, Yen CC, Tung SL, Chen PM. Toxic cardiogenic shock in a patient receiving weekly 24-h infusion of high-dose 5-fluorouracil and leucovorin. Jpn J Clin Oncol 1998;28:551–4.
17. Liss RH, Chadwick M. Correlation of 5-fluorouracil distribution in rodents with toxicity and chemotherapy in man. Cancer Chemother Rep 1974;58:777–86.
18. Suzuki T, Nakanishi H, Hayashi A, et al. Cardiac toxicity of 5- FU in rabbits. Jpn J Pharmacol 1972;27 (Suppl):137.
19. Matsubara I, Kamiya J, Imai S. Cardiotoxic effects of 5-fluorouracil in the guinea pig. Jpn J Pharmacol 1980;30:871–9.

20. Orditura M, De Vita F, Sarubbi B, Ducceschi V, Auriemma A, Infusino S, Iacono A, Catalano G. Analysis of recovery time indexes in 5-fluorouracil-treated cancer patients. Oncol Rep 1998;5:645–7.
21. Jakubowski AA, Kemeny N. Hypotension as a manifestation of cardiotoxicity in three patients receiving cisplatin and 5-fluorouracil. Cancer 1988;62:266–9.
22. Jeremic B, Jevremovic S, Djuric L, Mijatovic L. Cardiotoxicity during chemotherapy with 5-fluorouracil and cisplatin. J Chemother 1990;2:264–7.
23. Martin M, Diaz-Rubio E, Furio V, Blazquez J, Almenarez J, Farina J. Lethal cardiac toxicity after 5-fluorouracil and cisplatin chemotherapy: report of a case with necropsy study. Am J Clin Oncol Cancer Clin Trials 1989;12:229–34.
24. Kleiman NS, Lehane DE, Geyer Jr CE, Pratt CM, Young JB. Prinzmetal's angina during 5-fluorouracil chemotherapy. Am J Med 1987; 82:566–8.
25. Burger AJ, Mannino S. 5-Fluorouracil-induced coronary vasospasm. Am Heart J 1987;114:433–6.
26. Kohne C-H, Thuss-Patience P, Friedrich M, Daniel PT, Kretzschmar A, Benter T, Bauer B, Dietz R, Dorken B. Raltitrexed (Tomudex): an alternative drug for patients with colorectal cancer and 5-fluorouracil associated cardiotoxicity. Br J Cancer 1998;77:973–7.
27. Doll DC, Yarbro JW. Vascular toxicity associated with chemotherapy and hormonotherapy. Curr Opin Oncol 1994:6:345–50.
28. Papamichael D, Amft N, Slevin ML, D'Cruz D. 5-Fluorouracil-induced Raynaud's phenomenon. Eur J Cancer 1998;34:1983.
29. Fielding JW, Stockley RA, Brookes VS. Interstitial lung disease in a patient treated with 5-fluorouracil and mitomycin C. Br Med J 1978; 2:602.
30. Fielding JW, Crocker J, Stockley RA, Brookes VS. Interstitial fibrosis in a patient treated with 5-fluorouracil and mitomycin C. Br Med J 1979; 1:551–2.
31. Moertel CG, Reitemeier RJ, Bolton CF, et al. Cerebellar ataxia associated with fluorinated pyrimidine therapy. Cancer Chemother Rep 1964;41:15–18.
32. Tuxen M, Hansen S. Neurotoxicity secondary to antineoplastic drugs. Cancer Treat Rev 1994;20:191–214.
33. Ranuzzi M, Taddei A. Neurotoxicity of antineoplastic agents in chemotherapy. Nuova Riv Neurol 1996;6:55–63.
34. Lynch HT, Droszcz CP, Albano WA, Lynch JF. 'Organic brain syndrome' secondary to 5-fluorouracil toxicity. Dis Colon Rectum 1981; 24:130–1.
35. Adams JW, Bofenkamp TM, Kobrin J, Wirtschafter JD, Zeese JA. Recurrent acute toxic optic neuropathy secondary to 5-FU. Cancer Treat Rep 1984;68:565–6.
36. Weiss HD, Walker MD, Wiernik PH. Neurotoxicity of commonly used anti-neoplastic agents. New Engl J Med 1974;291:75-81, 127–33.
37. Shapiro WR, Young DF. Neurological complications of antineoplastic therapy. Acta Neurol Scand 1984:70 Suppl 100:125–32.
38. Fassas AB-T, Gattani A, Morgello S. Cerebral demyelination with 5-fluroruracil and levamisole. Cancer Invest 1994:12:379–83.
39. Bygrave HA, Geh JI, Jani Y, Glynne-Jones R. Neurological complications of 5-fluorouracil chemotherapy: case report and review of literature. Clin Oncol 1998;10:334–6.
40. Stein ME, Drumea K, Yarnitsky D, Benny A, Tzuk-Shina T. A rare event of 5-fluorouracil-associated peripheral neuropathy: a report of two patients. Am J Clin Oncol 1998;21:248–9.
41. El-Amrani M, Heinzlef O, Debroucker T, Roullet E, Bousser M-G, Amarenco P. Brain infarction following 5-fluorouracil and cisplatin therapy. Neurology 1998;51:899–901.
42. Koenig H, Patel A. Biochemical basis for fluorouracil toxicity; the role of the Krebs cycle inhibition by fluoroacetate. Arch Neurol 1970;23:155–60.
43. Weiss HD, Walker MD, Wiernik PH. Neurotoxicity of commonly used antineoplastic agents. New Engl J Med 1974:291:75–81.
44. Diasio RB, Beavers TL, Carpenter JT. Familial deficiency of dihydropyrimidine dehydrogenase. Biochemical basis for familial pyrimidinaemia and severe 5-fluorouracil-induced toxicity. J Clin Invest 1988;81:47–51.
45. Sadoff L. Overwhelming 5-fluorouracil toxicity in patients whose diabetes is poorly controlled. Am J Clin Oncol 1998:21:605–7.
46. Yeh KH Cheng AL. High-dose 5-fluorouracil infusional therapy is associated with hyperammonaemia, lactic acidosis and encephalopathy. Br J Cancer 1997;75:464–5.
47. Valik D, Yeh K-H, Cheng A-L. Encephalopathy, lactic acidosis, hyperammonaemia and 5-fluorouracil toxicity, Br J Cancer 1998;77:1710–12.
48. Yeh K-H, Cheng A-L. 5-Fluorouracil-related encephalopathy: at least two distinct pathogenetic mechanisms exist—reply. Br J Cancer 1998;77:1711–12.
49. Grem JL. Fluorinated pyrimidines. In: Chabner BA, Collins JM, eds. Cancer Chemotherapy: Principles and Practice. Philadelphia; Lippincoft, 1990:180–225.
50. Chabner BA, Myers CE. Clinical pharmacology of cancer chemotherapy. In: Devita VT, Hellman S, Rosenberg SA, eds. Cancer: Principles and Practice of Oncology, 3rd edn. Philadelphia: Lippincoft, 1990: 349–95.
51. Vaitevicius VK, Brennan MJ, Beckett VL, et al. Clinical evaluation of cancer chemotherapy with 5-FU. Cancer 1961;14:131–9.
52. Reitemeier RJ et al. Comparison of 5-fluorouracil (NSC-19893) and 2-deoxy-5-fluorouridine (NSC-27640) in the treatment of patients

with advanced adenocarcinoma of the colon or rectum. Cancer Chemother Rep 1965;44:39–43.
53. Piro AJ, Wilson RE, Hall TC, Aliapoulios MA, Nevinny HB, Moore FD. Toxicity studies of fluorouracil used with adrenalectomy in breast cancer. Arch Surg 1972;105:95–9.
54. Cohn I Jr. Complications and toxic manifestations of surgical adjuvant chemotherapy for breast cancer. Surg Gynecol Obstet 1968;127:1201–9.
55. Scott JM, Weir DG. Drug induced megaloblastic change. Clin Haematol 1980;9:587–606.
56. Seifert P, Baker LH, Reed ML, Vaitkevicius VK. Comparison of continuously infused 5-fluorouracil with bolus injection in treatment of patients with colorectal adenocarcinoma. Cancer 1975;36:123–8.
57. Lokich JJ Ahlgren JD, Gullo JJ, Philips JA, Fryer JG. A prospective randomised comparison of continuous infusion fluorouracil with a conventional bolus schedule in metastatic colorectal carcinoma: a Mid-Atlantic Oncology Programme Study. J Clin Oncol 1989;7:425–32.
58. Sotaniemi EA, Sutinen S, Arranto AJ, Sutinen S, Sotaniemi KA, Lehtola J, Pelkonen RO. Liver damage in nurses handling cytostatic agents. Acta Med Scand 1983;214:181–9.
59. Vestfrid MA, Castello L, Gimenez PO. Diffuse liver necrosis in treatment with 5-fluorouracil. Rev Clin Esp 1972;125:549–50.
60. Kemeny N, Seiter K, Martin D, Urmacher C, Neidzwiecki D, Kurtz RC, Costa P, Murray M. A new syndrome: ascites, hyperbilirubinaemia and hypoalbuminaemia after biochemical modulation of fluorouracil with N-phosphonacetyl-L-aspartate (PALA). Ann Intern Med 1991;115:946–51.
61. Lokich JJ, Bothe A, Fine N, Perri J. Phase I study of protracted venous infusion of 5-fluorouracil. Cancer 1981;48:2565–8.
62. McCarthy GM, Awde JD, Ghandi H, Vincent M, Kocha WI. Risk factors associated with mucositis in cancer patients receiving 5-fluouracil. Oral Oncol 1998;34:484–90.
63. Narsete T, Ansfield F, Wirtanen G, Ramirez G, Wolberg W, Jarrett F. Gastric ulceration in patients receiving intrahepatic infusion of 5-fluorouracil. Ann Surg 1977;186:734–6.
64. Rousselot LM, Cole DR, Grossi CE, et al. Gastro-intestinal bleeding as a sequel to cancer chemotherapy. Am J Gastroenterol 1965;43:311–16.
65. Biran S, Krasnokuki D, Brufman G. Life threatening gastro-intestinal toxicity during 5-fluorouracil therapy. Harefuah 1977;93:77.
66. Wadler S, Lyver A, Wiernik PH. Clinical toxicities of the combination of 5-fluorouracil and recombinant interferon alpha-2a: an unusual toxicity profile. Oncol Nurs Forum 1989;16(Suppl):12–15.
67. Barrett O Jr, Bourgeois C, Plecha FR. Fluorouracil toxicity following gastrointestinal surgery. Arch Surg 1965;91:1002–4.
68. Cudmore MA, Silva J Jr, Fekety R, Liepman MK, Kim KH. *Clostridium difficile* colitis associated with cancer chemotherapy. Arch Intern Med 1982;142:333–5.
69. Abe H, Tsunaga N, Yamashita S, Ishiguro K, Mitani I. Anticancer drug-induced colitis—case reports and review of the literature. Jpn J Cancer Chemother 1997;24:619–24.
70. Kronawitter U, Kemeny N, Blumgart L. Neutropenic enterocolitis in a patient with colorectal carcinoma: unusual course after treatment with 5-fluorouracil and leucovorin—a case report. Cancer 1997;80:656–60.
71. Trevisani F, Simoncini M, Alampi G, Bernardi M. Colitis associated to chemotherapy with 5-fluorouracil. Hepato-Gastroenterology 1997; 44:710–12.
72. Falkson C, Schultz E. Skin changes in patients treated with 5-fluorouracil. Br J Dermatol 1962;74:229–36.
73. Dunagin WO. Dermatologic toxicity. In: Perry MC, Yarbro JW, editors. Toxicity of Chemotherapy. Orlando: Grune and Stratton, 1984:125–54.
74. Hrushesky WJ. Unusual pigmentary changes associated with 5-fluorouracil therapy. Cutis 1980; 26:181–2.
75. Pujol RM, Rocamora V, Lopez-Pousa A, Taberner R, Alomar A. Persistent supravenous erythematous eruption: a rare local complication of intravenous 5-fluorouracil therapy. J Am Acad Dermatol 1998;39 (Suppl 2):839–42.
76. Sams WM. Untoward response with topical 5-fluorouracil. Arch Dermatol 1968;97:14–22.
77. Clemons DE. Dermatitis medicamentosa. A pitfall for the unwary. Arch Dermatol 1976; 112:1178–9.
78. Nixon DW, Pirozzi D, York RM, Black M, Lawson DH. Dermtologic changes after systemic cancer therapy. Cutis 1981;27:181–94.
79. Norton LA. Nail disorders. A Review. J Am Acad Dermatol 1980;2:451–67.
80. Katz ME, Hansen TW. Nail plate-nail bed separation. An unusual side-effect of systemic fluorouracil administration. Arch Dermatol 1979; 115:860–1.
81. Burnett JW. Two unusual complications of topical fluorouracil therapy. Arch Dermatol 1975; 111:398.
82. Curran F Luce JK. Fluorouracil and palmar-plantar erythrodysesthesia. Ann Intern Med 1989; 111:858.
83. Jorda E, Galan B, Betloch I, Ramon D, Revert A, Torres V. Painful, red hands: a side-effect of 5-fluorouracil by continuous perfusion. Int J Dermatol 1991;30:653.
84. Feldman LD, Ajani JA. Fluorouracil-associated dermatitis of the hands and feet. J Am Med Assoc 1985;254:3479.
85. Vukelja SJ, Lombardo FA, James WD, Weiss RB. Pyridoxine for palmar-plantar erythrodysesthesia syndrome. Ann Intern Med 1989;111:688–9.
86. Molina R, Fabian C, Slavik M, et al. Reversal of palmar-plantar erythrodysesthesia SPPE by B6 without loss of response in colon cancer patients receiving 200 mg/m^2/day continuous 5-FU. Proc Am Soc Clin Oncol 1987;6:90.

87. Bart BJ, Bean SF. Bullous pemphigoid following the topical use of fluorouracil. Arch Dermatol 1970;102:457–60.
88. Christophidis N, Vajda FJ, Lucas I, Louis WJ. Ocular side-effects with 5-fluorouracil. Aust NZ J Med 1979;9:143–4.
89. Hamersley J, Luce JK, Florentz TR, Burkholder MM, Pepper JJ. Excessive lacrimation from fluorouracil treatment. J Am Med Assoc 1973:225:747–8.
90. Griffin JD, Garnick MB. Eye toxicity of cancer chemotherapy. A review of the literature. Cancer 1981;48:1539–49.
91. Imperia PS, Lazarus HM, Lass JH. Ocular complications of systemic cancer chemotherapy. Surv Ophthalmol 1989;34:209–30.
92. Griffin JD, Garnick MB. Eye toxicity of cancer chemotherapy: a review of the literature. Cancer 1981;48:1539–49.
93. Straus DJ, Mausolf FA, Ellerby RA, McCracken JD. Cicatricial ectropion secondary to 5-fluorouracil therapy. Med Pediatr Oncol 1977; 3:15–19.
94. Haidak DJ, Hurwitz BS, Yeung KY. Tear duct fibrosis (dacryostenosis) due to 5-fluorouracil. Ann Intern Med 1978;88:657.
95. Product Information. 5-Fluorouracil injection, 1994.
96. Galentine P, Sloas H, Hargett N, Cupples HP. Bilateral cicatricial ectropion following topical administration of 5-fluorouracil. Ann Ophthalmol 1981;13:575–7.
97. Lee V, Bentley CR, Olver JM. Sclerosing canaliculitis after 5-fluorouacil breast cancer chemotherapy. Eye 1998;12(3A):343–9.
98. Hassan A, Hurwitz JJ, Burkes RL. Epiphora in patients receiving systemic 5-fluorouracil therapy. Can J Ophthalmol 1998;33:14–19.
99. Insler MS, Helm CJ. Ankyloblepharon associated with systemic 5-fluorouracil treatment. Ann Ophthalmol 1987;19:374–5.
100. Moroni M, Porta C. Possible efficacy of allopurinol vaginal washings in the treatment of chemotherapy induced vaginitis. Cancer Chemother Pharmacol 1998:41:171–2.
101. Nikula E, Kiviniitty K, Leisti J, Taskinen PJ. Chromosome aberration in lymphocytes of nurses handling cytostatic agents. Scand J Work Environ Health 1984;10:71–4.
102. DeBeer R, Kabakow B. Anaphylactoid reaction associated with intravenous administration of 5-fluorouracil. NY State J Med 1979;79:1750–1.
103. Stein BN, Petrelli NJ, Douglass HO, Driscoll DL, Arcangeli G, Meropol NJ. Age and sex are independent predictors of 5-fluorouracil toxicity. Analysis of a large scale phase III trial. Cancer 1995;75:11–17.
104. Harris BE, Carpenter JT, Diasio RB. Severe 5-FU toxicity secondary to dihyropyrimidine dehyrogenase deficiency: a potentially more common pharmacogenetic syndrome. Cancer 1991:68:499–501.
105. Shehata N, Pater A, Tang S-C. Prolonged severe 5-fluorouracil-associated neurotoxicity in a patient with dihydropyrimidine dehydrogenase deficiency. Cancer Invest 1999;17:201–5.
106. Levi F, Soussan A, Adam R, Caussanel JP, Metzger G, Jasmin C, Bismuth H, Smolensky M, Misset JL. A phase I-II trial of five-day continuous intravenous infusion of 5-fluorouracil delivered at circadian rhythm modulated rate in patients with metastatic colorectal carcinoma. J Infus Chemother 1995;5 (Suppl 1):153–8.
107. Chen MF, Chen LT, Boyce Jr HW. 5-Fluorouracil cytotoxicity in human colon HT-29 cells with moderately increased or decreased cellular glutathione level. Anticancer Res 1995;15:163–7.
108. Stephens JD, Golbus MS, Miller TR, Wilber RR, Epstein CJ. Multiple congential abnormalities in a fetus exposed to 5-fluorouracil during the first trimester. Am J Obstet Gynaecol 1980;137:747–9.
109. Shuey DL, Buckalew AR, Wilke TS, Rogers JM, Abbott BD: Early events following maternal exposure to 5-fluorouracil lead to dysmorphology in cultured embryonic tissues. Teratology 1994;50:379–86.
110. Remick SC, Grem JL, Fischer PH, Tutsch KD, Alberti DB, Nieting LM, Tombes MB, Bruggink J, Willson JKV, Trump DL. Phase I trial of 5-fluorouracil and dipyridamole administered by seventy-two-hour concurrent continuous infusion. Cancer Res 1990;50:2667–72.
111. Sullivan R, Young CW, Miller E, et al. The clinical effects of the continuous administration of fluorinated pyrimidines. Cancer Chemother Rep 1960;8:77–83.
112. Ardalan B, Singh C, Silberman H. A randomised phase I and II study of short-term infusion of high-dose fluorouracil with or without N-(phosphonoacetyl)-L-aspartic acid in patients with advanced pancreatic and colorectal cancers. J Clin Oncol 1988;6:1053–8.
113. Goldberg JA, Kerr DJ, Watson DC, Willmott N, Bates CD, McKillop JH, Mc Ardle CS. The pharmacokinetics of 5-fluorouracil administered by arterial infusion in advanced colorectal hepatic metastases. Br J Cancer 1990;61:913–15.
114. Speyer JL, Collins JM, Dedrick RL, Brennan MF, Buckpitt AR, Londer H, DeVita VT Jr, Myers CE. Phase I and pharmacologic studies of 5-fluorouracil administered intraperitoneally. Cancer Res 1980;40:567–72.
115. Schilsky RL, Choi KE, Grayhack J, Grimmer D, Guarnieri C, Fullem L. Phase I clinical and pharmacologic study of intraperitoneal cisplatin and fluorouracil in patients with advanced intra-abdominal cancer. J Clin Oncol 1990;8:2054–61.
116. Yoshida T, Araki E, Iigo M, Fujii T, Yoshino M, Shimada Y, Saito D, Tajiri H, Yamaguchi H, Yoshida S, Yoshino M, Ohkura H, Yoshimori M, Okazaki N. Clinical significance of monitoring serum levels of 5-fluorouracil by continuous infusion in patients with advanced colonic cancer. Cancer Chemother Pharmacol 1990;26:352–3.
117. Thyss A, Milano G, Renee N, Vallicioni J, Schneider M, Demard F. Clinical pharmacokinetic study of 5-FU in continuous 5-day infusions for

head and neck cancer. Cancer Chermother Pharmacol 1986;16:64–6.

118. Woolley PV, Ayoob MJ, Smith FP, Lokey JL, DeGreen P, Marantz A, Schein PS. A controlled trial of the effect of 4-hydroxypyrazolopyrimidine (allopurinol) on the toxicity of a single bolus dose of 5-fluorouracil. J Clin Oncol 1985;3:103–9.
119. Clark P1, Slevin ML. Allopurinol mouthwash and 5-FU-induced oral toxicity. Eur J Surg Oncol 1985;11:267–8.
120. Tsavaris NB, Komitsopoulou P, Tzannou I, Loucatou P, Tsaroucha Noutsou A, Kilafis G, Kosmidis P. Decreased oral toxicity with the local use of allopurinol in patients who received high dose 5-fluorouracil. Select Cancer Ther 1991;7:113–17.
121. Porta C, Moroni M, Nastasi G. Allopurinol mouthwashes in the treatment of 5-fluorouracil-induced stomatitis. Am J Clin Oncol 1994;17:246–7.
122. Loprinzi CL, Cianflone SG, Dose AM, Etzell PS, Burnham NL, Therneau TM, Hagen L, Gainey DK, Cross M, Athmann LM, et al. A controlled evaluation of an allopurinol mouthwash as prophylaxis against 5-fluorouracil-induced stomatitis. Cancer 1990;65:1879–82.
123. Howell SB, Pfeifle CE, Wung WE. Effect of allopurinol on the toxicity of high-dose 5-fluorouracil administered by intermittent bolus injection. Cancer 1983;51:220–5.
124. Harvey VJ, Slevin ML, Dilloway MR, Clark PI, Johnston A, Lant AF. The influence of cimetidine on the pharmacokinetics of 5-fluorouracil. Br J Clin Pharmacol 1984;18:421–30.
125. Elias L, Crissman HA. Interferon effects upon the adenocarcinoma 38 and HL-60 cell lines: antiproliferative responses and synergistic interactions with halogenated pyrimidine antimetabolites. Cancer Res 1988;48:4868–73.
126. Wadler S, Wiernik PH. Clinical update on the role of 5-fluorouracil and recombinant interferon alpha-2a in the treatment of colorectal carcinoma. Semin Oncol 1990;17(Suppl 1):16–21.
127. Schuller J, Czejka M, Miksche M, et al. Influence of interferon alpha-2b leucovorin on pharmacokinetics of 5-fluorouracil. Proc Am Soc Clin Oncol 1991;10:98.
128. DeLap RJ. The effect of leucovorin on the therapeutic index of 5-fluorouracil in cancer patients. Yale J Biol Med 1988;61:23–4.
129. Damon LE, Cadman E, Benz C. Enhancement of 5-fluorouracil antitumor effects by the prior administration of methotrexate. Pharmacol Ther 1989;43:155–85.
130. Bardakji Z, Jolivet J, Langelier Y, Besner JG, Ayoub J. 5-Fluorouracil-metronidazole combination therapy in metastatic colorectal cancer: clinical, pharmacokinetic and in-vitro cytotoxicity studies. Cancer Chemother Pharmacol 1986;18:140–4.
131. Fabian CJ, Molina R, Slavik M, Dahlberg S, Giri S, Stephens R. Pyridoxine therapy for palmar-plantar erythro-dysesthesia associated with continuous 5-fluorouracil infusion. Invest New Drugs 1990;8:57–63.
132. Beveridge RA, Kales AN, Binder RA, et al. Pyridoxine (86) and amelioration of hand/foot syndrome. Proc Am Soc Clin Oncol 1990;9:102.
133. Del Mastro L, Venturini M, Sertoli MR, Rosso R. Amenorrhea induced by adjuvant chemotherapy in early breast cancer patients: prognostic role and clinical implications. Breast Cancer Res Treat 1997;43:183–90.
134. Becker K, Erckenbrecht JF, Haussinger D, Frieling T. Cardiotoxicity of the antiproliferative compound fluorouracil. Drugs 1999;57:475–84.
135. Blackledge G. New developments in cancer treatment with the novel thymidylate synthase inhibitor raltitrexed ('Tomudex'). Br J Cancer 1998;77 (Suppl 2):29–37.
136. Bontenbal M, Anderson M, Wildiers J, Cocconi G, Jassem J, Paridaens R, Rotmensz N, Sylvester R, Mouridsen HT, Klijn JGM, Van Oosterom AT. Doxorubicin vs epirubicin, report of a second-line randomized phase II/III study in advanced breast cancer. Br J Cancer 1998;77:2257–63.
137. Levy E, Piedbois P, Buyse M, Pignon J-P, Rougier P, Ryan L, Hansen R, Zee B, Weinerman B, Pater J, et al. Toxicity of fluorouracil in patients with advanced colorectal cancer: effect of administration schedule and prognostic factors. J Clin Oncol 1998;16:3537–41.
138. Singer JM, Hartley JM, Brennan C, Nicholson PW, Souhami RL. The pharmacokinetics and metabolism of ifosfamide during bolus and infusional administration: a randomized cross-over study. Br J Cancer 1998;77:978–84.
139. Pronk LC, Schrijvers D, Schellens JHM, De Bruijn EA, Planting ASTh, Locci Tonnelli D, Groult V, Verweij J, Van Oosterom AT. Phase I study on docetaxel and ifosfamide in patients with advanced solid tumours. Br J Cancer 1998;77:153–8.
140. Glimelius B, Jackobsen A, Graf W, Berglund A, Gadeberg C, Hansen P, Kjaer M, Brunsgaard N, Sandberg E, Lindberg B, Sellstrom H, Lorentz T, Pahlman L, Gustavsson B. Bolus injection (2-4 min) versus short-term (10-20 min) infusion of 5-fluorouracil in patients with advanced colorectal cancer: a prospective randomised trial. Eur J Cancer 1998;34:674–8.
141. Wolmark N, Piedbois P, Buyse M, Carlson R, Rustum Y, Erlichman C. Efficacy of intravenous continuous infusion of fluorouracil compared with bolus administration in advanced colorectal cancer. J Clin Oncol 1998;16:301–8.
142. Zalcberg J, Kerr D, Seymour L, Palmer M. Haematological and non-haematological toxicity after 5-fluorouracil and leucovorin in patients with advanced colorectal cancer is significantly associated with gender, increasing age and cycle number. Eur J Cancer 1998;34:1871–5.
143. Suzuki T, Hayashi D, Yamazaki T, Mizuno T, Kanda Y, Komuro I, Kurabayashi M, Yamaoki K, Mitani K, Hirai H, Nagai R, Yazaki Y. Elevated B-type natriuretic peptide levels after anthracycline administration. Am Heart J 1998;136:362–3.

144. Simpson AB, Paul J, Graham J, Kaye SB. Fatal bleomycin pulmonary toxicity in the west of Scotland 1991-95: a review of patients with germ cell tumours, Br J Cancer 1998;78:1061–6.
145. Lesnik PG, Ciesielski KT, Hart BL, Benzel EC, Sanders JA. Evidence for cerebellar-frontal subsystem changes in children treated with intrathecal chemotherapy for leukemia: enhanced data analysis using an effect size model. Arch Neurol 1998;55:1561–8.
146. Schagen SB, Van Dam FSAM, Muller MJ, Boogerd W, Lindeboom J, Bruning PF. Cognitive deficits after postoperative adjuvant chemotherapy for breast carcinoma. Cancer 1999;85:640–50.
147. Wolff JEA, Hauch H, Kuhl J, Egeler RM, Jurgens H. Dexamethasone increases hepatotoxicity of MTX in children with brain tumors. Anticancer Res 1998;18(4B):2895–9.
148. Lyttelton MPA, Newlands ES, Giles C, Bower M, Guimaraes A, O'Reilly S, Rustin GJS, Samson D, Kanfer EJ. High-dose therapy including carboplatin adjusted for renal function in patients with relapsed or refractory germ cell tumour: Outcome and prognostic factors. Br J Cancer 1998;77:1672–6.
149. Skinner R, Pearson ADJ, English MW, Price L, Wyllie RA, Coulthard MG, Craft AW. Cisplatin dose rate as a risk factor for nephrotoxicity in children. Br J Cancer 1998;77:1677–82.
150. Judson I, Maughan T, Beale P, Primrose J, Hoskin P, Hanwell J, Berry C, Walker M, Sutcliffe F. Effects of impaired renal function on the pharmacokinetics of raltitrexed (Tomudex ZD1694). Br J Cancer 1998;78:1188–93.
151. Radaelli F, Calori R, Faccini P, Maiolo AT. Early cutaneous lesions secondary to hydroxyurea therapy. Am J Hematol 1998;58:82–3.
152. Best PJ, Daoud MS, Pittelkow MR, Petitt RM. Hydroxyurea-induced leg ulceration in 14 patients. Ann Intern Med 1998;128:29–32.
153. Cavaletti G, Bogliun G, Zincone A, Marzorati L, Melzi P, Frattola L, Marzola M, Bonazzi C, Cantu MG, Chiari S, Galli A, Bregni M,-Gianni MA. Neuro- and ototoxicity of high-dose carboplatin treatment in poor prognosis ovarian cancer patients. Anticancer Res 1998;18(5B):3797–802.
154. Bokemeyer C, Berger CC, Hartmann JT, Kollmannsberger C, Schmoll H-J, Kuczyk MA, Kanz L. Analysis of risk factors for cisplatin-induced ototoxicity in patients with testicular cancer. Br J Cancer 1998;77:1355–62.
155. Kunitoh H, Saijo N, Furuse K, Noda K, Ogawa N. Neuromuscular toxicities of paclitaxel 210 mg m^{-2} by 3-hour infusion. Br J Cancer 1998;77:1686–8.
156. Khalil A, Chammas M, Shamseddine A, Seoud M. Fatal acute tumor lysis syndrome following treatment of vulvar carcinoma: case report. Eur J Gynaecol Oncol 1998;19:415–16.
157. Goren MP, Houle JM, Bush DA, Li JT, Newman CE, Brade WP. Similar bioavailability of single-dose oral and intravenous mesna in the blood and urine of healthy human subjects. Clin Canc Res 1998;4:2313–20.
158. Wolff JEA, Egeler RM, Anderson R, Ujack E, Iceton S, Coppes MJ. Mesna inactivates platinum agents in vitro. Anticancer Res 1998;18:4077–81.

Sameh K. Morcos and Peter Brown

46 Radiological contrast agents

Intravascular radiological contrast agents include iodinated water-soluble contrast agents used for X-ray imaging, gadolinium-based contrast agents for magnetic resonance imaging (MRI), and contrast agents to enhance the diagnostic information provided by ultrasound imaging.

Four different classes of iodinated contrast media are currently available:

- high-osmolar ionic monomers;
- low-osmolar ionic dimers;
- low-osmolar non-ionic monomers;
- iso-osmolar non-ionic dimers.

These agents can also be given orally to image the gastrointestinal tract. Adverse reactions to all types of iodinated agents are usually few, and serious reactions are uncommon. Gadolinium-based contrast agents for MRI have even better tolerance and safety profiles than iodinated contrast agents. Ultrasound contrast agents, which use microbubbles to provide acoustic enhancement, are extremely safe.

INTRAVASCULAR IODINATED CONTRAST AGENTS

The four different classes of water-soluble iodinated contrast agents have essentially the same pharmacokinetics. Adverse reactions to these agents are more likely to occur in patients who are atopic or medically unstable, including those with renal insufficiency and severe cardiovascular or respiratory diseases. Acute reactions to contrast media are either idiosyncratic or toxic, although some reactions are difficult to categorize. Reactions can be minor, intermediate, or severe and life-threatening (SEDA-22, 498). Adverse reactions to low-osmolar contrast media are about five times less common than reactions to high-osmolar agents.

Side Effects of Drugs, Annual 23
J.K. Aronson, ed.

Acute reactions to iodinated contrast media *(SEDA-21, 476; SEDA-22, 498)*

Mild adverse reactions to iodinated radiograph contrast media are encountered in as many as 3.7% of patients who receive intravenous low-osmolar agents and 13% of patients who receive intravenous high-osmolar ionic agents. The majority of these reactions are mild and clinically insignificant. Severe and very severe reactions have been noted much less frequently, in only 0.04% and 0.004% of patients who receive intravenous low-osmolar media and 0.22% and 0.04% of patients who receive high-osmolar agents. Fatal reactions to both types of contrast media are exceedingly rare, and there is no significant difference between the two agents in the incidence of mortality.

At a time when reductions in the costs of medical care are critical, decisions about which classes of contrast media to use are not determined purely on clinical grounds, but by a consideration of the cost:benefit ratio. Concern about financial implications has been the major factor in preventing a universal conversion to non-ionic contrast agents, which are better tolerated but more expensive than high-osmolar ionic agents. In the US the Health Care Finance Administration (HCFA) has recommended that the use of the expensive non-ionic contrast media should be restricted only to patients with severe cardiac disease, a history of asthma, severe allergy, severe debility, sickle cell disease, or a previous severe adverse reaction to contrast media.

The results of a study in 1324 patients who underwent diagnostic arteriography have supported the selective use of non-ionic contrast agents following the HCFA guidelines. A cost saving of $41 per patient was possible without an increase in the incidence of complications (1[C]).

Anaphylactoid, allergic, and serious reactions to iodinated water-soluble contrast agents *(SEDA-20, 422)*

Iodinated contrast media were among the top ten drugs responsible for anaphylaxis in a recent study (161 cases due to contrast media out of 1338 reports of anaphylaxis) (2[CR]). Dextran was the most common cause of anaphylaxis (418 cases). The overall death rate was significantly higher in men than in women and increased with age. The report also suggested that since the introduction of low molecular weight dextran 1 the incidence of severe anaphylaxis to dextran has fallen markedly and that radiographic contrast media may now be the most common agents causing anaphylaxis. The majority of anaphylactic reactions and all the fatal cases were due to ionic agents.

Oral administration

Adverse effects can also follow the oral administration of water-soluble iodinated contrast agents. Most reactions are usually due to their physical effects. *Pulmonary edema* secondary to aspiration of high osmolar contrast media is well recognized and can be life-threatening. It is important to avoid these agents if there is a risk of vomiting and aspiration, and to substitute low osmolar agents.

Respiratory arrest occurred after aspiration of water-soluble contrast material in a 12-year-old girl who had been injured in a traffic accident. Gastrografin (2% diatrizoate meglumine) diluted with tap water (540 ml) was given into the stomach via a nasogastric tube as part of CT-enhanced contrast examination of the abdomen. She also received 150 ml of non-ionic contrast media (iopamidol, 300 mg I/ml) intravenously, which was followed by vomiting. She became irritable and had an acute fall in oxygen saturation and progressive respiratory distress, which required endotracheal intubation. The CT scan that was performed after she became stable showed contrast material in the lungs. The authors concluded that aspiration of contrast material can be life-threatening and that administration of oral contrast media in a trauma setting may increase the risk of aspiration of gastric contents (3[c]).

Allergic reactions are uncommon after oral administration of iodinated contrast media. However, oral administration should be used with caution in patients with a history of a previous allergic reaction to an intravascular injection of iodinated contrast.

Three cases of mild allergic-like reactions to oral water-soluble iodinated contrast media during CT examinations of the abdomen have been documented in a report from Australia (4[cR]). Two patients received Gastrografin (a high-osmolar ionic contrast medium) and the third received an oral contrast medium called Gastroview (the details of which were not provided in the report). The main reaction was a skin rash that resolved within 2 days. The author advised that clinicians and radiologists should be aware of the potential for adverse reactions to oral iodinated contrast agents. In a patient with known allergic reaction to iodinated contrast media it would be prudent to consider barium suspension in preference to an iodinated agent to outline the bowel.

Delayed reactions to iodinated water-soluble contrast media
(SEDA-20, 415; SEDA-21, 482; SEDA-22, 499)

Delayed reactions are usually defined as reactions that occur more than 1 h but within 3 days of contrast injection. These reactions are usually mild, and include *fever, rash, flushing, dizziness, pruritus, arthralgia, diarrhea, nausea, vomiting, headache,* and occasionally *hypotension.* They can occur after both ionic and non-ionic contrast media.

There are conflicting data on the prevalence of delayed reactions, comparing non-ionic monomers and iso-osmolar non-ionic dimers (iotrolan, iodixanol). European studies (5[CR]) have shown no significant difference (0.62% iotrolan, 0.82% non-ionic monomers), but studies from Japan and the US have suggested that delayed reactions are 2–5 times more common with iotrolan.

Racial differences could be a factor in the high incidence of *delayed skin reactions* in Japan, as 43% of Japanese are deficient in acetaldehyde dehydrogenase. This deficiency results in the accumulation of acetaldehyde, which potentiates the ability of contrast agents (especially dimers), to bridge proteins, which is a probable causative factor in many reactions to contrast agents (6[R]).

Occasionally there are serious delayed reactions and 26 such events have been reported from Germany and Japan (6[R]). Features *included shock, hypotension, angio-edema,* and *dyspnea.*

The Federal Institute of Drugs and Medical Devices in Germany has surveyed a total of 1135 adverse drug reactions (acute and late) associated with iotrolan 280 and 1354 reports associated with iodixanol at various iodine concentrations ([7C]). Late adverse reactions (observed later than 1 hour after injection) were observed in 757 cases (67%) associated with iotrolan 280 and 525 cases (39%) associated with iodixanol. Late reactions were observed mainly in the first 24 hours, with occasional reports at 24–72 hours after injection. Rarely, delayed contrast reactions have been reported more than 72 hours after injection, although they are difficult to substantiate. This study emphasizes the importance of extending the surveillance period for at least 72 hours after contrast administration. Most delayed reactions in this study were non-serious allergic-like reactions, with symptoms including *itching, urticaria, erythema, edema,* and *bronchospasm.* In a very few cases there were serious or life-threatening reactions, including *Quincke's edema* and *hypotension.* Because of the risk and consequences these serious reactions, which may occur when the patient is not under medical supervision, iotrolan has been withdrawn as an intravascular contrast agent.

The incidence of late adverse reactions to the iso-osmolar agent iodixanol has also been investigated in a retrospective comparison with the non-ionic monomer iohexol. Reactions after 3075 injections were reviewed. Patients were sent a written questionnaire to find out about the incidence of any acute or delayed reactions. Those who developed reactions were interviewed by telephone and specific second questionnaires were administered. The incidence of adverse reactions was low (2% for late adverse reactions and 2.3% for acute reactions). There was no significant difference in the incidence of acute or delayed adverse reactions to iohexol and iodixanol and there were no serious reactions ([8C]).

The efficacy and safety of iodixanol has also been documented in children. Iodixanol was well tolerated without any important adverse events in 25 children under 4 years old undergoing excretory urography ([9C]).

The incidence of delayed adverse reactions to various non-ionic monomers in Japanese patients undergoing contrast-enhanced CT has been compared with the incidence in control patients who did not receive contrast. Delayed reactions occurred in 12.4% of patients who received contrast compared with 10.3% in the control group. The authors concluded that the frequency of delayed reactions that can be attributed to contrast media is 2.1%. The most common reactions were *itching* and limited *urticaria* ([10C]). This report highlights the difficulty of verifying that adverse events that occur many hours after contrast administration are directly caused by the contrast agent.

There was no difference in the incidence of adverse effects between iotrolan 320 and iohexol 350 in cardiac angiography for ischemic heart disease in 120 patients ([11C]). There were no serious adverse events. One patient developed mild *urticaria* after iotrolan. Five patients in each group had mild delayed reactions. The nature of these reactions was not stated in the report. The authors concluded that iotrolan is a safe contrast agent for cardiac angiography.

Cardiovascular In a comparison of the effects of ioxaglate (a low-osmolar ionic dimer) with iopamidol (a non-ionic monomer), iopamidol caused fewer electrocardiographic changes and a reduction in ventricular excitability compared with ioxaglate ([12C]).

Nervous system Low-osmolar non-ionic monomers are widely used intrathecally for diagnostic procedures and neurotoxicity is low. Well known adverse effects in myelography with non-ionic agents are *nausea, vomiting, headache,* and *backache,* which are also associated with the procedure of lumbar puncture itself. Another case of *acute encephalopathy* after intrathecal administration of non-ionic media has been reported ([13c]).

Six hours after 10 ml of iohexol (Omnipaque, 240 mg of iodine per ml) had been injected into the left lateral ventricle during an operation on the thalamus of a 63-year-old man with Parkinson's disease, his level of alertness deteriorated and he became disorientated and confused. A CT scan of the head showed the surgical lesion and artifacts due to contrast medium, but no other abnormalities. After 24 hours he became more alert with coherent speech but there was still mild disorientation. These symptoms resolved within the next two days.

Acute encephalopathy after myelography with iohexol has been reported in a very few cases. According to the authors this was the first case of encephalopathy after iohexol ventriculography with the onset of symptoms several hours earlier than in myelography cases, probably owing to direct administration into the ventricular system. Awareness of this complication can be helpful in patient management after procedures in which iohexol is given intrathecally.

Cortical blindness after contrast media exposure has been reported to be as high as 1–4% in patients undergoing vertebral angiography, even with modern non-ionic low-osmolality contrast agents. It has been thought to be due to breakdown of the blood-brain barrier of the occipital cortex with subsequent direct neurotoxicity of the contrast medium. Repeated exposure to contrast media did not cause recurrent episodes of cortical blindness. The outcome seems to be favorable, with return of vision within 24–48 h and probably no increased risk on re-exposure. Occasionally cortical blindness can be caused by other procedures, e.g. coronary angiography (14[c]).

During coronary angiography a 55-year-old man was given 280 ml of non-ionic contrast media iomeprole (350 mg I/ml). Ten minutes later he became progressively confused and developed complete loss of vision. A CT scan of the head showed pronounced intracerebral enhancement of contrast media in the posterior third of the brain without evident relation to a vascular territory and a straight border towards normal brain tissue. Angiography of the right vertebral artery showed normal patency of the vertebrobasilar and venous systems, excluding thromboembolic events in the posterior cerebral circulation. Another CT scan of the head 1 day later showed clearing of the contrast medium. The neurological deficit resolved more slowly, but there was normal vision and minimal amnestic deficit after five days.

These findings were compatible with leakage of contrast medium through the blood-brain barrier, direct or indirect neurotoxicity of the contrast media being the most likely explanation for the neurological symptoms.

Endocrine, metabolic Contrast medium-induced *hyperthyroidism* is rare and usually occurs in patients with autonomous thyroid function. Treatment is exclusively symptomatic. Prophylaxis with sodium perchlorate should be considered in cardiac patients with a goiter and a subnormal concentration of thyroid stimulating hormone (THS).

In three women (aged 63, 72, and 75 years) with subclinical hyperthyroid goiters, hyperthyroidism developed after the intravenous administration of iodinated contrast medium (15[c]). There was a marked rise in the concentration of free T_4. The hyperthyroidism improved spontaneously in all three patients.

Hematological The effects of contrast media on blood coagulation and platelet aggregation have been extensively evaluated over the last decade. However, this issue remains contentious, and although non-ionic agents are viewed as being less anticoagulant than ionic contrast media, they are not considered to be procoagulant.

The *thrombotic complications* after angioplasty in patients with unstable angina have been investigated in a study from Canada (16[C]). There was no significant difference in the incidence of thrombotic complications between patients receiving the low-osmolar ionic dimer ioxaglate (n = 103) and those receiving the non ionic agent iopamidol (n = 102), although there was a non-significant trend towards more thrombus formation in the non-ionic group (21 of 129 patients) compared with the ionic group (15 of 141 patients). The two groups were well matched with respect to age, sex, class of unstable angina, and risk factors. There was no significant difference between the two groups with respect to clinical outcome in the first 24 h after percutaneous coronary angioplasty.

Thrombocytopenia and purpura after intravascular administration of contrast media is extremely rare. Acute thrombocytopenia has previously been observed after the injection of the non-ionic monomer iopamidol (SEDA-22, 501) and there has been the following further report (17[c]).

Thrombocytopenia occurred 24 h after 100 ml of iopamidol was given intravenously during cranial CT scanning to investigate a 9-month history of headache. The patient reported purpuric lesions on her legs, abdomen, and gingival bleeding within 24 h of the scan, and examination of the peripheral blood at 48 h confirmed severe thrombocytopenia. A bone-marrow smear showed a prominent increase in megakaryocytes and dysmegakaryopoiesis. The bleeding time was longer than 15 minutes. Other laboratory values were within normal limits. Within 10 days all the lesions disappeared spontaneously and the platelet count improved gradually and returned to normal within 2 months.

The pathogenesis of this complication is not understood but is most likely an immunological response to the contrast administration.

Liver *Hepatotoxicity* is uncommon with iodinated water-soluble contrast media but is occasionally reported (18[C]).

A 19-year-old woman without previous hepatic impairment developed abdominal pain and an acute rise in liver enzymes after an injection of iopromide. During intravenous infusion of iopromide she developed vomiting and hypotension, which resolved within a few hours. Repeat laboratory tests showed a rise in serum transaminases (AsT and AlT), which peaked on the second day and then rapidly fell. There was a slight prolongation of the prothrombin time and a moderate increase in total serum bilirubin. Serum gamma-glutamyltransferase activity was normal. Ultrasonography of the liver and biliary tree was normal and serological markers for viral hepatitis were negative. Two weeks later liver function tests were all in the normal range.

An acute rise in liver enzyme after intravascular iopromide is uncommon and has been previously reported only in some patients with concomitant hepatic impairment. The temporal association (rapid clinical onset and raised serum transaminases after the injection of iopromide) suggested that iopromide may have played a role in the occurrence of the hepatitis-like picture in this case.

Urinary system *Nephrotoxicity* due to contrast media is rare in patients with normal renal function before contrast administration. However, contrast injection may cause significant deterioration in renal function in patients with pre-existing renal insufficiency (19[cR]).

A 45-year-old man with aggressive hypertension underwent abdominal aortography to assess the possibility of renal artery stenosis. His baseline renal function was reduced and the serum creatinine was 210 mol/l. He received 1000 ml of saline solution intravenously as prophylaxis against contrast nephropathy. An unidentified high-osmolar contrast medium was injected into the abdominal aorta above the level of the renal arteries. There were atherosclerotic changes in the abdominal aorta and a discrete stenosis of left renal artery. Oliguria developed 24 hours later and the serum creatinine rose to 350 mol/l. He was given isotonic saline (2 l/day) with 100 mg of furosemide. After 2 days the serum creatinine concentration fell to 190 mol/l and his daily urine volume increased to 1.6 l/day.

The use of renal vasodilators to prevent contrast media-induced nephrotoxicity has been evaluated in the past. However, experience has been mixed and there is no conclusive evidence that these drugs are effective, particularly in patients with diabetic nephropathy who are at high risk of this complication (SEDA-19, 428). However, in a study from the US dopamine was effective in preventing further deterioration in renal function in patients with a raised serum creatinine undergoing angiography for lower limb ischemia (20[C]). Dopamine (2.5 mg/kg) was given to 28 patients beginning 1 h before injection of contrast medium (Omnipaque 300, mean volume about 140 ml) and continuing for a total of 12 h. Patients in the control group received an equal volume of isotonic saline. Serum creatinine was measured daily for 4 days after arteriography. Dopamine reduced the incidence of contrast nephrotoxicity (defined as an increase in the baseline serum creatinine concentration over 0.5 mg/dl (44 mol/l) from 44 to 18%. Previous studies have not shown any protective effect of dopamine against contrast-induced nephropathy, in spite of marked increase in renal blood flow shown in a study of patients undergoing cardiac catheterization (21[R]).

The lack of protective effect of prophylactic hemodialysis after contrast administration in patients with pre-existing renal impairment against the development of contrast nephropathy has previously been demonstrated in a report from Germany (SEDA-22, 502). The same group have now confirmed their previous observation in a bigger study in 30 patients with pre-existing renal impairment (22[C]). Hemodialysis did not influence the incidence or outcome of contrast-induced nephropathy, in spite of effective elimination of contrast medium from the circulation. The failure of hemodialysis to protect against the development of contrast nephropathy is due to the very rapid onset of renal injury after the administration of contrast medium.

Urinary enzymes are often raised after the administration of contrast media. However, no relation has been established between a reduction in glomerular filtration rate, a rise in serum creatinine (the characteristic features of contrast nephrotoxicity), and the presence of enzymuria. It has been argued that the detection of urinary enzymes is of little importance to the clinical assessment and management of contrast medium nephrotoxicity (21[R]).

Enzymuria has been reported after the intravascular administration of high-osmolar or low-osmolar contrast media (23[C]). The study suggested that the brush-border enzyme gamma glutamyltransferase is a better marker for tubular toxicity due to contrast media than alanine aminopeptidase.

Contrast media, particularly high-osmolar agents, can cause a significant *natriuresis and diuresis.* In a study of 42 patients who underwent cardiac angiography, the fractional excretion of sodium, the urinary excretion of the renal natriuretic peptide urodilatin, and the plasma concentration of atrial natriuretic peptide were measured before and after intravascular diatrizoate (an ionic high-osmolar contrast agent) 55 ml or the non-ionic agent iopamidol 200 ml (24[C]). None of the patients had diabetic nephropathy or multiple myeloma. Diuretics, angiotensin converting enzyme inhibitors, a non-steroidal anti-inflammatory drugs were withheld for at least 12 hours before the examination, and 11 patients received a mean of 600 ml of isotonic saline intravenously before and during angiography, because of mild chronic renal insufficiency. The other 31 received no volume expansion. Both groups received a similar volume of radiocontrast agent. After angiography the plasma concentration of atrial natriuretic peptide and the urinary excretion of urodilatin were both increased. Urinary urodilatin excretion correlated with an increase in the fractional excretion of sodium. There was no correlation between the serum concentration of atrial natriuretic peptide and urinary sodium excretion. This study suggests that the intravascular administration of contrast agents causes a natriuresis associated with the urinary excretion of urodilatin. This is consistent with the hypothesis that urodilatin may contribute to sodium excretion after radiocontrast administration in a paracrine manner.

Clinical experience has shown that non-ionic low-osmolar contrast media are less nephrotoxic compared with high-osmolar agents, particularly in patients with pre-existing renal impairment (SEDA-19, 428). However, renal tolerance of the different commercial formulations of non-ionic agents seems to be comparable.

The clinical and biological tolerance of iobitridol (Xenetix, a new non-ionic medium, osmolality 915 mOsm/kg at a concentration of 350 mg I/ml) has been assessed in a placebo-controlled study in 21 patients with chronic renal insufficiency (glomerular filtration rate less than 60 ml/minute) (25[C]). Serum creatinine and creatinine clearance remained stable 24 and 48 hours after the procedure. No patient had a nephrotoxic reaction or acute oliguria. Only one patient given iobitridol had an *increase in serum creatinine* of more than 15% from baseline; the serum creatinine normalized within 4 days of contrast administration. One patient given placebo had a similar increase in serum creatinine, which recovered within 48 hours. The author suggested that the use of non-ionic media such as iobitridol should result in a substantial decrease in the incidence of contrast nephropathy.

Interactions Recently concern has been expressed about the hazards of lactic acidosis after the use of intravascular iodinated contrast agents in patients taking *metformin.* Metformin is excreted through the kidneys, and renal insufficiency can lead to its retention, which can cause fatal lactic acidosis. The manufacturers have recommended that metformin should be withdrawn for 48 hours before and 48 hours after the administration of intravascular contrast media, which can cause renal damage, and treatment should not be restarted until normal renal function is confirmed. Reviews of reported cases of lactic acidosis after contrast administration have shown that there was pre-existing renal impairment in all cases. A retrospective evaluation of patients taking metformin who underwent contrast angiography has also confirmed this observation (26[C]). Of 33 patients, 29 had a normal serum creatinine before the angiographic procedure and none had a rise after angiography. Four had an abnormal serum creatinine before angiography; all four had a significant deterioration in renal function and died, two from unrelated causes and two from acute renal insufficiency and acidosis. The authors concluded that administration of contrast media is hazardous in diabetic patients with pre-existing renal impairment and that patients with normal renal function taking metformin are not at risk of lactic acidosis. They recommended that serum creatinine should be measured in all patients before angiography. In patients taking metformin with a normal serum creatinine intravascular contrast is not contraindicated.

Skin and appendages Cases of serious dermatological eruptions after the administration of contrast media have been reported, including a case of *fatal acute vasculitis, fatal Stevens-Johnson syndrome, and toxic epidermal necrolysis.*

Reticulated purpura has been reported after the use of diatrizoate meglumine, a high-osmolar water-soluble contrast agent, for hysterosalpingography (27[c]).

Within 48 hours of a hysterosalpingogram using diatrizoate meglumine a 34-year-old woman developed a burning sensation in her left leg, 4 days later developed tenderness and redness on the left posterior thigh and calf, and 4 days after that mottling of the skin of the thigh. Two weeks later she had marked tenderness and purpuric macules in a reticulated pattern on both legs. A skin biopsy showed changes suggestive of erythema multiforme. There was no evidence of vasculitis. The skin lesions persisted unchanged for about 1 week, after which they resolved without treatment.

This clinical picture of reticulated purpura with the formulation of a few bullae has not been previously reported in reaction secondary to the injection of contrast media. The histological changes supported the diagnosis of a drug reaction. Although some of the histological findings are seen in erythema multiforme the patient's clinical presentation did not support that diagnosis.

Subcutaneous extravasation of contrast media during rapid intravascular injection can cause *local irritation and inflammatory responses*. The severity of these effects depends on the volume and osmolality of the extravasated contrast medium. High-osmolality contrast media can cause skin ulceration and necrosis. Subcutaneous hyaluronidase, aspiration of fluid, elevation of the limb, and topical application of cold compresses are some of the measures used to treat this complication.

The frequency of *extravasation* of ionic and non-ionic contrast media during rapid bolus injection in 5106 CT contrast-enhanced scans was 0.9% (31 patients had extravasation of ionic media and 17 patients had extravasation of non-ionic media) (28[C]). There was no correlation between the injection rate and the frequency of extravasation. None of the patients who had extravasation had permanent damage.

THOROTRAST

Thorotrast was widely used in 1928–55 as an X-ray contrast medium. It contains thorium dioxide, which has a radioactive half-life of about 400 years. After intravenous administration it is deposited in the reticuloendothelial system, the majority being stored in the liver. Various *liver neoplasms* due to chronic α-ray irradiation have been reported, most notably angiosarcoma and cholangiocarcinoma. Multiple Thorotrast-induced primary tumors are rare but have been reported in a recent report from Japan (29[c]).

An 86-year-old man received intravenous Thorotrast to investigate a bullet wound to his shoulder in 1939. He presented in 1993 with jaundice, leading to liver failure and death. Autopsy showed four separate carcinomas: a cholangiocarcinoma in the left lobe of the liver, a well-differentiated tubular carcinoma of the antrum of the stomach, an invasive squamous carcinoma of the lung, and a well-differentiated adenocarcinoma of the ampulla of Vater. There were multiple mutations in the p53 tumor suppression gene caused by chronic alpha-ray irradiation.

There has also been a recent report of *nodular regenerative hyperplasia of the liver* associated with previous Thorotrast administration (30[c]).

GADOLINIUM

Gadolinium compounds used as contrast agents apart from MRI

Gadolinium can sufficiently attenuate X-rays to be visualized with digital subtraction angiography, although the quality of image is consistently inferior than with iodinated agents. Of 13 patients who underwent transplant angiography with 16–20 ml of either gadopentetate dimeglumine (0.5 mmol/ml) (Magnavist, Berlex Laboratories, Wayne, NJ) or gadolinium (0.5 mmol/ml) (Omniscan, Nycomed. Princeton, NJ), there was no significant deterioration in renal function in 11 patients (31[C]). In the other two there were significant increases that were not considered to be due to either gadolinium or the administration of CO_2. These findings are consistent with previous studies (SEDA-22, 504) showing that gadolinium compounds are not nephrotoxic.

MRI CONTRAST AGENTS

(SEDA-22, 503)

New non-gadolinium paramagnetic contrast agents have been developed to increase the diagnostic accuracy of MRI scans.

Mangafodipir trisodium

Mangafodipir trisodium (Mn DPDP; Teslascan, Nycomed, Oslo) has been developed for hepatobiliary imaging. Of 30 patients undergoing contrast enhanced MRI scanning for focal liver lesions only two complained of slight nausea during the injection of Mn DPDP (32^{C}). In all other cases the contrast agent was well tolerated.

Trifluoromethane

Animal studies have shown that the inhaled fluorine gas trifluoromethane (FC-23) can be used as an indicator of cerebral blood flow during MRI scans. However, a recent clinical study showed that FC-23 is not inert and that humans do not tolerate concentrations suitable for current MRI technology. Five healthy volunteers inhaled FC-23 at concentrations of 10–60% in a double-blind study (33^{C}). Concentrations over 30% produced *impairment of neuropsychological function.*

ULTRASOUND CONTRAST AGENTS

There have been further reports confirming the safety of these echo-enhancing agents. Several types of agent are being evaluated and various trials are reporting minimal adverse effects.

A phase 3 assessment of the accuracy of Levovist (SHU508A, Schering, Berlin), which contains galactose microparticles and palmitic acid, in investigating the portal system has been reported (34^{C}). It was injected into peripheral veins in 588 patients in concentrations of 200–400 mg/ml. During the 24 hours after the last injection, *pain at the site of injection, vasodilatation,* and *paresthesia* were the only adverse effects definitely related to the injection. There were 18 adverse events in 12 patients and the only severe reaction (fever) was not considered to have been related to Levovist.

A double-blind placebo-controlled evaluation of perflenapent emulsion as a contrast agent for the liver, kidneys, and vasculature has been reported in 151 patients of whom 12 had adverse effects compared with nine who received placebo (35^{C}). *Injection site pain, vasodilatation, rash,* and *rhinitis* occurred more often with perflenapent than placebo.

Albunex (a suspension of air-filled albumin microspheres) has been compared with Optison (albumin microspheres containing the gas perfluoropropane) in 203 patients undergoing echocardiography (36^{C}). There were no clinically significant changes in physical examination, vital signs, or electrocardiogram in either group. Adverse effects were few in each group and were most commonly related to *flushing, warmth,* or *taste disturbance.* Similar results have been reported from a comparison of Echogen (2% dodecafluoropentane emulsion) with Albunex (SEDA-22, 505; 36^{C}).

REFERENCES

1. Hartnell GG, Gates J, Underhill J. Implementing HCFA guidelines on appropriate use of non-ionic contrast for diagnostic arteriography: Effects on complication rates and management costs. Acad Radiol 1998;5(Suppl):S359–61.
2. Wang D-Y, Forslund C, Persson U, Wiholm B-E. Drug-attributed anaphylaxis. Pharmacoepidemiol Drug Saf 1998;7:269–74.
3. Donnelly LF, Frush DP, Frush KS. Aspirated contrast material contributing to respiratory arrest in a pediatric trauma patient. Am J Roentgenol 1998;171:471–3.
4. Ridley LJ. Allergic reactions to oral iodinated contrast agents: reactions to oral contrast. Australas Radiol 1998;42:114–17.
5. Niendorf HP. Delayed allergy like reactions to X-ray contrast media. Problem statement exemplified with iotrolan (Isovist) 280. Eur Radiol 1996;6 (Suppl):S8–10.
6. Thomsen HS, Muller RV, Mattery RF, editors. Trends in Contrast Media. Berlin: Springer-Verlag, 1999:71–2.
7. Pohly JP. Onset of late adverse drug reactions to dimeric non-ionic contrast media: iotrolan, iodixanol. Pharmacoepidemiol Drug Saf 1998;7(Suppl):S18–22.
8. Rydberg J, Aspelin P, Charles J. Late adverse reactions observed retrospectively after use of monomeric, dimeric X-ray contrast media. Pharmacoepidemiol Drug Saf 1998; 7 (Suppl): S16–17.
9. Dacher JN, Sirinelli D, Boscq M, Hassan M, Garel C. Iodixanol in paediatric excretory urography: efficiency and safety compared to iohexol. Pediatr Radiol 1998;28:112–14.
10. Yasuda R, Munechika H. Delayed adverse reactions to nonionic monomeric contrast-enhanced media. Invest Radiol 1998;33:1–5.

11. Mezilis N, Salame MY, Dyet JF, Arafa SO, Oakley GDG. Comparison of iotrolan 320 and iohexol 350 in cardiac angiography: a randomised double-blind clinical study. Eur J Radiol 1998; 28:171–5.
12. Altun A, Ozbay G. Effects of ionic versus nonionic contrast agents on dispersion of ventricular repolarization. Turk Kardiyol Dernegi Ars 1998; 26:362–7.
13. Schuurman PR, Speelman JD, Ongerboer De Visserz BW, Bosch D. Acute encephalopathy after iohexol ventriculography in functional stereotaxy. Acta Neurochir 1998;140:98–9.
14. Sticherling C, Berkefeld J, Auch-Schwelk W, Lanfermann H. Transient bilateral cortical blindness after coronary angiography. Lancet 1998; 351:570.
15. Van Guldener C, Blom DM, Lips P, Van Schijndel RJMS. Hyperthyroidism due to iodinated roentgen contrast media. Ned Tijdschr Geneeskd 1998;142:1641–4.
16. Malekianpour M, Bonan R, Lesperance J, Gosselin G, Hudson G. Comparison of ionic and nonionic low osmolar contrast media in relation to thrombotic complications of angioplasty in patients with unstable angina. Am Heart J 1998;135:1067–75.
17. Ural AU, Beyan C, Yalcin A. Thrombocytopenia following intravenous iopamidol. Eur J Clin Pharmacol 1998;54:575–6.
18. Re G, Lanzarini C, Melandri R. Liver injury after contrast-enhanced, computed tomography with iopromide. J Toxicol Clin Toxicol 1998;36:261–2.
19. Kolonko A, Kokot F, Wiecek A. Contrast-associated nephropathy—old clinical problem and new therapeutic perspectives. Nephrol Dial Transplant 1998;13:803–6.
20. Hans SS, Hans BA, Dhillon R, Dmuchowski C, Glover J. Effect of dopamine on renal function after arteriography in patients with pre-existing renal insufficiency. Am Surg 1998;64:432–6.
21. Morcos SK. Contrast media induced nephrotoxicity—questions and answers. Br J Radiol 1998;71:357–65.
22. Lehnert T, Keller E, Gondolf K, Schaffner T, Pavenstadt H. Effect of haemodialysis after contrast medium administration in patients with renal insufficiency. Nephrol Dial Transplant 1998; 13:358–62.
23. Donadio C, Tramonti G, Lucchesi A, Giordani R, Lucchetti A. Gamma-glutamyltransferase is a reliable marker for tubular effects of contrast media. Renal Failure 1998;20:319–24.
24. Haller C, Meyer M, Scheele T, Koch A, Forssmann WG, Kubler W. Radiocontrast-induced natriuresis associated with increased urinary urodilatin excretion. J Intern Med 1998;243:155–62.
25. Deray G, Bellin MF, Zamin S, Raymond F, Grellet J, Jacobs C. Evaluation of the renal tolerance of xenetix in patients with chronic renal failure. Nephron 1998;80:240.
26. Nawaz S, Cleveland T, Gaines PA, Chan P. Clinical risk associated with contrast angiography in metformin treated patients: a clinical review. Clin Radiol 1998;53:342–4.
27. Rinker MH, Sangueza OP, Davis LS. Reticulated purpura occurring with contrast medium after hysterosalpingography. Br J Dermatol 1998;138:919–20.
28. Federle MP, Chang PJ, Confer S, Ozgun B Frequency and effects of extravasation of ionic and nonionic CT contrast media during rapid bolus injection. Radiology 1998;206:637–40.
29. Iwamoyo KS, Mizuno T, Masuzawa M, Mori T. Seyama T. Multiple, unique, and common p53 mutations in a thorotrast recipient with four primary cancers. Hum Pathol 1998;29:412–16.
30. Beer TW, Cart NJ, Buxton PJ. Thorotrast associated nodular regenerative hyperplasia of the liver. J Clin Pathol 1998;51:941–2.
31. Spinosa DJ, Matsumo AH, Angle JF, Hagspiel KD, Issacs R. Gadolinium based contrast and carbon dioxide angiography to evaluate transplants for vascular causes of renal insufficiency and accelerated hypertension. J Vasc Intervent Radiol 1998;9:909–16.
32. Jung G, Heindel W, Krahe T, Kugel H, Walter C, Fischbach R. Influence of the hepatobiliary contrast agent mangafodipir trisodium (Mn-DPDP) on the imaging properties of abdominal organs. Magn Res Imaging 1998;16:925–31.
33. Rahill AA, Brown GG, Fagan SC, Ewing JR, Branch CA. Neuropsychological dose effects of a freon, trifloromethane (FC-23) compared to N_2O. Neurotoxicol Teratol 1998;20:617–26.
34. Gebel M, Caselitz M, Bowen-Davies PE, Weber S. A multicenter, prospective, open label, randomised, controlled phase IIIb study of SH U 508 A (Levovist) for Doppler signal enhancement in the vascular system. Ultraschall Med 1998;19:148–56.
35. Robbin ML, Eisenfeld AJ. Perflenapent emulsion: a US contrast agent for diagnostic radiology-multicenter, double-blind comparison with a placebo. Radiology 1998;207: 717–22.
36. Cohen JL, Cheirif J, Segar DS, Gillam LD, Gottdiener JS. Improved left ventricular endocardial border delineation and opacification with OPTISON (FS069), a new echocardiographic contrast agent; results of a phase 3 multicenter trial. J Am Coll Cardiol 1998; 32:746–52.

B.C.P. Polak

47 Drugs used in ocular treatment

Drugs used in ocular treatment are widely prescribed by growing numbers of eye-care professionals, increasingly by optometrists, opticians, and ophthalmic-trained nurses in addition to ophthalmologists and general practitioners. In some countries not only diagnostic ophthalmic drugs, but also therapeutic ophthalmic agents are used by professionals who have not received medical training: inadequate training can result in the prescription of potentially toxic drugs in patients at risk and a failure to associate a topical medication with a systemic condition, allowing an adverse effect to pass unrecognized. It is therefore of increasing importance to improve awareness of the potential dangers intrinsic in the use of topical eye medications.

DIAGNOSTIC DRUGS

Fluorescein

Local use *Pseudomonas aeruginosa* is an especially dangerous pathogenic micro-organism, likely to contaminate fluorescein eye-drops. Fluorescein is most safely dispensed in sterile single-dose units or as sterile fluorescein-impregnated strips (SED-13, 1425).

Topical fluorescein application is a routine component of the ophthalmological examination, especially to measure intraocular pressure by means of applanation tonometry. Recently a case of topical-fluorescein induced urticaria has been described (1[c]).

Systemic use The majority of the systemic reactions after intravenous fluorescein in fluorescein angiography are allergic, but some may be due to contamination with dimethylformamide, an industrial solvent. It is difficult to predict adverse effects by intracutaneous testing of the drug. A *delayed allergic response,* developing a few hours after intravenous fluorescein dye injection, can occur (2[c]). It is recommended that a complete allergy evaluation be performed in all patients who have adverse reactions to fluorescein, in order to differentiate true allergic reactions from other types of reactions (3[c]).

A study was undertaken to evaluate whether or not fluorescein interferes with erythrocyte properties during the angiographic procedure. In 37 patients, 26 with type II diabetes mellitus with and without retinopathy and 11 without diabetes mellitus, all undergoing fluorescein angiography, blood samples were drawn before and 30 minutes after fluorescein injection. The erythrocyte aggregation index, membrane lipid fluidity, and erythrocyte acetylcholinesterase activity were determined in both groups. After fluorescein injection there was no statistical change in erythrocyte aggregation index or erythrocyte membrane fluidity in either group. However, there was a significant *fall in erythrocyte acetylcholinesterase activity*, a marker of membrane protein integrity, in the diabetic patients. In other words, in diabetic patients fluorescein seems to interact with the erythrocyte membrane, and may interfere with the blood flow in the microcirculation (4[c]).

Fluorescein angiography using oral sodium fluorescein is generally effective and safe in standard practice. The solution used is 10 ml of 10% sodium fluorescein, the same material that is generally used for intravenous injection in conventional fluorescein angiography. Retinal photography starts 15 minutes after ingestion and continues for 1 h. The camera, the photography, and film processing techniques are the same as those used for conventional fluorescein angiography. In 97% of 2625 eyes adequate photographs for clinical use were obtained after oral fluorescein (5[C]). Only 1.7% of the patients

Side Effects of Drugs, Annual 23
J.K. Aronson, ed.

had minimal *itching, discomfort,* or *nausea* after oral sodium fluorescein. There were no anaphylactic or other severe adverse effects.

Phenylephrine

Phenylephrine was the drug that most often caused sensitization in patients with *contact allergy* after the application of mydriatic eye-drops: since several eye-drops are used in the same patient, it is always important to find out which drug or preservative is the allergen (6[c]–8[c]).

Systemic toxicity can result from topical application: *headache, raised blood pressure, extra beats, tachycardia, faintness,* and *strokes* have been reported (SED-13, 1422). The incidence of adverse effects is high with 10% phenylephrine, but is less with lower concentrations. Systemic reactions also increase with increased frequency of use and when phenylephrine is applied in a pledget. The package inserts for 10% phenylephrine in the US and Australia require that the drug should not be used more often than once an hour. A large number of severe systemic reactions, including death, have been reported in more than 20 articles in peer-reviewed ophthalmic journals. For this reason 10% phenylephrine eye-drops should be used with caution in patients with cardiac disease, significant hypertension, or advanced arteriosclerosis, and in the frail elderly.

Risk factors Phenylephrine eye-drops are contraindicated in *infants* and *patients with aneurysms.*

Interactions Phenylephrine should also be used with caution in patients taking *monoamine oxidase inhibitors, tricyclic antidepressants, propranolol, reserpine, guanethidine, methyldopa,* or *atropine-like drugs* (9[r]).

Tropicamide

Adverse reactions due to the administration of mydriatic eye-drops are not uncommon. The most commonly used are tropicamide, phenylephrine, and cyclopentolate hydrochloride. Tropicamide and phenylephrine are commonly used in the same patient, since these drugs act synergistically and give maximal pupillary dilatation greater than using either of the drugs alone.

Tropicamide tends to have a greater mydriatic than cycloplegic effect. It is a short-acting atropine-like derivative and has been regarded as an effective and safe mydriatic, used for pupillary dilatation by professionals, who are not always medical doctors.

Recently, however, a serious adverse reaction to topical tropicamide has been described: a *transient ischemic attack* in a 64-year-old patient with cardiovascular risk factors (10[c]).

Near fatal *anticholinergic intoxication* has been reported after routine fundoscopy (11[c]).

A 62-year-old man underwent fundoscopy after pharmacological pupillary dilatation with tropicamide eye-drops. Half an hour after fundoscopic examination he experienced two generalized seizures with respiratory arrest and required intubation and mechanical ventilation. He was treated with physostigmine and made a full recovery.

THERAPEUTIC DRUGS

The systemic effects of β-blocker eye-drops are described in Chapter 18.

Chloramphenicol

Local adverse effects *Allergic reactions* can occur, and consist of conjunctivitis, keratitis, and palpebral and periocular eczema (12[c]). Recently a case of erythema multiforme caused by local treatment with chloramphenicol eye-drops has been described (12[c]). The possible role of an allergic mechanism in this reaction was suggested, based upon a positive mast cell degranulation test (13[c]).

Systemic effects Chloramphenicol causes two types of *bone-marrow toxicity:*

- dose-related, reversible depression generally affecting erythroid cells;
- an idiosyncratic reaction that affects all three cell lines and is generally fatal.

Ocular chloramphenicol causes this idiosyncratic reaction only in genetically predisposed patients. Since topical administration achieves systemic effects by absorption through the conjunctival membrane or through drainage down the lacrimal duct, with eventual absorption from the gastrointestinal tract, the risk may be similar to that after oral administration of the antibiotic. Based on two international population-based case-control studies an association between ocular chloramphenicol and aplastic anemia cannot be excluded, but seems to be very small: less than one per million treatment courses (14[R], 15[R]). In one study the incidence of aplastic anemia among users of ocular chloramphenicol was 0.36 cases per million weeks of treatment, and the incidence among non-users was 0.04 cases per million weeks (16[R]). It remains difficult to justify subjecting patients to this small, potential risk, in view of the availability of other antibiotics for use in the eye. In the US the Physician Desk Reference emphasizes with repeated warnings the importance of not using ocular chloramphenicol unless there is no alternative, and this warning should be supported on both sides of the Atlantic (17[R]).

REFERENCES

1. Valvano MN, Martin TP. Periorbital urticaria and topical fluorescein. Am J Emerg Med 1998; 16:525–6.
2. Johnson RN, McDonald HR, Schatz H. Rash, fever and chills after intravenous fluorescein angiography. Am J Ophthalmol 1998;126:837–8.
3. Lopez Saez MP, Ordoqui E, Tornero P, Baeza A, Sainza T, Zubeldia JM. Fluorescein-induced allergic reaction. Ann Allergy Asthma Immunol 1998;81:428–30.
4. Sargento L, Zabala L, Saldanha C, Souza Ramalho P, Martins e Silva J. The effect of sodium fluorescein angiography on erythrocyte properties. Clin Hemorheol Microcirc 1998;18:135–9.
5. Hara T, Inami M, Hara T. Efficacy and safety of fluorescein angiography with orally administered sodium fluorescein. Am J Ophthalmol 1998;126:560–4.
6. Villarreal O. Reliability of diagnostic tests for contact allergy to mydriatic eyedrops. Contact Dermatitis 1998;38:150–4.
7. Wigger-Alberti W, Elsner P, Wuthrich B. Allergic contact dermatitis to phenylephrine. Eur J Allergy Clin Immunol 1998;53:217–18.
8. Rafael M, Pereira F, Faria MA. Allergic contact blepharoconjunctivitis caused by phenylephrine, associated with persistent patch test reaction. Contact Dermatitis 1998;39:143–4.
9. Fraunfelder FT. Pupil dilatation using phenylephrine alone or in combination with tropicamide. Ophthalmology 1999;106:4.
10. Vicedo CMF, Garcia MB, Bellver MJG, Bustamante AP. Conjunctival tropicamide and transitory ischemic accident (TIA). Farm Clin 1998;15:115–18.
11. Brunner GA, Fleck S, Pieber TR, Lueger A, Kaufmann P, Smolle KH, Brussee H, Krejs GJ. Near fatal anticholinergic intoxication after routine fundoscopy. Intensive Care Med 1998;24:730–1.
12. Le Coz CJ, Santinelli F. Facial contact dermatitis from chloramphenicol with cross-sensitivity to thiamphenicol. Contact Dermatitis 1998;38:108–9.
13. Amichai B, Grunwald MH, Halevy S. Erythema multiforme resulting from chloramphenicol in eye drops: confirmation by mast cell degranulation test. Ann Ophthalmol Glaucoma 1998;30:225–7.
14. Lancaster T, Swart AM, Jick H. Risk of serious haematological toxicity with use of chloramphenicol eye drops in a British general practice database. Br Med J 1998;316:667.
15. Wiholm BE, Kelly JP, Kaufman D, Issaragrisil S, Levy M, Anderson T. Relation of aplastic anaemia to use of chloramphenicol eye drops in two international case-control studies. Br Med J 1998;316:666.
16. Laporte JR, Vidal X, Ballarin E, Ibanez L. Possible association between ocular chloramphenicol and aplastic anemia—the absolute risk is very low. Br J Clin Pharmacol 1998;46:181–4.
17. Doona M, Walsh JB. Topical chloramphenicol is an outmoded treatment. Br Med J 1998; 316:1903.

E. Ernst

48 Treatments used in complementary medicine

Non-orthodox treatment, more commonly known as complementary or alternative medicine, is dramatically increasing in popularity. A set of surveys has shown that between 1990 and 1997 the 1-year prevalence in the US general population increased from 33 to 42% (1). This level of popularity is accompanied by more and more attention by the orthodox medical professions to complementary medicine. Most notably, in November 1998 all ten journals of the American Medical Association published theme issues on the subject. Other prominent articles focussed on the risks of complementary therapies. Angell and Kassierer expressed their fear that 'with the increased interest in alternative medicine, we see a reversion to irrational approaches to medical practice' (2). Others have summarized the reasons why traditional use is no reliable warranty for the safety of therapeutic interventions and have concluded that "the promotion of traditional remedies on the basis that they have passed the 'test of time' can be misleading, even dangerous". The potential risks are diverse and can be characterized as indirect or direct.

The most obvious danger lies in the fact that some patients (or their parents) elect to abandon conventional therapies for serious diseases in favor of alternative approaches. This can have fatal consequences (3[c]). Survey data suggest that a sizeable proportion of complementary practitioners advise their clients to reduce their prescribed medication (4). Risks are also brought about by the use of diagnostic techniques that are burdened with serious risks; an example is the apparent over-use of X-rays by chiropractors (5[R]).

The attitude of the consumer towards complementary medicine may also constitute a risk. When 515 users of herbal remedies were interviewed about their behavior vis a vis an adverse effect of a herbal versus a synthetic over-the-counter drug, a clear difference emerged. While 26% would consult their doctor for a serious adverse effect of a synthetic medication, only 0.8% would do the same in relation to a herbal remedy (6). A further risk might lie in the plethora of lay books on complementary medicine now available in every High Street bookstore. A pilot project has attempted to evaluate the value of a random selection of such books and concluded that the lay literature on complementary medicine is far from adequate and has the potential to put the health of the reader at risk (7).

Side Effects of Drugs, Annual 23
J.K. Aronson, ed.

WESTERN HERBALISM (PHYTOMEDICINE)

Several recent reviews have focussed on herbal medicines and have included sections on the toxicity of medicinal plants (8[R]–10[R]). Other reviews have been specifically dedicated to the safety of herbal products in general (11[R]–14[R]). Articles dealing with the safety of specific phytomedicines are summarized below.

Contamination is a notorious problem with herbal remedies. When 27 samples of commercially available camomile formulations were tested in Brazil, it was found that all of them contained contaminants and only 50% had the essential oils needed to produce anti-inflammatory activity (15).

Two cases have been reported of contamination of plantain (a plant of the genus *Plantago*) by *Digitalis lanata* (16). Both patients suffered from serious overdose of cardiac glycosides with toxic serum digoxin concentrations as a result.

When 62 samples of medicinal plant material and 11 samples of herbal tea were examined in Croatia, fungal contamination was found to be abundant (17). *Aspergillus flavus,* a known producer of aflatoxins was present in 11 and one sample respectively. Mycotoxins were found in seven of the samples analysed.

An outbreak of skin lesions affecting 20 patients from a village near Teheran has been reported (18[C]). The lesions were painless and had a central black necrotic area, marginal erythema, and severe peripheral edema. These clinical signs led to the suspicion of anthrax infection. It turned out that all patients had applied Kombucha mushroom locally as a painkiller. The skin lesions had developed 5–7 days after the application of the material. Cultures from the skin lesions confirmed the presence of *Bacillus anthracis.* Cultures of the Kombucha mushrooms were inconclusive, owing to multiple bacterial contamination and overgrowth, but it was shown that anthrax would grow on uncontaminated material. The patients all recovered on antibiotic therapy.

Arnica montana (Arnica)

(SED-13, 1430)

A 27-year-old woman presented with a rapidly enlarging necrotic lesion on her face and left leg together with malaise and high fever (19[c]). She reported that she had applied a 1.5% arnica cream to her face before these symptoms had occurred. The diagnosis was *Sweet's syndrome* elicited by pathergy to arnica. She was treated with prednisolone and her skin lesions disappeared within 3 weeks.

Caulophyllum thalictroides (Blue cohosh)

Heart failure has been attributed to blue cohosh (20[c]).

A 3.66 kg, 41-week-old boy developed respiratory distress, acidosis, and shock shortly after spontaneous vaginal delivery. The 36-year old mother had a history of adequately controlled hypothyroidism. She had taken tablets of blue cohosh for 1 month to induce uterine contractions. Subsequently she felt more contractions and less fetal activity. After delivery, the baby continued to be critically ill for several weeks and required treatment for respiratory failure and cardiogenic shock. He gradually improved and was extubated after 21 days. There were no congenital abnormalities or other reasons to explain the infant's problems. He remained in hospital for 31 days and an electrocardiogram at discharge was consistent with a resolving anterolateral myocardial infection. Two years later he had fully recovered, but cardiomegaly and impaired left ventricular function persisted.

Blue cohosh contains vasoactive glycosides and alkaloids known to produce toxic effects on the myocardium in animals. The authors believed that the consumption of this herbal preparation by the mother was the cause of the heart failure in the child.

Chelidonium majus (common celandine) *(SED-13, 1432)*

A further case of *toxic hepatitis* has been reported (21[C]).

A 42-year-old woman had been admitted twice to hospital with hepatitis. No toxic agent could be identified during the first episode, but detailed questioning during the second showed that in both cases she had self-prescribed a commercially available medication of common celandine. Discontinuation of this herbal remedy was followed by an unremarkable recovery.

Echinacea angustifolia (Echinacea)

(SED-13, 1434; SEDA-21, 490)

An *anaphylactic reaction* to *Echinacea angustifolia* has been reported (22[c]).

A 37-year-old woman who took various food supplements on an irregular basis self-medicated with 5 ml of an extract of *Echinacea angustifolia.* She had immediate burning of the mouth and throat followed by tightness of the chest, generalized urticaria, and diarrhea. She made a full recovery within 2 hours.

The basis for this anaphylactic reaction was hypersensitivity to *Echinacea,* confirmed by skin prick and RAST testing. However, others have challenged the notion of a causal relation in this case (23). Nevertheless, the author affirmed his belief that *Echinacea* was the causal agent and reported that at that time *Echinacea* had accounted for 22 of 266 suspected adverse reactions to complementary medicines reported to the Australian Adverse Drug Reaction Advisory Committee (24).

Eucalyptus spp *(SEDA-22, 512)*

Systemic effects of eucalyptus oil applied locally have been reported (25[c]).

A 6-year-old girl was treated with a home-made concoction mainly containing 50 ml of eucalyptus oil (consisting of 80–85% cineole oil) for pruritus. As the mixture seemed to relieve her symptoms the parents applied it more and more generously to the girl's skin. She subsequently developed symptoms of intoxication: slurred speech, unsteady gait, and drowsiness. Eventually she lost consciousness and was unrousable. She was admitted to hospital where several tests were negative, but her urine sample contained components of eucalyptus oil. She made a full recovery within 24 hours after withdrawal of the external herbal treatment.

Ginkgo biloba

Ginkgo biloba is a popular herbal remedy promoted for the enhancement of mental function. It has antiplatelet activity and could therefore interact with anticoagulants. A 78-year-old woman who had taken warfarin for 5 years started took *Ginkgo biloba* for 2 months, when she developed signs of a stroke which was diagnosed as intracerebral hemorrhage (26[c]). Even though it is impossible to establish causality in this case, it is conceivable that the stroke was the result of over-anticoagulation induced by the herbal medication.

Hypericum perforatum (St John's wort) *(SED-13, 1435; SEDA-20, 431; SEDA-21, 492;SEDA-22, 512)*

A review of all reported adverse effects associated with St John's Wort has shown that this herbal antidepressant has an encouraging safety profile (27[R]). Adverse effects reported in clinical trials were invariably mild and transient: *gastrointestinal symptoms* (8.5%), *dizziness/confusion* (4.5%), *tiredness/sedation* (4.5%), and *dry mouth* (4.0%). Synthetic drugs used in comparative trials were burdened with significantly higher rates of adverse effects. Data obtained from the WHO Collaborating Centre for International Drug Monitoring are summarized in Table 1.

Table 1. *Reports of adverse effects of formulations of St John's wort (up to May 1998)*

System	Number of cases
Cardiovascular (edema)	2
Cardiovascular (bradycardia)	1
Respiratory	4
Nervous system	5
Nervous system (stroke)	1
Psychiatric	15
Hematological (coagulation)	4
Liver	4
Gastrointestinal	2
Urinary system (interstitial nephritis)	1
Skin and appendages (allergic reactions)	16
Skin and appendages (conjunctivitis)	1
Reduced therapeutic response	1

Psychiatric *Hypomania* has been reported with St John's wort (28[c]).

A 47-year-old woman with an 8-year history of nocturnal panic attacks and a recent history of major depression had a poor response to SSRIs and instead took a 0.1% tincture of St John's wort. After 10 days she noted racing and distorted thoughts, increased irritability, hostility, aggressive behavior, and a reduced need for sleep. After discontinuing the herbal treatment, her symptoms resolved within 2 days.

The author suggested that St John's wort had caused this episode of hypomania.

Skin and appendages *Photosensitivity* has been attributed to St John's wort (29[c]).

A 35-year-old woman took ground whole St. John's wort (500 mg/day) for mild depression. After 4 weeks she developed stinging pain on her face and the backs of both hands, which worsened with sun exposure. She was seen after the area of pain had spread following exposure to the sun. After discontinuation of St John's wort, the symptoms gradually disappeared during the next 2 months.

The authors thought that photoactive hypericins had caused demyelination of cutaneous nerve axons. If they are correct, then this would be the first human case of photosensitivity after St. John's wort, a condition previously only reported in animals.

Use in pregnancy Like all herbal remedies, there is insufficient evidence that it is safe to take St John's wort during pregnancy. Two women who took St John's wort during pregnancy in order to avoid potential harmful effects of synthetic antidepressants to the fetus also discontinued their prescribed medications and did not discuss their decisions with their doctor (30[c]). Although the effects of St John's wort on the fetus are not known, the authors cautioned against the use of St John's wort under these circumstances and argued that tricyclic antidepressants or fluoxetine would be the safer form of antidepressive drug therapy.

Larrea tridentate (chaparral)

(SEDA-20, 249)

Chaparral-induced *hepatotoxicity* in 16 published cases has been summarized in the light of a further report (31[cr]).

A 27-year-old Hispanic man presented with nausea and vomiting, diarrhea, and upper abdominal pain 12 months after starting to take Chaparral capsules. A liver biopsy showed hepatocellular injury with necrosis and periportal inflammation. His liver function stabilized after withdrawal of chaparral.

Piper methysticum (kava)

(SED-13, 1438; SEDA-21, 491; SEDA-22, 513)

Another herbal anxiolytic drug is the increasingly popular kava root traditionally used as a recreational drug by the native inhabitants of the South Seas. It can cause *hepatitis* (21[c]).

A 39-year-old woman had been treated for toxic hepatitis of unknown cause. When she re-presented with hepatitis-like symptoms and high liver enzymes, toxic hepatitis was diagnosed. Other causes for the liver pathology were excluded and it was noted that before both exacerbations, she had self-prescribed kava. When the kava was withdrawn, the liver pathology normalized and she made an uneventful recovery.

Valeriana officinalis (valerian)

(SED-13, 1442; SEDA-20, 429)

Liver A French team has reported the case of a 13-year-old child with fulminant seronegative *liver failure* requiring liver transplantation (32[c]). Liver biopsy showed non-specific necrosis of more than 90% of the hepatocytes. Possible exogenous toxic factors were ruled out and it was thought that the most likely cause of the liver damage was self-medication with Euphytose, a herbal mixture of *Valeriana officinalis, Ballota nigra, Crategus oxyacantha, Passiflora incarnata,* and *Cola nitida.* The authors suggested that of these medicinal plants valerian was the most likely to have caused the liver damage.

Withdrawal effects *Delirium* has been attributed to valerian withdrawal (33[c]).

A 58-year-old man who had regularly taken excessive doses of valerian root extract for many years was given naloxone postoperatively and developed extreme tremulousness and worsening ventilation. His condition deteriorated and he became delirious. He was treated with midazolam, lorazepam and finally decreasing doses of clonazepam and made an uneventful recovery.

The authors suggested that the anxiolytic action of valerian is similar to that of benzodiazepines and that the patient had been suffering from a valerian withdrawal syndrome.

Viscum album (mistletoe)

(SED-13, 1437; SEDA-20, 429)

A 73-year-old man with a 5-year history of centrocytic non-Hodgkin's lymphoma presented with subcutaneous nodules in the abdominal wall at the sites where he had previously received subcutaneous injections of mistletoe, a widely used alternative treatment for cancer (34[c]). The nodules turned out to be infiltrations by the centrocytic lymphoma. The patient died 6 weeks later of bilateral pneumonia. The authors hypothesized that mistletoe has a growth-promoting action on lymphoma cells, mediated by high local concentrations of interleukin-6 liberated from the skin by mistletoe lectins.

ASIAN HERBALISM

The incidence of adverse drug reactions to Asian herbal remedies is largely unknown. A report from a German hospital specializing in Chinese herbalism is revealing in this context (35[C]). Of 145 patients who had been treated within a year at this establishment 53% reported having had at least one adverse effect attributable to Chinese herbal medicines. *Nausea, vomiting,* and *diarrhea* were the most common complaints. It should be noted that causality in these cases can only be suspected and not proven.

Contamination of Asian herbal products is a notorious problem. In Taipei, 319 children aged 1–7 years were screened for increased blood lead concentrations (36). The consumption of Chinese herbal medicines was significantly correlated with blood lead concentrations. In 2803 subjects from Taipei a history of herbal drug taking proved to be a major risk factor for *increased blood lead concentrations* (37).

Of 260 Asian patent medicines available in California, 7% contained undeclared pharmaceuticals. When 251 samples were tested for heavy metals, 24 products contained at least 10 parts per million of *lead,* 36 contained *arsenic,* and 35 contained *mercury* (38).

Wong et al. reported three cases of chronic arsenic poisoning with characteristic skin changes from Singapore (39[c]). All patients had taken Chinese herbal remedies for many years to treat their asthma. Two had cancers likely to be due to arsenic.

Aristolochia *(SED-13, 1430; SEDA-20, 429; SEDA-22, 515)*

Liver *Hepatitis* has been attributed to *Aristolochia* (40[C]).

A 49-year-old woman developed signs of hepatitis. All the usual causes were ruled out. The history revealed that she had recently started to use a Chinese herbal tea to treat her eczema. Examination of the herbal mixture showed that it contained *Aristolochia debilis* root and seven other medicinal plants.

Like *Aristolochia fangchi, Aristolochia debilis* contains the highly toxic aristolochic acid and was therefore the likely cause of the toxic hepatitis.

Urinary system At least 100 cases of extensive *interstitial fibrosis of the kidneys* have been observed in Belgium in women who had taken a Chinese herbal mixture for the purpose of weight loss. It is now assumed that in this formulation *Stephania tetrandra* was inadvertently replaced by *Aristolochia fangchi* (41[R], 42[R]). The remedy was apparently also distributed in France, and two cases have been reported from Toulouse and one possible case from Nice (43[c]).

Chinese herbal mixtures

A 36-year old woman was admitted to hospital because of general malaise (44[C]). She had lost 5 kg within 6 months. She was found to have interstitial renal fibrosis and irreversible renal insufficiency. She had taken a Chinese herbal mixture 'Jai Wey Guo Sao' to treat irregular menses. The formulation contained *Angelicae sinensis* root, *Rhemanniae* root and rhizome, *Ligustici* rhizome, *Paeoniae lactiflore* root, ginseng root, *Eucommiae* cortex, and honey. The pathological findings in this case were strikingly similar to the above-mentioned Belgian cases. The causative agent could not be identified beyond doubt.

Jin Bu Huan (*Lypocodium serratum*)

Jin Bu Huan can cause *liver damage* (45[c]).

A 49-year-old man developed signs of hepatitis after taking three tablets of Jin Bu Huan per day for 2 months for insomnia. No other potential causes for the liver damage could be identified. A liver biopsy showed chronic hepatitis with moderate portal and parenchymal lymphocytic inflammation and focal necrosis. The patient stopped taking the herbal remedy and his liver function normalized.

Since there had been previous reports of hepatotoxic effects of Jin Bu Huan, a drug that has been used in Chinese medicine for more than 1000 years, the authors concluded that Jin Bu Huan was the cause of the hepatitis.

Ma Huan ***(Ephedra)*** *(SED-13, 1434; SEDA-22, 512)*

Ma huan has been used in Chinese medicine for over 500 years to treat various ailments. More recently it has been advocated for asthma, enuresis, myasthenia gravis, nacrolepsy, and as a decongestant. Today it is contained in many herbal stimulants (e.g. Phen Fen or 'herbal ecstasy'). Ma huan contains ephedrine, which has well recognized toxic effects on the cardiovascular and central nervous systems. Between December 1993 and September 1995 more than 500 adverse events in patients taking Ma huan were registered (46).

Psychiatric A 40-year-old woman with bulimia presented with manic-like symptoms of an *acute dysphoric disorder* (47[c]). For about 1 year she had taken slimming aids containing Ma huan. She reported that after taking Ma huan she lost her appetite and slept only 2–3 hours a night. If she discontinued Ma huan she experienced hypersomnia, dysphoria, poor concentration, and fatigue. The authors believed that the effects of Ma huan self-medication had mimicked the symptoms of mania.

Urinary system A 27-year-old man with acute renal insufficiency had two obstructive *kidney stones* in his only kidney removed endoscopically. The stones were 95% composed of an ephedrine metabolite and 5% protein matrix. He had regularly used an 'energy supplement' (Pro Performance), which contained Ma huan extract 170 mg per tablet (corresponding to 6% ephedrine). He had taken 4–12 of these tablets

Table 2. *Reports of adverse events associated with acupuncture*

Indications	Adverse event	Site of acupuncture	Causality	Reference
Presumably local pain	A closed ankle fracture was converted to an open fracture and open joint by acupuncture	Local	Likely, but insufficient details reported	(51^C)
Intermittent claudication	Acclusion of the popliteal artery	Local	Likely	(52^C)
Back pain	Rupture of a pseudoaneurysm	Local	Likely	(53^C)
Arthritis	Pneumothorax	Area of the neck	Likely	(54^C)
Shoulder stiffness	High cervical epidural abscess and vertebral osteomyelitis	Posterior nuchal region	Fairly certain	(55^C)
Not stated	Peritemporomandibular abscess	Local	Fairly certain	(56^C)
Back pain	Unilateral septic sacroileitis	Local	Likely	(57^C)
Arthritis	Death due to streptococcal toxic shock-like syndrome	Right shoulder	Probable	(58^C)
Back pain	Argyria 10 years after acupuncture with a silver needle	Ear	Possible	(59^C)
Stroke (2 cases)	Angina pectoris during electroacupuncture	Scalp	Possible	(60^C)

Table 3. *Reports of adverse events associated with spinal manipulation*

Indication	Adverse event	Site of manipulation	Therapist	Causality	Reference
Back pain	Cauda equina syndrome	Lumbar	Traditional healer	Likely	(68^C)
Cervical pain	Brown-Séquard syndrome due to contusion of the spinal cord	Cervical	Chiropractor	Fairly certain	(69^C)
Neck pain	Vertigo, profuse vomiting	Cervical	Chiropractor	Certain	(70^C)

daily for about 1 year. The laboratory had previously analysed about 200 similar stones but could not identify the metabolite.

Both Jin Bu Huan and Ha huan have been in use for several hundred years. The above reports therefore serve as an appropriate reminder that the 'test of time' is an unreliable warranty for safety (48).

Shosaikoto

This Japanese kampo medicine has repeatedly been implicated in *interstitial or eosinophilic pneumonias* (49^c).

A 45-year-old woman developed a high fever, a non-productive cough, and severe dyspnea. Her chest X-ray showed bilateral alveolar infiltrates. Treatment with antibiotics was not successful and her condition deteriorated. She was finally put on mechanical ventilation and subsequently improved dramatically. It turned out that she had previously taken shosaikoto for liver dysfunction of unknown cause.

Based on a positive lymphocyte stimulation test, the authors were confident that this herbal remedy had caused pulmonary edema.

MISCELLANEOUS PROCEDURES

Acupuncture *(SED-13, 1447; SEDA-21, 492; SEDA-22, 516)*

In a rare prospective investigation of the adverse effects of Japanese acupuncture, all adverse effects experienced by patients in an acupuncture clinic seen between November 1992 and October 1997 were recorded (50). A total of 64 adverse events were noted. *Failure to remove the needles, dizziness, discomfort,* and *sweating* were the most frequent adverse reactions. No serious adverse events were noted. These data suggest that superficial needling as used in Japanese acupuncture is a relatively safe procedure.

A number of reports (51^C–60^C) of complications after acupuncture have been published. They are summarized in Table 2.

An epidemiological screening program in 2231 subjects in Japan was aimed at defining the risk factors of *hepatitis C infection* (61). It showed that the relative risk was increased (1.30, CI = 0.65–2.61) for those participants who had received acupuncture albeit not significantly. A newspaper article reported that 21 confirmed cases of hepatitis B were related to a London-based physician who practised an obscure variation of acupuncture (62).

Hypnosis

Hypnosis is not usually seen as a treatment burdened with adverse effects. Yet an authoritative review has reminded us that it is by no means completely safe (63[R]). Complications include amnesia, catharsis, paralysis, disorientation, literalness of response, accelerated transference, and memory contamination. A further unwanted effect of hypnosis is an inability to dehypnotize the patient. A review of the literature has shown several such cases and has contributed two new such incidents (64[cR]).

Spinal manipulation *(SED-13, 1448; SEDA-20, 431; SEDA-21, 494; SEDA-22, 516)*

Several surveys have addressed the safety of spinal manipulation. Lynch sent a questionnaire to all 13 consultant neurologists in the Republic of Ireland (65). The 11 who responded had seen a total of 16 patients with *neurological complications* after chiropractic spinal manipulation within 5 years. Strokes were the most frequently reported problem. In 13 cases, this had led to a persistent neurological deficit.

In a survey of UK physiotherapists trained in spinal manipulation, 19% reported having encountered complications of spinal manipulation (66). These related mostly to the upper spine and were mostly not serious. A further survey of 686 general practitioners in the UK disclosed 28 serious adverse effects related to spinal manipulation (67).

Several reports of adverse effects after spinal manipulation have been published (68[c]–70[c]). They are summarized in Table 3.

Finally, a report about malpractice suits in the US has shown that in 1990–6 claims against chiropractors have been constant (between 2.3 and 3.0 claims per 100 policy holders per year) (71). There were about four times more claims against primary care physicians. The percentage of claims paid varied between 46% and 57% for the chiropractors and 29% and 33% for the physicians. The three most frequent reasons for the claims against chiropractors were disc herniation, failure to diagnose, and bone fractures produced through treatment.

REFERENCES

1. Eisenberg D, David RB, Ettner SL, Appel S, Wilkey S, Van Rompay M, Kessler RC. Trends in alternative medicine use in the United States, 1990-1997. J Am Med Assoc 1998;280:1569–75.
2. Angell M, Kassirer JP. Alternative medicine—the risks of untested and unregulated remedies. New Engl J Med 1998;339:839–41.
3. Coppes MJ, Anderson RA, Egeler RM, Wolff JEA. Alternative therapies for the treatment of childhood cancer. New Engl J Med 1998;339:846.
4. Moody GA, Eaden JA, Bhakta P, Sher K, Mayberry JF. The role of complementary medicine in European and Asian patients with inflammatory bowel disease. Public Health 1998;112:269–71.
5. Ernst E. Chiropractors' use of X-rays. Br J Radiology 1998;71:249–51.
6. Barnes J, Mills SY, Abbot NC, Willoughby M, Ernst E. Different standards for reporting ADRs to herbal remedies and conventional OTC medicines: face-to-face interviews with 515 users of herbal remedies. Br J Clin Pharmacol 1998;45:496–500.
7. Ernst E, Armstrong NC. Lay books on complementary/alternative medicine: a risk factor for good health? Int J Risk Saf Med 1998;11:209–15.
8. Winslow LC, Droll DJ. Herbs as medicines. Arch Int Med 1998;158:2192–9.
9. Miller LG. Herbal medicinals. Selected clinical considerations focusing on known or potential drug-herb interactions. Arch Intern Med 1998;158:2200–11.
10. Mashour NH, Lin GI, Frishman WH. Herbal medicine for the treatment of cardiovascular disease. Arch Intern Med 1998;158:2225–34.
11. Saller R, Reichling J, Kristof O. Phytotherapie-Behandlung ohne Nebenwirkungen? Dtsch Med Wochenschr 1998;123:58–62.
12. Bateman J, Chapman RD, Simpson D. Possible toxicity of herbal remedies. Scott Med J 1998; 43:7–15.
13. Ernst E. Harmless herbs? A review of the recent literature. Am J Med 1998;104:170–8.
14. Shaw D. Risks or remedies? Safety aspects of herbal remedies in the UK. J R Soc Med 1998; 91:294–6.
15. Brandão MGL, Freire N, Vianna-Soares CD. Vigilância de fitoterápicos em Minas Gerais. Verificação da qualidade de diferentes amostras comerciais de camomila. Cad Saúde Pública Rio de Janeiro 1998;14:613–16.
16. Slifman NR, Obermeyer WR, Aloi BK, Musser SM, Correll WA, Cichowicz SM, Betz JM, Love LA. Contamination of botanical dietary supple-

ments by *Digitalis lanata.* New Engl J Med 1998;339:806–10.
17. Halt M. Moulds and mycotoxins in herb tea and medicinal plants. Eur J Epidemiol 1998;14:269–74.
18. Sadjadi J. Cutaneous anthrax associated with the Kombucha 'mushroom' in Iran. J Am Med Assoc 1998;280:1567–8.
19. Delmonte S, Brusati C, Parodi A, Rebora A. Leukemia-related Sweet's syndrome elicited by pathergy to arnica. Dermatology 1998;197: 195–6.
20. Jones TK, Lawson BM. Profound neonatal congestive heart failure caused by maternal consumption of blue cohosh herbal medication. J Pediatr 1998;132:550–2.
21. Strahl S, Ehret V, Dahm HH, Maier KP. Nedrotisierende Hepatitis nach Einnahme pflanzlicher Heilmittel. Dtsch Med Wochenschr 1998; 123:1410–14.
22. Mullins RJ. *Echinacea*-associated anaphylaxis. Med J Aust 1998;168:170–1.
23. Meyers SP, Wohlmuth H. *Echinacea*-associated anaphylaxis. Med J Aust 1998;168:583.
24. Mullins RJ. Reply: *Echinacea*-associated anaphylaxis. Med J Aust 1998;168:583–4.
25. Darben T, Cominos B, Lee CT. Topical eucalyptus oil poisoning. Aust J Dermatol 1998; 39: 265–7.
26. Matthews MK. Association of *Ginkgo biloba* with intracerebral haemorrhage. Neurology 1998;5:1933.
27. Ernst E, Rand JI, Barnes J, Stevinson C. Adverse effects profile of the herbal antidepressant St John's wort (*Hypericum perforatum* L.) Eur J Clin Pharmacol 1998;54:589–94.
28. Scheck, C. St John's wort and hypomania. J Clin Psychiatry 1998;59:689.
29. Bove GM. Acute neuropathy after exposure to sun in a patient treated with St John's wort. Lancet 1998;352:1121–2.
30. Grush LR, Nierengerg A, Keefe B, Cohen LS. St John's wort during pregnancy. J Am Med Assoc 1998;280:1566.
31. Grant KL, Boyer LV, Erdman BE. Chaparral-induced hepatotoxicity. Integrative Med 1998;1: 83–7.
32. Bagheri H, Broué P, Lacroix I, Larrey D, Olives JP, Vaysse PH, Ghisolfi J, Montastruc JL. Fulminant hepatic failure after herbal medicine ingestion in children. Thérapie 1998;53:77–83.
33. Garges HP, Varia I, Doraiswamy PM. Cardiac complications and delirium associated with valerian root withdrawal. J Am Med Assoc 1998; 280:1556–67.
34. Hagenah W, Dörges I, Gafumbegete E, Wagner T. Subkutane Manifestationen eines zentrozytischen Non-Hodgkin-Lymphoms an Injektionsstellen eines Mistelpräparats. Dtsch Med Wochenschr 1998;123:1001–4.
35. Melchart D, Hager S, Weidenhammer W, Liao JZ, Söllner C, Linde K. Tolerance of and compliance with traditional drug therapy among patients in a hospital for Chinese medicine in Germany. Int J Risk Saf Med 1998;11:61–4.
36. Cheng T, Wong R, Lin Y, Hwang Y, Horng J, Wang J. Chinese herbal medicine, sibship, and blood lead in children. Occup Environ Med 1998;55:573–6.
37. Chu N, Liou S, Wu T, Ko K, Chang P. Risk factors for high blood lead levels among the general population in Taiwan. Eur J Epidemiol 1998; 14:775–81.
38. Ko RJ. Adulterants in Asian patent medicines. New Engl J Med 1998;339:847.
39. Wong ST, Chan HL, Teo SK. The spectrum of cutaneous and internal malignancies in chronic arsenic toxicity. Singapore Med J 1998;39:171–3.
40. Levi M, Guchelaar H-J, Woerdenbag HJ, Zhu Y-P. Acute hepatitis in a patient using a Chinese herbal tea—a case report. Pharm World Sci 1998;20:43–4.
41. Vanherweghem JL. Misuse of herbal remedies: the case of an outbreak of terminal renal failure in Belgium (Chinese herbs nephropathy). J Alt/Comp Med 1998;4:9–13.
42. Van Ypersele De Strihou C. Chinese herb nephropathy or the evils of nature. Am J Kidney Dis 1998;32:2–3.
43. Stengel B, Jones E. Insuffisance rénale terminale associée à la consommation d'herbes chinoises en France. Néphrologie 1998;19:15–20.
44. Ng Y, Yu S, Chen T, Wu S, Yang A, Yang W. Interstitial renal fibrosis in a young woman: association with a Chinese preparation given for irregular menses. Nephrol Dial Transplant 1998;13:2115–17.
45. Picciotto A, Campo M, Brizzolara R, Giusto R, Guido G, Sinelli N, Lapertosa G, Celle G. Chronic hepatitis induced by Jin Bu Huan. J Hepatology 1998;28:165–7.
46. Powell T, Hsu FF, Turk J, Hruska K. Ma-Huang strikes again: ephedrine nephrolithiasis. Am J Kidney Dis 1998;32:153–9.
47. Emmanuel MP, Jones C, Lydiard RB. Use of herbal products and symptoms of bipolar disorder. Am J Psychiatry 1998;155:1627.
48. Ernst E, De Smet PAGM, Shaw D, Murray V. Traditional remedies and the 'test of time'. Eur J Clin Pharmacol 1998;54:99–100.
49. Miyazaki E, Ando M, Ih K, Matsumoto T, Kaneda K, Tsuda T. Pulmonary edema associated with the Chinese medicine Shosaikoto. Jpn J Respir Dis 1998;36:776–80.
50. Yamashita H, Tsukayama H, Tanno Y, Nishijo K. Adverse events related to acupuncture. J Am Med Assoc 1998;280:1563–4.
51. Kelsey JH. To the Editor. J Emerg Med 1998: 224–5.
52. Bergqvist D, Berggren A, Björck M, Boström A, Karacagil S. Akupunktur kan ge kärlskador. Lakartidningen 1998;95:180–1.
53. Matsuyama H, Nagao K, Yamakawa G, Akahoshi K, Naito K. Retroperitoneal hematoma due to rupture of a pseudoaneurysm caused by acupuncture therapy. J Urol 1998;159:2087–8.

54. Fulde GWO. Chest pain and breathlessness after acupuncture—again. Med J Aust 1998;169:64.
55. Yazawa S, Ohi T, sugimoto S, Satoh S, Matsukura S. Cervical spinal epidural abscess following acupuncture: successful treatment with antibiotics. Intern Med 1998;37:161–5.
56. Matsumura Y, Inui M, Tagawa T. Peritemporomandibular abscess as a complication of acupuncture: a case report. J Oral Maxillofac Surg 1998;56:495–6.
57. Lau S, Chou C, Huang C. Unilateral sacroiliitis as an unusual complication of acupuncture. Clin Rheumatol 1998;17:357–8.
58. Onizuka T, Oishi K, Ikeda T, Watanabe K, Senba M, Suga K, Nagatade T. A fatal case of streptococcal toxic shock-like syndrome probably caused by acupuncture. Kansenshogaku Zassi 1998;72:776–80.
59. Legat FJ, Goessler W. Argyria after short-contact acupuncture. Lancet 1998;352:241.
60. Chang-du L, Zhen-ya J. Angina pectoris induced by electric scalp acupuncture: report on two cases. Int J Clin Acupunct 1998;9:53–4.
61. Kayaba K, Igarashi M, Okamoto H, Tsuda F. Prevalence of anti-hepatitis C antibodies in a rural community without high mortality from liver disease in Niigata Prefecture. J Epidemiol 1998;8:250–5.
62. Burrell I. Acupuncture remedy linked to hepatitis outbreak. Independent Newspaper 1998;April 6.
63. Baber J. When hypnosis causes trouble. Int J Clin Exp Hypn 1998;46:157–70.
64. Gravitz MA. Inability to dehypnotize—implications for management. Hypnosis 1998;25: 93–7.
65. Lynch P. Incidence of neurological injury following neck manipulation. Irish Med J 1998; 91:130.
66. Adams G, Sim J. A survey of UK manual therapists' practice of and attitudes towards manipulation and its complications. Physiother Res Int 1998;3:206–27.
67. Abbot NC, Hill M, Barnes J, Hourigan PG, Ernst E. Uncovering suspected adverse effects of complementary and alternative medicine. Int J Risk Saf Med 1998;11:99–106.
68. Balblanc J-C, Pretot C, Ziegler F. Vascular complication involving the conus medullaris or cauda equina after vertebral manipulation for an L4–L5 disk herniation. Rev Rhum Engl Ed 1998;65:279–82.
69. Lipper MH, Goldstein JH, Do HM. Brown-Séquard syndrome of the cervical spinal cord after chiropractic manipulation. Am J Neuroradiol 1998;19:1349–52.
70. Hillier CEM, Gross MLP. Sudden onset vomiting and vertigo following chiropractic neck manipulation. J Postgrad Med 1998:567–8.
71. Studdert DM, Eisenberg DM, Miller FH, Curto DA, Kaptchuk TJ, Brennan TA. Medical malpractice implications of alternative medicine. J Am Med Assoc 1998;280:1610–15.

N.H. Choulis

49 Miscellaneous drugs, materials, and medical devices

BISPHOSPHONATES

The bisphosphonates are increasingly administered to treat bone diseases characterized by increased osteoclastic bone resorption (1[r]).

Etidronate

Etidronate, an alkylbisphosphonate, was the first to be introduced for the management of bone resorption disorders. In recent years, a cyclic regimen of etidronate followed by calcium supplementation has been established in the treatment of osteoporosis.

The safety of cyclic etidronate has been evaluated in 550 general practices in the UK in 7977 patients taking cyclic etidronate (7244 women) (2[R]). The findings were consistent with the conclusions of several reviews of the safety and tolerability of cyclic etidronate (3[r], 4[r]). The most common adverse effects reported in these review were minor gastrointestinal events, such *as diarrhea, nausea, and flatulence.* Etidronate has not been associated with an increased incidence of serious gastrointestinal adverse events.

In another study 72 postmenopausal women (mean age 65 years) with established osteoporosis took elemental calcium 1.0 g/day and vitamin D 400 units/day (5[C]). The Hormone Replacement Therapy group (n = 18) took cyclical estrogen and progesterone; the etidronate group (n = 17) took intermittent cyclical etidronate; and the combined therapy group (n = 19) took both HRT and etidronate. Three patients in the HRT group and two patients in the combined therapy group withdrew owing to *estrogen-related adverse effects.* One patient each from the control group and the etidronate group withdrew because of inability to tolerate the medications. Two patients each from the control and combined therapy groups, and one from the etidronate group withdrew owing to other medical problems. There was one death due to myocardial infraction in the etidronate group, and one patient in the control group was lost to follow-up. Six patients complained of *nausea* after etidronate, but symptoms improved with time.

Pamidronate

Pamidronate inhibits bone resorption but, unlike etidronate, does not impair bone mineralization at therapeutic dosages in patients with Paget's disease. Pamidronate inhibits osteoclast activity primarily by binding with hydroxyapatite crystals in the bone matrix, preventing the attachment of osteoclast precursor cells. Other mechanisms of action of matrix-bound pamidronate may include direct inhibition of mature osteoclast function, promotion of osteoclast apoptosis, and interference with osteoblast-mediated osteoclast activation.

Haworth et al. (6[c]) gave pamidronate to 12 patients (seven men, mean age 25 years) with osteoporosis associated with cystic fibrosis. None of the patients had undergone transplantation. Nine patients reported severe bone pain, starting at about 12 h after the infusion and lasting for up to 3 days. The bone pain typically started in the spine then migrated to the ribs and finally to the lower limbs. The pain was excruciating in seven patients, rendering them bed-bound and making sputum expectoration and physiotherapy difficult. Paracetamol and diclofenac were unsuccessful in preventing or relieving pain. Two of the nine patients also had febrile reactions and one developed phlebitis around the infusion site. None of the controls developed bone pain.

The high incidence of bone pain after intravenous pamidronate may be a novel drug reaction specific to cystic fibrosis. The pain may be

Side Effects of Drugs, Annual 23
J.K. Aronson, ed.

related to the abrupt reduction in bone turnover anticipated after intravenous pamidronate.

Of 300 patients, 221 (111 pamidronate, 110 placebo) withdrew prematurely (7[CR]). The majority of withdrawals (n = 115) were due to disease progression or death due to multiple myeloma. The number of patients who withdrew because of adverse experiences (n = 30) was small in both groups, and no deaths occurred due to the treatment. Adverse gastrointestinal events were reported in patients who received both pamidronate and placebo, but although the rates were not significantly different in the two groups there were more cases *of nausea, dysphagia/dyspepsia,* and *gastrointestinal ulceration* in the pamidronate group.

A 39-year-old normocalcemic patient with subclinical hypoparathyroidism and bone metastases from breast carcinoma was given pamidronate 60 mg parenterally and developed *hypocalcemia* (1.42 mmol/l) and carpopedal spasm (8[c]). Hypocalcemia due to latent hypoparathyroidism had been compensated by extensive osteolysis due to bone metastases.

OTHER DRUGS

Cremophor

Cremophor (polyoxyethyleneglycerol triricinoleate 35; BASF) is a non-ionic solubilizer and emulsifier that is made by reacting ethylene oxide with castor oil (9[r]). It is a pale yellow oily liquid consisting of a mixture of components, primarily polyethylene glycol conjugates of this triglyceride. Fatty acid esters of polyethyleneglycol are also present, as well as hydrophilic polyethylene glycols and ethoxylated glycerol. It is present in intravenous formulations of the anticancer drugs teniposide and paclitaxel. The paclitaxel formulation consists of 6 mg/ml in 50% ethanol and 50% cremophor. Thus, a patient receiving paclitaxel in the widely used dose of 175 mg/m^2 will also receive about 14 ml/m^2 of cremophor.

The hematological toxicity of cremophor has been evaluated after 74 cycles of doxorubicin in cremophor in 39 patients (10[C]). The principal hematological toxic effect was *neutropenia.* The incidence of grade 4 neutropenia increased with increasing doses of cremophor from 1 to 60 ml/m^2. Grade 4 neutropenia occurred in 0 of 3 patients at 1 ml/m^2, 1 of 4 patients at 7.5 ml/m^2, 4 of 6 patients at 15 ml/m^2, and 11 of 16 patients at 30 ml/m^2. When the dose of doxorubicin was reduced, grade 4 neutropenia occurred in 1 of 6 patients at 45 ml/m^2 and 2 of 4 patients at 60 ml/m^2. Febrile neutropenia occurred in one patient at 15 ml/m^2, three patients at 30 ml/m^2, one patient at 45 ml/m^2, and one patient at 60 ml/m^2. There was one death from neutropenic sepsis at 30 ml/m^2.

There were no major hypersensitivity reactions to cremophor, and no patients had their infusion discontinued or modified, while toxic effects considered potentially related to cremophor were cutaneous *(pruritus, flushing, or rashes), hypotension or dizziness,* and *headache.* Because of the subjective nature of some of these symptoms, they were classified as grade 1 (mild and not requiring treatment or interfering with function), grade 2 (moderate causing some impairment of function but not requiring hospitalization), or grade 3 (severe requiring hospitalization or causing significant interference with function). No grade 2 or 3 toxicity was recorded at the first three doses. One patient at level 4A had grade 2 dizziness, one patient at level 5 had grade 2 rash, one patient at level 5 had grade 3 headache and grade 3 pruritus, and one patient at level 6 had grade 3 hypotension and grade 3 rash. In no patient did these symptoms occur with doxorubicin alone, confirming their relation to cremophor. These symptoms began several hours to days after cremophor and persisted for 1–2 weeks, with the exception of the patient at level 5, whose pruritus gradually resolved over 3 months after discontinuing cremophor.

Disulfiram

Simultaneous abuse of *cocaine* and *alcohol* is common: alcohol reduces negative stimulant effects and potentiates ‘highs’. Disulfiram (Antabuse) has been used to treat cocaine dependence, with the rationale that an inability to modulate the effects of cocaine with alcohol may reduce cocaine use.

Six volunteers with cocaine dependence and alcohol abuse or dependence, mean age 32 years, took disulfiram 250 mg/day or placebo (11[r]). After 3 days they participated in cocaine administration sessions (one session daily for 3 days). Disulfiram study drugs were separated by at least 5 days, based on the time needed for enzyme regeneration (12[r]). After disulfiram, cocaine significantly increased heart rate, and blood pressure. These indices remained high when plasma cocaine concentrations were falling at later times and were greatest for cocaine 2 mg/kg. These findings contrast with those obtained when multiple doses of cocaine alone have been given to healthy volunteers, in whom there was evidence of acute tolerance to the cardiovascular effects of cocaine (13[c], 14[c]). Disulfiram therefore has potential as a treatment for cocaine-alcohol abuse, but could also increase the risk of toxicity as a result of its pharmacokinetic interaction with cocaine.

Mesna *(see also Chapter 16)*

Platinum agents are now combined with ifosfamide in the treatment of cancer. The possibility that mesna may interfere with the anticancer effects of platinum has been investigated using cultured malignant glioma cells (15[r]). Mesna protected tumor cell lines from the cytotoxic effect of the platinum agents. This in vitro study emphasizes the importance of specifying in detail the infusion schedules of mesna and platinum agents.

Methylene blue

Methylene blue has been used clinically for a variety of purposes, including marking of polyps, identification of sinus and fistula tracts, localizing islet cell tumors (16[R]), marking of skin incisions in plastic surgery (17[R]), labelling of vascular malformations, and the treatment of methemoglobinemia.

Methylene blue marking of a colonic polyp resulted in an *inflammatory mass* with small arteries showing both segmental and circumferential fibrinoid necrosis with thrombosis (18[c]).

A 68-year-old Hispanic woman had multiple polyps associated with recurrent episodes of hematochezia over several years. All but a single polyp were removed endoscopically. The region of the remaining polyp was labelled with 2 ml of methylene blue injected in divided doses to aid operative localization. Because surgery was postponed methylene blue was again injected. At surgery the polyp and a 5 cm perirectal indurated mass were identified, and there was a blue track from the submucosal to the outer portions of muscularis propria into the adjacent fat. Microscopically, the mucosa was intact and the submucosa was edematous. There were acute inflammatory cells in the submucosa and muscularis propria. Inflammation (acute and chronic), fibroblastic proliferation, and fat necrosis were seen in areas outside the muscularis propria and extending to the connective tissue margin. A prominent finding was fibrinoid necrosis of small arteries, in some cases segmental and in others circumferential. The internal elastic lamina was destroyed and there were thromboses and vessel wall inflammation. There was no evidence of infiltrating carcinoma in the adenomatous polyp or the adjacent colon. The inflammation and vascular changes were only in the mass defined grossly by induration; sections away from this area were unremarkable. The blue track contained blue-black pigment within macrophages.

The mechanisms of the tissue damage and vascular changes in this case were unclear.

Monofluorophosphate

There are currently no trial-based recommendations for the treatment of idiopathic osteoporosis in men. The effects of intermittent low-dose fluoride combined with continuous calcium supplementation on bone mass and future fracture events have been evaluated in 64 men with idiopathic osteoporosis (19[C]). They were randomized to intermittent treatment with monofluorophosphate plus calcium or calcium supplementation alone for 3 years. Seven of the patients given fluoride had *leg pain.* In most cases the pain, which was generally confined to the ankle, disappeared during the fluoride-free month. In a few cases, the fluoride-free month had to be prolonged to 7 or 8 weeks before the symptoms subsided. During fluoride therapy, two patients had mild *epigastric symptoms* and one had *diarrhea,* but these appeared to be related to calcium; seven of the patients who were given calcium alone complained of epigastric discomfort and two had diarrhea. All the adverse events were mild to moderate and transient, and none led to discontinuation of treatment.

Nicotine

Interactions The therapeutic effects of many drugs are less predictable in cigarette smokers, since smoking can potentially alter the pharmacokinetics of a drug by reducing its absorption, increasing its plasma clearance, or inducing the cytochrome P450 enzyme system. The enzyme induction is likely caused by the polycyclic aromatic hydrocarbons, as they are potent inducers of cytochrome P450 (20[R]).

Most such interactions appear to involve stimulation of hepatic drug metabolism by the constituents of cigarette smoke. Although rigorous data on the metabolism of antimalarial drugs is lacking, it appears from in vitro and in vivo studies that chloroquine is metabolized by cytochrome P450 (21[R]). It is therefore conceivable that cigarette smoking alters the hepatic metabolism of *antimalarial drugs.*

Antimalarial drugs (chloroquine, hydroxychloroquine, or quinacrine) were given to 36 patients with cutaneous lupus, 17 smokers and 19 non-smokers (22[C]). The median number of cigarettes smoked was one pack/day, with a median duration of 12.5 years. There was a reduction in the efficacy of antimalarial therapy in the smokers. Patients with cutaneous lupus should therefore be encouraged to stop smoking and consideration may be given to increasing the doses of antimalarial drugs in smokers with refractory cutaneous lupus before starting a cytotoxic agent.

Risk factors *Occlusive dressings* covering transdermal patches may increase the possibility of adverse effects (23[C]).

A 40-year-old man with renal carcinoma and extensive lung metastases who had smoked three packs per day for 25 years had two transdermal nicotine patches 21 mg placed on a clean hairless area of his body. Before he took a shower the next afternoon, the nursing staff covered the patches with Saranwrap. During the hot shower he felt nauseated, light-headed, and tremorous, and nearly lost consciousness. Removal of the patches and occlusive dressing alleviated the adverse effects.

The adverse effects experienced by this patient could have been due to the use of an occlusive dressing and exposure to a high temperature, in combination with a high nicotine dose. Absorption of nicotine through the skin is greater at high temperatures, because of increased blood flow to the skin. A high ambient temperature (77–84°C) significantly increases dermal absorption and plasma concentrations of nicotine in the first hour of heat exposure, starting 5 hours after application of nicotine patches (24[R]).

Polyethylene glycol

The safety and activity of outpatient-based continuous intravenous interleukin-2 (IL-2) or a modified-release, polyethylene glycol (PEG)-modified IL-2 have been studied in 115 HIV-positive patients with CD4 cell counts of 200–500 $\times$ 10^6/l randomized to antiretroviral therapy plus cyclical continuous intravenous IL-2 (n = 27), subcutaneous PEG IL-2 (n = 58), or no IL-2 (n = 30) (25[C]). The termination rates due to adverse events were 4% with continuous intravenous IL-2 and 7% with PEG IL-2. The frequency and severity of grade 3 and 4 adverse events were similar in both IL-2 groups, with the exception of *local erythema and induration* associated with subcutaneous PEG IL-2 injections. *Fever, fatigue, stomatitis, erythema, gastrointestinal symptoms,* and *mood alterations* constituted the majority of clinically significant toxic effects. Most of the adverse events resolved by 8–15 days of each cycle.

There were several unusual adverse effects of IL-2 that were not dose-related. These included worsening of pre-existing *diarrhea, cardiomyopathy* in a patient with a history of heroin abuse, and *attempted suicide* in a patient with a psychiatric history.

Trifluoromethane

Research in animals, including primates, has shown that the inhaled fluorine gas, trifluoromethane (FC-23) can be used as an indicator of cerebral blood flow measured by MRI (26[r], 27[r]). The development of a fluorinated indicator to measure cerebral blood flow with MRI would allow the interleaving of images of cerebral anatomy and metabolism with images of regional cerebral blood flow, all obtainable in one setting by magnetic resonance methods.

For human subject selection the criterion and physiological assessment to determine a maximum tolerated concentration of 30% trifluoromethane have been described (28[r]).

In five healthy men exposed to trifluoromethane, symptoms that occurred more often at higher doses included *tiredness, difficulty in concentrating, tingling, dry mouth, and loss of appetite* (29[c]).

EXCIPIENTS

Excipients are components of dosage formulations other than the therapeutic ingredients. They include lubricants, fillers, buffers, binders, antioxidants, disintegrants, and coating agents. They are considered to be inert, but may influence the quality of a product, owing to interactions with the drug substance. Adverse reactions can be caused by excipients, and some of the main reactions are *asthma, anaphylaxis,* and *local irritation* (30[R]).

Sulfites are often used as preservatives. They can cause hypersensitivity reactions, such as *asthma, generalized rash,* and *anaphylactic shock.* They have been withdrawn from the composition of several medicines intended for asthmatic patients, since these patients experience the most severe reactions to sulfites.

Benzalkonium chloride is used as a preservative in suspensions and solutions for nasal sprays and in eye-drops. In nasal sprays it can exacerbate *rhinitis* and in eye-drops it can cause *irritation* or *keratitis*.

Serious incidents can also occur when a product is administered by a route for which it is not intended and for which the excipient is not adapted. For example, drug addicts may crush tablets and then inject them; or a product containing benzyl alcohol that is not intended to be injected intrathecally may be given by this route (risk of *paraplegia*).

Teratogenicity A topical solution of erythromycin was recently withdrawn from the market because of its high content of 2-ethoxyethanol (ethylglycol), a substance that is easily absorbed by the skin and which is teratogenic in animals and alters spermatogenesis.

FRUITS

Avocado/soybean

Avocado/soybean unsaponifiables (ASU) (i.e. extracts) are made of unsaponifiable fractions containing one-third avocado oil and two-thirds soybean oil. Preclinical studies have shown some efficacy in the treatment of osteoarthritis. In vitro, ASU had an inhibitory effect on interleukin-1 (IL-1) and stimulated collagen synthesis in articular chondrocyte cultures (31[r]). In another in vitro model, ASU partially prevented the deleterious effect of IL-1 on human synovial cells and abolished its effects on rabbit articular chondrocytes (32[r]).

An open pilot study and a double-blind, placebo-controlled trial have suggested a beneficial delayed and prolonged effect of ASU on clinical symptoms of osteoarthritis of the knee and hip (33[r]).

In another placebo-controlled study of 164 patients (118 women, 46 men, mean age 64 years), 114 with osteoarthritis of the knee, and 50 with osteoarthritis of the hip, there were no severe treatment-related adverse reactions (34[c]). There were 33 adverse reactions in 23 patients (27%) taking ASU and 25 adverse reactions in 20 patients (26%) taking placebo. These adverse reactions were those usually expected, the most frequent being gastrointestinal, neurological, general, and cutaneous. Five patients taking ASU (6%) and two taking placebo (2.6%) withdrew because of an adverse event. Reasons for the withdrawal of patients from the ASU group were hemiplegia and low back pain (both thought not to be related to treatment), *and eczema, fever associated with migraine,* and *gastralgia and associated headache* (considered to be adverse effects). Other adverse reactions in those taking ASU were gastric disorders ($n = 5$), *pyrosis* ($n = 1$), *nausea* ($n = 1$), *vomiting* ($n = 1$), *febrile colitis* ($n = 1$), *headache* ($n = 2$), *drowsiness* ($n = 2$), a *flu-like illness* ($n = 2$), *allergy* ($n = 1$), *urticaria* ($n = 1$), and *pruritus* ($n = 2$). The intensity of these adverse reactions was judged to be slight or moderate in 79% of cases, and a relation to the study drug was judged to be excluded or doubtful in 88%, possible in 9%, and certain in only 3%. Most of these reactions resolved spontaneously.

Drug interactions with grapefruit juice R

Should I have orange juice or grapefruit juice with my breakfast? The answer to that question depends on whether you are taking medications that are metabolized by the cytochrome P-450 isozyme CYP3A4, since drug biotransformation by this enzyme is one of the most important systems for drug metabolism. Further to the above question it is interesting to note the wording used on a warning label in New Zealand, to alert patients to potential drug interactions with grapefruit: 'Do not take grapefruit or grapefruit juice while being treated with this medicine' (35[r]).

This cautionary and advisory label has been produced as a consequence of the discovery that grapefruit can significantly increase the plasma concentrations of many drugs. Of the several hundred chemical entities in grapefruit juice (36[R]), psoralens, mainly 6,7-dihydroxybergamottin, are thought to be the

Table 1. *Drug-grapefruit juice interactions*

Drug	Effect of grapefruit juice	Reference
Benzodiazepines	Pronounced CNS effects	(40[r])
Ciclosporin	Inhibits metabolism and increases concentration	(41[r], 42[r])
Coumarins	Interferes with the analysis of coumarins	(43[c])
Diazepam	Increases concentration	(44[r])
Felodipine	Enhances the effect and can cause increased BP and heart rate, headaches, flushing, light-headedness	(45[c])
Lovastatin	Greatly increases serum concentration	(46[C])
Nifedipine	Increases plasma concentration	(47[C])
Nisoldipine	Increases plasma concentration	(48[C])
Quinidine	Delays absorption and maximal effect on QT_c interval	(49[r])
Saquinavir	Dose-dependent increase in AUC and C_{max}	(50[r])
Terfenadine	Increase in systemic availability with possible cardiotoxicity at greater doses of grapefruit juice	(51[c])
Triazolam	Increases plasma concentration after oral administration	(52[c])

components in grapefruit that are responsible for these interactions, although the flavonoid naringenin, which was originally suspected, cannot be excluded and may have a minor role (37[r]).

The ability of grapefruit to increase the plasma concentrations of some drugs was accidentally discovered when grapefruit juice was used as a blinding agent in a drug interaction study of felodipine and alcohol (38[r]). It was noticed that plasma concentrations of felodipine were much higher when the drug was taken with grapefruit juice than those previously reported for the dose of drug administered.

In another study (39[c]) concurrent administration of grapefruit juice and felodipine increased the AUC (area under the curve) peak, a pharmacokinetic parameter associated with plasma concentration, causing increased heart rate and reduced diastolic blood pressure. Similarly, parallel administration of the juice with midazolam altered psychometric performance tests, while with nisoldipine or nitrendipine there was an increase in heart rate. Finally the concurrent administration of grapefruit juice with triazolam caused increased drowsiness.

Table 1 lists a number of other drugs whose effects are altered by grapefruit juice.

MEDICAL DEVICES

The year 2000 problem

Although by the time this volume is published, the problem of the year 2000 will have occurred, it is worth noting here, for the sake of the record, that during 1999 the Food and Drug Administration issued a document of guidance for industry, entitled ‘Guidance on FDA’s Expectations of Medical Device Manufacturers Concerning the Year 2000 Date Problem’ (53[r]).

Many medical devices use or incorporate computer systems or microprocessor controls as aspects of their design. Some of these computer systems and software applications, including embedded microprocessors, can experience problems in processing dates or date-related data, because they use two digits to represent the year. Problems may have occurred on or after 1 January 2000, when the year 2000 is represented as ‘00’ and the computer system or software cannot differentiate 1900 from 2000. Other date-related problems may have occurred, such as the failure to accurately address leap years (e.g. there will be a 29 February 2000) or the use of certain dates (e.g. 9 September 1999, i.e. 9/9/99) as 'flags' for specific computer actions.

Blood glucose meters

In early June 1998, the manufacturer of SureStep blood glucose meters (LifeScan), announced that it was replacing some of the meters used by diabetics to test their blood sugar concentration because they were giving confusing error readings. The FDA is concerned that some diabetics, wholesalers, and distributors who purchase these meters may not realize that this product replacement procedure concerns a potentially serious malfunction (54[r]). The FDA has therefore provided the following information:

LifeScan is recalling and replacing its SureStep home blood glucose meters manufactured before August 1997 because the meters may give an error message ('Er-1') instead of 'HI' (high) when a person's blood sugar is very high-500 mg/dl or greater. Such a level is very dangerous if not recognized and treated, and could result in hospitalization or death.

The FDA has received reports of two deaths in people whose glucose was very high but who repeatedly got error message readings from the SureStep blood glucose meters and delayed seeking medical care.

The FDA has classified LifeScan's recall as a Class I recall, that is a situation in which there is a reasonable probability that the use of the product will cause serious adverse health consequences or death.

People using the affected SureStep meters need to know that an 'Er-1' message may actually mean a very high concentration of blood glucose instead of an error. If users get an 'Er-1' message, they need to use the visual color change indicator to see if their blood glucose is too high. They must compare the blue dot on the test strip to the color chart on the test strip bottle. If the dot on the strip is as dark or darker than the color chart, it indicates very high blood glucose, and they should contact a health professional immediately.

Diabetics who use these SureStep brand glucose meters should not stop testing their blood glucose concentrations. They can continue to test with these meters as long as they know that an 'Er-1' message can actually mean a very high concentration. It is far more dangerous not to check blood glucose than to use a blood glucose meter that may give an unclear error message at high glucose concentrations.

Implantable insulin infusion pumps

See Chapter 44.

REFERENCES

1. Adami S, Zamberlan N. Adverse effects of bisphosphonates. Drug Saf 1996;14:158–70.
2. Van Staa TP, Leufkens H, Abenhaim L, Cooper C. Postmarketing surveillance of the safety of cyclic etidronate. Pharmacotherapy 1998;18:1121–8.
3. Fleisch H. Bisphosphonates in bone disease 1993. Berne: Stampflit Graphic Enterprise, 1993.
4. Papapoulos SE. Bisphosphonates: pharmacology and use in the treatment of osteoporosis. In: Marcus R, Feldman D, Kelsen J, editors. Osteoporosis, San Diego: Academic Press, 1996:1209–34.
5. Wimalawansa SJ. A four-year randomized controlled trial of hormone replacement and bisphosphonates, alone or in combination, in women with postmenopausal osteoporosis. Am J Med 1998; 104:219–26.
6. Haworth CS, Selby PL, Webb AK, Mawer EB, Adams JE, Freemont TJ. Severe bone pain after intravenous pamidronate in adult patients with cystic fibrosis. Lancet 1998;352:1753–4.
7. Brincker H, Westin J, Abildgaard N, Gimsing P, Turesson I, Hedenus M, Ford J, Kandra A. Failure of oral pamidronate to reduce skeletal morbidity in multiple myeloma: a double-blind placebo-controlled trial. Br J Haematol 1998;101:280–6.
8. Comlekci A, Biberoglu S, Hekimsoy, Okan I, Riskin O, Sekeloglu B, Alakavuklar M. Symptomatic hypocalcemia in a patient with latent hypoparathyroidism and breast carcinoma with bone metastasis following administration of pamidronate. Intern Med 1998;37:396–7.
9. Anonymous. Cremophor EL. BASF Technical Leaflet MEF, 1986:074e.
10. Millward MJ, Webster LK, Rischin D, Stokes KH, Toner GC, Bishop JF, Olver IN, Linahan BM, Linsemeyer ME, Woodcock DM, Phase I trial of Cremophor EL with bolus doxorubicin. Clin Cancer Res 1998;4:2321–9.
11. McCance-Katz EF, Kosten T,R, Jatlow P. Chronic disulfiram treatment effects on intranasal cocaine administration: initial results. Biol Psychiatry 1998;43:540–3.
12. Helander A, Carlsson S. Use of leukocyte aldehyde dehydrogenase activity to monitor inhibitory effect of disulfiram treatment. Alcohol Clin Exp Res 1990;14:48–52.
13. Fischman MW, Schuster CR, Hatano Y. A comparison of the subjective and cardiovascular effects of cocaine and lidocaine in humans. Pharmacol Biochem Behav 1983;18:123–7.

14. Fortin RW, Fischman MW. Smoked and intravenous cocaine in humans: Acute tolerance, cardiovascular and subjective effects of cocaine. J Pharmacol Exp Ther 1991;25:247–61.
15. Wolff JEA, Egeler RM, Anderson R, Ujack E, Iceton S, Coppes MJ. Mesna inactivates platinum agents in vitro. Anticancer Res 1998;18:4077–81.
16. Ko TC, Flisak M, Prinz RA Selective intraarterial methylene blue injection: a novel method of localizing gastrinoma. Gastroenterology 1992; 102:1062–4.
17. Granick MS, Heckler FR, Jones EW. Surgical skin-marking techniques. Plast Reconstr Surg 1987;79:573–80.
18. Borczuk AC, Petterino B, Alt E. Inflammatory mass with fibrinoid necrosis of vessels caused by methylene blue marking of a colonic polyp. Cardiovasc Pathol 1998;7:267–9.
19. Ringe JD, Dorst A, Kipshoven C, Rovati LC, Setnikar I. Avoidance of vertebral fractures in men with idiopathic osteoporosis by a three year therapy with calcium and low-dose intermittent monofluorophosphate. Osteoporosis Int 1998;8:47–52.
20. Shein J. Cigarette smoking and clinically significant drug interactions. Ann Pharmacol 1995; 29:1139–47.
21. Ducharme J, Farinotti R. Clinical pharmacokinetics and metabolism of chloroquine. Clin Pharmacokinet 1996;31:257–74.
22. Rahman P, Gladman DD, Urowitz MB. Smoking interferes with efficacy of antimalarial therapy in cutaneous lupus. J Rheumatol 1998; 25:1716–19.
23. Kratzer AM, Wolfgang SA. Nicotine patch needs to breathe. Am J Health-Syst Pharm 1998; 55:1413–15.
24. Vanakoski J, Seppala T, Sievi E. Exposure to high ambient temperature increase absorption and plasma concentrations of transdermal nicotine. Clin Pharmacol Ther 1996;60:308–15.
25. Carr A, Emery S, Lloyd A, Hoy J, Garcia R, French M, Stewart G, Fyfe G, Cooper DA. Outpatient continuous intravenous interleukin-2 or subcutaneous, polyethylene glycol-modified interleukin-2 in human immunodeficiency virus-infected patients: a randomized, controlled, multicenter study. J Infect Dis 1998;178:992–9.
26. Branch CA, Helpern JA, Ewing JR, Welch KMA. ^{19}F NMR imaging of cerebral blood flow. Magn Reson Med 1991;20:151–7.
27. Branch CA, Ewing JR, Helpern JA, Ordidge RJ, Butt S, Welch KMA. Atraumatic quantitation of cerebral perfusion in cats by ^{19}F magnetic resonance imaging. Magn Reson Med 1992;28:39–53.
28. Fagan SC, Rahill AA, Balakrishnan G, Ewing JR, Branch CA, Brown GG. Neurobehavioral and physiologic effects of trifluoromethane in humans. J Toxicol Environ Health 1995;45:221–9.
29. Rahill AA, Brown GG, Fagan SC, Ewing JR, Branch CA, Balakrishnan G. Neuropsychological dose effects of a freon, trifluoromethane (FC-23), compared to N_2O. Neurotoxicol Teratol 1998;20:617–26.
30. Anonymous. Excipients—review of adverse reactions. WHO Newsletter 1998;11/12:5.
31. Mauviel A, Daireaux M, Hartmann DJ, Galera P, Loyau G, Pujol JR. Effets des insaponificables d'avocat et de soja (PIAS) sur la production de collagène par des cultures de synoviocytes, chondrocytes articulaires et fibroblastes dermiques. Rev Rhum Mal Osteo Articul 1989;56:207–11.
32. Mauviel A, Loyau G, Pujol JR. Effet des insaponifiables d'avocat/soja (Piascledine) sur l'activitée collagenolytique de cultures de synoviocytes rhumatoïdes humains et de chondrocytes articulaires de lapin traités par l'interleukine. Rev Rhum Mal Osteo Artic 1991;58:241–5.
33. Maheu E, Les insaponifiables d'avocat/soja dans le traitement de la gonarthrose et de la coxarthrose. Synoviate 1992;9:31–8.
34. Maheu E, Mazieres B, Valat JP, Loyau G, Le Leet X, Bourgeois P, Grouin JM, Rosenberg S. Symptomatic efficacy of avocado/soyabean unsaponifiables in the treatment of osteoarthritis of the knee and hip. Arthritis Rheum 1998;41:81–91.
35. Anonymous. Grapefruit warning label: now official in some countries. Drugs Ther Perspect 1998; 12:12–13.
36. Rangana S, Govidarajan VS, Ramana KV. Citrus fruit—varieties, chemistry, technology, and quality evaluation. Chem Citr Rev Food Sci Nutr 1963;18:313–86.
37. Fuhr D. Drug interactions with grapefruit juice: extent, probable mechanism and clinical relevance. Drug Saf 1998;18:251–72.
38. Bailey DG, Spence JD, Edgar B, Bayliff CD, Arnold JMO. Ethanol enhances the hemodynamic effects of felodipine. Clin Invest Med 1989;12:357–62.
39. Rodvold KA, Meyer J. Drug-food interactions with grapefruit juice. Infect Med 1996;13:868–912.
40. Kupferschmidt HH, Ha HR, Ziegler WH. Interaction between grapefruit juice and midazolam in humans. Clin Pharmacol Ther 1995;58:20–8.
41. Hollander AAMJ, Van Rooij J, Lentjes EGWM, Arbow F, Van Bree JB, Schoemaker RC, Van Es LA, Van Der Woude FJ, Cohen AF. The effect of grapefruit juice on cyclosporine and prednisone metabolism in transplant patients. Clin Pharmacol Ther 1995;57:318–24.
42. Brunner LJ, Munar MY, Vallian J, Wolfson M, Stennett DJ, Meyer MM, Bennett WM. Interaction between cyclosporine and grapefruit juice requires long-term ingestion in stable renal transplant recipients. Pharmacotherapy 1998;18:23–9.
43. Runkel M, Tegtmeier M, Legrum W. Metabolic and analytical interactions of grapefruit juice and 1,2-benzopyrone (coumarin) in man. Eur J Clin Pharmacol 1996;50:225–30.
44. Ozdemir M, Aktan Y, Boydag BS, Cingi MI, Musmul A. Interaction between grapefruit juice and diazepam in humans. Eur J Drug Metab Pharmacol 1998;23:55–9.
45. Feldman EB. How grapefruit juice potentiates drug bioavailability. Nutr Rev 1997;55:398–400.

46. Kantola T, Kivisto KT, Neuvonen PJ. Grapefruit juice greatly increases serum concentrations of lovastatin and lovastatin acid. Clin Pharmacol Ther 1998;63:397–402.
47. Hashimoto Y, Kuroda T, Shimizu A, Hayakava M, Fukuzaki H, Morimoto S. Influence of grapefruit juice on plasma concentration of nifedipine. Jpn J Clin Pharmacol Ther 1996; 27:599–606.
48. Azuma J, Yamamoto I, Wafase T, Orii Y, Tinigawa T, Terashima S, Yoshikawa K, Tanaka T, Kawano K. Effects of grapefruit juice on the pharmacokinetics of the calcium channel blockers nifedipine and nisoldipine. Curr Ther Res Clin Exp 1998;59:619–34.
49. Min DI, Ku Y-M, Garaets DR, Lee H-C. Effects of grapefruit juice on the pharmacokinetics and pharmacodynamics of quinidine in healthy volunteers. J Clin Pharmacol 1996;36:469–76.
50. Fuhr U. Drug interactions with grapefruit juice. Extent, probable mechanism and clinical relevance. Drug Saf 1998;18:251–72.
51. Clifford CP, Adams DA, Murrays, Taylor GW, Wilkins MR, Boobies AR, Davies DS. The cardiac effects of terfenadine after inhibition of its metabolism by grapefruit juice. Eur J Clin Pharmacol 1997;52:311–15.
52. Hukkinen SK, Varhe A, Olkkola KT, Neuvonen PJ. Plasma concentrations of triazolam are increased by concomitant ingestion of grapefruit juice. Clin Pharmacol Ther 1995;58:127–31.
53. Anonymous. The year 2000 problem: guidance document. WHO Newsletter 1998;9/10: 17.
54. Anonymous. Blood glucose meters–recalled because of error reading. WHO Newsletter 1998;9/10:16.

S. Olsson and I.R. Edwards

50 The WHO international drug monitoring programme

History

The WHO International Drug Monitoring Programme was established in 1968 as a pilot project, with the participation of ten countries that had organized national pharmacovigilance systems at that time. The intent was to develop international collaboration in order to make it easier to detect rare adverse drug reactions not revealed during clinical trials. The Centre for International Drug Monitoring was moved from WHO headquarters in Geneva, Switzerland to a WHO Collaborating Centre for International Drug Monitoring in Uppsala, Sweden in 1978. This was the result of an agreement between WHO and the Swedish Government, by which Sweden assumed the operational responsibility for the Programme. WHO headquarters in Geneva retained responsibility for policy matters. The Collaborating Centre is often referred to as the Uppsala Monitoring Centre (UMC).

Current programme structure

At present 59 countries are active members of the WHO Programme. Another six countries have formally applied for membership; they are considered associated members while the issue of the technical compatibility of their reports with the requirements of WHO is established. Member countries and associated member countries are listed in Table 1.

In each country a national centre, designated by the competent health authority, is responsible for collecting, processing, and evaluating adverse reaction case reports submitted by health professionals. Information obtained from these reports is passed back to the professionals on a national basis, but is also submitted to the WHO Centre for inclusion in the international database. Collectively the centres annually provide 150 000–200 000 individual reports to WHO of reactions suspected of being drug-induced. The cumulative database of the WHO Programme now comprises over two million case reports.

Case reports submitted to the WHO Centre according to an agreed format, are checked for technical correctness and then incorporated into the international data base in a weekly routine. The material is screened at least four times a year for new and serious reactions, as well as the reporting frequencies of associations of particular interest. Many additional examinations of the data are made on an ad hoc basis

The WHO Centre in Uppsala currently has 20 staff members. Its Director is Professor I. Ralph Edwards, a clinical toxicologist. This staff is supported by people from various national centres, about 50 consultants of various kinds, as well as companies that provide particular specialist services. The Centre's strategy is to create a global network to tackle drug safety issues optimally.

Signal generation

A combination of automatic signalling devices and scanning by experienced medical personnel is considered most advantageous to successfully fulfil the original aim of the programme, i.e. the early identification of new adverse drug reactions. In 1998 a new set of methods (1), developed at the Uppsala Monitoring Centre, using a Bayesian Confidence Propagation Neural Network (BCPNN) in analysing the database, was put into routine use. This method provides a quantitative measure of the strength of association of a drug/reaction combination in the database. Combinations that occur more frequently than expected compared with the generality of the database are highlighted.

Side Effects of Drugs, Annual 23
J.K. Aronson, ed.

Table 1. *Members of the WHO International Drug Monitoring Programme and their year of entry*

Country	Year of entry	Country	Year of entry	Country	Year of entry
Argentina	1994	Hungary	1990	Romania	1976
Australia	1968	Iceland	1990	Russia	1998
Austria	1991	India	1998	Singapore	1993
Belgium	1977	Indonesia	1990	Slovak Republic	1993
Bulgaria	1975	Iran	1998	South Africa	1992
Canada	1968	Ireland	1968	Spain	1984
Chile	1996	Israel	1973	Sri Lanka	2000
China, PR	1998	Italy	1975	Sweden	1968
Costa Rica	1991	Japan	1972	Switzerland	1991
Croatia	1992	Korea, Republic of	1992	Tanzania	1993
Cuba	1994	Malaysia	1990	Thailand	1984
Cyprus	2000	Mexico	1998	Tunisia	1993
Czech Republic	1992	Morocco	1992	Turkey	1987
Denmark	1968	Netherlands	1968	United Kingdom	1968
Estonia	1998	New Zealand	1968	USA	1968
Fiji Islands	1999	Norway	1971	Venezuela	1995
Finland	1974	Oman	1995	Vietnam	1999
France	1986	Philippines	1995	Yugoslavia FR	2000
Germany	1968	Poland	1972	Zimbabwe	1998
Greece	1990	Portugal	1993		
Associated member countries					
Armenia				Macedonia	
Egypt				Pakistan	
Ghana				Netherlands Antilles	

When the new data have been processed and entered into the ADR database, a BCPNN scan is run to generate statistical measurements for each drug-ADR combination. The resulting Combinations Database (Combination: *Adverse drug reaction (ADR) data elements occurring together in ADR reports*) is made available to national centres and to pharmaceutical companies, in the latter case including only information on the company's own patented products. The database is presented in a computerized form which facilitates searching and sorting of the information.

An Associations Database (Association: *Combinations selected from a database on a quantitative basis.*) is generated by selecting those combinations that pass a pre-set threshold. Based on the results of the test runs of the BCPNN the threshold for associations is that of the lower 95% confidence limit of the IC value crossing zero when a new batch of reports is added.

All associations are followed automatically for 2 years, the data being checked at 6-monthly intervals. After the final listing, an association may be reintroduced for another 2-year follow-up. The associations are also copied to a cumulative log file (history file), which will serve as a filter to exclude combinations that have in previous quarters passed the threshold. This will prevent drug-ADR combinations with a confidence limit fluctuating around zero from being fed into the review process repetitiously.

A panel of experts has been established to analyse reactions pertaining to particular body systems. The associations database is sent to the expert review panel for evaluation. Before distributing the database, associations are checked against standard reference sources (e.g. the Physician's Desk Reference, Martindale's Extra Pharmacopoeia), and the published literature (using, for example, Medline and Reactions Weekly). This facilitates the review and identifies those associations that have been, if not generally known, at least identified previously.

Searching and sorting of the associations

data can be done, not only on drug, ADR, and the various statistical measurements, but also on System/Organ/Class (SOC) and on therapeutic drug groups using the Anatomical-Therapeutic-Chemical (ATC) classification. To ensure that there are at least two reviewers per SOC, we intend to extend the panel of reviewers from today's 30 experts to around the double over the next few years.

To the Associations stage, the process is purely quantitative, but clinical knowledge and judgement is necessary for the evaluation of associations, and is provided by the national centres and expert reviewers. Short summaries of their findings are circulated to participating national centres in a memorandum called SIGNAL®. An investigation has demonstrated that the WHO Programme is successful in finding new drug-ADR associations at an early stage and in providing useful information about them to national centres (2).

Individualized sections of the SIGNAL document will be provided to companies on a subscription basis (only on their patented products). To aid the expert reviewers, and also to facilitate interpretation of the information presented in the SIGNAL document, a set of guidelines is being established. As with the associations, all signals will be automatically reassessed on a 6-monthly basis for 2 years, with a possibility of re-introduction for follow-up, and also copied to a history file for easy tracking. With the new follow-up procedures we have introduced a mechanism by which signals can be re-evaluated following the acquisition of new information. This enables, for example, renewed consideration of associations for which there initially was not enough information to merit signalling. Signals that are later supported by new evidence can also be highlighted. The nature of the signal will determine what measures need be taken in terms of follow-up.

A larger numbers of variables than the routine drug-ADR combinations can also be considered using the Bayesian approach, as described above. For example, a specific pair of adverse reactions can be highly associated with a specific drug, or the effects can be determined of any other report variable or combination of variables on the 'information component' values. Also the effects of including drugs reported as 'concomitant medications' can be studied using the BCPNN. One of the outcomes of these analyses may be to identify patient subgroups that may be at particularly high risk of getting a specific adverse reaction when they have taken a specific drug. Another possibility is to establish that a drug safety problem is related to a particular country or region, or a certain time period. However, it should be pointed out that in order for these data to be useful there needs to be a substantial number of cases reported.

A reference source

The database of the WHO Programme is a unique reference source used in many different circumstances. When a national centre receives the first report of an unfamiliar drug-reaction association the WHO database is often consulted to find out whether a similar observation has been made elsewhere in the world. If so, the initial signal may be strengthened. National centres are provided with an annual reference document that provides summary figures of suspected drug-reaction associations reported to the WHO. On-line search facilities are also at the disposal of national centres, for up-to-date checking of the current status of reports.

From the database, cohorts of patients affected by similar kinds of drug associated reactions may be retrieved. By looking for common features in these reports, risk factors and hypotheses for underlying mechanisms may be revealed.

Quantification

There is a general need to quantify adverse drug reaction information. Under-reporting of adverse reactions in routine monitoring is the norm. However, the degree of under-reporting differs from time to time, from place to place, and between drugs. The WHO Centre is working jointly with IMS International to analyse adverse reaction reports together with drug use data from different countries. This allows national differences in reporting rates to be further analysed for reasons that may be due to differences in indications for use, medical practice, demographic differences, etc. (3), (4). It is hoped that this type of analysis of international data will serve as a guide to the need of more precise pharmacoepidemiological investigations.

A clearing house for information

The Uppsala Monitoring Centre has an important role to play as a communication centre—a clearing house for information on drug safety at the service of drug regulatory agencies, the pharmaceutical industry, researchers, and other groups in need of drug safety information. Each year about 275 requests for special database searches and investigations are received from these parties. In addition, flexible on-line retrieval programmes are made available, by which the database users can perform a variety of standardized searches by themselves. Access for non-member parties is subjected to confidentiality restrictions agreed by Programme members. Some countries maintain the right to refuse the release of their own information if they so wish. Use of the information released is subject to a caveat document as to its proper use. Detailed manuals for the on-line service and the customized retrievals on request are available from the Uppsala Centre.

National centres were provided with a three-monthly Adverse Reactions Newsletter from 1982 to 1999. The Newsletter contained reviews of national adverse drug reactions bulletins and news of drug problems being investigated in various countries, supplemented by figures from the WHO register. It was recently decided to incorporate this information into the WHO Pharmaceuticals Newsletter, distributed by the Health Technology & Pharmaceuticals Department of WHO headquarters, leading to a wider distribution of the information to all member countries of WHO.

Uppsala Reports® is the name of a bulletin that is made freely available to all interested parties by the UMC. It provides an easy-to-read account of news about pharmacovigilance, the WHO Programme, its members, and its services.

Communication within the WHO Programme has improved with the increasing use of electronic communications media. The Uppsala Monitoring Centre is maintaining an e-mail discussion group called 'Vigimed', which allows rapid exchange of information around the world on drug safety matters. Membership is restricted to persons connected to national pharmacovigilance centres.

The Internet home page of the WHO Programme (http://www.who-umc.org) was introduced in 1996. It is intended to be developed into a dynamic tool for communicating with all clients of the Uppsala Monitoring Centre. Recently internet-based seminars and training courses have been introduced on the UMC web site.

The Uppsala Monitoring Centre publishes a book 'National Pharmacovigilance Systems—Country Profiles and Overview' (2nd edition, 1999), in which the operating procedures of the national centres participating in the WHO Programme are described.

Terminologies and standards

The WHO Programme has assumed responsibility for developing a standardized adverse reactions terminology (WHO-ART) and a comprehensive index of reported drugs (WHO-DD), both of which have a utility beyond their importance to the monitoring system. These tools are used in the pre-marketing safety area, as well as for post-marketing studies by many pharmaceutical companies. WHO-ART has also been adopted by the International Programme on Chemical Safety as the medical terminology to describe poisoning incidents.

The WHO Drug Dictionary is unique in its coverage of drugs marketed throughout the world. It is available in paper print, as computer files, or on a CD-ROM together with user friendly software. The Uppsala Centre is developing it further to incorporate more detailed information and make it compatible with the pre-standard proposed by the European Committee for Standardization (CEN).

The Centre is also working with XML standards for its terminologies and dictionaries, as well as supporting such work with ICD10. The use of XML versions of terminologies will greatly enhance their combined utility and availability, for example by internet.

Within the WHO Programme definitions of commonly used terms like adverse reaction, side effect, adverse event, and signal, have been worked out (5). These definitions contribute to a harmonized way of communicating both inside and outside the Programme.

Education

In order to foster education and communication in pharmacovigilance, every other year the WHO Centre offers a 2-week training course in Adverse Reactions and Adverse Reactions Monitoring in Uppsala, to which 25 health-care professionals are accepted. The course is in three consecutive modules. The first offers some insight into the clinical aspects and diagnosis of adverse drug reactions. The second is about spontaneous monitoring and the practicalities of managing a drug monitoring centre; this section also offers hands-on experience in using the database of the WHO Programme. The final module is an introduction to wider issues in pharmacoepidemiology.

There is an increasing trend towards local and regional meetings and courses in pharmacovigilance. The WHO Programme often takes part in such meetings, particularly those organized in developing countries, to provide support and technical advise.

Annual meetings

Every year representatives of national centres are invited to a meeting arranged jointly by WHO and one of the participating countries. At these meetings technical issues are discussed, both in relation to how to improve global drug monitoring in general and concerning individual drug safety problems. Since the meetings have very high attendance rates, they are important for the establishment and maintenance of personal relationships, subsequently contributing to good communications.

Programme development

The Uppsala Monitoring Centre is currently exploring a number of leads to improve further the use of the information collected and to develop the services of the Programme.

- By further developing the method of Bayesian artificial neural networks (see above) for the analysis of the large amount of data in the WHO database it is expected that it will be possible to detect hitherto unrevealed risk factors for the development of drug-related ailments.
- In response to the challenge to safety monitoring offered by traditional herbal remedies, the WHO Centre has taken initiatives to improve the classification systems for such medicines. In a joint project with institutions in the UK and the Netherlands a system compatible with the ATC system used for modern synthetic medicines is being developed. Input from experts from all parts of the world, representing different therapeutic traditions, will be indispensable for this project.
- A new, extended adverse reactions database is being developed, based on the recommendations of the CIOMS 1A and the ICH E2B working parties. In this data model much more detailed information on each case may be stored and case reports can also, in principle, be received directly from drug companies. Other software to support the functions of national centres is also being developed.
- With the aim of improving communications in pharmacovigilance, initiatives have been taken to call together representatives of all major groups involved in the provision of drug safety information. The so-called Erice declaration on communicating drug safety information sets out the basis for further development in this area [6]. The Uppsala Monitoring Centre is collaborating with the Council for International Organizations of Medical Sciences (CIOMS) to work out detailed recommendations on good communication practices in pharmacovigilance.

Collaboration with other organizations

Co-operation with organizations interested in developing early signals of significance is of importance to achieve a safer drug therapy. The International Society for Pharmacoepidemiology (ISPE) is specifically interested in the science of pharmacovigilance, and the Council for International Organizations of Medical Sciences (CIOMS) is pivotal in bringing interested parties together to mount various collaborative projects. Much support has been given to the European Society of Pharmacovigilance (ESOP), which is gaining increasing international status. The Centre also supports the European Pharmacovigilance Research Group which has allowed regulators and drug safety specialists from a variety of European countries to come together to plan co-ordinated drug safety exercises. Initiatives like these may pave the way for a much more logical development and investigation of drug safety signals world wide.

Joining the WHO Programme

Considering the sensitive nature of the data being collected within the Programme, countries that contribute data to the scheme have agreed on certain requirements that should be complied with by countries who wish to join.

Collaborating with the WHO, an organization for cooperation between member states, also requires a certain administrative structure for drug monitoring activity. The basic requirements are:

- There must be a general acquaintance with the methods of spontaneous monitoring; a country that joins the WHO Programme must have in place a programme for collecting spontaneous adverse reactions reports.
- A national centre for pharmacovigilance must be designated and recognized by the country's Ministry of Health (or equivalent).
- There must be technical competence to fulfill reporting requirements to the WHO; case reports collected in the national drug monitoring programme must be submitted to the WHO Programme in a defined format.

The Uppsala Monitoring Centre has published 'Guidelines for Setting-up and Running a Pharmacovigilance Centre'.

Contact addresses

For further information please contact:

World Health Organization
Health Technology and Pharmaceuticals
CH-1211 Geneva 27
Switzerland
telephone: +41-22 7912111
telefax: +41-22 7910746
e-mail: couperm@who.int

WHO Collaborating Centre for
International Drug Monitoring
(the Uppsala Monitoring Centre)
Stora Torget 3
S-753 20 Uppsala
Sweden
telephone: +46-18 656060
telefax: +46-18 656080
e-mail: info@who-umc.org

REFERENCES

1. Bate A, Lindquist M, Edwards IR, Olsson S, Orre R, Lansner A, De Freitas RM. A Bayesian neural network method for adverse drug reaction signal detection. Eur J Clin Pharmacol 1998;54:315–21.
2. Fucik H, Edwards IR. Impact and credibility of the WHO adverse reaction signals. Drug Inf J 1996; 30:461–4.
3. Lindquist M, Sanderson J, Claesson C, Imbs J-L, Rohan A, Edwards IR. New pharmacovigilance information on an old drug; an international study of spontaneous reports on digoxin. Drug Invest 1994; 8:73–80.
4. Stahl MMS, Lindquist M, Pettersson M, Edwards IR, Sanderson JH, Taylor NFA, Fletcher AP, Schou J. Withdrawal reactions with selective serotonin re-uptake inhibitors as reported to the WHO system, Eur J Clin Pharmacol 1997;53: 163–9.
5. Biriell C, Edwards IR. Harmonisation in pharmacovigilance. Drug Saf 1994;10:93–102.
6. Olsson S. The Role of the WHO Programme on International Drug Monitoring in Coordinating Worldwide Drug Safety Efforts. Drug Saf 1998;19:1–10.

Address list of national centres that participate in the WHO drug monitoring programme

Argentina (ARG)
Dr. Mabel Teresa Foppiano
Tel: +54-1-340 0866
Fax: +54-1-340 0866
E-mail: snfvg@anmat.gov.ar

Administración Nacional de Medicamentos, Alimentos y Tecnologia Medica (ANMAT)
Sistema Nacional de Farmacovigilancia
Avenida de Mayo 869, piso 11o
(1084) Buenos Aires
Argentina

Australia (AUS)
Dr. Patrick Purcell
Tel: +61-2-6289 8671
Fax: +61-2-6232 8392
E-mail:
patrick.purcell@health.gov.au

Therapeutic Goods Administration
Dept of Community Services and Health
Australian Drug Evaluation Committee
P.O. Box 100
WODEN, A.C.T. 2606
Australia

Austria (AUT)
Ms. Eva Hofbauer
Tel: +43-1-711 72, ext 4641
Fax: +43-1-712 0823
E-mail: viiia3@bmg.gv.at

Federal Ministry of Health
Pharmacovigilance Department VIII/A/3
Stubenring 1
A-1010 VIENNA
Austria

Belgium (BEL)
Mr. Thierry Roisin
Tel: +32-2-227 5533
Fax: +32-2-227 5528

Ministry of Health
Pharmacy General Inspectorate
Centre National de Pharmacovigilance
Vesale Building, 20 rue Montagne de l'Oratoire
B-1010 BRUSSELS
Belgium

Bulgaria (BUL)
Dr. Iraida Bantutova
Tel: +359-2-446 566, 434 71
Fax: +359-2-442 697
E-mail: pharmacovig@ndi.bg400.bg

National Drug Institute
Committee on Adverse Drug Reactions
Yanko Sakazov Boulevard
BG-1504 SOFIA
Bulgaria

Canada (CAN)
Ms. Heather Sutcliffe
Acting Head
Tel: +1-613-946 1138
Fax: +1-613-957 0335
E-mail:
heather-sutcliffe@hc-sc.gc.ca

Health Canada
Bureau of Drug Surveillance
ADR Reporting Unit
Jackson Building, 122 Bank Street
OTTAWA, Ontario K1A 1B9
Canada

Canada (VAR)
Ms. Wikke Walop
Tel: +1-613-957 1340
Fax: +1-613-952 7948
E-mail: Wikke.Walop@hc-sc.gc.ca

Vaccine Safety Epidemiologist
VAAE Surveillance Section
Division of Immunization Laboratory
Centre for Disease Control
Tunney's Pasture 0603EI
Ottawa, Ontario K1A OL2
Canada

Chile (CHL)
Dr. Q F Cecilia Morgado – Cadiz
Tel: +56-2-239 8769, 1105
Fax: +56-2-239 8760, 6960
E-mail: cmorgado@ispch.cl

Instituto de Salud Publica de Chile
Centro Nacional de Información de Medicamentos y Farmacovigilancia-CENIMEF
Avenida Marathon 1000, 3 piso
Nuñoa-Casilla 48
SANTIAGO
Chile

China, People's Republic of (CHN)
Prof. Zhu Yonghong
Tel: +86-10-6701 7755, extension 339
Fax: +86-10-6701 3755, 6511 3987

National Centre for ADR Monitoring
National Institute for Drug Control
Temple of Heaven
BEIJING P.R.C. 100050
China, People's Rep of

Costa Rica (COR)
Dr. Albin Chaves Matamoros
Tel: +506-222 1878
Fax: +506-257 7004
E-mail: farmaco@info.ccss.sa.cr

Caja Costarricense de Seguro Social
Centro Nacional de Farmacovigilancia
Apartado 10-105
SAN JOSÉ 1000
Costa Rica

Croatia (CRO)
Prof. Bozidar Vrhovac
Tel: +385-1-213 861
Fax: +385-1-213 861
E-mail: vrhovac@rebro.mef.hr

National Adverse Drug Reactions Monitoring Centre
Section of Clinical Pharmacology
Department of Medicine
University Hospital Centre
Kispaticeva
ZAGREB
Croatia

Cuba (CUB)
Frank Debesa
Tel: +53-7-24 09 24
Fax: +53-7-24 72 27
E-mail: frank@mcdf.sld.cu

Pharmacoepidemiology Development Center
No 502 esq 5a Ave
Miramar, Playa
HAVANA CP 11300
Cuba

Cyprus (CYP)
Dr. Eftychios Kkolos
Tel: +357-2-302 001
Fax: +357-2-302 721

Ministry of Health
Pharmaceutical Services
Kimonos Street
NICOSIA 138
Cyprus

Czech Republic (CZE)
MUDr. Dana Stolbova
Tel: +420-2-732 335, 6708 1111
Fax: +420-2-7173 2377
E-mail: prazska@sukl.cz

Centre for Monitoring of Adverse Drug Reactions
State Institute for Drug Control
Státni ústav pro Kontrolu Léciv
Srobárova 48, post. prihr. 87
41 PRAHA 10
Czech Republic

Denmark (DEN)
Dr. Doris I Stenver
Tel: +45-44-889 111
Fax: +45-44-889 376
E-mail: dis@dkma.dk

Danish Medicines Agency
Department of Medicines Evaluation
Frederikssundsvej
DK-2700 BRONSHOJ
Denmark

Estonia (EST)
Dr. Maia Uusküla
Tel: +372-7-441 219
Fax: +372-7-441 549
E-mail: maia@sam.ee

Riigi Ravimiamet
State Agency of Medicines
Kalevi 4, PO Box 150
EE-2400 TARTU
Estonia

Fiji (FJI)
Mr. Abdul Ahjaz Azam
Tel: +679-315 022
Fax: +679-304 199
E-mail: aazam@govnet.gov.fj

Ministry of Health
GPO Box 106
SUVA
Fiji

Finland (FIN)
Dr. Erkki Palva
Tel: +358-9-4733 4288
Fax: +358-9-4733 4297
E-mail: erkki.palva@nam.fi

National Agency for Medicines-Lääkelaitos
Drug Information Centre
PO Box 55
Mannerheimintie 166
SF-00301 HELSINKI
Finland

France (FRA)
Dr. Anne Castot
Tel: +33-1-5587 3000
Fax: +33-1-5587 3532
E-mail:
fr-h.eudrawatch@fr-h.eudra.org

Agence du Médicament
Unité de Pharmacovigilance
143–145 boulevard Anatole France
F-93285 SAINT-DENIS, Cedex
France

Germany (GFR)
Dr. Jürgen Beckmann
Tel: +49-30-4548 3000, 4548 3311
Fax: +49-30-4548 3515
E-mail: j.beckmann@bfarm.de

Federal Institute for Drugs and Medical Devices
Bundesinstitut für Arzneimittel und Medizinprodukte
Seestrasse 10, D-13353 BERLIN
Germany

Germany (GFR)
Dr. Karl-Heinz Munter
Tel: +49-221-400 4525
Fax: +49-221-400 4539, 400 4510
E-mail: akdae@t-online.de

Drug Commission of the German Medical Profession
Arzneimittelkommission der Deutschen Ärzgeschaft
PO Box 41 01 25, Aachener Strasse 233-237
D-50931 KÖLN
Germany

Greece (GRC)
Ms. Antonia Pandouvaki
Tel: +30-1-654 9585
Fax: +30-1-654 9585
E-mail: padouvakia@eof.gr

National Drug Organization (EOF)
Adverse Drug Reactions Section
Messogion Avenue
GR-155 62 HOLARGOS
Greece

Hungary (HUN)
Dr. János Borvendég
Tel: +36-1-215 8977
Fax: +36-1-215 8977
E-mail: ogyiobgy@mail.elender.hu

National Institute of Pharmacy
Adverse Drug Reactions Monitoring Centre
Zrínyi u. 3-1051, PO Box 450
H-1372 BUDAPEST
Hungary

Iceland (ICE)
Dr. Olafur Olafsson
Tel: +354-5-627 555
Fax: +354-5-623 716

Director General of Public Health
Landlæknir
Laugavegi 116, IS-150 REYKJAVIK
Iceland

India (IND)
Prof. Suresh K Gupta
Tel: +91-11-686 4930
Fax: +91-11-686 2663
E-mail: skgupta@medinst.ernet.in

National Pharmacovigilance Centre
All India Institute of Medical Sciences
Ansari Nagar
NEW DELHI 110029
India

Indonesia (INO)
Dr. Lucky S Slamet
Tel: +62-21-424 5459
Fax: +62-21-426 5927
E-mail: regobpom@indo.net.id

Ministry of Health
Directorate General of Drug and Food Control
National Centre for Monitoring of Adverse Drug Reactions
Jalan Percetakan Negara 23
JAKARTA 10560
Indonesia

Iran, Islamic Republic of (IRN)
Dr. Mohammed Sharifzadeh
Tel: +98-21-640 5569, 641 9306
Fax: +98-21-675 868
E-mail: mosharifzad@yahoo.com

Ministry of Health and Medical Education
Iranian Drug Information Center, ADR unit
Under-secretary for Curative and Drug Affairs
Building number 3
Fakhre Razi Enghlab Ave
TEHRAN 13145,
Islamic Republic of Iran

Ireland (IRE)
Ms. Niamh Arthur
Tel: +353-1-676 4971
Fax: +353-1-676 7836
E-mail: niamh.arthur@imb.ie

Irish Medicines Board
Pharmacovigilance Unit
Earlsfort Centre
Earlsfort Terrace
DUBLIN 2
Ireland

Israel (ISR)
Dr. Dina Hemo
Tel: +972-2-568 1219
Fax: +972-2-672 58 20
E-mail: tal.lavy@moh.health.gov.il

Ministry of Health
Clinical Pharmacology Department
Drug Monitoring Center
Rivka Street 29
JERUSALEM 91010
Israel

Italy (ITA)
Dr. Nello Martini
Tel: +39-6-5994 3212
Fax: +39-6-5994 3365
E-mail:
dvf-uosi.sanita@interbusiness.it

Ministry of Health
National Pharmacovigilance Centre
Dipartimento per la valutazione dei medicinale e la farmacovigilanza
Via Civiltá Romana 7
I-00144 ROME
Italy

Japan (JPN)
Mr. Hirayam
Tel: +81-3-3508 4364
Fax: +81-3-3508 4364

Ministry of Health and Welfare
Pharmaceutical and Medical Safety Bureau
Safety Division
1-2-2 Kasumigaseki, Chiyoda-ku
TOKYO 100-8045,
Japan

Korea, Republic of (KOR)
Ms. Kyoung-Min Myoung
Tel: +82-2-380 1658
Fax: +82-2-383 2870
E-mail: kendy@kfda.go.kr

Korea Food and Drug Administration
Pharmaceutical Safety Division
Nokbun-dong, Eunpyong-ku
SEOUL 122-704
Republic of Korea

Malaysia (MAL)
Ms. Abida Haq Bt Syed M Haq
Tel: +60-3-757 3611, ext 258
Fax: +60-3-758 1312
E-mail: ah@bpfk.gov.my

Ministry of Health
National Pharmaceutical Control Bureau
Jalan University, PO Box 319
MA-46730 PETALING JAYA
Malaysia

Mexico (MEX)
Dr. Carmen Becerril Martinez
Tel: +52-5-203 4378
Fax: +52-5-203 4378
E-mail: cpfeum@mpsnet.com.mx

Ministry of Health
Gauss No 4, 7 piso
Col Casa Blanca
MEXICO CITY, DF CP 11590,
Mexico

Morocco (MOR)
Dr. Rachida Soulaymani-Bencheikh
Tel: +212-7-770 137, 772 225
Fax: +212-7-772 067

Institut National d'Hygiène
Centre Anti Poisons et de Pharmacovigilance
Avenue Ibn Batouta 27
BP 769, Agdal
M-11400 RABAT
Morocco

Netherlands (NET)
Dr. Arthur P Meiners
Tel: +31-70-356 7400
Fax: +31-70-356 7515
E-mail: ap.meiners@cbg-meb.nl

Medicines Evaluation Board
PO Box 16229
Kalvermarkt 53
NL-2500 BE THE HAGUE
The Netherlands

Netherlands (NET)
Dr. A C van Grootheest
Tel: +31-73-646 9700
Fax: +31-73-642 6136
E-mail: ac.vangrootheest@lareb.nl

Netherlands Pharmacovigilance Foundation LAREB
Goudsbloemvallei 7
NL-5237 MH S'HERTOGENBOSCH
The Netherlands

New Zealand (NEZ)
Dr. David Coulter
Tel: +64-3-479 7249
Fax: +64-3-477 0509
E-mail:
david.coulter@stonebow.otago.ac.nz

University of Otago Medical School
PO Box 913
DUNEDIN 9000
New Zealand

Norway (NOR)
Ms. Elena Kvan
Tel: +47-22-897 700
Fax: +47-22-897 799
E-mail: elena.kvan@slk.no

Norwegian Medicines Control Authority
Statens Legemiddelkontroll (SLK)
Adverse Drug Reaction Section
Sven Oftedals vei 6
N-0950 OSLO 9
Norway

Oman (OMN)
Dr. Ph Sawsan Ahmad Jaffar
Tel: +968-694 744
Fax: +968-602 287, 604 684

Ministry of Health
Directorate General of Pharmaceutical Affairs and Drug Control
PO Box 393, 113 MUSCAT
Oman

Philippines (PHL)
Dr. Kenneth Hartigan-Go
Tel: +63-2-743 8301
Fax: +63-2-781 2516
E-mail: hartigan@doh.gov.ph

Bureau of Food and Drugs
Department of Health
Filinvest Corporate City
Muntinlupa
METRO MANILA 1770
The Philippines

Poland (POL)
Ms. Anna Arcab
Tel: +48-22-841 6742
Fax: +48-22-851 4366
E-mail: amarcab@il.waw.pl

Drug Institute
Centre for Monitoring of Adverse Reactions to Drugs
30/34 Chelmska Street
PL-00725 WARSAW
Poland

Portugal (POR)
Dr. António M N Faria Vaz
Tel: +351-21-790 8558
Fax: +351-21-798 7155, 795 9069
E-mail: faria.vaz@infarmed.pt

Centro Nacional de Farmacovigilancia
Instituto Nacional da Farmácia e do Medicamento (INFARMED)
Parque de Saúde de Lisboa
Avenida do Brasil, 53
P-1700 LISBON
Portugal

Romania (ROM)
Dr. Juliana Daniela Stanciu
Tel: +40-1-224 1102, 224 1710
Fax: +40-1-230 5083
E-mail: anca.dragan@anm.kappa.ro

National Medicines Agency
Str Aviator Sanatescu no 48, Sector 1
R-71 324 BUCURESTI
Romania

Russia (RUS)
Prof. Cheltsov
Tel: +7-095-433 5600, 434 5244
Fax: +7-095-434 0292
E-mail: vlad@med.pfu.edu.ru

Department of Clinical Pharmacology
Miklucho-Maklaya str 8
MOSCOW
Russia

Singapore (SIN)
Ms. Cheng Leng Chan
Tel: +65-325 5604, 325 5610
Fax: +65-325 5448
E-mail:
chan_cheng_leng@moh.gov.sg

Ministry of Health
Adverse Drug Reaction Monitoring Unit
National Pharmaceutical Administration
No 2 Jalan Bukit Merah
SINGAPORE 169547
Singapore

Slovakia (SVK)
Dr. Pavol Gibala
Tel: +421-7-5293 17 35, 5493 17 32
Fax: +421-7-5293 17 34
E-mail: kevicka@IVZBA.sk

National Centre for Monitoring Adverse Reactions to Drugs
State Institute for Drug Control
Kvetná 11
08 BRATISLAVA
Slovakia

South Africa (SOA)
Ms. Ushma Mehta
Tel: +27-21-447 1618
Fax: +27-21-448 6181
E-mail: umehta@uctgsh1.uct.ac.za

National Adverse Drug Event Monitoring Centre
c/o Department of Pharmacology
Faculty of Medicine
University of Cape Town
OBSERVATORY 7925
South Africa

Spain (SPA)
Dr. Fransisco José de Abajo
Tel: +34-91-509 7947, 509 7902
Fax: +34-91-509 7948
E-mail: fabajo@agemed.es

Agencia Española del Medicamento
División de Farmacoepidemiología y Farmacovigilancia
Carretera a Pozuelo, Km 2
E-28220 MAJADAHONDA (MADRID)
Spain

Sweden (SWE)
Dr. Ingemar Persson
Tel: +46-18-17 46 00
Fax: +46-18-54 85 66
E-mail: ingemar.persson@mpa.se

Medical Products Agency
Div of Drug Epidemiology, Information & Inspection
Adverse Drug Reaction Section
PO Box 26, Husargatan 8
S-751 03 UPPSALA
Sweden

Switzerland (SCH)
Dr. Rudolf Stoller
Tel: +41-31-322 0348
Fax: +41-31-322 0418
E-mail: rudolf.stoller@iks.adwin.ch

Interkantonale Kontrollstelle für Heilmittel
Pharmacovigilance Centre
Erlachstrasse 8
CH-3000 BERN 9
Switzerland

Tanzania (TAN)
Ms. Mary Masanja
Tel: +255-51-450 512
Fax: +255-51-462 29
E-mail: tadatis@twiga.com

Tanzania Drug and Toxicology
Information Service (TADATIS)
PO Box 77150
Dar Es SALAAM
Tanzania

Thailand (THA)
Mrs Suboonya Hutangkabodee
Tel: +66-2-590 7281
Fax: +66-2-591 8497,590 7253
E-mail: suboonya@health.moph.go.th

Drug Information Center and NADRM, Technical Division
National Adverse Drug Reaction Monitoring Centre
Ministry of Public Health
Food and Drug Administration
Ti-wa-nondh Rd
NONTHABUREE 11000
Thailand

Tunisia (TUN)
Prof. Chelbi Belkahia
Tel: +216-1-562 098
Fax: +216-1-571 390
E-mail: chalbi.belkahia@rns.tn

Centre National de Pharmacovigilance
Sis Hôpital Charles Nicolle
TUNIS 1006
Tunisia

Turkey (TUR)
Ms. Eda Cindoglu
Tel: +90-312-230 1674, 230 2769
Fax: +90-312-230 1610
E-mail: tadmer@iegm.gov.tr

Ministry of Health
General Directorate of Drugs and Pharmacy
Ilkiz Sokak No 4, Sihhiye
ANKARA 06430
Turkey

United Kingdom (UNK)
Dr. June Raine
Tel: +44-207-273 0400
Fax: +44-207-273 0282, 273 0675

Medicines Control Agency
Pharmacovigilance, Department of Health
Market Towers, 1 Nine Elms Lane
Vauxhall
LONDON SW8 5NQ
United Kingdom

United States of America (USA)
Dr. Miles M Braun
Tel: +1-301-827 6079
Fax: +1-301-827 3529
E-mail: braunm@cber.fda.gov

US Department of Health and Human Services
Public Health Service, Food and Drug Administration
Center for Biologics Evaluation and Research
Division of Biostatistics and Epidemiology
Rockville Pike, HFM-225
ROCKVILLE, MD 20852-1448
United States of America

Venezuela (VEN)
Dr. Carman Lozada A
Tel: +58-2-662 4797
Fax: +58-2-662 4797, 693 1455

Instituto Nacional de Higiene "Rafael Rangel"
Sección de Farmacología Clinica Sanitaria
Centro Nacional de Vigilancia Farmacológia
Apartado Postal 60.412-Oficina del Este
Ciudad Universitaria
CARACAS
Venezuela

Vietnam (VNM)
Prof. Hoang Tich Huyên
Tel: +84-4-245 292
Fax: +84-4-823 1253

Adverse Drug Reaction Centre
Institute for Drug Quality Control
Ministry of Health
Hai Ba Trung Street
HANOI
Vietnam

Yugoslavia, Federal Republic of (YUG)
Prof. Vaso Antunovic
Tel: +381-11-361 5531
Fax: +381-11-361 5630

Clinical Centre of Serbia
National Centre for Adverse Drug Reactions
Visegradska 26
YU-11000 BELGRADE
Yugoslavia

Zimbabwe (ZWE)
Director General
Tel: +263-4-792 165
Fax: +263-4-736 980

Medicines Control Authority
PO Box UA 599, 106 Baines Avenue
Union Avenue
HARARE
Zimbabwe

Associate Member Countries

Armenia (ARM)
Dr. Samvel Azatyan
Tel: +374-2-584 020, 584 120
Fax: +374-2-151 697
E-mail: azatyan@pharm.am

Department of Pharmacovigilance and Rational Drug Use
Armenian Drug and Medical Technology Agency
Moskowian Street
YEREVAN 375001
Armenia

Egypt (EGY)
Dr. Gamila Mohamed Moussa
Tel: +20-2-354 9802
Fax: +20-2-354 2627

Ministry of Health
Directorate General of Drug Control
CAIRO
Egypt

Macedonia (MKD)
Ms. Vesna Nasteska-Nedanovska
Tel: +389-91-237 669
Fax: +389-91-230 857

Ministry of Health
Divizija BB
000 SKOPJE
Macedonia

Netherlands Antilles (ANT)
Msc Zjumira G M Wout
Tel: +599-9-614 877
Fax: +599-9-614 879
E-mail: zgwout@ibm.net

Bureau of Pharmaceutical Affairs
Fokkerweg #26
PO Box 3824
CURACAO
Netherlands Antilles

Pakistan (PAK)
Prof. Akhlaque Un-Nabi Khan
Tel: +92-21-588 2997, 589 2801
Fax: +92-21-589 3062, 588 7513
E-mail: whocpsp

College of Physicians & Surgeons Pakistan (CPSP)
Department of Clinical Pharmacology
th Central Street
Phase II, Defence Housing Authority
KARACHI 75500
Pakistan

Sri Lanka (LKA)
Dr. Bernadette M Rohini Fernandopulle
Tel: +94-1-695 230
Fax: +94-1-695 230
E-mail: phrm_cmb@slt.lk

Faculty of Medicine
University of Colombo
Kynsey Road, PO Box 271
COLOMBO 8
Sri Lanka

Institutions

EMEA
Ms. Priya Bahri
Tel: +44-207-418 8454
Fax: +44-207-418 8551
E-mail: priya.bahri@emea.eudra.org

EMEA-The European Agency for the Evaluation of Medicinal Products
Pharmacovigilance Section
Westferry Circus, Canary Wharf
LONDON E14 4HB
United Kingdom

EC
Emer Cooke
Tel: +32-2-296 7072
Fax: +32-2-296 1520
E-mail: Emer.Cooke@cec.eu.int

European Commission
Directorate General III-Industry
Rue de la Loi 200
B-1049 BRUSSELS
Belgium

FDA
Dr. Peter Honig
Tel: +1-301-827 1050
Fax: +1-301-827 1271
E-mail: honigp@cder.fda.gov

Food and Drug Administration
Office of Post-marketing Drug Risk Assessment
Center for Drug Evaluation and Research
Fishers Lane (HFD-400)
ROCKVILLE, MD 20857,
Unites States of America

WHO
Dr. Mary Couper
Tel: +41-22-791 3643
Fax: +41-22-791 4730
E-mail: couperm@who.ch

World Health Organization
Policy, Access and Rational Use, EDM-HTP
CH-1211 GENEVA 27
Switzerland

Index of drugs

Page numbers in **bold** indicate where the given drug is discussed in detail.

Index of side effects

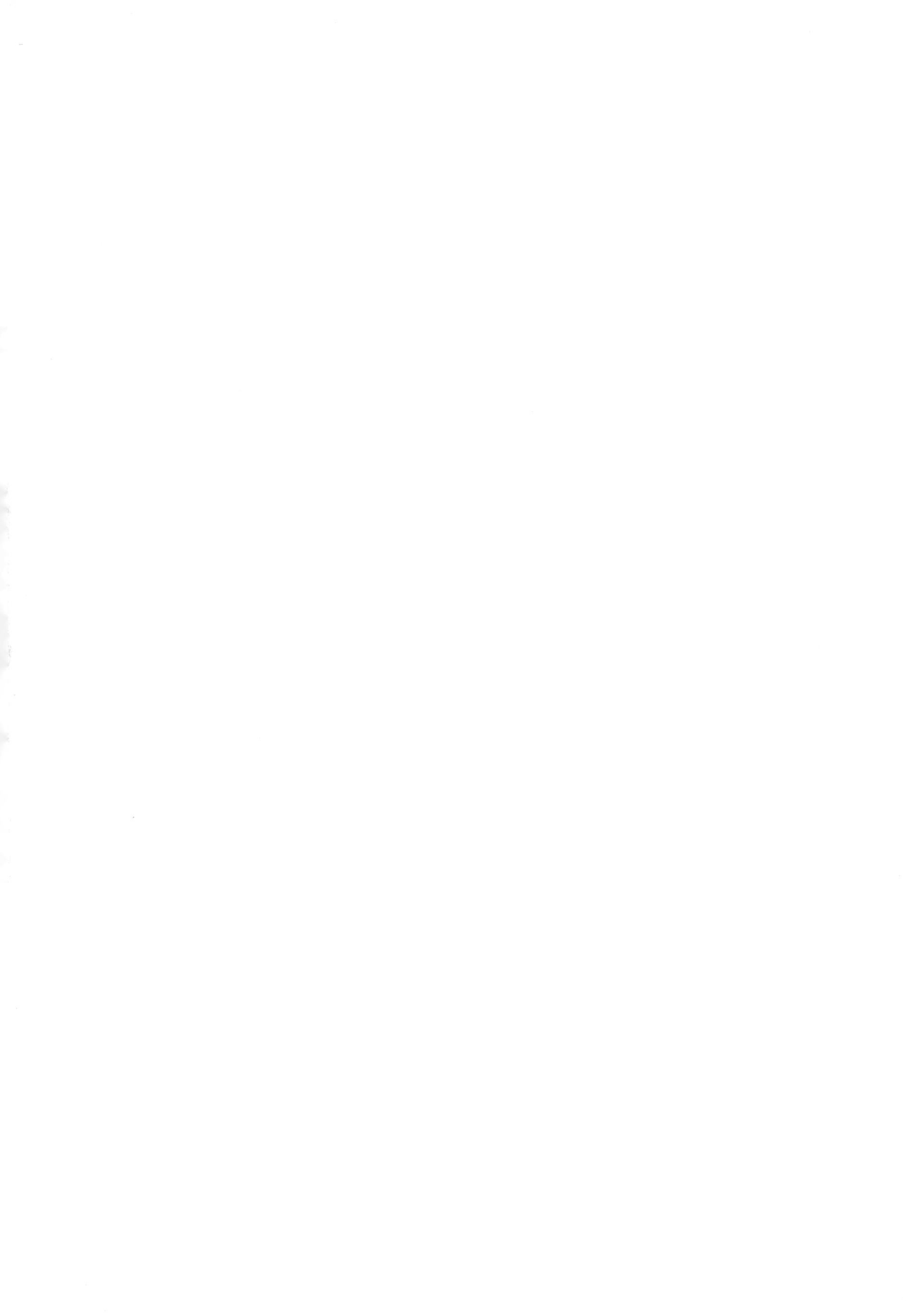